Clinical Obesity in Adults and Children

EDITED BY

PETER G. KOPELMAN MD, FRCP, FFPH

Principal
St George's, University of London
London, UK

IAN D. CATERSON AM, MBBS, BSc(med), PhD, FRACP

Boden Professor of Human Nutrition
Institute of Obesity Nutrition & Exercise (IONE)
University of Sydney
Sydney, New South Wales, Australia

WILLIAM H. DIETZ MD, PhD

Director
Division of Nutrition, Physical Activity, and Obesity
Centers for Disease Control and Prevention
Atlanta, Georgia, USA

THIRD EDITION

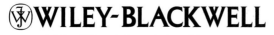
WILEY-BLACKWELL

A John Wiley & Sons, Ltd., Publication

This edition first published 2010, © 2010 Blackwell Publishing Limited
Previous editions: 1998, 2005

Blackwell Publishing was acquired by John Wiley & Sons in February 2007. Blackwell's publishing program has been merged with Wiley's global Scientific, Technical and Medical business to form Wiley-Blackwell.

Registered office: John Wiley & Sons Ltd, The Atrium, Southern Gate, Chichester, West Sussex, PO19 8SQ, UK

Editorial offices: 9600 Garsington Road, Oxford, OX4 2DQ, UK
                     The Atrium, Southern Gate, Chichester, West Sussex, PO19 8SQ, UK
                     111 River Street, Hoboken, NJ 07030-5774, USA

For details of our global editorial offices, for customer services and for information about how to apply for permission to reuse the copyright material in this book please see our website at www.wiley.com/wiley-blackwell.

Library of Congress Cataloging-in-Publication Data

Clinical obesity in adults and children / edited by Peter G. Kopelman, Ian D. Caterson, William H. Dietz. – 3rd ed.
    p. ; cm.
    Includes bibliographical references and index.
    ISBN 978-1-4051-8226-3
  1. Obesity.   I. Kopelman, Peter G.   II. Caterson, Ian D.   III. Dietz, William H.
    [DNLM: 1. Obesity.   2. Adult.   3. Child. WD 210 C64153 2010]
    RC628.C56 2010
    616.3′98–dc22
                                              2009004445

ISBN: 978-1-4051-8226-3

A catalogue record for this title is available from the British Library

Set in 9.25/12pt Minion by SNP Best-set Typesetter Ltd., Hong Kong

Printed and bound in Singapore by Fabulous Printers Pte Ltd

1   2010

Contents

Contents

List of Contributors

Sarah E. Anderson PhD
Assistant Professor, Division of Epidemiology
The Ohio State University
College of Public Health
Columbus, OH, USA

A. Colin Bell MD
Conjoint Associate Professor
School of Medicine and Public Health
University of Newcastle, NSW
Program Director, Good for Kids, Good for Life
Hunter New England Health
Wallsend, Australia

Graham Bentham MA
Centre for Diet and Activity Research (CEDAR)
School of Environmental Sciences
University of East Anglia
Norwich, UK

Neeraj Bhala MBChB MRCP (UK)
Clinical Sciences Research Institute
Warwick Medical School
University of Warwick, Coventry
Clinical Trial Service Unit & Epidemiological
Studies Unit (CTSU)
Nuffield Department of Clinical Medicine
University of Oxford
Oxford, UK

John E. Blundell PhD
Chair of Psychobiology
Institute of Psychological Sciences
Faculty of Medicine and Health
University of Leeds
Leeds, UK

George A. Bray MD
Boyd Professor, Pennington Biomedical Research
Center
Louisiana State University
Baton Rouge, LA, USA

Kelly D. Brownell PhD
Rudd Center for Food Policy & Obesity
Yale University
New Haven, CT, USA

Vicki L. Clark
Department of Psychiatry
University of Pennsylvania
School of Medicine
Philadelphia, PA, USA

Simon W. Coppack MD
Reader in Metabolic Medicine
Centre for Diabetes and Metabolic Medicine
Bart's and The London School of Medicine and
Dentistry
London, UK

Pippa Craig BSc, Dipl NutrDiet, MHPEd, PhD
Visiting Fellow, Muru Marri Indigenous Health
Unit
School of Public Health and Community Medicine
University of New South Wales
Sydney, NSW, Australia

Jean-Pierre Després PhD, FAHA
Professor and Director of Research, Cardiology
Quebec Heart and Lung Institute
Université Laval
Quebec, Canada

John B. Dixon MBBS, PhD, FRACGP
Head, Obesity Research Unit
School of Primary Health Care
Monash University
Melbourne, Victoria
Australia

Abdul G. Dulloo
Lecturer, Department of Medicine & Physiology
Institute of Physiology
University of Fribourg
Switzerland

Kristina Elfhag PhD
Lic. Psychologist
Obesity Unit
Karolinska University Hospital
Stockholm, Sweden

I. Sadaf Farooqi PhD, FRCP
Wellcome Trust Senior Clinical Fellow
Institute of Metabolic Science
Addenbrooke's Hospital
Cambridge, UK

Graham Finlayson PhD
Biopsychology Group
University of Leeds, UK

Janet Franklin PhD
Senior Dietitian, Metabolism & Obesity Services
Royal Prince Alfred Hospital
Sydney, NSW, Australia

Alessandra Gambineri MD
Endocrinology Unit
Department of Internal Medicine
S. Orsola-Malpighi Hospital
University Alma Mater Studiorum of Bologna, Italy

Matthew W. Gillman MD, SM
Director, Obesity Prevention Program
Professor, Department of Population Medicine
Harvard Medical School/Harvard
Pilgrim Health Care
Boston, MA, USA

Ronald R. Grunstein MBBS, FRACP, PhD, MD
Professor of Sleep Medicine and
Head, Sleep Research Group
Woolcock Institute of Medical Research
University of Sydney: Senior Staff Physician
Centre for Respiratory Failure and Sleep Disorders
Royal Prince Alfred Hospital
Sydney, NSW, Australia

Jason C.G. Halford PhD, CPsychol (Health)
Reader in Appetite and Obesity
Director, Kissileff Human Ingestive Behaviour
Laboratory
School of Psychology
University of Liverpool
Liverpool, UK

John Willy Haukeland MD, PhD
Unit for Diabetes and Metabolism
Clinical Sciences Research Institute
Warwick Medical School
University of Warwick
Coventry, UK;
Faculty Division
Aker University Hospital
University of Oslo
Oslo, Norway

Berit L. Heitmann PhD
Professor, Research Unit for Dietary Studies
Institute of Preventive Medicine
Centre for Health and Society
Copenhagen University Hospital
Denmark

Chelsea A. Heuer MPH
Rudd Center for Food Policy & Obesity
Yale University
New Haven, CT, USA

Rachel Jackson Leach
Center for Clinical Epidemiology and Biostatistics
University of Pennsylvania School of Medicine
Philadelphia, PA, USA

W. Philip T. James
Center for Clinical Epidemiology and Biostatistics
University of Pennsylvania School of Medicine
Philadelphia, PA, USA

Andy Jones PhD
Reader, The Centre for Diet and Activity Research
(CEDAR)
School of Environmental Sciences
University of East Anglia
Norwich, Norfolk, UK

Shiriki K. Kumanyika PhD, MPH
Professor of Epidemiology
Center for Clinical Epidemiology and Biostatistics
University of Pennsylvania School of Medicine
Philadelphia, PA, USA

Sudhesh Kumar MD FRCP FRCPath
Professor of Medicine, WISDEM
University Hospital Coventry and Warwickshire
Clinical Sciences Research Institute
Warwick Medical School
University of Warwick
Coventry, UK

Ioannis Kyrou MD
WISDEM, University Hospital Coventry and
Warwickshire
Clinical Sciences Research Institute
Warwick Medical School
University of Warwick
Coventry, UK;
Endocrinology, Metabolism and Diabetes Unit
Evgenidion Hospital
Athens University Medical School
Athens, Greece

Tim Lang PhD, FFPH
Professor of Food Policy
City University
Centre for Food Policy
London, UK

Jose Lara MSc, PhD
Research Fellow
University of Nottingham
School of Biomedical Sciences, UK

Tim Lobstein
Center for Clinical Epidemiology and Biostatistics
University of Pennsylvania School of Medicine
Philadelphia, PA, USA

Ian A. Macdonald PhD
Professor of Metabolic Physiology
University of Nottingham, UK

Yuji Matsuzawa MD, PhD
Director, Sumitomo Hospital
Professor Emeritus, Osaka University
Osaka, Japan

K. Ashlee McGuire MSc
School of Kinesiology and Health Studies
Queens University
Kingston, Ontario, Canada

Aviva Must
Professor, Department of Public Health and Family
Medicine
Tufts University School of Medicine
Boston, MA, USA

Paul E. O'Brien MD FRACS
Director, Centre for Obesity Research and
Education
Monash University
Melbourne
Victoria, Australia

Uberto Pagotto MD, PhD
Assistant Professor, Division of Endocrinology
Department of Clinical Medicine
S. Orsola-Malpighi Hospital
University Alma Mater Studiorum of Bologna, Italy

Divya Pamnani
Department of Psychiatry
University of Pennsylvania School of Medicine
Philadelphia, PA, USA

Renato Pasquali MD
Full Professor of Endocrinology
Director, Division of Endocrinology
S. Orsola-Malpighi Hospital
University Alma Mater Studiorum
University of Bologna, Italy

Joseph Proietto MBBS, FRACP, PhD
Professor of Medicine
University of Melbourne
Department of Medicine (AH/NH)
Repatriation Hospital
Heidelberg, Victoria
Australia

Rebecca M. Puhl PhD
Director of Research and Weight Stigma Initiatives
Rudd Center for Food Policy and Obesity
Yale University
New Haven, CT, USA

Geof Rayner PhD
Professor Associate in Public Health
Brunel University
Visiting Research Fellow
Centre for Food Policy
City University
London, UK

Neville Rigby
Center for Clinical Epidemiology and Biostatistics
University of Pennsylvania School of Medicine
Philadelphia, PA, USA

Robert Ross PhD
Professor, School of Kinesiology and Health Studies
Department of Medicine
Division of Endocrinology and Metabolism
Queen's University
Kingston, Ontario, Canada

Stephan Rössner
Professor of Health Behaviour Research, Obesity
Unit
Karolinska University Hospital
Huddinge, Stockholm
Sweden

Jacob C. Seidell MD, PhD
Professor of Nutrition and Health
Director, Institute of Health Sciences
EMGO Institute for Health and Care Research
VU University and VU University Medical Center
Amsterdam, The Netherlands

Marieke B. Snijder PhD
Institute of Health Sciences
VU University Amsterdam
Amsterdam, The Netherlands

Kate Steinbeck
Conjoint Professor, University of Sydney
and Endocrinology & Adolescent Medicine
Royal Prince Alfred Hospital
Sydney, NSW, Australia

Boyd Swinburn MB ChB, MD, FRACP
Professor of Population Health
School of Exercise and Nutrition Sciences
Deakin University
Melbourne, Australia

Moira A. Taylor PhD
Lecturer in Nutrition and Dietetics
University of Nottingham, UK

André Tchernof PhD
Professor, Laval University and
Laval University Medical Center
Quebec, Canada

Paul Trayhurn DSc FRSE
Professor of Nutritional Biology
University of Liverpool, UK

Marleen A. van Baak PhD
Professor, Nutrition & Toxicology Research Institute
Maastricht, The Netherlands

Valentina Vicennati MD
Specialist in Endocrinology
Division of Endocrinology
Department of Clinical Medicine
S. Orsola-Malpighi Hospital
University Alma Mater Studiorum of Bologna, Italy

Tommy L.S. Visscher PhD
Research Centre for Overweight Prevention
VU University/Windesheim Applied University
Zwolle, The Netherlands
Taskforce Prevention & Public Health
European Association for the Study of Obesity
London, UK

Thomas A. Wadden PhD
Director, Center for Weight and Eating Disorders
Professor, Department of Psychiatry
University of Pennsylvania School of Medicine
Philadelphia, PA, USA

Ian Wilcox MB BS BMedSci PhD FRACP FCCP
FCSANZ
Clinical Associate Professor
Sydney Medical School
Sydney University
NSW, Australia
Department of Cardiology
Royal Prince Alfred Hospital
Sydney, NSW, Australia

Brendon J. Yee MBChB, FRACP, PhD
Staff Physician, Centre for Respiratory Failure and
Sleep Disorders
Royal Prince Alfred Hospital
Senior Research Fellow
Woolcock Institute of Medical Research
Clinical Associate Professor
Department of Medicine
University of Sydney
Sydney, NSW, Australia

Preface

Overweight and obesity are diseases of modern society – indeed, the associated morbidities could be considered the doctor's dilemma for the 21st century. Since the first edition of *Clinical Obesity* in 1998, the prevalence of overweight and obese young people has continued to rise dramatically worldwide; the recent Foresight report in England predicts that approximately 70% of girls and 55% of boys will be overweight or obese by 2050 unless effective action is taken.

Clinical Obesity was conceived to address the need for a textbook that emphasized obesity as a disease entity by reviewing the more clinical and practical aspects of the condition as well as its scientific basis. The third edition follows the original objectives and expands them to include the impact on children and young people and the societal and environmental influences that are "fueling" the epidemic. There is also a greater focus on the prevention agenda. The book is aimed at a wide readership that includes clinicians, postgraduate and undergraduate medical students, and students of disciplines allied to medicine. This edition should also prove valuable to social scientists who are interested in factors, other than scientific, that are contributing to overweight and obesity across the globe.

The first two sections of the book include chapters on epidemiology, social consequences, biologic and genetic mechanisms and energy balance. The following section describes the disease consequences of obesity that unfortunately may be overlooked by many busy clinicians. The chapters on the management of overweight and obesity include the latest approaches to treatment and, importantly, maintenance of weight loss. The potential for pharmacotherapy is examined and the success of bariatric surgery for selected obese patients detailed. The final section flags the importance of modern society both in contributing to and in preventing obesity – the chapters highlight the importance of health and social policies that focus primarily on factors contributing to our sedentary existence and unhealthy eating.

We are indebted to Mike Stock who was the inspiration for the first edition. We suspect that Mike, if he had lived, would have been intrigued by the many advances in our scientific knowledge but shocked by the spiraling frequency of health and social problems as a consequence of obesity. We dedicate the third edition of *Clinical Obesity* to his memory.

P. G. Kopelman, I. D. Caterson & W. H. Dietz
London, Sydney and Atlanta

List of Abbreviations

ACTH	adrenocorticotropic hormone	DOHaD	developmental origins of health and disease
ADP	air displacement plethysmography	DEXA	dual-energy X-ray absorptiometry
AHI	Apnea/Hypopnea Index	EB	energy balance
AHO	Albright hereditary osteodystrophy	EBM	evidence-based medicine
AHS	*ad hoc* stomach	ED	erectile dysfunction
ART	assisted reproductive technology	EDS	excessive daytime sleepiness
ASP	acylation-stimulating protein	EE	energy expenditure
ATP	adenosine triphosphate	EI	energy intake
AgRP	agouti-related peptide	EMCL	extramyocellular lipid
BAT	brown adipose tissue	EMG	electromyogram
BDI	Beck Depression Inventory	EMR	electronic medical record
BED	binge-eating disorder	EOG	electro-oculogram
BGL	blood glucose levels	EPOC	postexercise oxygen consumption
BIA	bio-electrical impedance analysis	FABP	fatty acid binding proteins
BIH	benign intracranial hypertension	FDG-PET	fluorodeoxyglucose positron emission tomography
BMI	Body Mass Index		
BMR	basal metabolic rate	FFA	free fatty acids
BPD	biliopancreatic diversion procedure	FFM	fat-free mass
CART	cocaine and amphetamine-related transcript	FFQ	food frequency questionnaire
CBT	cognitive behavioral therapy	fMRI	functional magnetic resonance imaging
CKK	cholecystokinin	GERD	gastroesophageal reflux disease
CETP	cholesteryl ester transfer protein	GDM	gestational diabetes
CHD	coronary heart disease	GH	growth hormone
CHF	congestive heart failure	GHD	growth hormone deficiency
CI	confidence interval	GHS-R1a	growth hormone secretagog receptor 1a
CNS	central nervous system	GI	gastrointestinal; Glycemic Index
COH	controlled ovarian hyperstimulation	GIP	gastric inhibitory peptide
COPD	chronic obstructive pulmonary disease	GL	glycemic load
CPAP	continuous positive airway pressure	GLP-1	glucagon-like peptide-1
CPE	carboxypeptidase E	HCC	hepatocellular carcinoma
CPT1	carnitine palmitoyl transferase-1	HCG	human chorionic gonadotropin
CRH	corticotropin-releasing hormone	HD	hydrodensitometry
CRP	C-reactive protein	HDL	High-density lipoprotein
CT	computed tomography	HB-EGF	heparin-binding epidermal growth factor-like growth factor
CVD	cardiovascular disease		
DALY	disability-adjusted life-years	HSL	hormone-sensitive lipase
DC	direct calorimetry	IAPP	islet amyloid polypeptide
DIT	diet-induced thermogenesis	IBW	ideal body weight

IC	indirect calorimetry		OHS	obesity hypoventilation syndrome
IDF	International Diabetes Federation		OR	odds ratio
IGT	impaired glucose tolerance		OSA	obstructive sleep apnea
IHD	ischemic heart disease		PAI-1	plasminogen activator inhibitor-1
IMCL	intramyocellular lipid		PCOS	polycystic ovary syndrome
IOTF	International Obesity Task Force		PHT	pulmonary hypertension
IRS	insulin receptor substrates		PMF	protein-modified fast
IUGR	intrauterine growth restriction		POMC	pro-opiomelanocortin
IVF	*in vitro* fertilization		PP	pancreatic polypeptide
JIB	jejunoileal bypass		PSG	polysomnography
KO	knockout		PTP1B	protein tyrosine phosphatase 1B
LAGB	laparoscopic adjustable gastric banding		PUFA	polyunsaturated fatty acids
LAUP	laser-assisted uvulopalatoplasty		PVN	paraventricular nucleus
LDL	low-density lipoprotein		PWS	Prader–Willi syndrome
LBM	lean body mass		QOL	quality of life
LED	low-energy diets		R_a	rate of appearance
LH	lateral hypothalamic; luteinizing hormone		RBP-4	retinol binding protein-4
LPL	lipoprotein lipase		REE	resting energy expenditure
LV	left ventricular		REM	rapid eye movement
MAD	mandibular advancement devices		RMR	resting metabolic rate
MAS	McCune–Albright syndrome		ROS	reactive oxygen species
MC4R	melanocortin concentrating hormone receptor 4		RPE	rating of perceived exertion
			RQ	respiratory quotient
MCH	melanin-concentrating hormone		RR	relative risk
MCP-1	monocyte chemoattractant protein-1		RYGB	Roux-en-Y gastric bypass
MET	metabolic equivalent		SD	standard deviations
MI	myocardial infarction		SES	socio-economic status
MIF	migration inhibitory factor		SFA	saturated fatty acids
MMP	matrix metalloproteinase		SHGB	sex hormone-binding globulin
MRI	magnetic resonance imaging		SNP	single nucleotide polymorphisms
MRS	magnetic resonance spectroscopy		SNS	sympathetic nervous system
MS	metabolic syndrome		SPA	spontaneous physical activity
MSR	macrophage scavenger receptor		T1DM	type 1 diabetes mellitus
MUFA	monounsaturated fatty acid		T2DM	type 2 diabetes mellitus
NAFLD	nonalcoholic fatty liver disease		TCRFTA	temperature-controlled radiofrequency ablation to the tongue base and palate
NASH	nonalcoholic steatohepatitis			
NCD	noncommunicable diseases		TEF	thermic effect of food
NCEP	National Cholesterol Education Program		TG	triacylglycerol/triglyceride
NE	norepinephrine		TIMP	tissue inhibitor of metalloproteinase
NEAT	nonexercise activity thermogenesis		TRH	thyrotropin-releasing hormone
NEFA	nonesterified fatty acids		TSH	thyroid-stimulating hormone
NGF	nerve growth factor		UCP-1	uncoupling protein 1
NGT	normal glucose tolerance		UPPP	uvulopalatopharyngoplasty
NHLBI	National Heart, Lung, and Blood Institute		VBG	vertical banded gastroplasty
NMB	neuromedin B		VEGF	vascular endothelial growth factor
NMR	nuclear magnetic resonance		VLCD	very low-calorie diets
NPY	neuropeptide Y		VLDL	very low-density lipoprotein
NPY/AgRP	neuropeptide-Y/agouti-related protein		VLED	very low-energy diets
NREM	nonrapid eye movement		VMH	ventromedial hypothalamus (VMH
NST	nucleus of the solitary tract		WAT	white adipose tissue
NTS	nucleus tractus solitarius		WC	waist circumference
OFC	orbitofrontal cortex		WHO	World Health Organization
OGTT	oral glucose tolerance test		WHR	waist/hip ratio

1 Obesity

1 Epidemiology: Definition and Classification of Obesity

Tommy L.S. Visscher,[1-4] Marieke B. Snijder[2,3] and Jacob C. Seidell[1-4]

[1] Research Centre for Overweight Prevention, VU University/Windesheim Applied University, Zwolle, The Netherlands
[2] Institute for Health Sciences, VU University, Amsterdam, The Netherlands
[3] EMGO-Institute, VU Medical Centre, Amsterdam, The Netherlands
[4] Taskforce Prevention and Public Health, European Association for the Study of Obesity, London, UK

Introduction

The definition of obesity is a critical element in a book on the clinical aspects of obesity. Some may say that obesity is the equivalent of having "an excess of body fat." Others will argue that it is not the total fat mass that affects obesity and related health risks, but more an "excess of fat at certain locations." Clinicians benefit from clear definitions in protocols and clinical guidelines when identifying subjects who are candidates for treatment. Policy makers and researchers benefit from clear definitions when comparing subgroups between cities, countries or regions and when comparing obesity rates over time.

It is now clear that obesity has an important impact on the public (Fig. 1.1) [1,2]. Obesity-related healthcare costs are estimated at 1–10% of total healthcare costs, depending on obesity rates [3–6]. Obesity may have an even larger impact on indirect healthcare costs [7]. Sick leave-related productivity loss attributable to obesity has been estimated at around 10% in a Swedish study, when the obesity prevalence was less than 10% [8]. Further, obesity has a large societal impact. Obese subjects more often have social and physical disabilities and have therefore, on average, a lower quality of life [9]. Although obese subjects have a reduced life expectancy, they also have an increased number of unhealthy life-years [10].

Percentage of body fat versus location of excess fat

Since the pioneering work of Jean Vague in the 1940s it has slowly become accepted that different body morphology or types of fat distribution are independently related to the health risks associated with obesity [11]. Starting with Vague's brachiofemoral adipomuscular ratio as an index of fat distribution (which was based on ratios of skinfolds and circumferences of the arms and thighs), more recent indices were designed specifically to predict intra-abdominal fat. The most popular among all measures is the waist/hip circumference ratio (WHR). However, the simplest of these measures is the waist circumference, which appears to predict intra-abdominal fat at least as accurately as the waist/hip ratio [12] and to predict levels of cardiovascular risk factors and disease as well as Body Mass Index (BMI) and waist/hip ratio [13]. It has also been suggested that waist circumference could replace classifications based on BMI and the waist/hip circumference ratio [14]. More complex measures, such as the sagittal abdominal diameter, the ratio of waist/thigh circumference, the ratio of waist/height or the conicity index, may perform even better than waist circumference for one or more of these purposes. However, the differences among these measures are small and the use of ratios may complicate the interpretation of associations with disease and their consequences for public health measures.

Outline of this chapter

This chapter describes the literature regarding obesity measurements and clinical definitions of obesity. Specifically, the chapter describes:
• how to measure storage of body fat. This part will describe whether and how to measure the total fat mass or fat distribution
• how to define excess body fat. Cut-off points for different measures will be presented
• measured versus reported obesity status. It will be elucidated whether obesity measures should be measured by clinicians and researchers, and whether self-reported obesity measures can be used without correction factors
• obesity in clinical practice. This section will address the measurement of obesity status as an indicator of behavior and disease,

Clinical Obesity in Adults and Children, 3rd edition. Edited by Peter G. Kopelman, Ian D. Caterson and William H. Dietz.
© 2010 Blackwell Publishing, ISBN: 978-1-4051-8226-3.

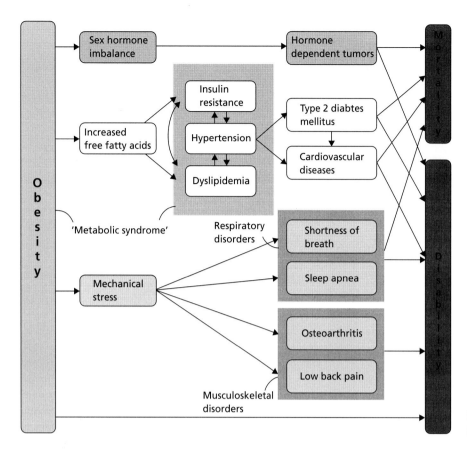

Figure 1.1 The public health impact of obesity. (Figure derived from Visscher and Seidell [1].)

and disability and mortality risk. Subgroups will be specified that require increased attention to assess obesity status.

How to measure storage of body fat

Numerous techniques are available for the measurement of "stored body fat" (Table 1.1). Sophisticated, precise measurements are often time-consuming and expensive and require trained personnel, and are therefore unlikely to be adopted at a large scale in clinical or monitoring settings. Examples of reliable techniques to obtain accurate measures of total body fat are underwater weighing (densitometry), dual-energy X-ray absorptiometry (DXA), and dilution techniques. Imaging techniques such as computed tomography (CT), and magnetic resonance imaging (MRI) are less useful to measure total body fat storage, but CT and MRI are highly accurate in defining local fat storage, and thus fat distribution. Bio-impedance analysis techniques are becoming widely available commercially, but they are of moderate use in estimating total body fat and cannot be used to estimate fat distribution.

Anthropometric measures
Although percentage body fat is best measured by underwater weighing or DXA, more feasible techniques are needed in clinical and monitoring settings. Anthropometric measures are

Table 1.1 Ability of different body fat measurements to estimate body fat and body fat distribution

Methods	Ability to measure total body fat	Ability to measure fat distribution	Applicability in large population studies
CT	Moderate	Very high	Low
MRI	High	Very high	Low
DXA	Very high	High	Moderate
Densitometry	Very high	Very low	Low
Dilution techniques	High	Very low	Moderate
BIA	Moderate	Very low	High

CT, computed tomography; MRI, magnetic resonance imaging; DXA, dual-energy X-ray absorptiometry; BIA, bio-electrical impedance analysis. Table adapted from Snijder et al. [89].

performed relatively easy and quickly, and are cheap and reliable, especially with trained personnel. One could argue whether the ideal anthropometric measure reflects total body mass or body fat distribution perfectly, but above all, the ideal anthropometric measurement should distinguish those at high risk of disability, morbidity or mortality.

The BMI is the measure most often used in children and adults. Numerically, waist/hip ratio is second, although it is now clear that interpreting waist circumference and hip circumference separately is more informative. Other measures include the sagittal abdominal diameter (waist depth) and the measurement of skinfold thickness.

Body Mass Index

The BMI is calculated as body weight (kg) divided by the square of body height (m). Body weight and height are measured with the participant standing without shoes and heavy outer garments. For the height measurement, participants are asked to push heels softly to the wall or the back of the stadiometer. Because some authors subtract 1 or 1.5 kg for light clothing, the basis for the measurement and calculation should be explicit. In practice, inclusion of patients for treatment programs may differ.

Because differences in weight between individuals are only partly due to variations in body fat, many people object to the use of weight or indices based on height and weight (such as the BMI) to discriminate between overweight and normal-weight people. There are always examples which illustrate its limitations, such as identical BMIs in a young male body builder and a middle-aged obese woman. However, despite these obvious extremes, BMI correlates well with the percentage of body fat in large populations. Deurenberg established that one can quite accurately estimate the body fat percentage in adults with the following equation:

$$\text{Body fat percent} = 1.2(\text{BMI}) + 0.23(\text{age}) - 10.8(\text{gender}) - 5.4$$

About 80% of the variation in body fat between Dutch individuals could be explained by this formula [15]. The standard error of estimate was about 4%. In this equation the value for gender is 1 for men and 0 for women. It follows from this equation that for a given height and weight, the body fat percentage is about 10% higher in women compared to men. In addition, people get fatter when they get older even when their body weights are stable because of the loss of lean body mass with age. The good correlation between BMI and fat percentage implies that in populations, BMI can be used to classify people in terms of excess body fat. In practice, people or populations are usually not classified on the basis of the body fat percentage but on the basis of their BMI.

Body Mass Index is probably linearly related to increased mortality in men and women. In many studies a U- or J-shaped association between BMI and mortality was observed [16] but some recent large studies have suggested that much of the increased mortality at low BMI is due to smoking and smoking-related disease as well as other clinical disorders causing weight loss [17–20]. It is clear that the U-shaped curve disappears after exclusion of women who were ill, had unstable weights or died early. The absolute mortality rates in women who were nonsmokers and had stable weights were much lower than the mortality rates in the total group. Allison et al explained the U-shaped BMI relation by the increased mortality associated with increased fat mass and the decreased mortality associated with increased lean mass [21].

Most epidemiologic studies of anthropometric measures as risk predictors relate values of BMI to the risk of early mortality. In adults, BMI predicts increased mortality, morbidity and disability, but the relationships between BMI and morbidity and disability are stronger than the relationship between BMI and mortality [1].

Skinfolds

In 1951, Brožek and Keys used skinfold thickness to estimate body fatness [22]. Although the skinfold measures the thickness of skin and subcutaneous fat, skinfold thickness also correlates with storage of visceral fat. The subscapular, triceps, biceps, and suprailiac skinfolds are used in the Durnin and Wormersley formula [23] and Siri's equation to calculate percentage body fat [24]. Calculators based on skinfolds for percentage body fat are found on the internet (www.bblex.de/en/calc/dw4folds.php). As suggested by Peterson, these calculations often underestimate the storage of body fat [25]. Although measurement of skinfolds may be useful in clinical studies and evaluation research, skinfold measures are not used in clinical guidelines and protocols to identify subjects with excess body fat.

Arguments against the use of skinfold measures in clinical or evaluation studies include the lack of reliability, and potential harm or inconvenience for participants. The use of skinfold measures in large population studies has shown that measuring skinfold thickness is feasible. A large subscapular skinfold predicted coronary heart disease in men independently of BMI and other cardiovascular risk factors [26]. The association between skinfolds and indicators of metabolic risk has been confirmed, but correlations of waist circumference with risk factors were either similar or stronger compared with those of the subscapular skinfold [27,28]. More research on the use of skinfold measures in clinical practice is warranted.

Waist circumference

Different scientific studies have measured the waist circumference at different sites. The original suggestions of cut-off points of 88 cm and 102 cm for women and men, respectively, were based on measurements of the waist circumference measured midway between the lower rib margin and the iliac crest with participants in standing position, without heavy outer garments and with emptied pockets, breathing out gently [14]. Without scientific rationale, other studies measured waist circumference as the minimal waist or at the umbilicus. An expert panel concluded that the location of the measurement does not affect the relationship between waist circumference and morbidity and mortality [29]. However, it is obvious that more at-risk individuals will be included for treatment when measurement is based on "maximum circumference" than when based on measurement at "umbilicus level" or "midway between iliac crest and lower rib."

Because definitions of large waist circumference promoted by the WHO [30] and NIH [31] are based on waist circumference measured midway between iliac crest and lower rib, this measurement seems the best option until scientific evidence proves otherwise. For research purposes it may well be valid and useful to use different sites. Enabling comparisons with other studies is a valid reason to choose one option. At the very least, authors should describe their measurement carefully and explain whether different measures could have lead to different conclusions.

The association of waist circumference with visceral fat storage is comparable to the abdominal sagittal diameter, which preceded the waist circumference as indicator of intra-abdominal fat storage. The sagittal abdominal diameter has a good correlation with insulin resistance, hypertension, type 2 diabetes mellitus, and dyslipidemia, and predicts increased mortality rates. This association appears stronger in relatively young adults [32]. A study of Dutch elderly showed no advantage of the sagittal abdominal diameter compared with other anthropometric measures as a correlate of components of the metabolic syndrome [33].

Han and Lean have explored the value of waist circumference. This measure is easy to perform, requires a tape measure only, and does not need to be calculated like the BMI [34]. Furthermore, Han et al showed that the relation between waist circumference and height was "not significant enough" to take into account body height when estimating fat storage [35]. An important advantage of waist circumference compared to BMI is that physical activity usually leads to reduction in waist circumference, whereas BMI may not decrease after physical activity, due to increased muscle mass. Interventions that do not affect BMI may prove effective when waist circumference is measured. Secular trends in waist circumference also appear stronger than the increase in BMI. High levels of waist circumference are associated with declines in quality of life and increased type 2 diabetes mellitus [9,36,37]. In longitudinal studies, waist circumference levels were clearly related to mortality [38,39].

Hip circumference

Hip circumference is most often recorded as the maximum circumference over the buttocks and has a strong association with leg fat mass, as well as leg lean mass. Lissner et al were among the first who showed that a small hip circumference predicted increased mortality, regardless of whether the waist circumference was taken into account [40]. This association has been replicated by more recent research [37]. A fair hypothesis is that if one has increased fat storage, the risk is lower if fat is stored in the hips and buttocks rather than the abdomen.

Waist/hip ratio

Waist/hip ratio is calculated as the ratio of waist to hip circumference. The different options for waist circumference (see above) will obviously lead to different values of the calculated waist/hip ratio.

Waist/hip ratio has been a popular marker for fat distribution in the last century. Some authors still present waist/hip ratio, because it may indeed be more strongly related to mortality than

waist circumference. Ratios, however, are hard to interpret [41]. For example, a high waist circumference may be a consequence of a large waist circumference or a small hip circumference.

New, promising measures

The BOD-POD and three-dimensional imaging techniques are expensive but highly feasible measures for large groups. They are reliable and provide innovative information.

The BOD-POD measures body composition through a sophisticated air displacement plethysmography technique [42]. The BOD-POD exists of two closed chambers. The participant is located in one chamber that is connected to a second chamber by a diaphragm. This diaphragm oscillates to create exactly the same volume perturbations in the two chambers. Software calculates the body's volume and density after weight has been measured [42].

Three-dimensional photography is now widely used in the fashion industry to study circumferences. Participants stand still for a few seconds and cameras take images from various positions. Software calculates circumferences of all sites requested by the researcher from these images and provides body volume estimates based on various circumferences.. The combination of body volume, body mass and lung volume enables the calculation of body density and thus percentage body fat. These calculations need to be agreed upon between researchers and companies delivering the software because these techniques are relatively new in obesity research.

How to define "excess" body fat

In adult men with an average weight the percentage body fat is in the order of 15–20%. In women this percentage is higher (about 25–30%). Based on percentage body fat, excess fat has been defined as exceeding 25% in men and 35% in women, although these definitions are not consensus based [42–45].

As stated before, accurate estimates of percentage body fat or amount of fat at certain locations are not feasible and can therefore not be used in clinical settings. Anthropometric measures provide valid alternatives for the definition of "excess fat" or "excess of fat at certain locations.". Because BMI and waist circumference are widely used and appear in guidelines for the prevention and treatment of obesity, this chapter is limited to the presentation of cut-off points for BMI and waist circumference. Furthermore, cut-off points for BMI and waist circumference have been validated in studies comparing subjects with levels below and above cut-off points with regard to disease, disability and mortality risk.

Cut-off points for measures other than BMI and waist circumference have not been studied with regard to health and mortality risk in prospective studies. Waist/hip ratio is the only exception, although cut-off points for waist/hip ratios are not consensus based. As stated before, waist/hip ratio itself is of limited use, due to difficulties in the interpretation of ratios [41] and the independent associations of waist and hip circumference with disease and mortality risk [37,40].

Table 1.2 Relative impact of overweight and obesity on coronary heart disease mortality in some recent large prospective studies in men and women

Authors	Jousilahti et al. [47]		Willett et al. [48]*		Seidell et al. [20]
Sex	Men	Women	Women	Men	Women
n	7740	8373	115,818	23,306	25,540
Follow-up (yrs)	15	15	14	12	12
Age at baseline (yrs)	30–59	30–59	30–55	30–54	30–54
% subjects with BMI ≥25 kg/m²	58	58	28	40	30
Relative risk BMI ≥25 vs <25 kg/m²	1.3	1.5	2.2	1.7	2.3
PAR (BMI ≥25 kg/m²)	15%	22%	25%	20%	28%
% subjects with BMI ≥30 kg/m²	11	20	11	4	6
Relative risk BMI ≥30 vs <30 kg/m²	1.4	1.3	2.6	2.5	2.3
PAR (BMI ≥30 kg/m²)	4%	6%	15%	6%	8%

*Fatal and nonfatal coronary heart disease combined.
PAR, population attributable risk.

Table 1.3 Relative impact of overweight and obesity on diabetes mellitus in some recent large prospective studies in men and women

Authors	Colditz et al. [50]	Chan et al. [49]
Sex	Women	Men
n	114,281	51,529
Follow-up (yrs)	14	5
Age at baseline (yrs)	30–55	40–75
% subjects with BMI ≥25 kg/m²	35	50
Relative risk BMI ≥25 vs <25 kg/m²	10.3	4.6
PAR (BMI ≥25 kg/m²)	77%	64%
% subjects with BMI ≥30 kg/m²	8	7
Relative risk BMI ≥30 vs <30 kg/m²	10.6	8.3
PAR (BMI ≥30 kg/m²)	44	33

PAR, population attributable risk.

Cut-offs for BMI

Until recently, anthropometry-based definitions of excess fat were most often based on BMI. Moderate overweight has long been classified as BMI between 25 and 29.9 kg/m² and obesity as BMI ≥30 kg/m² [30]. These cut-points apply to both men and women and to all adult age groups, and are based on the associations between BMI and mortality risk. Mortality risk is generally lowest in individuals with a BMI between 18.5 and 25 kg/m² [46]. Obesity based on BMI is related to diabetes mellitus and coronary heart disease in men and women. In addition, increasing degrees of overweight are associated with an increased incidence of osteoarthritis of knees and hips, gallbladder disease, sleep apnea and certain types of cancer (breast and endometrial cancer in women, colon cancer in men). In Tables 1.2 and 1.3 the relative impact of overweight (BMI ≥25 kg/m²) and obesity (BMI ≥30 kg/m²) is calculated for coronary heart disease [20,47,48] and diabetes mellitus [49,50]. In these studies performed in Finland, the United States and The Netherlands it can be shown that BMI in the range of 25–30 kg/m² is responsible for the major part of the impact of overweight on coronary heart disease mortality. If no one in these populations had a BMI greater than 25 kg/m², 15–30% of all deaths of coronary heart disease could theoretically have been prevented. It is difficult to see the impact of the increased prevalence of obesity on coronary heart disease (CHD) mortality because CHD mortality rates have been steadily decreasing in most rich countries since the 1970s due to improved diagnosis and treatment of CHD and its risk factors.

The impact of obesity on diabetes mellitus is much greater than for coronary heart disease (see Table 1.3). If these figures are correct then about 64% of male and 77% of female cases of type 2 diabetes mellitus could theoretically have been prevented if no person in these cohorts had a BMI over 25 kg/m². It is clear that the epidemic of obesity is closely followed by an epidemic of type 2 diabetes mellitus [51].

Recent literature has suggested that BMI 25–29.9 kg/m² was not associated with increased mortality risk [52]. However, there were methodologic explanations for not finding those relations, including inappropriate control for smoking and reverse causation [53,54]. More importantly, regardless of the mortality effects, BMI levels of ≥25 and ≥30 kg/m² are even more strongly related to morbidity and disability risks (Fig. 1.2). Thus, BMI 25–29.9 kg/m² does imply increased risk for individuals and public health and even exceeds costs of BMI ≥30 kg/m², at least in The Netherlands, due to high prevalence rates of BMI between 25 and 29.9 kg/m² [55]. When morbidity, disability and mortality are combined in analyses, both subjects with BMI 25–29.9 kg/m² and subjects with BMI ≥30 kg/m² have more unhealthy life-years than subjects with BMI 18.5–24.9 kg/m² [10].

Cut-offs for waist circumference

Lean et al defined action levels for waist circumference, based on a sample of 904 men and 1014 women participating in the Scottish MONICA sample. Waist circumference levels of 80 cm in women and 94 cm in men (action level 1) were associated with BMI of 25 kg/m². Waist circumference levels of 88 cm in women and 102 cm in men were in concordance with BMI ≥30 kg/m² [14]. These cut-off points are known as "action level 2" and identify subjects at increased risk for morbidity, disability, and mortality. No suggestions for other action levels are known, and although debated [56], waist circumference levels of 102 cm

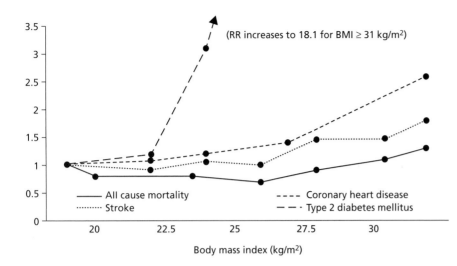

Figure 1.2 The relation of BMI to morbidity and mortality. (Figure derived from Visscher and Seidell [1]. Data based on the Nurses' Health Study [19,90–92].)

Table 1.4 Classification of overweight and obesity by cut-points of the BMI and the waist circumference, and related health risks (type 2 diabetes mellitus and cardiovascular diseases) [31]

	BMI	Normal waist circumference	Large waist circumference (>102 cm men, >88 cm women)
Underweight	<18.5	–	
Normal weight*	18.5–24.9	–	
Overweight	25–29.9	Increased	High
Obesity I	30–34.9	High	Very high
Obesity II	35–39.9	Very high	Very high
Extreme obesity	≥40	Extremely high	Extremely high

*Increased waist circumference can also be a marker for increased risk even in persons of normal weight.

for men and 88 cm for women have now reached the current WHO reports [30] and NIH guidelines [31] as indicators of increased health and mortality risk.

Waist circumference provides additional information on health and mortality risk independent of BMI. The NIH uses a combination of BMI and waist circumference to indicate individuals' health risk (Table 1.4) [31]. Note that large waist circumference is depicted as >102 and >88 cm for men and women, respectively, whereas Lean defined action level 2 as ≥102 and ≥88 cm, respectively [14]. Surgeons tend to use the terminology of super-obesity and super-super obesity for BMI levels of ≥50 and ≥60 kg/m², respectively.

Although the distribution of WHR categories is continuous, only dichotomous classifications have been proposed. No consensus has been reached regarding alternative cut-off points [56]. There are no commonly accepted cut-off points for high or low hip circumference or skinfolds.

The literature describes different categories of subjects with a different body composition or different body morphology, in which different levels of fat storage have a different link to risk of morbidity or premature risk. Conclusions that these relationships differ are often based on epidemiologic studies of subjects in whom BMI and not body fat has been measured. It could thus be questioned whether cut-off points that are presented here can be used in all individuals.

Measured versus self-reported obesity status

When identifying subjects who are candidates for treatment or prevention, measured rather than self-reported body weight should be used. When selection is based on self-reports a substantial proportion of subjects will be missed for appropriate treatment. Obese adults tend to under-report their body weight. This is understandable if patients do not routinely weigh themselves because body weight increases by 300–500 grams per year [57].

Four reviews have compared measured and reported body weight and height among adults [58–61], of which the review by Gorber et al. [60] was the most recent and most comprehensive. All concluded that there is a tendency to over-report body height and under-report body weight.

Large-scale studies that utilize BMI levels are often based on self-reported body weight and height. This could lead to underestimates of obesity prevalence rates, because adults also tend to under-report their body weight, especially the obese, and subjects tend to over-report body height. The significance of underreporting has been questioned, and some authors argue that mean levels of BMI may be estimated relatively well by use of self-reported data.

Measured body weight and height are generally most valuable when monitoring body weight and obesity prevalence rates, but there are alternatives. Measuring body weight and height consumes more time and money than self-reported height and weight. Reporting body weight and height is less time consuming. Therefore, people are more likely to participate.

Size of under-reporting

Gorber et al. [60] identified 28 studies that provided mean differences between both measured and reported body height. Mean difference between self-reported and measured body height varied between −1.3 cm (underestimation) to 5.0 cm (overestimation) among men and between − 1.7 cm to 5.0 cm among women. One study on both men and women exceeded the 5.0 cm difference. Hill and Roberts found a mean difference of 7.5 cm between measured and reported body height [62].

A total of 14 studies were found by Gorber et al. that presented difference in mean body weight when based on measured and reported body weight, and 24 studies provided these data for either men or women. Body weight was overestimated in all but two studies on both men and women; one was a sample of anorectics. All but three studies of women showed body weight was underestimated (range: 0.1–6.5 kg). The largest mean underestimation occurred in a study of women with BMIs between 35 and 40 kg/m^2. One study of women did not find a difference, and one of the two studies showing an overestimation was a study of women with BMI <20 kg/m^2. Twenty-four of 27 studies of men showed that body weight was underestimated (range: 0.1–3.2 kg).

Underestimation of BMI was calculated from those studies that included both reported and measured weight and height. In studies that combined men and women, underestimates ranged from 0.2 to 2.3 kg/m^2. Fourteen of 16 studies of men showed underestimates of BMI, ranging from −0.3 to −1.1 kg/m^2. Fifteen of 16 studies of women showed underestimates of BMI ranging from −0.1 to −2.4 kg/m^2. The largest underestimates occurred among women with BMI >40 kg/m^2. One study of the general Scottish population aged 25–64 years showed an overestimation

by 0.2 kg/m^2 with standard deviations of 1.4 and 1.3 kg/m^2 in men and women, respectively [63]. In the Spanish general population aged 15 years and over, BMI was overestimated by 0.5 and 0.9 kg/m^2 among men and women, respectively [64].

Under-reports of mean body weight and BMI may be regarded as relatively small, and about 97% of men and 95% of women report a body weight within 10% of their measured body weight. About 80% of men and 77% of women reported a body weight within 5% of their measured body weight [61]. Mean body height was 0.5 cm and 0.6 cm higher, and mean BMI was 0.4 kg/m^2 and 0.6 kg/m^2 lower among men and women respectively, when based on self-reported data [61]. Prevalence rates of overweight and obesity, however, were significantly lower when based on reported rather than measured body weight and height (Fig. 1.3) [61]. The prevalence of obesity was 3.0% and 3.3% lower among men and women, respectively, when based on self-reported data. As a percentage of the measured prevalence, obesity was underestimated by 26.1% among men and by 30.0% among women, when based on reported data.

The variance in difference between measured and reported obesity prevalence rates varies between studies, from 0.0% to 49.6% as a percentage of the true obesity prevalence rate (Fig. 1.4) [62–71]. In one study, where underestimation of obesity was nearly absent, the questionnaire to report body weight was sent out 2 weeks before the clinic appointment date [63]. There was no relationship between the reported obesity prevalence rate and the size of underestimation.

A few studies have presented linear regression equations to estimate "true" obesity prevalence rates from reported body weight and height [63,68,72–75]. Some of these estimates appeared valid within the sample from which the linear regression equation was formulated [63,68,73]. One study (NHANES II) developed linear regression equations from half of the sample to test the validity of the equations in the other half of the sample,

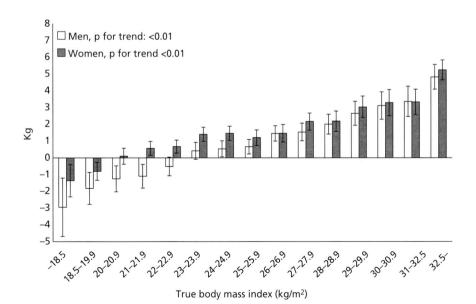

Figure 1.3 Under-reporting of body weight (kg) among Dutch men (full bars) and women (open bars) aged 20–59 years by measured BMI. (Figure derived from Visscher et al. [61]. Data from the National Institute for Public Health and the Environment, and Statistics Netherlands.)

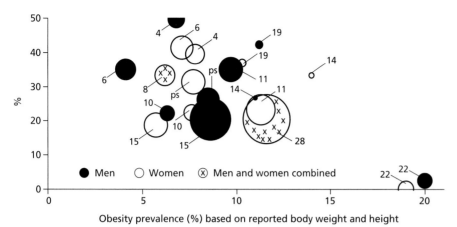

Figure 1.4 Underestimation of obesity prevalence rates as a percentage of the "true" obesity prevalence rate in various studies. Larger data points represent larger studies. Numbers denote references. 4: Hill and Roberts [62]. 6: Boström and Diderichsen [65]. 8: Stewart [93]. 10: Roberts [67]. 11: Spencer et al. [68]. 14: Flood et al. [69]. 15: Niedhammer et al. [70]. 19: Alvarez-Torices et al. [64]. 22: Bolton-Smith et al. [63].

and concluded that self-reported BMI is difficult or impossible to correct by the use of such equations [23]. Furthermore, when different correction equations are applied to a single database, a large variety of estimations for percentage of obesity is found [61].

Frequent weighing, at least once per month, reportedly leads to more accurate reporting of body weight [69]. Although self-reported body weight and height may not be valid alternatives for measuring body weight and height, it seems advisable to ask subjects to weigh themselves before they report their body weight and height in an interview or questionnaire. Spencer et al. hypothesized that an alternative may be to measure a few subjects per quantile of the BMI distribution [68].

Reporting body weight and body height is not a valid alternative for measuring body weight and height when estimating the obesity prevalence in a population or an individual's obesity status. Adjusting prevalence rates that are based on reported body weight and height does not lead to valid estimates. In addition, formulas used to calculate prevalence rates from reported data do not lead to valid estimates. Measuring body weight and height is costly and time consuming, but valuable efforts for monitoring and evaluating prevention and treatment studies do require direct measurements of body weight and height. As the most important determinant of under-reporting body weight is true body weight, we propose that monitoring efforts should include measured values of body weight and height once in every 3–5 years.

Obesity in clinical practice

Clinicians have two good reasons for discussing overweight or obesity with their patients. First, as described, obesity is not only a major risk factor but also a precursor for chronic diseases, disabilities, and premature mortality. Recent guidelines for the treatment of obesity suggest that body weight be measured and discussed only when co-morbidities are present. Second, obesity is the result of an overconsumption of energy, reduced activity or excess inactivity. Overweight alone is not the only reason for discussing nutrition and physical activity patterns, but body weight status provides an opportunity to discuss determinants of obesity.

Determinants of obesity

Diminished physical activity, high-calorie diets and inadequate adjustments of energy intakes to the diminished energy requirements are likely to be major determinants of weight changes. Prentice and Jebb [76] have proposed that, on a population level, limited physical activity may be more important than energy or fat consumption in explaining the time-trends of obesity in the UK. Their analyses were based on aspects of physical activity (such as number of hours spent watching television) and household consumption survey data. Although such data may be suggestive, they may also be biased. For example, under-reporting of fat consumption increases with the degree of overweight [77]. Changes in smoking behavior may also contribute to changes in body weight on a population level. Data from the United States showed that although smoking cessation could explain some of the increase in the prevalence of overweight, smoking cessation alone could not account for the major portion of the increase [78]. Other studies have also shown that the increase in obesity prevalence may be independent of smoking status [79,80].

Very little is known about the factors that may explain the large differences between populations in the distributions of BMI. Obviously, overweight in individuals in any population is the result of a long-term positive energy balance. The conclusion that overweight is attributable to physical inactivity or ingestion of large quantities of food is an oversimplification. Several epidemiologic studies have shown that the following factors are associated with overweight in the population.

Demographic factors
• *Age:* obesity increases with age at least up until age 50–60 years in men and women. Figure 1.5 shows the relation between age and prevalence of obesity in The Netherlands [81].
• *Gender:* the prevalence of obesity is generally higher in women compared to men especially when older than 50 years of age.

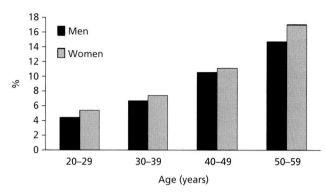

Figure 1.5 Prevalence of obesity by age in The Netherlands. (Data derived from Visscher et al. [81], National Institute of Public Health and the Environment.)

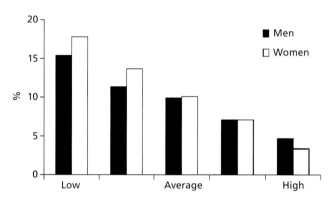

Figure 1.6 Obesity prevalence according to educational level. (Data derived from Visscher et al. [81], National Institute of Public Health and the Environment.)

• *Ethnicity:* large variations between ethnic groups are often not explained by socio-economic status measured by level of education and or income.

Sociocultural factors

• *Educational level and income:* in many industrialized countries there is a higher prevalence in those with lower education and/or income. Figure 1.6 illustrates the inverse association between the level of education and the prevalence of obesity in adults in The Netherlands.
• *Marital status:* obesity usually increases after marriage.

Biologic factors

It has been claimed that BMI increases with increasing number of children but recent evidence suggests that this contribution is, on average, likely to be small, less than 1 kg per pregnancy. Many study designs confound the changes in weight with aging with changes in weight with parity [82].

Obesity rates are increased in certain categories which deserve increased attention, as well as the absolute risks of morbidity, disability and mortality. Important subcategories that need further attention are men/women, elderly populations, children, and disabled persons.

Men/women

Usually, the same cut-off points are applied to men and women and to different age groups. This is done because the relationships between BMI and mortality are similar (i.e. the relative mortality associated with obesity is similar in men and women). In most age groups the absolute mortality among women is much lower. The same relative risk and lower absolute risk associated with overweight and obesity among women compared to men implies that women tolerate body fat better than men. Excess body fat in women is usually distributed as subcutaneous fat and mainly peripherally (thighs, buttocks, breasts) whereas in men there is a relative excess of body fat stored as visceral and subcutaneous abdominal fat.

Elderly

Body Mass Index levels are associated with increased mortality risk in the elderly, although relative risks decline with aging [10,83] and the optimal BMI with lowest mortality risk seems to increase with age [84]. The reasons why older people seem to tolerate excess body fat better than younger people are manifold and range from selective survival to decreased lipolysis of adipose tissue in older people.

Although BMI is still the most often used estimate of total body fat storage in older adults, there are limitations to its use as a single estimate for body fat. Body composition is changing in the elderly, muscle mass is decreasing, fat mass is increasing and becoming more centralized to the abdominal region. Health behaviors in the elderly differ from younger populations; undernutrition is more common and physical activity levels decline. Some have suggested the use of height measured at a younger age to calculate BMI in older adults, but this does not solve the problem of changing body composition and sarcopenia – losing muscle mass.

Waist circumference at age 55 has shown a fair association with risk factors for cardiovascular diseases and type 2 diabetes mellitus in both men and women. In never-smoking men, a large waist circumference identified more men with an increased risk of mortality than did high BMI. Changes in waist and hip circumference were better anthropometric predictors of changes in body fat storage over a 10-year period compared with changes in skinfold thickness [85]. High BMI in persons aged 70–79 years, however, had a stronger association with total body fat than did waist circumference.

Disabled persons

Disabled persons have an increased risk of developing obesity [86]. Some categories of physical disabilities prevent patients standing for measurement of body weight, waist and hip circumference or skinfold thickness. It is still unclear whether and which correction factors can be used for body height measures that are taken in standing and sitting or lying position. Suggestions have been made, however, to use knee height as proxy for body height in children and adults [87]. It should be noted that these studies have been performed in nondisabled persons and thus may not be necessarily valid for specific disability categories. Upper arm length, tibial length, and knee height have been suggested as proxies for body height in children with disorders such as cerebral palsy [88].

Conclusion

All European ministers of public health have now committed themselves to appropriate monitoring of overweight and obesity levels in children and adults. These efforts will lead to a further understanding of the increase in obesity and of measurement issues of obesity. Validation studies based on large-scale studies using innovative measures such as BOD-POD and three-dimensional imaging will lead to a further understanding of the value of definitions for the identification of individuals with "excess body fat" or at "increased risk." Research is especially needed in the elderly.

Clinicians can play an important role in the identification of individuals with overweight or obesity. Although their role will be further specified in the near future, measuring obesity status is already part of standard procedures when co-morbidities are presented or when patients have questions regarding their weight, nutrition or physical activities.

References

1. Visscher TLS, Seidell JC. The public health impact of obesity. Annu Rev Public Health 2001;22:355–75.
2. Kopelman P. Health risks associated with overweight and obesity. Obes Rev 2007;8(suppl 1):13–17.
3. Caterson ID, Franklin J, Colditz GA. Economic costs of obesity. In: Bray GA, Bouchard C, James WPT (eds) *Handbook of Obesity*. New York: Marcel Dekker, 2004:149–56.
4. Knai C, Suhrcke M, Lobstein T. Obesity in Eastern Europe: an overview of its health and economic implications. Econ Hum Biol 2007;5(3):392–408.
5. Wolf AM, Colditz GA. Current estimates of the economic cost of obesity in the United States. Obes Res 1998;6(2):97–106.
6. McTigue KM, Harris R, Hemphill B, et al. Screening and interventions for obesity in adults: summary of the evidence for the U.S. Preventive Services Task Force. Ann Intern Med 2003;139(11):933–49.
7. Trogdon JG, Finkelstein EA, Hylands T, et al. Indirect costs of obesity: a review of the current literature. Obes Rev 2008;9(5):489–500.
8. Narbro K, Jonsson E, Larsson B, et al. Economic consequences of sick-leave and early retirement in obese Swedish women. Int J Obes 1996;20(10):895–903.
9. Han TS, Tijhuis MA, Lean ME, et al. Quality of life in relation to overweight and body fat distribution. Am J Public Health 1998;88(12):1814–20.
10. Visscher TL, Rissanen A, Seidell JC, et al. Obesity and unhealthy life-years in adult Finns: an empirical approach. Arch Intern Med 2004;164(13):1413–20.
11. Vague J. The degree of masculine differentiation of obesities: a factor determining predisposition to diabetes, atherosclerosis, gout, and uric calculous disease. Am J Clin Nutr 1956;4(1):20–34.
12. Pouliot M-C, Després J-P, Lemieux S, et al. Waist circumference and abdominal sagittal diameter: best simple anthropometric indexes of abdominal visceral adipose tissue accumulation and related cardiovascular risk in men and women. Am J Cardiol 1994;73(7):460–8.
13. Han TS, Leer EM, Seidell JC, et al. Waist circumference action levels in the identification of cardiovascular risk factors: prevalence study in a random sample. BMJ 1995;31:1401–5.
14. Lean MEJ, Han TS, Morrison CE. Waist circumference as a measure for indicating need for weight management. BMJ 1995;311:158–61.
15. Deurenberg P, Weststrate JA, Seidell JC. Body mass index as a measure of body fatness: age- and sex-specific prediction formulas. Br J Nutr 1991;65(2):105–14.
16. Troiano RP, Frongillo EA, Sobal J, et al. The relationship between body weight and mortality: a quantitative analysis of combined information from existing studies. Int J Obes 1996;20:63–75.
17. Jousilahti P, Tuomilehto J, Vartiainen E, et al. Body weight, cardiovascular risk factors, and coronary mortality: 15-year follow-up of middle-aged men and women in eastern Finland. Circulation 1996;93(7):1372–9.
18. Lee I-M, Manson JE, Hennekens CH, et al. Body weight and mortality: a 27-year follow-up of middle-aged men. JAMA 1993;270(23):2823–8.
19. Manson JE, Willett WC, Stampfer MJ, et al. Body weight and mortality among women. N Engl J Med 1995;333(11):677–85.
20. Seidell JC, Verschuren WMM, Leer EM, et al. Overweight, underweight, and mortality: a prospective study of 48 287 men and women. Arch Intern Med 1996;156:958–63.
21. Allison DB, Faith MS, Heo M, et al. Hypothesis concerning the U-shaped relation between body mass index and mortality. Am J Epidemiol 1997;146(4):339–49.
22. Brožek J, Keys A. The evaluation of leanness–fatness in man: norms and interrelationships. Br J Nutr 1951;5(2):194–206.
23. Durnin JVGA, Womersley J. Body fat assessed from total body density and its estimation from skinfold thickness: measurements on 481 men and women aged from 16 to 72 years. Br J Nutr 1974;32:77–97.
24. Siri WAS. The gross composition of the body. In: Tobias CA & Lawrence JH, ed. In: Advantages in biological and medical physics. New York: The Academic Press; 1956.
25. Peterson MJ, Czerwinski SA, Siervogel RM. Development and validation of skinfold-thickness prediction equations with a 4-compartment model. Am J Clin Nutr 2003;77(5):1186–91.
26. Donahue RP, Abbott RD. Central obesity and coronary heart disease in men. Lancet 1987;2:1215.
27. Seidell JC, Cigolini M, Charzewska J, et al. Indicators of fat distribution, serum lipids, and blood pressure in European women born in 1948 – the European Fat Distribution Study. Am J Epidemiol 1989;130(1):53–65.
28. Seidell JC, Cigolini M, Deslypere J-P, et al. Body fat distribution in relation to serum lipids and blood pressure in 38-year-old European men: the European fat distribution study. Atherosclerosis 1991;86:251–60.
29. Ross R, Berentzen T, Bradshaw AJ, et al. Does the relationship between waist circumference, morbidity and mortality depend on measurement protocol for waist circumference? Obes Rev 2008;9(4):312–25.

30. World Health Organization. Obesity: preventing and managing the global epidemic. WHO Technical Report Series #894. Geneva: World Health Organization, 2000.

31. National Institutes of Health. Guidelines on the identification evaluation, and treatment of overweight and obesity in adults. Bethesda, MD: National Institutes of Health, 1998.

32. Seidell JC, Andres R, Sorkin JD, et al. The sagittal waist diameter and mortality in men: the Baltimore longitudinal study in aging. Int J Obes 1994;18:61–7.

33. Mukuddem-Petersen J, Snijder MB, van Dam RM, et al. Sagittal abdominal diameter: no advantage compared with other anthropometric measures as a correlate of components of the metabolic syndrome in elderly from the Hoorn Study. Am J Clin Nutr 2006;84(5):995–1002.

34. Han TS, Lean MEJ. Self-reported waist circumference compared with the 'Waist watcher' tape-measure to identify individuals at increased health risk through intra-abdominal fat accumulation. Br J Nutr 1998;80:81–8.

35. Han TS, Seidell JC, Currall JEP, et al. The influences of height and age on waist circumference as an index of adiposity in adults. Int J Obes 1997;21:83–9.

36. Han TS, Williams K, Sattar N, et al. Analysis of obesity and hyperinsulinemia in the development of metabolic syndrome: San Antonio Heart Study. Obes Res 2002;10(9):923–31.

37. Snijder MB, Zimmet PZ, Visser M, et al. Independent and opposite associations of waist and hip circumferences with diabetes, hypertension and dyslipidemia: the AusDiab Study. Int J Obes 2004;28(3):402–9.

38. Visscher TLS, Seidell JC, Molarius A, et al. A comparison of body mass index, waist-hip ratio and waist circumference as predictors of all-cause mortality among the elderly: the Rotterdam study. Int J Obes 2001;25(11):1730–5.

39. Wannamethee SG, Shaper AG, Lennon L, et al. Decreased muscle mass and increased central adiposity are independently related to mortality in older men. Am J Clin Nutr 2007;86(5):1339–46.

40. Lissner L, Bjorkelund C, Heitmann BL, et al. Larger hip circumference independently predicts health and longevity in a Swedish female cohort. Obes Res 2001;9(10):644–6.

41. Allison DB, Paultre F, Goran MI, et al. Statistical considerations regarding the use of ratios to adjust data. Int J Obes 1995;19(9):644–52.

42. Heymsfield SB, Baumgartner RN, Allison DB, et al. Evaluation of total and regional adiposity. In: Bray GA, Bouchard C, James WPT (eds) *Handbook of Obesity*. New York: Marcel Dekker, 2004:33–80.

43. Nooyens AC, Koppes LL, Visscher TL, et al. Adolescent skinfold thickness is a better predictor of high body fatness in adults than is body mass index: the Amsterdam Growth and Health Longitudinal Study. Am J Clin Nutr 2007;85(6):1533–9.

44. Gallagher D, Heymsfield SB, Heo M, et al. Healthy percentage body fat ranges: an approach for developing guidelines based on body mass index. Am J Clin Nutr 2000;72(3):694–701.

45. Taylor RW, Jones IE, Williams SM, et al. Body fat percentages measured by dual-energy X-ray absorptiometry corresponding to recently recommended body mass index cutoffs for overweight and obesity in children and adolescents aged 3–18 y. Am J Clin Nutr 2002;76(6):1416–21.

46. Lew EA, Garfinkel L. Variations in mortality by weight among 750,000 men and women. J Chron Dis 1979;32:563–76.

47. Jousilahti P, Tuomilehto J, Vartiainen E, et al. Body weight, cardiovascular risk factors, and coronary mortality: 15-year follow-up of middle-aged men and women in eastern Finland. Circulation 1996;93(7):1372–9.

48. Willett WC, Manson JE, Stampfer MJ, et al. Weight, weight change, and coronary heart disease in women: risk within the "normal" weight range. JAMA 1995;273(6):461–5.

49. Chan JM, Rimm EB, Colditz GA, et al. Obesity, fat distribution, and weight gain as risk factors for clinical diabetes in men. Diabetes Care 1994;17(9):961–9.

50. Colditz GA, Willett WC, Rotnitzky A, et al. Weight gain as a risk factor for clinical diabetes mellitus in women. Ann Intern Med 1995;122(7):481–6.

51. Seidell JC. Obesity, insulin resistance and diabetes – a worldwide epidemic. Br J Nutr 2000;83(suppl 1):S5–S8.

52. Flegal KM, Graubard BI, Williamson DF, et al. Excess deaths associated with underweight, overweight, and obesity. JAMA 2005;293(15):1861–7.

53. Manson JE, Stampfer MJ, Hennekens CH, et al. Body weight and longevity: a reassessment. JAMA 1987;257(3):353–8.

54. Lawlor DA, Hart CL, Hole DJ, et al. Reverse causality and confounding and the associations of overweight and obesity with mortality. Obesity (Silver Spring) 2006;14(12):2294–304.

55. Seidell JC. The impact of obesity on health status: some implications for health care costs. Int J Obes 1995;19(suppl 6):S13–S16.

56. Molarius A, Seidell JC. Selection of anthropometric indicators for classification of abdominal fatness – a critical review. Int J Obes 1998;22:719–27.

57. Nooyens AC, Visscher TL, Verschuren WM, et al. Age, period and cohort effects on body weight and body mass index in adults: The Doetinchem Cohort Study. Public Health Nutr 2008; Jul 24:1–9.

58. Bowman RL, DeLucia JL. Accuracy of self-reported weight: a meta-analysis. Behav Ther 1992;23:637–55.

59. Engstrom JL, Paterson SA, Doherty A, et al. Accuracy of self-reported height and weight in women: an integrative review of the literature. J Midwifery Womens Health 2003;48(5):338–45.

60. Gorber SC, Tremblay M, Moher D, et al. A comparison of direct vs. self-report measures for assessing height, weight and body mass index: a systematic review. Obes Rev 2007;8(4):307–26.

61. Visscher TL, Viet AL, Kroesbergen IH, et al. Underreporting of BMI in adults and its effect on obesity prevalence estimations in the period 1998 to 2001. Obesity (Silver Spring) 2006;14(11):2054–63.

62. Hill A, Roberts J. Body mass index: a comparison between self-reported and measured height and weight. J Public Health Med 1998;20(2):206–10.

63. Bolton-Smith C, Woodward M, Tunstall-Pedoe H, et al. Accuracy of the estimated prevalence of obesity from self reported height and weight in an adult Scottish population. J Epidemiol Commun Health 2000;54(2):143–8.

64. Alvarez-Torices JC, Franch-Nadal J, Alvarez-Guisasola F, et al. Self-reported height and weight and prevalence of obesity: study in a Spanish population. Int J Obes 1993;17(11):663–7.

65. Boström G, Diderichsen F. Socioeconomic differentials in misclassification of height, weight and body mass index based on questionnaire data. Int J Epidemiol 1997;26(4):860–6.

66. Stewart AW, Jackson RT, Ford MA, et al. Underestimation of relative weight by use of self-reported height and weight. Am J Epidemiol 1987;125(1):122–6.

67. Roberts RJ. Can self-reported data accurately describe the prevalence of overweight? Public Health 1995;109(4):275–84.

68. Spencer EA, Appleby PN, Davey GK, et al. Validity of self-reported height and weight in 4808 EPIC-Oxford participants. Public Health Nutr 2002;5(4):561–5.

69. Flood V, Webb K, Lazarus R, et al. Use of self-report to monitor overweight and obesity in populations: some issues for consideration. Aust NZ J Public Health 2000;24(1):96–9.

70. Niedhammer I, Bugel I, Bonenfant S, et al. Validity of self-reported weight and height in the French GAZEL cohort. Int J Obes 2000;24(9): 1111–18.

71. Nieto-Garcia FJ, Bush TL, Keyl PM. Body mass definitions of obesity: sensitivity and specificity using self-reported weight and height. Epidemiology 1990;1(2):146–52.

72. Rowland ML. Self-reported weight and height. Am J Clin Nutr 1990;52(6):1125–33.

73. Kuskowska-Wolk A, Karlsson P, Stolt M, et al. The predictive validity of body mass index based on self-reported weight and height. Int J Obes 1989;13(4):441–53.

74. Kuskowska-Wolk A, Bergstrom R, Bostrom G. Relationship between questionnaire data and medical records of height, weight and body mass index. Int J Obes 1992;16(1):1–9.

75. Plankey MW, Stevens J, Flegal KM, et al. Prediction equations do not eliminate systematic error in self-reported body mass index. Obes Res 1997;5(4):308–14.

76. Prentice AM, Jebb SA. Obesity in Britain: gluttony or sloth? BMJ 1995;311:437–9.

77. Seidell JC. Dietary fat and obesity: an epidemiologic perspective. Am J Clin Nutr 1998;67(suppl):546S–550S.

78. Flegal KM, Trolano RP, Pamuk ER, et al. The influence of smoking cessation on the prevalence of overweight in the United States. N Engl J Med 1995;333(18):1165–70.

79. Boyle CA, Dobson AJ, Egger G, et al. Can the increasing weight of Australians be explained by the decreasing prevalence of cigarette smoking? Int J Obes 1994;18(1):55–60.

80. Wolk A, Rössner S. Effects of smoking and physical activity on body weight: development in Sweden between 1980 and 1989. J Intern Med 1995;237(3):287–91.

81. Visscher TL, Kromhout D, Seidell JC. Long-term and recent time trends in the prevalence of obesity among Dutch men and women. Int J Obes 2002;26(9):1218–24.

82. Williamson DF, Madans J, Pamuk E, et al. A prospective study of childbearing and 10-year weight gain in US white women 25 to 45 years of age. Int J Obes 1994;18(8):561–9.

83. Stevens J, Cai J, Pamuk ER, et al. The effect of age on the association between body-mass index and mortality. N Engl J Med 1998;338(1):1–7.

84. Andres R, Elahi D, Tobin JD, et al. Impact of age on weight goals. Ann Intern Med 1985;103(6 part 2):1030–3.

85. Hughes VA, Roubenoff R, Wood M, et al. Anthropometric assessment of 10-y changes in body composition in the elderly. Am J Clin Nutr 2004;80(2):475–82.

86. Bandini LG, Curtin C, Hamad C, et al. Prevalence of overweight in children with developmental disorders in the continuous national health and nutrition examination survey (NHANES) 1999–2002. J Pediatr 2005;146(6):738–43.

87. Chumlea WC, Guo SS, Steinbaugh ML. Prediction of stature from knee height for black and white adults and children with application to mobility-impaired or handicapped persons. J Am Diet Assoc 1994;94(12):1385–8, 1391; quiz 1389–90.

88. Stevenson RD. Use of segmental measures to estimate stature in children with cerebral palsy. Arch Pediatr Adolesc Med 1995;149(6): 658–62.

89. Snijder MB, van Dam RM, Visser M, et al. What aspects of body fat are particularly hazardous and how do we measure them? Int J Epidemiol 2006;35(1):83–92.

90. Carey VJ, Walters EE, Colditz GA, et al. Body fat distribution and risk of non-insulin-dependent diabetes mellitus in women: the Nurses' Health Study. Am J Epidemiol 1997;145(7):614–19.

91. Manson JE, Colditz GA, Stampfer MJ, et al. A prospective study of obesity and risk of coronary heart disease in women. N Engl J Med 1990;322(13):882–9.

92. Rexrode KM, Hennekens CH, Willett WC, et al. A prospective study of body mass index, weight change, and risk of stroke in women. JAMA 1997;277(19):1539–45.

93. Stewart AL. The reliability and validity of self-reported weight and height. J Chron Dis 1982;35:295–309.

2   Measuring Body Composition in Adults and Children

K. Ashlee McGuire[1] and Robert Ross[1,2]

[1] School of Kinesiology and Health Studies
[2] Medicine, Division of Endocrinology and Metabolism, Queens University, Kingston, Ontario, Canada

Introduction

The dramatic rise in overweight and obesity over the past several years in both the adult and pediatric populations has sparked immense interest in the measurement of body composition. Although the immediate consequences of obesity have been more extensively studied in adults, longitudinal studies indicate that childhood obesity is associated with obesity in adulthood which in turn is associated with increased risk of cardiovascular disease, type 2 diabetes and other metabolic complications [1]. These observations underline the importance of advancing our knowledge of the connection between excess weight gain and risk of obesity-related metabolic disorders. The purpose of this chapter is to provide an update on recent advances in body composition measurement techniques and to describe how these measures relate to the more commonly used anthropometric measures in clinical use.

Field methods: bio-electric impedance and densitometry

Several field methods, including bio-electric impedance and hydrodensitometry, are employed to measure body composition. Common to these methods in field settings is the use of a two-compartment model which is best explained using the formula developed by Heymsfield and associates [2]:

$C_i = f(P_A)$, where C_i is the unknown component, P_A is the measureable property and f is the mathematical function that links C_i to P_A.

Clinical Obesity in Adults and Children, 3rd edition. Edited by Peter G. Kopelman, Ian D. Caterson and William H. Dietz.
© 2010 Blackwell Publishing, ISBN: 978-1-4051-8226-3.

For example, body density (a measureable property) can be used to estimate total body fat (unknown component) using a regression equation (mathematical function). The ability of the equation to estimate body fat accurately is determined by: a "criterion" or "reference" method such as whole-body magnetic resonance imaging (MRI) being used to measure the component of interest; the component of interest being measured in a well-characterized group of participants such as premenopausal overweight women; and the development of a prediction equation by regression analysis. Problems occur (e.g. underestimation of body fat) when, for example, an equation developed in young adults is utilized to predict body fat in the elderly or a poor reference method is used to validate the field method (e.g. the given equation). Thus, it is critical to understand that the ability of the equation to provide accurate estimations is heavily dependent on the above criteria being rigorously followed and the equation being applied appropriately.

Bio-electric impedance analysis

Bio-electric impedance analysis (BIA) is a field method used to estimate body fat and/or lean mass. BIA is quick and noninvasive, making it a popular device. Detailed reviews have been published previously [3,4] and only a brief review will be provided here. BIA applies the principle that fat is a poor conductor of an applied current and fat-free tissues are good conductors. Thus, measures of electrical conductivity are proportional to total body water and fat-free mass and are converted to estimates of body fat and fat-free mass using population-specific equations. Conductivity is also affected by numerous other factors, such as hydration or temperature; therefore preassessment guidelines must be followed with rigor. Comparisons of BIA to other methods have reported inconsistent results. BIA may underestimate or overestimate body fat mass in individuals of all ages [5–7].

Hydrodensitometry and air displacement plethysmography

The procedures for hydrodensitometry (HD) and air displacement plethysmography (ADP) estimate body composition from body density [8] or volume [9]. Population-specific formulas have been derived to calculate percentage body fat using these two methods. The validity and accuracy of any equation depend on whether assumptions are appropriate for the individual being measured. HD has traditionally been considered the "gold standard" measurement of body composition and has often been utilized as the criterion method to validate new body composition assessment tools. In recent years ADP has become a popular alternative, due to its ease of administration. Despite the widespread use and acceptable precision and accuracy of these techniques in most groups, numerous limitations are associated with methods of densitometry [8]. Excellent reviews have previously been conducted [8]. Measurements obtained from HD and ADP generally provide information regarding percentage body fat in the population studies but rarely describe how this relates to health outcomes.

Dual-energy X-ray absorptiometry (DXA)

Dual-energy X-ray absorptiometry is used to measure total and regional body composition, including the estimation of lean soft tissue mass, fat-free mass, fat mass and bone mineral content [10]. DXA is associated with low radiation exposure, is relatively quick and requires little effort from the participant, making it ideal for use in youth [11]. Body composition is assessed by measuring the attenuation of X-rays emitted using pencil- or-fan-beam technology at two energy levels as it traverses the body [10]. Measures of fat and fat-free mass may be affected by scanner type (pencil or fan), software used (algorithms), sagittal diameter, hydration status, tissue thickness and subject size but measurements are highly repeatable. Measurements of fat-free mass, appendicular fat mass and total abdominal fat correlate highly with measures of computed tomography (CT) and MRI. However, DXA can only assess body composition two-dimensionally. Thus, it is unable to differentiate subcutaneous fat from visceral fat [12]. Also, DXA may overestimate percentage body fat in subjects with higher percentage body fat and underestimate body fat percentage in subjects with lower percentage body fat [13].

Imaging techniques for assessing body composition

The most accurate measurements currently available for *in vivo* quantification of body composition at the tissue level are imaging methods such as MRI and CT. These noninvasive tools are able to measure skeletal muscle, adipose tissue and internal tissues, and organs *in vivo* in both adults and youth. These tools are ideal in youth, since there are no age-related assumptions [14]. Thus, although these devices are associated with high cost and time-consuming analyses, they are used extensively in body composition research. In addition, they provide accurate tools for

which anthropometric measures can be validated as proxy measurements for internal adipose depots. These measures can then be applied in clinical settings.

Computed tomography

Computed tomography uses X-rays that are attenuated as they pass through tissues to construct images of the body. The X-ray attenuation, determined primarily by physical density, is expressed as a linear attenuation coefficient relative to air and water (−1000 and 0, respectively) known as CT numbers or, more commonly, Hounsfield units (HU). Cross-sectional CT images are composed of picture elements, or pixels, each of which has a CT number or HU on a gray scale to reflect the composition of the tissue. The lower the density of the tissue, the lower the HU values for the pixels that construct the tissue [15].

Magnetic resonance imaging

Magnetic resonance imaging is based on the interaction between hydrogen nuclei (protons) and the magnetic fields generated by the MRI system's instrumentation to construct cross-sectional images [15]. Since MRI does not use harmful ionizing radiation such as CT, it is generally the method of choice for assessing whole-body tissue composition. Although MRI data acquisition is more time consuming, advances in MRI instrumentation now allow for a series of whole-body images to be acquired in less than 30 minutes [16].

Image analysis: quantifying tissue area, tissue volume and mass

The approach used for quantifying body components, such as adipose tissue, skeletal muscle, bone, visceral organs, and brain, using CT and MRI images is similar. One of two techniques can be utilized to determine tissue area (cm^2):

1 The perimeter of the tissue of interest can be traced using a light pen or a trackball-or mouse-controlled pointer [17] and then the area within the perimeter can be calculated by multiplying the number of pixels in the highlighted region by their known area.

2 Image segmentation algorithms can be used that highlight all pixels within a selected range of intensities believed to be representative of a specific tissue [18].

The latter approach is more problematic in MRI than CT for the following three reasons: the distribution of pixel intensity (gray scale) values for different tissues overlap more for MRI than for CT images; noise from respiratory motion blurs the borders between tissues in the abdomen to a greater extent in MRI than in CT; and inhomogeneity in the magnetic field can produce "shading" at the peripheries of MRI images [19].

When multiple CT or MRI images are obtained, tissue volumes can be calculated by integrating the cross-sectional area data from consecutive slices. Since data acquisition and analysis of contiguous images are time consuming and expensive, axial images are usually collected with gaps ranging from 20 to 40 mm between the top of one image and the bottom of the next image. Volumes can then be calculated using geometric models based on the tissue areas in the images and the distance between adjacent images [15]. Currently three models are being used: a "parallel trapezium" model [20]; a "truncated cone" model [16]; and the "two-column" model [21]. Tissue densities for adipose tissue, skeletal muscle, and organs are quite constant from person to person. Therefore CT and MRI volume measures for these tissues can be converted to mass units by multiplying the volume by the assumed density values for that tissue. Density values for the brain and visceral organs vary from organ to organ but reference values are available [22].

Measurement of visceral adipose tissue

The only *in vivo* methods available to quantify visceral fat are MRI and CT. The ability to measure visceral adipose tissue using these noninvasive methods is representative of major advancements in understanding the relationship between fat distribution and health risk. Visceral fat is known to be strongly associated with the metabolic syndrome and cardiovascular disease risk, [23,24] and is an independent predictor of morbidity [25,26] and mortality [27] in adults. Similar to adults, visceral fat in children (especially obese children [1]) is positively associated with a host of metabolic complications such as impaired insulin sensitivity and increased total and low-density lipoprotein cholesterol [28–30]. Currently, there is debate as to the optimal location for visceral fat measurement. It has been suggested that the gold standard measurement protocol is contiguous images from T10–T11 to L5–S1, but due to time and radiation exposure (with CT), single MRI or CT images at L4–L5 are typically utilized. Visceral fat measures taken using a single image at any anatomic level within the abdomen are highly correlated with multiple image protocols despite substantial differences in the absolute amount of fat [31,32]. Traditionally visceral fat was measured at L4–L5 but recently, Kuk and colleagues [31] reported that the L1–L2 level may be the landmark that predicts total visceral fat mass and the metabolic syndrome the strongest in Caucasian men. It is unclear whether this is also true in women, men of other ethnicities or youth.

Growth and gender are known to influence the quantity of visceral adipose tissue present in youth [14]. Beginning at a baseline of 8 years of age, the general increase in visceral adipose tissue occurs at a more rapid rate than abdominal subcutaneous adipose tissue and is approximately 5.2 cm^2/year over a 5-year period [33]. Adolescent boys preferentially deposit fat in the intra-abdominal region whereas adolescent girls deposit more total fat, and a higher percentage of this fat is found in the subcutaneous region of the abdomen [34].

Measurement of abdominal subcutaneous fat

As with visceral adipose tissue, there is presently no consensus on the ideal measurement protocol for abdominal subcutaneous fat. Abdominal subcutaneous fat is usually measured on the single image being used to acquire visceral fat in adults and youth.

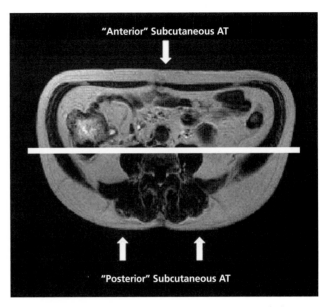

Figure 2.1 Subdivision of abdominal subcutaneous adipose tissue (AT) into anterior and posterior depots.

Substantial differences exist in the absolute amount of abdominal subcutaneous fat measured in different locations across the abdomen. However, the relationship between abdominal subcutaneous fat and the metabolic syndrome seems to be similar across all measurement sites in adults [31] but this is unknown in youth. It has been suggested that there are metabolic differences in subcutaneous adipocytes located throughout the abdomen. The deep abdominal subcutaneous adipose tissue is thought to function as a metabolically active tissue whereas the superficial abdominal subcutaneous adipose tissue functions primarily as a storage depot or thermoinsulatory layer. Consequently, health may be affected differently by a greater amount of fat in one area as opposed to the other. Unfortunately, the anatomic boundaries that separate the regions of abdominal adipose tissue are presently unclear (see Fig. 2.1 for examples) and the results describing the relationship between the different fat depots and health risk are controversial in adults [15].

In youth, the role of subcutaneous adipose tissue in metabolic dysfunction is inconsistent in the literature and is affected by ethnicity, gender and weight status. In African-American children, increased subcutaneous abdominal adipose tissue is associated with increased indicators of metabolic disturbances [35,36] but in Caucasian obese adolescent girls there is no relationship between subcutaneous adipose tissue and markers of the metabolic syndrome [28]. Goran and Gower [1] report that in lean, but not obese, children and adolescents, subcutaneous adipose tissue predicts lower insulin sensitivity. Further research is warranted in this area.

Measurement of thigh subcutaneous adipose tissue

Measurements of thigh subcutaneous adipose tissue can be obtained using the seven images distal to the femoral head from

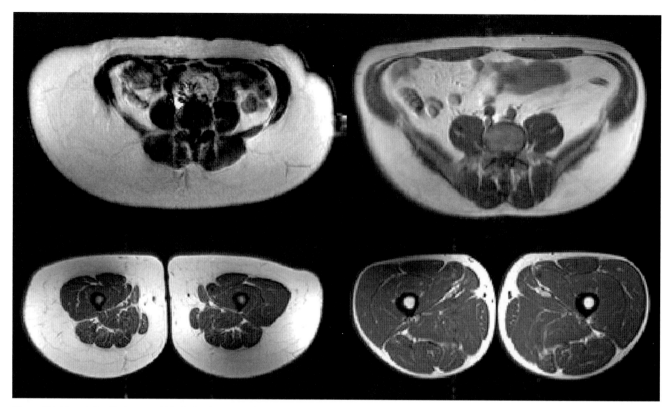

Figure 2.2 The relationship between high thigh subcutaneous fat and subcutaneous abdominal fat (*left*) and low thigh subcutaneous fat and high visceral abdominal fat (*right*) as measured by MRI is demonstrated in two individuals classified as high risk by waist circumference.

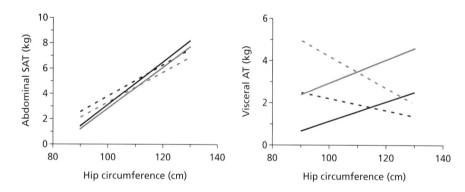

Figure 2.3 Associations between hip circumference and abdominal subcutaneous tissue (SAT) and visceral adipose tissue (AT) before (*solid lines*) and after (*dotted lines*) control for waist circumference in men (*gray lines*) and women (*black lines*). (Reproduced from reference [37] with permission from the American Society for Nutrition.)

an MRI scan [37]. Using MRI to distinguish between fat depots in the abdomen, a negative relationship between visceral fat and thigh circumference, and a positive relationship between abdominal subcutaneous fat and thigh circumference in both middle-aged men and women has been detected [37] (Fig. 2.2). Regardless of measurement technique used for the acquisition of thigh size (CT or anthropometry), increased total thigh adipose tissue area (reported in cm²) and increased thigh circumference (reported in cm) are associated with more favorable glucose and lipid levels in men and lipid levels in women independent of all other fat depots and ethnicity [38]. Further, in adults aged 50–75 years, Snijder et al. [39] found that a larger thigh circumference in women is associated with a lower risk of diabetes. These data

demonstrate that the use of thigh circumference alone provides useful information regarding metabolic health. In addition, Kuk and associates [37] recently reported that for a given waist circumference, male and female individuals with increased hip or thigh circumference have greater amounts of subcutaneous adipose tissue and decreased visceral adipose tissue within the abdomen (Fig. 2.3). Both the hip and the thigh circumference can provide additional health-related information to either the waist circumference alone without regard for the lower body or the lower body circumference alone without regard for the waist circumference. This also demonstrates the utility of imaging techniques in enhancing our ability to interpret simple anthropometric measurements.

This phenotype has not yet been explored extensively in children and adolescents but Freedman and colleagues [40] report that its prognostic value is limited and does not show the same negative correlations with intra-abdominal fat as in adults [34].

Measurement of skeletal muscle quantity

Magnetic resonance imaging and CT are presently the only measures available for *in vivo* quantification of body composition at the tissue level and therefore are the tools of choice to measure skeletal muscle mass. Measurement of skeletal muscle mass is important for assessing change in muscle with training programs or in older adults for assessing skeletal muscle loss. Generally, a single image located mid-thigh is used as a proxy measure of whole-body skeletal muscle in adults [41] and youth [42]. This measure of mid-thigh muscle mass correlates strongly (Pearson correlation, r = 0.97) with results from cadaver sections [43]. When volume measures are acquired using multiple images, the error associated with MRI is <1%; however, this process is both time consuming and costly. Abdominal muscle mass measured by MRI at L4–L5 has been reported to be a significant predictor of whole-body muscle mass in middle-aged men and women as well but does not correlate as strongly to whole-body skeletal muscle mass as the measurement at the thigh [41]. Since this is a common measurement location for abdominal adipose tissue, this location may have great potential in clinical practice because it would decrease cost by decreasing time associated with measurement and analysis.

Measurement of skeletal muscle tissue quality

Fat deposition within the muscle is of interest due to the inverse relationship between intramyocellular lipid (IMCL) and insulin sensitivity in sedentary or untrained adults and youth, thus supporting a role for IMCL in the pathogenesis of skeletal muscle insulin resistance and type 2 diabetes [44,45]. However, in endurance-trained individuals, high IMCL levels are associated with high insulin sensitivity compared with healthy sedentary subjects. This paradox requires further investigation, but imaging methods provide opportunities with which to gain considerable information regarding fat metabolism within the muscle. Previously, muscle biopsies were the method of choice used to determine accumulation of fat within the muscle but due to limitations using this protocol, the use of noninvasive measures such as CT, MRI and magnetic resonance spectroscopy (MRS) has become common for examining the relationship between IMCL and obesity-related metabolic disorders.

Magnetic resonance spectroscopy is based on principles similar to those of MRI and can usually be performed with the same MR machine. In contrast to MRI, MRS investigates the chemical composition of the tissue at a lower spatial resolution than MRI [46], and uses the differing proton resonance signals from the fatty acyl groups within the muscle to quantify skeletal muscle fat [47]. The two lipid pools present in skeletal muscle – extramyocellular lipid (EMCL), located outside the muscle cell and defined as compact portions of adipose tissue in subcutaneous or interstitial layers,

and IMCL, located within the muscle cell and stored in close contact with mitochondria in spheroid droplets – present different geometrical arrangements which result in different MR characteristics. Thus, proton MRS (^{1}H-MRS) is able to partition the lipid signal into IMCL and EMCL components in the skeletal muscle [46,48].

Recently, CT has been applied to measure tissue composition. The lower the average skeletal muscle HU value or the greater the number of low-density skeletal muscle pixels, the higher the skeletal muscle lipid content. Muscle attenuation values determined by CT reflect both IMCL and EMCL content and therefore cannot be directly compared to IMCL values obtained by skeletal muscle biopsy or ^{1}H-MRS [15].

MRI may also be used to measure the quality of skeletal muscle by applying "chemical shift" techniques such as the Dixon method [49]. This method separates the water and fat signals from the region of interest in order to create the potential to determine water and fat contents of skeletal muscle. Similar to CT, MRI cannot be used to partition the IMCL and EMCL into separate compartments.

Although quantification of IMCL is usually obtained from a single muscle, it is not homogeneous between different muscles in one individual or identical muscles in different individuals [48]. For example, in a trained swimmer, IMCL levels are high in m. rectus femoris whereas in a trained orienteer, IMCL levels are high in m. tibialis anterior. In trained and untrained individuals, there are greater amounts of IMCL in the soleus muscle as compared to the tibialis anterior muscle [50], tibialis posterior and gastrocnemius. This difference in IMCL between muscle groups occurs due to the fiber orientation [48] and primary fiber type of each muscle group. For example, the soleus is composed primarily of type 1 or slow-twitch fibers whereas the tibialis anterior is primarily composed of type 2 or fast-twitch fibers [50]. It has also been reported that numerous other factors such as age, training, oxygenation, diet or pennation angle (the angle formed by the individual muscle fibers with the line of action of the muscle) may influence IMCL in the muscle [44]. Despite providing important information regarding metabolic health, this technique has limited utility in clinical practice due to the high cost and difficult assessment.

Measurement of liver tissue

Hepatic steatosis or "fatty liver" is associated with the pathogenesis of liver disease, diabetes mellitus and features of the metabolic syndrome such as insulin resistance and hypertriglyceridemia [51]. Currently hepatic steatosis has been proposed as a core feature of the metabolic syndrome in adults and possibly in children and adolescents [52]. Liver biopsy is considered the "gold standard" measurement of liver fat, but it can be painful [51] and has a notable risk of mortality [53]. Thus, the use of noninvasive devices to measure liver fat and further explore obesity-related health complications of fatty liver is important.

Computed tomography has been utilized to determine liver density in a manner similar to that of skeletal muscle tissue density. As with skeletal muscle, lower mean liver HU values are associated with lower densities and therefore greater fat content. However, an overlap exists between normal and abnormal liver HU values [54] indicating that, using an absolute liver density, CT may not be sensitive enough to predict an abnormal liver. In individuals with normal livers, there is a constant relationship between liver and spleen attenuation. Therefore, the ratio of mean liver to spleen attenuation values is used as an index of liver fat [54]. Because the attenuation values within the liver and spleen are fairly homogeneous throughout, it has recently been suggested that the whole liver and spleen surface areas be used to derive attenuation values. This method reduces the interobserver coefficient of variation from 5.1% to 2.9% [55]. Davidson et al. [55] proposed that a single axial image at the T12–L1 intervertebral space may be the optimal landmark for the assessment of both liver and spleen attenuation. Both organs were identified approximately 90% of the time at this location in the men and women studied. In addition, it is recommended that the index of liver and spleen attenuation be derived from a mean score of the entire image to avoid potential bias introduced by variable placement of a region of interest [55].

Magnetic resonance imaging can also be used to estimate liver fat. A liver fat index can be created by examining the signal intensity in a region of interest within the right lobe of the liver and comparing this to the signal intensity of a same-sized region of interest within the adjacent subcutaneous adipose tissue [56]. To quantify hepatic fat content in children and adolescents, the fast MRI technique, using the modified Dixon method, can be completed during a single 15-second breath hold [57]. The method is described in detail elsewhere [49,52]. Fast MRI has been validated in lean and obese individuals against hepatic fat measured by ^{1}H-NMR (r = 0.93, p < 0.001) and liver biopsy [58].

The quantification of liver fat by ^{1}H-MRS is easy because unlike skeletal muscle, there is no EMCL in the liver. Liver spectra will only have one peak to reflect the IMCL component (methylene signal) which is measured at 0–3.0 ppm, and another peak from the water signal between 3.0 and 7.8 ppm. The percentage of liver fat is derived from the ratio of the area under the curve for fat and compared with the area under the curve for water [51,59,60]. The values obtained using ^{1}H-MRS correlate well with liver biopsy results and this is considered to be the optimal noninvasive method to assess fatty liver [51]. This technique has recently allowed for the assessment of fatty liver in the general population (inclusive of both adults and youth) [51,61].

The correlation between body composition and liver fat is controversial. In women, hepatic fat is not related to body mass index (BMI), percentage body fat, fat mass, waist-to-hip ratio (WHR), intra- or subcutaneous abdominal fat [62]. Some researchers [63,64] reported that both visceral and subcutaneous fat depots and anthropometric indices are strong correlates of liver fat. Others [65] reported no differences in body fat between obese individuals with or without increased hepatic triglyceride content.

In adolescents, a hepatic fat fraction of >5.5% has been defined as the cut-off to denote steatosis [52]. Recently it has been shown using ^{1}H-MRS that in obese adolescents with normal glucose tolerance, hepatic steatosis is associated with a less healthy lipoprotein profile and an increase in indicators of the metabolic syndrome [52,58,66]. Obese adolescents with hepatic steatosis also have increased visceral fat and higher IMCL and are more insulin resistant than obese adolescents without hepatic steatosis [52,58,67]. Interestingly, fatty liver has not been found to correlate with BMI in obese adolescents [68].

Although the literature regarding the use of imaging techniques in children and adolescents is just emerging, there is potential to expand our understanding of the relationship between fatty liver and obesity-related metabolic disorders in this population. However, these techniques currently have limited clinical utility and are more prominent in the research setting.

Other ectopic fat depots

Imaging methods are widely used to examine small ectopic fat depots, such as those surrounding or within the heart and blood vessels. These methods have replaced the need for autopsy and animal studies, making data acquisition much easier and relationships simpler to explore [69,70]. The most persuasive evidence proving that lipid overaccumulation occurs in human organs has been obtained noninvasively using MRS [71] as well as MRI and CT. Localized MRS is a precise and reproducible tool for *in vivo* quantification of ectopic fat in humans. This method is able to distinguish between depots of triglyceride in adipose tissue cells (fat surrounded by fat) and triglyceride droplets stored in the cytosol of parenchymal cells (fat surrounded by cytosol) [72]. Quantification of lipid surrounding the heart is difficult because the heart is always in motion [73]. The MRS technique has been validated in *ex vivo* and *in vivo* rodent studies [74,75].

Epicardial, myocardial and pericardial fat

Epicardial fat lies on the surface of the heart, especially around the epicardial coronary vessels, and can extend into the heart and be interspersed with myocardial muscle fibres [76]. Pericardial fat is located on the external surface of the parietal pericardium and differs from epicardial fat in location and blood supply. The strength of the relationship between epicardial, myocardial or pericardial fat and various measurements of body composition is controversial [69] but in general, these ectopic fat depots are associated with excess body weight [73,77,78]. Based on autopsy studies, epicardial fat is not correlated to subcutaneous abdominal fat [77]; *in vivo* studies report correlations with visceral fat of varying strength [69,79]. Visceral fat is reported to be an independent predictor of myocardial fat [80] and strongly correlated to pericardial fat [81]. Furthermore, epicardial, pericardial and myocardial fat are correlated with components of the metabolic syndrome such as elevated waist circumference (WC), increased fasting insulin [82,83], type 2 diabetes mellitus [80], elevated triglycerides and hypertension [78]. Evidence suggests that excess epicardial and pericardial fat may contribute to the pathogenesis of coronary artery disease [69,77,78] and that myocardial fat contributes to impaired ventricular function [71]. Figure 2.4 illustrates a heart with and without increased epicardial fat.

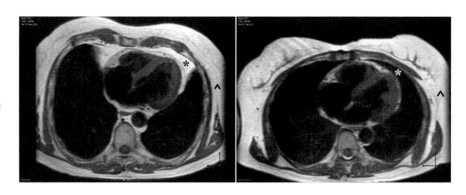

Figure 2.4 Visceral cardiac fat (*) and subcutaneous fat (^) identified by cardiovascular magnetic resonance. The left image is a subject with visceral cardiac fat stores while the subject on the right displays little visceral cardiac fat. (Reproduced from Mathieu P, Pibarot P, Larose E, et al. Int J Biochem Cell Biol 2008;40(5):821–36, with permission from Elsevier.)

Utility of anthropometric measurement tools as assessed by imaging techniques

Due to the high cost, technical expertise required to analyze data, and difficulty in using imaging tools in field situations, anthropometric measurements such as WC or BMI are commonly used to estimate body fatness and assess body fat distribution. Currently, imaging techniques are the most accurate methods available to examine body composition; thus they have been used to assess the ability of various anthropometric measurements to estimate body fatness.

Body mass index is the anthropometric measurement most widely used to assess total body fatness and is highly correlated with total fat mass as assessed by MRI in both men and women (r = 0.78–0.92 and r = 0.92–0.93, respectively) [84–87] and in children as measured by DXA (r = 0.50–0.83)[88]. Although skinfold thickness measurements provide a better estimate of body fat than BMI [89], they are more time consuming and require greater expertise for accurate data acquisition than BMI. In addition, skinfold measurements are difficult to attain and reproduce in the more overweight individuals[88]. WC is also significantly associated with total fat mass in both genders [86,87] but is more commonly utilized to assess body fat distribution as opposed to total body fatness.

Due to the strong association between abdominal obesity and health risk, there is strong interest in obtaining accurate measures of fat depots, primarily visceral fat, in this region. Despres and colleagues [87] reported that in a sample of men with a large variation in body fatness, all anthropometric measurements of body fatness (BMI and skinfold thickness) and body fat distribution (WC and WHR) were highly correlated with abdominal measurements obtained from CT. However, when examining only the obese participants (defined as having BMI ≥28), WC and WHR were the only anthropometric measurements significantly associated with CT measurements. This suggests that some degree of caution should be exercised when interpreting correlations between field and laboratory methods of body fat assessment. Regardless of body composition, WC is the best anthropometric indicator of visceral fat in both adults (r = 0.46–0.82 in men and r = 0.60–0.96 in women) [84–87,90] and youth (r = 0.80–0.84)

[91–93]. Significant correlations have also been found between both BMI and WHR and visceral fat [84,92,94]. It is important to note that WC is also a good indicator of subcutaneous adipose tissue in all populations [84–87,91–93] and it is unable to differentiate between the subcutaneous and visceral adipose tissue [89]. BMI is more strongly associated with subcutaneous adipose tissue than WC in both males and females of all ages [84,91,92].

Conclusion

Advances in body composition measurement have improved our understanding of the complex relationship between total adipose tissue or specific adipose tissue depots and obesity-related health complications. More research has been conducted in adults than youth, but consequent to the rising obesity prevalence in children and adolescents, measurement techniques are being adjusted for use in younger populations and knowledge is advancing rapidly. Simple and inexpensive anthropometric measures, such as WC or BMI, can be employed within a clinical setting to identify individuals at increased health risk. Sophisticated methods such as MRI or CT will continue to be employed in research settings to help ensure that we continue to advance our understanding of the relationship between body composition, morbidity and mortality.

References

1. Goran M, Gower B. Relation between visceral fat and disease risk in children and adolescents. Am J Clin Nutr 1999;70(suppl):149S–56S.
2. Heymsfield S, Wang Z, Visser M, Gallagher D, Pierson RJ. Techniques used in the measurement of body composition: an overview with emphasis on bioelectrical impedance analysis. Am J Clin Nutr 1996;64(suppl):478S–84S.
3. Jebb S, Wells J. Measuring body composition in adults and children. In: Kopelman P, Caterson I, Dietz W (eds) *Clinical Obesity in Adults and Children*, 2nd edn. Massachusetts: Blackwell Publishing, 2005.
4. Chumlea W, Sun S. Bioelectrical impedance analysis. In: Heymsfield S, Lohman T, Wang Z, Going S (eds) *Human Body Composition*, 2nd edn. Windsor, ON: Human Kinetics, 2005.

5. Fogelholm M, van Marken Lichtenbelt W. Comparison of body composition methods: a literature analysis. Eur J Clin Nutr 1997; 51:495–503.

6. Hosking J, Metcalf B, Jeffery A, Voss L, Wilkin T. Validation of foot-to-foot bioelectrical impedance analysis with dual-energy X-ray absorptiometry in the assessment of body composition in young children: the EarlyBird cohort. Br J Nutr 2006;96:1163–8.

7. Eisenmann J, Heelan K, Welk G. Assessing body composition among 3- to 8-year-old children: anthropometry, BIA, and DXA. Obes Res 2004;12:1633–40.

8. Going S. Hydrodensitometry and air displacement plethysmography. In: Heymsfield S, Lohman T, Wang Z, Going S (eds) *Human Body Composition*, 2nd edn. Windsor, ON: Human Kinetics, 2005:15–33.

9. Fields D, Goran M, McCrory M. Body-composition assessment via air-displacement plethysmography in adults and children: A review. Am J Clin Nutr 2002;75:453–67.

10. Lohman T, Chen Z. Dual-energy X-ray absorptiometry. In: Heymsfield S, Lohman T, Wang Z, Going S (eds) *Human Body Composition*, 2nd edn. Windsor, ON: Human Kinetics, 2005.

11. Fu W, Lee H, Ng C, et al. Screening for childhood obesity: international vs population-specific definitions. Which is more appropriate? Int J Obes 2003;27:1121–6.

12. Kamel E, McNeil G, Han T, et al. Measurement of abdominal fat by magnetic resonance imaging, dual-energy X-ray absorptiometry and anthropometry in non-obese men and women. Int J Obes 1999;23:686–92.

13. Sopher A, Shen W, Pietrobelli A. Pediatric body composition methods. In: Heymsfield S, Lohman T, Wang Z, Going S (eds) *Human Body Composition*, 2nd edn. Windsor, ON: Human Kinetics, 2005:129–39.

14. Pietrobelli A, Malavolti M, Fuiano N, Faith M. The invisible fat. Acta Paediatrica 2006;96:35–8.

15. Ross R, Janssen I. Computed tomography and magnetic resonance imaging. In: Heymsfield S, Lohman T, Wang Z, Going S (eds) *Human Body Composition*, 2nd edn. Windsor, ON: Human Kinetics, 2005:89–108.

16. Ross R. Magnetic resonance imaging provides new insights into the characterization of adipose and lean tissue distribution. Can J Physiol Pharmacol 1996;74:778–85.

17. Abate N, Burns D, Preshock R, Garg A, Grundy S. Estimation of adipose tissue mass by magnetic resonance imaging: validation against dissection in human cadavers. J Lipid Res 1994;35:1490–6.

18. Mourier A, Gautier J, de Kerviler E, et al. Mobilization of visceral adipose tissue related to the improvement in insulin sensitivity in response to physical training in NIDMM. Effects of branched-chain amino acid supplements. Diabetes Care 1997;20:385–91.

19. Ross R, Leger L, Morris D, de Guise J, Guardo R. Quantification of adipose tissue by MRI: relationship with anthropometric variables. J Appl Physiol 1992;72:787–95.

20. Kvist H, Sjostrom L, Tylen U. Adipose tissue volume determinations in women by computed tomography: technical considerations. Int J Obes Res 1986;10:53–67.

21. Shen W, Wang Z, Tang H, et al. Volume estimates by imaging methods: model comparisons with visible women as the reference. Obes Res 2003;11:217–25.

22. Gallagher D, Belmonte D, Deurenberg P, et al. Organ-tissue mass measurement allows modeling of REE and metabolically active tissue mass. Am J Physiol 1998;275:E249–E58.

23. Despres J, Moorjani S, Lupien P, Tremblay A, Nadlau S, Bouchard C. Regional distribution of body fat, plasma lipoproteins, and cardiovascular disease. Arteriosclerosis 1990;10:497–511.

24. Kissebah A, Peiris A. Biology of regional body fat distribution: relationship to non-insulin-dependent diabetes mellitus. Diabetes Metab Rev 1989;15:83–109.

25. Carr D, Utzschneider K, Hull R, et al. Intra-abdominal fat is a major determinant of the National Cholesterol Education Program Adult Treatment Panel 3 Criteria for the metabolic syndrome. Diabetes 2004;53:2087–94.

26. Kuk J, Nichaman M, Church T, Blair S, Ross R. Liver fat is not a marker of metabolic risk in lean premenopausal women. Metabolism 2004;53(8):1066–71.

27. Kuk J, Katzmarzyk P, Nichman M, Church T, Blair S, Ross R. Visceral fat is an independent predictor of all-cause mortality in men. Obesity 2006;14:336–41.

28. Caprio S. Relationship between abdominal visceral fat and metabolic risk factors in obese adolescents. Am J Hum Biol 1999;11:259–66.

29. Brambilla P, Manzoni P, Sironi S, et al. Peripheral and abdominal adiposity in childhood obesity. Int J Obes 1994;18:795–800.

30. Gower B, Nagy T, Goran M. Visceral fat, insulin sensitivity, and lipids in prepubertal children. Diabetes 1999;48:1515–21.

31. Kuk J, Church T, Blair S, Ross R. Does measurement site for visceral and abdominal subcutaneous adipose tissue alter associations with the metabolic syndrome? Diabetes Care 2006;29:679–84.

32. Siegel M, Hildeboit C, Bae K, Hong C, White N. Total and intra-abdominal fat distribution in preadolescents and adolescents: measurement with MR imaging. Radiology 2007;242:846–56.

33. Huang T, Johnson M, Figueroa-Colon R, Dwyer J, Goran M. Growth of visceral fat, subcutaneous abdominal fat, and total body fat in children. Obes Res 2001;9:283–9.

34. Fox K, Peters D, Sharpe P, Bell M. Assessment of abdominal fat development in young adolescents using magnetic resonance imaging. Int J Obes 2000;24:1653–9.

35. Gower B, Nagy T, Trowbridge C, Dezenberg C, Goran M. Fat distribution and insulin response in prepubertal African American and white children. Am J Clin Nutr 1998;67:821–7.

36. Yanovski J, Yanovski S, Filmer K, et al. Differences in body composition of black and white girls. Am J Clin Nutr 1996;64:833–9.

37. Kuk J, Janiszewski P, Ross R. Body mass index and hip and thigh circumferences are negatively associated with visceral aipose tissue after control for waist circumference. Am J Clin Nutr 2007;85:1540–4.

38. Snijder M, Visser M, Dekker J, et al. Low subcutaneous thigh fat is a risk factor for unfavourable glucose and lipid levels, independently of high abdominal fat. The Healthy ABC Study. Diabetologia 2005;48:301–8.

39. Snijder M, Dekker J, Visser M, et al. Larger thigh and hip circumferences are associated with better glucose tolerance: the Hoorn Study. Obes Res 2003;11:104–11.

40. Freedman D, Serdula M, Srinivasan S, Berenson G. Relation of circumferences and skinfold thicknesses to lipid and insulin concentrations in children and adolescents: the Bogalusa Heart Study. Am J Clin Nutr 1999;69:308–17.

41. Lee S, Janssen I, Heymsfield S, Ross R. Relation between whole-body and regional measures of human skeletal muscle. Am J Clin Nutr 2004;80:1215–21.

42. Tylavsky F, Lohman T, Dockrell M, et al. Comparison of the effectiveness of 2 dual-energy X-ray absorptiometers with that of total body water and computed tomography in assessing changes in body composition during weight change. Am J Clin Nutr 2003; 77:356–63.

43. Mitsiopoulos N, Baumgartner R, Heymsfield S, Lyons W, Gallagher D, Ross R. Cadaver validation of skeletal muscle measurement by magnetic resonance imaging and computerized tomography. J Appl Physiol 1998;85(1):115–22.

44. Boesch C, Machann J, Vermathen P, Schick F. Role of proton MR for the study of muscle lipid metabolism. NMR Biomed 2006;19: 968–88.

45. Goodpaster B, Wolf D. Skeletal muscle lipid accumulation in obesity, insulin resistance, and type 2 diabetes. Pediatr Diabetes 2004;5: 219–26.

46. Boesch C, Kreis R. Observation of intramyocellular lipids by 1H-magnetic resonance spectroscopy. Ann NY Acad Sci 2000;904: 25–31.

47. Schick F, Eismann B, Jung W, Bongers H, Bunse M, Lutz O. Comparison of localized proton NMR signals of skeletal muscle and fat tissue in vivo: two lipid compartments in muscle tissue. Magn Reson Med 1993;29:158–67.

48. Vermathen P, Kreis R, Boesch C. Distribution of intramyocellular lipids in human calf muscles as determined by MR spectroscopic imaging. Magn Reson Med 2004;51:253–62.

49. Lee J, Dixon W, Ling D, Levitt R, Murphy WJ. Fatty infiltration of the liver: demonstration by proton spectroscopic imaging. Preliminary observations. Radiology 1984;157:195–201.

50. Hwang J, Pan J, Heydari S, Hetherington H, Stein D. Regional differences in intramyocellular lipids in humans observed by in vivo 1H-MR spectroscopic imaging. J Appl Physiol 2001;90: 1267–74.

51. Szczepaniak L, Nuremberg P, Leonard D, et al. Magnetic resonance spectroscopy to measure hepatic triglyceride content: prevalence of hepatic steatosis in the general population. Am J Physiol Endocrinol Metab 2005;288:E462–E8.

52. Burgert T, Taksali S, Dziura J, et al. Alanine aminotransferase levels and fatty liver in childhood obesity: associations with insulin resistance, adiponectin, and visceral fat. J Clin Endocrinol Metab 2006;91:4287–94.

53. Gilmore I, Burroughs A, Murray-Lyon I, Williams R, Jenkins D, Hopkins A. Indications, methods, and outcomes of percutaneous liver biopsy in England and Wales: an audit by the British Society of Gastroenterology and the Royal College of Physicians of London. Gut 1995;36:437–41.

54. Piekarski J, Goldberg H, Royal S, Axel L, Moss A. Difference between liver and spleen CT numbers in the normal adult: its usefulness in predicting the presence of diffuse liver disease. Radiology 1980;137:727–9.

55. Davidson L, Kuk J, Church T, Ross R. Protocol for measurement of liver fat by computed tomography. J Appl Physiol 2006;100:864–8.

56. Marks S, Moore N, Ryley N, et al. Measurement of liver fat by MRI and its reduction by dexfenfluramine in NIDDM. Int J Obes 1997;21:274–9.

57. Fishbein M, Stevens W. Rapid MRI using a modified Dixon technique: a non-invasive and effective method for detection and monitoring of fatty metamorphosis of the liver. Pediatr Radiol 2001;31:806–9.

58. Cali A, Zern T, Taksali S, et al. Intrahepatic fat accumulation and alterations in lipoprotein composition in obese adolescents. Diabetes Care 2007;30(12):3093–8.

59. Tiikkainen M, Tamminen M, Hakkinen A, et al. Liver-fat accumulation and insulin resistance in obese women with previous gestational diabetes. Obes Res 2002;10:859–67.

60. Longo R, Ricci C, Masutti F, et al. Fatty infiltration of the liver. Quantification by 1H localized magnetic resonance spectroscopy and comparison with computed tomography. Invest Radiol 1993;28: 297–302.

61. Browning J, Szczepaniak L, Dobbins R, et al. Prevalence of hepatic steatosis in an urban population in the United States: impact of ethnicity. Hepatology 2004;40:1387–95.

62. Tiikkainen M, Bergholm R, Vehkavaara S, et al. Effects of identical weight loss on body composition and features of insulin resistance in obese women with high and low liver fat content. Diabetes 2003;52:701–7.

63. Nguyen-Duy T, Nichaman M, Church T, Blair S, Ross R. Visceral fat and liver fat are independent predictors of metabolic risk factors in men. Am J Physiol Endocrinol Metab 2003;284:E1065–E71.

64. Westerbacka J, Corner A, Tiikkainen M, et al. Women and men have similar amounts of liver and intra-abdominal fat, despite more subcutaneous fat in women: implications for sex differences in markers of cardiovascular risk. Diabetologia 2004;47:1360–9.

65. Vega G, Chandalia M, Szczepaniak L, Grundy S. Metabolic correlates of nonalcoholic fatty liver in women and men. Hepatology 2007;46:716–22.

66. Liska D, Dufour S, Zern T, et al. Interethnic differences in muscle, liver and abdominal fat partitioning in obese adolescents. PLOS One 2007;2(6):e569.

67. Fishbein M, Mogren C, Gleason T, Stevens W. Relationship of hepatic steatosis to adipose tissue distribution in pediatric nonalcoholic fatty liver disease. J Pediatr Gastroenterol Nutr 2006;42: 83–8.

68. Fishbein M, Miner M, Mogren C, Chalekson J. The spectrum of fatty liver in obese children and the relationship of serum aminotransferases to severity of steatosis. J Pediatr Gastroenterol Nutr 2003;36:54–61.

69. Sacks H, Fain J. Human epicardial adipose tissue: a review. Am Heart J 2007;153:907–17.

70. Abbara S, Desai J, Ricardo C, Butler J, Nieman K, Vivek R. Mapping epicardial fat with mult-detector computed tomography to facilitate percutaneous transepicardial arrhythmia ablation. Eur J Radiol 2006;57:417–22.

71. Szczepaniak L, Victor R, Rorci L, Unger R. Forgotten but not gone: the rediscovery of fatty heart, the most common unrecognized disease in America. Circ Res 2007;101:759–67.

72. Boesch C, Slothboom J, Hoppeler H, Kreis R. In vivo determination of intra-myocellular lipids in human muscle by means of localized 1H-MR-spectroscopy. Magn Reson Med 1997;37:484–93.

73. McGavock J, Victor R, Unger R, Szczepaniak L. Adiposity of the heart, revisited. Ann Int Med 2006;144(7):517–24.

74. Szczepaniak L, Dobbins R, Metzger G, et al. Myocardial triglycerides and systolic function in humans: in vivo evaluation by localized proton spectroscopy and cardiac imaging. Magn Reson Med 2003;49:417–23.

75. Reingold J, McGavock J, Kaka S, Tillery T, Victor R, Szczepaniak L. Determination of triglyceride in the human myocardium by

magnetic resonance spectroscopy: reproducibility and sensitivity of the method. Am J Physiol Endocrinol Metab 2005;289:E935–E9.

76. Williams P (ed). *Cardiovascular System.* Edinburgh: Churchill Livingstone, 1995.

77. Rabkin S. Epicardial fat: properties, function and relationship to obesity. Obes Rev 2007;8:253–61.

78. Taguchi R, Takasu J, Itani Y, et al. Pericardial fat accumulation in men as a risk factor for coronary artery disease. Atherosclerosis 2001;157:203–9.

79. Iacobellis G, Assael F, Ribaudo M, et al. Epicardial fat from echocardiography: a new method for visceral adipose tissue prediction. Obes Res 2003;11:304–10.

80. McGavock J, Lingvay I, Zib I, et al. Cardiac steatosis in diabetes mellitus. A 1H-magnetic resonance spectroscopy study. Circulation 2007;116:1170–5.

81. Wheeler G, Shi R, Beck S, et al. Pericardial and visceral adipose tissues measured volumetrically with computed tomography are highly associated in type 2 diabetic families. Invest Radiol 2005;40:97–101.

82. Iacobellis G, Ribaudo M, Assael F, et al. Echocardiographic epicardial adipose tissue is related to anthropometric and clinical paramters of metabolic syndrome: a new indicator of cardiovascular risk. J Clin Endocrinol Metab 2003;88:5163–8.

83. Iacobellis G, Leonetti F. Epicardial adipose tissue and insulin resistance in obese subjects. J Clin Endocrinol Metab 2005;90:6300–2.

84. Janssen I, Heymsfield S, Allison D, Kotler D, Ross R. Body mass index and waist circumference independently contribute to the prediction of nonabdominal, abdominal subcutaneous, and visceral fat. Am J Clin Nutr 2002;75:683–8.

85. Kuk J, Ross R. Measurement of body composition in obesity. In: Kushner R, Bessesen D (eds) *Contemporary Endocrinology: Treatment of the Obese Patient.* Totowa, NJ: Humana Press, 2007.

86. Ross R, Shaw K, Martel Y, de Guise J, Avruch L. Adipose tissue distribution measured by magnetic resonance imaging in obese women. Am J Clin Nutr 1993;57:470–5.

87. Despres J, Prud'homme D, Pouliot M, Tremblay A, Bouchard C. Estimation of deep abdominal adipose-tissue accumulation from simple anthropometric measurements in men. Am J Clin Nutr 1991;54:471–7.

88. Dietz W, Bellizzi M. Introduction: the use of body mass index to assess obesity in children. Am J Clin Nutr 1999;70(suppl):123S–5S.

89. Janssen I, Heymsfield S, Ross R. Application of simple anthropometry in the assessment of health risk: implications for the Canadian Physical Activity, Fitness and Lifestyle Appraisal. Can J Appl Physiol 2002;27:396–414.

90. van der Kooy K, Leenan R, Seidell J, Deurenberg P, Visser M. Abdominal diameters as indicators of visceral fat: comparison between magnetic resonance imaging and anthropometry. Br J Nutr 1993;70:47–58.

91. Goran M, Gower B, Treuth M, Nagy T. Prediction of intraabdominal and subcutaneous abdominal adipose tissue in healthy pre-pubertal children. Int J Obes 1998;22:549–58.

92. Benfield L, Fox K, Peters D, et al. Magnetic resonance imaging of abdominal adiposity in a large cohort of British children. Int J Obes 2008;32:91–9.

93. Brambilla P, Bedogni G, Moreno L, et al. Crossvalidation of anthropometry against magnetic resonance imaging for the assessment of visceral and subcutaneous adipose tissue in children. Int J Obes 2006;30:23–30.

94. van der Kooy K, Leenen R, Seidell J, Deurenberg P, Droop A, Bakker C. Waist-hip ratio is a poor predictor of changes in visceral fat. Am J Clin Nutr 1993;57:327–33.

3   Stigma and Social Consequences of Obesity

Rebecca M. Puhl, Chelsea A. Heuer and Kelly D. Brownell

Rudd Center for Food Policy and Obesity, Yale University, New Haven, CT, USA

Introduction

"My mother told me that I won't find a boyfriend/husband being fat. She said that no one could fit their arms around me, that I was the biggest person she's ever seen, and swears I get bigger each time she looks at me."

"My mother used to sing the 'too fat polka' (lyrics: I don't want her, you can have her, she's too fat for me ...) to me as a way of encouraging me to lose weight. All this did was make me want to eat more."

"I remember one incident when I was in the sixth grade and my teacher was looking at my latest handwriting assignment and she announced to the whole class that my handwriting was just like me – 'fat and squatty' ... The pain and humiliation aimed at you as an innocent child never leaves you!"

The consequences of obesity reach far beyond detriments to physical health. Research has documented evidence of weight-based stigma, discrimination, and negative outcomes for obese individuals in areas of education, employment, socio-economic status, healthcare, interpersonal relationships, and psychologic health. With obesity now a national public health priority, it is fundamental to understand and prevent these social disadvantages to improve the health and well-being of overweight and obese adults, children, and adolescents. This chapter provides a review of the literature describing the social consequences of obesity, and highlights strategies to reduce weight stigma including avenues for future research in this area.

Evidence of stigma and bias against obese individuals

Over the past several decades, increasing research evidence has demonstrated that obese individuals face systematic and

Clinical Obesity in Adults and Children, 3rd edition. Edited by Peter G. Kopelman, Ian D. Caterson and William H. Dietz.
© 2010 Blackwell Publishing, ISBN: 978-1-4051-8226-3.

widespread stigma in the form of negative stereotyping, discrimination, and unequal treatment. Studies have documented commonly held perceptions that obese people possess negative attributes ranging from laziness and lack of self-control to flaws in competence, attractiveness, and even moral character. Research evidence further indicates that this stigmatization results in negative social consequences for both obese adults and children [1,2].

Documentation of weight stigma began several decades ago [3] and has had a resurgence in recent years. In 2001, Puhl and Brownell reviewed the literature documenting discriminatory attitudes and behaviors against obese individuals, concluding that there was sufficient evidence of clear and consistent weight-related stigmatization within domains of employment, education, and healthcare [4]. Since then, evidence has continued to accumulate to support these conclusions, and has documented additional contexts where weight bias occurs, including socio-economic status, interpersonal relationships, and psychologic health.

The high prevalence of obesity might suggest that weight tolerance should in turn increase, but evidence from several large-scale studies in recent years indicates that weight bias remains pervasive and widespread. Using an online sample of 4283 adults from the general population, Schwartz and colleagues found significant anti-fat bias among participants across all weight categories (underweight, normal weight, overweight, obese, and extremely obese) [5]. In addition, 46% of participants indicated that they would rather give up at least 1 year of life than be obese, one-third reported that they would rather be divorced than be obese, and one-fourth of respondents reported that they would rather be unable to have children than be obese. Thinner respondents were even more likely to endorse these trade-offs than heavier respondents [5]. Puhl and Brownell surveyed 2671 overweight and obese adults who reported multiple instances of weight stigmatization across a variety of settings. Moreover, stigmatizing experiences increased in frequency as weight increased [1]. A 2005 study analyzed data from a nationally representative sample of 3000 men and women and found that obese individuals perceived themselves as targets of multiple forms of discrimination, and that weight discrimination negatively affected their psychologic well-being [6]. Puhl et al. (n = 2290) demonstrated that the incidence of weight discrimination in American society is relatively close to reported rates of racial discrimination, particularly among women [7]. Similar research indicates that prevalence of weight-based discrimination has increased in the last decade [8].

A smaller qualitative study (n = 13) demonstrated that obese individuals reported frequent experiences of weight-based stigmatization and discrimination from family members, peers, healthcare providers, and strangers [9]. The authors concluded that the pattern of denigration was so pervasive that it constituted civilized oppression. Hebl and Mannix, using an experimental design (n = 196), found obesity stigma to be so profound that a person who was perceived to be associated with an obese individual or even in close physical proximity to an obese individual was judged more negatively than someone who was seen with a thin person [10].

Some studies suggest that the stigma of obesity is worse for women than men, especially in areas of education, employment, and interpersonal relationships [7,11–14]. However, Hebl and Turchin found that men are also stigmatized for being overweight and demonstrated that while black men are more accepting of larger body sizes in women than white men, black men are also stigmatized themselves for being overweight, although to a lesser degree than white men [15]. While other research demonstrates that the social stigma of obesity may be more prominent among whites than among African-Americans [16], some studies yield contrary results [7,17,18]. In order to better understand the social consequences of obesity for African-Americans, Latinos, and other racial/ethnic groups, future obesity research should target more diverse samples.

Regardless of race, gender or age, weight stigma remains an acceptable form of discrimination in our society. Derogatory weight-related stereotypes abound in popular culture and negative portrayals of overweight characters are abundant in television programs and movies [19]. One study examined 56 different television series and found that heavier characters were underrepresented compared to the actual population [20]. They also found heavier characters more likely to be in minor roles, less likely to be in romantic relationships, and more likely to be seen eating and to be the objects of humor. The conventional nature of "fat jokes" and weight-related stereotyping in the media contributes to the social acceptability of weight stigma. Overweight people are one of the few remaining groups that can be openly ridiculed without public backlash. Unfortunately, this disrespect is a reality for increasing numbers of overweight people who are confronted with stereotypes and social denigration on a daily basis.

Why does weight stigma occur?

Weight stigma has roots in perceptions of personal responsibility for health, which can result in blaming individuals for their excess weight. This explanation comes from attribution theory, which is the primary theoretical model used to explain weight stigma. This research, conducted primarily by Crandall and colleagues, highlights perceptions of controllability when making judgments about social groups, and suggests that when we encounter a person with a stigmatized trait, we search for its cause and form our reactions to the person using this causal information [21–24].

Crandall and colleagues propose that negative attitudes towards obese people result from particular attributional tendencies of blame [21,25]. Specifically, traditional conservative North American values of self-determination and individualism provide a foundation for weight stigma through beliefs that people get what they deserve, and that the fates of others are due to internal, controllable factors [23].

Consistent with this theory, research suggests that stigma is more likely to occur when individuals perceive obese people to be responsible for their weight because of controllable factors such as laziness, overeating or low self-discipline [26–30]. Some studies also show that obese people are less likely to be denigrated when explanations are provided that their obesity is beyond personal control (e.g. due to a thyroid condition) compared to when controllable causes (like overeating) are perceived to be responsible [26,29,31,32].

Despite the commonly held belief that obesity is a personally controllable condition and that body weight is easily modifiable, current scientific evidence shows that obesity is determined by an interplay of biologic, genetic, and environmental factors that are not readily controllable by the individual [33–37]. In addition, efforts to lose weight through dieting and weight loss programs rarely result in lasting and significant weight reduction [38–40]. Maintaining existing assumptions about the personal causes of obesity may only lead to more stigmatization and could impede scientifically based efforts to prevent and treat obesity. Some experimental research has also demonstrated that providing individuals with information that emphasizes the "controllable" aspects of obesity increases negative weight-based stereotypes [41].

Consequences of obesity and weight stigma

Obesity is associated with stigma and negative outcomes across multiple aspects of life. Existing literature documents negative outcomes for obese individuals in areas of education, employment, socio-economic status, healthcare, interpersonal relationships, and psychologic health. This research is summarized below.

Education

Several studies have documented disparities in educational attainment between obese and nonobese groups. Some research suggests that weight bias within educational institutions and among teachers may prevent obese individuals from achieving the same educational goals of their normal-weight counterparts. A study conducted by Canning and Mayer in 1966 was the first to document weight bias in education. The researchers examined high school records and college applications of 2506 high school students, and found that obese students were less likely to be accepted to college, despite having equivalent application rates and academic performance to nonobese peers [42]. Moreover, only 31% of obese women were accepted compared to 41% of obese males.

In the 40 years since, several other studies have documented educational disparities for obese individuals. A 2006 study of more than 700,000 Swedish men found that those who were obese at age 18 had a lower chance of attaining higher education than their normal-weight peers, even after adjustments for intelligence and parental socio-economic position [43]. The authors concluded that discrimination in the educational system may explain these results. A 2007 study using data from the National Longitudinal Study of Adolescent Health ($n = 10,829$) reported that obesity undermined the educational attainment of female students. Obese girls had a 50% lower chance of attending college than nonobese girls. However, obese girls who attended schools where female obesity was more prevalent had a 50% greater chance of attending college than obese girls who attended schools in which they were the only obese girl [12].

There have also been cases of obese students who were dismissed from college because of their weight. One case that reached the US Supreme Court involved an obese nursing student who was dismissed from Salve Regina College 1 year before obtaining her nursing degree for failing to lose weight [44]. Although the school did not object to the student's obesity at her admission, she was later asked to sign a contract agreeing that she could remain in her program if she lost 2 pounds a week. A year later she was dismissed from the school for her inability to lose weight. After her dismissal, she transferred to another college, successfully completed her degree, and attained licensure as a registered nurse. Ms Russell then sued Salve Regina and after a 7-year legal battle, was awarded monetary damages.

Studies suggest that educators' biased attitudes towards obese students may affect perceptions of performance among obese students or that unequal treatment may interfere with the ability of obese students to succeed. One self-report study of 115 junior and senior high school teachers and school health workers indicated that these educators perceived obesity to be primarily under individual control, and 20% agreed that obese persons are untidy, 19% perceived them to be more emotional, and 17% believed them less likely to succeed at work [45]. In addition, 28% agreed that becoming obese is one of the worst things that could happen to a person. A study examining the beliefs about the causes of obesity of over 200 elementary school principals found that 59% attributed obesity to a lack of self-control, 57% to psychologic problems, and 47% to lack of parental concern [46]. Other research has demonstrated negative attitudes towards obese youth among physical education teachers that resulted in students' avoidance of physical education classes [47–49].

Surprisingly, parental biases may also affect educational outcomes for obese students. Crandall surveyed over 3000 high school seniors about their weight, college aspirations, financial support, grades, and parental political attitudes. Overweight students were under-represented in those who attended college, with overweight females being least likely to receive financial support from their families [50].

Although some research has pointed to an association between obesity and lower intelligence as an explanation for unfavorable educational outcomes [51–53], there is insufficient evidence to conclude that obese individuals are at an intellectual disadvantage compared to nonobese persons. Alternatively, research in this area suggests that the social stigma of obesity, its influence on the school climate for obese students, and the resulting psychosocial and academic consequences may account for these educational disparities. More research in this area is needed.

Employment

Studies find inequalities in employment status, wages, position, and benefits eligibility for obese workers compared to nonobese workers, which may be explained by weight-related bias and discrimination in the workplace. Research using data from a nationwide prospective cohort ($n = 4290$) to estimate the effect of obesity on future employment found that, after adjusting for sociodemographic characteristics, smoking status, exercise, and self-reported health, obesity was associated with reduced employment at follow-up for both men and women [54]. A similar study in Canada ($n = 73,531$) also found obesity associated with lower workforce participation, independent of associated co-morbidity and sociodemographic factors [55]. A British prospective cohort study of 8490 participants found that women who were obese in both childhood and adulthood were half as likely to have ever been gainfully employed or ever married compared with those who were never obese [56].

Obesity has been found to negatively affect wages. A study of over 2000 women and men (aged 18 years and older) reported that obesity lowered wage growth rates by almost 6% in 1982–1985 [57]. More recent research ($n = 12,686$) indicates that the wage penalty faced by obese employees is persistent over the first two decades of employees' careers, and ranges from 1.4% to 4.5%, after controlling for socio-economic and familial variables [13]. In a study using a cross-national dataset covering countries in the European Union, it was observed that a 10% increase in the average Body Mass Index (BMI) reduced the hourly wages of males by 1.86% and that of females by 3.27%. In southern European countries, where citizens are reportedly more concerned with weight gain, the effect is much larger [58].

Both obese men and women face wage-related obstacles, but are affected differently by wage penalties. An analysis from the National Longitudinal Survey Youth Cohort examined earnings in over 8000 men and women aged 18–25 years, which indicated that obese women earned 12% less than their nonobese female counterparts [59]. This study parallels other investigations that show that the economic penalty of obesity is greater for females.

For example, longitudinal research examined data on 12,686 workers (50% female) and found that the obesity wage penalty was greater for obese women (6.2%) than for obese men (2.6%) [13]. The effect of ethnicity on wages for obese women has been documented in studies of labor market outcomes which reported that body weight lowered wages for white women, but not for Hispanic or black women [18]. Among white women, a weight increase of two standard deviations (approximately 65 pounds) decreased their pay by 7%, which is equivalent to 3 years of work experience.

Employment consequences are also evident from research showing that fewer obese employees are hired in high-level positions. Data on earnings of 7000 males and females from the National Longitudinal Survey of Youth showed that obese females are more likely than thinner women to hold low-paying jobs [60]. Obese men are similarly under-represented and paid less than nonobese men in managerial and professional occupations, and are over-represented in transportation occupations, suggesting that obese men engage in occupational sorting to counteract a wage penalty [60].

Obese employees may also be less likely to be eligible for employer-sponsored health insurance or may be asked to pay more than nonobese employees for the same benefits. A self-report study of 445 obese workers found that 26% of individuals who were 50% or more above ideal weight indicated they were denied benefits such as health insurance because of their weight, and 17% reported being fired or pressured to resign because of their weight [61]. More recent evidence of this phenomenon has surfaced in the news media [62,63] but additional research is needed to assess the proportion of obese employees who are affected by these policies, as well as the consequences for their employment and health outcomes.

Legal case findings indicate that employment termination against obese persons due to weight does exist, and that it occurs in a variety of employment positions that are not necessarily compromised by body weight. Recent wrongful termination cases have been filed by obese employees who were city laborers [64,65], state troopers [66,67], teachers [68], and office managers [69], many of whom had been commended for good job performance or maintained excellent employment records. Several of these cases also involved suspended work without pay or demotion until the obese employee lost weight.

The existence of legal cases does not prove that weight discrimination is widespread, but does show that many perceive their obesity to be the reason for unfair treatment. Recent research using data from a nationally representative sample of over 2000 adults found that overweight and obese men and women reported weight-related employment discrimination [7,70]. In addition, overweight respondents were 12 times more likely than normal-weight respondents to report weight-related employment discrimination, obese respondents were 37 times more likely, and severely obese respondents were 100 times more likely [70]. Puhl and Brownell found that 54% of overweight or obese respondents ($n = 2671$) reported being stigmatized because of their weight by co-workers or colleagues and 43% reported experiencing stigma from their employers or supervisors [1]. In addition, very obese persons working in professional jobs are more likely than obese nonprofessionals to report job discrimination [6].

Experimental research provides further evidence of the existence of weight-related employment discrimination and demonstrates that overweight applicants face biased hiring decisions. This research typically asks participants to evaluate a fictional applicant's qualifications for a job, where the employee's weight has been manipulated (through written vignettes, videos, photographs or computer morphing). Participants consistently evaluate overweight applicants more negatively and rate them less likely to be hired than average-weight employees, despite having identical qualifications [71–73]. This bias may be especially salient in jobs like sales positions, where obese people are perceived to be inappropriate for face-to-face interactions [74–77]. In a recent study, New Zealand researchers presented fictitious CVs with photographs of either overweight or normal-weight women to 56 human resource consultants and asked them to rank the job candidates based on suitability for a specified position. Normal-weight applicants were ranked significantly higher than overweight applicants, despite the fact that the CVs were identical [78].

Survey research shows that negative stereotypes about obese employees are common. These stereotypes may lead to inaccurate perceptions about obese employees' performance, resulting in discrimination. Three decades ago, Larkin and Pines documented beliefs that obese workers are less neat, productive, ambitious, disciplined and determined compared to nonobese employees [79]. More recent studies indicate this pattern has worsened and that people perceive overweight employees to be sloppy, lazy, less competent, poor role models, lacking in self-discipline, disagreeable, unattractive, unsuccessful, and emotionally unstable compared to average-weight employees or job applicants [80–82]. Other work reveals perceptions that obese workers have low supervisory potential, and poor personal hygiene and professional appearance [77]. Despite a lack of evidence showing any truth to these stereotypes, obese employees remain vulnerable to negative evaluations because of their weight. Interestingly, some research shows that obese job applicants who acknowledge their stigma in an interview are evaluated more negatively than those who do not mention their weight [83].

Clearly there is a compelling need for laws to protect obese individuals from discrimination in the workplace. In the United States, overweight individuals have depended on the Rehabilitation Act of 1973 (RA) and the Americans with Disabilities Act of 1990 (ADA). However, whether obesity qualifies as a disability under the ADA has caused much debate. Overweight people who are not "morbidly obese" but who experience weight discrimination cannot file claims under the ADA because they are not considered disabled. These unresolved issues, along with public perceptions that blame obese people for their own negative experiences, result in inconsistent court rulings and deter other overweight people from seeking legal recourse at all [84].

Socio-economic status

Numerous studies show that obesity is more prevalent among lower socio-economic groups [85–87]. While the relationship between obesity and socio-economic status (SES) is bidirectional [86], it difficult to determine causality and highlight the complexity of this relationship. Research suggests, however, that negative outcomes in domains such as education, employment, and income contribute to negative socio-economic consequences for obese individuals, especially for obese women.

A longitudinal study that examined obesity and SES among over 10,000 adolescents who were followed for 7 years established that women who had been overweight in adolescence completed less education, were less likely to be married, and had lower incomes and higher rates of poverty compared to those who had not been overweight. This relationship remained after controlling for socio-economic origins and academic test scores [88]. This study also demonstrated that individuals with chronic health conditions did not have lower socio-economic attainment than nonoverweight participants, indicating that these outcomes were not due to health problems. Other prospective research ($n = 12,537$) found that girls in the top 10% of BMI earned 7.4% less income 7 years later than girls who were not overweight [89]. In a study of 15,061 respondents to the 1996 Health Survey for England, lower educational attainment and lower socio-economic status were associated with a higher risk of obesity in both men and women [87]. A 2004 study of adults at or near retirement age ($n = 8733$) found overweight and obesity to be associated with lower net worth for women, but not for men [90]. Other studies, however, have found no differences in SES outcomes between obese individuals and nonobese individuals, particularly for men [56,91].

The mixed findings of existing studies may in part reflect different methods used to define and measure socio-economic variables. Nevertheless, there is sufficient evidence that obese individuals suffer from negative socio-economic consequences, especially in areas of education and employment. These socio-economic challenges may create significant barriers for the health and well-being of obese individuals.

Healthcare

Because obesity is associated with numerous co-morbidities, it is critical for obese individuals to obtain necessary preventive care and medical treatment. Research finds evidence of negative attitudes toward obese patients and questionable obesity management practices among providers. Weight stigma in healthcare settings may interfere with the frequency and quality of care received by obese patients and contribute to the negative health consequences associated with obesity.

A number of studies demonstrate that physicians, dietitians, psychologists, nurses, and medical students hold negative attitudes towards obese patients [92–99]. Schwartz and colleagues assessed 389 health professionals attending a national obesity conference and found them to exhibit significant implicit and explicit anti-fat bias, including associations that obese persons are

lazy, stupid and worthless [100]. Foster et al. examined attitudes toward obese patients among 620 primary care physicians and found that they viewed obesity as a largely behavioral problem and expressed negative stereotypes of obese individuals [101]. Other self-report studies show that healthcare providers perceive obese patients to be unsuccessful, unpleasant, unintelligent, dishonest, lacking in self-control, overindulgent, weak-willed, and lazy [93–95,102,103]. One study of RN graduate female nurses ($n = 107$) reported that 24% of nurses agreed that caring for an obese patient repulsed them, and 12% reported that they preferred not to even touch an obese patient [104]. Other work shows that people overestimate the likelihood that obese patients are noncompliant with their physician's advice, despite the absence of data to suggest this relationship exists [105].

Additional research shows that healthcare providers may engage in questionable obesity management practices. Bertakis and Azari investigated the impact of obesity on primary care by analyzing videotapes of 506 first-time patient visits with 105 physicians [106]. Physicians in the study failed to document obesity in 63% of obese patients. Physicians also spent relatively less time providing health education to obese patients, while spending more time providing health education to patients who had better physical health and higher economic status. Another study examining attitudes and weight management practices among 752 general practitioners found that physicians reported positive views about their roles in managing obesity, but underutilized practices that promoted lifestyle changes in patients, described weight management as professionally unrewarding, and reported their most common frustrations in treating obesity to be poor patient compliance and motivation [107].

Healthcare providers' attitudes and practices are often reflected in the perceptions of their obese patients. In a survey of 2671 overweight and obese women, Puhl and Brownell [1] found that 69% of participants reported experiencing weight stigma from a doctor and 52% felt stigmatized by doctors multiple times. In addition, doctors were reported to be the second most frequent source of weight bias among over 20 potential sources provided to them. Other research has documented reports by obese individuals of stigmatizing experiences with healthcare providers [9], and expectations of confronting negative stereotypes in primary care [108]. Additional work examining women's perceptions of their physicians' weight management attitudes found that almost 50% of participants ($n = 259$) reported that their physicians had not recommended any common weight loss methods, and nearly 60% of participants reported that most doctors do not understand how difficult it is to lose weight [109].

These experiences of stigma and questionable weight management practices in healthcare may lead obese individuals to avoid or delay seeking preventive health services. A 2006 study found that obesity is a barrier to obtaining preventive healthcare services among women. Specifically, obese women ($n = 498$) reported that they delay cancer screenings, and their reasons for avoiding care included receiving disrespectful treatment, embarrassment about being weighed, negative attitudes of providers, unsolicited advice to lose weight, and medical equipment that was too small to be functional [110]. The percentage of women who reported these barriers increased with BMI. This parallels other research demonstrating a positive association between BMI and delay or avoidance of healthcare [111], and findings that obese women are less likely to undergo routine breast, cervical and colorectal cancer screening [111–115]. This is especially concerning because obesity increases their risk for developing these types of cancers. One self-report study of 310 hospital-employed women found that 12% indicated that they delayed or cancelled physician appointments due to weight concerns, 55% of those with a BMI over 35 delayed or cancelled visits because they knew they would be weighed, and in the 33% of women who had discussed weight with their physicians, discussions were described as negative [116]. The most common reason cited for delaying appointments was embarrassment about weight.

It is important to determine how weight stigma among health professionals affects their care of obese patients, such as time spent with patients, quality of patient–provider interactions, optimism about improvement, and willingness to provide support [117]. Hebl and Xu conducted an experimental study to examine how a patient's body weight influences both the attitudes that physicians hold as well as the treatments they prescribe [118]. Findings showed that physicians ($n = 122$) indicated that they would spend less time with heavier patients and viewed them significantly more negatively on 12 of 13 indices, including how self-disciplined they perceived the patient to be and the likelihood that the patient would comply with medical advice. Notably, only 42% of physicians chose to discuss weight loss with obese patients and only 31% would refer an obese patient to a nutrition counselor.

Considering the serious and costly co-morbidities associated with obesity, it is important to determine the extent to which weight bias affects the quality and frequency of care received by obese patients. Efforts to reduce weight stigma in healthcare settings may ameliorate some of these health consequences and improve obese patients' functional well-being.

Interpersonal relationships

Obese individuals may experience negative consequences in their social lives and interpersonal relationships with peers, family, and romantic partners. Some research finds that obese individuals are often perceived as less desirable candidates for any of these roles, and are viewed as being unpopular and having few friends [119,120]. These perceptions may be true in some cases, as studies have indicated that obese women are more dissatisfied with family relationships, partner relationships, and social activities than thinner women [121] and have fewer close friends than thinner women [122]. Other studies have found obesity positively associated with loneliness [123,124], and that obese individuals believe their weight has interfered in their participation in social activities [14,125].

Obese individuals may confront heightened consequences in family relationships. For example, some work has documented

significantly lower levels of support for severely obese persons in their family relationships [126], and that family members are reported to be the most frequent sources of weight stigma by obese individuals [1].

Obese individuals also appear to experience some difficulties in romantic partnerships. A 2005 study found that overweight women were less likely to be dating than their normal-weight peers. While heavier women found their relationships less satisfying, heavier men were more satisfied with their relationships [127]. Harris et al. found that weight was negatively associated with likelihood and frequency of dating for Caucasian women, and that Caucasian men were more likely than African-American men to have refused to date a woman because of her weight [128]. Sitton and Blanchard found that fewer men responded to a personal advertisement in which the woman was identified as obese compared to an advertisement in which a woman disclosed having a history of drug problems [129]. Regan found that subjects rated obese women as less sexually attractive, skilled, warm, and responsive, and less likely to experience sexual desire than normal-weight women; this difference did not hold when the target stimulus was male [130].

Few studies have examined the effect of obesity on sexual relationships. One study asked college students to rank order six drawings of potential sexual partners, including an obese partner, a healthy partner, and partners with various disabilities [131]. Both men and women ranked the obese person as the least desirable sexual partner; however, men ranked the obese partner as significantly less preferable than women did. Both men and women ranked figures described as having a mental illness and a history of sexually transmitted diseases as more preferred than an obese partner [131]. Another study found that obese individuals reported a high frequency of sexual difficulties attributed to their weight, which was more pronounced for women than for men, and that higher BMIs were associated with greater impairments in sexual quality of life [132].

Despite these findings, more work is needed in this area as some studies have reported no differences in degree of loneliness or romantic relationships between obese and nonobese persons [122]. For example, a recent study investigated social skills, social support, and subjective well-being in a sample of 226 obese individuals from the general population and found no differences between obese and comparison groups [133]. Similarly, a survey of 3000 adults found no significant differences between obese and nonobese participants in reported quality of relationships with friends, co-workers and spouses [126]. Other work has found no difference across weight groups in self-reported social support, size of social networks, socially based self-esteem [134] or popularity with peers [135,136].

While negative stereotypes about the relationship skills and desirability of obese individuals are common, some research supports the contention that obese individuals do, indeed, experience negative outcomes in the interpersonal domain, while other research finds that they fare similarly to their normal-weight counterparts. The subgroup most impacted by the negative stereotypes appears to be Caucasian women. Additional research is needed to help clarify whether true differences exist between obese and nonobese individuals, and how gender influences these outcomes.

Psychologic health and coping

A large body of research exists on the psychologic health of obese people, yielding mixed findings. It appears that the psychologic consequences of obesity may be mediated by several variables, such as gender, degree of obesity, and experiences of weight-related stigma. The main variables that have received attention in the literature are psychopathology, depression, risk for suicide, self-esteem, body esteem, quality of life, and coping strategies in response to stigma. This literature is briefly summarized below.

Early studies indicated lower levels of depression and anxiety in some obese demographic groups, giving rise to the "jolly fat" stereotype [137–143]. Other researchers have found no such relationship [144–147]. In their review of this literature, Friedman and Brownell found little consistent evidence that obese individuals as a group suffer greater psychopathology than their thinner counterparts [148]. Still others report small to moderate relationships between weight and depression across a variety of obese samples, especially for women [149–153]. A recent study of 44,800 respondents from the 2001 Behavioral Risk Factor Surveillance Survey demonstrated that young obese women were significantly more likely than nonobese women to have a sustained depressive mood [154].

Specific subpopulations of obese people may be more vulnerable to psychologic distress, most notably binge-eaters, obesity treatment-seeking populations, and certain social strata groups [155–160]. Wadden and colleagues found that extremely obese individuals who seek bariatric surgery are more vulnerable to depression and psychosocial complications than nontreatment-seeking individuals, with approximately 25–30% reporting clinically significant levels of depression [161]. The authors concluded that emotional stress associated with the physical complications and experiences of weight-related prejudice and discrimination can lead extremely obese individuals to seek medical attention.

One criticism of the early research in this area is the use of cross-sectional data. Roberts et al. reported findings from a large prospective study of adults (n = 1739) over the age of 50 [162]. Cross-sectionally, obese individuals were more likely to report poorer perceived mental health, less optimism, greater life dissatisfaction, and greater depression. Longitudinally, obesity predicted risk for subsequent depression, pessimism, and unhappiness 5 years later, even when controlling for baseline mental health problems. Two recent prospective studies, however, yielded mixed results. Sachs-Ericsson et al. (n = 2406) found that BMI moderately predicted depressive symptoms, and that this relationship was greater for African-Americans than for whites [163]. In contrast, a large prospective study of over 15,000 men and women found that obesity was associated with reduced subsequent risk of hospital admission for psychoses, depression, and anxiety, even after adjusting for related variables [164]. Faith

et al. reviewed this literature and concluded that the relationship between obesity and depression will likely prove to be a complex pattern of mediated and moderated relationships [165]. Two recent studies found the relationship between weight and psychologic health to be mediated by weight and shape concerns and weight cycling [166,167].

Miller and Downey published a meta-analysis of the relationship between weight and self-esteem [168]. They found a moderate relationship, which was stronger for women, individuals of higher SES, those of nonminority status, and those seeking treatment. This relationship does not hold across all studies [169]. As with obesity and depression, obesity and self-esteem appear more strongly related in certain subpopulations, such as binge-eaters and treatment-seeking populations [170]. It also appears to be moderated by body esteem. Body esteem has been of interest both as a variable in its own right and, more recently, as a moderator and/or mediator of the relationship between weight and other psychologic variables such as depression and global self-esteem. The relationship between body dissatisfaction and overweight is well established [169,171–173].

Recent studies have investigated the role of weight stigma in mediating the relationship between psychologic functioning and obesity. A 2007 study of morbidly obese surgery-seeking adults found depressed mood to be most related to weight stigma, rather than other factors such as BMI, gender, binge-eating status, and physical disability [174]. Similarly, a study of obese treatment-seeking adults found frequency of stigmatizing experiences to be associated with depression, general psychiatric symptoms, body image disturbance, and low self-esteem. Interestingly, participants' personal anti-fat attitudes moderated the relationship between stigma and body image [175]. Other research has reported that a history of appearance-based teasing while growing up is associated with body dissatisfaction, depression, low self-esteem, and higher frequency of binge eating [176–178]. Carr and Friedman [6] found that very obese persons who perceived they were discriminated against because of their weight reported lower levels of self-acceptance and self-esteem. Importantly, a 2007 study found that after controlling for common obesity-related stressors (e.g. poor physical health, interpersonal discrimination, and problematic relationships with family members) the effects of obesity on psychologic functioning attenuated and even reversed so that obese persons actually enjoyed better psychologic functioning than their thinner peers [179]. These findings suggest that reducing the weight stigma will significantly help to improve the psychologic health of obese individuals.

While the data on psychosocial outcomes in obesity are mixed, studies examining the relationship between weight stigma and psychologic impairments encourage increased attention toward efforts to reduce weight-related prejudice. One particularly sobering finding from a large US population-based sample ($n = 40,086$) is that BMI is associated with suicidal ideation in women, and with both suicide attempts and suicidal ideation in men [152]. More research is needed to establish causality and to pinpoint the particular aspects of obesity to target for intervention.

There is a range of strategies that obese individuals use to cope with stigmatizing experiences [180]. Some coping methods may improve well-being, while others may impair emotional and physical health. Certain coping responses, such as the adoption of unhealthy eating behaviors in reaction to stigma, may particularly exacerbate health consequences of obesity and interfere with attempts to lose weight. A study surveying over 2000 overweight and obese adults found that 79% of adults reported coping with weight stigma by eating more food, and 75% reported refusing to diet in response to weight stigma [1]. Other coping responses reported included heading off negative comments, using positive self-talk, coping through prayer, and seeking social support from others. Puhl and colleagues also found that obese individuals ($n = 1013$) who internalize negative weight-related stereotypes were particularly vulnerable to the psychologic consequences of stigma, including more frequent binge eating and refusal to diet [181]. The literature on coping strategies for weight bias remains scant, and more work is needed in this area to identify adaptive versus maladaptive responses to bias.

Special consideration: weight stigma in youth

As childhood obesity rates continue to rise [182], an increasing number of young people are vulnerable to the social consequences of obesity. Research shows that overweight and obese youth experience weight stigma from multiple sources, including peers, educators, and parents. In their 2007 review of research on weight stigma in children and adolescents, Puhl and Latner conclude that the scientific literature is clear in demonstrating that stigmatization directed at obese children is pervasive and often unrelenting, and that as a result of weight bias and discrimination, obese children suffer psychologic, social, and health-related consequences [2].

Numerous studies have documented children's negative attitudes toward obese individuals, which often result in weight-related victimization and teasing of overweight peers. In a classic 1961 study, Richardson and colleagues found that 10–11 year olds reported that they would prefer to be friends with children who had disabilities (e.g. children in a wheelchair or with a facial disfigurement) rather than an overweight child, whom they ranked last in their friendship preferences [183]. A 2003 replication of this study suggests that weight stigma among children has worsened over the last 40 years [184]. Brylinsky and Moore demonstrated that children as young as age 3 described a "chubby" target as mean, stupid, loud, ugly, lazy, sad, and lacking in friends [185]. This finding is supported by research spanning several decades demonstrating that children associate negative stereotypes with overweight individuals [184,186–196]. As a result of these negative attitudes, a number of studies have found that overweight and obese children report being teased, bullied, verbally abused, rejected, and isolated because of their weight [197–203].

Overweight and obese youth are not only stigmatized by their peers; teachers and parents also express negative weight-related attitudes. As mentioned above, research shows that teachers exhibit biased attitudes towards obesity [45,95], with the most recent work demonstrating negative attitudes towards obese students by physical education (PE) teachers who also have higher expectations for "normal-weight" students than overweight students [48,49]. In addition, Bauer and colleagues found that middle school students reported receiving negative comments from teachers about their athletic abilities that in turn led them to avoid participating in PE classes [47]. This finding is discouraging considering the importance of physical activity for promoting the health of obese children.

Studies find that parents can be additional sources of biased attitudes towards weight, which can be communicated to their children in both subtle and overt ways [204,205]. Self-report studies further reveal that overweight and obese individuals report experiencing weight-based teasing from their parents [1,200,206].

For children, the impact of obesity and weight-related stigma can be severe, having negative psychologic, interpersonal, academic, and physical health consequences. Wardle and Cooke reviewed empiric evidence on the relationship between childhood obesity and psychologic well-being [207]. They found that while clinical samples of obese youth typically report poorer psychologic health than population-based samples, research in community samples suggests that few obese children are depressed or have low self-esteem. The exception to this finding is that some studies find obese children to have moderate levels of body dissatisfaction [208–211]. As with the literature on adults, Wardle and Cooke conclude that a number of mediators and moderators influence the relationship between obesity and well-being, including weight-based teasing [207].

Several studies have documented evidence that weight-based teasing is associated with poorer psychologic outcomes among both male and female adolescents [202,212,213]. In a sample of 4746 adolescents, Eisenberg and colleagues [206] found that teasing about weight was consistently associated with body dissatisfaction, low self-esteem, high depressive symptoms and suicidal ideation. Weight category was not related to these outcomes after controlling for teasing, suggesting that teasing itself, rather than weight, may be most relevant in predicting emotional well-being. Other research has found weight teasing to be associated to body dissatisfaction, regardless of weight category [214,215]. One of the most alarming consequences of obesity and weight-related teasing is the increased risk for suicidal behaviors. Several large population-based studies have demonstrated that obese adolescents are more likely to consider or attempt suicide than their nonobese peers [216–218], while obese adolescents who are teased because of their weight may be at an even higher risk [200,206].

Weight stigma is particularly harmful for overweight children when it interferes with the formation of social relationships and friendships. Overweight children in elementary school have been shown to be less liked and more often rejected than their nonoverweight peers [194]. Data from 90,118 adolescents in the National Longitudinal Study of Adolescent Health found that overweight adolescents were more likely to be socially isolated and were less likely to be chosen by their peers as friends [209]. Another study of almost 10,000 adolescents found that obese boys and girls were less likely to spend time with friends than their thinner peers [218]. There is also evidence that overweight youth report that their weight is the reason for their social isolation [202,219].

Obesity and weight stigma also appear to interfere with academic success and educational achievement. In 1994, the National Education Association's report on size discrimination observed: "For fat students, the school experience is one of ongoing prejudice, unnoticed discrimination, and almost constant harassment. From nursery school through college, fat students experience ostracism, discouragement, and sometimes violence" [220]. Additional research with adolescents supports these conclusions. A 2007 study using data from the National Longitudinal Study of Adolescent Health reported that obesity undermined the educational attainment of female students. Obese girls experienced higher levels of self-rejection, suicidal ideation, substance use and academic failures, and had a 50% lower chance of attending college, suggesting that the negative social climate for obese girls may have disrupted their academic attention and their future academic success [12].

Similar to the coping strategies obese adults may use in response to stigmatizing experiences, obese youth who experience weight stigma may engage in disordered eating behaviors in response to stigmatizing situations. Several studies have documented weight-related teasing to be associated with unhealthy behaviors in adolescents, such as binge eating, vomiting, bulimia, and the use of diet pills or laxatives [198,214,215,221–223]. In a study assessing associations with weight-based teasing among 4746 adolescents, Neumark-Sztainer and colleagues reported that overweight boys and girls who experienced frequent weight-related teasing were more likely to engage in unhealthy weight control behaviors and binge eating than overweight adolescents who were not teased about their weight [200]. Even after controlling for socio-economic status and BMI, the relationship between teasing and disordered eating remained. Prospective research following these adolescents also found that weight-related teasing predicted binge eating and extreme weight control behaviors 5 years later [224,225].

The evidence is clear that a growing proportion of overweight children face stigmatization in multiple aspects of their lives. Not only does this stigmatization affect their psychologic well-being, but it damages their social relationships, hinders their academic success, and triggers unhealthy behaviors that can harm their physical health, making their struggles with weight more difficult. Furthermore, there is no evidence to suggest that weight teasing directed at children is a positive motivator for weight loss. Thus, successful efforts to prevent and reduce childhood obesity should include programs to reduce weight stigma and help children to effectively cope with its deleterious effects.

Strategies for weight stigma reduction

Weight stigma reduction is clearly an important goal to improve both the social consequences related to obesity and the quality of health for obese children and adults. Although attribution research provides important insights about the origins of obesity stigma, only a handful of published studies have addressed attributions of controllability and causality of obesity in direct attempts to improve attitudes. Some experimental research has improved attitudes towards obese people by providing information to participants about biologic, genetic, and noncontrollable causes of obesity [21,41]. However, other studies providing explanations for obesity outside one's personal control did not lead to attitude change [226,227]. Thus, more work is needed to determine the utility of attribution theory to reduce weight bias, and it is important to examine other stigma reduction methods.

A school-based intervention improved weight tolerance among elementary students through a curriculum designed to promote size acceptance, although children's attitudes were not directly assessed, making it difficult to determine whether actual changes occurred [228]. Negative attitudes were also reduced in a study of medical students following an intervention that used videos of obese people, role-play exercises, and written materials about the causes of obesity [96]. One-year follow-up results indicated that students endorsed fewer negative stereotypes compared to their preintervention attitudes. An experimental study evaluated a web-based intervention to reduce weight stigma among educators [229]. The online module, covering topics such as obesity, the consequences of obesity stigma, and sociocultural pressures on young people to be thin, successfully improved attitudes towards obesity and maintained these improvements at 6-month follow-up. Interestingly, participants' attitudes improved more when there was an overweight female presenter for the online course compared to a thin female presenter.

Studies designed to evoke empathy towards obese people have also attempted to reduce stigma, but have produced discouraging findings. This research instructed participants to read stories about weight discrimination or watch empathic videos of obese women, neither of which changed negative associations about obese people [227,230]. Another study was unable to improve negative attitudes among medical students by increasing their direct interpersonal contact with obese patients [102]. There is extensive research support for the effectiveness of increased interpersonal contact on attitude change [231], but certain types of stigmas, like obesity, may resist these strategies.

A relatively new stigma reduction strategy targeting perceptions of social consensus about obesity has successfully decreased negative attitudes and increased positive attitudes towards obese people. The perceived social consensus model suggests that stereotypes and stigma are a function of their perceptions of others' stereotypical or stigmatizing beliefs [232]. Puhl et al. conducted three experimental studies in which students completed self-report measures of attitudes towards obese people prior to and following manipulated feedback depicting the attitudes of other students [41]. University students who received favorable consensus feedback (suggesting that others held more favorable beliefs about obese people than they did) reported significantly fewer negative attitudes and more positive attitudes toward obese persons compared to their reported attitudes prior to feedback. In addition, students shifted their reported beliefs about the causes of obesity following favorable consensus feedback to beliefs that obesity is due to factors outside, rather than within, personal control. This social consensus approach remained predictive of positive attitude change when it was compared to other methods of stigma reduction (such as providing causal information about obesity).

Few published studies have attempted to reduce weight stigma among children and adolescents. Bell and Morgan attempted to reduce weight stigma among children in grades 3–6 by addressing perceptions of the controllability of body weight [226]. Providing medical information to explain the causes of obesity improved attitudes among younger children, but not among older children, who displayed more negative behavioral intentions toward obese targets. A similar study presented information to students about the uncontrollability of body size, but was unable to improve negative weight-based stereotyping [233]. Other research suggests that the media may be a promising avenue for stigma reduction strategies in children [2]. Considering the role of television in perpetuating children's endorsement of obesity stereotypes [234], future research should examine the potential for the media to improve weight-related attitudes among youth through specific programming and more positive depictions of overweight characters.

Many questions remain about how to overcome negative attitudes towards obese people. There is clearly a need for additional research to identify key factors that are necessary for effective stigma reduction interventions, and to determine whether there are particular approaches that may work better than others in certain circumstances. It will also be useful to test the social consensus framework with more diverse samples and to compare its utility with attribution approaches of attitude modification, in both adults and children.

Conclusion

Weight stigma negatively impacts multiple aspects of life including education, employment, healthcare, and social relationships. These obstacles can significantly impair overall quality of life for obese adults and children. While other forms of bias, such as racism and sexism, are prohibited by federal legislation, weight bias is rarely challenged, often ignored, and offers no legal recourse for obese individuals who experience weight discrimination.

In order to establish effective strategies to improve society's negative attitudes, research efforts must focus on the development, testing and implementation of stigma reduction

interventions. The lack of research in this area and the mixed findings of existing work indicate the need to integrate current theories of weight bias and to find new conceptual approaches to guide efforts aimed at improving negative attitudes towards obese people. Attribution and social consensus perspectives provide promising avenues for research, but both require further testing to determine whether attitude change resulting from these methods reliably translates into less biased behavior toward obese individuals.

Educational programs aimed at increasing diversity and reducing bias must also be tested to offer parents and teachers ways of helping obese children cope with prejudice, and to ensure that there are equal opportunities for overweight and obese children to succeed. Within medical settings, clinicians and healthcare professionals have a responsibility to assist obese patients in managing their stigma experiences, take steps to reduce weight bias in their practice, and improve the healthcare environment for obese patients. Given that obese individuals are at increased risk for a wide variety of medical problems, facilitating their participation in preventive services and treatment is paramount. This requires that healthcare is delivered with sensitivity and free of bias.

The damaging social consequences of obesity for both adults and children are significant, and the impact of bias and discrimination on public health could be considerable. Major shifts in societal attitudes are needed to combat weight bias. The national obesity research agenda must do its part to address this important social issue. Clinicians, obesity researchers, and healthcare professionals have a responsibility to improve the well-being of obese adults and children, which requires us to address not only physical but also emotional, social, and psychologic indices of health.

References

1. Puhl RM, Brownell KD. Confronting and coping with weight stigma: an investigation of overweight and obese adults. Obesity 2006;14(10):1802–15.
2. Puhl RM, Latner JD. Stigma, obesity, and the health of the nation's children. Psychol Bull 2007;133:557–80.
3. Allon N. The stigma of overweight in everyday life. In: Woldman BB (ed) *Psychological Aspects of Obesity*. New York: Van Nostrand Reinhold, 1982:130–74.
4. Puhl RM, Brownell KD. Bias, discrimination, and obesity. Obes Res 2001;9(12):788–905.
5. Schwartz MB, Vartanian LR, Nosek BA, Brownell KD. The influence of one's own body weight on implicit and explicit anti-fat bias. Obesity 2006;14:440–7.
6. Carr D, Friedman MA. Is obesity stigmatizing? Body weight, perceived discrimination, and psychological well-being in the United States. J Health Soc Behav 2005;46(3).
7. Puhl RM, Andreyeva T, Brownell KD. Perceptions of weight discrimination: prevalence and comparison to race and gender discrimination in America. Int J Obes 2008;32(6):992–1000.

8. Andreyeva T, Puhl RM, Brownell KD. Changes in perceived weight discrimination among Americans: 1995–1996 through 2004–2006. Obesity 2008;16(5):1129–34.

9. Rogge MM, Greenwald M, Golden A. Obesity, stigma, and civilized oppression. Adv Nurs 2004;27(4):301–15.

10. Hebl MR, Mannix LM. The weight of obesity in evaluating others: a mere proximity effect. Person Soc Psychol Bull 2003;29:28–38.

11. Falkner NH, French SA, Jeffery RW, Neumark-Sztainer D, Sherwood NE, Morton M. Mistreatment due to weight: prevalence and sources of perceived mistreatment in women and men. Obes Res 1999;7:572–6.

12. Crosnoe R. Gender, obesity, and education. Sociol Educ 2007; 80:241–60.

13. Baum CL, Ford WF. The wage effects of obesity: a longitudinal study. Health Econ 2004;13:885–99.

14. Tiggemann M, Rothblum ED. Gender differences in social consequences of perceived overweight in the United States and Australia. Sex Roles 1988;18:75–86.

15. Hebl MR, Turchin JM. The stigma of obesity: what about men? Basic Appl Soc Psychol 2005;27:267–75.

16. Hebl MR, Heatherton TF. The stigma of obesity in women: the difference is black and white. Person Soc Psychol Bull 1998; 24(4):417–26.

17. Wang SS, Brownell KD, Schwartz MB. The influence of the stigma of obesity on overweight individuals. Int J Obes 2004;28:1333–7.

18. Cawley J. *Body Weight and Women's Labor Market Outcomes*. Report No. 7841. Cambridge, MA: National Bureau of Economic Research, 2000.

19. Himes SM, Thompson JK. Fat stigmatization in television shows and movies: a content analysis. Obesity 2007;15:712–18.

20. Greenberg BS, Eastin M, Hofshire L, Lachlan K, Brownell KD. The portrayal of overweight and obese persons in commercial television. Am J Pub Health 2003;93(8):1342–8.

21. Crandall CS. Prejudice against fat people: ideology and self-interest. J Person Soc Psychol 1994;66:882–94.

22. Crandall CS, Cohen C. The personality of the stigmatizer: cultural world view, conventionalism, and self-esteem. J Res Person 1994;28:461–80.

23. Crandall CS, Martinez R. Culture, ideology, and anti-fat attitudes. Person Soc Psychol Bull 1996;22:1165–76.

24. Crandall CS, Reser AH. Attributions and weight-based prejudice. In: Brownell KD, Puhl RM, Schwartz MB, Rudd L (eds) *Weight Bias: Nature, Consequences, and Remedies*. New York: Guilford Press, 2005.

25. Crandall CS, Schiffhauer KL. Anti-fat prejudice: beliefs, values, and American culture. Obes Res 1998;6:458–60.

26. Weiner B, Perry RP, Magnusson J. An attributional analysis of reactions to stigmas. J Person Soc Psychol 1988;55(5):738–48.

27. Crandall CS. Ideology and lay theories of stigma: the justification of stigmatization. In: Heatherton TF, Kleck RE, Hebl MR, Hull JG (eds) *The Social Psychology of Stigma*. New York: Guilford Press, 2000:126–52.

28. Crandall CS, Moriarty D. Physical illness stigma and social rejection. Br J Soc Psychol 1995;34:67–83.

29. Menec VH, Perry RP. Reactions to stigmas among Canadian students: testing an attributional-affect-help judgment model. J Soc Psychol 1988;138:443–54.

30. Rodin M, Price JH, Sanchez F, McElliot S. Derogation, exclusion, and unfair treatment of persons with social flaws: controllability of stigma and the attribution of prejudice. Person Soc Psychol Bull 1989;15:439–51.

31. DeJong W. Obesity as a characterological stigma: the issue of responsibility and judgements of task performance. Psychol Rep 1993;73:963–70.

32. DeJong W. The stigma of obesity: the consequences of naive assumptions concerning the causes of physical deviance. J Health Soc Behav 1980;21(1):75–87.

33. Rashad I. Assessing the underlying economic causes and consequences of obesity. Gender Issues 2003;21:17–29.

34. Swinburn B, Egger G. The runaway weight gain train: too many accelerators, not enough brakes. BMJ 2007;329:736–9.

35. Booth KM, Pinkston MM, Poston WSC. Obesity and the built environment. J Am Diet Assoc 2005;105(suppl):110–17.

36. Walley AJ, Blakemore AIF, Froguel P. Genetics of obesity and the prediction of risk for health. Hum Mol Genet 2006;15: R124–R30.

37. Friedman JM. Modern science versus the stigma of obesity. Nat Med 2004;10:563–9.

38. Curioni CC, Lourenco PM. Long-term weight loss after diet and exercise: a systematic review. Int J Obes 2005;29:1168–74.

39. Mann T, Tomiyama AJ, Westling E, Lew A-M, Samuels B, Chatman J. Medicare's search for effective obesity treatments. Am Psychol 2007;62:220–33.

40. Tsai AG, Wadden TA. Systematic review: an evaluation of major commercial weight loss programs in the United States. Ann Intern Med 2005;142:56–66.

41. Puhl RM, Schwartz MB, Brownell KD. Impact of perceived consensus on stereotypes about obese people: a new approach for reducing bias. Health Psychol 2005;24:517–25.

42. Canning H, Mayer J. Obesity – its possible effect on college acceptance. N Engl J Med 1966;275:1172–4.

43. Karnehed N, Rasmussen F, Hemmingsson T, Tynelius P. Obesity and attained education: cohort study of more than 700,000 Swedish men. Obesity 2006;14:1421–8.

44. Weiler K, Helms LB. Responsibilities of nursing education: the lessons of Russell v Salve Regina. J Prof Nurs 1993;9:131–8.

45. Neumark-Sztainer D, Story M, Harris T. Beliefs and attitudes about obesity among teachers and school health care providers working with adolescents. J Nutr Educ 1999;31:3–9.

46. Price JH, Desmond SM, Stelzer CM. Elementary school principals' perceptions of childhood obesity. J School Health 1987;57:367–70.

47. Bauer KW, Yang YW, Austin SB. "How can we stay healthy when you're throwing all this in front of us?" Findings from focus groups and interviews in middle schools on environmental influences on nutrition and physical activity. Health Educ Behav 2004; 31:34–6.

48. Greenleaf C, Weiller K. Perceptions of youth obesity among physical educators. Soc Psychol Educ 2005;8:407–23.

49. O'Brien KS, Hunter JA, Banks M. Implicit anti-fat bias in physical educators: physical attributes, ideology, and socialization. Int J Obes 2007;31:308–14.

50. Crandall CS. Do parents discriminate against their heavyweight daughters? Person Soc Psychol Bull 1995;21:724–35.

51. Li X. A study of intelligence and personality in children with simple obesity. Int J Obes 1995;19:355–7.

52. Sorenson TI, Sonne-Holm S. Intelligence test performance in obesity in relation to educational attainment and parental social class. J Biosoc Sci 1985;17:379–87.

53. Elias MF, Elias PK, Wolf PA, d'Agostino RB. Lower cognitive function in the presence of obesity and hypertension: the Framingham Heart Study. Int J Obes 2003;27:260–80.

54. Tunceli K, Li K, Williams LK. Long-term effects of obesity on employment and work limitations among U.S. adults, 1986–1999. Obesity 2006;14:1637–46.

55. Klarenbach S, Padwal R, Chuck A, Jacobs P. Population-based analysis of obesity a workforce participation. Obesity 2006;14:920–7.

56. Viner RM, Cole TJ. Adult socioeconomic, educational, social, and psychological outcomes of childhood obesity: a national birth cohort study. BMJ 2005;330:1354.

57. Loh ES. The economic effects of physical appearance. Soc Sci Q 1993;74:420–37.

58. Brunello G, d'Hombres B. Does body weight affect wages? Evidence from Europe. Econ Hum Biol 2007;5:1–19.

59. Register CA, Williams DR. Wage effects of obesity among young workers. Soc Sci Q 1990;71:130–41.

60. Pagan JA, Davila A. Obesity, occupational attainment, and earnings. Soc Sci Q 1997;78:756–70.

61. Rothblum ED, Brand PA, Miller CT, Oetjen HA. The relationship between obesity, employment discrimination, and employment-related victimization. J Vocat Behav 1990;37:251–66.

62. Celizic M. Company to workers: Shape or pay up. 2007, Available from: www.msnbc.msn.com/id/20212332/

63. Weight matters. San Francisco Chronicle, July 31, 2007.

64. Civil Service Commission v. Pennsylvania Human Relations Commission, 1991.

65. Perroni PJ. Cook v. Rhode Island, Department of Mental Health, Retardation, & Hospitals: the first circuit tips the scales of justice to protect the overweight. N Engl Law Rev 1996;30:993–1018.

66. Frisk AM. Obesity as a disability: an actual or perceived problem? Army Lawyer 1996:3–19.

67. Smaw v. Virginia Department of State Police, 1994.

68. Nedder v. Rivier College, 1995.

69. Gimello v. Agency Rent-A-Car Systems, Inc.: N.J. Super Ct. App. Div., 1991.

70. Roehling MV, Roehling PV, Pichler S. The relationship between body weight and perceived weight-related employment discrimination: the role of sex and race. J Vocat Behav 2007;71:300–18.

71. Bellizzi JA, Hasty RW. Territory assignment decisions and supervising unethical selling behavior: the effects of obesity and gender as moderated by job-related factors. J Person Selling Sales Manage 1998;XVIII:35–49.

72. Decker WH. Attributions based on managers' self-presentation, sex, and weight. Psychol Rep 1987;61:175–81.

73. Klassen ML, Jasper CR, Harris RJ. The role of physical appearance in managerial decisions. J Bus Psychol 1993;8:181–98.

74. Everett M. Let an overweight person call on your best customers? Fat chance. Sales Marketing Manage 1990;142:66–70.

75. Jasper CR, Klassen ML. Perceptions of salespersons' appearance and evaluation of job performance. Percept Motor Skills 1990;71:563–6.

76. Pingitoire R, Dugoni R, Tindale S, Spring B. Bias against overweight job applicants in a simulated employment interview. J Appl Psychol 1994;79:909–17.

77. Rothblum ED, Miller CT, Garbutt B. Stereotypes of obese female job applicants. Int J Eating Disord 1988;7:277–83.

78. Ding VJ, Stillman JA. An empirical investigation of discrimination against overweight female job applicants in New Zealand. NZ J Psychol 2005;34:139–48.

79. Larkin JC, Pines HA. No fat persons need apply: experimental studies of the overweight stereotype and hiring preference. Sociol Work Occup 1979;6:312–27.

80. Paul RJ, Townsend JB. Shape up or ship out? Employment discrimination against the overweight. Employee Responsibilities Rights J 1995;8:133–45.

81. Polinko NK, Popovich PM. Evil thoughts but angelic actions: responses to overweight job applicants. J Appl Soc Psychol 2001;31:905–24.

82. Roehling MV. Weight-based discrimination in employment: psychological and legal aspects. Personnel Psychol 1999;52:969–1017.

83. Hebl MR, Kleck RE. Acknowledging one's stigma in the interview setting: effective strategy or liability? J Appl Soc Psychol 2002;32:223–49.

84. Theran EE. Legal theory on weight discrimination. In: Brownell KD, Puhl RM, Schwartz MB, Rudd L (eds) *Weight Bias: Nature, Consequences, and Remedies*. New York: Guilford Press, 2005.

85. Sobal J, Stunkard AJ. Socioeconomic status and obesity: a review of the literature. Psychol Bull 1989;105:260–75.

86. Stunkard AJ, Sorenson TI. Obesity and socioeconomic status: a complex relation. N Engl J Med 1993;329:1036–7.

87. Wardle J, Volz C, Jarvis MJ. Sex differences in the association of socioeconomic status with obesity. Am J Pub Health 2002;92:1299–304.

88. Gortmaker SL, Must A, Perrin JM, Sobol AM, Dietz WH. Social and economic consequences of overweight in adolescence and young adulthood. N Engl J Med 1993;399:1008–12.

89. Sargent RG, Blanchflower DG. Obesity and stature in adolescents and earnings in young adulthood: analysis of a British cohort. Arch Pediatr Adolesc Med 1994;148:681–7.

90. Fonda SJ, Fultz NH, Jenkins KR, Wray LA. Relationship of body mass and net worth for retirement-aged men and women. Res Aging 2004;26:153–76.

91. Patt MR, Yanek LR, Moy TF, Becker DM. Sociodemographic, behavioral, and psychological correlates of current overweight and obesity in older, urban African American women. Health Educ Behav 2004;31:57.

92. Davis-Coelho K, Waltz J, Davis-Coelho B. Awareness and prevention of bias against fat clients in psychotherapy. Prof Psychol: Res Pract 2000;31:682–4.

93. Maddox GL, Liederman V. Overweight as a social disability with medical implications. J Med Educ 1969;44:214–20.

94. Maroney D, Golub S. Nurses' attitudes toward obese persons and certain ethnic groups. Percept Motor Skills 1992;75:387–91.

95. Price JH, Desmond SM, Krol RA, Snyder FF, O'Connell JK. Family practice physicians' beliefs, attitudes, and practices regarding obesity. Am J Prev Med 1987;3:339–45.

96. Wiese HJ, Wilson JF, Jones RA, Neises M. Obesity stigma reduction in medical students. Int J Obes 1992;16:859–68.

97. McArthur L, Ross J. Attitudes of registered dietitians toward personal overweight and overweight clients. J Am Diet Assoc 1997;97:63–6.

98. Berryman D, Dubale G, Manchester D, Mittelstaedt R. Dietetic students possess negative attitudes toward obesity similar to nondietetic students. J Am Diet Assoc 2006;106:1678–82.

99. Oberrieder H, Walker R, Monroe D, Adeyanju M. Attitudes of dietetic students and registered dietitians toward obesity. J Am Diet Assoc 1995;95:914–6.

100. Schwartz MB, Chambliss HO, Brownell KD, Blair SN, Billington C. Weight bias among health professionals specializing in obesity. Obes Res 2003;11(9):1033–9.

101. Foster GD, Wadden TA, Makris AP, et al. Primary care physicians' attitudes about obesity and its treatment. Obes Res 2003;11(10):1168–77.

102. Blumberg P, Mellis LP. Medical students' attitudes toward the obese and morbidly obese. Int J Eating Disord 1980:169–75.

103. Klein D, Najman J, Kohrman AF, Munro C. Patient characteristics that elicit negative responses from family physicians. J Fam Pract 1982;14:881–8.

104. Bagley CR, Conklin DN, Isherwood RT, Pechiulis DR, Watson LA. Attitudes of nurses toward obesity and obese patients. Percept Motor Skills 1989;68:954.

105. Madey SF, Ondrus SA. Illusory correlations in perceptions of obese and hypertensive patients' noncooperative behaviors. J Appl Soc Psychol 1999;29:1200–17.

106. Bertakis KD, Azari R. The impact of obesity on primary care visits. Obes Res 2005;13(9):1615–22.

107. Campbell K, Engel H, Timperio A, Cooper C, Crawford D. Obesity management: Australian general practitioners' attitudes and practices. Obes Res 2000;8:459–66.

108. Brown I, Thompson J, Tod A, Jones G. Primary care support for tackling obesity: a qualitative study of the perceptions of obese patients. Br J Gen Pract 2006;56:666–72.

109. Wadden TA, Anderson DA, Foster GD, Bennet A, Steinberg C, Sarwer DB. Obese women's perceptions of their physician's weight management attitudes and practices. Arch Fam Med 2000;9:854–60.

110. Amy NK, Aalborg A, Lyons P, Keranen L. Barrier to routine gynecological cancer screening for White and African-American obese women. Int J Obes 2006;30:147–55.

111. Drury CAA, Louis M. Exploring the association between body weight, stigma of obesity, and health care avoidance. J Am Acad Nurse Pract 2002;14(12):554–60.

112. Wee CC, McCarthy EP, Davis RB, Phillips RS. Obesity and breast cancer screening: the influence of race, illness burden, and other factors. J Gen Intern Med 2004;19:324–31.

113. Rosen AB, Schneider EC. Colorectal cancer screening disparities related to obesity and gender. J Gen Intern Med 2004;19(332–338).

114. Meisinger C, Heier M, Loewel H. The relationship between body weight and health care among German women. Obes Res 2004;23:1473–80.

115. Heo M, Allison DB, Fontaine KR. Overweight, obesity, and colorectal cancer screening: disparity between men and women. BMC Public Health 2004;4:53.

116. Olson CL, Schumaker HD, Yawn BP. Overweight women delay medical care. Arch Fam Med 1994;3:888–92.

117. Schwartz MB, Puhl RM. Childhood obesity: a societal problem to solve. Obes Rev 2003;4:57–71.

118. Hebl MR, Xu J. Weighing the care: physicians' reactions to the size of a patient. Int J Obes 2001;25:1246–52.

119. Harris MB, Harris RJ, Bochner S. Fat, four-eyed, and female: stereotypes of obesity, glasses, and gender. J Appl Soc Psychol 1982;12:503–16.

120. Harris MB, Smith SD. The relationships of age, sex, ethnicity, and weight to stereotypes of obesity and self-perception. Int J Obes 1983;7:361–71.

121. Ball K, Crawford D, Kenardy J. Longitudinal relationships among overweight, life satisfaction, and aspirations in young women. Obes Res 2004;12:1019–30.

122. Sarlio-Lahteenkorva S. Weight loss and quality of life among obese people. Social Indicators Res 2001;54:329–54.

123. Lauder W, Mummery K, Jones M, Caperchione C. A comparison of health behaviors in lonely and non-lonely populations. Psychol Health Med 2006;11:233–45.

124. Schumaker JF, Krejci RC, Small L, Sargent RG. Experience of loneliness by obese individuals. Psychol Rep 1985;57:1147–54.

125. Bullen BA, Monello LF, Cohen H, Mayer J. Attitudes towards physical activity, food, and family in obese and nonobese adolescent girls. Am J Clin Nutr 1963;12:1–11.

126. Carr D, Friedman MA. Body weight and the quality of interpersonal relationships. Soc Psychol Q 2006;2006:127–49.

127. Sheets V, Ajmere K. Are romantic partners a source of college students' weight concern? Eating Behav 2005;6:1–9.

128. Harris MB, Walters LC, Waschull S. Gender and ethnic differences in obesity-related behaviors and attitudes in a college sample. J Appl Soc Psychol 1991;21:1545–66.

129. Sitton S, Blanchard S. Men's preferences in romantic partners: obesity vs. addiction. Psychol Rep 1995;77:1185–1186.

130. Regan PC. Sexual outcasts: the perceived impact of body weight and gender on sexuality. J Appl Soc Psychol 1996;26:1803–15.

131. Chen EY, Brown M. Obesity stigma in sexual relationships. Obes Res 2005;13:1393–7.

132. Kolotkin RL, Binks M, Crosby RD, Ostbye T, Gress RE, Adams TD. Obesity and sexual quality of life. Obesity 2006;14:472–9.

133. Dierk J-M, Conradt M, Rauh E, Schlumberger P, Hebebrand J, Rief W. What determines well-being in obesity? Associations with BMI, social skills, and social support. J Psychosom Res 2006;60:219–27.

134. Miller CT, Rothblum ED, Brand PA, Felicio D. Do obese women have poorer social relationships than nonobese women? Reports by self, friends, and co-workers. J Person 1995;63:65–85.

135. Jarvie GJ, Lahey B, Graziano W, Framer E. Childhood obesity and social stigma: what we know and what we don't know. Dev Rev 1983;3:237–73.

136. Sallade J. A comparison of the psychological adjustment of obese vs. non-obese children. J Psychosom Res 1973;17:89–96.

137. Crisp AH, McGuiness B. Jolly fat: relation between obesity and psychoneurosis. BMJ 1975;1:7–9.

138. Crisp AH, Queenan M, Sittampaln Y, Harris G. "Jolly fat" revisited. J Psychosom Res 1980;24:233–41.

139. Kittel F, Rustin RM, Dramaix M, Debacker G, Kornitzer M. Psycho-socio-biological correlates of moderate overweight in an industrial population. J Psychosom Res 1978;22:145–58.

140. Palinkas LA, Wingard DL, Barrett-Connor E. Depressive symptoms in overweight and obese older adults: a test of the "jolly fat" hypothesis. J Psychosom Res 1996;40:59–66.

141. Silverstone JT. Psychological aspects of obesity. Proc Roy Soc Med 1968;61:371.

142. Simon RI. Obesity and depressive equivalent. JAMA 1963;183:208–10.

143. Stewart A, Brook RH. Effects of being overweight. Am J Pub Health 1983;73:171–8.

144. Faubel M. Body image and depression in women with early and late onset obesity. J Psychol 1989;12:385–95.

145. Hallstrom T, Noppa H. Obesity in women in relation to mental illness, social factors, and personality traits. J Psychosom Res 1981;25:75–82.

146. Hayes D, Ross CE. Body and mind: the effect of exercise, overweight, and physical health on psychological well-being. J Health Soc Behav 1986;27:387–400.

147. Moore ME, Stunkard AJ, Strole L. Obesity, social class, and mental illness. JAMA 1962;181:138–42.

148. Friedman MA, Brownell KD. Psychological correlates of obesity: moving to the next research generation. Psychol Bull 1995; 117:3–20.

149. Anderson SE, Cohen P, Naumova EN, Jacques PF, Must A. Adolescent obesity and risk for subsequent major depressive disorder: prospective evidence. Psychosom Med 2007;69:740–7.

150. Istvan J, Zavela K, Weidner G. Body weight and psychological distress in NHANES I. Int J Obes 1992;19:999–1003.

151. Homer TN, Utermohlen V. A multivariate analysis of psychological factors related to body mass index and eating preoccupation in female college students. J Am Coll Nutr 1993;12:459–65.

152. Carpenter KM, Hasin DS, Allison DB, Faith MS. Relationships between obesity and DSM-IV major depressive disorder, suicide ideation, and suicide attempts: results from a general population study. Am J Pub Health 2000;90:251–7.

153. Roberts RE, Kaplan GA, Shema SJ, Strawbridge WJ. Are the obese at greater risk of depression? Am J Epidemiol 2000;152:163–70.

154. Heo M, Pietrobelli A, Fontaine KR, Sirey JA, Faith MS. Depressive mood and obesity in U.S. adults: comparison and moderation by sex, age, and race. Int J Obes 2006;30:513–19.

155. Black DS, Goldstein RB, Mason EE. Prevalence of mental disorder in 88 morbidly obese bariatric clinic patients. Am J Psychiatr 1992;149:227–34.

156. Fitzgibbon ML, Stolley MR, Kirschenbaum DS. Obese people who seek treatment have different characteristics than those who do not seek treatment. Health Psychol 1993;12:346–53.

157. Goldsmith SJ, Anger-Friedfeld K, Beren S, Rudolph D, Boeck M, Arrone L. Psychiatric illness in patients presenting for obesity treatment. Int J Eating Disord 1992;12:63–71.

158. Kuehnel RH, Wadden TA. Binge eating disorder, weight cycling, and psychopathology. Int J Eating Disord 1994;26:205–10.

159. Musante GJ, Costanzo PR, Friedman KE. The co-morbidity of depression and eating dysregulation processes in a diet-seeking obese population: a matter of gender specificity. Int J Eating Disord 1998;23:65–75.

160. Telch CF, Agras WF. Obesity, binge eating and psychopathology: are they related? Int J Eating Disord 1994;15:53–61.

161. Wadden TA, Sarwer DB, Fabricatore AN, Jones L, Stack R, Williams NS. Psychosocial and behavioral status of patients undergoing bariatric surgery: what to expect before and after surgery. Med Clin North Am 2007;91:451–69.

162. Roberts RE, Strawbridge WJ, Deleger S, Kaplan GA. Are the fat more jolly? Ann Behav Med 2002;24:169–80.

163. Sachs-Ericsson N, Burns AB, Gordon KH, et al. Body mass index and depressive symptoms in older adults: the moderating roles of race, sex, and socioeconomic status. Am J Geriatr Psychiatr 2007;15(9):815–25.

164. Lawlor DA, Hart CL, Hole DJ, Gunnell D, Smith GD. Body mass index in middle life and future risk of hospital admission for psychoses or depression: findings from the Renfrew/Paisley study. Psychol Med 2007;37:1151–61.

165. Faith MS, Matz PE, Jorge MA. Obesity-depression associations in the population. J Psychosom Res 2002;53:935–42.

166. Mond JM, Rodgers B, Hay PJ, et al. Obesity and impairment in psychosocial functioning in women: the mediating role of eating disorder features. Obesity 2007;15:2769–79.

167. Petroni ML, Villanova N, Avagnina S, et al.. Psychological distress in morbid obesity in relation to weight history. Obes Surg 2007;17:391–9.

168. Miller CT, Downey KT. A meta-analysis of heavyweight and self-esteem. Person Soc Psychol Rev 1999;3:68–84.

169. Sarwer DB, Wadden TA, Foster GD. Assessment of body image dissatisfaction in obese women: specificity, severity, and clinical significance. J Consult Clin Psychol 1998;66:651–4.

170. Miller PM, Watkins JA, Sargent RG, Rickert EJ. Self-efficacy in overweight individuals with binge eating disorder. Obes Res 1999;7(6):552–5.

171. Cash TF, Winstead BW, Janda LH. The great American shape-up: body image survey report. Psychol Today 1986;20:30–7.

172. Friedman KE, Reichmann SK, Costanzo PR, Musante GJ. Body image partially mediates the relationship between obesity and psychological distress. Obes Res 2002;10:33–41.

173. Rosen JC. Improving body image in obesity. In: Thompson JK (ed) *Body Image, Eating Disorders, and Obesity*. Washington, DC: American Psychological Association, 1996: 425–40.

174. Chen EY. Depressed mood in class III obesity predicted by weight-related stigma. Obes Surg 2007;17:669–71.

175. Friedman KE. Weight stigmatization and ideological beliefs: relation to psychological functioning in obese adults. Obes Res 2005;13:907–16.

176. Jackson TD, Grilo CM, Masheb RM. Teasing history, onset of obesity, current eating disorder psychopathology, body dissatisfaction, and psychological functioning in binge eating disorder. Obes Res 2000;8:451–8.

177. Rosenberger PH, Henderson KE, Bell RL, Grilo CM. Associations of weight-based teasing history and current eating disorder features and psychological functioning in bariatric surgery patients. Obes Surg 2007;17:470–7.

178. Annis NM, Cash TF, Hrabosky JI. Body image and psychosocial differences among stable average weight, currently overweight, and formerly overweight women: the role of stigmatizing experiences. Body Image 2004;1:155–67.

179. Carr D, Friedman MA, Jaffe K. Understanding the relationship between obesity and positive and negative affect: the role of psychosocial mechanisms. Body Image 2007;4:165–77.

180. Puhl RM, Brownell KD. Ways of coping with obesity stigma: conceptual review and analysis. Eating Behav 2003;4:53–78.

181. Puhl RM, Moss-Racusin CA, Schwartz MB. Internalization of weight bias: implications for binge eating and emotional well-being. Obesity 2007;15(1):19–23.

182. Ogden CL, Carroll MD, Curtin LR, McDowell MA, Tabak CJ, Flegal KM. Prevalence of overweight and obesity in the United States, 1999–2004. JAMA 2006;295(13):1549–55.

183. Richardson SA, Goodman N, Hastorf AH, Dornbusch SM. Cultural uniformity in reaction to physical disabilities. Am Sociol Rev 1961:241–7.

184. Latner JD, Stunkard AJ. Getting worse: the stigmatization of obese children. Obes Res 2003;11:452–6.

185. Brylinski JA, Moore JC. The identification of body build stereotypes in young children. J Res Person 1994;28:170–81.

186. Caskey SR, Felker DW. Social stereotyping of female body image by elementary school age girls. Res Q 1971;42:251–5.

187. Kilpatrich SW, Sanders DM. Body image stereotypes: a developmental comparison. J Gen Psychiatr 1978;132:87–95.

188. Lerner RM, Korn SJ. The development of body-build stereotypes in males. Child Dev 1972;43:908–20.

189. Staffieri JR. Body build and behavioral expectancies in young females. Dev Psychol 1972;6:125–7.

190. DeJong W, Kleck RE. The social psychological effects of overweight. In: Herman CP, Zanna MP, Higgins ET (eds) *Physical Appearance, Stigma and Social Behavior: The Ontario Symposium*. Hillsdale, NJ: Lawrence Erlbaum, 1986:65–88.

191. Goldfried A, Chrisler JC. Body stereotyping and stigmatization of obese persons by first graders. Percept Motor Skills 1995; 81:909–10.

192. Greenleaf C, Chambliss HO, Rhea DJ, Martin SB, Morrow JR. Weight stereotypes and behavioral intentions toward thin and fat peers among White and Hispanic adolescents. J Adolesc Health. 2006;39:546–52.

193. Kraig KA, Keel PK. Weight-based stigmatization in children. Int J Obes 2001;25:1661–6.

194. Strauss CC, Smith K, Frame C, Forehand R. Personal and interpersonal characteristics associated with childhood obesity. J Pediatr Psychol 1985;10:337–43.

195. Wardle J, Volz C, Golding C. Social variation in attitudes to obesity in children. Int J Obes 1995;19:562–9.

196. Musher-Eizenman DR, Holub SC, Miller AB, Goldstein SE, Edwards-Leeper L. Body size stigmatization in preschool children: the role of control attributions. J Pediatr Psychol 2004;29:613–20.

197. Griffiths LJ, Wolke D, Page AS, Horwood JP, Team AS. Obesity and bullying: different effects for boys and girls. Arch Dis Child 2006;91:121–5.

198. Hayden-Wade HA, Stein RI, Ghaderi A, Saelens BE, Zabinski MF, Wilfey DE. Prevalence, characteristics, and correlates of teasing experiences among overweight children vs. non-overweight peers. Obes Res 2005;13:1381–92.

199. Janssen I, Craig WM, Boyce WF, Pickett W. Associations between overweight and obesity and bullying behaviors in school-aged children. Pediatrics 2004;113:1187–93.

200. Neumark-Sztainer D, Falkner N, Story M, Perry C, Hannan PJ, Mulert S. Weight-teasing among adolescents: correlations with weight status and disordered eating behaviors. Int J Obes 2002; 26:123–31.

201. Pearce MJ, Boergers J, Prinstein MJ. Adolescent obesity, overt and relational peer victimization, and romantic relationships. Obes Res 2002;10:386–93.

202. Pierce JW, Wardle J. Cause and effect beliefs and self-esteem of overweight children. J Child Psychol Psychiatr All Discip 1997; 38:645–50.

203. Neumark-Sztainer D, Story M, Faibisch L. Perceived stigmatization among overweight African-American and Caucasian adolescent girls. J Adolesc Health 1998;23:264–70.

204. Adams GR, Hicken M, Salehi M. Socialization of the physical attractiveness stereotype: parental expectations and verbal behaviors. Int J Psychol 1988;23:137–49.

205. Davison KK, Birch LL. Predictors of fat stereotypes among 9-year-old girls and their parents. Obes Res 2004;12:86–94.

206. Eisenberg ME, Neumark-Sztainer D, Story M. Associations of weight-based teasing and emotional well-being among adolescents. Arch Pediatr Adolesc Med 2003;157:733–8.

207. Wardle J, Cooke L. The impact of obesity on psychological well-being. Best Pract Res Clin Endocrincol Metab 2005;19:421–44.

208. French SA, Story M, Perry CL. Self-esteem and obesity in children and adolescents: a literature review. Obes Res 1995;3:479–90.

209. Strauss RS, Pollack HA. Social marginalization of overweight children. Arch Pediatr Adolesc Med 2003;157:746–52.

210. Davison KK, Markey CN, Birch LL. A longitudinal examination of patterns in girls' weight concerns and body dissatisfaction from ages 5–9 years. Int J Eating Disord 2003;33:320–32.

211. Ricciardelli LA, McCabe MP. Children's body image concerns and eating disturbance: a review of the literature. Clin Psychol Rev 2001;21:325–44.

212. Davison KK, Birch LL. Processes linking weight status and self-concept among girls from ages 5 to 7 years. Dev Psychol 2002; 38:735–48.

213. Young-Hyman D, Schlundt DG, Herman-Wenderoth L, Bozylinski K. Obesity, appearance, and psychosocial adaptation in young African American children. J Pediatr Psychol 2003;28:463–72.

214. Thompson JK, Coovert MD, Richards KJ, Johnson S, Cattarin J. Development of body image, eating disturbance, and general psychological functioning in female adolescents: covariance structure modeling and longitudinal investigations. Int J Eating Disord 1995;18:221–36.

215. Keery H, Boutelle K, van den Berg P, Thompson JK. The impact of appearance-related teasing by family members. J Adolesc Health 2005;37:120–7.

216. Ackard DM, Neumark-Sztainer D, Story M, Perry C. Overeating among adolescents: prevalence and associations with weight-related characteristics and psychological health. Pediatrics 2003;111: 67–74.

217. Eaton DK, Lowry R, Brener ND, Galuska DA, Crosby AE. Associations of body mass index and perceived weight with suicide ideation and suicide attempts among US high school students. Arch Pediatr Adolesc Med 2005;159:513–19.

218. Falkner N, Neumark-Sztainer D, Story M, Jeffery RW, Beuhring T, Resnick MD. Social, educational, and psychological correlates of weight status in adolescents. Obes Res 2001;9:32–42.

219. Monello LF, Mayer J. Obese adolescent girls: unrecognized "minority" group? Am J Clin Nutr 1963;13:35–49.

220. National Education Association. *Report on Discrimination Due to Physical Size*. Report No. 11. Washington, DC: National Education Association, 1994.

221. Garner DM, Olmsted MP, Polivy J. Development of a multidimensional eating disorder inventory for anorexia nervosa and bulimia. Int J Eating Disord 1983;2:15–34.

222. Fabian LJ, Thompson JK. Body image and eating disturbance in young females. Int J Eating Disord 1989;8:63–74.

223. Kaltiala-Heino R, Rissanen A, Rimpela M, Rantanen P. Bulimia and bulimic behavior in middle adolescence: more common than thought? Acta Psychiatr Scand 1999;100:33–9.

224. Neumark-Sztainer DR, Wall MM, Haines J, Story M, Sherwood NE, van den Berg P. Shared risk and protective factors for overweight and disordered eating in adolescents. Am J Prev Med 2007;33: 359–69.

225. Haines J, Neumark-Sztainer D, Eisenberg ME, Hannan PJ. Weight teasing and disordered eating behaviors in adolescents: longitudinal

findings from Project EAT (Eating Among Teens). Pediatrics 2005;117:209–15.

226. Bell SK, Morgan SN. Children's attitudes and behavioral intentions toward a peer presented as obese: does a medical explanation for the obesity make a difference? J Pediatr Psychol 2000;25:137–45.

227. Teachman BA, Gapinski KD, Brownell KD, Rawlins M, Jeyaram S. Demonstrations of implicit anti-fat bias: the impact of providing causal information and evoking empathy. Health Psychol 2003; 22:68–78.

228. Irving LM. Promoting size-acceptance in elementary school children: the EDAP puppet program. Eating Disord Treat Prev 2000; 8:221–32.

229. Hague AL, White AA. Web-based intervention for changing attitudes of obesity among current and future teachers. J Nutr Educ Behav 2005;37:58–66.

230. Gapinski KD, Schwartz MB, Brownell KD. Can television change anti-fat attitudes and behavior? J Appl Biobehav Res 2006;11: 1–28.

231. Pettigrew TF, Tropp LR. Does intergroup contact reduce prejudice: recent meta-analytic findings. In: Oskamp S (ed) *Reducing Prejudice and Discrimination: The Claremont Symposium on Applied Social Psychology*. Hillsdale, NJ: Lawrence, Erlbaum, 2000:93–114.

232. Stangor C, Sechrist GB, Jost JT. Changing beliefs by providing consensus information. Person Soc Psychol Bull 2001;27:486–96.

233. Anesbury T, Tiggemann M. An attempt to reduce negative stereotyping of obesity in children by changing controllability beliefs. Health Educ Res 2000;15:145–52.

234. Harrison K. Televisions viewing, fat stereotyping, body shape standards, and eating disorder symptomatology in grade school children. Commun Res 2000;27:617–40.

4 Obesity and Culture

Pippa Craig

Indigenous Health Unit, School of Public Health and Community Medicine, University of New South Wales, Sydney, Australia

Obesity has become one of the most discussed topics of our time [1], particularly in recent years. Obesity has also become highly newsworthy with a roughly fivefold increase in media attention since 1992 [2]. The majority of the 750 articles on obesity published in the *New York Times* alone between 1990 and 2001 have appeared since 1998 [3], and reported US news items on obesity grew from 62 articles in 1980 to 6500 in 2004 [4].

This observation is also confirmed by both medical and sociologic databases, although the approaches of these two sources differ. Medical texts focus on prevalence, perceptions, preferences and the consequences, complications and management of obesity. Initially focused on the increasing size of bodies in Westernized societies, more recently the export of obesity to the rapidly developing world has become a concern. The sociologic literature, on the other hand, concentrates primarily on the significance of body size across and within societies and the consequences of the export of Western cultural norms. There has also been a growing interest in the "social body" and the "medicalization" of obesity. These different foci reflect the philosophic divide between the body and mind, and between biologic and social science that has influenced Western thought for several centuries.

Definition of culture

Culture is largely a way of perceiving, feeling, and believing, and consists of a body of learned behaviors which shape ways of thinking and doing from generation to generation [5]. Culture influences both human interactions and expectations. It interacts with biology, and biologic functioning is modified by cultural norms, whether these manifest as products (such as clothing and body ornamentation) or processes (ways of doing or reacting).

Although many aspects of culture are explicit, many are implicit. Each culture is composed of many overlapping subcultures that may be defined on the basis of region, economic status, occupation or subgroup membership [6].

Obesity and culture inter-relate in a nonrandom way [7] and it is this relationship that will be explored in this chapter. An evolutionary perspective on obesity and culture will outline how the cultural environment has shaped the body over time. Various aspects of the surroundings in which humans find themselves influence levels of obesity, and at any point in time obesity prevalence differs between and within social and ethnic groups to an extent that cannot be fully explained by genetic variation. Obesity is largely concentrated in affluent and stratified societies [7] and those undergoing cultural change towards a more Westernized lifestyle commonly demonstrate rapid increases in obesity. The ways in which those in Western societies respond to large bodies is consistent with Western philosophic thought, and thus the cultural context influences ways of thinking and feeling about obesity and being obese.

Culture and obesity over time

Evolution of human culture and obesity
Both food and economy played pivotal roles in the etiology of obesity [7]. The current environment, dominated by abundant variety of readily available food contrasts starkly with one where a society focused attention on acquiring food for survival. The transition from using only what was required from the environment to survive to the present-day prodigious choice has fashioned human body size and shape and human culture.

Anthropologists have used an evolutionary perspective to show how both genetic and cultural predispositions have contributed to the etiology of obesity [8]. Those with a genetic propensity for obesity were selected because they were more likely to survive. Those with the fatter bodies then became the culturally preferred symbol of social prestige and good health [8].

Food was acquired by means of hunting and gathering for most of human history. Cultural evidence from archeologic remains and ethnographic studies of the social organization and cultural

Clinical Obesity in Adults and Children, 3rd edition. Edited by Peter G. Kopelman, Ian D. Caterson and William H. Dietz.
© 2010 Blackwell Publishing, ISBN: 978-1-4051-8226-3.

traditions of the few remaining hunter-gatherers suggest they lived in small semi-nomadic groups, enjoyed high-quality diets, and distributed food equitably within the group [9]. Hunters and gatherers ate a diet based on uncultivated plants and wild game and lived highly active lifestyles. There are neither reported cases of obesity in remaining hunter-gatherer groups [7] nor evidence of obesity from archeology, but as traditional societies adopt a Western lifestyle, whether by migration or acculturation, levels of obesity increase dramatically [10].

Domestication of plants and animals and development of food preservation techniques occurred with the introduction of agriculture approximately 12,000 years ago [11]. Although it is generally believed that hunter-gatherers were frequently hungry while the agriculturalist enjoyed a stable food supply supplemented with stored reserves for times of need, ethnographic and archeologic evidence suggests the contrary [12]. Hunter-gatherers were comparatively healthy and only needed to forage for food every few days whereas ancient agriculturalists and modern peasant villagers lived relatively shorter lives, had higher rates of infant mortality, shorter stature, more infections and higher levels of tooth decay [8,12]. With settlement, food acquisition became less efficient, cereal monoculture reduced food variety, and crop failures in bad seasons led to general food shortages and consequent dietary deficiencies [8,11]. Although it seems surprising that settlement ever took place in these circumstances the impetus for change was cultural; only settlement allowed development of more culturally complex societies [12].

Following the Industrial Revolution, a rapid increase in cultural complexity occurred, allowing the emergence of social stratification. Stratified societies enabled the ruling elites to overcome the succession of "feasts and famines" and ensured access to food at all times. Although today obesity is not just a disease of civilization, it commonly occurs in socially stratified societies that have sufficient affluence and surplus food [7].

It has been proposed that our hunter-gatherer ancestors consumed the diet for which they were originally adapted (high protein, lower fat, limited carbohydrate, with no cereal grains, dairy products or refined foods), and that present chronic disease patterns can be explained by a "discordance" between human genes and modern lifestyle [10,11]. Chronic diseases resulted from an interaction of genetically controlled metabolism and biocultural influences; lifestyle and culture have moved ahead in leaps and bounds from a hunter-gatherer nomadic tradition to a modern way of life, outpacing genetic adaptation [10].

Explorations of the acculturation of food patterns among both Native American and Canadian Arctic populations identified significantly higher intakes of carbohydrate, fat and sucrose in the form of least-cost, low nutrition-density manufactured foods. The tendency to add manufactured foods to traditional staples, rather than displacing staples, triggered the massive increase in obesity [13,14].

Different modernization patterns occurred in other groups undergoing rapid rural-to-urban transitions. Obesity was more prevalent among children and adolescents in urban areas in China but evidenced primarily in rural areas in Russia [15]. In China, higher-income urban populations consumed more fat, sweet foods and animal protein, and reduced carbohydrate and fiber [16]. In all cases the decreased physical activity accompanying modernization contributed to increased obesity rates. The way in which these changes have influenced cultural perceptions and preferences of body size will be discussed in more depth later in this chapter.

Humans have undergone cultural modifications over thousands of years to adapt to the environment in which they found themselves, resulting in vastly different eating and activity patterns and social structures. This adjustment to the environment was culturally driven as human groups explored and found unique ways to survive. Present-day widespread acculturation to a Western lifestyle is the antithesis to this adaptation. Instead, an infinite variety of lifestyles uniquely suited to myriad particular situations have converged towards norms that may not be well suited to the human body.

Evolution of fat storage and fat distribution

The "thrifty genotype" hypothesis proposed 40 years ago in relation to type 2 diabetes was modified by its author to include genes for obesity and hypertension, characterized by their familial nature and slow onset and referred to as "civilization syndromes" [17]. Obesity results from incremental changes over a long period of time, and the complex interplay of genetic and environmental factors. Because there is no evidence for a strong ethnic predisposition for obesity among native populations pursuing a traditional lifestyle, increased prevalence must predominantly reflect lifestyle changes or "cultural engineering" [17].

Accumulation of lower body fat is a human female characteristic that developed because of a need to carry an infant while foraging to meet the energy demands of lactation [11]. Lower body fat is positively related to fertility [18] and a characteristic sign of female beauty in the majority of human societies [8].

All animals favor storage of the more metabolically active but more pathologic upper body fat in optimal conditions [11]. Famines occurred regularly throughout most of human history and storage of excess energy for lean times was essential for survival. Overconsumption in times of plenty became the social norm, with bigness the conspicuous marker of prosperity in societies based on social hierarchy [9,19].

This brief anthropologic and evolutionary perspective on obesity shows how cultural and societal development can explain the increase in obesity over time [8]. Obesity is the consequence of cultural changes occurring more rapidly than genetic adaptation [10]. Plumpness in women, particularly as lower body fat, evolved to ensure survival of the human race and thus became a rational cultural preference supporting a biologic norm. Economic factors were also of etiologic importance with the increasing prevalence of obesity accompanying growing cultural complexity and social stratification. As affluence and abundance became widespread, so did obesity. Within this environment, a uniquely human creation, culture, has been crucial in shaping human bodies.

Culture, obesity and place

It has been estimated that approximately one-half of the contribution to fatness and fat distribution is genetic, but it is the environment that determines whether obesity is realized [11,20–22].

Although environment suggests physical circumstances, it also embraces the social and cultural context in which people live. Numerous social and cultural factors impinge on a whole society and in differing ways on subgroups within that society. Some of these factors may be explicit and measurable, but many are implicit and difficult to quantify. If a perceived normative way of acting and/or reacting is reinforced, it will be strengthened and may gradually become characteristic of the group. Many studies described such norms and beliefs in relation to obesity between and within societies, and there have been many attempts to explain them. One particular area of interest has been how social gradients and Westernization shape obesity prevalence, beliefs, practices and preferences.

Differences between societies
Desirable body size in developed and developing societies
Populations, conceived of as cultural groups, differ in their concept of desirable body size. Obesity may be considered a disease and is socially stigmatized in Western cultures [23], but elsewhere large body size signifies health and beauty [8,24]. These differences relate to the core value system of the particular society, with body sizes and shapes sending powerful cultural messages [25].

The discourse on body size and culture has largely been the province of anthropologists and sociologists. Despite evidence for an impact of socio-economic variables and disease states on body size and shape, body dimensions may also be manipulated to some extent by means of bodily adornments or deliberate action in response to perceived cultural values, ideals or myths [25].

Large body size is still, on the whole, preferred in developing countries [12]. The Human Relation Area Files, founded at Yale University in 1949, is a central dataset of information on 127 cultures studied by ethnographers and historians, now web based [26]. Less than half of those represented in the database include data on characteristics of ideal body type [8,27]. Of these, none preferred extreme obesity, 81% preferred plumpness or moderate fat levels in women, and only 19% preferred thinness [8,27]. For those societies with specific details, peripheral fatness was preferred, in particular large hips and legs [8].

Preference for bigness
Bigness can mean taller, more muscular or fatter, and physical bigness can symbolize abundance, acceptance, power, success or fecundity [12].

Tallness has long been a symbol of power and dominance [24,28]. "Big men" are cultural institutions in New Guinea and West Africa [8]. The majority of US presidents were taller than the average American male at the time they were in office [28]. Australia has had its share of statuesque prime ministers (such as Malcolm Fraser, and Gough Whitlam who measured 193 cm). Despite Napoleon's traditional portrayal as a short man, at 163 cm he was unusually tall for a Corsican and of average height for northern France [28]. Polynesian chiefs were "almost without exception" taller and heavier than their subjects, due to "different treatment in infancy, (and) superior and regular diet" [29].

The few societies registered in the Human Relation Area Files with information on preferred size and shape of men predominantly preferred a muscular physique and moderate to tall stature [8]. There has been a trend towards a more muscular cultural ideal in Western societies over the past 25 years [30–32].

Plumpness is admired in a woman in the context of food scarcity, reflecting well on her male provider [8,28], and signifying the increased likelihood of fertility and reproductive success [18].

Large, even fat, bodies have traditionally been considered a positive attribute in the Pacific [19], although attitudes are undergoing some change with Western influence [33]. Co-operation in the production and distribution of food in Polynesian society was a rational response to an environment constantly under the threat of hurricanes and famines [34]. People ate irregularly and consumed large feasts organized by chiefs to gain prestige and reinforce communal attachment [35]. Now ritual feasting occurs with more regularity and accompanies Sunday church services in predominantly Christian societies.

Nancy Pollock has described traditional Nauruan fattening practices. A young woman of rank was provided with large quantities food and made to rest when experiencing her first menses and during pregnancy. A wide network of relatives was expected to assist in providing food in exchange for reciprocal support. These patterns of reciprocity, and the cultural reverence for plumpness as a symbol of well-being and social pride, served to maintain the society. Ritual fattening was also practiced among Tahitians and Cook Island Maori [19,36].

Examples of preference for fatness in men are rare but do exist. Sumo wrestling in Japan has a 2000-year-old history. With a Body Mass Index (BMI) of around 45 kg/m^2, top-league *sekitori* provide a striking contrast to the slight physique of the average Japanese male [37].

The Massa of West Africa participate in the practice of *guru*, with the purpose of making men plump or obese. *Guru* can take the form of collective fattening where groups of men live with the cattle herd, drink large quantities of milk and are preferentially fed by the villagers, or takes place as individual fattening sessions. The esteemed male body shape is one with a protruding stomach and full figure, with smooth shiny skin [38]. Energy balance studies of nine lean young Massa men found that they gained a mean of 17 kg, 64–75% as fat, in 2 months [39].

Preference for smallness
Most non-Western peoples value large body size, particularly at certain life stages. Slenderness is nonetheless admired by a

number of Southeast Asian, South Asian and North African societies where austerity, self-denial and control of appetite form part of the moral tradition for women [24], possibly as a cultural response to chronic food shortages. The Gurage of Ethiopia were expected to eat in moderation to preserve supplies although gorging at festivals was accepted and expected. Constant overeating was considered a measure of bad upbringing [24].

Western cultures prefer slimness but not necessarily small stature in women, requiring a lengthening and narrowing of the female body. While lengthening is consistent with secular trends, narrowing is more problematic. Weight concerns and dieting behaviors in young Canadian university students were influenced more by the deviation of their skeletal structure (frame size measured with bone calipers) from the ideal than by their degree of adiposity (measured with skinfolds) [40].

Cultural predictors of ideal female body shape

Anderson and colleagues [27] conducted a detailed analysis of the 62 cultures for which information on female preferred body shape was available in the Human Relations Area Files, testing a number of existing hypotheses which were developed to explain differing cross-cultural ideals of female body size and shape. Attitudes towards fatness related to the reliability of the food supply, climate, the relative social dominance of women, the value placed on women's work, and likely consequences of the expression of female adolescent sexuality. Cultural groups preferring plump women were located in colder climates, were male dominated, experiencing food insecurity, had low adolescent stress and expected women's role to be predominantly in reproduction and homemaking [27].

Differences within societies
Social factors and obesity

The Midtown Manhattan Study first raised the profile of social factors and obesity [41]. This study found that the prevalence of obesity fell as socio-economic status (SES) rose and with increasing length of time a migrant family had been in the US, particularly among women. Upwardly mobile females were less obese than those who moved in the opposite direction. Trends, although similar for men, were less marked [41]. These trends were confirmed by a longitudinal study of British women [42].

Using social networks of over 12,000 people from the Framingham Heart Study, Christakis and Fowler illustrated how social connections can explain individual weight gain in relation to the weight gain in others. This obesity influence reached a distance of three degrees of social separation. Geographic separation did not have the same effect, suggesting that local environmental factors were less explanatory than social factors [43]. The effect occurred irrespective of educational level [44].

Major reviews of socio-economic status and obesity in 1989 and 2007 confirmed the strong inverse relationship between obesity and socio-economic status in women from developed societies but found the opposite in developing countries [45,46], in particular when education was used as an indicator of social class [42]. The relationship was the same for men as for women in least developed countries, with the indicators of income and occupation both positively associated with obesity [46]. The direct relationship between obesity and socio-economic status in developing societies was attributed to lower dietary intake and higher energy output among those of low status. The association between socio-economic status and obesity in men in developed societies was inconsistent or nonsignificant [45,46].

The unique relationship of socio-economic status and obesity among women in developed societies has been attributed to greater pressure to comply with the cultural norms of thinness and more opportunities to exercise, eat well and invest in appearance by higher status women [42,45–47]. A positive relationship between socio-economic position and height may also contribute to lower BMI. Those in the highest social class were taller, and the upwardly mobile were taller than those in the class they had left [48,49]. US research suggests that ethnicity may explain some of the inconsistencies in men. Although a reverse association between socio-economic status and obesity was found in Caucasian men, the relationship was positive in African and Mexican Americans [50].

Obesity and poverty

Social and cultural factors play a significant role in the relationship between obesity and poverty, particularly among women. Although extreme poverty is associated with undernutrition, the pattern of obesity common in developed countries is gradually spreading to those countries experiencing demographic and epidemiologic transition, such as Latin America and the Caribbean, particularly in urban areas [51,52]. A significant trend for higher rates of obesity with increasing deprivation among children has been reported in southern England [53]. In the US, the prevalence of overweight was higher among families with incomes below, compared with those above the poverty threshold, although this relationship was mediated by ethnicity [54].

During transition, obesity prevalence increases among lower socio-economic segments of the population as GNP increases. This occurs earlier among women than among men, and is still kept somewhat in check by overall food shortages, the greater ability of those with higher SES to acquire food, and cultural preferences for large body sizes [55]. Urbanization resulted in reduced physical activity and increased consumption of an energy-dense diet as food became more available and inappropriate aspects of the Western lifestyle were adopted [51,52,56]. Women were home based and engaged in limited physical activity whereas men are more likely to work outside the home and participate in sporting activities [57]. Purchasing energy-dense fatty meats and processed carbohydrates that "fill" but may not "nourish" in preference to less energy dense foods, was a cost-effective way of providing food energy on a limited budget [57–59]. Among the poorest in Argentina, processed, mass-produced, energy-dense foods with high fat and sugar content and "Western" appeal were targeted towards those with low purchasing power [57]. The poor faced a conflict between their capacity to provide and the ideal cultural images with which they were constantly bombarded, as these were beyond their means [60].

The poor woman needs a strong body to work, to nurture others or just to survive [57,61,62]. It was not acceptable for overweight disadvantaged African women from Cape Town, familiar with food insecurity, to voluntarily regulate intake when food was available. For these women, weight gain reflected marital harmony and well-being, and plump children indicated that they had sufficient food to eat [63]. Mothers of overweight low-income preschool children from Cincinnati, Ohio, described their children as "solid" or "big boned," attributing their size to familial predisposition [64]. Having a child with a good appetite was their highest priority; only when obesity resulted in inactivity or low self-esteem did it warrant attention. On the other hand, women of high SES voluntarily restrict their food intake; the body of the upper-income woman is valued for its slimness, and higher income allows access to resources for obesity prevention [47,61].

Childhood obesity may vary significantly across countries with different levels of socio-economic development. In Russia, low- and high-income adolescents (as opposed to those in the middle-income range), particularly in rural areas were at increased risk of obesity; in China, high-income, urban children and adolescents were more at risk [15]. Not only does this suggest the importance of considering socio-economic factors, but also that different ethnic groups may respond differently to interventions targeting obesity [50].

Ethnic differences

Numerous studies have shown that perceptions and preferences of body size differ between ethnic groups. These studies confirmed slim cultural preference, widespread body size dissatisfaction, and likelihood for body size overestimation among Caucasians compared with African-Americans, Caribbeans, Hispanics, First Nation Canadians, South Asians, Ugandan Africans and Polynesians [33,65–73]. In the few instances where no ethnic differences were found, comparisons were made between groups within the same country and perceptions and preferences may have been influenced by the cultural values of the adopted home [74,75]. Oriental Asian females were reported to prefer smaller body sizes [71,76], while males preferred larger sizes than did Caucasians [76].

Views and expectations of children's body sizes reflected those of adults. African-American children were reported to have different attitudes about weight, body size and attractiveness and to accept larger body proportions than Caucasian-Americans [74,77]. Young migrants readily adopted a preoccupation with dieting and other weight-related concerns. Despite being lighter, British South Asian girls reported similar dieting levels to British Caucasian girls [78].

The process of Westernization

Hispanic immigrants' length of stay in the US was associated with increasing levels of obesity, even after statistical adjustment for socio-economic and demographic characteristics, smoking and health status, differential access to health services and psychologic well-being [79]. However, Mexican women migrants weighed less and men weighed more as they advanced up the social strata, reflecting their adopted culture. This resulted in a complete reversal of the body size norms in Mexico (where women weighed more than men). The changed association of SES with weight could not be explained by biologic and genetic means, but only by social and cultural changes [80].

A number of large studies indicated some influence of cultural norms and environment on body size. Differences between African-American and Caucasian-American women, men and children from the US National Health Examination and National Health and Nutrition surveys (NHANES) suggested that there may be cultural set points and norms of acceptable body size determined by ethnicity, gender, age and SES [54,81]. An exploration of the association between neighborhood context and BMI confirmed that the strength and patterns varied with ethnicity, particularly for females. These differences may relate to opportunities for exercising and access to "healthy" foods, but also to reinforced social norms of body size resulting from the concentration of people from the same ethnic group within a neighborhood [82]. Hodge and Zimmet [83] attributed their observations, that ethnicity and poverty were independent predictors of obesity in women in the USA and Australia, to different attitudes towards obesity. Both ethnicity and SES were shown to predict obesity in Caucasian and African-Americans [84].

Although Polynesians prefer larger body sizes than Caucasians [33,68,85], these preferences change with increasing Westernization [33]. The invasiveness of Western social and cultural influences on body size has been confirmed by comparing similar subjects in different settings. Western Samoan women living in New Zealand [85], South Asians from Kenya and India living in Britain [65] and more acculturated First Nation [69] and Inuit Canadians [86] preferred smaller female body sizes than did those remaining at home.

An examination of Samoan populations at differing stages of Westernization showed sex-specific interactions between modernity and obesity. Traditionally, men and women had clearly defined roles with men being more physically active. Men were the first to become wage earners, often engaging in relatively labor-intensive work which provided some compensation for their changed diet. With increasing Western influence, they moved into occupations with reduced energy expenditure and gained weight. The activity level of women was reduced as they took up lower activity employment. As a consequence of the traditional division of labor, women were likely to develop obesity earlier in the modernization process than men [87].

Thus, accepted cultural norms can shape both the perceptions and preferences of body size and ultimately actual body size within cultural groups and subgroups. There is also convincing evidence that Westernization changes these cultural norms towards the norm of slimness, particularly in women.

Culture and obesity in Western societies
The changing cultural context and emergence of the slim ideal

Significant changes occurred in the perception of the ideal woman in Western culture and in cultural reactions to body fatness during the 20th century. Slimness became a virtue in the 1920s and received increasing emphasis from the 1950s onwards. A frequently cited study by Garner and colleagues provided evidence of the acceptance of gradually diminishing female dimensions between 1959 and 1978, documented by Miss America pageant winners and *Playboy* centerfolds [88]. Follow-up studies confirmed the continued trend over subsequent years [89–92]. The changes in preferred body size and shape for Western women between 1959 and 2001 are summarized in Table 4.1.

As the socially approved Western feminine figure became more and more cylindrical, female peripheral fatness, the naturally occurring component of female bodies favored in the majority of traditional societies, became increasingly disparaged. Women are expected to remain sexual (but not too sexual), to reproduce and nurture (but not overnurture themselves), and to succeed in a masculine world [93]. The ideal became increasingly distant from the average, resulting in wide dissatisfaction among Western women [94]. It is considered "normal" for women to be vigilant about their weight, with chronic dietary restraint an accepted way of life [93,95]. Dieting is widespread among adolescents, and girls learn from an early age that they will be judged by their appearance. The widely quoted aphorism "A woman can never be too rich or too thin," attributed to Wallis Simpson, typifies Western culture [95]. The female body is socially constructed as an object, and slimness has become so internalized as to appear natural [93]. Fat people are seen as morally bad and held responsible for their condition [96]. Women themselves perpetuate the system

Table 4.1 Changes in preferred body size and shape for Western women 1959–2001

Year	Playboy centerfolds			Miss America pageant contestants		Fashion models	
	1959–78[1]	1979–88[2]	1953–2001[3]	1959–78[1]	1979–88[2]	1967–87[4]	1997[5]
Number	240	120	577	–	–	256	300
Weight change	No change	No change	No change	Decreased $r = -0.83$ ($p < 0.001$)	Decreased $r = -0.77$ ($p < 0.01$)	–	–
Height	Mean = 1.66 m	–	–	–	–	–	Mean = 1.77 m
Height change	Increased $r = 0.22$ ($p < 0.01$)	–	Increased $r = 0.36$ ($p < 0.001$)	–	–	Increased $F = 17.02$ ($p < 0.001$)	–
Wgt/hgt change	Decreased $r = -0.22$ ($p < 0.001$)	–	–	–	–	–	–
BMI change	–	–	Decreased $r = -0.46$ ($p < 0.001$)	–	Decreased $r = -0.46$ ($p < 0.001$)	–	–
Waist change	Increased $r = 0.41$ ($p < 0.001$)	–	Increased $r = 0.27$ ($p < 0.001$)	–	–	Increased $F = 3.36$ ($p < 0.002$)	–
Hips change	Decreased $r = -0.12$ ($p < 0.05$)	–	Decreased $r = -0.29$ ($p < 0.001$)	–	Decreased $r = -0.87$ ($p = 0.01$)	No change	–
Population mean	Mean weight gain = 0.14 kg/year	–	–	Subjects differed from pop mean $r = 6.20$ ($p < 0.001$)	–	–	Mean hgt = 1.66 m Mean BMI = 21.9 kg/m^2
Compared with population mean	–	69% subjects had weight >15% below pop. wgt/hgt	–	87.6% of pop. mean (pre 1970); 84.6% of mean (post 1970)	60% subjects had weight >15% below pop. wgt/hgt	–	–

Sources: [1]Garner et al 1980 [88]; [2]Wiseman et al. 1992 [90]; [3]Voracek and Fisher 2002 [92]; [4]Morris et al. 1989 [89]; [5]Tovee et al. 1997 [91].
r, correlation between measured anthropometric values with time; F, change in measured anthropometric values over time.

by condemning their overweight peers [95,97]. Characteristics of this moral paradigm of obesity are summarized in the first column of Table 4.3.

The Western media have had a significant role in promoting images of women's bodies as "objects," with consequent increasing anxiety among women unable to attain a virtually impossible ideal. Historically, media images of men have presented the "body as process," valuing the ability of the male body to perform. Striving towards this cultural standard has generally had a positive effect on self-attitude of men [98]. More recently, there has been a trend towards media portrayal of male bodies for their physical attractiveness ("body as object") [99,100]. Furthermore,

the ideal male body being marketed to men in men's magazines is more muscular than male images presented in women's magazines [31]. Studies of *Playgirl* centerfolds [30], the portrayal of men in *Men's Health*, *Men's Fitness* and *Muscle & Fitness* [31], and the disproportionate leanness and muscularity of current action figures compared with their counterparts produced 25 years ago [32] all showed that men's bodies were becoming more muscular (Table 4.2). In the past, boys have been less concerned with body image than girls, but increasing levels of dissatisfaction are now being reported [77,101–103], with increasing danger of at-risk behaviors [99].

Table 4.2 Changes in preferred body size and shape for Western men 1964–2005

| Year | Playgirl centerfolds | Action toys[a] | | | Magazine images | |
	1973–97[1]	1973–94[2,b]	1964–2004[3,c]	1973/80–2004[3]	2006[4,d]	1975–2005[5,e]
Number	115	–	–	–	–	–
Height	–	1.78 m	1.78 m	1.78 m	–	–
Chest change	–	Little change	Unchanged 44.4 to 43.2 cm	Increased $t(4) = 5.15$ $p = 0.007$	–	–
Biceps change	–	Increased	Increased 12.2 to 16.4 cm	Increased $t(4) = 3.49$ $p = 0.025$	–	–
Waist change	–	Unchanged	Decreased 31.7 to 29.2 cm	Unchanged $t(4) = 1.66$ $p = 0.173$	–	–
BMI change	Increased $r = 0.29$ $(p < 0.01)$	–	–	–	–	–
Body fat change	Decreased $r = -0.34$ $(p < 0.01)$	–	–	–	–	Decreased $(p < 0.05)$
Muscularity change	Increased $r = 0.38$ $(p < 0.01)$	–	–	–	Increased as male audience increased $(p < 0.001)$	Increased $(p < 0.05)$
Fat-free mass index (FFMI)	8/115 had FFMI >25	–	–	–	–	–
Population mean	Mean FFMI = 20	–	Australian soccer players: Waist = 29.6 cm Chest = 36.3 cm Biceps = 11.8 cm Hgt = 170.2 cm	–	–	–

Sources: [1]Leit et al. 2001 [30]; [2]Pope et al. 1999 [153]; [3]Baghurst et al. 2006 [32]; [4]Frederick et al. 2005 [31]; [5]Farquhar and Wasylkiw 2007 [99].
Footnotes:
[a]Action toys adjusted up to the height of a 1.78 cm human male.
[b]Selection of action toys include GI Joe, Star Wars and Star Trek characters, Superman, Spiderman, and Batman.
[c]Comparing original GI Joe to current GI Joe.
[d]Images arranged in order of increasing male audience (*Cosmopolitan*, *Men's Health*, *Men's Fitness*, and *Muscle & Fitness*).
[e]Images in *Sports Illustrated*.
r, correlation between measured anthropometric values with time; t, t-test between original and current measurements.

The social/biologic body divide

Medicine and the biologic sciences understand the physical body independently from the social body (the mind and emotions), which belongs to the social sciences. Bryan Turner attributed this division and the dichotomies of nature–culture or body–mind to the philosophy of Descartes [104]. It was not until the second half of the 20th century that social scientists began to consider social aspects of the body, recognizing that the perceived opposition between nature and culture was a product of Western thought and rejecting the conception of the body as a purely natural phenomenon. Instead, society exerts regulation or control over the body, and the way the body is presented by an individual. This can signify belonging to, or alternatively rejection by, a particular society or cultural group. When considered as a social entity, the body is not seen as stable, universal and comparable regardless of its setting, but as culturally contextualized [105,106].

Control and surveillance of the body

In his exploration of dieting, Turner [104] draws a parallel between the strong morality of religious constraint and the medical dietary regimen; both focus on disciplining the body. Abstemiousness is consistent with the biologic basis of the civilized society, as is the metaphor of the body as a machine that can be controlled and repaired [107]. Modern medical dieting probably began in the 17th century with Cheyne, a Scottish doctor who attributed all major illnesses to eating habits. Excessively obese himself, he succeeded in trimming his own size and then proposed a system of dietary management for the London elite as a remedy for the diseases of civilization [104].

The French philosopher Foucault has profoundly influenced anthropologic representations of the body, particularly the concept of surveillance over that which is institutionalized within a culture [105]. This concept of surveillance and control is an important one in Western societies and has been applied to the preoccupation of American females with dieting and slimness [106,108]. Although efforts to control body size taken out of context appear to be both an ideology and paradox, they can be understood as part of Western culture characterized by a continuous cycling of control and release (Puritanism and hedonism). The body becomes both the object of punishment and the site of pleasure, the Protestant ethic espousing hard work and control (self-control, dietary restraint, regular exercise) and in turn permitting reward or indulgence (such as sweet or fatty foods). The individual is called upon to balance these oppositions to maintain a culturally acceptable weight, creating yet another dichotomy between the forces of good (slimness) and evil (fatness) [108].

The supportive cultural context for the slim ideal

The pursuit of slimness by dietary restraint tempered by indulgence is a culturally acceptable way of thinking and behaving in Western societies. It is sustained because it is consistent with and reinforced by norms, values and interests within the wider cultural context. Although it is claimed that Western culture today places undue emphasis on the esthetics of the human body [109], every culture has a concept of what is beautiful. What is unprecedented is the persistent diminution of the ideal female body, concurrent with relentless expansion of the actual body.

Crandall and colleagues applied a prejudice model to current attitudes about obesity across samples from six countries. They showed that anti-fat prejudice occurred towards those who possessed the negative attribute (fatness) for which they were held responsible. These two attributes worked together to produce a particularly virulent form of prejudice in individualistic countries (such as the USA, Australia and Poland), whereas in collectivist countries (represented by India, Turkey and Venezuela) fat individuals were considered less responsible for their condition [110].

These norms and values are reinforced by many vested interests in the "business of thinness." The corporate dieting industry, the fitness industry, manufacturers of diet products, women's fashion and cosmetics, women's beauty magazines and cosmetic surgeons all benefit financially from perpetuation of a slim ideology [95]. The majority of those purchasing weight loss products and attending weight loss centers are women, further reinforcing their concern with weight. Preference for thinness in women has also been related to the value placed on youth and the greater participation of women in the workforce, which coincided with lower acceptance of the more rounded maternal image preferred in the past.

Present understanding of and approaches towards obesity and eating disorders are socially constructed and reflect the shared values, beliefs and practices of Western culture. Conceptualizing slimness as control over one's body and the converse, obesity, as lack of control, fits well with modern Western perceptions of control and release [108] and religio-moral management of the body [111]. These shared meanings of obesity are that it is a serious health problem and costly in both economic and personal terms; self-induced and amenable to change by personal sacrifice.

Cultural influences on medical definitions of obesity

The downward trend in recommended weight for women in the USA demonstrated the influence of the culturally defined desire for thinness on the medical definition of obesity. Recommended female weight declined steadily through various revisions of recommended weight/height tables between 1943 and 1980. At the same time evidence was mounting for larger body size as a health risk for young and middle-aged adults, particularly men, but not necessarily women [112]. More recently, the downward trend has applied to male recommended body size.

Defining the limits of obesity remains controversial. Studies have repeatedly illustrated that many perceive "normal" weight as the socially desirable ideal, well below medically recommended normal weight. Achieving this "normal" level is unlikely and may be unnecessary, given the health benefits of moderate weight reduction in the obese [96]. The reduction of the cut-off point for "ideal" healthy weight ranges from 27 to 25 kg/m^2 in 1994

[113] increased the number of overweight and obese people in the USA by 29 million [114], and dramatically raised the profile of obesity as a cause for concern. Application of an international uniform standard for healthy weight ranges to the global diversity of body types has been questioned from both the slight and the more robust extremes of the body size spectrum [115,116].

The medicalization of obesity

"Medicalization" is the process of reclassifying "badness" to "sickness" that thrives in a cultural context where religious faith has declined, and faith in science and preferences for individual and technologic solutions has increased [117]. The medicalization of obesity during the 20th century has been investigated by a number of social scientists. Despite much evidence that obesity is a major health problem, there has been some selective use or misrepresentation of scientific data supporting the risks of obesity at the expense of data portraying less clear evidence of risk [118–121]. Underutilized data show the negative consequences of dieting, the failure of restrictive dieting to produce long-term weight loss, the psychologic toll of weight regain, and the potential health risks of weight fluctuation. The economic costs of obesity have been well publicized, but seldom the cost of the pursuit of thinness. The importance of changing other risk factors, and the role of genetics and biology in determining body weight, are not part of the core beliefs surrounding cultural knowledge about obesity. The confounding effect of fitness and impact of social factors on health has been downplayed. The stigma of being obese is firmly placed among the cultural values in Western societies and multifarious perceptions of obesity do not fit well with these values [118,120,121]. There is evidence for perceived and actual size discrimination and pressure to conform resulting in disordered eating patterns and low self-esteem, particularly among adolescents [121–123].

Although obesity has been claimed as unhealthy for centuries, the medicalization of obesity really began in the 1950s. It occurred slowly at first as the concept changed within the medical framework, growing dramatically during the 1960s and 1970s [96]. Obesity became classified as a disease in the *International Classification of Diseases* in 1990 [96]. Chang and Christakis documented these developments through their analysis of entries in *Cecil's Textbook of Medicine* between 1927 and 2000 [124]. During this time, obesity was transformed from a moral deviance and the responsibility of the fat individual to a disease with reduced individual responsibility, thus providing a rationale for therapeutic intervention (see Table 4.3, column 2, for characteristics of the medical paradigm of obesity). As a consequence, the importance of structural conditions (sociocultural, environmental and material context) was diminished and individual factors (lifestyle, personal behavior) became the focus of explanation, diagnosis and intervention. Even the mass public health campaigns promoting healthy lifestyles in the 1970s and 1980s directed action towards changes in individual behavior, minimizing the significance of the broader sociocultural and environmental constraints [124,125]. The so-called self-help weight loss organizations were established by nonmedical groups but many applied a medical model that legitimized the need for external assistance to achieve weight loss [96].

Within the wider society, the moral overtones surrounding obesity remain, with obese people still considered largely responsible for their own condition. Even the health care community is not immune; health professionals specializing in obesity surveyed at an international conference exhibited a significant pro-thin, anti-fat implicit bias [126]. Technologic or psychobehavioral interventions by medical or health professionals engaged only a small proportion of the obese population in the developed world [96] and even fewer in societies undergoing rapid transition.

In the last decade, a different theoretical has paradigm emerged which acknowledges the importance of the environment in promoting and perpetuating obesity [127–129]. Certain food producers have always enjoyed subsidies or protection from governments, an action directly affecting the availability of foods for purchase. Human bodies of increasing size in Western societies can be considered as products of an environment of "fattening food systems" which consist of increasingly available and affordable energy-dense food in easily acquired forms [130,131].

The cultural and social context for medicalized obesity

The medicalization of obesity involved the conceptual transfer of perceived control and supervision of solutions to the biomedical model. This change neither necessarily nor solely depended on actions of medical personnel, but was facilitated by compatibility with other cultural norms and activities within the wider society [124,132].

The ideology of systems of surveillance and control focused on the body [132]. Subordination of desire to reason, religious moral authority transferred to secular institutions such as the medical profession, and wide-scale dieting were all concordant with the capitalist ideology so central to 20th-century Western societies [124]. At the same time, there was a growing tendency towards measuring and categorizing, whether by insurance companies, physical anthropologists, anthropometrists, elite sporting bodies or scientific researchers.

Powerful groups benefit from obesity as a medical problem, the most obvious being the healthcare, pharmaceutical and fitness industries. More broadly, medicalization increased dependence on other industries producing various consumer goods compatible with this form of social control and associated with individualized treatment of obesity. Medicalized obesity thus forms a part of the wider system of disciplinary techniques, or the "technologies of power," that regulated and normalized the population [132].

Within the wider Western cultural context, there are a multitude of subcultures whose perception of their own risks associated with obesity is bound up with their cultural beliefs, moral values and life circumstances [132]. At one end of the socioeconomic continuum the perceived risk of obesity may be relative to the standard of a slim trim body and addressed by joining a

Table 4.3 The four paradigms of obesity

Paradigm characteristics	Moral	Medical	Sociopolitical	Globopolitical
Paradigm reach	Wide	Medium	Small and select	Global
Perception of body fat	Bad, sinful, ugly	Promotes illness	A fact	Present in epidemic proportions
Perception of fat person	Weak	Have an illness beyond their	Member of society	Disdain
	Lacks willpower	control		Discrimination
Relationship with society	Burden on society	Society a source of harm (e.g. excess calories)	Confrontational	Affliction of the century
Responsibility for fat condition	Personal blame	An illness	None	Maladaption
		Neutral but not value free		All are at risk
Language	Fat, corpulent, plump	Obese, adipose, overweight	Large, ample, of size	Fat, socially/sexually unattractive (female)
				Slob, "fat bastard" (male)
Eating	Gluttony, gorging	Acoria, polyphagia, hyperorexia	A pleasurable social activity	Vigilance required
				All are at risk
Activity	Sloth, laziness	Lethargy, listlessness	Neutral	Sedentary
Reaction to fat person	Stigmatization	Stigma of sickness and disability	Accept large people as	Mortality risk
	Discrimination	Dependent on medical expertise	normal	Drain on health budget
	Distain			
Legitimizing experts	Religious or traditional	Scientific or clinical	Selected scientists and social scientists	Medical and other clinical obesity specialists
Organizations/industries supporting paradigm	Fashion, cosmetic	Healthcare	Selected magazines, books	Medical and other clinical obesity specialists
	Weight loss	Pharmaceutical	Specialized fashions	
	Sport, activity	Weight loss		Pharmaceutical
		Sport, activity		Weight loss
				Fashion, cosmetic
				Media
Solution focus	Fat person's willpower and determination	Treatment with medical supervision	Change society's attitudes Fat liberation	Preventive focus, especially for children Realistic expectations

Sources: Sobal 1995, 1999 [96,134]; Chang and Christakis 2002 [124]; Kersh and Morone 2002 [146]; Campos et al. 2006 [4]; Orbach 2006 [154]; Boero 2007 [3].

fitness club, attending a health farm or hiring a personal trainer. In contrast, the primary concern of poor mothers from Ohio and Cape Town may be a child with a good appetite and their own ability to provide a regular supply of food and an occasional treat [64], while those in Argentina select energy-dense foods as a cost-effective way of filling their family's stomachs [57].

Thus the pursuit of the thin ideal woman and the change in the meaning of obesity from a moral to a medical issue has been consistent with a number of Western cultural norms and values, supported by many powerful interests. At the same time, there is evidence that more males than females in the USA and Australia have body sizes above the medically accepted normal weight range, and many women who diet are within the medically acceptable weight range [97,133].

Obesity as a social and cultural issue

The medicalized approach, with its associated reduction in individual moral responsibility and increased dependence on individualized therapeutic action [124], cannot address the burgeoning epidemic of obesity alone. Furthermore, the social science discourses on the body presented here have demonstrated how the Western context strives to maintain a culturally defined ideal body and systems for its monitoring, measurement and control. But change is possible, and some changes have occurred. These newer paradigms include resistance to the restrictive nature of ideal body size, a shift towards a self-care model of body maintenance, and an orientation to the social and environmental causes of obesity, and the concept of the "obesity epidemic".

Resistance to the normalizing process

Crandall and colleagues recommend two changes to address anti-fat prejudice: a change in the cultural norm to a larger, or at least more liberal, ideal body size; and a reduction in attributing personal responsibility for body size [110]. While there have been attempts to liberalize the cultural norm, this chapter has argued that individual blame remains a particularly robust value in Western societies.

The size acceptance movement developed in reaction to intolerance of fat people, dissatisfaction with the cultural emphasis on thinness and widespread promotion of dieting as a solution to the problem of obesity, and aimed to promote size diversity and tolerance in a size-neutral society [134]. The US National Association to Advance Fat Acceptance (NAAFA), which commenced in 1969, is the original and largest size acceptance organization. Similar groups exist in Canada, Britain, Australia, Israel, Iceland and Sweden [97,134]. NAAFA sees obesity as a political problem rather than a moral or medical one, and emphasizes the possible psychologic harms of dieting over medical claims of the health risk [96] (see the third column in Table 4.3 for this paradigm). Rather than considering themselves victims, members accept their size and learn to respond to the pressure to conform to the slim ideal [97]. Despite the Big Man's Special Interest Group, membership of NAAFA is small, mostly female, and largely from upper socio-economic groups. Another group, the Health at Every Size movement, includes membership from the health promotion field who are focusing on becoming fit and healthy rather than on weight [97].

Some changes are occurring in the fashion industry. The UK established a Model Health Inquiry [135] and Spain banned models whose BMI fell below 18 from Madrid's 2006 Fashion Week. Other countries, however, have proved less eager to follow these examples [136]. The size of mannequins, at "six inches (15 cm) taller and six sizes smaller than the average American woman," continues to perpetuate unrealistic ideals [137].

The increased use of the internet, with pro-anorexia websites and direct advertising to consumers, serves both as a resistance to medicalization and a means of perpetuating the norm of slimness as a desirable goal [117]. The 2006 winner of the UK's "Make Me a Supermodel" (at size 12, 177 cm and 70 kg), was criticized for being too fat [138].

Body maintenance, health and fitness

Health promotion and fitness focusing on body maintenance has become increasingly important in Western culture [107]. Simultaneous changes have taken place in the relationship between modern medicine and the public, a growing scepticism about the limits of medicinal capabilities, and a movement towards self-care [132]. Although the obsession with "keeping to a diet" has diminished, the change is a conceptual one and involves a transfer from an externally defined and imposed diet regimen to self-regulation and self-monitoring of healthy eating [139]. The health promotion and fitness movement still adheres to the "control and release" metaphor and the imperatives of production and consumption; disciplinary power has moved from institutionalized surveillance to "technologies of self" [140]. Obese people are still held responsible for their body status, but the fitness, health food, weight loss and beauty industries are there to assist them in their endeavors to achieve culturally acceptable bodies.

A renewed social and environmental orientation on obesity

At the same time there has been growing attention to the role played by the environment. A wide variety of readily available, energy-enhanced foods exploit the human predilection for sweet and fatty flavors. Nutrient-dense low-energy foods remain comparatively expensive, and consumption of relatively cheap fast foods is increasing. Human food consumption behavior has been shown to respond to environmental stimuli, such as occasion to eat and portion size, rather than adjusting to maintain a constant weight [141]. More labor-saving devices, fewer manual jobs, increasing use of motor vehicles, poor town planning, the perceived danger surrounding outside activity, and appealing technologic entertainment have all encouraged sedentary behavior [7,129].

The sheer weight provided by the increasing proportion and number of obese people in Western societies has tipped the scales towards greater consideration of the structural aspects of obesity [124,127,128]. Obesity results from the accumulation of small incremental weight gains and is a normal response to an abnormal environment [7,17,127,128]. This new perspective goes beyond interpreting obesity simply as the moral concern of the individual failing to measure up to the cultural ideal, or a medical condition corrected by individual lifestyle change, but envisages environmental causes which suggest a reorientation to address obesity [124].

Sociocultural implications of the obesity epidemic

Morbid obesity continues to increase, as does the collective weight of those in Western countries and progressively, those in countries undergoing transition. In response, the social sciences are paying growing attention to the "obesity crisis" [2–4].

This increased attention has both coincided with and suggested a new paradigm for addressing obesity. At the same time, the increasing concern has raised more fundamental questions about how best to respond to the "obesity epidemic." These sociologic explorations of how the obesity epidemic is being presented may offer some useful insights. (The obesity epidemic paradigm is summarized in column 4 of Table 4.3.)

The explosion in attention paid to obesity, both by the media and via the internet, has assisted in transmitting medical and scientific knowledge, and helped to promote the concept of an obesity epidemic [3,121]. Despite dependence on the biomedical narrative, some have argued that the increase in attention does not necessarily reflect an increase of substantive evidence and the strength of the relationships between health, body size and weight may be less clear-cut than suggested [4,121]. In addition, the media have often presented the obesity epidemic in an oversimplified way [120], with a relatively simple message that counsels weight loss by consuming less (in the context of abundance) and exercising more (in the context of increased use of labor-saving and technologic devices and entertainment).

These presentations are not value free and add to the discriminatory perception of the place of the obese in the society. A continued focus on weight fuels concerns about the body [100,121] and media representations contribute to the perception of who is and who is not acceptable [102,121,123]. Anti-fat feeling is primarily driven by "social fitness" rather than health and fitness [120] and, if anything, has increased person anxiety. Although weight loss maintenance has improved in the medium term [142], reported success rates after 5 or more years continue to be in the order of 15–20% [143,144], and repeated weight loss attempts may engender unhealthy relationships with food [145].

The element of "moral panic" engendered by the obesity epidemic is associated more with the concept of beauty than with health [131]; it remains socially acceptable to show prejudice towards obese people [130]. The reality television program *The Biggest Loser* features obese contestants in a weight loss competition and is the embodiment of the stigmatization of obesity in Western societies. The series began in the USA in 2004 and is now screened in nine other countries.

A new approach

Nevertheless there is growing recognition that addressing the obesity epidemic requires some political response in addition to changes in food consumption and activity levels. Kersh and Morone identified a number of triggers that traditionally occur when personal health issues become of sufficient concern to warrant political action, assess whether society is yet sufficiently ready for political mobilization against obesity. These triggers included social disapproval, medicalization of the condition, the presence of self-help organizations, demonization of both those with the condition and of an industry "peddling poison" to the human race, and the development of a groundswell of public opinion demanding action, with involvement by advocacy groups formulating the issues and outlining policy solutions [146]. Considerable evidence is available for the first four of these conditions, all of which have been discussed in this chapter. There is also a good deal of evidence of targeted attacks on fast food exemplified by popular literature such as Eric Schlosser's *Fast Food Nation* [147]; and the concepts of a "toxic food environment" [125] promulgated by a demon industry from which the public requires protection [121]. However the multinational food industry remains a significant stakeholder with powerful lobbyists well integrated into the current political system, and a difficult target unless some evidence emerges of deliberate deception of the public about the health effects of their products [2].

Thus the debate as to whether the obesity epidemic requires a political or a personal solution remains somewhat equivocal. Despite an increased interpretation of obesity in terms of the social environment, ingrained cultural norms of individual responsibility are difficult to eradicate and cultural and individual explanations and solutions are still repeatedly applied [2,3].

The media's portrayal of obesity has been summarized as "problematic bodies, problematic individuals and problematic populations," in which obesity is presented as a problem of culture, gender, race and ethnicity [3]. Western culture has fashioned an inactive way of life in the presence of plenty and created a situation in which people are able to become fat, particularly children. The relationship between nature and culture has become confused. Women and those who are the victims of inequality have then been portrayed, to some extent, as responsible. Despite

women's perceived connection to nature, their cultural responsibility for the socialization of children suggests an implicit role in spreading obesity. The association has been applied particularly to working mothers who have failed to monitor eating habits and television viewing, and relied too much on convenience foods [3]. Members of ethnic groups with a higher prevalence of obesity are exemplars of maladaption to the wider culture.

Viewing obesity as a threat to all of us is a newer concept that has not yet been readily acknowledged. For obesity as a risk for all to become accepted, demonization of the obese will need to be curtailed because it will apply not to "them" but to "us." The current focus on childhood obesity, in which children can be seem as victims in an environment created by adults, may help to shift the focus away from individual blame and even modify the strict cultural norms [2]. However, the impending sense of doom implied by the obesity "crisis" will have to be handled with care to avoid a sense of chaos implied by "moral panic" [3,4].

These three approaches to the obesity epidemic (the personal, the environment and the universal threat) run counter to the growing evidence of the major role of health inequality in the current proliferation of obesity [148]. Those most likely to become obese are those who are most likely to lack the resources to become thin.

Conclusion

From the social and cultural perspective, there are a number of ways forward that are both practical and policy driven.

Firstly, acceptance of a wider body diversity in place of "the current negative social, cultural and medical attitudes about fatness" [121]. Although the possibility of "fat and beautiful" or "fat and healthy" is unlikely to receive wide currency, avoiding negative stereotypes in preference to a more rational approach to body size and shape as "normal" may reduce body anxieties and diminish pressure towards eating disorders. An exploration of some of the existing positive aspects of slight plumpness could begin to redress the current imbalance in information available on obesity [149].

The second is to avoid "pathologizing" most of the adult population and refocus on metabolic health, fitness and well-being rather than weight loss as a method of achieving health. Once a problem is as prevalent in Western cultures as obesity, it is no longer simply a medical problem but a social one. Strategies to address so prevalent an issue, particularly among those with least control over their circumstances, must consider the social determinants of health and be mindful of the cultural context in which it occurs.

Thirdly, and linked with the previous concern, is to consider social inequalities. Individualistic interventions are less available to the socially and economically marginalized [120]. Social inequality probably the most critical and the most intransigent issue to be addressed.

It will be important to avoid falling back on old remedies, such as relying on individual lifestyle solutions to fight the "war on obesity" [3]. Health Canada's Vitality and ParticipACTION programs, stressing health rather than weight loss and "social acceptance of a wider range of healthy weights and body sizes," is a more positive approach [150].

Considering the body within its social and environmental context will help to focus on the structural aspects of obesity, and there is some evidence that this is beginning to take place [2]. A deeper understanding of how the cultural and social context contributes to and supports the "obesogenic" or "toxic" environment can assist in devising more successful strategies to address obesity as a social issue. The Western cultural environment is one of excess, with an abundance of highly processed foods in ever increasing portion sizes. Strategies that tackle some ingrained norms in modern Western culture may benefit from observing and listening to other cultural groups who have a greater respect for and more sophisticated relationship with food [24].

Rising obesity levels are occurring at the same time as other psychopathologies such as increasing alcohol abuse, drug misuse, eating disorders, self-harm and suicide [151]. This is not a new concept in the social sciences; over 40 years ago Mary Douglas proposed that individual bodies may reflect the anxieties of the social body. Thus fatness "may function as a site for social reflection, or social diagnosis, an index of our relation to consumption in advanced consumer capitalism" [152]. The obese society as a whole may signify that the present-day Western capitalist culture itself is in need of remedy.

Western society, grounded in the separation of body and mind [105,111], has focused on changing the obese body, reducing the mind to second-class status. Renewed interest by the social sciences in a broader concept of the body may result in a greater understanding of the place of the body in Western culture, provide insight into the ways in which the cultural context influences thinking and feeling about obesity, and suggest some constructive ways to approach the obesity epidemic.

Acknowledgment

I would like to thank Gayl Galbraith for reviewing a draft of this chapter.

References

1. Blair SN, LaMonte MJ. Commentary: current perspectives on obesity and health: black and white, or shades of grey? Int J Epidemiol 2006;35:69–72.
2. Lawrence RG. Framing obesity: the evolution of news discourse on a public health issue. Harvard Int J Press/Politics 2004;9:56–75.
3. Boero N. All the News that's fat to print: the American "obesity epidemic" and the media. Qual Sociol 2007;30:41–60.
4. Campos P, Saguy A, Ernsberger P, et al. The epidemiology of overweight and obesity: public health crisis or moral panic? Int J Epidemiol 2006;35:55–60.
5. Kluckhohn C. *Mirror for Man.* New York: McGraw-Hill, 1949:23.
6. Kroeber AL. *Culture.* New York: Vintage Books, 1963.
7. Brown PJ, Krick SV. Culture and economy in the etiology of obesity: diet, television and the illusions of personal choice. Working paper 003-01. Atlanta, GA: MARIAL Center, Emory University, 2001. Available from: www.emory.edu/COLLEGE/MARIAL/ pdfs/wp003-01obesity.pdf
8. Brown PJ, Konner M. An anthropological perspective on obesity. Ann NY Acad Sci 1987;499:29–46.
9. Brown PJ. The biocultural evolution of obesity: an anthropological view. In: Bjorntorp P, Brodoff BN (eds) *Obesity.* Philadelphia: JB Lippincott, 1992:320–9.
10. Eaton SB, Shostak M, Konner M. Stone agers in the fast lane: chronic degenerative diseases in evolutionary perspective. In: Brown PJ (ed) *Understanding and Applying Med Anthropol.* Mountainview, CA: Mayfield, 1998:21–33.
11. Lev-Ran A. Human obesity: an evolutionary approach to understanding our bulging waistline. Diabetes/Metab Res Rev 2001; 17:347–62.
12. Cassidy CM. Nutrition and health in agriculturalists and hunter-gatherers. In: Jerome NW, Kandel RF, Pelto HP (eds) *Nutritional Anthropology: Contemporary Approaches to Diet and Culture.* New York: Redgrave, 1980:117–45.
13. Szathmary EJE. Diabetes in Amerindian populations: the Dogrib studies. In: Swedland AC, Armelagos GJ (eds) *Disease in Populations in Transition: Anthropological and Epidemiological Perspectives.* New York: Bergin and Garvey, 1990:75–104.
14. Kuhnlein HV, Receveur O, Soueida R, et al. Artic indigenous peoples experience the nutrition transition with changing dietary patterns and obesity. J Nutr 2004;124:1447–53.
15. Wang Y. Cross-national comparison of childhood obesity: the epidemic and the relationship between obesity and socioeconomic status. Int J Epidemiol 2001;30:1129–36.
16. Popkin BM. Nutrition in transition: the changing global nutrition challenge. Asia Pacific J Clin Nutr 2001;10(suppl):S13–S18.
17. Neel JV. The "thrifty genotype" in 1998. Nutr Rev 1999;57(5 Pt 2):S2–S9.
18. Norgan NG. The beneficial effects of body fat and adipose tissue in humans. Int J Obes 1997;21:738–46.
19. Pollock NJ. Social fattening patterns in the Pacific – the positive side of obesity. A Nauru case study. In: de Garine I, Pollock NJ (eds) *Social Aspects of Obesity.* Luxembourg: Gordon and Breach Publishers, 1995:87–109.
20. Weinsier RL, Hunter GR, Heini AF, et al. The etiology of obesity: relative contribution of metabolic factors, diet, and physical activity. Am J Med 1998;105:145–50.
21. Katzmarzyk PT, Perusse L, Rao DC, et al. Familial risk of obesity and central adipose tissue distribution in the general Canadian population. Am J Epidemiol 1999;149:933–42.
22. Rebato E, Salces I, Jelenkovic A, et al. Familial resemblance in fatness and fat distribution in nuclear families from Biscay (Basque Country). Hum Ecol Special Issue 2007;15:23–9.
23. Cahnman WJ. The stigma of obesity. Sociol Q 1968;9:294–7.
24. Messer E. Small but healthy? Some cultural considerations. Hum Organiz 1989;48:39–52.
25. Ritenbaugh C. Body size and shape: a dialogue of culture and biology. Med Anthropol 1991;13:173–80.
26. eHRAF (Human Relation Area Files). Collection of ethnography (database on the internet). Available from: www.yale.edu/hraf/index.html.

27. Anderson JL, Crawford CB, Nadeau J, et al. Was the Duchess of Windsor right? A cross-cultural review of the socioecology of ideals of female body shape. Ethol Sociobiol 1992;13:197–227.

28. Cassidy CM. The good body: when bigger is better. Med Anthropol 1991;13:181–213.

29. Cook J. *Captain Cook's Voyages Round the World*. London: Ward, Lock Bowden, 1886:1150.

30. Leit RA, Pope HG, Gray JJ. Cultural expectations of muscularity in men: the evolution of Playgirl centerfolds. Int J Eat Disord 2001;29:90–3.

31. Frederick DA, Fessler DMT, Haselton MG. Do representations of male muscularity differ in men's and women's magazines? Body Image 2005;2:81–6.

32. Baghurst T, Hollander DB, Nardella B, et al. Change in sociocultural ideal male physique: an examination of past and present action figures. Body Image 2006;3:87–91.

33. Craig PL, Swinburn BA, Matenga-Smith T, et al. Do Polynesians still believe that big is beautiful? NZ Med J 1996;109:200–3.

34. Wright St-Clair RE. Diet of the Maoris of New Zealand. In: Robson JRK (ed) *Food Ecology and Culture*. New York: Gordon and Breach, 980:35–45.

35. Graves NB, Graves TD. The impact of modernization on the personality of a Polynesian people. Hum Organiz 1978;37:115–35.

36. Buck PH. *Ethnology of Manahiki and Ragahanga*. Bernice P Bishop Museum Bulletin 99. Honolulu, Hawaii: BP Bishop Museum, 1932.

37. Hattori K. Physique of Sumo wrestlers in relation to some cultural characteristics of Japan. In: de Garine I, Pollock NJ (eds) *Social Aspects of Obesity*. Luxembourg: Gordon and Breach, 1995:31–43.

38. de Garine I. Sociocultural aspects of the male fattening sessions among the Massa of Northern Cameroon. In: de Garine I, Pollock NJ (eds) *Social Aspects of Obesity*. Luxembourg: Gordon and Breach, 1995:45–70.

39. Pasquet P, Brigant L, Froment A, et al. Massive overfeeding and energy balance in men: the Guru Walla model. Am J Clin Nutr 1992;56:483–90.

40. Davis C, Durnin JVGA, Gurevich M, et al. Body composition correlates of weight dissatisfaction and dietary restraint in young women. Appetite 1993;20:197–207.

41. Goldblatt PB, Moore ME, Stunkard AJ. Social factors in obesity. JAMA 1965;192:97–102.

42. McLaren L, Kuh D. Women's body dissatisfaction, social class, and social mobility. Soc Sci Med 2004;58:1575–84.

43. Christakis NA, Fowler JH. The spread of obesity in a large social network over 32 years. N Engl J Med 2007;357:370–9.

44. Christakis NA, Fowler JH. The spread of obesity in a social network: authors reply to letters to the editor. N Engl J Med 2007; 357:1867–8.

45. Sobal J, Stunkard AJ. Socioeconomic status and obesity: a review of the literature. Psychol Bull 1989;105:260–75.

46. McLaren L. Socioeconomic status and obesity. Epidemiol Rev 2007;29:29–48.

47. Ball K, Mishra G, Crawford D. What aspects of socioeconomic status are related to obesity among men and women? Int J Obes 2002;26:559–65.

48. Komlos J, Kriwy P. Social status and adult heights in the two Germanies. Ann Hum Biol 2002;9:641–8.

49. Power C, Manor O, Li L. Are inequalities in height underestimated by adult social position? Effects of changing social structure and height selection in a cohort study. BMJ 2002;325:131–4.

50. Zhang Q, Wang Y. Socioeconomic inequality of obesity in the United States: do gender, age, and ethnicity matter? Soc Sci Med 2004;58:1171–80.

51. Pena M, Bacallao J. Obesity and the poor: an emerging problem. In: Pena M, Bacallao J (eds) *Obesity and Poverty*. Pan American Health Organisation Scientific Publication No. 576. Washington, DC: Pan American Health Organization, 2000:3–10.

52. Filozof C, Gonzalez C, Sereday M, et al. Obesity prevalence and trends in Latin-American countries. Obes Rev 2001;2: 99–106.

53. Kinra S, Nelder RP, Lewendon GJ. Deprivation and childhood obesity: a cross sectional study of 20973 children in Plymouth, United Kingdom. J Epidemiol Commun Health 2000;54: 456–60.

54. Freedman DS, Ogden CL, Flegal KM, et al. Childhood overweight and family income. Medscape Gen Med 2007;9:26. Available from www.medscape.com/viewarticle/552148.

55. Monteiro CA, Moura EC, Conde WL, et al. Socioeconomic status and obesity in adult populations in developing countries: a review. Bull WHO 2004;82:940–6.

56. Caballero B. Introduction to symposium: obesity in developing countries: biological and ecological factors. J Nutr 2001; 131:866S–870S.

57. Aguirre P. Socioanthropological aspects of obesity in poverty. In: Pena M, Bacallao J (eds) *Obesity and Poverty*. Pan American Health Organisation Scientific Publication No. 576. Washington, DC: Pan American Health Organization, 2000:11–22.

58. Wrigley N, Warm D, Margetts B, et al. Assessing the impact of improved retail access on diet in a "food desert": a preliminary report. Urban Studies 2002;39:2061–82.

59. Drewnowski A, Darmon N. Food choices and diet costs: an economic analysis. J Nutr 2005;135:900–50.

60. Pena, M., Bacallao, J. Malnutrition and poverty. Annu Rev Nutr 2002;22:241–53.

61. Olson CM. Nutrition and health outcomes associated with food insecurity and hunger. J Nutr 1999;192(2S suppl): 521S–524S.

62. Townsend MS, Peerson J, Love B, et al. Food insecurity is positively related to overweight in women. J Nutr 2001;131:1738–45.

63. Mvo Z, Dick J, Steyn K. Perceptions of overweight African women about acceptable body size of women and children. Curationis 1999;22:27–31.

64. Jain A, Sherman SN, Chamberlain LA, et al. Why don't low income mothers worry about their preschoolers being overweight? Pediatrics 2001;107:1138–46.

65. Furnham A, Alibhai N. Cross-cultural differences in the perception of female body shapes. Psychol Med 1983;13:829–37.

66. Dawson DA. Ethnic differences in female overweight: data from the 1985 National Health Interview Survey. Am J Publ Health 1888; 78:1326–9.

67. Furnham A, Baguma P. Cross-cultural differences in the evaluation of male and female body shapes. Int J Eat Disord 1994;15: 81–9.

68. Wilkinson J, Ben-Tovim DI, Walker MK. An insight into the personal and cultural significance of weight and shape in large Samoan women. Int J Obes 1994;18:602–6.

69. Gittelsohn J, Harris SB, Thorne-Lyman AL, et al. Body image concepts differ by age and sex in an Ojibway-Cree community in Canada. J Nutr 1996;126:2990–3000.

70. Mossavar-Rahmani Y, Pelto GH, Ferris AM, et al. Determinants of body size perceptions and dieting behavior in a multiethnic group of hospital staff women. J Am Diet Assoc 1996;96:252–6.

71. Altabe M. Ethnicity and body image: quantitative and qualitative analysis. Int J Eat Disord 1998;23:–9.

72. Craig P, Halavatau V, Comino E, et al. Perception of body size in the Tongan community: differences from and similarities to an Australian sample. Int J Obes 1999;23:1288–94.

73. Bush HM, Williams RGA, Lean MEJ, et al. Body image and weight consciousness among South Asian, Italian and the general population. Appetite 2001;37:207–15.

74. Miller MN, Pumariega AJ. Culture and eating disorders: a historical and cross-cultural review. Psychiatry 2001;64:93–110.

75. Cachelin FM, Rebeck RM, Chung GH, et al. Does ethnicity influence body-size preference? A comparison of body image and body size. Obes Res 2002;10:158–66.

76. Sharps MJ, Price-Sharps JL, Hanson J. Body image preferences in the United States and rural Thailand: an exploratory study. J Psychol 2001;135:518–26.

77. Ricciardelli LA, McCabe MP. Children's body image concerns and eating disturbance: a review of the literature. Clin Psychol Rev 2001; 21:325–44.

78. Hill AJ, Bhatti R. Body shape perception and dieting in preadolescent British Asian girls – links with eating disorders. Int J Eat Disord 1995;17:175–83.

79. Kaplan MS, Huguet N, Newsom JT, et al. The association between length of residence and obesity among Hispanic immigrants. Am J Prev Med 2004;27:323–6.

80. Ross CE, Mirowsky J. Social epidemiology of overweight: a substantive and methodological investigation. J Health Soc Behav 1983;24:288–98.

81. Flegal KM, Harlan WR, Landis JR. Secular trends in body mass index and skinfold thickness with socioeconomic factors in young adult women. Am J Clin Nutr 1988;48:535–43.

82. Do DP, Dubowitz T, Bird CE, et al. Neighbourhood context and ethnicity differences in body mass index: a multilevel analysis using the NHANES III survey (1988–1994). Econ Hum Biol 2007; 5:179–203.

83. Hodge AM, Zimmet PZ. The epidemiology of obesity. In: Caterson ID (ed) *Clinical Endocrinology and Metabolism*. London: Baillière Tindall, 1994:577–599.

84. Woodward JR. An examination of the effects of race and socioeconomic status on health behaviours. Dissertation. Abstracts Int 2001;61:2934A–2935A.

85. Brewis AA, McGarvey ST, Jones J, et al. Perceptions of body size in Pacific Islanders. Int J Obes 1998;22:185–9.

86. Young TK. Sociocultural and behavioural determinants of obesity among Inuit in the Central Canadian Arctic. Soc Sci Med 1996;43:1665–71.

87. Bindon JR. Polynesian responses to modernization: overweight and obesity in the South Pacific. In: de Garine I, Pollock NJ (eds) *Social Aspects of Obesity*. Luxembourg: Gordon and Breach, 1995: 227–51.

88. Garner DM, Garfinkel PE, Schwartz E, Thompson M. Cultural expectations of thinness in women. Psychol Rep 1980;47:483–91.

89. Morris A, Cooper T, Cooper PJ. The changing shape of female fashion models. Int J Eat Disord 1989;8:593–96.

90. Wiseman CV, Gray JJ, Mosimann JE, et al. Cultural expectations of thinness in women: an update. Int J Eat Disord 1992;11:85–9.

91. Tovee, MJ, Mason SM, Emery JL, et al. Supermodels: stick insects or hourglasses? Lancet 1997;350:1474–5.

92. Voracek M, Fisher ML. Shapely centerfolds? Temporal change in body measures: trend analysis. BMJ 2002;325:1447–8.

93. McKinley NM. Ideal weight/ideal women. In: Sobal J, Maurer D (eds) *Weighty Issues: Fatness and Thinness as Social Problems*. New York: Aldine de Gruyter, 1999:97–115.

94. Rodin J, Silberstein L, Striegel-Moore R. Women and weight: a normative discontent. In: Sonderegger TB (ed) *Nebraska Symposium on Motivation, Psychology And Gender*, 1984, Vol 32. Lincoln, NE: University of Nebraska Press, 1985:267–307.

95. Way K. Never too rich … or too thin: the role of stigma in the social construction of anorexia nervosa. In: Maurer D, Sobal J (eds) *Eating Agendas: Food and Nutrition as Social Problems*. New York: Aldine de Gruyter, 1995:91–113.

96. Sobal J. The medicalization and demedicalization of obesity. In: Maurer D, Sobal J (eds) *Eating Agendas: Food and Nutrition as Social Problems*. New York: Aldine de Gruyter, 1995:67–90.

97. Williams L, Germov J. Body acceptance: exploring women's experiences. In: Germov J, Williams L (eds) *A Sociology of Food and Nutrition*, 2nd edn. Melbourne: Oxford University Press, 2004; 401–26.

98. Franzoi SL. The body-as-object versus the body-as-process: gender differences and gender considerations. Sex Roles 1995;33:417–37.

99. Farquhar JC, Wasylkiw L. Medical images of men: trends and consequences of body conceptualisation. Psychol Men Masculinity 2007;8:145–60.

100. McCabe MP, Butler K, Watt C. Media influences on attitudes and perceptions toward the body among adult men and women. J Appl Biobehav Res 2007;12:101–18.

101. McCabe MP, Ricciardelli LA. Sociocultural influences on body image and body changes among adolescent boys and girls. J Soc Psychol 2003;143:5–26.

102. Agliata D, Tantleff-Dunn S. The impact of media exposure on males' body image. J Soc Clin Psychol 2004;23:7–22.

103. Cafri G, Thompson JK, Ricciardelli L, et al. Pursuit of the muscular ideal: physical and psychological consequences and putative risk factors. Clin Psychol Rev 2005;25:215–39.

104. Turner BS. The government of the body: medical regimens and the rationalization of diet. Br J Sociol 1982;33:254–69.

105. Lock M. Cultivating the body: anthropology and epistemologies of bodily practice and knowledge. Annu Rev Anthropol 1993;22: 133–55.

106. Lupton D. The body, medicine and society. In: Germov J (ed) *Second Opinion: an Introduction to Health Sociology*, 3rd edn. Melbourne: Oxford University Press, 2005:195–207.

107. Featherstone M. The body in consumer culture. In: Featherstone M, Hepworth M, Turner BS (eds) *The Body: Social Process and Cultural Theory*. London: Sage Publications, 1991:170–96.

108. Nichter M, Nichter M. Hype and weight. Med Anthropol 1991;13:249–84.

109. Cash TF, Roy RE. Pounds of flesh. In: Sobal J, Maurer D (eds) *Interpreting Weight*. New York: Aldine de Gruyter, 1999:209–28.

110. Crandall CS, d'Anello S, Sakalli N, et al. An attribution model of prejudice: anti-fat attitudes in six nations. Person Soc Psychol Bull 2001;130–7.

111. Turner BS. The discourse of diet. In: Featherstone M, Hepworth M, Turner BS (eds) *The Body: Social Process and Cultural Theory*. London: Sage Publications, 1991:157–69.

112. Ritenbaugh C. Obesity as a culture-bound syndrome. Culture Med Psychiatr 1982;6:347–61.

113. American Institute of Nutrition. Report of the American Institute of Nutrition (AIN) Steering Committee on Healthy Weight. J Nutr 1994;124:2240–3.

114. Kettle M. Fat is a mathematical issue – as 29m Americans find out. Guardian Weekly, June 14, 1998, p4.

115. Deurenberg P, Deurenberg-Yap M. Ethnic and geographical influences on body composition. In: Bray GA, Bouchard C (eds) *Handbook of Obesity: Etiology and Pathophysiology*, 2nd edn. New York: Marcel Dekker, 2004:1–108.

116. Craig P, Colagiuri S, Hussain Z, et al. Identifying cut-points in anthropometric indexes for predicting previously undiagnosed diabetes and cardiovascular risk factors in the Tongan population. Obes Res Clin Pract 2007;1:17–25.

117. Conrad P. The medicalization of society: on the transformation of human conditions into treatable disorders. Baltimore, MD: Johns Hopkins University Press, 2007.

118. Cogan JC. Re-evaluating the weight-centred approach towards health. In: Sobal J, Maurer D (eds) *Interpreting Weight*. New York: Aldine de Gruyter, 1999: 229–53.

119. Aphramor L. Is a weight-centred health framework salutogenic? Some thoughts on unhinging certain dietary ideologies. Social Theory Health 2005;3:315–40.

120. Monaghan LF. Discussion piece: a critical take on the obesity debate. Social Theory Health 2005;3:302–14.

121. Rich E, Evans J. "Fat ethics" – the obesity discourse and body politics. Social Theory Health 2005;3:341–58.

122. Jones DC. Body image among adolescent girls and boys: a longitudinal study. Dev Psychol 2004;40:823–35.

123. Klaczynski PA, Goold KW, Mudry JJ. Culture, obesity stereotypes, self-esteem, and the "thin ideal": a social identity perspective. J Youth Adolesc 2004;33:307–17.

124. Chang VW, Christakis NA (eds). Medical modeling of obesity: the transition from action to experience in a 20th century American medical textbook. Sociol Health Illness 2002;24:151–77.

125. Battle EK, Brownell KD. Confronting a rising tide of eating disorders and obesity: treatment vs prevention and policy. Addict Behav 1996;21:755–65.

126. Schwartz MB, Chamblis HO'N, Brownell KD, et al. Weight bias among health professionals specializing in obesity. Obes Res 2003;11:1033–9.

127. Eggar G, Swinburn B. An "ecological" approach to the obesity pandemic. BMJ 1997;315:477–80.

128. Hill JO, Peters JC. Environmental contributions to the obesity epidemic. Science 1998;280:1371–4.

129. Nestle M, Jacobson MF. Halting the obesity epidemic: a public health policy approach. Public Health Rep 2000;115: 12–24.

130. Sobal J. Sociological analysis of the stigmatisatoin of obesity. In: Germov J, Williams L (eds) *A Sociology of Food and Nutrition*, 2nd edn. Melbourne: Oxford University Press, 2004;383–402.

131. Williams L, Germov J. The social appetite: a sociological approach to food and nutrition. In: Germov J (ed) *Second Opinion: an Introduction to Health Sociology*, 3rd edn. Melbourne: Oxford University Press, 2005:129–46.

132. Williams SJ, Calnan M. The "limits" of medicalization? Modern medicine and the lay populace in "late" modernity. Soc Sci Med 1996;42:1609–20.

133. Chang VW, Christakis NA. Self-perception of weight appropriateness in the United States. Am J Prev Med 2003;24:332–9.

134. Sobal J. The size acceptance movement and the social construction of body weight. In: Sobal J, Maurer D (eds) *Weighty Issues: Fatness and Thinness as Social Problems*. New York: Aldine de Gruyter, 1999:231–49.

135. Kingsmill D (chair). *Model Health Enquiry. Fashioning a Healthy Future: the Report of the Model Health Inquiry*. London: British Fashion Council, 2007. Available from: www.modelhealthinquiry.com/docs/The%20Report%20of%20the%20Model% 20Health%20 Inquiry,%20September%202007.pdf.

136. British Fashion Council. Model Health Inquiry, update on 07-02-2008. Available from: www.modelhealthinquiry.com/docs/Hilary %20Riva's%20Open%20Letter%20re%20MHI.pdf.

137. Meierdierks-Lehman S. Fighting dummies: the crusade against ultrathin body ideals. Columbia News Service, April 10, 2007. Available from: http://jscms.jrn.columbia.edu/cns/2007-04-10/meierdierkslehman-mannequinbodyimage.

138. Foster J. Available from: www.diet-blog.com/archives/2007/09/21/is_this_woman_plus_size.php.

139. Chapman GE. From "dieting" to "healthy eating". In: Sobal J, Maurer D (eds) *Interpreting Weight*. New York: Aldine de Gruyter, 1999:73–87.

140. Foucault M. Technologies of self: a seminar with Michel Foucault. In: Chang VW, Christakis NA (eds) Medical modeling of obesity: the transition from action to experience in a 20th century American medical textbook. Sociol Health Illness 2002;24:151–77.

141. Stunkard A, Allison KC. Socioeconomic status and the obesity epidemic. In: Medeiros-Neto G, Halpern A, Bouchard C (eds) *Progress in Obesity Research, 9*. Montrouge, France: John Libbey Eurotext, 2003:485–98.

142. Avenell A, Brown TJ, McGee MA, et al. What interventions should we add to weight reducing diets in adults with obesity? A systematic review of randomized controlled trials of adding drug therapy, exercise, behaviour therapy or combinations of these interventions. J Hum Nutr Dietet 2004;17:293–316.

143. Ayyad C, Anderson T. Long-term efficacy of dietary treatment of obesity: a systematic review of studies published between 1931 and 1999. Obes Rev 2000;1:113–19.

144. Anderson T. Is there a place for dietary treatment of obesity given a 5-year 85 per cent relapse? In: Medeiros-Neto G, Halpern A, Bouchard C (eds) *Progress in Obesity Research, 9*. Montrouge, France: John Libbey Eurotext, 2003:387–91.

145. Green GC, Buckroyd J. Disordered eating cognitions and behaviours among slimming organization competition winners. J Hum Nutr Diet 2008;21:31–8.

146. Kersh R, Morone J. How the personal becomes political: prohibitions, public health and obesity. Stud Am Polit Dev 2002; 16:162–75.

147. Schlosser E. *Fast Food Nation*. Boston: Houghton Mifflin, 2001.

148. Kivimaki M, Head J, Ferrie JE, et al. Work stress, weight gain and weight loss: evidence for bidirectional effects of job strain on body mass index in the Whitehall II study. Int J Obes 2006; 30:982–7.

149. Bradley PJ. Is obesity an advantageous adaptation? Int J Obes 1982;6:43–52.

150. Gingras J. Throwing their weight around: Canadians take on Health At Every Size. Health At Every Size 2006;19:195–206.

151. Cottam R. Obesity and culture. Lancet 2004;364:941, 1202–3.

152. Douglas, M. Purity and danger: an analysis of concepts of pollution and taboo. In: Chang VW, Christakis NA (eds) Medical modelling of obesity: the transition from action to experience in a 20th century American medical textbook. Sociol Health Illness 2002;24:151–77.

153. Pope HG, Olivardia R, Gruber A, Borowiecki J. Evolving ideals of male body image as seen through action toys. Int J Eat Disord 1999; 26: 65–72.

154. Orbach S. There is a public health crisis – it's not fat on the body but fat in the mind and the fat of profits. Int J Epidemiol 2006;35:67–9.

5 Obesity and Gender

Berit L. Heitmann

Research Unit for Dietary Studies, Institute of Preventive Medicine, Centre for Health and Society, Copenhagen University Hospital, Denmark

Gender differences in obesity development

Data from most countries all over the world suggest that obesity prevalence is increasing among men, women, children, adolescents and adults, and poor and rich [1,2]. As a consequence, obesity has become a greater threat to public health than more traditional health concerns, such as infection or undernutrition [1,2]. Worldwide, more than 1.6 billion are estimated to be overweight, of which at least 300 million are obese [2]. However, even if general obesity is spreading fast throughout the world, a large heterogeneity exists between and within countries, and patterns of development seem different for men and women, for young and for old, for rich and poor, and for urban and rural groups of individuals. For instance, differences in prevalence are extreme worldwide, and among Pacific Islander women, almost 80% are severely obese in middle age compared to less than 1% among rural Chinese men. However, variations are seen even within more heterogeneous areas such as Europe, where prevalences are lower in northern compared to southern or eastern regions [2].

In general, there are more obese women than men, but gender differences may become smaller with time, because the incidence of obesity seems greater for men than women [1]. If the current developmental trends for obesity among men and women continue, some of the observed gender differences in occurrence may in fact disappear [3]. Indeed, in many countries, during the 1980s and 1990s the increase in severe obesity was generally greater for men than for women and hence men may, in the near future, present similar obesity prevalences as women, if these trends continue [2]. Certainly, European gender differences in obesity prevalence have already diminished. More recent data, collected around 2000, show that several European countries now display a similar prevalence in the two genders [2].

It is interesting to note, however, that the development of severe obesity in the two genders is also heterogeneous among countries. For instance, trend data from Denmark [4] show that over the 30 years between 1964 and 1994, the prevalence of obesity increased for all men and older women, and to different degrees for different age groups. In contrast, prevalence was decreasing for middle-aged women and was stable for younger women. The same pattern of development was seen for middle-aged Finnish, Norwegian and Swedish women [5–7] but not middle-aged Nordic men or middle-aged women elsewhere. The study proposed that the identification of those determinants responsible for the differing trends in obesity for men and women would be of great value for understanding causes behind the current obesity epidemic [4]. However, this study suggested that changes in the lifestyle factors generally assumed to be associated with increasing trends for obesity could not explain the observed heterogeneous trends. For instance, even if all four countries had decreasing trends for obesity among the middle-aged women, changes over time in dietary intakes, smoking habits or physical activity varied more between the four Nordic countries than between men and women or between the Nordic countries and other Western societies, and could not explain the gender differences [4]. It was concluded that only the increase in the proportion of women entering the labor force had changed in comparable ways in the four Nordic countries. Hence, it was proposed that the declining trends among middle-aged women were explained by the rise in the socio-economic status women experienced during the period. This rise in social class for women, prompted by their entry to the labor force, was generally larger in the Nordic countries than elsewhere during this period (Box 5.1). The decline in the trends for obesity among middle-aged women seems to have ceased after 1990, and since then obesity seems to be on the increase among middle-aged Nordic women. In Nordic countries, as well as elsewhere, prevalence data for obesity have never been greater.

Clinical Obesity in Adults and Children, 3rd edition. Edited by Peter G. Kopelman, Ian D. Caterson and William H. Dietz.
© 2010 Blackwell Publishing, ISBN: 978-1-4051-8226-3.

Gender differences in fat distribution

Fat localized peripherally and subcutaneously on hips and thighs is labeled gynoid, or female-type fat patterning, whereas centralized fat on the trunk, particularly viscerally, is labeled android, or male-type fat patterning. This distribution is largely determined by hormones and therefore the differences in the typical fat patterns tend to fade with age, particularly when women enter menopause and develop a more android pattern (Table 5.1).

Circumference measurements of hips, waists and thighs, and ratios of these, are often used to determine fat distribution. Most data will show only marginal overlap in the ranges of the waist or the waist-to-hip ratios between men and women, whereas hip circumferences generally are more similar for men and women [8].

Box 5.1 Socio-economic conditions: female labor force as a percentage of total labor force 1960–1990

Denmark	31 → 45%
Finland	39 → 47%
Norway	23 → 41%
Sweden	30 → 47%
Austria	40 → 40%
Germany	37 → 37%
Italy	25 → 32%
Netherlands	22 → 31%
United Kingdom	32 → 39%
Portugal	18 → 37%
Spain	20 → 24%
Greece	33 → 27%

Adapted from Niemi [67].

Gender differences in risk associated with fat distribution

Both total fat mass in general and the specific fat mass localizations are related to excess morbidity and mortality. For fat distribution, early studies by Larsson et al. [9] showed that the different fat distribution patterns among middle-aged men and women largely seemed to explain observed differences in mortality between the two genders. The study compared 12-year mortality risk to fat distribution in men and women, and found an almost sixfold difference in the crude odds ratio, favoring the women. The difference was eliminated when the associations were adjusted for differences between men and women in fat distribution. Adjustment for overall obesity, smoking, blood pressure or cholesterol only reduced the odds ratio slightly. These data clearly suggested that at similar fat distributions, mortality risk was alike for men and women.

More recent research has suggested that the apparent health disadvantage related to android-type fat distribution may relate to harmful effects of substances produced by the visceral fat, a tissue that has been found to be particularly lipolytic and productive of proatherosclerotic and inflammatory peptides. However, recent studies also suggest health advantages associated with gynoid-type fat distribution that may relate to the production of protective substances produced primarily in peripheral fat, such as adiponectins that possess anti-inflammatory and antiatherosclerotic properties [10]. In addition, the size of the peripheral lean tissue, particularly on the lower body and extremities, may provide protection by regulating insulin sensitivity [11]. Therefore, the recent discovery that gynoid fat distribution, e.g. the more female type of fat distribution with wide hips and narrow waists, seems to offer health protection and to be independently related to longevity for *both* men and women. This finding is surprising, and warrants further studies to elucidate whether the fat, lean or *both* may carry the health benefit [12,13] (Fig. 5.1).

Table 5.1 Median values and 10th and 90th percentile of waist and hip circumference, as well as waist-to-hip ratio by age among 1527 Danish men and 1467 Danish women

	Men				Women			
	35 years	45 years	55 years	65 years	35 years	45 years	55 years	65 years
Waist circumference (cm)	87.5	90.0	93.0[a]	94.0	73.5	76.0	79.0[a]	80.5
10th percentile	78.0	80.0	82.0	82.1	66.5	67.5	67.2	68.0
90th percentile	100.5	103.5	108.0	107.0	86.3	92.1	95.0	96.0
Hip circumference (cm)	97.0	98.0[a,b]	99.0[a,b]	98.0[b]	94.0	97.0	98.8[a]	99.0
10th percentile	90.0	92.0	91.5	92.0	87.0	89.5	90.2	89.5
90th percentile	105.5	106.0	107.6	108.0	105.8	109.6	111.0	112.5
W/H ratio	0.90	0.92	0.95[a]	0.95	0.79[a]	0.79[a]	0.79	0.81
10th percentile	0.84	0.86	0.88	0.88	0.73	0.73	0.73	0.74
90th percentile	0.98	1.00	1.02	1.02	0.86	0.88	0.89	0.90

[a]No difference between values of one age group and the following.
[b]No difference between men and women of the same age group.
Adapted from Heitmann [8].

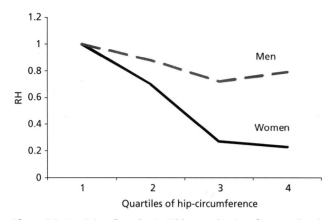

Figure 5.1 Associations (hazard ratio, HR) between hip circumference and total mortality among Danish men and women. (Adapted from Heitmann et al. [12].)

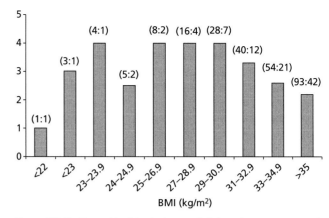

Figure 5.2 The 8-year risk of developing type 2 diabetes for women compared to men at the same BMI. (Adapted from Colditz et al. [16] and Chan et al. [17].)

Gender differences in risk associated with general obesity

Obesity is closely linked to development of diabetes, and most health authorities agree that the current obesity epidemic has initiated a diabetes epidemic that is expected to culminate in 10–15 years [14]. Furthermore, type 2 diabetes mellitus, which was hitherto found only among adults, now is occurring among children and adolescents [15]. The close association between diabetes and cardiovascular disease is creating a great fear that trends in heart disease, for which most Western countries have observed a decline since the 1960s, may reverse if the obesity epidemic and the consequent diabetes epidemic cannot be arrested quickly.

However, the relationships between obesity and diabetes and between diabetes and heart disease are different for men and women. This fact is not well recognized, but is supported by large and well-conducted studies showing that obesity seems to be a greater health disadvantage to women than to men. Data from studies of the relation between Body Mass Index (BMI) and the incidence of type 2 diabetes document, for instance, that for the same degree of overweight and obesity, the risk of developing diabetes is much higher for women than for men [16,17] (Fig. 5.2). Furthermore, for a BMI of around 30 kg/m², a woman with no previous history of diabetes had an 8-year risk of developing diabetes that was 28-fold greater than that of a women with a BMI <22 kg/m² [16]. The excess risk among obese men was sevenfold only [17] and hence, the diabetes risk for obese women was fourfold higher than that of a man with similar BMI.

In addition, this gender difference in risk seems to carry over in the relation to developing heart disease [18]. In fact, a recent meta-analysis, which included 37 studies and a total of almost 500,000 patients with type 2 diabetes, found that not only was the rate of fatal coronary heart disease associated with diabetes higher in patients with diabetes than in those without (5.4 v 1.6%), the overall summary relative risk for fatal coronary heart disease in patients with diabetes compared with no diabetes was

significantly greater among women (relative risk (RR) 3.5, 95% confidence interval (CI) 2.70–4.53) than it was among men (RR 2.06, 95% CI 1.81–2.34). Even after the exclusion of eight studies that had adjusted only for age, the difference in risk between the sexes was substantially reduced but still highly significant, suggesting that the excess risk of coronary death associated with diabetes is substantially (50%) higher in women than in men. This difference may be a consequence of the diabetic disease inducing a more adverse cardiovascular risk profile in women than in men, combined with possible disparities in treatment that may favor men [18].

Differences in attitudes towards male and female obesity

The medical profession

Despite the fact that cardiovascular disease kills a higher percentage of women (56%) than men (43%) [19], a reduced likelihood that women receive similar standard treatment for their heart disease is well documented. Women with cardiovascular disease are both underdiagnosed and undertreated by a medical profession [20] that may perceive that cardiovascular disease is a male disease. Women are also under-represented in clinical trials of treatment effects for acute myocardial infarct or other coronary diseases. Additionally, mortality following acute myocardial infarction (MI) is higher among women, even after adjusting for age [21]. Swedish studies show that women with acute MI waited on average 1 hour longer than men from onset of pain to reach the hospital [20], in part because acute MI among women had lower ambulance priority than acute MI among men [20]. In addition, women also waited 20 minutes longer between arrival and treatment [21].

Likewise, studies show that the medical profession takes female obesity less seriously than male obesity, and that obese women have less chance of being referred to treatment for obesity than a man with the same degree of obesity [22–24]. Paradoxically, a

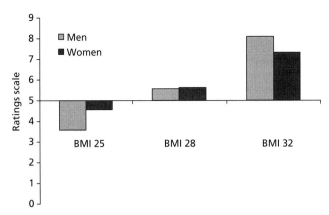

Figure 5.3 Association between physician attitudes towards treatment referrals for weight loss and BMI of male and female patients. Based on ratings scale of 1–9: 1, strongly disagree; 5, neither agree nor disagree; 9, strongly agree. (Adapted from Anderson et al. [23].)

normal-weight woman is more likely to be erroneously encouraged by her general practitioner to lose weight despite no medical indication than a normal-weight man [22–24] (Fig. 5.3). Other studies show that complaints from obese female patients are taken less seriously by health professionals than complaints from normal-weight women whereas this pattern is not documented for men. For instance, one study documented that doctors spend less time with their obese patients' problems [25], and that obese women were less likely to be screened for cervical and breast cancer than normal-weight women [26].

Relatives, educators and employers

Discrimination by the medical profession is not the only type of discrimination that occurs more frequently among obese women than obese men. The international literature contains abundant reports on stigmatization of obese girls and women [27,28]. Societal pressures against obesity are strong and many studies document that overweight is considered self-inflicted, a sign of weakness and lack of character. Several reports suggest that quality of life is grossly reduced among obese people [27]. The obese are discriminated against by peers, relatives, educators and employers, and obese women are affected more than obese men. For example, obese women marry less often than obese men, are less likely to obtain education than obese men, and more likely to live under poverty levels or in households with a low income, independent of differences in their baseline socio-economic status [27]. However, even with equal education, overweight women are discriminated against. In this regard, a Finnish study showed that overweight, well-educated women seem to have lower incomes and poorer jobs than normal-weight women of similar high education [28,29] whereas among men, job opportunities and income were only related to education.

Many studies document that obese children are stigmatized, and that the negative attitudes towards obesity start at a very early age. Peers view their obese mates as different and undesirable,

and the obese suffer much teasing, bullying and social exclusion [30–33]. Already at the age of 3 years, children hold negative attitudes towards their obese peers, and these attitudes develop and amplify as the children grow older [34]. Consistent with an earlier study conducted among 3–5 year old children, overweight children ranked lowest in the social hierarchy and were excluded from peer interaction. The other children preferred children with scars or various physical handicaps to the overweight children [35]. Other studies show that overweight children more often are called names, threatened, or made fun of than normal-weight children, but studies also document that girls seem to suffer the most [31,32,36,37].

Biased attitudes toward obese girls and women have also been noted from family members and teachers [38]. For instance, some studies document that obese girls are more often excluded from education than obese boys, because they are provided with fewer grants and scholarships for their future studies. Overweight girls, but not overweight boys, are under-represented at prestigious universities [39,40].

Gender differences in depressive symptoms associated with obesity

Overweight women also display a stronger association between stigmatization and lower psychologic well-being than overweight men. Obese women suffer from lower self-esteem than obese men [41–44], and one study reported that mental well-being was worse among obese than among chronically ill or injured persons [45]. The prevalence of depressive mood seems to vary with degree of obesity for women at all ages, but not for men, with more depression among obese than normal-weight women. In men, depressive mood and obesity seemed unrelated [46]. Consistent with this observation, overweight girls and women have a higher rate of suicidal thoughts compared to overweight boys and men [41,42,44]. It is possible that women are more influenced psychologically by stigmatization because women may base their self-esteem more on appearance than men [47,48]. The female body is partly valued based on attraction, whereas the male body may be viewed more in terms of effective performance in external environments [47].

Stigmatization of the obese in itself may contribute to a higher prevalence of obesity, because of the association between stigmatization and a negative body image, body dissatisfaction and low self-esteem, which may cause more overeating and an inactive lifestyle [48,49]. Likewise, studies have shown that bullying may lead to an inactive lifestyle [50] and/or to the development of eating disorders [51]. In accordance, a high self-esteem may prevent weight gain among adolescents [52]. Surprisingly, despite the rising prevalence of obesity, stigmatization has not apparently decreased. This observation suggests that obesity has not yet become a social norm [48].

Understanding that overweight occurs as a consequence of a complicated interaction between our genes and our lifestyle, and is influenced by social, psychosocial and cultural factors, rather than just a simple consequence of too much food and too little exercise, may help to prevent further stigmatization of the obese, irrespective of gender.

Female diseases and obesity

Obesity has consequences for several female diseases. Female cancers in the endometrium, the uterus, the ovary, the cervix and the breast, at least after menopause, are all related to obesity [1]. The relative risk of menstrual cycle irregularity and ovulatory failure is higher among obese than normal-weight women, and the Nurses' Health Study has shown that the risk of ovulatory infertility was about doubled among obese women with a BMI above 32 kg/m^2 compared to women with a normal BMI below 25 kg/m^2 [53]. Pregnancy rates in obese women with assisted reproduction treatment are half those in normal-weight women [54]. Polycystic ovary syndrome (PCOS), which is the most common endocrine disorder in women of reproductive age, is a condition characterized by hyperandrogenic chronic anovulation. Polycystic ovary syndrome affects around 6.5% of all women, but 30–75% of the obese [55]. Abdominal obesity occurs in 50–60% of women with PCOS [56]. Polycystic ovary syndrome causes problems with fertility and menstruation and the obese often suffer reduced fertility. Furthermore, if the obese woman conceives, she has a fourfold greater risk of miscarriage than normal-weight women [57], a 40–100% greater risk of stillbirth [58], and a higher risk of a planned or acute cesarean delivery. Cesarean deliveries are more complicated in obese women due to an increased risk of excessive blood loss, thrombosis and postoperative infection. [59]. Pregnancy complications, such as gestational hypertension, pre-eclampsia or gestational diabetes, are also common. The risk of gestational diabetes is doubled among overweight women, and is six times greater among obese women [60]. The subsequent risk of type 2 diabetes after gestational diabetes is doubled but, depending on ethnic origin, may be as high as 60% over 5–16 years. Finally, polycystic ovary syndrome independently increases metabolic and cardiovascular risk factors, and is a significant risk factor for later heart disease [61].

Intergenerational effects of obesity

The increase in the number of obese women has impacts on the coming generations. Maternal obesity predicts a fourfold increased risk of obesity in the offspring [62,63]. Overall, increased birth weight is a risk factor for child and adult obesity [64], and obese mothers tend to experience gestational diabetes more than normal-weight mothers. This reduced insulin sensitivity among obese mothers increases the availability of glucose to the fetus, and thereby potentially affects fetal growth [65]. Gestational diabetes also predisposes to macrosomia, congenital abnormalities, and prenatal mortality and morbidity in the offspring, as well as

an increased risk of impaired glucose tolerance. For instance, one study found a 10 times higher risk of impared glucose tolerance among 10–16 year old children of mothers with gestational diabetes, compared to same aged children of mothers without diabetes [66]. Similarly, maternal diet during pregnancy, and possibly during lactation, can influence the later risk of obesity and chronic diseases, because the fetal period is a critical period for disturbance in programming. New data gathered over long periods of time among Pima Indians furthermore suggest that the risk of developing gestational diabetes also depends on the pregnant woman's own mother's birth weight. It appears that nutritional programming during fetal life in one generation can influence disease risk in the following generation [67]. Hence, the generally increasing BMI among young women during the past 30–40 years may be a concern not only for the woman herself but also for her children and grandchildren.

Conclusion

Women not only display a higher obesity prevalence, but also seem to suffer more somatic and psychosocial health consequences than do obese men. The obesity epidemic is a major threat to individual and public health that may be a particular burden to girls and women.

References

1. World Health Organization. *Obesity – Preventing and Managing the Global Epidemic.* WHO Technical Report Series No. 894. Geneva: World Health Organization, 2000.
2. www.iotf.org/globalepidemic.asp
3. Heitmann BL. Gender, obesity and health. Sborník lékařský 1999;103(4):465–70
4. Heitmann BL Strøger U, Mikkelsen KL, et al. Large heterogeneity of the obesity in Danish adults Public Health Nutr 2003;7(3): 453–60.
5. Tverdal A. [Height, weight and body mass index of men and women aged 40–42 years.] Tidsskrift for den Norske Laegeforening 1996;116:2152–6.
6. Lissner L, Björkelund C, Heitmann BL, Lapidus L, Bjorntorp P, Bengtsson C. Secular increases in waist–hip ratio among Swedish women. Int J Obes Relat Metab Disord 1998;22:1116–20.
7. Pietinen P, Vartiainen E, Männistö S. Trends in body mass index and obesity among adults in Finland from 1972 to 1992. Int J Obes Relat Metab Disord 1996;20:114–20.
8. Heitmann BL. Body fat in the adult Danish population aged 35–65 years: an epidemiological study. Int J Obes 1991;15:535–45.
9. Larsson B, Svärdsudd K, Welin L, et al. Abdominal adipose tissue distribution, obesity, and risk of cardiovascular disease and death: 13 year follow up of participants in the study of men born in 1913. BMJ Clin Res 1984;188:1401–4.
10. ESHRE Capri Workshop Group. Nutrition and reproduction in women. Hum Reprod Update 2006;12(3):1993.

11. Sacchetti M, Olsen DB, Saltin B, et al. Heterogeneity in limb fatty acid kinetics in type 2 diabetes. Diabetologia 2005;48(5): 938–45.

12. Heitmann BL, Frederiksen P, Lissner L. Hip circumference and cardiovascular morbidity and mortality in men and women. Obes Res 2004;12(3):482–7.

13. Bigaard J, Frederiksen K, Tjonneland A. Waist and hip circumferences and all-cause mortality: usefulness of the waist-to-hip ratio? Int J Obes 2004;28(6):741–7.

14. James PT, Rigby N, Leach R, International Obesity Taskforce. The obesity epidemic, metabolic syndrome and future prevention strategies. Eur J Cardiovasc Prev Rehabil 2004;11(1):3–8.

15. Ehtisham S, Barrett TG. The emergence of type 2 diabetes in childhood. Ann Clin Biochem 2004;41(pt 1)10–16.

16. Colditz GA, Willett WC, Rotnitzky A, et al. Weight gain as a risk factor for clinical diabetes mellitus in women. Ann Intern Med 1995;122:481–6.

17. Chan JM, Rimm EB, Colditz GA, et al. Obesity, fat distribution, and weight gain as risk factors for clinical diabetes in men. Diabetes Care 1994;17(9):961–9.

18. Huxley R, Barzi F, Woodward M. Excess risk of fatal coronary heart disease associated with diabetes in men and women: meta-analysis of 37 prospective cohort studies. BMJ 2006;332:73–8.

19. World Health Organization Statistical Information System 2004. www.who.int/whosis/

20. Herlitz J, Starke M, Hansson E, et al. Characteristics and outcome among women and men transported by ambulance due to symptoms arousing suspicion of acute coronary syndrome. Med Sci Monit 2002;8:CR251–CR256.

21. Coutinho WF. The obese older female patient: CV risk and the SCOUT study. Int J Obes 2007;31:S26–S30.

22. Hølund U, Boysen G, Charles P, et al. Sygdomsforebyggelse i almen praksis. Gøres der forskel på kvinder og mænd? En spørgeskemaundersøgelse. Ugeskr Læger 1999;161(1):43–8. Hølund U, Boysen G, Charles P, et al. Praktiserende lægers holdning til kønnets og kostens betydning ved sygdomsforebyggelse. Ugeskr Læger 1999;161(1): 40–3.

23. Anderson C, Peterson CB, Fletcher L, et al. Weight loss and gender: an examination of physician attitudes. Obes Res 2001;9:257–63.

24. Wee CC, McCarthy EP, Davis RB, et al. Screening for cervical breast cancer: is obesity an unrecognized barrier to preventive care? Ann Intern Med 2000;132:697–704.

25. Brandsma L. Physician and patient attitudes toward obesity. Eating Disord 2005;13:201–11.

26. Gortmaker SL, Must A, Perrin JM, et al. Social and economic consequences of overweight in adolescence and young adulthood. N Engl J Med 1993;329(14):1008–12.

27. Sarlio-Lahteenkorva S, Lahelma E. The association of body mass index with social and economic disadvantage in women and men. Int J Epidemiol 1999;28(3):445–9.

28. Sarlio-lähteenkorva S. Relative weight and income at different levels of socioeconomic status. Am J Pub Health 2004;94(3):468–72.

29. Janssen I, Craig WM, Boyce WF, et al. Associations between overweight and obesity with bullying behaviors in school-aged children. Pediatrics 2004;113(5):1187–94.

30. Neumark-Sztainer D, Falkner N, Story M, et al. Weight-teasing among adolescents: correlations with weight status and disordered eating behaviors. Int J Obes 2002;26(1):123–31.

31. Pearce MJ, Boergers J, Prinstein MJ. Adolescent obesity, overt and relational peer victimization, and romantic relationships. Obes Res 2002;10(5):386–93.

32. Strauss RS, Pollack HA. Social marginalization of overweight children. Arch Pediatr Adolesc Med 2003;157(8):746–52.

33. Schwartz MB, Puhl R. Childhood obesity: a societal problem to solve. Obes Rev 2003;4(1):57–71.

34. Latner JD, Stunkard AJ. Getting worse: the stigmatization of obese children. Obes Res 2002;11(3):452–6.

35. Hayden-Wade HA, Stein RI, Ghaderi A, et al. Prevalence, characteristics, and correlates of teasing experiences among overweight children vs. non-overweight peers. Obes Res 2005;13(8):1381–92.

36. Franklin J, Steinbeck KSS, Booth M, Hill AJ, Caterson IDC. Obes Rev 2006;7(suppl 2):77.

37. Falkner NH, French SA, Jeffery RW, et al. Mistreatment due to weight: prevalence and sources of perceived mistreatment in women and men. Obes Res 1999;7(6):572–6.

38. Crandall CS. Do parents discriminate against their heavyweight daughters? Person Soc Psychol Bull 1995;21(7):724–35.

39. Crandall CS. Do heavy-weight students have more difficulty paying for college? Person Soc Psychol Bull 1991;17(6):606–11.

40. Falkner NH, Neumark-Sztainer D, Story M, et al. Social, educational, and psychological correlates of weight status in adolescents. Obes Res 2001;9(1):32–42.

41. Fabricatore AN, Wadden TA. Psychological aspects of obesity. Clin Dermatol 2004;22(4):332–7.

42. Stunkard AJ, Faith MS, Allison KC. Depression and obesity. Biol Psychiatr 2003;54:330–7.

43. Strauss RS. Childhood obesity and self-esteem. Pediatrics 2000;105(1):e15.

44. Sullivan M, Karlsson J, Sjöström L, et al. Swedish Obese Subjects (SOS). An intervention study of obesity. Baseline evaluation of health and psychosocial functioning in the first 1743 subjects examined. Int J Obes 1993;17:503–12.

45. Heo M, Allison DB, Faith MS, et al. Obesity and quality of life: Mediating effects of pain and comorbidities. Obs Res 2003;11: 209–16.

46. Currie C, Roberts C, Morgan A. *Young People's Health in Context. Health Behaviour in School-Aged Children: A WHO Cross-National Collaborative Study (HBSC)*. Copenhagen: WHO, 2004.

47. Heitmann BL, Tang-Peronard J. Psychosocial issues in female obesity. Women's Health 2007;3:271–3.

48. Puhl RM, Brownell KD. Psychosocial origins of obesity stigma: toward changing a powerful and pervasive bias. Obes Rev 2003;4:213–27.

49. Storch EA, Milsom VA, Debraganza N, et al. Peer victimization, psychosocial adjustment, and physical activity in overweight and at-risk-for-overweight youth. J Pediatr Psychol 2006;32(1):80–9.

50. Eisenberg ME, Neumark-Sztainer D, Story M. Associations of weight-based teasing and emotional well-being among adolescents. Arch Pediatr Adolesc Med 2003;157(8):733–8.

51. French SA, Story M, Perry CL. Self-esteem and obesity in children and adolescents: a literature review. Obes Res 1995;3(5):479–90.

52. Rich-Edwards JW, Goldman MB, Willett WC, et al. Adolescent body mass index and infertility caused by ovulatory disorder. Am J Obstet Gynecol 1994;171:171–7.

53. Wang JX, Davies M, Norman RJ. Body mass and probability of pregnancy during assisted reproduction treatment: retrospective study. BMJ 2000;321:1320–1.

54. Ehrmann DA. Polycystic ovary syndrome. N Engl J Med 2005;352:1223–36.
55. Azziz R, Carmina E, Dewailly D, et al. Criteria for defining polycystic ovary syndrome as a predominantly hyperandrogenic syndrome: an androgen excess society guideline. J Clin Endocrinol Metab 2006;91:4237–45.
56. Bellver J, Rossal LP, Bosch E. Obesity and the risk of spontaneous abortion after oocyte donation. Fertil Steril 2003;79:1136–40.
57. Sebire NJ, Jolly M, Harris JP, et al. Maternal obesity and pregnancy outcome: a study of 287 213 pregnancies in London. Int J Obes 2001;25:1175–82.
58. Nuthalampaty FS, Rouse DJ. The impact of obesity on obstetrical practice and outcome. Clin Obstet Gynecol 2004;47:898–913.
59. Cnattingius S, Lambe M. Trends in smoking and overweight during pregnancy: prevalence, risks of pregnancy complications, and adverse pregnancy outcomes. Semin Perinatol 2002;26:286–95.
60. Diamanti-Kandarakis E. Insulin resistance in PCOS. Endocrine 2006;30:13–17.
61. Reilly JJ, Armstrong J, Dorosty AR, et al. Avon early life risk factors for obesity in childhood: cohort study. BMJ 2005;330:1357–9.
62. Ryan D. Obesity in women: a life cycle of medical risk, Int J Obes 2007;31:S3–S7.
63. Eriksson J, Forsen T, Toumilehto J. Size at birth, childhood growth and obesity in adult life. Int J Obes 2001;25:735–40.
64. Surkan PJ, Hsieh CC, Joansson ALV, et al. Reasons for increasing trends in large for gestational age births. Obstet Gynecol 2004;104:720–6.
65. Silverman BL, Metzger BE, Cho NH. Impaired glucose tolerance in adolescent offspring of diabetic mothers. Relationship to fetal hyperinsulinism. Diabetes Care 1995;18:611–17.
66. Pettitt DJ, Baird HR, Aleck KA. Excessive obesity in offspring of Pima Indian women with diabetes during pregnancy. N Engl J Med 1983;308:242–5.
67. Niemi I (ed). *Time Use of Women in Europe and North America*. New York: United Nations, 1995;1–22.

2 Biology of Obesity

Energy Balance and Body Weight Homeostasis

Abdul G. Dulloo

Department of Medicine and Physiology, Institute of Physiology, University of Fribourg, Switzerland

Introduction

Obesity is often considered to result from the failure of homeostatic mechanisms that regulate body weight to cope with an environment that encourages overeating and sedentary. In addressing the issue of the "biology of obesity," it is therefore pertinent to raise the question of whether body weight is indeed a regulated variable. Because large variations in body fat can be observed both between and within individuals, it could be argued that body weight is a poorly regulated variable. By contrast, the fact that in many individuals, body weight remains relatively constant over years and decades, in spite of large day-to-day variations in the amount of food consumed, might instead suggest that body weight is precisely regulated in these individuals. But constancy of body weight *per se* is not evidence for regulation. A critical feature of any regulated system is that disturbance of the regulated variable results in compensatory responses that tend to attenuate the disturbance and to restore the system to its "set" or "preferred" value. The direct application of this approach to testing whether body weight is regulated in human beings is difficult because of ethical and practical reasons, but observations on adults recovering from food shortages during postwar famine or from experimental starvation indicates that a return to normal body weight is eventually achieved. Conversely, excess weight gained during experimental overeating or during pregnancy is subsequently lost, and most individuals return to their initial body weight. There is therefore little doubt that regulation of body weight occurs, albeit with varying degrees of precision.

How such long-term weight regulation is achieved in humans is the focus of this chapter. To address this question, it is first important to underscore the basic concepts and principles about the flux of energy transformations through which body weight is regulated.

Clinical Obesity in Adults and Children, 3rd edition. Edited by Peter G. Kopelman, Ian D. Caterson and William H. Dietz.
© 2010 Blackwell Publishing, ISBN: 978-1-4051-8226-3.

Basic concepts and principles in human energetics

Energy balance and laws of thermodynamics

Life exists in a flux of energy transformations which are governed by the laws of thermodynamics. According to the *first law*, energy cannot be created or destroyed but can only be transformed from one form into another. Biologic systems, like machines, depend on the transformation of some form of energy in order to perform work. The chemical energy obtained from foods (plant or animal in origin) is used to perform a variety of work, such as in the synthesis of new macromolecules (*chemical work*), in muscular contraction (*mechanical work*) or in the maintenance of ionic gradients across membranes (*electrical work*). The intermediate steps in this flux of energy transformations between food and heat production are illustrated in Figure 6.1, and are embodied in the following energy balance equation:

Energy intake = Energy expenditure + Δ Energy stores

where energy intake refers to the metabolizable energy intake, i.e. the energy available to perform work after taking into account losses in feces and urine (see Fig. 6.1) and Δ Energy stores represents any change in the body's store of energy.

Thus, if the total energy contained in the body (as fat, protein and glycogen) of a given individual is not altered (i.e. Δ Energy stores = 0), then energy expenditure must be equal to energy intake, in keeping with the first law of thermodynamics. In this case, the individual is said to be in a *state of energy balance*. If the intake and expenditure of energy are not equal, then a change in body energy content will occur, with *negative energy balance* resulting in the degradation of the body's energy stores (glycogen, fat and protein) or *positive energy balance* resulting in an increase in body energy stores, primarily as fat. The first law of thermodynamics, however, overlooks the possible inter-relationships between energy intake and energy expenditure. It does not illustrate that voluntary energy intake may rise with intense physical

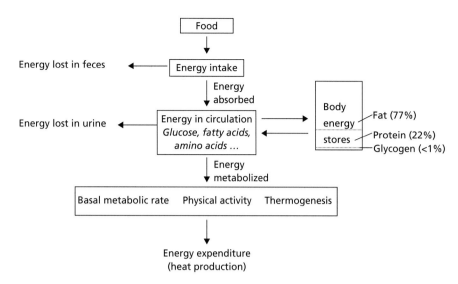

Figure 6.1 Principles of energy balance, within a schematic framework that depicts the transformation of energy from food to heat through the body. Note that on diets typically consumed in developed countries, the total energy losses in feces and urine are small (about 5%), so that the metabolizable energy available from these diets is about 95%.

activity (competition athletes eat more than sedentary clerks), that energy expenditure may increase in response to increased food intake, nor that both energy intake and energy expenditure can be influenced by changes in body energy stores. It is merely concerned with initial and final states.

The *second law* of thermodynamics, by contrast, makes a subtle distinction between the potential energy of food, useful work and heat. It states that when food is utilized in the body, whether for muscular contraction, synthesis of new tissues or maintenance of electrolyte equilibrium across membranes, these processes must be accompanied inevitably by a loss of heat. In thermodynamic terms, some energy is degraded, and such heat energy which is no longer available for work is termed "entropy." In other words, the conversion of available food energy is not a perfectly efficient process: about 75% of the chemical energy contained in foods may be ultimately dissipated as heat because of the inefficiency of intermediary metabolism in transforming food energy into a form (e.g. adenosine triphosphate, ATP) which can be used for work, whether it be the internal work required to maintain structure and function or external physical work (i.e. work performed on the environment). Thus, all the energy used by the body at rest is ultimately lost as heat, and physical (external) work will also be eventually degraded as heat. These theoretical considerations constitute the framework of a biologic system in which changes in energy intake and expenditure can oppose changes in energy balance and body weight.

Pattern of food intake and energy expenditure

Humans eat food in a discontinuous mode, and the amount of food eaten can range from zero to up to 21 MJ/day in highly active individuals or during acute episodes of hyperphagia. This contrasts with energy expenditure which is continuous irrespective of the conditions encountered. This irregularity of food behavior occurs within-day and between-days, the latter explaining the 2–3 times greater coefficient of variation for energy intake (15–20%) than for energy expenditure (5–8%). This also explains the

difficulties with which food intake is assessed in order to obtain a representative picture of "habitual" food (energy) intake. In addition, the wide variety of feeding behavior makes it tremendously difficult to track adequately both of these factors and this jeopardizes the interpretation of data on food intake. Since many factors can lead to underestimation or overestimation of energy intake, and hence lead to a bias in energy balance, it is therefore not surprising that energy requirements are based preferentially on estimates of energy expenditure rather than on energy intake.

Components of energy expenditure

It is customary to consider human energy expenditure as being made up of three components: the energy spent for basal metabolism (or basal metabolic rate), the energy spent on physical activity, and the increase in resting energy expenditure in response to a variety of stimuli (including food, cold, stress and drugs). These three components are depicted in Figure 6.1 and are described below.

Basal metabolic rate (BMR)

This is the largest component of energy expenditure for most individuals. Typically in developed countries, BMR accounts for 60–75% of daily energy expenditure. It is measured under standardized conditions, i.e. in an awake subject lying in the supine position, in a state of physical and mental rest in a confortable warm environment, and in the morning in the postabsorptive state, usually 10–12 hours after the last meal. These conditions are referred to as "basal" as they should reflect the energy needed for the work of vital functions (maintaining electrolyte equilibrium across cell membranes, cell and protein turnover, respiratory and cardiovascular functions, etc.). BMR is greater than the metabolic rate during sleep by 5–20%, this difference between BMR and sleeping metabolic rate being explained by the effect of arousal.

By far the most important determinant of BMR is body size, and in particular the fat-free mass of the body which is influenced by weight, height, age and gender. On average, men have greater

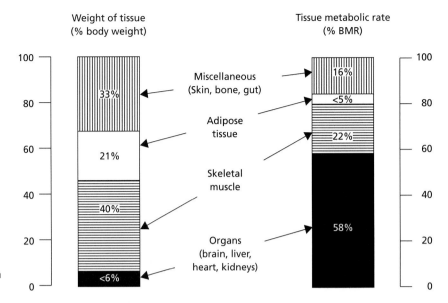

Weight of tissue
(% body weight)

Tissue metabolic rate
(% BMR)

Miscellaneous
(Skin, bone, gut)

Adipose
tissue

Skeletal
muscle

Organs
(brain, liver,
heart, kidneys)

Figure 6.2 Contribution of organ/tissues to BMR) of a nonobese man. Note that the organs contribute <6% of body weight but that their contribution to BMR is disproportionately high (>50% BMR). (Adapted from Elia [67].)

fat-free mass and BMR than women even for the same age, weight and height, and older people have lower fat-free mass and BMR than young adults. Most, but not all, of the differences in BMR between these groups disappear when BMR is expressed as a function of fat-free-mass. This is not surprising since fat-free mass contains tissues and organs which have high metabolic activities such as liver, kidneys, heart, and to a lesser extent the resting muscles (Fig. 6.2). In contrast, the contribution of adipose mass to BMR is small. In a non-obese subject, adipose tissue contributes to 3–5% of the total resting energy expenditure, although it represents 20–30% of total body weight. The majority of the heat production (about 60%) comes from the active organs (liver, kidney, heart and brain), although they account for only 5 to 6% of total body weight. The resting heat production of skeletal muscle per unit mass is 15–40 times lower than that of metabolically organs, but because of its large size (more than half of the total fat-free mass) it makes a significant contribution (~20%) to BMR.

Energy expenditure due to physical activity

The energy spent on physical activity depends on the type and intensity of the physical activity and on the time spent in different activities. Physical activity is often considered to be synonymous with "muscular work" which has a strict definition in physics, i.e. force x distance, during which external work is performed on the environment. During muscular work (muscle contraction), the muscle produces 3–4 times more heat than mechanical energy. There is a wide variation in the energy cost of any activity both within and between individuals. The latter variation is due to differences in body size and in the speed and dexterity with which an activity is performed. In order to adjust for differences in body size, the energy costs of physical activities are expressed as multiples of BMR [1]. These generally range from 1 to 5 for most activities, but can reach values between 10 and 14

during intense exercise. In terms of daily energy expenditure, physical activity can represent up to 70% of daily energy expenditure in an individual involved in heavy manual work or competition athletics. For most individuals in industrialized societies, however, the contribution of physical activity to daily energy expenditure is much lower −10–25% of daily energy expenditure.

Energy expenditure in response to various thermogenic stimuli

This component of energy expenditure – often referred to as "thermogenesis" – is best described by the various forms in which it can exist. These have been described by Miller [2] as follows.

• *Isometric thermogenesis:* this is due to increased muscle tension; no physical work is done in the physical sense. The differences in energy expenditure in a person who is lying, sitting or standing are due mainly to changes in muscle tone.

• *Dynamic thermogenesis:* the term "negative work" is used to describe heat production of stretched muscle, with heat being again produced without any work (being performed on the environment). For example, when someone goes down a ladder, heat production increases but there is no work inn the physical sense of work. Contracting muscles produce heat because of their inefficiency, but tensed and stretched muscles are simply thermogenic.

• *Psychological thermogenesis:* the psychologic state may affect energy expenditure, as anxiety, anticipation and stress stimulate adrenaline (or epinephrine) secretion, leading to increased heat production. A twofold difference can be found in the energy cost of sitting at ease and sitting playing chess, a difference that cannot entirely be attributed to muscular movement. The best evidence comes from a study on pilots whose energy expenditure increased when they were under air traffic control, with the rise being inversely related to their level of experience [3].

• *Cold-induced thermogenesis:* humans rarely need to increase heat production for the purpose of thermal regulation because they are able to seek an equitable environment or wear suitable clothing, i.e. their bodies are generally kept at thermoneutrality. At low temperatures, their resting metabolic rate (and hence heat production) increases. For example, normal-weight women maintained in identical clothing in a calorimeter room adjusted their 24-hour heat production by about 7% when the temperature in the calorimeter room was lowered from 28 to 22 °C [4]. It is customary to distinguish between two forms of cold-induced thermogenesis – shivering and nonshivering. Shivering is rhythmic muscle contraction, while nonshivering thermogenesis is increased heat production not associated with muscle contraction, and is due to increased activity of the sympathetic nervous system (particularly in brown adipose tissue (BAT) in small mammals). Nonshivering thermogenesis is inversely correlated with body size, age and ambient temperature and has been demonstrated to exist in adult human beings chronically exposed to extreme temperatures [5]. Recent evidence, albeit circumstantial, suggests that BAT may also contribute to nonshivering thermogenesis in adult humans.

• *Diet-induced thermogenesis:* heat production increases following the consumption of a meal, and this thermic effect of food is classically termed "specific dynamic action." Heat production also increases on a high plane of nutrition, the so-called "luxus-consumption." These two forms of thermogenesis related to food have been regrouped under the term "diet-induced thermogenesis" or DIT and are often divided into an *obligatory* component (related to the energy costs of absorption and metabolic processing of nutrients or the energy cost of tissue synthesis during overfeeding) and a *facultative* component which in part results from the sensory aspects of foods and in part from stimulation of the sympathetic nervous system.

• *Drug-induced thermogenesis:* the consumption of caffeine, nicotine and alcohol may form an integral part of daily life for many individuals, and all three "drugs of everyday life" stimulate thermogenesis. A cup of coffee (containing 60–80 mg caffeine) can increase BMR by 5–10% over an hour or two. Oral intake of 100 mg caffeine every 2 hours during the day and smoking a packet of 20 cigarettes increase daily energy expenditure by 5% and 15%, respectively. Furthermore, the thermogenic effects of nicotine are potentiated by caffeine. The cessation of elevated thermogenesis induced by nicotine or nicotine and caffeine is an important factor that contributes to the average weight gain of 7 kg after cessation of smoking.

Spontaneous physical activity and nonexercise activity thermogenesis

Another way to look at the components of energy expenditure is shown in Figure 6.3 where energy expenditure is divided into resting and nonresting expenditure, but also into voluntary and involuntary energy expenditure. Resting energy expenditure comprises all measurements of energy expenditure made at rest – BMR and the thermic effect of food – and which are beyond voluntary control. Nonresting energy expenditure is divided into voluntary and involuntary physical activities. Voluntary physical activity comprises volitional activities such as exercise and sports as well as occupational activities (going to work and performing work duties) and leisure activities (e.g. gardening). Involuntary physical activity comprises spontaneous and subconscious fidgeting and posture maintenance, and is referred to as spontaneous physical activity (SPA). SPA is an important component of "nonexercise activity thermogenesis" or NEAT – the latter being defined as the energy expended for all physical activities other than volitional exercise and sports activities. NEAT is therefore not limited solely to SPA but also includes energy expended for "voluntary" occupational and leisure-time activities [6,7]. The potential importance of variations in SPA and NEAT in body weight regulation is discussed below.

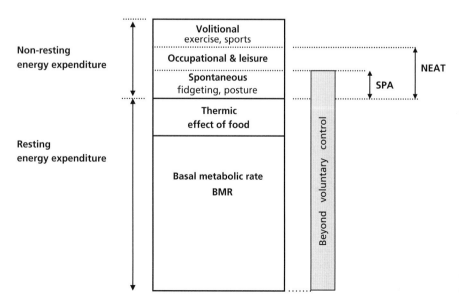

Figure 6.3 Components of energy expenditure contributing to voluntary and involuntary control of energy expenditure (see text for details). SPA, spontaneous physical activity; NEAT, nonexercise activity thermogenesis.

Timescale of energy balance

As mentioned in the introduction, there is little doubt that regulation of body weight occurs in human beings (albeit with varying degrees of precision), although the time-scale over which it occurs is not clear. In this context, it is important to emphasize the cardinal features of human energy balance and weight regulation.

• Human beings do not balance energy intake and energy expenditure on a day-to-day basis nor is positive energy balance one day spontaneously compensated by negative energy balance the next day. Near equality of intake and expenditure most often appears over 1–2 weeks. Longer measurements are difficult to conduct and impractical because of cumulative errors, but there is no doubt that over months and years, total energy intake and expenditure must be very close in any individual whose body weight and body composition have remained relatively constant.

• This matching of long-term energy intake and energy expenditure must be extremely precise since a theoretical error of only 1% between input and output of energy, if persistent, will lead to a gain or loss of about 10 kg per decade. But this does not occur for many individuals, whose weights remain relatively constant within a few kg over several decades.

• Even in adults who apparently maintain a stable body weight over months, years and decades, there is in reality no "absolute" constancy of body weight. Instead, when examined over years and decades, body weight tends to fluctuate or oscillate around a constant mean value.

Understanding how these short-term deviations in body weight are corrected through changes in energy intake, in energy expenditure, or in both, still remains a challenging issue for human research today. In such a dynamic state within which weight homeostasis occurs, it is likely that long-term constancy of body weight is achieved through a highly complex network of autoregulatory control systems and subsystems through which changes in food intake, body composition and energy expenditure are interlinked.

Control of food intake

Hunger and satiety

Research into the control of energy intake in humans is very difficult, primarily because habitual intake is not easy to measure and because the intake of foods is altered by the experiments themselves. Because of these difficulties, much of the work carried out in humans has been concerned with short-term hunger and appetite studies or with short-term satiety and satiation [8,9].

It is important to differentiate between these terms. Hunger may be defined as a "demand for calories" (e.g. after starvation), while appetite refers to "a demand for a particular food." In laboratory animals allowed *ad libitum* access to standard laboratory chow, energy intake is controlled mainly by the sensations of hunger and satiety. If (like human beings) the laboratory rat has access to a variety of palatable foods rather than to a monotonous

diet, it may be stimulated to eat something delicious by appetite rather than by hunger. The physiologic mechanisms which control energy intake in the rat certainly exist in humans. If a person is deprived of food, they become hungry, and if they have eaten a lot, they become satiated. *Satiation* refers to processes involved in the termination of a meal, and is studied by providing individuals with test meals and measuring the amount consumed when the food is freely available. *Satiety* refers to the ongoing inhibition of further intake of a food after eating has ended. However, lifestyle factors ensure that appetite is a powerful but poorly controlled stimulus to eat even when an individual is not hungry because feeding patterns are influenced strongly by psychologic, economic and social factors. Even though subjects may feel satiated by one particular food, they will continue to eat when a new food is presented – a phenomenon that is referred to as "sensory-specific satiety." Conversely, when subjects are presented with a monotonous diet, their intakes are usually low. Among some communities living in developing countries, the major part of energy intake derives from one staple food, which together with low fat intakes constitutes a bland and monotonous diet, so that even when supplies are adequate, obesity is rarely seen. These observations suggest that when the psychosocial incentives to eat are removed, human beings (like the laboratory rat fed a chow diet) can control food intake quite precisely.

Hunger and satiety control centers in the brain

Much of our understanding about centers in the brain that are involved with the control of food intake derives from studies conducted in laboratory animal models. As a result of numerous experiments involving ablation, electrical and chemical stimulation of specific areas in the brain, it has been proposed that "centers" localized in the hypothalamus are involved in the control of feeding behavior. In particular, the ventromedial hypothalamic (VMH) region has been implicated in satiety, the lateral hypothalamic (LH) region in the initiation of feeding, and the paraventricular nucleus (PVN) of the rostral hypothalamus is thought to be important in initiating the cessation of the meal. These "centers" serve to analyze and integrate afferent signals that are neural (via the vagal nerve) or circulatory (via nutrients and hormones). Although these centers have received a great deal of attention, it is now apparent that this approach represents a rather simplistic view because many other hypothalamic and extrahypothalamic areas also play a major role in the control of food intake [10]. Nonetheless, the molecular and genetic studies which followed the discovery of leptin in 1994 have led to major advancements in elucidating the neurochemical basis for the activities of some of these centers [11,12]. In particular, the identification of the two subpopulations of neurons in the arcuate (ARC)–PVN pathway (NPY/AgRP neurons and POMC/CART neurons) and the identification of melanin-concentrating hormone (MCH) and orexin in the LH neurons have provided neurochemical insight into the function of these sites (depicted in Fig. 6.4), as follows:

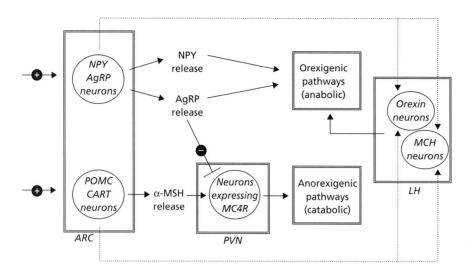

Figure 6.4 Hypothalamic circuits implicated in the control of food intake depicting (see text for details): ARC, arcuate nucleus; PVN, paraventricular nucleus; LH, lateral hypothalamus.

• The NPY/AgRP neurons, which co-express NPY (neuropeptide Y) and AgRP (agouti-related peptide) are orexigenic, i.e. their activation stimulates food intake.

• By contrast, the POMC/CART neurons are anorexigenic, i.e. their activation reduces food intake. POMC (pro-opiomelanocortin) is cleaved into melanocortins, including α-melanocyte stimulating hormone (α-MSH), which exerts anorexigenic action via melanocortin-4 receptors (Mc4r) and, to a lesser extent, via Mc3r. Most arcuate nucleus POMC neurons also express cocaine and amphetamine-related transcript (CART).

• All these neurons project to other regions of the hypothalamus where further signal processing occurs, and in particular in the LH area to populations of neurons expressing melanin-concentrating hormone (MCH) and orexins A and B, all peptides that are orexigenic.

There are also extensive reciprocal connections between the hypothalamus and the brainstem, and food intake is co-ordinated on the basis of information received by both regions. In the brainstem, the nucleus of the solitary tract (NST), area postrema, and dorsal motor nucleus of the vagus have all been implicated in the control of food intake and weight homeostasis [10]. These pathways respond to afferent signals from other hypothalamic/extrahypothalamic regions and from the periphery.

Hunger and satiety signals from the periphery

The sensations of hunger and satiety result from the central integration of numerous signals originating from a variety of peripheral tissues and organs, including the gastrointestinal tract, liver, pancreas, adipose tissue, and perhaps also skeletal muscle. The putative hunger and satiety signaling systems that have generated the most interests are outlined below.

Signals from the gastrointestinal tract

The progression of food through the stomach and small intestine, which can be considered as a short-term nutrient reservoir,

initiates a number of sequential peripheral satiety signals that are thought to be important in influencing meal-to-meal feeding responses [13,14]. Signals from stretch- and mechano-receptors that respond to gatric distension or from chemoreceptors that respond to the products of digestion (sugars, fatty acids, amino acids and peptides) are transmitted via vagal afferent nerves to the brainstem [14]. These neural signals are centrally integrated with those transmitted by a number of hormones released from the gastrointestinal system. These gut hormones then stimulate afferent (ascending) vagal pathways from the gut to the brainstem or act directly on neurons in the brain to mediate short-term feelings of hunger and satiety [13]. Among endocrine signals from the gut that are believed to exert important influences on food intake are:

• *cholecystokinin* (CCK) (the first gut hormone shown to influence food intake), which is released from the small intestine into the circulation in response to luminal nutrients; it decreases meal size

• *peptides* that are released postprandially and reduce appetite in humans, including gastric inhibitory peptide (GIP), glucagon-like peptide-1 (GLP-1) and PYY, the peptide YY(3-36)

• ghrelin, which is secreted by the stomach, and whose concentration increases after food deprivation and decreases in response to the presence of nutrients in the stomach.

Ghrelin is the only known circulating factor to increase hunger. This "hunger hormone" is a powerful stimulator of feeding and can induce obesity when given chronically to rodents through its modulation of NPY, AgRP and melanocortin systems in the arcuate–PVN axis [12]. Like ghrelin, GLP-1 and PYY(3-36) can also directly stimulate anorexigenic pathways in the hypothalamus and brainstem. In contrast, CCK reduces food intake and inhibits gastric emptying through action on CCK1 receptors and afferent vagal information passing to the brainstem regions of the central nervous system (CNS). A physiologic role for CCK1 in the control of meal size is suggested by the hyperphagia and obesity seen in rats that have a natural deletion of the gene for

CCK1 [15]. Although there is some evidence that ghrelin, GLP-1 and PYY (3-36) can also signal to the brainstem through the vagal nerve, the physiologic relevance of such vagal signalling by gut hormone systems other than CCK is less certain.

Aminostatic or protein-static signals

A link between fluctuations in serum amino acids and food intake was proposed nearly 50 years ago [16] and this topic has been reviewed more recently by Bray [17]. Dietary protein induces satiety in the short term, and consumption of low-protein diets leads to increased appetite for protein-containing foods. Administration of amino acids such as phenylalanine and tryptophan (which are precursors of monoamine neurotransmitters) leads to reduced food intake, and the ratio of plasma tryptophan to other amino acids affects brain serotonin, which is known to have an inhibitory influence on food intake. These observations lead to an *aminostatic* theory which states that food intake is determined by the level of plasma amino acids, and that this could be related to the regulation of lean body mass, which is known to be rigorously defended against experimental or dietary manipulation. A "protein-stat" mechanism for the regulation of lean body mass has been proposed by Millward [18] and draws support from the fact that food intake during growth is known to be dominated by the impetus for lean tissue deposition.

Glucostatic and glycogenostatic signals

A glucostatic theory for the regulation of feeding behavior was also proposed some 50 years ago [19]. It suggested that there were chemoreceptors in the hypothalamic satiety center which would be sensitive to the arteriovenous difference in glucose or to the availability and utilization of glucose. The arguments in favor of this hypothesis in humans include the small decreases of blood glucose observed prior to spontaneous meal consumption, the suppression of food intake induced by infusion of glucose, and the spontaneous decrease in total energy intake observed when dietary carbohydrate content is increased. These same arguments in support of the glucostatic theory of food intake also form the basis of the proposal of Flatt [20] that the control of food intake, via the prevention of hypoglycemia and maintainance of adequate glycogen levels, primarily serves the maintenance of the carbohydrate balance.

Lipostatic and adiposity signals

A lipostatic theory of food intake control, first proposed by Kennedy [21], postulates that substances released from the fat stores function as satiety signals. This theory is based on a set-point control system with body fat (rather than body weight) acting as the regulated variable and energy intake the controlled variable. Body fat is thus maintained at a set value, and any deviation from this value is detected by the controller of the system (the hypothalamus) via a circulating metabolite (the error signal) which is related to the size of the fat stores. Having detected such a deviation, the controller elicits compensatory changes in energy intake and hence restores the system to its preset or preferred level. The lipostatic hypothesis is perhaps the one that provides the most plausible explanation for long-term regulation of the fat stores. Many experiments support this theory, leading to the suggestion that humans who are predisposed to obesity may have a homeostatic mechanism in which the set-point for weight regulation is set at a higher level than those who are more resistant to obesity. The nature of the various components, such as the set-point and feedback signal(s), involved in the lipostatic theory as yet remains unclear.

A major advance came in the mid 1990s following the cloning of the *ob* gene, whose protein product (leptin) is primarily produced by adipocytes, released into the circulation and acts on hypothalamic receptors to induce satiety by inhibiting the orexigenic NPY/AgRP neurons and stimulating the anorexigenic POMC/CART neurons [11,12] (see Fig. 6.4; Fig. 6.5). Brain-specific deletion of the leptin receptor, like in leptin-deficient *ob/ob* mice, leads to obesity [22]. Conversely, the obesity phenotype of the *db/db* mice, which lack functional leptin receptors, is rescued by brain-specific re-expression of leptin receptors [23]. Rare people with mutations causing complete leptin deficiency,

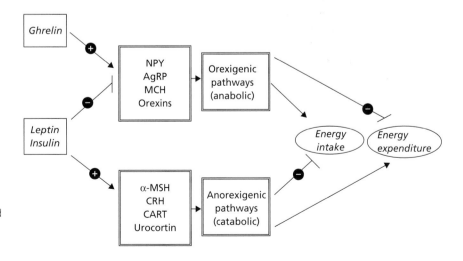

Figure 6.5 Neuropeptides implicated in co-ordinated effects on both energy intake and energy expenditure (see text for details).

as in the *ob/ob* mice, show marked hyperphagia and severe obesity, which can be reversed by administration of small doses of leptin. The rare people with mutations affecting the leptin receptor mechanism, like the *db/db* mice, also show hyperphagia and severe obesity but do not respond to the administration of leptin. In other rare cases of severe childhood-onset obesity, single gene defects have been identified for genes which code for proteins that act downstream to leptin receptor in the hypothalamic neural circuits (see Fig. 6.4), in particular for POMC and MC4R [24].

In the vast majority of humans tested, however, the blood concentration of leptin was found to be proportional to the adipose mass. Its elevation in the obese has led to the hypothesis that resistance to the action of leptin is a factor in obesity, possibly because of diminished access of circulating leptin to target areas of the brain and impairments in intracellular leptin signaling [25]. However, because blood leptin concentration varies widely in individuals with the same degree of obesity, the possibility arises that subpopulations might have relative leptin deficiency. Support for this notion can be derived from the fact that relatives of leptin-deficient patients, who are heterozygous for leptin deficiency, exhibit modest obesity and leptin levels below that expected for their increased fat mass [26]. With more recent data in animals suggesting that leptin actions go beyond known hypothalamic targets to modulate the sensitivity of taste receptor cells in the oral cavity, vagal mechanoreceptors in the gut, olfactory detection in the olfactory bulb, and visual perception of food, it thus appears that leptin can gate food-related sensory input signals even at early stages of processing [27].

There has also been considerable interest in the role of insulin as an adiposity signal (since it is secreted by the pancreas in proportion to adiposity) in the control of food intake via the CNS. Insulin stimulates leptin release from adipose tissue and leads to postprandial increases in circulating leptin [28]. Like leptin, insulin also circulates at levels proportional to body fat content and enters the CNS (in proportion to its plasma level) where it interacts with autonomic circuits which control meal size, including, as indicated in Figure 6.5, via inhibition of NPY/AgRP neurons and stimulation of POMC/CART neurons [11]. Targeted deletion of the insulin receptor in neurons leads to obesity in mice [29], albeit to a much lesser extent compared to the severe obesity resulting from deletion of leptin receptors [22].

It should be noted that although leptin/insulin levels and fat mass are correlated in the fed state, their rapid fall in starvation and rapid restoration on refeeding suggest that changes in circulating leptin and insulin are independent of the dynamics of acute changes in body fat content. Their circulating levels may therefore be a function of changes in the flux of energy intake (coupled with fat mobilization/storage) rather than a "lipostatic" signal whose level is altered as a function of the degree of depletion and repletion of the fat stores. Within the context of food intake control based upon the defense of the fat stores, both the feedback signal(s) on food intake and the nature of the set-point (if it exists) remain elusive.

Hepatic nutrient metabolism signals

A role for hepatic metabolism in the control of food intake was advocated in the 1960s [30] and it now appears that a common pathway leading from nutrient metabolism to ATP production and cell membrane polarity changes may be involved in the signaling mechanism [31,32]. The notion that hepatic oxidation of fatty acids plays a role in the control of food intake is based upon studies in rat, mouse and humans showing that pharmacologic inhibition of fatty acid oxidation leads to an increase in food intake which, in the rat, has been shown to be attenuated by hepatic branch vagotomy [33]. It would appear therefore that a feeding modulatory signal derived from fatty acid oxidation in abdominal tissues (like in the liver) is conveyed to the brain by vagal afferents. However, in contrast to the stimulatory effect of feeding produced by inhibition of fatty acid oxidation, the evidence for a suppressive effect of feeding by stimulation of fatty acid oxidation is inconsistent and comparatively weak.

Exercise-related signals

More recently, a role for exercise in the control of food intake has been proposed on the basis of studies in rats indicating that signals generated by the exercising body can feed back on the brain to regulate central neuropeptide systems involved in the control of hunger and appetite [34]. Unlike the changes in gene expression of NPY and POMC observed during caloric restriction of sedentary rats which brings them to levels of adiposity seen in exercising rats, the reduced adiposity associated with exercise fails to alter the expression of these peptides despite considerable lowering of plasma leptin levels. These data suggest that exercise provides some unknown signal/s to the brain that allow rats to over-ride the usually potent stimulation of orexigenic NPY and inhibition of anorexigenic POMC expression provided by the lowering of leptin levels during weight loss. As a result, they fail to compensate for reduced adiposity by increasing their caloric intake, and they defend their adiposity at a new lower set-point. In humans, the few who succeed in maintaining weight after slimming report high levels of physical activity, but whether such exercises may, in addition to their effects in raising energy expenditure, also have a direct role in limiting the hyperphagic drive that follows weight loss is unknown. Similarly, the peripheral exercise-related signals that feed back to brain centers that control food intake remain ill defined, although muscle-derived interleukin-6 and lactate, as well as adipose-derived fatty acids, may be implicated [34].

Impact of peripheral signals on brain higher centers

Although the classic signals from the periphery, such as leptin, insulin, gut hormones, and circulating nutrients themselves, act mainly on a few specific areas of the brain such as the hypothalamus and brainstem, recent studies suggest that these metabolic signals have a much broader influence on brain function [10,35]. The adiposity signals leptin and insulin can also act directly on mesolimbic dopamine neurons to modulate wanting of food and reward signals. The gut hormone PYY(3-36), which suppresses food intake in humans and rodents, also modulates activity in the ventral tegmental area and ventral striatum, and hence impinges upon the brain pleasure and reward circuits. Ghrelin also appears to facilitate foraging behavior and increases reward processing as part of its orexigenic actions. Furthermore, modern neuroimaging studies support the importance of a balance in distinct areas of the prefrontal cortex in the control of food intake. As reviewed by Zheng and Berthoud [35], successful dieters who have higher levels of dietary restraint compared to nondieters show increased neural activity in the right dorsolateral prefrontal cortex in response to food consumption. In contrast, obese subjects show less activation of the left dorsolateral prefrontal cortex in response to food, while patients with the Prader–Willi syndrome, who show severe disturbances in appetite control resulting in hyperphagia and obesity, show increased activity in the ventromedial prefrontal cortex when viewing pictures of food after glucose consumption. Thus, it is clear that leptin and gut hormones do not only act on the "energy balance" control circuits in the hypothalamus and brainstem, but in addition impinge on corticolimbic systems involved in cognitive, reward, and executive brain functions important for ingestive and exercise behavior, particularly in our modern environment.

Integrated models of food intake control

The various hunger and satiety signals from the periphery can be integrated into models in which the control of food intake is considered in three phases, each with a distinct goal.

1. *Short-term* (hour to hour): blood glucose homeostasis by dampening episodes of hypoglycemia or hyperglycemia.

2. *Medium-term* (day-to-day): maintenance of adequate hepatic stores of glycogen which, consistent with Flatt's glycogenostatic theory [20], would imply corrective responses to offset deviations from carbohydrate balance during the previous day.

3. *Long-term* (weeks, months or years): maintenance of the body's fat and protein compartments, i.e. fat mass and fat-free mass. Periods of food deprivation that lead to substantial reductions in body weight are normally followed by increased food intake (hyperphagia). Indeed, the reanalysis of data on food intake and body composition in humans subjected to experimental semi-starvation and refeeding in the classic Minnesota Experiment [36] suggests that the duration and magnitude of such compensatory hyperphagia is determined by three independent factors: the magnitude of fat loss, the magnitude of fat-free mass loss, and the severity of energy deprivation [37]. These findings are consistent with the existence of powerful signals that relate food intake to body composition as well as to psychobiologic reactions to the state of food deprivation. Conversely, in human overfeeding trials, subjects often report great difficulty in maintaining high levels of food intake over long periods of time, and they spontaneously lose weight over subsequent weeks and months, apparently by eating less.

The nutrient balance model

According to the model proposed by Flatt [20], the long-term stability of body weight and body composition requires not only that energy expenditure is equal to energy intake, but also that the composition of the fuel mix which is oxidized relates to that which is ingested. Since the protein and carbohydrate stores in the body are limited, they tend to be modulated by an autoregulatory process, allowing an increase in their own oxidation in response to an increase in exogenous supply. In contrast, the stores of fat are not well regulated by fat oxidation since an increase in dietary fat does not promote its own oxidation. Hence (unlike carbohydrate and protein) fat balance is not precisely regulated. The failure to adjust fat oxidation in response to excess intake will contribute to depletion of glycogen stores by increasing carbohydrate oxidation, with consequent negative feedback on total energy intake. In other words, the size of carbohydrate stores exerts negative feedback on total energy intake, so that high-fat diets (containing little carbohydrate) will promote excess energy intake to reach an appropriate level of carbohydrate intake. This energy imbalance would persist until the fat stores build up sufficiently to provide a greater supply for fat oxidation. When the higher fat oxidation matches the higher intake, the individual would then be both in fat balance and in energy balance, but at a higher percentage of body fat. Indeed, many obese individuals have a significantly lower respiratory quotient (RQ) than lean people [38] and hence a greater proportion of their elevated energy expenditure is met by fat oxidation. The interpretation of this concept of nutrient balance is that the control of food intake can be viewed as both glycogenic (short-term) and lipostatic (long-term) and tends to integrate control of food intake via glycogenostatic and lipostatic signaling. Furthermore, it also explains the role of alcohol in substrate metabolism; alcohol disrupts nutrient balance by sparing fat from oxidation. It may also lead to overconsumption of energy since alcohol is generally consumed in addition to normal food intake.

This nutrient balance theory, which centers upon the need to maintain specific carbohydrate (glycogen) stores as a determinant of appetite, has been challenged by Stubbs [39]. In people fed a very low-carbohydrate (high-fat) diet to deplete the glycogen stores, appetite did not increase, and fat oxidation increased to meet energy needs. Furthermore, in human studies in which fat content was altered from 24% to 47% but the energy density of the diet maintained constant, there was no evidence of high-fat induced hyperphagia relative to high-carbohydrate feeding, indicating that the hyperphagia often associated with high-fat diets may not be due to the fat *per se*, but to the higher energy density (and hence lower volume and weight) that fat contributes to the diet. As Frayn [40] has argued, it is too simplistic to argue that protein, carbohydrate and fat balance can be considered independently, and that the complex relationships between fat and other constituents of foods in the control of appetite cannot be ignored.

Autoregulatory adjustments in energy expenditure

Whatever mechanisms operate for the control of food intake, however, this control is not by itself sufficient to explain long-term regulation of body weight and body composition. There is also ample evidence that autoregulatory adjustments in energy expenditure also play an important role in correcting deviations in body weight and body composition.

Beyond adaptation through mass action

There is in fact a built-in stabilizing mechanism in the overall homeostatic system for body weight. Any imbalance between energy intake and energy requirements will result in a change in body weight which, in turn, will alter the maintenance energy requirements in a direction tending to counter the original imbalance. This change would hence be stabilizing. The system thus exhibits *dynamic equilibrium*. For example, an increase in body weight will be predicted to increase metabolic rate (on the basis of the extra energy cost for synthesis and subsequent maintenance of extra lean and fat tissues), which will tend to produce a negative energy balance and hence a subsequent decline in body weight towards its set or preferred value. Similarly, a reduction in body weight would result in a reduction in metabolic rate due to the loss in lean and fat tissues, which will tend to produce a positive balance and hence a subsequent return towards the set or preferred weight.

But in reality, the homeostatic system is much more complex than this simple effect of *mass action* since the efficiency of metabolism (or metabolic efficiency) may also alter in response to the alterations in body weight. Indeed, subjects forced to maintain body weight at a level 10% above their initial body weight showed an increase in daily energy expenditure even after adjusting for changes in body weight and body composition [41]. Conversely, in subjects maintaining weight at a level 10% below the initial body weight, daily energy expenditure was also lower after adjusting for losses in weight and lean tissues. These compensatory changes in energy expenditure (~15% above or below predicted values) reflect changes in metabolic efficiency that oppose the maintenance of a body weight that is above or below the set or preferred body weight.

Interindividual variability in metabolic adaptation

These experiments of forced changes in body weight have also revealed that there is a large interindividual variability in the ability to readjust energy expenditure. Some individuals show little or no evidence for altered metabolic efficiency, while others reveal a marked capacity to decrease or increase energy expenditure through alterations in metabolic efficiency.

Indeed, the most striking feature of virtually all experiments of human overfeeding (lasting from a few weeks to a few months) is the wide range of individual variability in the amount of weight gain per unit of excess energy consumed. Some of these differences in the efficiency of weight gain could be attributed to interindividual variability in the gain of lean tissue relative to fat tissue (i.e. variability in the composition of weight gain), but most is in the ability to convert excess calories to heat, i.e. in the large interindividual capacity for DIT.

A detailed reanalysis of data from some 150 human beings participating in the various overeating experiments conducted

between 1965 and 1999 suggested that at least 40% of these overfed subjects must have exhibited an increase in DIT, albeit to varying degrees [42]. Genes do play an important role in variability in metabolism and underlie such susceptibility to weight gain and obesity and this has been established from overfeeding experiments in identical twins [43]. Conversely, a role for genotype in human variability in both the composition of weight loss (i.e. ratio of lean to fat tissue) as well as in the enhanced metabolic efficiency (i.e. adaptive reduction in thermogenesis) during weight loss has been suggested from studies in which identical twins underwent slimming therapy on a very low-calorie diet [44]. Taken together, it is evident that in addition to the control of food intake, changes in the composition of weight changes (via partitioning between lean and fat tisues) and in metabolic efficiency (via adaptive thermogenesis) all play an important role in the regulation of body weight and body composition, and that the magnitude of these adaptive changes is strongly influenced by the genetic make-up of the individual.

Adaptive thermogenesis at rest and during movements

The quantitative assessment of adaptive thermogenesis in the regulation of body weight and body composition is hampered by difficulties in pinpointing which component(s) of energy expenditure could be contributing in a major way to the changes in metabolic efficiency. As depicted in Figure 6.3, energy expenditure in the resting state is measured as BMR or as thermic effect of foods. Changes in the thermic effect of food (as % of calories ingested) or resting energy expenditure (after adjusting for changes in fat-free mass and fat mass) can be quantified, and reflect changes in metabolic efficiency and hence in adaptive thermogenesis. Such decreases in mass-adjusted BMR in response to weight loss and increases in mass-adjusted BMR in response to weight gain have often been demonstrated in humans and other mammals, and hence reflect the operation of adaptive changes in thermogenesis in the compartment of resting energy expenditure [45].

By contrast, any changes in heat production from what is generally clustered under nonresting energy expenditure – the most variable component of energy expenditure – are more difficult to quantify. The efficiency of muscular contraction during exercise is low (~25%) but that of SPA, including fidgeting, muscle tone and posture maintenance, and other low-level physical activities of everyday life, is even lower since these essentially involuntary activities comprise a larger proportion of isometric work which is simply thermogenic. Since actual work done on the environment during SPA is very small compared to the total energy spent on such activities, the energy cost associated with SPA has been referred to as movement-associated thermogenesis or SPA-associated thermogenesis. It has also been argued that since SPA is essentially subconscious and hence beyond voluntary control, a change in the *level* or *amount* of SPA in a direction that defends body weight also constitutes autoregulatory changes in energy expenditure. In this context, an increase in the amount of SPA in response to overfeeding, or a decrease during starvation, also constitutes adaptive changes in thermogenesis.

Spontaneous physical activity

To date, the most direct evidence that changes in SPA contribute to autoregulatory changes in energy expenditure in humans derives from data obtained from the eight men and women who participated in the Biosphere 2 experiment, a self-contained ecologic "miniworld" and prototype planetary habitat built in Arizona [46]. As a result of unexpected shortage of food, their losses in body weight (8–25%) over a 2-year period were found to be accompanied by a major reduction in SPA (assessed by a radar system in a calorimeter chamber). Such a reduction in SPA, like their reduced daily energy expenditure, persisted several months after the onset of weight recovery and was associated with a disproportionate recovery of fat mass. Whether interindividual variability in the *amount* of SPA during overfeeding contributes to variability in resistance or susceptibility to obesity has also been the focus of a few human studies of energy expenditure. The importance of SPA-associated thermogenesis in human weight regulation was in fact underscored by the findings that even under conditions where subjects were confined to a metabolic chamber, the 24-hour energy expenditure attributed to SPA was found to vary between 100 and 700 kJ/day, and to be a predictor of subsequent weight gain [47].

In fact, a main conclusion of early overfeeding experiments conducted in the late 1960s was that most of the extra heat dissipation in some of the individuals resisting obesity by increased DIT could not be accounted for by an increase in resting metabolic rate but could be due to an increased energy expenditure associated with simple (low-level) activities of everyday life [48]. This notion has recently gained much support from the findings that more than 60% of the increase in total daily energy expenditure in response to an 8-week overfeeding period could be attributed to SPA, and that interindividual variability in energy expenditure associated with SPA – an important component of NEAT – was the most significant predictor of the resistance or susceptibility to obesity [6]. A role of SPA in obesity was more recently highlighted by the observation that NEAT differs between obese and lean individuals. Using microsensors that subjects wore under their clothes and allowed body postures and movements to be accurately measured every half-second for 10 days, Levine et al. [7] have shown that obese participants were seated for 2 hours longer per day than lean participants. Moreover, this difference in posture allocation (corresponding to about 350 kcal per day) is not altered after weight gain in lean individuals or weight loss in obese individuals, indicating that increased sedentariness is not secondary to the increased body mass in the obese subjects, and that SPA and NEAT might be biologically determined.

The preponderance of evidence indicates that SPA and NEAT are major factors in the ability of individuals to prevent or reverse weight gain. Furthermore, in addition to the suppression of thermogenesis in the compartment of resting energy expenditure [49], reduced SPA and NEAT may play a role in the conservation of energy in response to caloric restriction, and hence are counteractive to the efficacy of slimming regimens [50].

Efficiency of muscle work

There is, however, no consistent evidence to suggest that change in SPA is always the major component in adaptive changes in nonresting energy expenditure. Indeed, in the experiments of forced changes in weight whereby subjects maintained body weight at 10% above or below their habitual body weight [41], the autoregulatory increases or decreases in nonresting energy expenditure could not be explained by the amount of time spent in physical activity. Instead, changes in muscle work efficiency could account for one-third of the change in daily energy expended in physical activity. These findings are consistent with other reports of an increase in skeletal muscle work efficiency (i.e. decreased thermogenesis) after experimentally induced weight reduction or in chronically undernourished subjects (see Dulloo et al. [45] for review).

Interactions between resting and nonresting energy expenditure

It must be emphasized that the separation of adaptive thermogenesis between resting and nonresting is artificial, given the possibilities of their interactions across the various energy expenditure compartments. For example, energy expenditure during sleep, which is generally nested under "resting" energy expenditure, also comprises a "nonresting" component due to spontaneous movement (or SPA) occurring during sleep, the frequency of which seems to be highly variable between individuals. Furthermore, nonresting energy expenditure or NEAT could also include heat production resulting from the impact of physical activity (exercise or SPA) on postabsorptive metabolic rate or postprandial thermogenesis. There is in fact some evidence that relatively low-intensity exercise can lead to potentiation of the thermic effect of food and that the effect of physical activity on energy expenditure can persist well after the period of the physical activity (postexercise or post-SPA stimulation of thermogenesis). Reduction in postexercise stimulation of metabolic rate has also been put forward as a mechanism for energy conservation in individuals who are considered to be chronically energy deficient since childhood. Thus, any changes in metabolic efficiency in resting or nonresting state that would tend to attenuate energy imbalance or to restore body weight and body composition towards its set or preferred value would constitute adaptive changes in thermogenesis.

Mechanisms of thermogenesis

Ever since studies on the mechanisms of DIT started in the 1960s, the focus of attention on the neurohormonal control of thermogenesis has been on the pivotal role played by the sympathetic nervous system (SNS) which, via its neurotransmitter norepinephrine (NE), acts upon α- and β-adrenoceptors to influence heat production. Although many hormones are also known to exert important control over thermogenesis (notably thyroid hormones, insulin, glucagon, adrenocorticotropic hormone (ACTH), glucocorticoids, leptin and ghrelin), they are thought to play a more permissive or facilitatory role in SNS-mediated

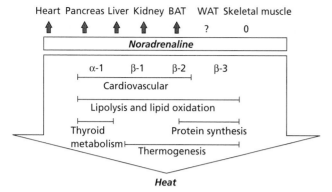

Figure 6.6 Sympathetic nervous system (SNS) activity in various organs/tissues in response to food. The thick arrows imply marked increases in SNS activity, as assessed by techniques for measuring 24-hour NE turnover rates, in rat heart, pancreas, liver, kidney, BAT, white adipose tissue (WAT) and skeletal muscle; the symbols "0" and "?" indicate no significant, or unknown, changes, respectively. Through the release of its neurotransmitter norepinephrine (NE) which acts on some or all of various adrenoceptors (α, β1, β2 and β3) present in these tissues/organs, the activated SNS might then co-ordinate cardiovascular and metabolic events that converge towards increased production of heat, i.e. diet-induced thermogenesis (DIT). (Adapted from Dulloo [68]).

thermogenesis, either by altering peripheral adrenergic responsiveness to the thermogenic effects of NE or by acting as peripheral signals for central control of SNS activity to peripheral tissues (Fig. 6.6). Indeed, as depicted in Figure 6.5 the interaction of several of the peripheral signals (e.g. insulin, ghrelin, leptin) that control feeding behavior and satiety in animals, via inhibition of orexigenic NPY/AgRP neurons and stimulation of anorexigenic POMC/CART neurons in the hypothalamus, also result in altered SNS activity and thermogenesis [12,51].

Peripheral effectors of thermogenesis

Of particular interest for SNS-mediated thermogenesis is the potential control by NE over biochemical mechanisms, the activation of which leads either to an increased use of ATP (e.g. ion pumping and substrate cycling) or to a high rate of mitochondrial oxidation with poor coupling of ATP synthesis. The net result of either is an increase in heat production. It was not until the demonstration that SNS activity in a variety of tissues is increased during overfeeding and decreased during starvation (a state of energy conservation) that the SNS was considered as a potentially pivotal efferent system linking diet and thermogenesis [52]. In fact, recent studies in mice lacking genes coding for all β-adrenoceptors ($β_1$AR, $β_2$AR and $β_3$AR) show the pivotal role of the SNS in the mediation of DIT [53]. In contrast to wild-type mice which resist obesity by activating DIT during overfeeding, mice lacking βARs (or β-less mice) are incapable of increasing thermogenesis and develop massive obesity despite similar food intake to wild-type controls. Furthermore, the β-less mice are intolerant to cold exposure, emphasizing the overlapping role of SNS via βAR signaling in the control of heat production in response to both diet and cold.

It was indeed proposed some 30 years ago [54] that these two forms of thermogenesis have a common origin in brown adipose tissue (BAT). The thermogenic activity of BAT, which is abundant in small animals and human infants, is under SNS control and is primarily mediated in brown adipocytes by a mitochondrial protein (UCP1) which allows protons to leak back across the inner mitochondrial membrane [55]. The resulting dissipation of the proton electrochemical gradient (a phenomenon referred to as "proton leak") allows substrate oxidation to occur without concomitant capture of some of the useful energy via the synthesis of ATP. The net effect during activation of UCP1 (by cold or diet) is that substrate oxidation is effectively uncoupled from phosphorylation with a resultant increase in heat production.

Although in humans, several lines of evidence are consistent with an important role for the SNS in the regulation of thermogenesis [52,56], demonstrating the importance of BAT as a site of adaptive thermogenesis in the adult human proved to be elusive. However, recent morphologic and scanning studies have raised the possibility that BAT in humans may not be as rare as once believed [57]. Indeed, the use of fluorodeoxyglucose positron emission tomography (FDG-PET) scans has visualized areas of uptake that correspond to BAT, with main depots occurring primarily in the supraclavicular and neck regions, with some additional locations in the axillary and paravertebral regions of normal individuals. It is now clear that these BAT-like depots express UCP1 – the unique identifying characteristic of BAT. The demonstration that the activity of these BAT-like depots (as assessed by uptake of FDG) is stimulated by acute exposure to mild cold and inhibited by β-adrenoceptor blockade is indicative of a tissue that is under direct sympathetic neural control. These findings have regenerated interest in pharmacologic activation of BAT in anti-obesity therapy.

Nonetheless, doubts about the physiologic importance and/or recruitability of BAT or $β_3$-adrenoceptors in adult human beings have shifted more attention to the skeletal muscle, which by its sheer size (30–40% of body weight) and important contribution to daily metabolic rate (>20% even in "sedentary" humans) has long been advocated as the major site for adaptive thermogenesis in large mammals. A report in the mid-1990s [58], that the phenomenon of mitochondrial "proton leak" is not unique to BAT (as originally thought) but also exists in other tissues and could contribute as much as 50% of the skeletal muscle heat production at rest, prompted the search for uncoupling protein(s) in this tissue. Several new members of the "uncoupling" protein family which have a high sequence homology to BAT-UCP1 have been found in skeletal muscle and named UCP2 and UCP3. There are still considerable doubts about whether these UCP1 homologs have physiologically relevant uncoupling properties in the context of adaptive thermogenesis and weight homeostasis [45].

Leptin and other adipokines as thermogenic hormones

The discovery of leptin provided the first adipokine signal implicated in the link between diet, white adipose tissue and SNS-mediated thermogenesis. In humans, this thermogenic role of leptin has been demonstrated to occur primarily in the nonresting component of energy expenditure involving diminished skeletal muscle work efficiency [59] and possibly also increased spontaneous physical activity [60], associated with alterations in SNS activity and thyroid hormones. In rodents, most attention has been directed at the thermogenic action of leptin through sympathetic control of UCP1 in BAT, but skeletal muscle is also likely to be an important site for leptin-induced thermogenesis. Indeed, studies in mice and rats indicate that leptin therapy promotes SPA or movement-induced thermogenesis, possibly through a specific subset of hypothalamic neurons and neuropetides. Also it seems to work through the modulation of mesolimbic dopamine neurons important for the regulation of reward signals, motivated behaviors that influence appetite, and locomotor activity [61,62]. In addition to the central effects of leptin in controlling SNS-mediated BAT thermogenesis as well as SPA and NEAT, there is also evidence that leptin has peripheral thermogenic effects in skeletal muscle by exerting direct actions on skeletal muscle, possibly through the stimulation of "futile" substrate cycling between *de novo* lipogenesis and lipid oxidation. This is a thermogenic effector that requires both PI3K and AMPK signaling [63].

Besides leptin, several other adipokines are currently under investigation for any potential role in thermogenesis. Interleukin 6 (IL-6), a multifunctional cytokine that is produced and released by a wide variety of cell types, including adipocytes, has generated interest following the demonstration that mice lacking IL-6 developed obesity in the absence of hyperphagia, apparently through diminished sympathetic control of thermogenesis, and that the secretion of IL-6 from adipose tissue is enhanced by adrenergic activation, and hence may represent an auxiliary mechanism through which the SNS might influence thermogenesis. Another prime candidate adipokine in the control of thermogenesis is adiponectin which, like leptin, can act directly on skeletal muscle to stimulate both glucose and lipid oxidation, and hence potentially could activate substrate cycling between *de novo* lipogenesis and lipid oxidation [63]. Furthermore, recent studies indicate that adiponectin can exert direct peripheral control on mitochondrial biogenesis in skeletal muscle [64], and that it can act in the brain to decrease body weight apparently without affecting appetite [65]. This central action of adiponectin on energy expenditure is accompanied by an increase in BAT thermogenesis, and involves hypothalamic corticotropin-releasing hormone (CRH) and the melanocortin pathway.

Despite these advancements in the identification of "hormone-like" factors secreted by adipose tissue with potential implications for both central and peripheral control of thermogenesis, there is still no adipokine that has been shown to display the characteristics of a lipostatic signal. There is still no *adipose-specific* signal whose blood concentrations will alter in proportion to *dynamic* changes in the adipose tissue fat stores, and which would trigger compensatory changes in thermogenesis (or food intake) in a direction that would restore deviation of the fat store to its preset or preferred value.

Models for body composition regulation via adaptive thermogenesis

Despite major gaps in our understanding of the various components of the regulatory loop controlling adaptive thermogenesis, the available evidence, based on studies in rodents and in humans [45], strongly suggests the existence of two distinct control systems underlying adaptive thermogenesis.

One control system is a direct function of energy imbalance and responds rapidly to attenuate the impact of changes in food intake on changes in body weight through alterations in the activity of the SNS. It is suppressed during starvation and increased during overfeeding. The other control system has a much slower time-constant since it operates as a feedback loop between the size of the fat stores and thermogenesis (i.e. a lipostatic or adipose-specific control of thermogenesis). Whereas its suppression during weight (and fat) losses is to reduce the overall rate of fuel utilization during starvation, its sustained suppression until body fat is recovered during refeeding serves to accelerate the replenishment of the fat stores. Conversely, during periods of excess fat gain, its activation will serve to oppose the maintenance of the excess fat and hence to restore body fat to its set or preferred level.

These autoregulatory control systems operating through adjustments in heat production or thermogenesis play a crucial role in attenuating and correcting deviations of body weight from its set or preferred value. The extent to which these adjustments through adaptive thermogenesis are brought about is dependent upon the environment (e.g. diet composition), and is highly variable from one individual to another, largely because of variations in genetic make-up. In societies where food is plentiful all year round and physical activity demands are low, the resultant subtle variations among individuals in adaptive thermogenesis can, in dynamic systems and over the long term, be important in determining long-term constancy of body weight in some, and in provoking the drift towards obesity in others [45].

Integrating intake and expenditure

The modern Western lifestyle has led to drastic changes in what food is eaten and in the amount of physical activity done, leading to an environment where the precise matching between energy intake and energy expenditure is difficult. Yet, there are many individulas living in the same "obesogenic" environment who manage to resist obesity. How they achieve energy balance is likely to be determined by highly complex neuroendocrine systems and subsystems, some of which could be integrated as in the simple model presented in Figure 6.7. However, it needs to be pointed out that despite the advances of the past decade in our understanding of molecular pathways and control systems underlying the regulation of body weight and body composition, the explanation for an accurate regulation of long-tem body weight in the face of poor short-term control still remains a challenging issue for human research. When attempting to explain the actual responses in energy balance and weight regulation in real life, it

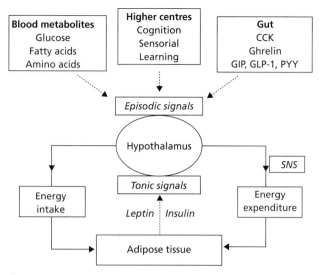

Figure 6.7 Integrating energy intake and energy expenditure in an overview of energy balance. (Adapted from Arch [69].)

is important to recognize that several factors may be operating simultaneously on both sides of the energy balance equation. In order to achieve long-term constancy of body weight, compensatory adjustments occur in both energy intake and energy expenditure, so that unraveling the importance of one or other is difficult, if not impossible.

Models of body weight regulation have primarily focused on physiologically induced *autoregulatory* adjustments in energy intake and in energy expenditure, i.e those beyond voluntary control. However, the range of variation in body weight is large enough to be detected consciously and there is certainly some degree of cognitive control. As pointed out by Garrow [66], a change of several kilograms in body weight can hardly be ignored since clothes which formerly fit will no longer do so, and there will be changes in appearance, exercise tolerance, and general well-being. When such chronic energy imbalance occurs during adolescence or adult life, it is also corrected by more or less conscious effort when the individual decides, for efficient survival, cultural or health reasons, that the change in body weight is no longer acceptable. In response, they control or attempt to control food intake or energy expenditure via changes in physical activity. In many individuals, such cognitive (conscious) controls over food intake and energy expenditure can be as important as nonconscious physiologic controls in achieving energy balance and weight homeostasis.

References

1. Durnin JVGA. Practical estimates of energy requirements. J Nutr 1991;121:1907–13.
2. Miller DS. Factors affecting energy expenditure. Proc Nutr Soc 1982;41:193–202.
3. Corey E. Pilot metabolism and respiratory activity during varied flight tasks. J Appl Physiol 1948;1:35–44.
4. Dauncey MJ. Influence of mild cold on 24 hour energy expenditure, resting metabolism and diet-induced thermogenesis. Br J Nutr 1981;45:257–67.
5. Jessen K. An assessment of human regulatory nonshivering thermogenesis. Acta Anaesth Scand 1980;24:138–43.
6. Levine JA, Eberhardt NL, Jensen MD. Role of nonexercise activity thermogenesis in resistance to fat gain in humans. Science 1999;283:212–14.
7. Levine JA, Lanningham-Foster LM, McCrady, et al. Interindividual variation in posture allocation: possible role in human obesity. Science 2005;307:584–6.
8. Blundell JE, Lawton CL, Cotton JR, Macdiarmid JI. Control of human appetite: implications for the intake of dietary fat. Ann Rev Nutr 1996;16:285–319.
9. Stubbs RJ. Appetite, feeding behaviour and energy balance in humans. Proc Nutr Soc 1998.57:341–56.
10. Berthoud HR. Multiple neural systems controlling food intake and body weight. Neurosci Biobehav Rev 2002;26:393–428.
11. Schwartz MW, Woods SC, Porte D, Seeley R, Baskin D. Central nervous system control of food intake. Nature 2000;404:661–71.
12. Flier JF. Obesity wars: molecular progress confronts an expanding epidemic. Cell 2004;116:337–50.
13. Murphy KG, Bloom SR. Gut hormones and the regulation of energy homeostasis. Nature 2006;444:854–9.
14. Havel PJ. Peripheral signals conveying metabolic information to the brain: short-term and long-term regulation of food intake and energy homeostasis. Exp Biol Med 2001;226:963–77.
15. Moran TH. Cholecystokinin and satiety: current perspectives. Nutrition 2000;16:858–65.
16. Mellinkoff SM, Franklund M, Bouyle D, Greipel M. Relationships between serum amino acid concentration and fluctuations in appetite. J Appl Physiol 1956;8:535–8.
17. Bray GA. Amino acids, protein and body weight. Obes Res 1997;5:373–9.
18. Millward DJ. A protein-stat mechanism for the regulation of growth and maintenance of the lean body mass. Nutr Res Rev 1995;8: 93–120.
19. Mayer J. Glucostatic mechanism of regulation of food intake. N Engl J Med 1953;249:13–16.
20. Flatt JP. Diet, lifestyle and weight maintenance. Am J Clin Nutr 1995;62:820–36.
21. Kennedy AG. The role of the fat depot in the hypothalamic control of food intake in the rat. Proc Roy Soc Lond B Biol Sci 1953; 140:578–92.
22. Cohen P, Zhao C, Cai X, et al. Selective deletion of leptin receptor in neurons leads to obesity. J Clin Invest 2001;108:1113–21.
23. Kowalski TJ, Liu SM, Leibel RL, Chua SC Jr. Transgenic complementation of leptin-receptor deficiency. I. Rescue of the obesity/diabetes phenotype of LEPR-null mice expressing a LEPR-B transgene. Diabetes 2001;50:425–35.
24. Farooqi IS. Monogenic human obesity syndromes. Prog Brain Res 2006;153:119–25.
25. Badman MK, Flier JS. The adipocyte as an active participant in energy balance and metabolism. Gastroenterology 2007;132: 2103–15.
26. Farooqi IS, Keogh JM, Kamath S, et al. Partial leptin deficiency and human obesity. Nature 2007;414:34–5.
27. Zheng H, Berthoud HR. Eating for pleasure or calories. Curr Opin Pharmacol 2007;7:607–12.

28. Lee MJ, Fried SK. Multilevel regulation of leptin storage, turnover, and secretion by feeding and insulin in rat adipose tissue. J Lipid Res 2006;47:1984–93.

29. Bruning JC, Gautam D, Burks DJ, et al. Role of brain insulin receptor in control of body weight and reproduction. Science 2000;289:2122–5.

30. Russek M. An hypothesis on the participation of hepatic glucoreceptors in the control of food intake. Nature 1963;197:79–80.

31. Langhans W. Metabolic and glucostatic control of feeding. Proc Nutr Soc 1996;55:497–515.

32. Friedman MI. An energy sensor for control of energy intake. Proc Nutr Soc 1997;56:41–50.

33. Langhans W. Role of the liver in the control of glucose-lipid utilization and body weight. Curr Opin Clin Nutr Metab Care 2003;6:449–55.

34. Patterson CM, Levin BE. Role of exercise in the central regulation of energy homeostasis and in the prevention of obesity. Neuroendocrinology 2008;87:65–70.

35. Zheng H, Berthoud HR. Neural systems controlling the drive to eat: mind versus metabolism. Physiology 2008;23:75–83.

36. Keys A, Brozek J, Hanschel A, Mickelson O, Taylor HL. *The Biology of Human Starvation*. Minneapolis: University of Minnesota Press, 1950.

37. Dulloo AG, Jacquet J, Girardier L. Poststarvation hyperphagia and body fat overshooting in humans: a role for feedback signals from lean and fat tissues. Am J Clin Nutr 1997;65:717–23.

38. Schutz Y. Macronutrients and energy balance in obesity. Metabolism 1995;44(suppl 3):7–11.

39. Stubbs FJ. Macronutrient effects on appetite. Int J Obes 1995;19(suppl 5):S11-S19.

40. Frayn KN. Physiological regulation of macronutrient balance. Int J Obes 1995;19(suppl 5):S4–10.

41. Leibel RL, Rosenbaum M, Hirsch J. Changes in energy expenditure resulting from altered body weight. N Engl J Med 1995;332:621–8.

42. Stock MJ. Gluttony and thermogenesis revisited. Int J Obes 1999;23:1105–17.

43. Bouchard C, Tremblay A, Després JP, et al. The response to long-term overfeeding in identical twins. N Engl J Med 1990;322:1477–82.

44. Hainer V, Stunkard AJ, Kunesova M, Parizkova J, Stich V, Allison DB. A twin study of weight loss and metabolic efficiency. Int J Obes 2001;25:533–7.

45. Dulloo AG, Seydoux J, Jacquet J. Adaptive thermogenesis and uncoupling proteins: a reappraisal of their roles in fat metabolism and energy balance. Physiol Behav 2004;83:587–602.

46. Weyer C, Walford RL, Harper IT, et al. Energy metabolism after 2 y of energy restriction: the Biosphere 2 experiment. Am J Clin Nutr 2000;72:946–53.

47. Ravussin E, Lillioja S, Anderson TE, Christin L, Bogardus C. Determinants of 24-hour energy expenditure in man. Methods and results using a respiratory chamber. J Clin Invest 1986;78:1568–78.

48. Miller DS, Mumford P, Stock MJ. Gluttony 2. Thermogenesis in overeating man. Am J Clin Nutr 1967;20:1223–9.

49. Major GC, Doucet E, Trayhurn P, Astrup A, Tremblay A. Clinical significance of adaptive thermogenesis. Int J Obes 2007;31:204–12.

50. Dulloo AG. Suppressed thermogenesis as a cause for resistance to slimming and obesity rebound: adaptation or illusion? Int J Obes 2007;31:201–3.

51. Castaneda TR, Jürgens H, Wiedmer P, et al. Obesity and the neuroendocrine control of energy homeostasis: the role of spontaneous locomotor activity. J Nutr 2005;135:1314–19.

52. Landsberg L, Saville ME, Young JB. The sympathoadrenal system and regulation of thermogenesis. Am J Physiol 1984;247:E181–9.

53. Bachman ES, Dhillon H, Zhang CY, et al. betaAR signaling required for diet-induced thermogenesis and obesity resistance. Science 2002;297:843–5.

54. Rothwell NJ, Stock MJ. A role for brown adipose tissue in diet-induced thermogenesis. Nature 1979;281:31–5.

55. Cannon B, Nedergaard J. Brown adipose tissue: function and physiological significance. Physiol Rev 2004;84:277–359.

56. Snitker S, Macdonald I, Ravussin E, Astrup A. The sympathetic nervous system and obesity: role in aetiology and treatment. Obes Rev 2000;1:5–15.

57. Nedergaard J, Bengtsson T, Cannon B. Unexpected evidence for active brown adipose tissue in adult humans. Am J Physiol Endocrinol Metab 2007;293:E444–52.

58. Rolfe DF, Brand MD. Contribution of mitochondrial proton leak to skeletal muscle respiration and to standard metabolic rate. Am J Physiol 1996;271:1380–9.

59. Rosenbaum M, Goldsmith R, Bloomfield D, et al. Low-dose leptin reverses skeletal muscle, autonomic, and neuroendocrine adaptations to maintenance of reduced weight. J Clin Invest 2005;115:3579–86.

60. Licinio J, Caglayan S, Ozata M, et al. Phenotypic effects of leptin replacement on morbid obesity, diabetes mellitus, hypogonadism, and behavior in leptin-deficient adults. Proc Natl Acad Sci (USA) 2004;101:4531–6.

61. Fulton S, Pissios P, Manchon RP, et al. Leptin regulation of the mesoaccumbens dopamine pathway. Neuron 2006;51:811–22.

62. Kotz CM, Teske JA, Billington CJ. Neuropeptidergic mediators of spontaneous physical activity and non-exercise activity thermogenesis. Neuroendocrinology 2008;87:71–90.

63. Dulloo AG, Gubler M, Montani JP, Seydoux J, Solinas G. Substrate cycling between de novo lipogenesis and lipid oxidation: a thermogenic mechanism against skeletal muscle lipotoxicity, glucolipotoxicity. Int J Obes 2004;28(suppl 4):S29–37.

64. Civitarese AE, Ukropcova B, Carling S, et al. Role of adiponectin in human skeletal muscle bioenergetics. Cell Metab 2006;4:75–87.

65. Qi Y, Takahashi Ni, Hileman SM, et al. Adiponectin acts in the brain to decrease body weight. Nat Med 2004;10:524–9.

66. Garrow JS. *Energy Balance and Obesity in Man*. Amsterdam: North-Holland, 1974.

67. Elia M. Fuel of the tissues. In: Garrow JS, James WPT, Ralph A (eds) *Human Nutrition and Dietetics*, 10th edn. Edinburgh: Churchill Livingstone, 1996:37–59.

68. Dulloo AG. A sympathetic defense against obesity. Science 2002;297:780–1.

69. Arch JRS. Lessons in obesity from transgenic animals. J Endocrinol Invest 2002;25:867–75.

7 Genes and Obesity

I. Sadaf Farooqi

Institute of Metabolic Science, Addenbrooke's Hospital, Cambridge, UK

Introduction

Obesity is determined by an interaction between genetic, environmental and behavioral factors acting through the physiologic mediators of energy intake and energy expenditure. Body weight is the archetypal polygenic trait, a quantitative phenotype that usually fails to display a mendelian pattern of inheritance because it is influenced by many different regions of the genome. The concept that environmental factors operate on an underlying pool of genes that contribute to obesity susceptibility has important implications for our approach to the prevention and treatment of obesity. If some environmental variables manifest themselves only on certain genotypes, efforts to prevent obesity at a public health level can be focused on recognition and counseling of susceptible individuals. In addition, appreciating the importance of genetic variation as an underlying cause helps to dispel the notion that obesity represents an individual defect in behavior with no biologic basis, and provides a starting point for efforts to identify the genes involved.

Much of the recent excitement about understanding and treating obesity is based on the identification of genes responsible for existing murine obesity syndromes, and the subsequent realization that several of these genes uncover fundamental physiologic pathways that were unappreciated previously. As the endocrinologic, metabolic and behavioral features of monogenic rodent obesities have been well characterized, these provide considerable insight into the biology that underlies each mutation. In the last 10 years seven single gene defects causing severe human obesity have been identified. Studies of patients with mutations in these molecules have shed light on the physiologic role of these molecules in the regulation of body weight in humans.

Clinical Obesity in Adults and Children, 3rd edition. Edited by Peter G. Kopelman, Ian D. Caterson and William H. Dietz.
© 2010 Blackwell Publishing, ISBN: 978-1-4051-8226-3.

Historical perspective

Obesity, defined as an excess of body fat, is frequently considered to be a "modern" disease – a reflection of the excesses of Western urbanized society. However, artefacts dating from the Palaeolithic Stone Age clearly represent subjects with an excess of body fat and descriptions of obese individuals have emerged in manuscripts and medical texts from many of the ancient civilizations, from Mesopotamia to Arabia, China to India. This historical evidence suggests that, independent of diet and geographical region, throughout history some individuals have harbored the propensity to store excess energy as fat.

Gene–environment interactions

The increase in the prevalence of obesity in the last 30 years suggests the importance of changing environmental factors, in particular the increasing availability of energy-dense, high-fat foods and a reduction in physical activity. Further evidence for the critical role of environmental factors in the development of obesity comes from migrant studies and the "westernization" of diet and lifestyles in developing countries. A marked change in Body Mass Index (BMI) is frequently witnessed in migrant studies, where subjects with a common genetic heritage live under new and different environmental circumstances. Pima Indians, for example, living in the United States are on average 25 kg heavier than Pima Indians living in Mexico [1]. A similar trend is seen for Africans living in the United States and Asians living in the United Kingdom. Moreover, within some ethnic groups the prevalence of obesity has increased very dramatically not only amongst migrants but also amongst the indigenous population. In fact, the prevalence of obesity is currently more than 60% in Nauruan men and women in Micronesia and amongst Polynesians in Western Samoa. This observation suggests that subjects from these ethnic groups are more susceptible to developing obesity and that environmental factors have varying effects depending upon genetic background.

82

Evidence for the heritability of fat mass

There is considerable evidence to suggest that, like height, weight is a heritable trait. Genetic epidemiologic studies in different populations can attribute the underlying phenotypic variance of a trait to genetic and/or environmental sources. Longitudinal data from one of the largest family studies, the Quebec Family Study of over 400 families, suggest a significant cross-trait familial resemblance for parent–offspring (0.20–0.25) and sibling relationships (0.25–0.35) [2]. However, in traditional nuclear families, family members generally share both genes and environment to some degree, so it is difficult to assess the contribution of each component.

Adoption studies

Complete adoption studies are useful in separating the common environmental effects since adoptive parents and their adoptive offspring share only environmental sources of variance, whilst the adoptees and their biologic parents share only genetic sources of variance. One of the largest series, based on over 5000 subjects from the Danish adoption register which contains complete and detailed information on the biologic parents, showed a strong relationship between the BMI of adoptees and biologic parents across the whole range of body fatness but none when compared with the adoptive parents [3]. The Danish group has also shown a close correlation between BMI of adoptees and their biologic full siblings who were reared separately by the biologic parents of the adoptees, and a similar, but weaker relationship with half-siblings [4].

Twin studies

Traditionally the most favored model for separation of the genetic component of variance is based on studies of twins, as monozygotic co-twins share 100 percent of their genes and dizygotes 50% on average. Heritability estimates the proportion of the total variance attributable to genetic variation under a polygenic model by comparing the similarity of a trait within monozygotic twins with the similarity within dizygotic twins. Heritability is a function of both the number of genes influencing a phenotype and the proportion of phenotypic variation accounted for by each of these genes. The advantage of studies of the heritability of BMI is that age-dependent influences of genes or environmental factors are the same for both twins. Genetic contribution to the BMI has been estimated to be 64–84% [5].

The most powerful genetic epidemiologic design is the study of monozygotic twins reared apart, which has all the advantages of a twin study but does not rely on the equal environmental exposure assumption. Correlation of monozygotic twins reared apart is virtually a direct estimate of the heritability, although monozygotic twins do share the intrauterine environment, which may contribute to lasting differences in body mass in later life. Estimates vary from 40% to 70%, depending on age at separation of twins and the length of follow-up. Longitudinal data from Virginia looking at adult twins and their offspring have reported a heritability of 69% [6]. Studies of Swedish twins have suggested a heritability of 0.70 for men and 0.66 for women [7], whilst a heritability of 0.61 was observed in a cohort of UK twins [8]. In a meta-analysis of results derived from Finnish, Japanese and American archival twins, Allison observed similar correlations [9]. In addition, Price and Gottesman have shown that these correlations did not differ significantly between twins reared apart and twins reared together, and between twins reared apart in relatively more similar (i.e. with relatives) versus less similar environments [8].

Familial resemblance in nutrient intake has been reported in parents and their children [10] although the extent to which this is genetically determined is unclear. Twin data suggest that there are notable genetic influences on the overall intake of nutrients, size and frequency of meals and intake of particular foods. Bouchard and Tremblay have shown that about 40% of the variance in resting metabolic rate, thermic effect of food and energy cost of low to moderate intensity exercise may be explained by inherited characteristics [11]. In addition, significant familial resemblance for level of habitual physical activity has been reported in a large cohort of healthy female twins [12].

Pleiotropic obesity syndromes

It is well established that obesity runs in families, although the vast majority of cases do not segregate with a clear mendelian pattern of inheritance. There are about 30 mendelian disorders with obesity as a clinical feature but often associated with mental retardation, dysmorphic features and organ-specific developmental abnormalities (i.e. pleiotropic syndromes). A number of families with these rare pleiotropic obesity syndromes have been studied by linkage analysis and the known chromosomal loci for obesity syndromes are summarized in Table 7.1. For a comprehensive list of syndromes in which obesity is a recognized part of the phenotype, see Online Mendelian Inheritance in Man (OMIM), www.ncbi.nlm.nih.gov/omim/

Prader–Willi syndrome

The Prader–Willi syndrome is the most common syndromal cause of human obesity with an estimated prevalence of about 1 in 25,000. It is an autosomal dominant disorder and is caused by deletion or disruption of a paternally imprinted gene or genes on the proximal long arm of chromosome 15. The Prader–Willi syndrome (PWS) is characterized by diminished fetal activity, obesity, hypotonia, mental retardation, short stature, hypogonadotropic hypogonadism, and small hands and feet [13]. The diagnostic criteria arrived at by a consensus group were based on a point system: one point each was allowed for each of five major criteria, such as feeding problems in infancy and failure to thrive, and half a point each for seven minor criteria, such as hypopigmentation. A minimum of 8.5 points was considered necessary for the clinical diagnosis of PWS [14]. There is mild prenatal growth retardation with a mean birth weight of about 6 lbs

Table 7.1 Human pleiotropic obesity syndromes

Syndrome	Additional clinical features	Locus	Reference
Autosomal dominant			
Ulnar–mammary syndrome	Ulnar defects, delayed puberty, hypoplastic nipples	12q24.1	Bamshad et al. (1995) [56]
Autosomal recessive			
Alstom syndrome	Retinal dystrophy, neurosensory deafness, diabetes	2p13	Collin et al. (2002) [57]
Cohe syndrome	Prominent central incisors, ophthalmopathy, microcephaly	8q22	Tahvanainen et al. (1994) [58]
X-linked			
Borjeson–Forssman– Lehmann syndrome	Mental retardation, hypogonadism, large ears	Xq26	Turner et al. (1989) [59]
Mehmo syndrome	Mental retardation, epilepsy, hypogonadism, microcephaly	Xp22.13	Steinmuller et al. (1998) [60]
Simpson–Golabi– Behmel, type 2	Craniofacial defects, skeletal and visceral abnormalities	Xp22	Brzustovic et al. (1999) [61]
Wilson–Turner syndrome	Mental retardation, tapering fingers, gynecomastia	Xp21.1	Wilson et al. (1991) [62]

(2.8 kg) at term, hyporeflexia and poor feeding in neonatal life due to diminished swallowing and sucking reflexes; infants often require assisted feeding for about 3–4 months. Feeding difficulties generally improve by the age of 6 months. From 12–18 months onward, uncontrollable hyperphagia results in severe obesity invariably associated with abdominal striae. Diabetes mellitus is not a diagnostic criterion for PWS but is often found in older PWS patients.

Whilst hyperphagia is a dominant feature in PWS subjects, the eating behavior in PWS might be due to decreased satiation as well as increased hunger. One suggested mediator of the obesity phenotype in PWS patients is the novel enteric hormone ghrelin, which is implicated in the regulation of mealtime hunger in rodents and humans and is also a potent stimulator of growth hormone secretion. Fasting plasma ghrelin levels are 4.5-fold higher in PWS subjects than equally obese controls and thus may be implicated in the pathogenesis of hyperphagia in these patients [15].

Children with PWS display diminished growth, reduced muscle mass (lean body mass) and increased fat mass, body composition abnormalities resembling those seen in growth hormone (GH) deficiency. Diminished GH responses to various provocative agents, low insulin-like growth factor-I levels, and the presence of additional evidence of hypothalamic dysfunction support the presence of true GH deficiency (GHD) in many children with PWS. GH treatment in these children decreases body fat and increases linear growth, muscle mass, fat oxidation and energy expenditure.

Prader-Willi syndrome is caused by deficiency of one or more paternally expressed imprinted transcripts within chromosome 15q11-q13, a region that includes *SNURF-SNRPN* and multiple small nucleolar RNAs (snoRNAs). The molecular pathophysiology of PWS remains unclear although several candidate genes in this region have been studied and their expression shown to be absent in postmortem brains of PWS patients [16]. Balanced translocations that leave the *SNURF-SNRPN* promoter and coding regions intact [17] suggest that disruption of *SNURF-SNRPN* is less important, whereas a recently reported microdeletion of the HBII-85 snoRNAs in a child with PWS provides strong evidence that deficiency of HBII-85 snoRNAs plays a major role in the key characteristics of the PWS phenotype [18]. However, some atypical features in the latter patient suggest that other genes in this region may also be important.

Diagnosis

Loss of the paternal chromosomal segment 15q11.2-q12 (usually *de novo*) is principally responsible for PWS. There are two mechanisms by which such a loss can occur: either through deletion of the paternal "critical" segment (75%) or through loss of the entire paternal chromosome 15 with presence of two maternal homologs (uniparental maternal disomy) in approximately 22% of patients. The opposite, i.e. maternal deletion or paternal uniparental disomy, causes another characteristic phenotype, the Angelman syndrome. In rare instances, imprinting errors due to a sporadic or inherited microdeletion in the imprinting center (3% of patients) or a paternal imprinted translocation (<1%) are observed.

Deletions account for 70–80% of cases, many of which can be visualized by standard prometaphase banding examination. A minority consist of unbalanced translocations which are easily detected by routine chromosome examination. The remainder of cases are the result of maternal uniparental disomy where cytogenetic examinations yield normal results. However, there are distinct differences in DNA methylation at the D15S9 locus on 15q11-q13 according to the parent of origin, so DNA methylation can be used as a reliable postnatal diagnostic tool in PWS patients with a normal karyotype.

Treatment

Traditionally, the mainstay of management has centered on early institution of a low-calorie diet with regular exercise, rigorous supervision, restriction of food and money, and appropriate psychologic and behavioral counseling of the patient and family, often in the context of group homes for PWS adolescents and adults.

In PWS children, therapy with GH significantly improves the rate of growth and final height. Long-term studies show that the final height is in the average range for age and GH is now licensed for use in PWS.

Albright hereditary osteodystrophy

Gs is the ubiquitously expressed heterotrimeric G protein that couples receptors to the effector enzyme adenylyl cyclase and is required for receptor-stimulated intracellular cAMP generation. Inactivating and activating mutations in the gene encoding Gs α (GNAS1) are known to be the basis for two well-described contrasting clinical disorders, Albright hereditary osteodystrophy (AHO) and McCune–Albright syndrome (MAS). AHO is an autosomal dominant disorder due to germline mutations in GNAS1 that decrease expression or function of Gs α protein. Heterozygous loss-of-function mutations lead to AHO, a disease characterized by short stature, obesity, skeletal defects, and impaired olfaction. Maternal transmission of GNAS1 mutations leads to AHO plus resistance to several hormones (e.g. parathyroid hormone) that activate Gs in their target tissues (pseudohypoparathyroidism type IA), while paternal transmission leads only to the AHO phenotype (pseudopseudohypoparathyroidism). Studies in both mice and humans demonstrate that GNAS1 is imprinted in a tissue-specific manner, being expressed primarily from the maternal allele in some tissues and biallelically in most other tissues; thus multihormone resistance occurs only when Gs α mutations are inherited maternally [19].

Fragile X syndrome

Fragile X syndrome is characterized by moderate to severe mental retardation, macro-orchidism, large ears, prominent jaw, and high-pitched jocular speech associated with mutations in the FMR1 gene [20]. Expression is variable, with mental retardation being the most common feature. A PWS-like subphenotype of the fragile X syndrome has been described. The features were extreme obesity with a full, round face, small, broad hands and feet, and regional skin hyperpigmentation. Behavioral characteristics such as hyperkinesis, autistic-like behavior, and apparent speech and language deficits may help point toward the diagnosis of the fragile X. It has been suggested that a reasonable estimate of frequency is 0.5 per 1000 males.

Bardet–Biedl syndrome

Bardet–Biedl syndrome (BBS) is a rare (prevalence <1/100,000), autosomal recessive disease characterized by obesity, mental retardation, dysphormic extremities (syndactyly, brachydactyly or polydactyly), retinal dystrophy or pigmentary retinopathy, hypogonadism or hypogenitalism (limited to male patients) and structural abnormalities of the kidney or functional renal impairment. The differential diagnosis includes Biemond syndrome II (iris coloboma, hypogenitalism, obesity, polydactyly, and mental retardation) and Alstrom syndrome (retinitis pigmentosa, obesity, diabetes mellitus and deafness).

Bardet–Biedl syndrome is a genetically heterogeneous disorder. Although BBS was originally thought to be a recessive disorder, Katsanis and colleagues demonstrated that clinical manifestation of some forms of BBS requires recessive mutations in one of the six loci plus an additional mutation in a second locus [21].

Recent studies strongly indicate that most of the genes implicated in BBS are involved in the structure and/or function of the basal body, a modified centriole which is essential for the function of nonmotile cilia, subcellular organelles whose importance for intercellular communication is becoming increasingly evident [22]. Some BBS proteins are involved in noncanonical Wnt and sonic hedgehog signaling within the cilium, suggesting that BBS proteins may contribute to disease pathogenesis through multiple molecular mechanisms.

BDNF and TrkB deficiency

A single patient has been reported with a *de novo* missense mutation in the neurotropin receptor TrkB associated with severe hyperphagia and obesity, delayed speech and language development, impaired short-term memory and loss of nociception [23]. A *de novo* chromosomal inversion on the short arm of chromosome 11 which disrupts the expression of brain-derived neurotropic factor (BDNF), which signals through TrkB, also gives a comparable obesity and neurobehavioral phenotype [24]. The neurotropins are involved in the development and maintenance of neurons and in mediating synaptic plasticity in the brain and peripheral nervous system.

Molecular mechanisms involved in energy homeostasis

The first description of hypothalamic injury associated with obesity was published by Mohr in 1840 [25] but remained unsupported until two landmark papers by Babinski in 1900 [26] and by Frohlich in 1901 [27] describing tumous in the region of the hypothalamus that were associated with obesity, gonadal atrophy, decreased vision and short stature. In 1940, Hetherington and Ranson published their first report demonstrating that electrolytic lesions in rodents involving, but not restricted to, the ventromedial region of the hypothalamus (VMH) were associated with hyperphagia (increased food intake), hyperinsulinemia and obesity [28]. However, the precise nature of these hypothalamic pathways and the nature of their inputs and outputs were only clarified with the identification and characterization of single gene defects in rodent models of obesity.

Rodent models of obesity

Since the early 1900s, a number of obese inbred strains of mice, both dominant (yellow, *Ay/a*) and recessive (*ob/ob, db/db, fa/fa, tb/tb*), had been studied. In the 1990s, the genes responsible for these syndromes were identified mostly by positional cloning techniques and these observations have given substantial insights into the physiologic disturbances that can lead to obesity, the metabolic and endocrine abnormalities associated with the obese phenotype, and the more detailed anatomic and neurochemical pathways that regulate energy intake and energy expenditure [29]. These studies provide the basic framework upon which the understanding of the more complex mechanisms in humans can be built.

Leptin–melanocortin pathway

The initial observations in this field were made as a result of positional cloning strategies in two strains of severely obese mice (*ob/ob* and *db/db*). Severely obese *ob/ob* mice were found to harbor mutations in the *ob* gene resulting in a complete lack of its protein product, leptin [30]. Administration of recombinant leptin reduced the food intake and body weight of leptin-deficient *ob/ob* mice and corrected all their neuroendocrine and metabolic abnormalities. The signaling form of the leptin receptor is deleted in *db/db* mice, which are consequently unresponsive to endogenous or exogenous leptin. The identification of these two proteins established the first components of a nutritional feedback loop from adipose tissue to the brain. However, it is considered that the physiologic role of leptin in humans and rodents might be to act as a signal for starvation because as fat mass increases, further rises in leptin have a limited ability to suppress food intake and prevent obesity [31].

Considerable attention has focused on deciphering the hypothalamic pathways that co-ordinate the behavioral and metabolic effects downstream of leptin. The first-order neuronal targets of leptin action in the brain are anorectic (reducing food intake) pro-opiomelanocortin (POMC) and orexigenic (increasing food intake) neuropeptide-Y/agouti-related protein (NPY/AgRP) neurons in the hypothalamic arcuate nucleus, where the signaling isoform of the leptin receptor is highly expressed [32]. Forty percent of POMC neurons in the arcuate nucleus express the mRNA for the long form of the leptin receptor and POMC expression is regulated positively by leptin. POMC is sequentially cleaved by prohormone convertases to yield peptides including α-melanocyte-stimulating hormone (MSH) that have been shown to play a role in feeding behavior. There is clear evidence in rodents that α-MSH acts as a suppressor of feeding behavior, probably through the melanocortin 4 receptor (MC4R). In fact, targeted disruption of MC4R in rodents leads to increased food intake, obesity, severe early hyperinsulinemia and increased linear growth; heterozygotes have an intermediate phenotype compared to homozygotes and wild-type mice [33].

Human monogenic obesity syndromes

Congenital leptin deficiency

In 1997, we reported two severely obese cousins from a highly consanguineous family of Pakistani origin [34]. Both children had undetectable levels of serum leptin and were found to be homozygous for a frameshift mutation in the *ob* gene (ΔG133), which resulted in a truncated protein that was not secreted. We have since identified three further affected individuals from two other families who are also homozygous for the same mutation in the leptin gene [35]. All the families are of Pakistani origin but not known to be related over five generations. A large Turkish family who carry a homozygous missense mutation have also been described [36]. All subjects in these families are characterized by severe early-onset obesity and intense hyperphagia

[35,37,38] with food-seeking behavior and an inability to discriminate between appetizing and bland foods [39]. Hyperinsulinemia and an advanced bone age are also common features. Some of the Turkish subjects are adults with hypogonadotropic hypogonadism [36]. Although normal pubertal development did not occur, there was some evidence of a delayed but spontaneous pubertal development in one person [38].

We demonstrated that children with leptin deficiency had profound abnormalities of T cell number and function [35], consistent with high rates of childhood infection and a high reported rate of childhood mortality from infection in obese Turkish subjects. Most of these phenotypes closely parallel those seen in murine leptin deficiency. However, there are some phenotypes where the parallels between human and mouse are not as clearcut. Thus, while *ob/ob* mice are stunted, it appears that growth retardation is not a feature of human leptin deficiency [35], although abnormalities of dynamic growth hormone secretion have been reported in one human subject [38]. *ob/ob* mice have marked activation of the hypothalamic pituitary adrenal axis with very elevated corticosterone levels. In humans, abnormalities of cortisol secretion, if present at all, are much more subtle [37]. The contribution of reduced energy expenditure to the obesity of the *ob/ob* mouse is reasonably well established [40]. In leptin-deficient humans we found no detectable changes in resting or free-living energy expenditure [35], although it was not possible to examine how such systems adapted to stressors such as cold. Ozata et al reported abnormalities of sympathetic nerve function in leptin-deficient humans consistent with defects in the efferent sympathetic limb of thermogenesis [38].

Response to leptin therapy

In 2002 we reported the dramatic and beneficial effects of daily subcutaneous injections of leptin in reducing body weight and fat mass in three congenitally leptin-deficient children [35]. We have also commenced therapy in the other two children and seen comparably beneficial results. All children showed a response to initial leptin doses designed to produce plasma leptin levels at only 10% of those predicted by height and weight (i.e. approximately 0.01 mg/kg of lean body mass). The most dramatic example of leptin's effects was with a 3-year-old boy, severely disabled by gross obesity (wt 42 kg), who now weighs 32 kg (75th centile for weight) after 48 months of leptin therapy (Fig. 7.1) [35].

The major effect of leptin was on appetite, with normalization of hyperphagia. Leptin therapy reduced energy intake during an 18 MJ *adlibitum* test meal by up to 84% (Fig. 7.2a). We were unable to demonstrate a major effect of leptin on basal metabolic rate or free-living energy expenditure (Fig. 7.2b) but, as weight loss by other means is associated with a decrease in basal metabolic rate (BMR) [41], the fact that energy expenditure did not fall in our leptin-deficient subjects is notable.

The administration of leptin permitted progression of appropriately timed pubertal development in the single child of appropriate age and did not cause the early onset of puberty in the

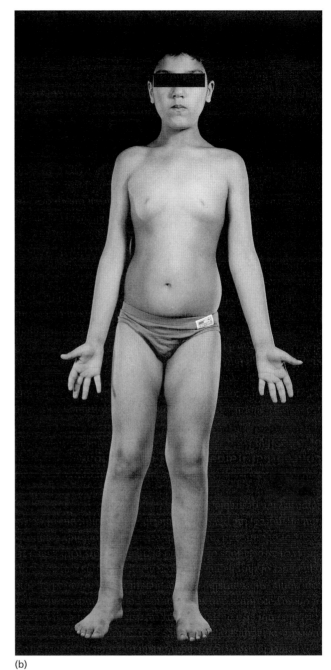

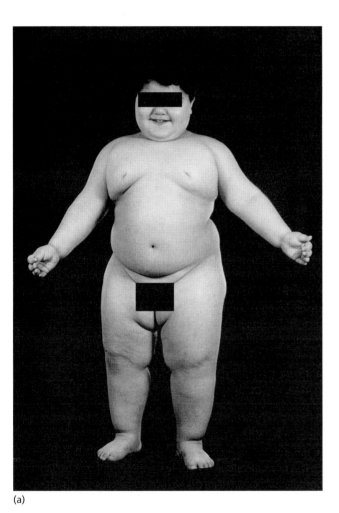

(a)   (b)

Figure 7.1 Clinical response to leptin therapy in congenital leptin deficiency.

younger children (Fig. 7.3) [35]. Free thyroxine and thyroid-stimulating hormone (TSH) levels, although in the normal range before treatment, had consistently increased at the earliest post-treatment time point and subsequently stabilized at this elevated level [35]. These findings are consistent with evidence from animal models that leptin influences thyrotropin-releasing hormone (TRH) release from the hypothalamus [42] and from studies illustrating the effect of leptin deficiency on TSH pulsatility in humans [43].

Throughout the trial of leptin administration, weight loss continued in all subjects, albeit with refractory periods which were overcome by increases in leptin dose. The families in the UK harbor a mutation which leads to a prematurely truncated form of leptin and thus wild-type leptin is a novel antigen to them. Thus, all subjects developed anti-leptin antibodies after ~6 weeks of leptin therapy, which interfered with interpretation of serum leptin levels and in some cases were capable of neutralizing leptin in a bio-assay. These antibodies are the likely cause of refractory

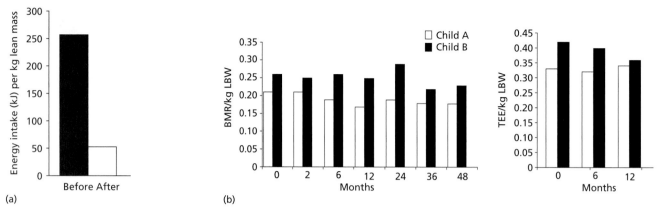

Figure 7.2 (a) Change in ad libitum food intake with leptin therapy in congenital leptin deficiency. (b) Changes in energy expenditure in response to leptin. BMR, basal metabolic rate; TEE, total energy expenditure.

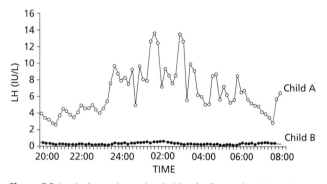

Figure 7.3 Leptin therapy is associated with pulsatile gonadotropin secretion at an appropriate developmental age in child (a) (age 11 yrs) compared to child (b) (age 5 yrs).

periods occurring during therapy. The fluctuating nature of the antibodies probably reflects the complicating factor that leptin deficiency is itself an immunodeficient state and administration of leptin leads to a change from the secretion of predominantly Th2 to Th1 cytokines, which may directly influence antibody production. Thus far, we have been able to regain control of weight loss by increasing the dose of leptin.

Partial leptin deficiency

The major question with respect to the potential therapeutic use of leptin in more common forms of obesity relates to the shape of the leptin dose–response curve. We have clearly shown that at the lower end of plasma leptin levels, raising leptin levels from undetectable to detectable has profound effects on appetite and weight. Supraphysiologic doses (0.1–0.3 mg/kg body weight) of leptin have been administered to obese subjects for 28 weeks [44]. On average, subjects lost significant weight, but the extent of weight loss and the variability between subjects has led many to conclude that the leptin resistance of common obesity cannot be usefully overcome by leptin supplementation, at least when administered peripherally. However, on scientific rather than

pragmatic grounds, it is of interest that there was a significant effect on weight, suggesting that plasma leptin can continue to have a dose–response effect on energy homeostasis across a wide plasma concentration range. To test this hypothesis, we studied the heterozygous relatives of our leptin-deficient subjects. Serum leptin levels in the heterozygous subjects were found to be significantly lower than expected for % body fat and they had a higher prevalence of obesity than seen in a control population of similar age, sex and ethnicity [45]. Additionally, % body fat was higher than predicted from their height and weight in the heterozygous subjects compared to control subjects of the same ethnicity. These findings closely parallel those in heterozygous *ob-* and *db/-* mice [46]. These data provide further support for the possibility that leptin can produce a graded response in terms of body composition across a broad range of plasma concentrations. Recently, leptin has been used in combination with other drugs with some success in common forms of obesity.

Leptin receptor deficiency

Up to 3% of patients with severe obesity have been found to harbor mutations in the leptin receptor gene that are associated with a loss of function *in vitro* [47]. Whilst heterozygosity for LEP or LEPR mutations is associated with an increase in body weight, severe obesity requires the loss of two alleles due to homozygous or compound heterozygous mutations. Serum leptin levels are not disproportionately elevated in LEPR deficiency, although particular mutations located near the transmembrane domain can result in a truncated extracellular domain that may act as a false binding protein and result in abnormally elevated leptin levels [48,49]. The clinical phenotype of congenital leptin receptor deficiency is similar to that of leptin deficiency with hyperphagia, severe early-onset obesity, hypogonadism and frequent infections.

POMC deficiency

Several unrelated obese children with homozygous or compound heterozygous mutations in POMC have been reported [50]. These children were hyperphagic, developing early-onset obesity as a result of impaired melanocortin signaling in the hypothalamus. They presented in neonatal life with adrenal crisis due to isolated adrenocorticotropic hormone (ACTH) deficiency (POMC is a precursor of ACTH in the pituitary) and had pale skin and red hair due to the lack of MSH function at melanocortin 1 receptors in the skin, although hypopigmentation may be less obvious in children from different ethnic backgrounds. A number of groups have identified a heterozygous missense mutation (Arg236Gly) in POMC that disrupts the dibasic amino acid processing site between β-MSH and β-endorphin [51]. This mutation results in an aberrant β-MSH/β-endorphin fusion peptide which binds to MC4R with an affinity identical to that of α- and β-MSH but has a markedly reduced ability to activate the receptor. Thus this cleavage site mutation in POMC may confer susceptibility to obesity through a novel molecular mechanism [51].

Prohormone convertase 1 deficiency

Further evidence for the role of the melanocortin system in the regulation of body weight in humans comes from the description of three patients with severe childhood obesity, abnormal glucose homeostasis, very low plasma insulin but elevated levels of proinsulin, hypogonadotropic hypogonadism and hypocortisolemia associated with elevated levels of POMC. These subjects were found to be compound heterozygote/homozygous for mutations in prohormone convertase 1, which cleaves prohormones at pairs of basic amino acids, leaving C-terminal basic residues which are then excised by carboxypeptidase E (CPE) [52]. Although failure to cleave POMC is a likely mechanism for the obesity in these patients, prohormone convertase 1 (PC1) cleaves a number of other neuropeptides in the hypothalamus, such as glucagon-like peptide 1, which may influence feeding behavior. Intriguingly, the second patient suffered from severe small intestinal absorptive dysfunction as well as the characteristic severe early-onset obesity, impaired prohormone processing and hypocortisolemia. We hypothesized that the small intestinal dysfunction seen in this patient, and to a lesser extent in the first patient we described, may be the result of a failure of maturation of propeptides within the enteroendocrine cells and nerves that express PC1 throughout the gut. The finding of elevated levels of progastrin and proglucagon provided *in vivo* evidence that, indeed, prohormone processing in enteroendocrine cells was abnormal [53].

MC4R deficiency

Mutations in MC4R have been reported in up ~6% of patients with severe early-onset obesity and are found at a frequency of approximately 1 in 1000 in the general UK population, making this one of the most common human monogenic diseases. While we found a 100% penetrance of early-onset obesity in heterozygous probands, others have described obligate carriers who were not obese. Given the large number of potential influences on body weight, it is perhaps not surprising that both genetic and environmental modifiers will have important effects in some pedigrees. Taking account of all these observations, co-dominance,

with modulation of expressivity and penetrance of the phenotype, is the most appropriate descriptor for the mode of inheritance.

Detailed phenotypic studies of patients with MC4R mutations reveal that this syndrome is characterized by an increase in lean body mass and bone mineral density, increased linear growth throughout childhood, hyperphagia and severe hyperinsulinemia [54]. These features are similar to those seen in MC4R knockout mice, suggesting the preservation of the relevant melanocortin pathways between rodents and humans. Of particular note is the finding that the severity of receptor dysfunction seen in *in vitro* assays can predict the amount of food ingested at a test meal by the subject harboring that particular mutation [54]. An elevated respiratory quotient (ratio of carbohydrate to fat oxidation) in MC4R deficiency is consistent with an impaired ability to mobilize fat seen in MC4R knockout mice. Linear growth of these subjects is striking, with affected children having a height standard deviation score (SDS) of +2 compared to population standards and adults have an increased final height when compared to equally obese adults with a normal MC4R genotype. MC4R-deficient subjects also have higher levels of fasting insulin than age- and BMI SDS-matched children.

We have studied in detail the signaling properties of many of these mutant receptors and this information should help to advance the understanding of structure/function relationships and potentially provide *in vitro* support for the use of MC4R agonists in this group of patients [55]. Importantly, we have been unable to demonstrate evidence for dominant negativity associated with these mutants, which suggests that MC4R mutations are more likely to result in a phenotype through haploinsufficiency.

Energy expenditure genes

Although several lines of evidence suggest that obesity in humans may be in part determined by reduced energy expenditure, molecular insights into the pathways for energy expenditure have lagged behind those related to altered appetite. In most well-identified syndromes of obesity, such as those involving defects in leptin and the melanocortin pathway, obesity results from both increased feeding and decreased energy expenditure in rodents, suggesting that the leptin and melanocortin pathways are upstream of effector mechanisms that regulate both appetite and energy expenditure and thus disruption of these pathways is likely to have subtle effects on energy expenditure in humans too.

Future perspectives

Although monogenic syndromes are rare, an improved understanding of the precise nature of the inherited component of severe obesity has undoubted medical benefits. For individuals at highest risk of the complications of severe obesity, such findings provide a starting point for providing more rational mechanism-based therapies, as has successfully been achieved for congenital leptin deficiency. Thus in patients with severe obesity, a history of hyperphagia, age of onset and family history should be sought. As congenital leptin deficiency is a treatable condition, it is plausible that all children with features of a recessive disorder should have a serum leptin measurement. Additional features such as hypogonadism, severe hyperinsulinemia, postprandial hypoglycemia and developmental delay should be sought as genetic counseling of families with monogenic disorders is important.

For common polygenic obesity, a number of recent advances are likely to make significant contributions to the search for obesity genes, including the completion of a draft of the human genome sequence and the discovery and cataloguing of single nucleotide polymorphisms (SNPs), the most prevalent source of sequence variation throughout the human genome. These efforts promise to enhance our ability to identify risk-conferring genes for complex traits such as obesity. In this way it is hoped that genetics will continue to make a significant contribution to understanding the pathophysiology of obesity, the identification of potential drug targets and the development of more rational mechanism-based interventions at both the individual and population levels.

References

1. Kopelman PG. Obesity as a medical problem. Nature 2000; 404(6778):635–43.
2. Rice T, Perusse L, Bouchard C, Rao DC. Familial aggregation of body mass index and subcutaneous fat measures in the longitudinal Quebec family study. Genet Epidemiol 1999;16(3):316–34.
3. Stunkard AJ, Sorensen TI, Hanis C, Teasdale TW, Chakraborty R, Schull WJ, et al. An adoption study of human obesity. N Engl J Med 1986;314(4):193–8.
4. Sorensen TI, Price RA, Stunkard AJ, Schulsinger F. Genetics of obesity in adult adoptees and their biological siblings. BMJ 1989;298(6666):87–90.
5. Stunkard AJ, Foch TT, Hrubec Z. A twin study of human obesity. JAMA 1986;256(1):51–4.
6. Maes HH, Neale MC, Eaves LJ. Genetic and environmental factors in relative body weight and human adiposity. Behav Genet 1997; 27(4):325–51.
7. Stunkard AJ, Harris JR, Pedersen NL, McClearn GE. The body-mass index of twins who have been reared apart. N Engl J Med 1990; 322(21):1483–7.
8. Price RA, Gottesman, II. Body fat in identical twins reared apart: roles for genes and environment. Behav Genet 1991;21(1):1–7.
9. Allison DB, Kaprio J, Korkeila M, Koskenvuo M, Neale MC, Hayakawa K. The heritability of body mass index among an international sample of monozygotic twins reared apart. Int J Obes 1996; 20(6):501–6.
10. Perusse L, Tremblay A, Leblanc C, Cloninger CR, Reich T, Rice J, et al. Familial resemblance in energy intake: contribution of genetic and environmental factors. Am J Clin Nutr 1988;47(4):629–35.
11. Bouchard C, Tremblay A. Genetic effects in human energy expenditure components. Int J Obes 1990;14(suppl 1):49–55; discussion 55–8.
12. Samaras K, Kelly PJ, Chiano MN, Spector TD, Campbell LV. Genetic and environmental influences on total-body and central abdominal fat: the effect of physical activity in female twins. Ann Intern Med 1999;130(11):873–82.
13. Butler M. Prader–Willi syndrome: current understanding of cause and diagnosis. Am J Med Genet 1990;35(3):319–32.
14. Holm VA CS, Butler MG, Hanchett JM, Greenswag LR, Whitman BY, Greenberg F. Prader–Willi syndrome: consensus diagnostic criteria. Pediatrics 1993;91(2):398–402.
15. Cummings DE CK, Purnell JQ, Vaisse C, et al. Elevated plasma ghrelin levels in Prader Willi syndrome. Nat Med 2002;8(7): 643–4.
16. Swaab DF, Purba JS, Hofman MA. Alterations in the hypothalamic paraventricular nucleus and its oxytocin neurons (putative satiety cells) in Prader–Willi syndrome: a study of five cases. J Clin Endocrinol Metab 1995;80(2):573–9.
17. Schulze A, Hansen C, Skakkebaek NE, Brondum-Nielsen K, Ledbeter DH, Tommerup N. Exclusion of SNRPN as a major determinant of Prader–Willi syndrome by a translocation breakpoint. Nat Genet 1996;12(4):452–4.
18. Sahoo T, del Gaudio D, German JR, Shinawi M, Peters SU, Person RE, et al. Prader–Willi phenotype caused by paternal deficiency for the HBII-85 C/D box small nucleolar RNA cluster. Nat Genet 2008;40(6):719–21.
19. Weinstein LS, Chen M, Liu J. Gs(alpha) mutations and imprinting defects in human disease. Ann NY Acad Sci 2002;968:173–97.
20. Kaplan G, Kung M, McClure M, Cronister A. Direct mutation analysis of 495 patients for fragile X carrier status/proband diagnosis. Am J Med Genet 1994;51(4):501–2.
21. Katsanis N, Lupski JR, Beales PL. Exploring the molecular basis of Bardet–Biedl syndrome. Hum Mol Genet 2001;10(20):2293–9.
22. Mykytyn K, Sheffield VC. Establishing a connection between cilia and Bardet–Biedl syndrome. Trends Mol Med 2004;10(3):106–9.
23. Yeo GS, Connie Hung CC, Rochford J, Keogh J, Gray J, Sivaramakrishnan S, et al. A de novo mutation affecting human TrkB associated with severe obesity and developmental delay. Nat Neurosci 2004;7(11):1187–9.
24. Gray J, Yeo GS, Cox JJ, Morton J, Adlam AL, Keogh JM, et al. Hyperphagia, severe obesity, impaired cognitive function, and hyperactivity associated with functional loss of one copy of the brain-derived neurotrophic factor (BDNF) gene. Diabetes 2006;55(12):3366–71.
25. Mohr B. Hypertrophie der hypophysis cerebri und dadurchbedingter druck auf die hirngrundflache, insbesndere auf die Schnerven, das chiasma deselben und den linkseitigen. Hirnschenkel Wschr Ges Heilk 1840;6:565–571.
26. Babinski MJ. Tumeur du corps pituitaire sans acromegalie et avec de developpement des organes genitaux. Rev Neurol 1900;8: 531–3.
27. Frolich A. Ein fall von tumor der hypophysis cerebri ohne akromegalie. Wien Klin Rund 1901;15:883–6.
28. Hetherington AW, Ranson SW. Hypothalamic lesions and adiposity in the rat. Anat Rec 1940;78:149–72.
29. Leibel RL, Chung WK, Chua SC Jr. The molecular genetics of rodent single gene obesities. J Biol Chem 1997;272(51):31937–40.
30. Zhang Y, Proenca R, Maffei M, Barone M, Leopold L, Friedman JM. Positional cloning of the mouse obese gene and its human homologue. Nature 1994;372(6505):425–32.
31. Flier JS. Clinical review 94: what's in a name? In search of leptin's physiologic role. J Clin Endocrinol Metab 1998;83(5):1407–13.

32. Schwartz MW, Woods SC, Porte D Jr., Seeley RJ, Baskin DG. Central nervous system control of food intake. Nature 2000;404(6778): 661–71.

33. Huszar D, Lynch CA, Fairchild-Huntress V, Dunmore JH, Fang Q, Berkemeier LR, et al. Targeted disruption of the melanocortin-4 receptor results in obesity in mice. Cell 1997;88(1):131–41.

34. Montague CT, Farooqi IS, Whitehead JP, Soos MA, Rau H, Wareham NJ, et al. Congenital leptin deficiency is associated with severe early-onset obesity in humans. Nature 1997;387(6636):903–8.

35. Farooqi IS, Matarese G, Lord GM, Keogh JM, Lawrence E, Agwu C, et al. Beneficial effects of leptin on obesity, T cell hyporesponsiveness, and neuroendocrine/metabolic dysfunction of human congenital leptin deficiency. J Clin Invest 2002;110(8):1093–103.

36. Strobel A, Issad T, Camoin L, Ozata M, Strosberg AD. A leptin missense mutation associated with hypogonadism and morbid obesity. Nat Genet 1998;18(3):213–15.

37. Farooqi IS, Jebb SA, Langmack G, Lawrence E, Cheetham CH, Prentice AM, et al. Effects of recombinant leptin therapy in a child with congenital leptin deficiency. N Engl J Med 1999;341(12):879–84.

38. Ozata M, Ozdemir IC, Licinio J. Human leptin deficiency caused by a missense mutation: multiple endocrine defects, decreased sympathetic tone, and immune system dysfunction indicate new targets for leptin action, greater central than peripheral resistance to the effects of leptin, and spontaneous correction of leptin-mediated defects. J Clin Endocrinol Metab 1999;84(10):3686–95.

39. Farooqi IS, Bullmore E, Keogh J, Gillard J, O'Rahilly S, Fletcher PC. Leptin regulates striatal regions and human eating behavior. Science 2007;317(5843):1355.

40. Trayhurn P, Thurlby PL, James WPT. Thermogenic defect in pre-obese ob/ob mice. Nature 1977;266:60–2.

41. Rosenbaum M, Murphy EM, Heymsfield SB, Matthews DE, Leibel RL. Low dose leptin administration reverses effects of sustained weight-reduction on energy expenditure and circulating concentrations of thyroid hormones. J Clin Endocrinol Metab 2002;87(5):2391.

42. Harris M, Aschkenasi C, Elias CF, Chandrankunnel A, Nillni EA, Bjoorbaek C, et al. Transcriptional regulation of the thyrotropin-releasing hormone gene by leptin and melanocortin signaling. J Clin Invest 2001;107(1):111–20.

43. Mantzoros CS, Ozata M, Negrao AB, Suchard MA, Ziotopoulou M, Caglayan S, et al. Synchronicity of frequently sampled thyrotropin (TSH) and leptin concentrations in healthy adults and leptin-deficient subjects: evidence for possible partial TSH regulation by leptin in humans. J Clin Endocrinol Metab 2001;86(7):3284–91.

44. Heymsfield SB, Greenberg AS, Fujioka K, Dixon RM, Kushner R, Hunt T, et al. Recombinant leptin for weight loss in obese and lean adults: a randomized, controlled, dose-escalation trial. JAMA 1999;282(16):1568–75.

45. Farooqi IS, Keogh JM, Kamath S, Jones S, Gibson WT, Trussell R, et al. Partial leptin deficiency and human adiposity. Nature 2001; 414(6859):34–5.

46. Chung WK, Belfi K, Chua M, Wiley J, Mackintosh R, Nicolson M, et al. Heterozygosity for Lep(ob) or Lep(rdb) affects body composition and leptin homeostasis in adult mice. Am J Physiol 1998;274(4 Pt 2):R985–90.

47. Farooqi IS, Wangensteen T, Collins S, Kimber W, Matarese G, Keogh JM, et al. Clinical and molecular genetic spectrum of congenital deficiency of the leptin receptor. N Engl J Med 2007;356(3): 237–47.

48. Clement K, Vaisse C, Lahlou N, Cabrol S, Pelloux V, Cassuto D, et al. A mutation in the human leptin receptor gene causes obesity and pituitary dysfunction [see comments]. Nature 1998;392(6674): 398–401.

49. Lahlou N, Clement K, Carel JC, Vaisse C, Lotton C, Le Bihan Y, et al. Soluble leptin receptor in serum of subjects with complete resistance to leptin: relation to fat mass. Diabetes 2000;49(8): 1347–52.

50. Krude H, Biebermann H, Luck W, Horn R, Brabant G, Gruters A. Severe early-onset obesity, adrenal insufficiency and red hair pigmentation caused by POMC mutations in humans. Nat Genet 1998;19(2):155–7.

51. Challis BG, Pritchard LE, Creemers JW, Delplanque J, Keogh JM, Luan J, et al. A missense mutation disrupting a dibasic prohormone processing site in pro-opiomelanocortin (POMC) increases susceptibility to early-onset obesity through a novel molecular mechanism. Hum Mol Genet 2002;11(17):1997–2004.

52. Jackson RS, Creemers JW, Ohagi S, Raffin-Sanson ML, Sanders L, Montague CT, et al. Obesity and impaired prohormone processing associated with mutations in the human prohormone convertase 1 gene [see comments]. Nat Genet 1997;16(3):303–6.

53. Jackson RS, Creemers JW, Farooqi IS, Raffin-Sanson ML, Varro A, Dockray GJ, et al. Small-intestinal dysfunction accompanies the complex endocrinopathy of human proprotein convertase 1 deficiency. J Clin Invest 2003;112(10):1550–60.

54. Farooqi IS, Keogh JM, Yeo GS, Lank EJ, Cheetham T, O'Rahilly S. Clinical spectrum of obesity and mutations in the melanocortin 4 receptor gene. N Engl J Med 2003;348(12):1085–95.

55. Yeo GS, Lank EJ, Farooqi IS, Keogh J, Challis BG, O'Rahilly S. Mutations in the human melanocortin-4 receptor gene associated with severe familial obesity disrupts receptor function through multiple molecular mechanisms. Hum Mol Genet 2003;12(5):561–74.

56. Bamshad M, Krakowiak PA, Watkins WS, Root S, Carey JC, Jorde LB. A gene for ulnar-mammary syndrome maps to 12q23-q24.1. Hum Mol Genet 1995;4:1973–7.

57. Collin GB, Marshall JD, Cardon LR, Nishina PM. Homozygosity mapping at Alstrom syndrome to chromosome 2p. Hum Mol Genet 1997;6:213–19.

58. Tahvanainen E, Norio R, Karila E, et al. Cohen syndrome gene assigned to the long arm of chromosome 8 by linkage analysis. Nat Genet 1994;7:201–4.

59. Turner G, Gedeon A, Mulley J, et al. Borjeson-Forssman-Lehmann syndrome: clinical manifestations and gene localization to Xq26-27. Am J Med Genet 1989;34:463–69.

60. Steinmuller R, Steinberger D, Muller U. MEHMO (mental retardation, epileptic seizures, hypogonadism and -genitalism, microcephaly, obesity), a novel syndrome: assignment of disease locus to xp21.1-p22.13. Eur J Hum Genet 1998;6:201–6.

61. Brzustowicz LM FS, Khan MB, Weksberg R. Mapping of a new SGBS locus to chromosome Xp22 in a family with a severe form of Simpson-Golabi-Behmel syndrome. Am J Hum Genet 1999;65:779–83.

62. Wilson M, Mulley J, Gedeon A, Robinson H, Turner G. New X-linked syndrome of mental retardation, gynecomastia, and obesity is linked to DXS255. Am J Med Genet 1991;40:406–13.

8 Fetal and Infant Origins of Obesity

Matthew W. Gillman

Department of Population Medicine, Harvard Medical School, Boston, MA, USA

Introduction

The worldwide obesity epidemic has existed for several decades in upper- and middle-income countries, and is emerging along with the epidemiologic transition in most developing countries. The epidemic includes all ages, even very young children. Among infants, as well as older children, the prevalence of obesity has increased substantially over the past 2–3 decades (Figs 8.1, 8.2) [1–3].

Excess weight in children can cause type 2 diabetes mellitus [4–6], hypertension and dyslipidemia [7,8], sleep apnea [9], early maturation [10] and psychosocial stress, and is associated with increased risk of asthma, the only childhood chronic disease that rivals obesity in prevalence, morbidity, and cost [11–14]. Obesity in children, especially older children, also predicts adult obesity and its morbid consequences [15,16]. Once present, obesity is hard to treat, not only because of entrenched behaviors but also because physiologica mechanisms tend to resist weight loss [17,18].

For these reasons it is highly desirable to begin prevention efforts as early as possible, even before birth. This chapter therefore focuses on factors in the prenatal period and in infancy that determine obesity and its consequences later in life.

Measurement of obesity in young children

Because many studies of pre- and perinatal origins of obesity employ outcomes assessed during childhood, it is important to consider relevant measures of adiposity. From the age of 2 years

onwards, Body Mass Index (BMI, kg/m^2) is the standard measure of adiposity for clinical and public health purposes. BMI has the advantage of being relatively easily measured, as long as one obtains accurate measures of height, and the US Centers for Disease Control and Prevention (CDC) and the International Obesity Taskforce (IOTF) have widely disseminated growth charts using BMI [19,20].

In the US, the recommended ranges for overweight and obesity are age- and sex-specific 85th–95th percentile and >95th percentile, respectively [21]. The reference population for these percentile calculations is based on nationally representative surveys primarily from the 1970s, when the population was much thinner as a whole. Many other countries use growth curves of the IOTF [20] which define overweight and obesity by age- and sex-specific cutpoints that predict the adult cutpoints of 25 and $30 \, kg/m^2$, respectively. In adolescence, the CDC curves tend to overestimate these adult ranges, so the IOTF standards have advantages at that stage. But for young children, the CDC growth curves are adequate.

For children 0–2 years of age, the definitions of overweight and obesity are based on the CDC's weight-for-length standards rather than BMI. Like the standards for older children, the definitions are based on the 85th and 95th percentile cutpoints. But the definitions are less certain because fewer nationally representative data exist to create the reference population. For infants and young children, some researchers and clinicians are now using the newer WHO charts based on breast-fed infants [22–25].

It is also important to note that errors in length measurement in clinical practice are common and lead to false inferences. In a validation study of 160 children aged 0–23 months in a primary care practice, Rifas-Shiman et al [26] showed that clinical length measures overestimate research-standard measures by a reliably predictable amount, an average of over 1 cm across this age range (Fig. 8.3).

This overestimation of length results in weight-for-length measures that markedly underestimate obesity prevalence. Thus clinicians currently underdetect overweight among their very young patients, and should therefore adopt and use accurate measurement equipment and technique. Researchers using

Clinical Obesity in Adults and Children, 3rd edition. Edited by Peter G. Kopelman, Ian D. Caterson and William H. Dietz.
© 2010 Blackwell Publishing, ISBN: 978-1-4051-8226-3.

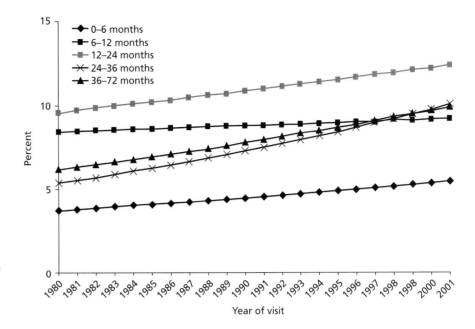

Figure 8.1 Age-specific predicted prevalence of overweight from 1980 through 2001 among 120,680 children 0–71.9 months seen at 366,109 well-child care visits at a Massachusetts HMO, according to age group. (Reproduced with permission from Kim et al. [1].)

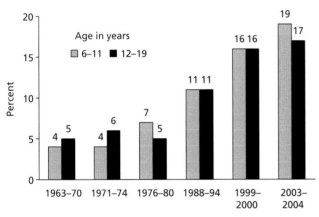

Figure 8.2 The rising prevalence of obesity (BMI >95th percentile for age and sex) among children 6–19 years old, from US national data. (Adapted from Ogden et al. [2] and Hedley et al. [3].)

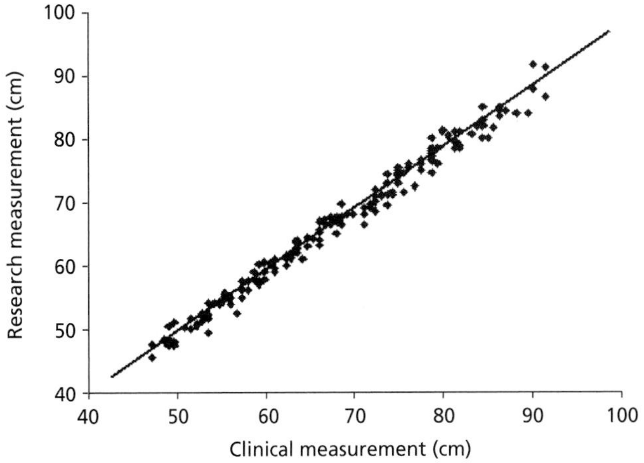

Figure 8.3 Relationship between clinical and research measurements of length among 160 children age 0–23 months of age. Research measurement = clinical measurement × 0.953 + 1.88 cm. (Reproduced with permission from Rifas-Shiman et al. [132].)

clinical databases to estimate length, and thus weight-for-length or BMI, must be aware of this limitation and may consider using a regression equation (as given in Fig. 8.3) to correct length measurements.

The situation in 2–3 year olds is even more confusing. Depending on how well the child can stand, clinicians may measure recumbent length or standing height. Even with research-standard measurement, standing height is about 0.5–0.75 cm lower than recumbent length [27,28]. Thus researchers need to know which type of measure applies to an individual, and use the appropriate growth chart. In the US, the CDC provides charts for weight-for-length for 0–36 month olds, and BMI (which assumes standing height) for 24 months or older.

Even if one measures length or height accurately, both BMI and weight-for-length have the inherent limitation of not measuring body composition directly. While BMI >95th percentile appears to be a valid measure of excess adiposity, the lower the percentile, the lower the correlation between BMI and fatness [29].

In a research setting, direct measures of body composition are feasible starting at birth. These include dual-energy X-ray absorptiometry (DXA) [30–32] and the PEAPOD, which uses air displacement plethysmography [33,34]. Both DXA and PEAPOD measure total body fat. DXA can also estimate regional fat as well as lean body mass and bone density and content, but emits a small amount of radiation. Skinfold thicknesses are a much cheaper alternative, but require strict attention to technique and thus highly skilled operators. Bio-impedance techniques may not be reliable in very young children because of divergence from assumptions that underlie the equations to determine fat mass [35,36].

Whether to use weight/length/height measures or a more direct measure of adiposity in any research study rests not only on feasibility but also purpose. Many current studies of early origins of obesity are limited to simple anthropometric indices, and they contribute substantially to the literature. As reviewed in the remainder of the chapter, however, many questions remain about observed associations of pre- and perinatal factors with later adiposity or obesity, and for these, direct measures of body composition or, indeed, the physiologic/metabolic concomitants of excess adiposity are desirable.

Conceptual framework of early origins of obesity

Two recent paradigms offer useful conceptual frameworks. One is termed the life course approach to chronic disease [37]. Factors may act in the preconceptional phase through the prenatal period, into infancy, childhood and beyond, to determine risk of chronic disease. Orthogonal to the time axis, influencing factors can range from the social/built/natural environment (macro) through behavior, physiology, and genetics (micro). Factors interact with each other over the life course, with different determinants being more or less important at different life stages.

Under this paradigm, some factors may be more deterministic than others. "Programming" refers to insults at critical or sensitive periods of development that have lifelong, sometimes irreversible consequences. An example from a rat model is that a low-protein maternal diet consumed *only* during the embryonic period can cause lifelong hypertension in the offspring [38]. The mechanism underlying this finding appears to involve reduced activity of the placental enzyme that normally protects the fetus from excess exposure to glucocorticoids, which are stress hormones. Other factors may contribute to chronic disease through accumulation of risk. For example, chronic exposure to elevated lipid levels is associated with preatherosclerotic coronary lesions among adolescents [39].

A second, related paradigm is called developmental origins of health and disease (DOHaD). Based on similar principles, DOHaD focuses primarily on the prenatal period and infancy as determinants of long-term health [40]. Both of these frameworks call attention to the period of developmental plasticity in determining lifelong trajectories of health. This plastic period is different for different organs and systems, but is generally complete by birth or the first years of life [40]. Factors that occur later in life, e.g. childhood or adult risk factors, modify the trajectories started during early life.

One epidemiologic pattern consistently observed across ages and geography supports this theory: the highest risk of cardiometabolic outcomes occurs among individuals with the combination of lower birth weight and higher Body Mass Index later in life, mediated through accelerated weight gain during childhood [41–47]. This particular pattern has been termed the "thrifty phenotype" [48]. Animal models of energy deprivation during pregnancy followed by energy excess in the offspring clearly demonstrate that such patterns are the result of changes in the fetal environment: that is, they are not due to variation in the fetal genome [49–51].

Observational designs to study developmental origins of health and disease

Animal experiments provide compelling data that early developmental perturbations shape lifelong health [52]. Long-term effects on body composition, hypertension, and cardiometabolic outcomes are relatively easy to induce by interventions ranging from the nutritional – typically protein or energy restriction – to administration of hormones such as glucocorticoids, mechanical disruption such as uterine artery ligation, and by inducing anemia or hypoxia [40]. While these experiments are proof of principle, translation to the human condition is not straightforward. Obtaining physiologic data from the maternal-placental-fetal unit is most often indirect. Also, the majority of animal interventions are not feasible or too extreme for humans. Thus one needs to make judicious inferences from well-designed epidemiologic studies.

The first generation of epidemiologic studies were historical, and took advantage of recorded or recalled data on birth size. Professor David Barker from Southampton and his colleagues, by taking advantage of perinatal information meticulously recorded by health visitors in Hertfordshire, were among the first to demonstrate that birth weight is associated with cardiovascular disease and its risk factors many decades later [53]. Birth weight, however, is not an etiologic factor itself and so cannot lead to an understanding of mechanism or public health implication. For example, both lower and higher birth weight are associated with later adiposity-related outcomes, probably representing different underlying pathways [54]. DOHaD researchers now recognize that birth weight, as well as its components fetal growth and length of gestation, are proxy measures for many determinants of lifelong health, and it is essential to identify and quantify these determinants themselves [55]. Thus other types of studies, with data on potentially etiologic pre- and postnatal factors, are required.

A second type of study takes advantage of cohort studies of pregnant women and their children that were begun decades ago. In the US, examples are the National Collaborative Perinatal Project (NCPP) and Child Health and Development Study, both cohort studies with prenatal recruitment in the 1950s and 1960s and initial follow-up until school age. Several investigators have now recontacted and followed up subcohorts in adulthood, and publications on obesity and other health outcomes are beginning to appear [56–61]. The UK's Boyd Orr study is another example [62]. This type of study has the advantages of research-quality data collection during pregnancy and early childhood, but it can lack some key data elements in which researchers are now interested. For example, the NCPP collected no maternal dietary data, and blood samples were stored at −20C, not the current standard of −80C or lower.

A third type of epidemiologic study is creating new prospective cohorts of pregnant women and their children. These prebirth cohort studies have the advantage of collecting more current information, especially the opportunity to collect and store biosamples. But one has to be patient; a long period of time needs to elapse before hard clinical outcomes occur. Fortunately, obesity and its cardiometabolic sequelae have a relatively large number of accepted surrogate outcomes in childhood. In the US, the National Children's Study offers an example of such a design on a large scale [63].

Identifying modifiable developmental determinants

Prenatal determinants: maternal smoking during pregnancy, gestational weight gain, gestational diabetes

Because severe protein or energy restriction in pregnant animal species causes adverse offspring outcomes reproducibly, maternal "undernutrition" is a useful construct for experimental physiologists. In the human, a more helpful concept is "fetal nutrition," which is the entire supply line of nutrients, oxygen, hormones, etc., to the growing embryo and fetus. Thus one considers not only maternal diet, but also other maternal behaviors. Moreover, both more proximal influences such as uteroplacental blood flow and placental and fetal metabolism, and distal influences such as maternal preconceptional health and even the mother's own intrauterine and early life experiences, may be important.

Using this conceptual basis, investigators have begun to identify modifiable prenatal determinants of offspring obesity and its consequences. Maternal smoking during pregnancy is one example. While maternal smoking causes reduced fetal growth, more than a dozen studies now confirm that it is associated with offspring obesity. In a recent meta-analysis of 14 studies, Oken et al. [64] estimated that maternal smoking during pregnancy conferred increased odds of 50% (adjusted odds ratio 1.50, 95% confidence interval (CI) 1.36–1.65) for offspring obesity across an age range of 3–33 years (Fig. 8.4). Adjustment for factors related to social and economic position did not markedly affect estimates, but residual confounding is still possible. Animal studies of this phenomenon are few; one in rats indicates that nicotine administration in the puerperal period leads to higher weight through early adulthood [65].

If this relationship is causal, the public health implications could be considerable in developing countries in which maternal smoking is rising with the obesity epidemic. The small fetus, obese child phenotype of maternal smoking is not only characteristic of the epidemiologic transition from acute to chronic disease [66] but as noted above ("thrifty phenotype"), it also confers the highest risk for cardiometabolic health outcomes [41–46].

Another example is gestational weight gain. As summarized in a recent report from the US National Academy of Sciences [67], more mothers are entering pregnancy overweight or obese than in the past, and excessive weight gain during pregnancy is also probably more frequent than in previous decades. In Project Viva, a modern US-based prebirth cohort study, Oken et al. [68] showed that excessive gestational weight gain, as defined by the 1990 Institute of Medicine guidelines [69], was associated with higher BMI and risk of obesity in the offspring at the age of 3 years (Fig. 8.5). This pattern is also evident in analyses of participants in the NCPP, an older US study [70]. Remarkably little is

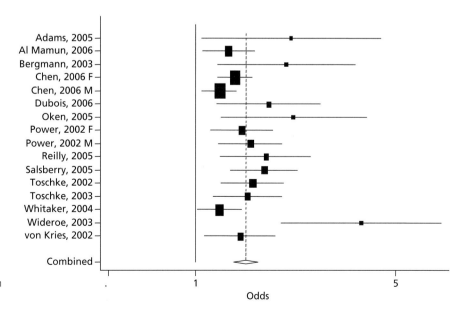

Figure 8.4 Results of meta-analysis of maternal smoking during pregnancy and child overweight. The pooled adjusted odds ratio was 1.50 (95% CI 1.36–1.65). (Reproduced with permission from Oken et al. [64].)

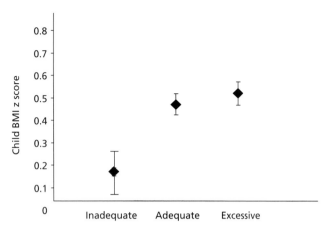

Figure 8.5 Adjusted mean child BMI z-score (95% CI) at age 3 years, according to the maternal gestational weight gain category recommended by the Institute of Medicine [69]. Data from Project Viva. (Reproduced with permission from Oken et al. [133].)

Table 8.1 Association of varying levels of glucose tolerance in pregnancy with offspring overweight at age 5–7 years

Pregnancy result	Weight-for-age at age 5–7 years, Odds ratio (95% CI)	
	>85th percentile	>95th percentile
Normal screening glycemic test	1.0 (ref)	1.0 (ref)
Normal follow-up oral glucose tolerance test	0.98 (0.81–1.17)	0.97 (0.77–1.24)
Impaired glucose tolerance	1.37 (1.01–1.84)	1.30 (0.89–1.90)
Gestational diabetes, not treated	1.89 (1.30–2.76)	1.82 (1.15–2.88)
Gestational diabetes, treated	1.29 (0.85–1.97)	1.38 (0.84–2.27)

Data from 9439 members of Kaiser Permanente in Hawaii, Oregon, and Washington. Adapted from Hillier et al. [78].

known about either the mechanisms of these effects or about modifiable determinants of gestational weight gain. Because women gained less in earlier eras, however, hope exists that new behavior change interventions can moderate excessive weight gain. In the current era of epidemic obesity, more evidence is urgently needed on identifying optimal weight gain during pregnancy for both maternal and child health as well as on strategies to induce pregnant women to gain within recommended ranges.

Higher maternal BMI at the start of pregnancy is a strong risk factor for many adverse outcomes, including offspring obesity [71], but it is not part of this chapter because it is not modifiable once pregnancy begins. Nevertheless, ensuring optimal BMI at the start of pregnancy is one of the most important goals for intergenerational prevention of obesity.

One major disorder that is strongly related to maternal pre-pregnancy obesity is gestational diabetes (GDM). GDM is associated with higher fetal growth, and thus birth weight, and many studies now show that birth weight is directly related to later BMI [72–74]. Thus it makes sense to consider GDM as a potential determinant of offspring obesity. Animal studies of induced GDM suggest that this relationship holds, as do epidemiologic studies in areas of high GDM prevalence, including the methodologically strong within-family (sib-pair) approach [75,76].

However, some other studies, in more general population samples, are equivocal [72,77]. One reason may be that these studies likely include both untreated and successfully treated cases of GDM. In one study, offspring of untreated GDM had higher weights at school age than offspring of treated GDM (Table 8.1) [78], suggesting that the natural history of GDM is to cause offspring obesity. It is important to understand this association. Given that obesity and diabetes are rising around the world [79], the intergenerational vicious cycle of obesity leading to GDM leading to offspring obesity could contribute to the amplification of the obesity epidemic.

Many challenges also remain in studying causes and consequences of GDM. While physical activity both before and during pregnancy appears to reduce the risk of impaired glucose tolerance and GDM [80–82], only dietary factors before, but not during, pregnancy seem to play a preventive role [83,85]. In addition, studies of body composition and cardiometabolic outcomes in childhood and adulthood, not just BMI, are important to understand more fully the intergenerational consequences of GDM.

Maternal dietary intakes during pregnancy represent another potential cause of offspring obesity. Perhaps surprisingly, the literature reveals no consistent findings. Part of the issue is methodologic, as the combination of accurate dietary data collected during pregnancy and offspring follow-up long enough to detect salient outcomes is scarce. Current research focuses on the role of micronutrients (e.g. vitamin D), macronutrient quantity and quality (e.g. glycemic load), and dietary patterns. Novel work in a mouse model indicates that maternal diet around the time of conception that is replete with methyl donors such as folate, vitamin B12, betaine and choline can lower the risk of offspring obesity and diabetes through epigenetic mechanisms [86]. Analogous studies in humans are yet to surface because of difficulties surrounding tissue and species specificity in epigenetic research as well as the need for longitudinal studies with accurate periconceptional diet, biomarker, and outcome data.

Postnatal determinants: infant weight gain, feeding, sleep

In the first year of life, at least three factors play a role in determining later obesity. One is infant growth. It is critical to distinguish linear growth from weight gain. Because weight gain accompanies linear growth, weight gain in excess of linear growth is more interesting than weight gain alone. As noted above, obtaining accurate length measures is crucial. Most studies to date do not have accurate lengths, and therefore resort to examining weight gain alone. Future studies would benefit from having longitudinal measures of body composition in addition to accurate weights and lengths.

Meta-analyses now show that accelerated weight gain during the first weeks or months of life is associated with higher BMI or obesity later in life [87,88]. For example, Baird et al. [87] reviewed 10 studies that assessed the relationship of infant growth with subsequent obesity. Compared with other infants, among infants with more rapid growth the odds ratios (OR) and relative risks of later obesity ranged from 1.17 to 5.70. Associations were consistent for obesity at different ages and for people born over a period from 1927 to 1994.

One study of formula-fed infants in the US suggests that weight gain even in the first week of life predicts obesity at age 20–32 years old [89]. After adjustment for confounding factors, each 100 g increase in weight gain during the first week of life was associated with a 28% increased odds of adult overweight (OR 1.28, 95% CI 1.08–1.52). Follow-up of UK-born infants, either premature or small for gestational age, who had experienced higher rates of weight gain in early infancy from being allocated higher-energy infant formula, showed higher BMI, blood pressure, insulin and leptin levels in later childhood or adolescence [90,91]. In one of the few studies employing accurate length measures, Belfort et al. [92] showed that gain in weight-for-length from birth to 6 months was associated with higher systolic blood pressure among 3-year-old participants in Project Viva.

Despite the seeming consistency of these studies, one must also be aware of counter examples. Among Finnish men, those who eventually developed coronary heart disease, compared with the cohort as a whole, appeared to have experienced declining height, weight, and BMI during the first year of life before increasing dramatically after the age of 2 years [47]. Indian men and women who developed impaired glucose tolerance or type 2 diabetes in young adulthood appeared to follow the same pattern [46]. In the Finnish cohort, gain in BMI in the first 2 years of life was associated with adult lean mass but not fat mass [93]. In contrast, BMI gain from 2 to 7 years was associated with higher fat as well as lean mass. These discrepancies in the role of infant weight gain may be due to differing measurements or participant experiences across time or geography, but the true explanations are as yet unclear. Disentangling them is critical for public health and clinical medicine. In addition, the apparent cardiometabolic harms of rapid infant weight gain need to be balanced against its potential benefit for neurocognitive outcomes, especially in babies born preterm and in the developing world, where some studies question the link between weight gain in infancy and later fatness [94–96].

One determinant of infant weight gain is infant feeding. Having been breast fed at all, or for a longer duration, may lower risk for subsequent obesity. In a meta-analysis of duration of breast feeding, Harder et al. [97] estimated a 4% decreased odds for each additional month of breast feeding. Two meta-analyses of breast versus bottle feeding showed 13–22% reductions in odds of later obesity [98,99]. The two largest US studies with racial/ethnic information, however, showed that effects were limited to whites [100,101]. One potential explanation is different breast-feeding traditions in different cultural groups (e.g. complementary bottle feeding along with nursing), but evidence is lacking. Also, one additional meta-analysis that employed individual-level data, rather than combining published group results, did not show a protective effect of having been breast fed on mean BMI as a continuous variable [102]. One explanation for the null findings could be different outcomes. The studies with dichotomous outcomes appear to show an effect, while the ones with mean BMI do not. Effects at the extreme of the BMI distribution could be larger than those at the mean. An alternative explanation could be better adjustment for social and economic confounding factors in the individual-level meta-analysis. Six-year follow-up of children in a large randomized trial of breast-feeding promotion in the Republic of Belarus showed no intervention effect on anthropometric outcomes, supporting this inference [103]. One should note, however, that all children in the Belarussian trial were breast fed. Also, in the Growing Up Today Study, Gillman et al. [104] found similar odds ratios for a within-family and an overall cohort analysis of breast-feeding duration, suggesting that residual socio-economic confounding did not play a major role. In addition, some recent studies have taken into account a range of potentially confounding variables, and still confirm an association [105]. The best evidence indicates that having been breast fed does not increase the risk of obesity, and may reduce it to a moderate degree.

A third factor during infancy is sleep duration, an issue of great importance to many new parents. Lack of sleep among adults is associated with excess weight gain and development of obesity [106]. Although the data are still few, the same relationship appears to exist in early childhood. For example, in the Project Viva cohort, Taveras et al. [107] showed that infant sleep of less than 12 hours per day was associated with an OR of 2.20 (95% CI 1.16–4.19) for overweight at age 3 years. Sleep quality, and possibly duration, appear modifiable in infancy [108–110].

Combination of pre- and postnatal factors

The life course approach to chronic disease [37] proposes that combinations of factors at different life stages influence health trajectories. Using data from Project Viva, Gillman et al. [111] examined predicted probabilities of obesity at age 3 years according to covariate-adjusted levels of four potentially modifiable risk factors in pregnancy and infancy. These factors were maternal smoking during pregnancy, gestational weight gain, breast-feeding duration, and infant sleep. Given optimal levels of all four factors, the predicted probability of obesity was 6%, whereas the predicted probability associated with adverse levels of all four was 29% (Fig. 8.6). This wide range of predicted probabilities suggests that interventions to modify these factors during pregnancy and infancy could have a substantial impact on reducing childhood obesity rates.

Applying newer analytical methods may help in disentangling complex pathways. Analyses involving growth in particular are challenging because, for example, weight gain in one period of life typically entrains weight gain in the next. Isolating one or more critical periods of weight gain is difficult [112], as is

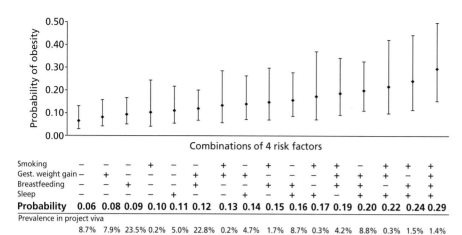

Smoking	–	–	–	+	–	–	+	–	+	–	+	+	–	+	+	+
Gest. weight gain	–	+	–	–	–	+	+	+	–	–	–	+	+	+	–	+
Breastfeeding	–	–	+	–	–	+	–	–	+	+	+	–	+	+	–	+
Sleep	–	–	–	–	+	–	–	+	–	+	+	+	+	–	+	+
Probability	**0.06**	**0.08**	**0.09**	**0.10**	**0.11**	**0.12**	**0.13**	**0.14**	**0.15**	**0.16**	**0.17**	**0.19**	**0.20**	**0.22**	**0.24**	**0.29**
Prevalence in project viva	8.7%	7.9%	23.5%	0.2%	5.0%	22.8%	0.2%	4.7%	1.7%	8.7%	0.3%	4.2%	8.8%	0.3%	1.5%	1.4%

Figure 8.6 Predicted probability of obesity (BMI > 95th percentile) at 3 years of age for 16 combinations of four modifiable risk factors during pregnancy and infancy. Bars show 95% confidence limits. Also shown is prevalence for each depicted combination of factors among 1110 mother–child pairs participating in Project Viva. Probabilities are adjusted for maternal education and BMI, household income, and child race/ethnicity.

Table 8.2 Definitions of risk factors in Figure 8.6

Smoking in pregnancy	Yes	No
Gestational weight gain*	"Excessive"	"Adequate or inadequate"
Breast-feeding duration	<12 m	≥12 m
Daily sleep in infancy	<12 h/d	≥12 h/d

*Gestational weight gain categories per 1990 recommendations of Institute of Medicine [69]. Adapted from Gillman et al. [111].

combining growth with other parameters in one analysis. De Stavola [113] suggests use of structural equation modeling, a promising but unproven technique for these issues. In addition, for growth analyses, newer studies with serial prenatal ultrasound measurements will allow more direct measures of prenatal growth parameters than merely measuring anthropometry at birth.

Clinical and public health implications; future research

While much more work is needed on identifying and quantifying pre- and perinatal determinants of obesity and its consequences, some implications are already clear. The first is that intervening to change birth weight is likely to be ineffective, if not harmful. Birth weight is a proxy for many determinants, not an etiologic factor itself. Efforts should focus on the etiologic factors themselves, each of which may or may not affect birth weight. We review many of these factors in this chapter.

While having decreased in recent decades in the developed world, rates of maternal smoking during pregnancy are probably rising in developing countries, owing to marketing practices by tobacco companies [114–118]. The combination of policy, environmental, and individual behavior change strategies that have been successful in Western societies to reduce rates of smoking may be more difficult to plan and implement in the developing parts of the world [119–122]. Nevertheless, preventing smoking

among girls and women of reproductive age is a health priority worldwide, only one reason for which is to potentially prevent offspring obesity.

Prevention of gestational diabetes is also a priority. GDM causes many perinatal complications as well as offspring obesity [72,77]. The most important prevention measure is the least attainable at present: to ensure that women enter pregnancy at a normal BMI. However, promotion of light to moderate physical activity during pregnancy appears to be a promising strategy [80].

It is not known whether treatment of GDM will reduce risk of offspring obesity. Following up children whose mothers participated in successful short-term trials of GDM treatment [123] represents a robust study design to answer this question as well as to solidify the causal link between GDM and offspring obesity.

Modifying gestational weight gain appears to be an attractive public health goal at this time. But some caution is warranted, as too little weight gain is associated with reduced fetal growth and neonatal morbidity [69]. The Institute of Medicine and other authoritative groups need more data on the balance of short- and long-term risks and benefits of various amounts of gestational weight gain in general, and according to groups defined by pre-pregnancy BMI. In addition, the best strategies to modify gestational weight gain are unknown, as its determinants are yet to be clarified. Fortunately, pregnancy appears to be one period of a woman's life during which behavior change may be readily achievable [124].

Breast-feeding initiation and maintenance benefit many health outcomes in children, including atopy and gastrointestinal illness [125]. While confounding is still an issue, the best evidence to date suggests that having been breast fed may also lower the risk of later obesity. Therefore it is reasonable for clinicians and public health officials to include obesity prevention as one of the benefits in programs to increase breast-feeding rates. Breast-feeding behavior is surely modifiable, as both initiation and maintenance rates have increased in the US substantially in the past 30–40 years [126].

Not enough is known yet about infant weight gain or sleep duration to include them in clinical or public health programs to prevent childhood obesity. Over and above the effects of infant feeding, determinants of infant weight gain that are related to later obesity are obscure. Therefore it is not known whether (or how) moderating infant weight gain will lower obesity rates later in childhood or adulthood. Further, at least among premature infants, weight gain that is too low is associated with adverse neuropsychologic outcomes [96,127]. Therefore, more information is needed about optimal levels of infant weight gain, as well as its modifiability, before anyone should make clinical recommendations.

Similarly, recommendations about sleep duration for obesity prevention are premature. More data are required about the underlying association, its mechanisms and potential determinants. In the meantime, however, clinicians and parents may wish to employ evidence-based sleep hygiene techniques to improve sleep quality and perhaps increase sleep duration [128–130].

Future research should take advantage of longitudinal study designs to explore new pre- and perinatal determinants and pathways leading to offspring adiposity and its consequences. For example, analogous to animal models, Gillman et al. [131] reported that maternal second-trimester levels of corticotropin-releasing hormone, a proxy for fetal glucocorticoid exposure, were associated with lower BMI but higher ratio of subscapular:triceps skinfold ratio, a measure of central adiposity, among 3-year-old children. This result raises the possibility that maternal stress, irrespective of any lifestyle behavior choice, may program offspring metabolic dysfunction.

In addition, more refined measurement techniques and new analytic methods, as discussed in this chapter, will provide more insight into underlying pathways. Through these approaches, researchers are becoming more and more likely to find modifiable etiologic factors that lend themselves to judicious clinical and public health interventions. Ultimately, the hope is that interventions during pregnancy and early childhood that are developmentally appropriate, and that employ strategies to change both environmental and behavioral factors, will contribute substantially to preventing obesity and its consequences throughout the life course.

References

1. Kim J, Peterson KE, Scanlon KS, et al. Trends in overweight from 1980 through 2001 among preschool-aged children enrolled in a health maintenance organization. Obesity (Silver Spring) 2006; 14(7):1107–12.

2. Ogden CL, Carroll MD, Curtin LR, McDowell MA, Tabak CJ, Flegal KM. Prevalence of overweight and obesity in the United States, 1999–2004. JAMA 2006;295(13):1549–55.

3. Hedley AA, Ogden CL, Johnson CL, Carroll MD, Curtin LR, Flegal KM. Prevalence of overweight and obesity among US children, adolescents, and adults, 1999–2002. JAMA 2004; 291(23):2847–50.

4. Liese AD, d'Agostino RB Jr, Hamman RF, et al. The burden of diabetes mellitus among US youth: prevalence estimates from the SEARCH for Diabetes in Youth Study. Pediatrics 2006;118(4): 1510–18.

5. Haines L, Wan KC, Lynn R, Barrett TG, Shield JP. Rising incidence of type 2 diabetes in children in the United Kingdom. Diabetes Care 2007;30(5):1097–101.

6. Molnar D. The prevalence of the metabolic syndrome and type 2 diabetes mellitus in children and adolescents. Int J Obes 2004; 28(suppl 3):S70–S74.

7. Freedman DS, Serdula MK, Srinivasan SR, Berenson GS. Relation of circumferences and skinfold thicknesses to lipid and insulin concentrations in children and adolescents: the Bogalusa Heart Study. Am J Clin Nutr 1999;69(2):308–17.

8. Morrison JA, Sprecher DL, Barton BA, Waclawiw MA, Daniels SR. Overweight, fat patterning, and cardiovascular disease risk factors in black and white girls: The National Heart, Lung, and Blood Institute Growth and Health Study. J Pediatr 1999;135(4):458–64.

9. Daniels SR. The consequences of childhood overweight and obesity. Future Child 2006;16(1):47–67.

10. Lee JM, Appugliese D, Kaciroti N, Corwyn RF, Bradley RH, Lumeng JC. Weight status in young girls and the onset of puberty. Pediatrics 2007;119(3):E624–E630.

11. Gold DR, Damokosh AI, Dockery DW, Berkey CS. Body-mass index as a predictor of incident asthma in a prospective cohort of children. Pediatr Pulmonol 2003;36(6):514–21.

12. Akinbami L. The state of childhood asthma, United States, 1980–2005. Adv Data 2006:381:1–24.

13. Lozano P, Sullivan SD, Smith DH, Weiss KB. The economic burden of asthma in US children: estimates from the National Medical Expenditure Survey. J Allergy Clin Immunol 1999;104(5):957–63.

14. Wang G, Dietz WH. Economic burden of obesity in youths aged 6 to 17 years: 1979–1999. Pediatrics 2002;109(5):e81.

15. Whitaker RC, Wright JA, Pepe MS, Seidel KD, Dietz WH Jr. Predicting obesity in young adulthood from childhood and parental obesity. N Engl J Med 1997;337:869–73.

16. Baker JL, Olsen LW, Sorensen TI. Childhood body-mass index and the risk of coronary heart disease in adulthood. N Engl J Med 2007;357(23):2329–37.

17. Rosenbaum M, Leibel RL. The physiology of body weight regulation: relevance to the etiology of obesity in children. Pediatrics 1998;101(3 Pt 2):525–39.

18. Rosenbaum M, Goldsmith R, Bloomfield D, et al. Low-dose leptin reverses skeletal muscle, autonomic, and neuroendocrine adaptations to maintenance of reduced weight. J Clin Invest 2005;115(12):3579–86.

19. Centers for Disease Control and Prevention. CDC growth charts: United States, 2000. Available at: www.cdc.gov/nchs/about/major/nhanes/growthcharts/datafiles.htm.

20. Cole TJ, Bellizzi MC, Flegal KM, Dietz WH. Establishing a standard definition for child overweight and obesity worldwide: international survey. BMJ 2000;320(7244):1240–3.

21. Barlow SE. Expert committee recommendations regarding the prevention, assessment, and treatment of child and adolescent overweight and obesity: summary report. Pediatrics 2007;120(suppl 4):S164-S192.

22. World Health Organization. New growth charts, 2007. Available at: www.who.int/nutrition/media_page/en/index.html

23. de Onis M, Onyango AW. The Centers for Disease Control and Prevention 2000 growth charts and the growth of breastfed infants. Acta Paediatr 2003;92(4):413–19.

24. Wright CM. Growth charts for babies. BMJ 2005;330(7505): 1399–400.

25. de Onis M, Garza C, Onyango AW, Borghi E. Comparison of the WHO child growth standards and the CDC 2000 growth charts. J Nutr 2007;137(1):144–8.

26. Rifas-Shiman SL, Rich-Edwards JW, Scanlon KS, Kleinman KP, Gillman MW. Misdiagnosis of overweight and underweight children younger than 2 years of age due to length measurement bias. Medscape Gen Med 2005;7(4):55.

27. World Health Organization. Child growth standards based on length/height, weight and age. Acta Paediatr 2006;450(76, suppl):85.

28. Buyken AE, Hahn S, Kroke A. Differences between recumbent length and stature measurement in groups of 2- and 3-y-old children and its relevance for the use of European body mass index references. Int J Obes 2005;29(1):24–8.

29. Daniels SR, Khoury PR, Morrison JA. The utility of body mass index as a measure of body fatness in children and adolescents: differences by race and gender. Pediatrics 1997;99(6):804–7.

30. Goran MI. Measurement issues related to studies of childhood obesity: assessment of body composition, body fat distribution, physical activity, and food intake. Pediatrics 1998;101;505–18.

31. Eisenmann JC, Heelan KA, Welk GJ. Assessing body composition among 3- to 8-year-old children: anthropometry, BIA, and DXA. Obes Res 2004;12(10):1633–40.

32. Fors H, Gelander L, Bjarnason R, Albertsson-Wikland K, Bosaeus I. Body composition, as assessed by bioelectrical impedance spectroscopy and dual-energy X-ray absorptiometry, in a healthy paediatric population. Acta Paediatr 2002;91(7):755–60.

33. Ellis KJ, Yao M, Shypailo RJ, Urlando A, Wong WW, Heird WC. Body-composition assessment in infancy: air-displacement plethysmography compared with a reference 4-compartment model. Am J Clin Nutr 2007;85(1):90–5.

34. Ma G, Yao M, Liu Y, et al. Validation of a new pediatric airdisplacement plethysmograph for assessing body composition in infants. Am J Clin Nutr 2004;79(4):653–60.

35. Dung NQ, Fusch G, Armbrust S, Jochum F, Fusch C. Body composition of preterm infants measured during the first months of life: bioelectrical impedance provides insignificant additional information compared to anthropometry alone. Eur J Pediatr 2007;166(3): 215–22.

36. Mast M, Sonnichsen A, Langnase K, et al. Inconsistencies in bioelectrical impedance and anthropometric measurements of fat mass in a field study of prepubertal children. Br J Nutr 2002;87(2): 163–75.

37. Kuh D, Ben-Shlomo Y. *A Life Course Approach to Chronic Disease Epidemiology: Tracing the Origins of Ill-Health from Early to Adult Life*, 2nd edn. Oxford: Oxford Medical Publications, 2004.

38. Kwong WY, Wild AE, Roberts P, Willis AC, Fleming TP. Maternal undernutrition during the preimplantation period of rat development causes blastocyst abnormalities and programming of postnatal hypertension. Development 2000;127(19):4195–202.

39. PDAY Research Group. Relationship of atherosclerosis in young men to serum lipoprotein cholesterol concentrations and smoking. A preliminary report from the Pathobiological Determinants of Atherosclerosis in Youth (PDAY) Research Group. JAMA 1990;264:3018–24.

40. Gluckman P, Hanson M. *Developmental origins of health and disease*. New York: Cambridge University Press, 2006.

41. Bavdekar A, Yajnik CS, Fall CHD, et al. The insulin resistance syndrome in eight-year-old Indian children; small at birth, big at eight years or both? Diabetes 1999;48:2422–9.

42. Adair LS, Cole TJ. Rapid child growth raises blood pressure in adolescent boys who were thin at birth. Hypertension 2003;41(3): 451–6.

43. Valdez R, Mitchell BD, Haffner SM, et al. Predictors of weight change in a bi-ethnic population. The San Antonio Heart Study. Int J Obes 1994;18(2):85–91.

44. Frankel S, Elwood P, Sweetnam P, Yarnell J, Davey Smith G. Birthweight, body-mass index in middle age, and incident coronary heart disease. Lancet 1996;348:1478–80.

45. Rich-Edwards JW, Kleinman K, Michels KB, et al. Longitudinal study of birth weight and adult body mass index in predicting risk of coronary heart disease and stroke in women. BMJ 2005; 330(7500):1115.

46. Bhargava SK, Sachdev HS, Fall CH, et al. Relation of serial changes in childhood body-mass index to impaired glucose tolerance in young adulthood. N Engl J Med 2004;350(9):865–75.

47. Barker DJP, Osmond C, Forsen TJ, Kajantie E, Eriksson JG. Trajectories of growth among children who later have coronary events. N Engl J Med 2005;353(17):1802–9.

48. Hales CN, Barker DJP. Type 2 (non-insulin-depedent) diabetes mellitus: the thrifty phenotype hypothesis. Diabetologia 1992;35: 595–601.

49. Ikenasio-Thorpe BA, Breier BH, Vickers MH, Fraser M. Prenatal influences on susceptibility to diet-induced obesity are mediated by altered neuroendocrine gene expression. J Endocrinol 2007;193(1): 31–7.

50. Vickers MH, Breier BH, McCarthy D, Gluckman PD. Sedentary behavior during postnatal life is determined by the prenatal environment and exacerbated by postnatal hypercaloric nutrition. Am J Physiol Regul Integr Comp Physiol 2003;285:R271–R273.

51. Vickers MH, Gluckman PD, Coveny AH, et al. Neonatal leptin treatment reverses developmental programming. Endocrinology 2005;146(10):4211–16.

52. McMillen IC, Robinson JS. Developmental origins of the metabolic syndrome: prediction, plasticity, and programming. Physiol Rev 2005;85(2):571–633.

53. Barker DJP. *Mothers, Babies, and Disease in Later Life*, 2nd edn. London: BMJ Publishing, 1998.

54. Oken E, Gillman MW. Fetal origins of obesity. Obes Res 2003;11:496–506.

55. Gillman MW. Developmental origins of health and disease. N Engl J Med 2005;353:1848–50.

56. Stettler N, Kumanyika SK, Katz SH, Zemel BS, Stallings VA. Rapid weight gain during infancy and obesity in young adulthood in a cohort of African Americans. Am J Clin Nutr 2003;77:1374–8.

57. Monuteaux MC, Blacker D, Biederman J, Fitzmaurice G, Buka SL. Maternal smoking during pregnancy and offspring overt and covert conduct problems: a longitudinal study. J Child Psychol Psychiatr 2006;47(9):883–90.

58. Martin LT, Fitzmaurice GM, Kindlon DJ, Buka SL. Cognitive performance in childhood and early adult illness: a prospective cohort study. J Epidemiol Commun Health 2004;58(8):674–9.

59. Buka SL, Shenassa ED, Niaura R. Elevated risk of tobacco dependence among offspring of mothers who smoke during pregnancy: a 30-year prospective study. Am J Psychiatr 2003; 160(11):1978–84.

60. Susser ES, Schaefer CA, Brown AS, Begg MD, Wyatt RJ. The design of the prenatal determinants of schizophrenia study. Schizophr Bull 2000;26(2):257–73.

61. Insel BJ, Brown AS, Bresnahan MA, Schaefer CA, Susser ES. Maternal-fetal blood incompatibility and the risk of schizophrenia in offspring. Schizophr Res 2005;80(2–3):331–42.

62. van der Pols JC, Bain C, Gunnell D, Smith GD, Frobisher C, Martin RM. Childhood dairy intake and adult cancer risk: 65-y follow-up of the Boyd Orr cohort. Am J Clin Nutr 2007;86(6): 1722–9.

63. Transande L, Cronk C, Durkin M, et al. Environment and obesity in the National Children's Study. Environ Health Perspect 2009; 117(2):159–66.

64. Oken E, Levitan EB, Gillman MW. Maternal smoking during pregnancy and child overweight: systematic review and meta-analysis. Int J Obes 2008;32(2):201–10.

65. Gao YJ, Holloway AC, Zeng ZH, et al. Prenatal exposure to nicotine causes postnatal obesity and altered perivascular adipose tissue function. Obes Res 2005;13(4):687–92.

66. Rivera JA, Barquera S, Gonzalez-Cossio T, Olaiz G, Sepulveda J. Nutrition transition in Mexico and in other Latin American countries. Nutr Rev 2004;62(7 Pt 2):S149-S157.

67. Committee to Reexamine IOM Pregnancy Weight Guidelines. *Weight gain during Pregnancy: reexamining the guidelines.* Washington, DC: The National Academies Press, 2009.

68. Oken E, Taveras EM, Kleinman K, Rich-Edwards JW, Gillman MW. Gestational weight gain and child adiposity at age 3 years. Am J Obstet Gynecol 2007;196(322e1):322e8.

69. Institute of Medicine. *Nutrition During Pregnancy*. Washington, DC: Institute of Medicine, 1990.

70. Wrotniak BH, Shults J, Butts S, Stettler N. Gestational weight gain and risk of overweight in the offspring at age 7y in a multicenter, multiethnic cohort study. Am J Clin Nutr 2008;87(6): 1587–9.

71. Whitaker RC, Whitaker RC. Predicting preschooler obesity at birth: the role of maternal obesity in early pregnancy. Pediatrics 2004;114(1):e29–e36.

72. Gillman MW, Rifas-Shiman SL, Berkey CS, Field AE, Colditz GA. Maternal gestational diabetes, birth weight, and adolescent obesity. Pediatrics 2003;111:e221–e226.

73. Rogers I. The influence of birthweight and intrauterine environment on adiposity and fat distribution in later life. Int J Obes 2003; 27:755–77.

74. Parsons TJ, Powers C, Logan S, Summerbell CD. Childhood predictors of adult obesity: a systematic review. Int J Obes 1999;23: S1–107.

75. Silverman BL, Cho NH, Rizzo TA, Metzger BE. Long-term effects of the intrauterine environment. Diabetes Care 1998;21(2S): B142–B148.

76. Dabelea D, Hanson RL, Lindsay RS, et al. Intrauterine exposure to diabetes conveys risks for type 2 diabetes and obesity: a study of discordant sibships. Diabetes 2000;49(12):2208–11.

77. Whitaker RC, Pepe MS, Seidel KD, Wright JA, Knopp RH. Gestational diabetes and the risk of offspring obesity. Pediatrics 1998;101(2), e9.

78. Hillier TA, Pedula KL, Schmidt MM, Mullen JA, Charles MA, Pettitt DJ. Childhood obesity and metabolic imprinting: the ongoing effects of maternal hyperglycemia. Diabetes Care 2007;30(9): 2287–92.

79. Wild S, Roglic G, Green A, Sicree R, King H. Global prevalence of diabetes: estimates for the year 2000 and projections for 2030. Diabetes Care 2004;27(5):1047–53.

80. Oken E, Ning Y, Rifas-Shiman SL, Radesky JS, Rich-Edwards JW, Gillman MW. Associations of physical activity and inactivity before and during pregnancy with glucose tolerance. Obstet Gynecol 2006;108:1200–17.

81. Zhang C, Solomon CG, Manson JE, Hu FB. A prospective study of pregravid physical activity and sedentary behaviors in relation to the risk for gestational diabetes mellitus. Arch Intern Med 2006; 166(5):543–8.

82. Dempsey JC, Butler CL, Sorensen TK, et al. A case-control study of maternal recreational physical activity and risk of gestational diabetes mellitus. Diabetes Res Clin Pract 2004;66(2):203–15.

83. Zhang C, Liu S, Solomon CG, Hu FB. Dietary fiber intake, dietary glycemic load, and the risk for gestational diabetes mellitus. Diabetes Care 2006;29(10):2223–30.

84. Zhang C, Schulze MB, Solomon CG, Hu FB. A prospective study of dietary patterns, meat intake and the risk of gestational diabetes mellitus. Diabetologia 2006;49(11):2604–13.

85. Radesky JS, Oken E, Rifas-Shiman SL, Kleinman KP, Rich-Edwards JW, Gillman MW. Diet during early pregnancy and development of gestational diabetes. Paediatr Perinat Epidemiol 2008;22(1): 47–59.

86. Waterland RA, Jirtle RL. Early nutrition, epigenetic changes at transposons and imprinted genes, and enhanced susceptibility to adult chronic diseases. Nutrition 2004;20(1):63–8.

87. Baird J, Fisher D, Lucas P, Kleijnen J, Roberts H, Law C. Being big or growing fast: systematic review of size and growth in infancy and later obesity. BMJ 2005;331(7522):929–34.

88. Ong KK, Loos RJ. Rapid infancy weight gain and subsequent obesity: systematic reviews and hopeful suggestions. Acta Paediatr 2006;95(8):904–8.

89. Stettler N, Stallings VA, Troxel AB, et al. Weight gain in the first week of life and overweight in adulthood: a cohort study of European American subjects fed infant formula. Circulation 2005; 111(15):1897–903.

90. Singhal A, Lucas A. Early origins of cardiovascular disease: is there a unifying hypothesis? Lancet 2004;363(9421):1642–5.

91. Singhal A, Cole TJ, Fewtrell M, et al. Promotion of faster weight gain in infants born small for gestational age: is there an adverse effect on later blood pressure? Circulation 2007;115(2):213–20.

92. Belfort MB, Rifas-Shiman SL, Rich-Edwards JW, Kleinman KP, Gillman MW. Size at birth, infant growth, and blood pressure at 3 years of age. J Pedratr 2007;151(6):670–74.

93. Yliharsila H, Kajantie E, Osmond C, Forsen T, Barker DJP, Eriksson JG. Body mass index during childhood and adult body composition in men and women aged 56 to 70 years. Am J Clin Nutr 2008;87(6): 1769–75.

94. Horta BL, Sibbritt DW, Lima RC, Victora CG. Weight catch-up and achieved schooling at 18 years of age in Brazilian males. Eur J Clin Nutr 2009;63(3):369–74.

95. Victora CG, Sibbritt D, Horta BL, Lima RC, Cole T, Wells J. Weight gain in childhood and body composition at 18 years of age in Brazilian males. Acta Paediatr 2007;96(2):296–300.

96. Casey PH, Whiteside-Mansell L, Barrett K, Bradley RH, Gargus R. Impact of prenatal and/or postnatal growth problems in low birth weight preterm infants on school-age outcomes: an 8-year longitudinal evaluation. Pediatrics 2006;118(3):1078–86.

97. Harder T, Bergmann R, Kallischnigg G, Plagemann A. Duration of breastfeeding and risk of overweight: a meta-analysis. American Journal of Epidemiology, Am J Epidemiol 2005;162(5):397–403.

98. Arenz S, Ruckerl R, Koletzko B, von Kries R. Breast-feeding and childhood obesity–a systematic review. Int J Obes 2004;28(10):1247–56.

99. Owen CG, Martin RM, Whincup P, Davey Smith G, Cook DG. Effect of infant feeding on the risk of obesity across the life course: a quantitative review of published evidence. Pediatrics 2005;115:1367–77.

100. Bogen DL, Hanusa BH, Whitaker RC. The effect of breast-feeding with and without formula use on the risk of obesity at 4 years of age. Obes Res 2004;12(9):1527–35.

101. Grummer-Strawn LM, Mei Z. Does breastfeeding protect against pediatric overweight? Analysis of longitudinal data from the Centers for Disease Control and Prevention Pediatric Nutrition Surveillance System. Pediatrics 2004;113(2):e81–e86.

102. Owen CG, Martin RM, Whincup PH, Davey-Smith G, Gillman MW, Cook DG. The effect of breastfeeding on mean body mass index throughout life: a quantitative review of published and unpublished observational evidence. Am J Clin Nutr 2005;82(6):1298–307.

103. Kramer MS, Matush L, Vanilovich I, et al. Effects of prolonged and exclusive breastfeeding on child height, weight, adiposity, and blood pressure at age 6.5 y: evidence from a large randomized trial. Am J Clin Nutr 2007;86(6):1717–21.

104. Gillman MW, Rifas-Shiman SL, Berkey CS, et al. Breastfeeding and overweight in adolescence: within-family analysis. Epidemiology 2006;17(1):112–14.

105. Taveras EM, Rifas-Shiman SL, Scanlon KS, Sherry BL, Grummer-Strawn LM, Gillman MW. To what extent is the protective effect of breastfeeding on future overweight explained by decreased maternal feeding restriction? Pediatrics 2006;118(6):2341–8.

106. Patel S, Hu FB. Short sleep deprivation and weight gain: a systematic review. Obesity (Silver Spring) 2008;16(3):643–53.

107. Taveras EM, Rifas-Shiman SL, Oken E, Gunderson EP, Gillman MW. Short sleep duration in infancy and risk of childhood overweight. Arch Pediatr Adolesc Med 2008;162(4):305–11.

108. Ferber R. *Solve Your Child's Sleep Problems*. New York:Simon Schuster, 2006.

109. Eckerberg B. Treatment of sleep problems in families with young children: effects of treatment on family well-being. Acta Paediatr 2004;93(1):126–34.

110. Mindell JA, Kuhn B, Lewin DS, Meltzer LJ, Sadeh A. Behavioral treatment of bedtime problems and night wakings in infants and young children. Sleep 2006;29(10):1263–76.

111. Gillman MW, Rifas-Shiman SL, Kleinman KP, Taveras EM, Oken E. Developmental origins of childhood overweight: potential public health impact. Obesity 2008;16(7):1651–6.

112. Cole TJ. Modeling postnatal exposures and their interactions with birth size. J Nutr 2004;134:201–4.

113. de Stavola BL, Nitsch D, dos Santos SI, et al. Statistical issues in life course epidemiology. Am J Epidemiol 2006;163(1):84–96.

114. Mackay J, Amos A. Women and tobacco. Respirology 2003;8(2):123–30.

115. CDC. Tobacco Control State Highlights 2002: Impact and Opportunity. Atlanta, GA: US Department of Health and Human Services, CDC, 2002.

116. Orleans CT, Barker DC, Kaufman NJ, Marx JF. Helping pregnant smokers quit: meeting the challenge in the next decade. Tob Control 2000;9(suppl 3):III6–11.

117. Taylor T, Lader D, Bryant A, Keyse L, McDuff TJ. Smoking-related behavior and attitudes. Newport, South Wales: National Statistics, 2005.

118. The World Health Organization. Women and the tobacco epidemic: Challenges for the 21st century. Canada: WHO, 2001.

119. Jha P, Chaloupka F. Tobacco control in developing countries. Oxford: Oxford University Press, 2000.

120. Abdullah AS, Husten CG. Promotion of smoking cessation in developing countries: a framework for urgent public health interventions. Thorax 2004;59(7):623–30.

121. Mackay J. The tobacco problem: commercial profit versus health – the conflict of interests in developing countries. Prev Med 1994;23(4):535–8.

122. Lumley J, Oliver SS, Chamberlain C, Oakley L. Interventions for promoting smoking cessation during pregnancy. Cochrane Database Syst Rev (4), CD001055, 2004.

123. Crowther CA, Hiller JE, Moss JR, McPhee AJ, Jeffries WS, Robinson JS. Effect of treatment of gestational diabetes mellitus on pregnancy outcomes. N Engl J Med 2005;352(24):2477–86.

124. Oken E, Kleinman KP, Berland WE, Simon S, Rich-Edwards JW, Gillman MW. Decline in fish consumption after a national mercury advisory. Obstet Gynecol 2003;102:346–51.

125. Kramer MS, Chalmers B, Hodnett ED, et al. Promotion of Breast-feeding Intervention Trial (PROBIT): a randomized trial in the Republic of Belarus. JAMA 2001;285(4):413–20.

126. Ryan AS, Wenjun Z, Acosta A. Breastfeeding continues to increase into the new millennium. Pediatrics 2002;110:1103–9.

127. Ehrenkranz RA, Dusick AM, Vohr BR, Wright LL, Wrage LA, Poole WK. Growth in the neonatal intensive care unit influences neurodevelopmental and growth outcomes of extremely low birth weight infants. Pediatrics 2006;117(4):1253–61.

128. Taheri S. The link between short sleep duration and obesity: we should recommend more sleep to prevent obesity. Arch Dis Child 2006;91(11):881–4.

129. Stremler R, Hodnett E, Lee K, MacMillan S, Mill C, Ongcangco L, Willan A. A behavioral-educational intervention to promote maternal and infant sleep: a pilot randomized, controlled trial. Sleep 2006;29(12):1609–15.

130. Hiscock H, Wake M. Randomised controlled trial of behavioural infant sleep intervention to improve infant sleep and maternal mood. BMJ 2002;324(7345):1062–5.

131. Gillman MW, Rich-Edwards JW, Huh S, et al. Maternal corticotropin-releasing hormone levels during pregnancy and offspring adiposity. Obesity 2006;14(9):1647–53.

132. Rifas-Shiman SL, Rich-Edwards JW, Scanlon KS, Kleinman KP, Gillman MW. Misdiagnosis of overweight and underweight children younger than 2 years of age due to length measurement bias. Med Gen Med 2005;7(4):56.

133. Oken E, Taveras EM, Kleinman KP, Rich-Edwards JW, Gillman MW. Gestational weight gain and child adiposity at age 3 years. Am J Obstet Gynecol 2007;196(4):322–8.

9 Adipocyte Biology

Paul Trayhurn

Obesity Biology Research Unit, School of Clinical Sciences, University of Liverpool, Liverpool, UK

Introduction

White adipose tissue (WAT), or white fat, is at the epicenter of obesity; indeed, its expansion is the defining characteristic of the obese state. However, for many years the tissue was viewed as something of a Cinderella in energy regulation and obesity research, the main focus being on the biological mechanisms associated with appetite and the adaptive components of energy expenditure. This is despite the fact that in the obese, white fat is the major component of body composition, amounting to up to half or more of total tissue mass. Even in those individuals who are lean (Body Mass Index (BMI) <25), adipose tissue accounts for up to 25% of body weight. The tissue is in effect the main variable in body composition, the amount varying by an order of magnitude between lipodystrophy at one end of the spectrum and obesity at the other. WAT is, of course, the main site of fuel storage in mammals, energy being deposited in the form of triacylglycerols which are mobilized during periods of fasting or starvation. Triacylglycerols allow fuel to be stored at a high energy density, since the energy content of lipid is twice that of carbohydrate and lipids can be deposited with minimal associated water.

Over the past 15 years there has been a radical change in perspective on the physiological role of WAT and the disease links between the tissue and obesity. WAT is now recognized as a major endocrine and secretory organ which plays an active role in physiological and metabolic regulation [1–5]. White fat is actually one part of what Cinti has termed the "adipose organ," the other being brown adipose tissue [6]. Not only do these tissues appear different histologically, but they have fundamentally different physiological roles. The main focus of this chapter is on white adipocytes and white fat, but first the key features of brown adipocytes will be briefly considered.

Brown adipose tissue and brown adipocytes

Brown adipose tissue (BAT), originally described as the "hibernating gland," is found only in mammals. Physiologically, the primary function of brown fat is to produce heat without shivering, by the process of nonshivering thermogenesis [7,8]. Traditionally, this has been associated with thermal physiology and the need to generate heat for the maintenance of body temperature. Thus BAT is prominent in small mammals (such as rodents) adapted to the cold, in hibernating species (such as ground squirrels) and in the neonate of a number of species (particularly ruminants) [8]. There are several distinct brown fat depots in rodents, the most accessible of which is the interscapular depot which is located between the shoulder blades.

Ruminants such as sheep, goats and deer have large quantities of BAT at birth, especially around the kidneys; indeed, brown fat may be the only form of adipose tissue present in the newborn of these animals [9,10]. However, there is a rapid loss of brown adipocytes and a transition to white fat over the first days and weeks of postnatal life. BAT is also present in humans, but this has been generally considered to be the case only during the early months, or first year or two, of postnatal life. This is despite evidence indicating that immunoreactive uncoupling protein (uncoupling protein-1) is present in adults and is stimulated in patients with pheochromocytoma [11–14]. A recent set of studies employing fluorodeoxyglucose positron emission tomography has, however, provided further evidence that BAT is in practice widely present in adult humans [15].

Classically, brown fat has been differentiated from WAT at the histological level primarily through the arrangement of the lipid droplets within the adipocytes. In brown adipocytes there are multiple lipid droplets, which serve to maximize the surface area available for rapid lipolysis; this contrasts with white adipocytes

Clinical Obesity in Adults and Children, 3rd edition. Edited by Peter G. Kopelman, Ian D. Caterson and William H. Dietz.
© 2010 Blackwell Publishing, ISBN: 978-1-4051-8226-3.

in which there is normally a single lipid droplet (unilocular structure) [6,8]. The total amount of triacylglycerol stored in brown adipocytes is generally rather lower than in white adipocytes – approximately 20–40% of cell weight compared with up to 85% in the case of white fat cells. The second key histological feature differentiating brown and white adipocytes is the number and structure of the mitochondria. In the case of brown adipocytes, there are many more mitochondria than in white adipocytes and in thermogenically active tissue they have a much denser cristae structure.

Brown fat is extensively innervated by the sympathetic nervous system and the tissue is highly vascularized [8]. These factors further distinguish it from WAT in which the sympathetic innervation and the degree of vascularization are more modest. Heat, the principal "product" of brown adipocytes, is generated by a cascade which begins with the release of noradrenaline from the sympathetic nerve endings. The noradrenaline then binds to β-adrenoceptors on the plasma membrane which in the case of rodents is predominantly of the β 3 subtype [8,16]. In humans, however, the β 1 and β 2 subtypes are more important [17,18]. β-adrenoceptor activation leads to the stimulation of both lipolysis and the direct heat-generating mechanism within the mitochondria [16]. Heat is generated in brown fat mitochondria through a regulated uncoupling of the proton conductance pathway across the inner mitochondrial membrane so that adenosine triphosphate (ATP) synthesis is bypassed [7,8]. This occurs through the localization within BAT mitochondria of a specific uncoupling protein (uncoupling protein-1), the original member of the uncoupling protein gene family [7,8,19].

Uncoupling protein-1 (UCP1) is a 32,000 M_r moiety which in effect acts as a proton pore across the inner mitochondrial membrane. The presence of UCP1 is the critical diagnostic feature of brown fat, providing a molecular marker for distinguishing the major forms of adipose tissue. Two other members of the uncoupling protein gene family, UCP2 and UCP3, are also expressed in brown fat mitochondria and this argues against these proteins functioning as immediate uncouplers given the presence of UCP1. The physiological role of UCP2 and UCP3 remains uncertain, but the possibilities center on a fatty acid transporter function and protection against reactive oxygen species (ROS) [19,20]. UCP2 is expressed in a number of cell types and tissues, including white adipocytes, while UCP3 is particularly expressed in skeletal muscle [21,22]. Exposure to a cold environment leads to an acute stimulation of thermogenesis in brown fat through the activation of the mitochondrial proton conductance [8]. Long-term exposure to the cold results in an increase in thermogenic capacity of BAT, involving a stimulation of mitochondriogenesis and an increase in the concentration of UCP1 in the mitochondrial inner membrane.

Brown fat first became linked to obesity in the late 1970s when reduced thermogenic activity of the tissue was demonstrated in genetically obese (*ob/ob*) mice [23]. Shortly after this, activation of heat production in the tissue was reported in rats exhibiting diet-induced thermogenesis following voluntary overfeeding through the provision of a "cafeteria" diet [24,25]. This led to the proposition that BAT is an important component of adaptive energy expenditure in mammals, playing a role in the regulation of energy balance [26]. The studies on *ob/ob* mice and cafeteria-fed rats was subsequently followed by investigations on other rodent models of obesity, both genetic and experimentally induced, and in specific physiological conditions where energy balance is altered, such as fasting and lactation [8,26–28]. Although the evidence in support of the view that BAT is a significant component of the regulation of energy balance is strong in rodents, it has remained at best speculative in the case of humans.

White adipose tissue: general characteristics

In addition to the histological differences described above, WAT is functionally quite distinct from brown fat. It is not involved in thermogenesis *per se*, but has in practice a multiplicity of functions. The classic role is that of fuel storage, as indicated in the Introduction, while additional roles include thermal and mechanical insulation. Thermal insulation is most clearly exhibited in the case of marine mammals, such as seals and whales, the blubber of which helps minimize heat loss. WAT exists in multiple depots in the body, with both subcutaneous and internal locations. In addition, groups of adipocytes may infiltrate other organs such as skeletal muscle.

Mature adipocytes can be very large cells, reaching up to 150 μm or even 200 μm in diameter in obese individuals [29]. Histologically, the large, central, unilocular lipid droplet (see Fig. 9.1) is surrounded by a thin rim of cytoplasm which includes the nucleus and a modest number of mitochondria. The large size of the mature fat cell has resulted in a misplaced assumption that adipocytes are by far the most prevalent cell within adipose tissue. However, depending upon depot, age and physiological state, the proportion of cells within WAT that are mature adipocytes varies from between 25% to 60%. Thus, in most cases around half of the total cell content is made up of nonadipocytes; these cells, which constitute what is termed the stromal vascular fraction, include fibroblastic preadipocytes, endothelial cells, mast cells and in many circumstances macrophages [30]. Recent work has highlighted the importance of macrophages in modulating adipocyte function in obesity [31,32], but it is likely that there is cross-talk between several of the cell types within WAT.

Although WAT has a more limited sympathetic innervation than brown fat, sympathetic nerves are present and in contrast to what was considered to be the case, they appear to be in close contact with the plasma membrane of adipocytes as well as with the blood vessels [6]. The vasculature is also less extensive than in brown fat, although the tissue is generally regarded as being well vascularized. Certainly, the oxygen tension within the tissue in lean animals is similar to that of other well-oxygenated tissues [33,34].

It is clear that the various adipose tissue depots are not functionally identical. Indeed, there is considerable functional

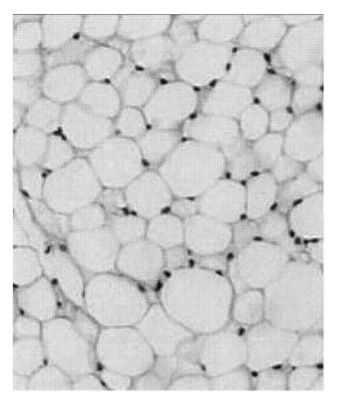

Figure 9.1 Histological view (light microscopy) of mouse white adipose tissue showing mature adipocytes and illustrating the apparent simplicity of the tissue.

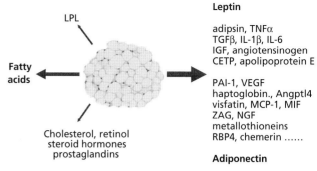

Figure 9.2 The secretome of white adipocytes. The major secretory products are illustrated, both those that are lipids and the major adipokines. The total number of recognized adipokines numbers is in excess of 60. CETP, cholesteryl ester transfer protein; Angptl4, angiopoietin-like protein 4 (also known as fasting-induced adipose factor); IGF, insulin-like growth factor; IL, interleukin; LPL, lipoprotein lipase; MCP-1, monocyte chemoattractant protein-1; MIF, macrophage migration inhibitory factor; NGF, nerve growth factor; PAI-1, plasminogen activator inhibitor-1; RBP4, retinol binding protein-4; TGF-β, transforming growth factor-β; VEGF, vascular endothelial growth factor; ZAG, zinc-α2-glycoprotein.

heterogeneity, with visceral fat in humans in particular being strongly linked to the diseases associated with obesity [35,36]. Several factors have been proposed as underlying this depot specificity, and with visceral adipose tissue the proximity to the portal outflow has been widely considered to be significant.

Triacylglycerol storage and release

The general mechanisms by which lipid is stored and released are well documented and only the key elements are described here. Nevertheless, there have been some important recent developments relating to lipid mobilization. Adipose tissue can in principle derive its stored fatty acids through three main routes. They may be obtained from circulating lipoproteins, being released through the action of lipoprotein lipase, or be derived directly from the circulation following release from the liver. Fatty acids obtained by both these routes are then re-esterified within the cell for storage as triacylglycerols. The third route for the production of fatty acids is by *de novo* synthesis from glucose (and possibly other substrates) and this process of lipogenesis occurs predominantly on a low-fat/high-carbohydrate diet. Consumption of a high-fat diet is generally associated with low rates of lipogenesis, as occurs during the consumption of a normal "Western diet", containing as it does some 35–40% of calories as lipid.

Fatty acids are released in adipose tissue via the action of the classic and extensively characterized enzyme, hormone-sensitive lipase, and through the recently discovered adipocyte triglyceride

lipase (ATGL) [37]. Together, these two enzymes account for almost all triacylglycerol breakdown in adipose tissue [38]. Further insight into the lipolytic system has also emerged from the recognition of the important regulatory role of the perilipin family of lipid-coating proteins, the most prominent of which is perilipin itself [39,40]. Perilipin is localized on the surface of lipid droplets, which are now viewed as dynamic organelles, and facilitates maximal lipolysis when lipid mobilization is required [39–41]. However, perilipin also acts to limit lipolysis in nutritional excess when there is net triacylglycerol deposition.

A number of hormonal and other external signals have been identified, largely from studies of cells *in vitro*, which may stimulate lipolysis in white adipocytes [42]. However, it seems probable that the sympathetic nervous system is the major physiological regulator [42,43]. In fasting and cold exposure, for example, noradrenaline turnover studies have demonstrated marked activation of the sympathetic innervation of white fat [44,45], although there are some depot-specific responses [46]. In the case of fasting, the changes are highly selective to WAT, there being a decrease in noradrenaline turnover in tissues such as BAT and the heart [45,47].

Secretory function of white adipocytes

Adipose tissue has always been recognized as a major secretory organ by virtue of the release of large quantities of fatty acids from adipocytes. Fatty acid release is, of course, most obvious during fasting and other periods of negative energy balance, or when there is a need for increased energy flux such as during the response to cold environments. Other lipid moieties are also released as part of the *secretome* of fat cells (Fig. 9.2). Some of these, such as cholesterol and prostaglandins (e.g. PGD_2, PGE_2), are synthesized *de novo* within the adipocyte [4]. A substantial amount of retinol is stored within adipocytes, but this is taken up from the circulation and subsequently released rather than being synthesized *de novo* in the cells. Thus adipose tissue acts as a retinol store and may also store other lipidic moieties, including environmental pollutants such as organochlorine pesticides [48,49].

WAT is also the site of production of key steroid hormones, converting inactive circulating 11-keto steroids into active glucocorticoids through the presence in adipocytes of the enzyme 11β-hydroxysteroid dehydrogenase type 1 [50]. The activity of the enzyme in adipose tissue is increased in obesity and plays an important role in the raised local production of active glucocorticoids such that there is glucocorticoid excess [50]. This excess has been linked to the development of the metabolic syndrome.

A radical shift in our understanding of the secretory role of white fat and the physiological function of adipose tissue occurred in 1994 with the identification of leptin, a key protein hormone [51]. Leptin, which is the product of the *ob* gene, was identified during the search for the mutant gene which results in the obesity of the *ob/ob* mouse – possibly the most widely used animal model in obesity research. The discovery of leptin resulted in white fat being recognized as a major endocrine organ. Indeed, the size of the fat depots is such that the tissue is much the largest endocrine organ in obese humans. One of the *a priori* consequences of this is that even small perturbations in the metabolic activity of WAT would be expected to have a considerable impact at the whole-body level.

Prior to the discovery of leptin, a small number of other protein factors had been shown to be released from fat cells, but the broader significance of this in terms of the secretory function of WAT went largely unappreciated. The enzyme lipoprotein lipase was, of course, known to be released by adipocytes in order to facilitate the breakdown of triacylglycerols in circulating lipoproteins. The complement-related factor, adipsin, was discovered in the latter part of the 1980s [52,53]. However, once it was found not to be the anticipated signaling factor from adipocytes to the brain in the regulation of energy balance (contrary to the initial expectation), interest in this protein waned. In the early 1990s, the pleiotrophic proinflammatory cytokine TNF-α was shown to be synthesized and released by adipocytes, the amount increasing markedly with cell size [54]. TNF-α production by adipocytes was linked to the development of insulin resistance in adipocytes, but the concept that fat cells might synthesize and secrete a key cytokine was initially met with some scepticism.

Adipokines – secreted proteins from adipocytes

In the decade and a half following the discovery of leptin, a wide and diverse range of other protein factors secreted by white adipocytes have been identified [1–5]. These secreted proteins were initially given the collective name of "adipocytokines" but this

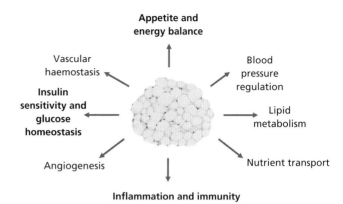

Figure 9.3 Physiological and metabolic processes with which white adipocytes are involved through the secretion of adipokines. Major processes are illustrated, with those that have received most interest shown in bold. (Adapted from Trayhurn and Wood [4].)

has been largely replaced by the expression "adipokine." This reflects the fact that the term "adipocytokine" carries the inference that the proteins secreted from adipocytes are cytokines. While this is certainly true for some, it is not so for the majority. The recognition that adipocytes secrete a multiplicity of protein factors and signals indicates that adipose tissue communicates extensively with other organs and tissues; the classic view of WAT as effectively only a lipid storage organ has been replaced by a much more dynamic view.

In excess of 60 different adipokines have now been identified, together constituting the *adipokinome* [4]. It is important to emphasize that adipokines are protein molecules secreted specifically from adipocytes, rather than from the other cells within adipose tissue. It would, for example, be inappropriate to describe a cytokine secreted from a macrophage as an "adipokine" when that macrophage was passing through adipose tissue but as a "normal" cytokine once the immune cell had exited the tissue. The adipokines are varied in molecular size and protein structure and are also very diverse in terms of physiological function (see Fig. 9.2; Fig. 9.3). They include factors involved in appetite and energy balance (primarily leptin), angiogenesis (e.g. vascular endothelial growth factor), lipid metabolism (e.g. apolipoprotein E), blood pressure regulation (angiotensinogen), vascular hemostasis (e.g. plasminogen activator inhibitor-1), insulin sensitivity (e.g. adiponectin, interleukin-6) and inflammation and immunity (e.g. interleukin-1β, tumor necrosis factor-α) [1–5]. Recent additions to the list of adipokines include chemerin [55–57], which has been implicated in adipogenesis and the potentiation of insulin-stimulated glucose uptake in adipocytes [58].

It is in practice difficult to think of a cell type that is currently known to be as rich in the nature of the proteins that it secretes as the adipocyte. Nevertheless, several other cells secrete multiple protein factors, including chondrocytes [59]. The adipokine concept has recently been mirrored by the emerging family of proteins secreted from myocytes – the *myokines* [60,61]. This followed the discovery that substantial quantities of IL-6 are synthesized and released from skeletal muscle following exercise [62].

The various adipokines can act in an autocrine, paracrine or endocrine manner, or a combination thereof. It is increasingly evident from the range of adipokines that there is cross-talk between the various cell types within adipose tissue as well as extensive communication between WAT and other organs, especially skeletal muscle and the brain, through the secretion of adipokines. Although, as emphasized above, adipokines have been linked to a range of physiological processes, most emphasis has been placed on two particular areas – energy balance and insulin sensitivity (see Fig. 9.3).

Energy balance

The lipostatic theory introduced by Kennedy in the 1950s [63] suggested that there was a factor released from adipocytes to the brain signaling the size of the fat stores, which led to the modulation of appetite and energy balance. Until the discovery of leptin, there was no clear candidate molecule which fulfilled the criteria for such a signal. Leptin is a powerful anorectic factor, food intake being substantially reduced by administration of the recombinant protein to *ob/ob* mice which lack the functional hormone [64–66]. Leptin also greatly decreases food intake, with an accompanying reduction in body weight, in humans with mutations in the *OB* (leptin) gene [67]. Studies on rodents have identified a number of central hypothalamic neuroendocrine systems with which leptin interacts, including orexigenic neurons expressing neuropeptide Y (NPY) and agouti-related peptide (AgRP), and anorexigenic neurons including those expressing pro-opiomelanocortin (POMC) and cocaine- and amphetamine-regulated transcript (CART) [66,68,69]. In essence, leptin induces an inhibition of orexigenic pathways and an upregulation of anorexigenic systems, such that there is a powerful integrated signal to reduce intake.

The effect of exogenous leptin on normal mice, or as a potential antiobesity agent in obese humans, is very limited and this may reflect either a state of "resistance" in the case of the obese, or the possibility that only a limited amount of the hormone is required for the maximal effect on intake to be realized. This does not, of course, necessarily mean that higher levels of leptin are without effect on the other, multiple, processes with which the hormone is involved.

One of the earliest observations with leptin was that the expression and circulating levels, in both rodents and humans, are elevated in obesity, there being a direct correlation between body fat and the plasma concentration of the hormone [70–72]. Although white adipocytes are the most important site of production of leptin, as indicated by the relationship between body fat content and the circulating level, the hormone is also synthesized in a number of other cell types and tissues, including the stomach, placenta, and osteoblasts [73–76]. While leptin was originally considered as a satiety factor, it rapidly became evident that it is a pleiotrophic hormone and this is, of course, consistent with the multiple sites of synthesis and the wide distribution of its

receptors [76]. In terms of energy balance, leptin also appears to affect energy expenditure, as well as food intake [65,76,77].

Other adipokines have also been linked with a central role in the regulation of energy balance, particularly interleukin-6 (IL-6) and adiponectin [66]. In the case of IL-6, weight loss as well as insulin resistance in adipocytes is induced by this cytokine and the IL-6 receptor is expressed in neurons of hypothalamic nuclei that regulate body composition [78], implying a role in the central modulation of energy homeostasis. Indeed, chronic intracerebroventricular volume administration of IL-6 reduces body fat through an upregulation of energy expenditure, while IL-6 knockout mice have been shown to develop late-onset obesity [79,80]. However, the extent to which these effects are dependent on IL-6 emanating from adipocytes (or from WAT as a whole) is currently difficult to assess, given the multiplicity of sites of production of this cytokine. There is a similar argument in relation to any putative role for IL-1β and TNF-α. Chronic administration of apelin has also now been reported to lead to a reduction of adiposity and an increase in UCP1 expression and protein content in BAT, suggesting that this adipokine may stimulate energy expenditure associated with thermogenesis [81].

Adiponectin is perhaps the most interesting of the other adipokines that have been implicated in the control of energy balance. Like leptin, it is synthesized predominantly in adipocytes and both adipokines are considered to be only expressed after the induction of adipocyte differentiation, being markers of differentiation. Adiponectin is a highly expressed transcript in adipocytes and was identified as an adipokine by several groups more than a decade ago [82–84]. As a consequence, it has multiple names, but adiponectin is much the most commonly used descriptor, with the term Acrp30 also occasionally being employed. In marked contrast to leptin, and to most other adipokines, the circulating levels of adiponectin fall in obesity [85,86]. Several key functions have been described for this hormone, including in insulin sensitivity, vascular function and inflammation [87–90].

Adiponectin also appears to be a direct signal in appetite and energy balance control, a view that is supported by several recent studies [91,92]. For example, peripheral administration of the hormone has been reported to reduce body weight through increased energy expenditure, without effects on feeding [89,90,93]. On the other hand, sustained peripheral expression of adiponectin through a viral vector inhibits food intake and reduces body weight in diet-induced obese rats [91]. The adiponectin receptors, AdipoR1 and AdipoR2, are expressed in the brain [94] and recent knockout studies have shown that they have opposing effects on energy balance [95]. AdipoR1 knockout mice have increased body fat and decreased energy expenditure, while AdipoR2 knockout animals are lean, and are resistant to obesity when fed a high-fat diet and exhibit higher levels of energy expenditure. Importantly, adiponectin appears to cross the blood–brain barrier and stimulates hypothalamic corticotropin-releasing hormone synthesis [92], providing at least one target neuroendocrine system.

Insulin sensitivity

The association between obesity and the metabolic syndrome and type 2 diabetes has led to much emphasis on adipose tissue in relation to insulin sensitivity. It is important to note that too little adipose tissue (as with too much) leads to insulin resistance and other metabolic derangements, as is evident in lipodystrophy or lipoatrophy. There are also circumstances such as cachexia where a major loss of adipose tissue may occur with profound metabolic disruptions [96]. While fatty acids have been implicated in the reduction of insulin sensitivity in the obese, most focus in recent years has been on the role of various adipokines. As already implied, several adipokines have been specifically linked to insulin sensitivity. These include leptin and adiponectin, and the administration of either of these adipokines to lipodystrophic animals leads to a partial restoration of normal glycemia and the combination of the two will largely restore normal glycemia [90,97,98]. Initially on its discovery, resistin was thought to be a key factor in the development of insulin resistance in obesity, at least in experimental animals [99], but this view has not been sustained, particularly in humans.

Several other adipokines are considered to be candidates in the modulation of insulin sensitivity and its loss in obesity. The factor visfatin was reported to be more strongly expressed in visceral fat than elsewhere and to act as an insulin mimetic, binding to the insulin receptor [100]; however, as with resistin, the picture has become less clear. Apelin may also have a role in the modulation of insulin sensitivity [101], but this may be indirect through an apelin-induced increase in circulating adiponectin [81]. Perhaps the most interesting recent candidate is retinol binding protein-4 (RBP4), a factor that has been directly linked to insulin resistance and which is secreted by the liver as well as by adipocytes [102]. Circulating RBP4 levels are increased in obesity and type 2 diabetes, and administration of the protein to normal animals, either by injection of the recombinant protein or by transgenic overexpression, is reported to induce insulin resistance, while deletion, or reduction in the plasma level, improves insulin sensitivity and glucose tolerance [102]. Interestingly, RBP4 is more highly expressed in visceral than in subcutaneous adipose tissue, and in obese as compared to lean individuals. From these observations, it has been suggested that visceral fat may be a major source of RBP4 in insulin-resistant states and that the serum levels are a marker of intra-abdominal fat mass [103].

A group of adipokines that are also linked to the loss of insulin sensitivity in obesity are the inflammation-related factors TNF-α, IL-6 and monocyte chemoattractant protein-1 (MCP-1), reflecting the inflammatory response in WAT. These adipokines are considered in the next section.

Inflammation in adipose tissue

One of the key developments in obesity research in recent years is the recognition that the disorder is characterized by a state of chronic, low-grade inflammation [104–106]. This is based on an increase in the circulating level of several inflammatory markers, including C-reactive protein (CRP), IL-6, MCP-1 haptoglobin, serum amyloid A and plasminogen activator inhibitor-1 (PAI-1). WAT appears central to this inflammatory response, the raised circulating levels reflecting in several cases release or spillover from adipose tissue itself. The inflammatory response in adipose tissue is now considered to be pivotal in the development of obesity-associated diseases [5,104,105]. Thus type 2 diabetes mellitus, cardiovascular disease, and the other components of the metabolic syndrome may relate to either specific or general changes in the production of some adipokines. Certain cancers, such as breast and colon, have also been linked to inflammation in adipose tissue. In the case of breast cancer, the close proximity between adipose tissue and the mammary ducts means that local inflammatory changes in the tissue may impact very strongly on the ductal tissue [107].

A substantial number of adipokines are involved in immunity and inflammation, and this encompasses classic cytokines, chemokines, acute-phase proteins and other inflammation-related factors such as those involved in angiogenesis [1–5,34]. The list of cytokines and chemokines produced by adipocytes is now extensive and includes IL-1β, IL-6, IL-8. IL-10 and IL-18, as well as MCP-1, macrophage migration inhibitory factor (MIF), transforming growth factor-β and TNF-α (Fig. 9.4). Major acute-phase proteins released by adipocytes are PAI-1, haptoglobin and serum amyloid A, while other key inflammation-related adipokines include nerve growth factor (NGF) and adiponectin.

Not only does WAT, and adipocytes in particular, secrete a wide range of inflammation-related proteins but the production and release of these factors increase markedly as fat mass expands

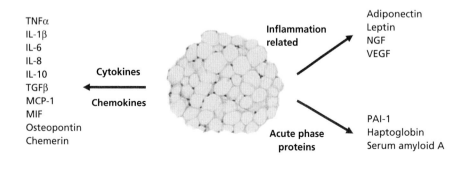

Figure 9.4 Major inflammatory and inflammation-related adipokines secreted from white adipocytes. TNF-α, which has a key role in inflammation, is highlighted, as is adiponectin with its anti-inflammatory action. IL, interleukin; MCP-1, monocyte chemoattractant protein-1; MIF, macrophage migration inhibitory factor; NGF, nerve growth factor; PAI-1, plasminogen activator inhibitor-1; TGF-β, transforming growth factor-β; VEGF, vascular endothelial growth factor.

in obesity, thereby creating an inflammatory state within the tissue [4,105,106]. An important exception is adiponectin, with its anti-inflammatory action, whose expression and secretion fall in obesity, as noted earlier [85]. The proinflammatory cytokine TNF-α may play a central role in the inflammatory response in obesity since not only does its own production increase, but it has a wide regulatory effect on the synthesis and release of other adipokines, stimulating IL-6, MCP-1 and NGF production, while inhibiting adiponectin expression [108,109]. TNF-α appears to play a pervasive role in adipocyte function since it also, for example, stimulates apoptosis and lipolysis [110,111].

A recent major finding is the discovery that in obesity, macrophages infiltrate adipose tissue and this appears to be an important part of the inflammatory response [31,32]. Macrophages secrete, of course, a wide range of cytokine and chemokines such as TNF-α and IL-6 and these would be expected to stimulate the adipocytes, amplifying their inflammatory state. Adipocyte-derived factors may in turn feed back to the macrophages as part of an inflammatory cascade within WAT. In addition to macrophages and the adipocytes themselves, preadipocytes may be an important source of secreted factors and a significant component of the inflammatory response within WAT in obesity. Indeed, preadipocytes have been suggested to be highly inflammatory and to signal directly to the adipocyte, leading to the induction of insulin resistance [112]. From this perspective, preadipocytes are important regulators of the adipocyte. Certainly, the response by preadipocytes to challenge with lipopolysaccharide is greater than that of adipocytes [112] and the secretion of some cytokines, such as IL-6, is much greater than in mature fat cells.

These interactions highlight the extent and importance of cellular cross-talk within adipose tissue. While this concept evolved with the recognition that macrophages infiltrate WAT in obesity and are involved in the inflammatory response, communication between different cell types is much wider than this. In addition to adipocytes, macrophages and preadipocytes, it is likely to involve other cells, such as those of the vascular endothelium as well. Conversations also occur between adipocytes and other tissues, the most obvious case being the CNS through leptin. However, cross-talk between adipocytes and organs such as skeletal muscle and the adrenal cortex [113–116] also occurs through the action of adipokines such as adiponectin, with myocyte-derived IL-6 being a factor in the stimulation of lipolysis in adipocytes [62].

While at least three different cell types within WAT are able to mount an inflammatory response, the extent to which each contributes quantitatively to the overall production of inflammatory mediators by the tissue is unclear. From *in vitro* studies it is suggested that mature adipocytes are less important than the non-adipocyte fraction in the production and release of most cytokines and chemokines [117,118]. However, quantitative comparisons between cell types is fraught with difficulty since the preparation and incubation of different cell fractions may alter their relative rate of adipokine production. Importantly, although large adipocytes show the highest rates of production of inflammatory

adipokines [29], because of their fragility they are likely to be under-represented in most WAT fractionations.

Hypoxia: a key influence on adipocytes

While there has been a considerable, and growing, focus on the mechanistic basis of the link between inflammation-related adipokines and the development of the diseases associated with obesity, there has been only limited interest in the factors that cause adipocytes to mount an inflammatory response as WAT mass expands. Three general propositions have been advanced – that it is a response to endoplasmic reticulum stress [119,120], to oxidative stress [121] or to hypoxia [4,34]. There is evidence in support of each of the proposals; however, in practice they may well be linked since underlying hypoxia can lead both to endoplasmic reticulum stress and to the generation of reactive oxygen species [122,123].

In 2004 we put forward the view that inflammation in WAT is the consequence of hypoxia in regions of the tissue distant from the vasculature as adipocyte size and mass expand in obesity [4]. The "goal" of the inflammatory response is presumed to be to increase the blood flow to adipose tissue and to stimulate angiogenesis. It was further proposed that the response to hypoxia was transmitted through the recruitment of the hypoxia inducible transcription factor, HIF-1, the so-called master regulator of oxygen deprivation [124], via stabilization of the HIF-1α subunit [4]. There is now growing evidence from studies on experimental animals that adipose tissue is indeed hypoxic in obesity. Low O_2 tension has been demonstrated in the tissue in three different obese models, namely *ob/ob* and KKAy mice and mice with diet-induced obesity [33,125,126]. Recruitment of HIF-1α is evident in WAT of obese animals, together with increased expression of a number of genes that are hypoxia sensitive through HIF-1, such as the GLUT1 facilitative glucose transporter (a commonly employed marker of hypoxia) and the key angiogenic signal vascular endothelial growth factor (VEGF) [33,125,126].

Importantly, in addition to VEGF, the expression of several other hypoxia-sensitive genes encoding proteins linked to inflammation is increased in WAT of the obese models, including leptin, IL-6, matrix metalloproteinase 2, MIF and PAI-1 [33,125]. There have also been several studies on the response to hypoxia of adipocyte systems in cell culture, both murine and human [33,125,127–129]. These have directly demonstrated that the expression of a number of inflammation-related adipokine genes is hypoxia sensitive in fat cells, and in addition to those investigated in the *ex vivo* studies such as leptin, IL-6, PAI-1 and VEGF, they include angiopoietin-like protein 4 which is a highly hypoxia-inducible gene. The cell culture studies have further shown that the increases in gene expression are accompanied by parallel changes in the secretion of the encoded adipokine into the medium [128,129]. Of particular significance is that both the expression and release of adiponectin are inhibited by low O_2 tension [128,129].

These observations are consistent with the concept that hypoxia underlies the inflammatory response in adipose tissue in obesity and the well-documented changes in leptin and adiponectin production in the obese state may be essentially a direct consequence of the hypoxic environment for adipocytes. One gene that is particularly hypoxia sensitive in human adipocytes is metallothionein-3, the expression of which is dramatically and rapidly increased in response to low O_2, and this may reflect a protective response to stress [130]. Hypoxia has other effects on adipocytes, including the inhibition of differentiation from preadipocytes, and the stimulation of glucose uptake [131]. With regard to glucose transport, the expression of the genes encoding the GLUT1, GLUT3 and GLUT5 facilitative glucose transporters are each stimulated by hypoxia in human adipocytes, and both GLUT1 protein level and the uptake of 2-deoxy-D-glucose are markedly increased [131].

Overall, it is likely that hypoxia has a pervasive influence on adipocyte function in obesity, as well as on the metabolism of the other cell types within adipose tissue. Hypoxia as a probable key influence on adipocytes is only now beginning to be recognized.

Conclusion

Adipocytes, the major cells within adipose tissue, are now regarded as major endocrine and secretory cells, with white fat being by far the largest endocrine organ in the obese. Not only do adipocytes act as key fuel storage cells through the deposition and release of fatty acids, but they also synthesize and secrete a wide range of protein signals and factors. These adipokines are involved in a multiplicity of physiological and metabolic functions, leading to extensive communication with other tissues and organs, including the hypothalamus and skeletal muscle.

There is also cross-talk between adipocytes and the other cell types within WAT, involving both adipokines and fatty acids. This is especially significant in relation to the inflammatory state that develops in WAT as adipose tissue mass expands in obesity. Inflammation is a characteristic of obese adipose tissue, with the production and release of a series of inflammation-related adipokines. The inflammatory response in adipose tissue is viewed as central to the development of obesity-associated diseases and may be a consequence of hypoxia as tissue mass expands and large fat cells become distant from the vasculature. Low O_2 tension may be a feature of the environment to which adipocytes are exposed in obesity and a key driver of the metabolic and physiological functions of fat cells. Finally, adipocytes are undoubtedly critical to many aspects of obesity and to overall homeostasis.

Acknowledgments

I am grateful to my colleagues in the Obesity Biology Research Unit (University of Liverpool) for their support. I am also grateful to the agencies who have funded our research program on adipose tissue, and particularly the Biotechnology and Biological Sciences Research Council (UK). The author is a member of COST BM0602.

References

1. Trayhurn P, Beattie JH. Physiological role of adipose tissue: white adipose tissue as an endocrine and secretory organ. Proc Nutr Soc 2001;60:329–39.
2. Rajala MW, Scherer PE. The adipocyte – at the crossroads of energy homeostasis, inflammation, and atherosclerosis. Endocrinology 2003;144:3765–73.
3. Kershaw EE, Flier JS. Adipose tissue as an endocrine organ. J Clin Endocrinol Metab 2004;89:2548–56.
4. Trayhurn P, Wood IS. Adipokines: inflammation and the pleiotropic role of white adipose tissue. Br J Nutr 2004;92:347–55.
5. Rosen ED, Spiegelman BM. Adipocytes as regulators of energy balance and glucose homeostasis. Nature 2006;444:847–53.
6. Cinti S. The adipose organ: morphological perspectives of adipose tissues. Proc Nutr Soc 2001;60:319–28.
7. Ricquier D, Bouillaud F. Mitochondrial uncoupling proteins: from mitochondria to the regulation of energy balance. J Physiol 2000;529:3–10.
8. Cannon B, Nedergaard J. Brown adipose tissue: function and physiological significance. Physiol Rev 2004;84:277–359.
9. Soppela P, Nieminen M, Saarela S, Keith JS, Morrison JN, Macfarlane F, et al. Brown fat-specific mitochondrial uncoupling protein in adipose tissues of newborn reindeer. Am J Physiol Reg Integr Comp Physiol 1991;260:R1229–R1234.
10. Trayhurn P, Thomas ME, Keith JS. Postnatal development of uncoupling protein, uncoupling protein mRNA, and GLUT4 in adipose tissues of goats. Am J Physiol Reg Integr Comp Physiol 1993;265:R676–R682.
11. Ricquier D, Néchad M, Mory G. Ultrastructural and biochemical characterization of human brown adipose tissue in pheochromocytoma. J Clin Endocrin Metab 1982;54:803–7.
12. Lean MEJ, James WPT, Jennings G, Trayhurn P. Brown adipose tissue uncoupling protein content in human infants, children and adults. Clin Sci 1986;71:291–7.
13. Lean MEJ, James WPT, Jennings G, Trayhurn P. Brown adipose tissue in patients with phaeochromocytoma. Int J Obes 1986;10:219–27.
14. Garruti G, Ricquier D. Analysis of uncoupling protein and its messenger RNA in adipose tissue deposits of adult humans. Int J Obes 1992;16:383–90.
15. Nedergaard J, Bengtsson T, Cannon B. Unexpected evidence for active brown adipose tissue in adult humans. Am J Physiol Endocrinol Metab 2007;293:E444–E452.
16. Arch JR. β(3)-Adrenoceptor agonists: potential, pitfalls and progress. Eur J Pharmacol 2002;440:99–107.
17. Lafontan M, Berlan M. Fat cell adrenergic receptors and the control of white and brown fat cell function. J Lipid Res 1993;34:1057–91.
18. Hagstrom-Toft E, Enoksson S, Moberg E, Bolinder J, Arner P. β-adrenergic regulation of lipolysis and blood flow in human skeletal muscle in vivo. Am J Physio Endocrinol Metab 1998;38:E909–E916.

19. Ricquier D, Bouillaud F. The uncoupling protein homologues: UCP1, UCP2, UCP3, StUCP and AtUCP. Biochem J 2000;345: 161–79.

20. Rousset S, Alves-Guerra MC, Mozo J, Miroux B, Cassard-Doulcier AM, Bouillaud F, et al. The biology of mitochondrial uncoupling proteins. Diabetes 2004;53(suppl 1):S130–S135.

21. Fleury C, Neverova M, Collins S, Raimbault S, Champigny O, Levi-Meyrueis C, et al. Uncoupling protein-2: a novel gene linked to obesity and hyperinsulinemia. Nat Genet 1997;15:269–72.

22. Boss O, Samec S, Paoloni Giacobino A, Rossier C, Dulloo A, Seydoux J, et al. Uncoupling protein-3: a new member of the mitochondrial carrier family with tissue-specific expression. FEBS Lett 1997;408:39–42.

23. Himms-Hagen J, Desautels M. A mitochondrial defect in brown adipose tissue of the obese (ob/ob) mouse: reduced binding of purine nucleotides and a failure to respond to cold by an increase in binding. Biochem Biophys Res Commun 1978;83: 628–34.

24. Rothwell NJ, Stock MJ. A role for brown adipose tissue in diet-induced thermogenesis. Nature 1979;281:31–5.

25. Brooks SL, Rothwell NJ, Stock MJ, Goodbody AE, Trayhurn P. Increased proton conductance pathway in brown adipose tissue mitochondria of rats exhibiting diet-induced thermogenesis. Nature 1980;286:274–6.

26. Himms-Hagen J. Brown adipose tissue thermogenesis and obesity. Prog Lipid Res 1989;28:67–115.

27. Himms-Hagen J. Brown adipose tissue thermogenesis – interdisciplinary studies. FASEB J 1990;4:2890–8.

28. Trayhurn P. Brown adipose tissue – from thermal physiology to bioenergetics. J Biosci 1993;18:161–73.

29. Skurk T, Alberti-Huber C, Herder C, Hauner H. Relationship between adipocyte size and adipokine expression and secretion. J Clin Endocrinol Metab 2007;92:1023–33.

30. Hausman GJ. The comparative anatomy of adipose tissue. In: Cryer A, Van RLR (eds) *New Perspectives in Adipose Tissue: Structure, Function and Development.* London: Butterworths, 1985: 1–21.

31. Weisberg SP, McCann D, Desai M, Rosenbaum M, Leibel RL, Ferrante AW Jr. Obesity is associated with macrophage accumulation in adipose tissue. J Clin Invest 2003;112:1796–808.

32. Xu H, Barnes GT, Yang Q, Tan G, Yang D, Chou CJ, et al. Chronic inflammation in fat plays a crucial role in the development of obesity-related insulin resistance. J Clin Invest 2003;112:1821–30.

33. Ye J, Gao Z, Yin J, He Q. Hypoxia is a potential risk factor for chronic inflammation and adiponectin reduction in adipose tissue of ob/ob and dietary obese mice. Am J Physiol Endocrinol Metab 2007;293:E1118–1128.

34. Trayhurn P, Wang B, Wood IS. Hypoxia in adipose tissue: a basis for the dysregulation of tissue function in obesity? Br J Nutr 2008;100:227–35.

35. Björntorp P. Adipose tissue distribution and function. Int J Obes 1991;15:67–81.

36. Björntorp P. Regional fat distribution – implications for type-II diabetes. Int J Obes 1992;16:S19–S27.

37. Zimmermann R, Strauss JG, Haemmerle G, Schoiswohl G, Birner-Gruenberger R, Riederer M, et al. Fat mobilization in adipose tissue is promoted by adipose triglyceride lipase. Science 2004;306: 1383–6.

38. Schweiger M, Schreiber R, Haemmerle G, Lass A, Fledelius C, Jacobsen P, et al. Adipose triglyceride lipase and hormone-sensitive lipase are the major enzymes in adipose tissue triacylglycerol catabolism. J Biol Chem 2006;281:40236–41.

39. Brasaemle DL. Adipocyte biology. The perilipin family of structural lipid droplet proteins: stabilization of lipid droplets and control of lipolysis. J Lipid Res 2007;48:2547–59.

40. Ducharme NA, Bickel PE. Lipid droplets in lipogenesis and lipolysis. Endocrinology 2008;149:942–9.

41. Blanchette-Mackie EJ, Dwyer NK, Barber T, Coxey RA, Takeda T, Rondinone CM, et al. Perilipin is located on the surface-layer of intracellular lipid droplets in adipocytes. J Lipid Res 1995;36: 56–60.

42. Hales CN, Luzio JP, Siddle K. Hormonal control of adipose tissue lipolysis. Biochem Soc Trans 1978;43:97–135.

43. Bartness TJ, Bamshad M. Innervation of mammalian white adipose tissue: implications for the regulation of total body fat. Am J Physiol Reg Integr Comp Physiol 1998;275:R1399–R1411.

44. Garofalo MAR, Kettelhut IC, Roselino JES, Migliorini RH. Effect of acute cold exposure on norpinephrine turnover rates in rat white adipose tissue. J Autonom Nervous System 1996;60:206–8.

45. Migliorini RH, Garofalo MAR, Kettelhut IC. Increased sympathetic activity in rat white adipose tissue during prolonged fasting. Am J Physiol Reg Integr Comp Physiol 1997;41:R656–R661.

46. Brito NA, Brito MN, Bartness TJ. Differential sympathetic drive to adipose tissues after food deprivation, cold exposure or glucoprivation. Am J Physiol Reg Integr Comp Physiol 2008;294: R1445–R1452.

47. Young JB, Landsberg L. Suppression of sympathetic nervous system during fasting. Science 1976;196:1473–5.

48. Bigsby RM, Caperell-Grant A, Madhukar BV. Xenobiotics released from fat during fasting produce estrogenic effects in ovariectomized mice. Cancer Res 1997;57:865–9.

49. Chevrier J, Dewailly E, Ayotte P, Mauriege P, Despres JP, Tremblay A. Body weight loss increases plasma and adipose tissue concentrations of potentially toxic pollutants in obese individuals. Int J Obes 2000;24:1272–8.

50. Seckl JR, Morton NM, Chapman KE, Walker BR. Glucocorticoids and 11β-hydroxysteroid dehydrogenase in adipose tissue. Recent Prog Horm Res 2004;59:359–93.

51. Zhang YY, Proenca R, Maffei M, Barone M, Leopold L, Friedman JM. Positional cloning of the mouse obese gene and its human homolog. Nature 1994;372:425–32.

52. Cook KS, Min HY, Johnson D, Chaplinsky RJ, Flier JS, Hunt CR, et al. Adipsin: a circulating serine protease homolog secreted by adipose tissue and sciatic nerve. Science 1987;237:402–5.

53. Flier JS, Cook KS, Usher P, Spiegelman BM. Severely impaired adipsin expression in genetic and acquired obesity. Science 1987;237:405–8.

54. Hotamisligil GS, Shargill NS, Spiegelman BM. Adipose expression of tumor necrosis factor-alpha - direct role in obesity-linked insulin resistance. Science 1993;259:87–91.

55. Bozaoglu K, Bolton K, McMillan J, Zimmet P, Jowett J, Collier G, et al. Chemerin is a novel adipokine associated with obesity and metabolic syndrome. Endocrinology 2007;148:4687–94.

56. Goralski KB, McCarthy TC, Hanniman EA, Zabel BA, Butcher EC, Parlee SD, et al. Chemerin, a novel adipokine that regulates adipogenesis and adipocyte metabolism. J Biol Chem 2007;282: 28175–88.

57. Roh S-G, Song S-H, Choi K-C, Katoh K, Wittamer V, Parmentier M, et al. Chemerin – a new adipokine that modulates adipogenesis

via its own receptor. Biochem Biophys Res Commun 2007;362: 1013–18.

58. Takahashi M, Takahashi Y, Takahashi K, Zolotaryov FN, Hong KS, Kitazawa R, et al. Chemerin enhances insulin signaling and potentiates insulin-stimulated glucose uptake in 3T3-L1 adipocytes. FEBS Lett 2008;582:573–8.

59. de Ceuninck F, Dassencourt L, Anract P. The inflammatory side of human chondrocytes unveiled by antibody microarrays. Biochem Biophys Res Commun 2004;323:960–9.

60. Akerstrom T, Steensberg A, Keller P, Keller C, Penkowa M, Pedersen BK. Exercise induces interleukin-8 expression in human skeletal muscle. J Physiol (Lond) 2005;563:507–16.

61. Pedersen BK. IL-6 signalling in exercise and disease. Biochem Soc Trans 2007;35:1295–7.

62. Pedersen BK, Steensberg A, Fischer C, Keller C, Keller P, Plomgaard P, et al. The metabolic role of IL-6 produced during exercise: is IL-6 an exercise factor? Proc Nutr Soc 2004;63:263–7.

63. Kennedy GC. The role of depot fat in the hypothalamic control of food intake in the rat. Proc Roy Soc Lond B Biol Sci 1953;140:578–92.

64. Friedman JM, Halaas JL. Leptin and the regulation of body weight in mammals. Nature 1998;395:763–70.

65. Harris RB. Leptin – much more than a satiety signal Annu Rev Nutr 2000;20:45–75.

66. Trayhurn P, Bing C. Appetite and energy balance signals from adipocytes. Philos Trans R Soc Lond B Biol Sci 2006;361:1237–49.

67. Farooqi IS, Jebb SA, Langmack G, Lawrence E, Cheetham CH, Prentice AM, et al. Effects of recombinant leptin therapy in a child with congenital leptin deficiency. N Engl J Med 1999;341:879–84.

68. Ahima RS, Saper CB, Flier JS, Elmquist JK. Leptin regulation of neuroendocrine systems. Front Neuroendocrinol 2000;21: 263–307.

69. Schwartz MW, Woods S, Porte DJ, Seeley RJ, Baskin DG. Central nervous system control of food intake. Nature 2000;404:661–71.

70. Maffei M, Halaas J, Ravussin E, Pratley RE, Lee GH, Zhang Y, et al. Leptin levels in human and rodent – measurement of plasma leptin and ob RNA in obese and weight-reduced subjects. Nat Med 1995;1:1155–61.

71. Considine RV, Sinha MK, Heiman ML, Kriauciunas A, Stephens TW, Nyce MR, et al. Serum immunoreactive leptin concentrations in normal-weight and obese humans. N Engl J Med 1996;334: 292–5.

72. Ostlund RE, Yang JW, Klein S, Gingerich R. Relation between plasma leptin concentration and body fat, gender, diet, age, and metabolic covariates. J Clin Endocrinol Metab 1996;81:3909–13.

73. Hoggard N, Hunter L, Duncan JS, Williams LM, Trayhurn P, Mercer JG. Leptin and leptin receptor mRNA and protein expression in the murine fetus and placenta. Proc Natl Acad Sci USA 1997;94:11073–8.

74. Bado A, Levasseur S, Attoub S, Kermorgant S, Laigneau JP, Bortoluzzi MN, et al. The stomach is a source of leptin. Nature 1998;394:790–3.

75. Reseland JE, Syversen U, Bakke I, Qvigstad G, Eide LG, Hjertner O, et al. Leptin is expressed in and secreted from primary cultures of human osteoblasts and promotes bone mineralization. J Bone Mineral Res 2001;16:1426–33.

76. Rayner DV, Trayhurn P. Regulation of leptin production: sympathetic nervous system interactions. J Mol Med 2001;79:8–20.

77. Doring H, Schwarzer K, Nuesslein-Hildesheim B, Schmidt I. Leptin selectively increases energy expenditure of food-restricted lean mice. Int J Obes 1998;22:83–8.

78. Shizuya K, Komori T, Fujiwara R, Miyahara S, Ohmori M, Nomura J. The expressions of mRNAs for interleukin-6 (IL-6) and the IL-6 receptor (IL-6R) in the rat hypothalamus and midbrain during restraint stress. Life Sci 1998;62:2315–20.

79. Wallenius V, Wallenius K, Ahren B, Rudling M, Carlsten H, Dickson SL, et al. Interleukin-6-deficient mice develop mature-onset obesity. Nat Med 2002;8:75–9.

80. Wallenius K, Wallenius V, Sunter D, Dickson SL, Jansson JO. Intracerebroventricular interleukin-6 treatment decreases body fat in rats. Biochem Biophys Res Commun 2002;293:560–5.

81. Higuchi K, Masaki T, Gotoh K, Chiba S, Katsuragi I, Tanaka K, et al. Apelin, an APJ receptor ligand, regulates body adiposity and favors the messenger ribonucleic acid expression of uncoupling proteins in mice. Endocrinology 2007;148:2690–7.

82. Scherer PE, Williams S, Fogliano M, Baldini G, Lodish HF. A novel serum protein similar to C1q, produced exclusively in adipocytes. J Biol Chem 1995;270:26746–9.

83. Hu E, Liang P, Spiegelman BM. AdipoQ is a novel adipose-specific gene dysregulated in obesity. J Biol Chem 1996;271:10697–703.

84. Maeda K, Okubo K, Shimomura I, Funahashi T, Matsuzawa Y, Matsubara K. cDNA cloning and expression of a novel adipose specific collagen-like factor, apM1 (AdiPose Most abundant Gene transcript 1). Biochem Biophys Res Commun 1996;221:286–9.

85. Arita Y, Kihara S, Ouchi N, Takahashi M, Maeda K, Miyagawa J, et al. Paradoxical decrease of an adipose-specific protein, adiponectin, in obesity. Biochem Biophys Res Commun 1999;257:79–83.

86. Hotta K, Funahashi T, Arita Y, Takahashi M, Matsuda M, Okamoto Y, et al. Plasma concentrations of a novel, adipose-specific protein, adiponectin, in type 2 diabetic patients. Arterioscl Thromb Vasc Biol 2000;20:1595–9.

87. Ouchi N, Kihara S, Arita Y, Maeda K, Kuriyama H, Okamoto Y, et al. Novel modulator for endothelial adhesion molecules – adipocyte-derived plasma protein adiponectin. Circulation 1999;100:2473–6.

88. Yokota T, Oritani K, Takahashi I, Ishikawa J, Matsuyama A, Ouchi N, et al. Adiponectin, a new member of the family of soluble defense collagens, negatively regulates the growth of myelomonocytic progenitors and the functions of macrophages. Blood 2000;96: 1723–32.

89. Berg AH, Combs TP, Du X, Brownlee M, Scherer PE. The adipocyte-secreted protein Acrp30 enhances hepatic insulin action. Nat Med 2001;7:947–53.

90. Yamauchi T, Kamon J, Waki H, Terauchi Y, Kubota N, Hara K, et al. The fat-derived hormone adiponectin reverses insulin resistance associated with both lipoatrophy and obesity. Nat Med 2001;7: 941–6.

91. Shklyaev S, Aslanidi G, Tennant M, Prima V, Kohlbrenner E, Kroutov V, et al. Sustained peripheral expression of transgene adiponectin offsets the development of diet-induced obesity in rats. Proc Natl Acad Sci USA 2003;100:14217–22.

92. Qi Y, Takahashi N, Hileman SM, Patel HR, Berg AH, Pajvani UB, et al. Adiponectin acts in the brain to decrease body weight. Nat Med 2004;10:524–9.

93. Tomas E, Tsao TS, Saha AK, Murrey HE, Zhang Cc C, Itani SI, et al. Enhanced muscle fat oxidation and glucose transport by ACRP30

globular domain: acetyl-CoA carboxylase inhibition and AMP-activated protein kinase activation. Proc Natl Acad Sci USA 2002;99:16309–13.

94. Yamauchi T, Kamon J, Ito Y, Tsuchida A, Yokomizo T, Kita S, et al. Cloning of adiponectin receptors that mediate antidiabetic metabolic effects. Nature 2003;423:762–9.

95. Bjursell M, Ahnmark A, Bohlooly-Y M, William-Olsson L, Rhedin M, Peng X-R, et al. Opposing effects of adiponectin receptors 1 and 2 on energy metabolism. Diabetes 2007;56:583–93.

96. Bing C, Trayhurn P. Regulation of adipose tissue metabolism in cancer cachexia. Curr Opin Clin Nutr Metab Care 2008;11:201–7.

97. Ebihara K, Ogawa Y, Masuzaki H, Shintani M, Miyanaga F, Aizawa-Abe M, et al. Transgenic overexpression of leptin rescues insulin resistance and diabetes in a mouse model of lipoatrophic diabetes. Diabetes 2001;50:1440–8.

98. Oral EA, Simha V, Ruiz E, Andewelt A, Premkumar A, Snell P, et al. Leptin-replacement therapy for lipodystrophy. N Engl J Med 2002;346:570–8.

99. Steppan CM, Brown EJ, Wright CM, Bhat S, Banerjee RR, Dai CY, et al. A family of tissue-specific resistin-like molecules. Proc Natl Acad Sci USA 2001;98:502–6.

100. Fukuhara A, Matsuda M, Nishizawa M, Segawa K, Tanaka M, Kishimoto K, et al. Visfatin: a protein secreted by visceral fat that mimics the effects of insulin. Science 2005;307:426–30.

101. Boucher J, Masri B, Daviaud D, Gesta S, Guigne C, Mazzucotelli A, et al. Apelin, a newly identified adipokine up regulated by insulin and obesity. Endocrinology 2005;146:1764–71.

102. Yang Q, Graham TE, Mody N, Preitner F, Peroni OD, Zabolotny JM, et al. Serum retinol binding protein 4 contributes to insulin resistance in obesity and type 2 diabetes. Nature 2005;436:356–62.

103. Kloting N, Graham TE, Berndt J, Kralisch S, Kovacs P, Wason CJ, et al. Serum retinol-binding protein is more highly expressed in visceral than in subcutaneous adipose tissue and is a marker of intra-abdominal fat mass. Cell Metab 2007;6:79–87.

104. Yudkin JS. Adipose tissue, insulin action and vascular disease: inflammatory signals. Int J Obes 2003;27(suppl 3):S25–S28.

105. Hotamisligil GS. Inflammation and metabolic disorders. Nature 2006;444:860–7.

106. Wellen KE, Hotamisligil GS. Inflammation, stress, and diabetes. J Clin Invest 2005;115:1111–19.

107. Pischon T, Nothlings U, Boeing H. Obesity and cancer. Proc Nutr Soc 2008;67:128–45.

108. Wang B, Jenkins JR, Trayhurn P. Expression and secretion of inflammation-related adipokines by human adipocytes differentiated in culture: integrated response to TNF-α. Am J Physiol Endocrinol Metab 2005;288:E731–E740.

109. Wang B, Trayhurn P. Acute and prolonged effects of TNF-alpha on the expression and secretion of inflammation-related adipokines by human adipocytes differentiated in culture. Pflügers Archiv Eur J Physiol 2006;452:418–27.

110. Prins JB, Niesler CU, Winterford CM, Bright NA, Siddle K, Orahilly S, et al. Tumor necrosis factor-α induces apoptosis of human adipose cells. Diabetes 1997;46:1939–44.

111. Ryden M, Arvidsson E, Blomqvist L, Perbeck L, Dicker A, Arner P. Targets for TNF-α-induced lipolysis in human adipocytes. Biochem Biophys Res Commun 2004;318:168–75.

112. Chung S, LaPoint K, Martinez K, Kennedy A, Boysen Sandberg M, McIntosh MK. Preadipocytes mediate lipopolysaccharide-induced

inflammation and insulin resistance in primary cultures of newly differentiated human adipocytes. Endocrinology 2006;147: 5340–51.

113. Ehrhart-Bornstein M, Lamounier-Zepter V, Schraven A, Langenbach J, Willenberg HS, Barthel A, et al. Human adipocytes secrete mineralocorticoid-releasing factors. Proc Natl Acad Sci USA 2003;100:14211–16.

114. Sell H, Eckardt K, Taube A, Tews D, Gurgui M, van Echten-Deckert G, et al. Skeletal muscle insulin resistance induced by adipocyte-conditioned medium: underlying mechanisms and reversibility. Am J Physiol Endocrinol Metab 2008;294:E1070–E1077.

115. Sell H, Dietze-Schroeder D, Kaiser U, Eckel J. Monocyte chemotactic protein-1 is a potential player in the negative cross-talk between adipose tissue and skeletal muscle. Endocrinology 2006;147: 2458–67.

116. Sell H, Dietze-Schroeder D, Eckel J. The adipocyte-myocyte axis in insulin resistance. Trends Endocrinol Metab 2006;17: 416–22.

117. Fain JN, Madan AK, Hiler ML, Cheema P, Bahouth SW. Comparison of the release of adipokines by adipose tissue, adipose tissue matrix, and adipocytes from visceral and subcutaneous abdominal adipose tissues of obese humans. Endocrinology 2004;145: 2273–82.

118. Fain JN. Release of interleukins and other inflammatory cytokines by human adipose tissue is enhanced in obesity and primarily due to the nonfat cells. Vitam Horm 2006;74:443–77.

119. Ozcan U, Cao Q, Yilmaz E, Lee AH, Iwakoshi NN, Ozdelen E, et al. Endoplasmic reticulum stress links obesity, insulin action, and type 2 diabetes. Science 2004;306:457–61.

120. Gregor MF, Hotamisligil GS. Adipocyte stress: the endoplasmic reticulum and metabolic disease. J Lipid Res 2007;48:1905–14.

121. Houstis N, Rosen ED, Lander ES. Reactive oxygen species have a causal role in multiple forms of insulin resistance. Nature 2006;440:944–8.

122. Koumenis C, Naczki C, Koritzinsky M, Rastani S, Diehl A, Sonenberg N, et al. Regulation of protein synthesis by hypoxia via activation of the endoplasmic reticulum kinase PERK and phosphorylation of the translation initiation factor eIF2α. Mol Cell Biol 2002;22:7405–16.

123. Carriere A, Carmona M-C, Fernandez Y, Rigoulet M, Wenger RH, Penicaud L, et al. Mitochondrial reactive oxygen species control the transcription factor CHOP-10/GADD153 and adipocyte differentiation: a mechanism for hypoxia-dependent effect. J Biol Chem 2004;279:40462–9.

124. Brahimi-Horn MC, Pouysségur J. Oxygen, a source of life and stress. FEBS Lett 2007;581:3582–91.

125. Hosogai N, Fukuhara A, Oshima K, Miyata Y, Tanaka S, Segawa K, et al. Adipose tissue hypoxia in obesity and its impact on adipocytokine dysregulation. Diabetes 2007;56:901–11.

126. Rausch ME, Weisberg SP, Vardhana P, Tortoriello DV. Obesity in C57BL/6J mice is characterised by adipose tissue hypoxia and cytotoxic T-cell infiltration. Int J Obes 2008;32:451–63.

127. Lolmède K, Durand de Saint Front V, Galitzky J, Lafontan M, Bouloumie A. Effects of hypoxia on the expression of proangiogenic factors in differentiated 3T3-F442A adipocytes. Int J Obes 2003;27:1187–95.

128. Chen B, Lam KSL, Wang Y, Wu D, Lam MC, Shen J, et al. Hypoxia dysregulates the production of adiponectin and plasminogen

activator inhibitor-1 independent of reactive oxygen species in adipocytes. Biochem Biophys Res Commun 2006;341:549–56.

129. Wang B, Wood IS, Trayhurn P. Dysregulation of the expression and secretion of inflammation-related adipokines by hypoxia in human adipocytes. Pflügers Archiv Eur J Physiol 2007;455:479–92.

130. Wang B, Wood IS, Trayhurn P. PCR arrays identify metallothionein-3 as a highly hypoxia-inducible gene in human adipocytes. Biochem Biophys Res Commun 2008;368:88–93.

131. Wood IS, Wang B, Lorente-Cebrián S, Trayhurn P. Hypoxia increases expression of selective facilitative glucose transporters (GLUT) and 2-deoxy-d-glucose uptake in human adipocytes. Biochem Biophys Res Commun 2007;361:468–73.

10 Metabolic Fuels and Obesity

Simon W. Coppack

East London Obesity Service, Barts and The London School of Medicine and Dentistry, London, UK

Introduction

Metabolism and fuel selection vary between different tissues and between different physiologic conditions. This is true of both obese and lean subjects. However, when one compares like-with-like conditions, obesity is associated with multiple changes in metabolism. Some of these changes appear to be adaptive and others maladaptive.

Because energy metabolism undergoes marked changes to adapt to everyday life, it is necessary to consider separately the different physiologic conditions that determine energy balance. Thereafter we will consider the ways in which obese patients respond to situations of energy imbalance and mention some metabolic theories for the propensity to obesity. Finally we will summarize the concept of metabolic inflexibility as it applies in obesity and some of its consequences.

There are good reviews of the metabolism (and its regulation) of whole-body, skeletal muscle [1,2] and adipose tissue [3–5]. The theme of this chapter will be the main fluxes of energy-bearing fuels in these tissues, and their contributions to whole-body energy fluxes. Because the emphasis will be on fuels and energy metabolism, little will be said about amino acid and protein metabolism.

We will discuss the normal metabolic contributions of these tissues in the whole body, in lean and obese subjects, and how the changes of obesity lead in turn to many of the adverse metabolic characteristics associated with obesity.

An important conceptual issue is the difference between "absolute" and "relative" changes in metabolism. By virtue of simply being larger people, obese subjects have absolute increases in many parameters. But a different impression arises when one

makes allowance for the different body sizes. An example might be glucose disposal. "Whole-body glucose uptake per minute" is typically greater in obese than smaller leaner people, but if one considers either "glucose uptake rate per kilogram of body weight" or "fractional clearance rate of plasma glucose" then the obese usually show reduced glucose disposal. This issue is further discussed below.

Physiologic conditions encountered in weight-stable patients

General considerations

During the "typical" day, free-living subjects will go through times during which their metabolic physiology might be characterized as (1) fasting (also called postabsorptive), (2) postprandial and (3) exercise. Figure 10.1 shows the transition between postabsorptive and postprandial states as normal weight and obese subject spend 24 hours in a metabolic study unit. Unfortunately, the subjects in Figure 10.1 were relatively inactive throughout the study period. As can be seen, the transitions between these states may occur within minutes (e.g. after eating, starting exercise) or may be more gradual (e.g. returning to a postabsorptive state after eating) and hence a significant portion of the 24 hours is spent in transition. However, for convenience, we will primarily discuss the ends of the spectrum. Unless otherwise stated, exercise in this chapter means endurance, aerobic exercise at 50–60% VO_{2max}. Although other forms of exercise (e.g. anaerobic sprinting) can have entirely different metabolic characteristics, most subjects spend little or none of their usual lifestyle in these conditions.

Fuller information about body composition is given in Chapter 2. However, it is obvious that an expanded adipose tissue mass will potentially increase the release of nonesterified fatty acids (NEFA) from the whole-body adipose organ or that the expanded muscle mass of athletes can increase uptake of glucose into muscle. Technically, of course, subjects may be "obese" according to World Health Organization criteria by virtue of an expanded

Clinical Obesity in Adults and Children, 3rd edition. Edited by Peter G. Kopelman, Ian D. Caterson and William H. Dietz.
© 2010 Blackwell Publishing, ISBN: 978-1-4051-8226-3.

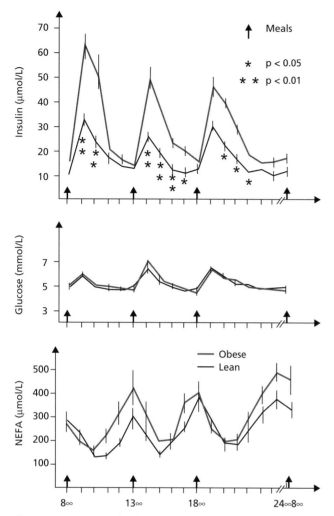

Figure 10.1 Systemic insulin, glucose and NEFA concentrations in healthy lean and obese subjects studied whilst in clinical research center for 24 hours. (Data from Chen et al. [176].)

muscle mass. In this chapter, we will use the term "obesity" to mean adiposity, i.e. an expanded adipose tissue mass and increased body fat content ("percent body fat").

Both skeletal muscle and white adipose tissue are distributed in discrete sites throughout the body. These sites are not homogeneous in their histology or metabolic characteristics. Different muscles (e.g. soleus compared to gastrocnemius) have different oxidative capacity, histology and stores of glycogen and triglyceride, although in humans (as opposed to rodents) all skeletal muscles are of mixed fiber type [6]. Clearly, during exercise, there are muscle-specific differences in metabolism, as different muscles are recruited to different extents, and this implies that there is local regulation of skeletal muscle metabolism, but even at rest there may be significant differences. In the case of adipose tissue, the differences between depots in their metabolic characteristics may be quite marked and may be relevant to their role in whole-body energy metabolism [7]. Some site-specific properties will be discussed later in this chapter, but it is important to note the large

body of evidence that links the accumulation of abdominal, and especially intra-abdominal, adipose tissue with adverse metabolic changes in obesity [8–13]. Unfortunately, because the intra-abdominal fat depots are not accessible for direct study, our knowledge of them comes almost entirely from *in vitro* studies on the metabolic properties of samples removed at operation. Most of the metabolic properties of adipose tissue discussed below are therefore based on studies of subcutaneous adipose tissue, which is accessible for study *in vivo* [14,15].

When discussing obesity, one needs to be aware of the "denominator question" whereby a metabolic flux can be increased, "normal" or decreased depending upon the units in which it is expressed [16]. An example of this point is lipolysis in obesity which produces an elevation of the plasma NEFA concentration [17]. This has been attributed to the increased adipose tissue mass [18]. Obese subjects have increased basal rates of lipolysis when the whole-body rate of appearance (R_a) is expressed in absolute amounts (i.e. mmoles of NEFA per minute) or per lean body mass units (i.e. mmoles of NEFA per minute per kg LBM) but have a reduced basal NEFA R_a when expressed per kg of body fat (i.e. mmoles of NEFA per minute per kg fat mass)[16,19]. Equivalent "denominator issues" can arise for carbohydrate fuels.

The metabolic changes of obesity in weight-stable subjects are summarized in Table 10.1.

Fasting/postabsorptive conditions

People awake in a fasted or postabsorptive metabolic state. Most meals will be completely absorbed and their nutrients dealt with metabolically within 2–6 hours (depending on size and composition of the meal). As a consequence, normal healthy subjects eating typical diets spend up to 8–12 hours per day in a postabsorptive state (see Fig. 10.1).

Whole-body postabsorptive metabolism

Over a 24-hour period during a day of net energy balance, the respiratory quotient (RQ) of the whole body will be the same as that of the food absorbed [20]. This will closely resemble the food eaten although metabolic effects of gut bacteria (and indeed, the consequences of incomplete food digestion) may affect this.

In fasting conditions, whole-body RQ drops towards 0.70, suggesting that lipid is the predominant fuel. The RQ after an overnight fast would be typically 0.80, but as the subjects continued to fast this would drop progressively to reach 0.72 by 48 hours.

Postprandially, obese subjects will tend to have a higher resting energy expenditure (REE) and will tend to have a lower RQ than lean subjects [21]. The higher REE is a consequence of the greater lean body mass which is present in obesity (as well as the expanded adipose tissue mass). The lower RQ presumably reflects the higher fat content of the diet (to the extent that one can be sure the subjects were weight stable). If the subjects were not weight stable, the expanded triglyceride stores in adipose and other tissues in obesity could explain this observation. The association between obesity and high-fat diets [22] can make it difficult to distinguish the effects of the two.

Table 10.1 Overview of metabolic fuels in weight-stable obese

	Absolute	"Corrected" for increased body mass
Resting metabolic rate	Increased	Normal per kg lean body mass
Energy expenditure related to activity	Normal	Usually low per kg lean body mass
Respiratory quotient (RQ)	Depends on diet Tends to be increased	
Fasting glucose concentration	Increased	
Hepatic glucose output	Increased	
Total body glucose uptake (R_d)	Normal or increased	Usually low per kg lean body mass
NEFA concentration	Slightly increased postaborptively Does not suppress postprandially	
Total NEFA production (R_a)	Increased	Increased per kg lean body mass, reduced per kg adipose mass
Triglyceride concentration	Slightly increased postabsorptively More markedly increased postprandially	
VLDL triglyceride secretion rate	Increased	Increased per kg lean body mass
VO_{2max}	Reduced	Reduced

For abbreviations, please see text.

Muscle (resting) postabsorptive metabolism

Skeletal muscle makes up 40% of body weight in "reference man" and 30% in "reference woman" [23]. In trained athletes, skeletal muscle may contribute up to 65% of body mass [24]. Even at rest, skeletal muscle metabolism plays a major role in whole-body energy fluxes because of muscle mass [25].

Skeletal muscle is the body's major reservoir of carbohydrate, in the form of glycogen. Typically liver glycogen content in the fed state is around 100 g, whereas whole-body skeletal muscle contains about 400 g, and may contain much more during high-carbohydrate feeding [26]. It is therefore evident that skeletal muscle plays a major role in the regulation of the metabolic disposal of carbohydrate in the body.

In the 1950s, Baltzan et al. [27] showed that the main oxidative fuel of skeletal muscle after an overnight fast at rest must be lipid; the RQ measured across the forearm is around 0.76. Plasma glucose disposal by skeletal muscle in that state is therefore small. The rate of anaerobic glycolysis of glucosyl units from both plasma glucose and muscle glycogen also appears to be small: net release of lactate from resting skeletal muscle after an overnight fast is inconsistent, and close to zero [28]. Figure 10.2 indicates the sources of circulating fuel taken up by forearm skeletal muscle in this state.

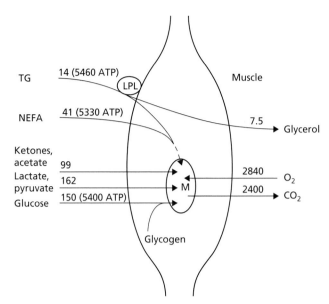

Figure 10.2 Fluxes of metabolic fuels and gases in and out of forearm muscle of lean subjects in fasting, resting state (values are nmole/100 g tissue/min). For some metabolic fuels the equivalent ATP value of the fuel is indicated. (Data from Coppack et al. [90].)

Because of its large mass, skeletal muscle is one of the most important organs in the removal from the bloodstream of NEFA both at rest and during exercise. It is also an important site for the removal of plasma triacylglycerol (TG). Both NEFA and plasma TG are quantitatively important contributors to the energy uptake of resting postaborptive muscle.

The size of the intramuscular TG store does not fluctuate greatly during normal daily life, except during exercise. Although it may turn over, it is not therefore a net contributor to muscle fatty acid oxidation at rest. In muscle (and adipose tissue), lipoprotein lipase (LPL) is the key enzyme regulating plasma TG extraction and hence uptake of its fatty acid content. Active LPL is bound to the capillary endothelium. This enzyme is more active in oxidative than glycolytic muscles, and it is activated by training. Selective venous catheterization clearly demonstrates that TG extraction does occur [29,30].

Extraction of plasma NEFA by muscle has also been studied, usually by a combination of tracer infusion and selective venous catheterization [31,32]. At rest, in the overnight fasted state, NEFA extraction from plasma appears to provide most of the fatty acids required for oxidation. Whether these fatty acids pass through an intramyocellular TG pool before oxidation is not clear: older evidence for such a pathway [33] has been challenged [34].

On a high-fat diet, plasma TG-derived fatty acid oxidation is increased, suggesting that although plasma NEFA remain the main source of fat oxidation, diet composition may affect the contribution of both sources to some extent [35]. The rate of fatty acid extraction from the plasma by skeletal muscle appears to be affected by their delivery in plasma, i.e. by the product of muscle blood flow and the plasma NEFA concentration [36]. Additionally, evidence from *in vitro* and whole-animal studies supports the existence of transmembrane transport of NEFA, which is likely to co-exist with passive diffusional uptake. There is also concerted action between the membrane and cytoplasmic fatty acid binding proteins (FABP) that allow for efficient regulation of NEFA transport and metabolism [37].

The rate of uptake of fatty acids by skeletal muscle is linked to their oxidation, as the muscle TG pool is of relatively constant size. The oxidation of fatty acids has been proposed to be linked to that of glucosyl units by mechanisms described by Randle and colleagues [38]. This concept postulates that products of fatty acid oxidation (acetyl-CoA, cytosolic citrate) exert inhibitory feedback control over the rate of glucose uptake and oxidation via inhibition of phosphofructokinase (a key regulatory enzyme in glycolysis) and pyruvate dehydrogenase. This link has received most attention with respect to insulin resistance and type 2 diabetes mellitus, although there is also evidence for it operating in normal daily life [39]. Although there is consistent evidence that increased NEFA concentrations are associated with insulin resistance, there are also studies that argue for mechanisms additional to those proposed by Randle and colleagues [38]. In this respect, an early NEFA-induced decline in glucose-6-phosphate concentration has been reported, suggesting that NEFA primarily inhibit glucose transport/phosphorylation [40,41].

The concept of competition between carbohydrate and lipid fuels is reinforced by indications that the intracellular availability of glucose (rather than NEFA alone) may determine the nature of substrate oxidation in human subjects by controlling fatty acid transport into the mitochondria [42,43]. This may occur via the inhibitory effect of malonyl-CoA (formed under conditions of high glucose and insulin) on carnitine palmitoyl transferase-1 (CPT1), a key regulatory enzyme in fatty acid oxidation [44].

Skeletal muscle plays an important role in amino acid metabolism. Intracellular concentrations of some amino acids are several-fold greater than those in plasma, and again, by virtue of its mass, skeletal muscle constitutes the largest reservoir of free amino acids in the body [45]. Skeletal muscle also contains the largest amount of protein of any single tissue in the body, and although its rate of protein turnover is slower than that of some smaller organs, the absolute rate of turnover is greater than from any other tissue/organ [46].

Within muscle, one of the most obvious changes that occur in obesity is the accumulation of excess triglyceride. Some of this triglyceride is within adipocytes in the muscles. These intramuscular adipocytes [47] may release NEFA and adipokines (see Chapter 9) that influence muscle metabolism in a "portal" or "paracrine" manner. However, other triglyceride accumulates within the myocytes themselves. This intramyocellular triglyceride appears to cause insulin resistance [48], high lipid oxidation in the muscles and "metabolic inflexibility" (discussed below). For many years there has been uncertainty about the importance of the intramyocellular triglyceride as elevated quantities are also seen in trained athletes whose muscle shows none of these

characteristics. Recently it has been suggested that obesity-related intramyocellular triglyceride is histologically in larger droplets which may have different phospholipid content, different enzymes associated with the droplets and an increased propensity to induce local production of metabolically active cytokines such as TNF-α [49]. These features are not seen with intramyocellular triglyceride in athletes.

Adipose tissue postabsorptive metabolism

As the body's main energy store, the contribution of white adipose tissue to whole-body energy fluxes is of obvious importance. White adipose tissue contributes about 20% of body weight in a "reference" (nonobese) man and 30% in a "reference woman" [23]. In trained athletes, the proportion of adipose tissue is smaller than in nonathletes (typically 9–12%) of body weight in men and women [50] but it still plays a key role in the supply of energy (NEFA) to exercising muscle. In obesity, the amount of adipose tissue may, of course, increase enormously. Although this excessive adipose tissue may not be as metabolically active (per kg) as in lean subjects, by virtue of its expanded mass it exerts powerful influences on some whole-body energy fluxes. An athlete may have a total adipose tissue mass of <10 kg, whilst his morbidly obese age- and height-matched colleague is likely to be carrying >60 kg.

Despite its mass, adipose tissue plays only a small (5–10%) role in postabsorptive whole-body glucose disposal [51–53]. The role of glucose and other fuel fluxes is shown in Figure 10.3.

Adipose tissue is mainly concerned with lipid fuel metabolism. The rate of release of NEFA from adipose tissue is the major determinant of the systemic plasma NEFA concentration and thus of the delivery of NEFA to other tissues [54,55]. As shown in Figures 10.1 and 10.4, this is a highly regulated process, switching in a short time from its high postabsorptive rate in the normal daily pattern to almost zero in lean subjects. These rapid changes in NEFA release reflect regulation of the key enzyme in the

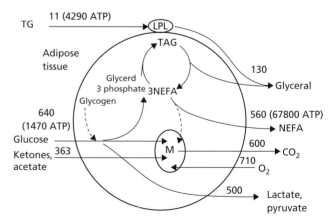

Figure 10.3 Fluxes of metabolic fuels and gases in and out of adipose tissue of lean subjects in fasting, resting state (values are nmole/100 g tissue/min). For some metabolic fuels the equivalent ATP value of the fuel is indicated. (Data from Coppack et al. [90].)

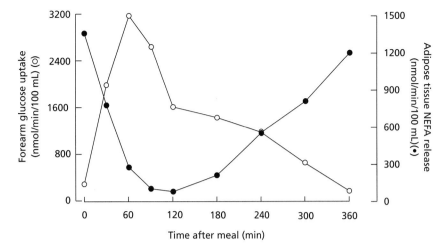

Figure 10.4 Major metabolic fluxes in skeletal muscle (glucose uptake, ●) and white adipose tissue (NEFA release, ○) in the overnight fasted state, and their responses to ingestion of a mixed meal. Changes of several-fold are observed within 60–90 min of meal ingestion. Fluxes were estimated by selective venous catheterization with measurement of arteriovenous differences and blood flow. (Data taken from the studies reported in Coppack et al. [90,109] with the addition of further subjects by Frayn.)

hydrolysis of adipocyte TG, the intracellular enzyme hormone-sensitive lipase (HSL). Regulation of HSL is co-ordinated (inversely) with regulation of fatty acid esterification: when HSL is suppressed by insulin, fatty acid esterification is stimulated and fatty acids are effectively trapped in adipocytes.

In normal daily life, most of the regulation of NEFA delivery from adipose tissue [56] is determined by the inhibitory effect of insulin on HSL (reviewed by Coppack et al. [16]). HSL is stimulated by agents that raise the cellular cyclic AMP concentration, particularly β-adrenergic agents, and in the longer term by a number of hormones, including growth hormone and cortisol, which may either affect enzyme expression or modify the sensitivity to catecholamines (e.g. by regulation of adrenoceptor expression). In normal subjects fasted overnight, local introduction of propranolol into subcutaneous adipose tissue has no effect on lipolysis, suggesting that adrenergic stimulation of lipolysis is not operative in this state [57]. Instead the lipolytic "tone" against which insulin acts may be set by the normal early morning rise in cortisol [58] and perhaps by overnight growth hormone pulses [59,60].

Despite the primacy of HSL in lipolysis, adipose tissue lipolysis is maintained in HSL-deficient animals, although sensitivity to catecholamine stimulation is reduced [61,62]. This is due to the presence of at least one other TG lipase expressed in adipose tissue, although this other lipase (known as adipose triglyceride lipase, PNPLA2) is usually much less active than HSL [63]. It has also been appreciated that the acute regulation of lipolysis is achieved only in part through reversible phosphorylation of HSL and consequent changes in its enzyme activity.

Perilipin is a protein that coats the fat droplet in white adipocytes [64]. Perilipin, like HSL, is phosphorylated in response to elevation of cellular cyclic AMP. Phosphorylation of perilipin causes it to move away from the fat droplet, whereas HSL translocates from a cytoplasmic location onto the surface of the lipid droplet [65].

Adipose tissue plays an important part in the regulation of fasting plasma TG concentrations, in two ways. The rate of NEFA delivery plays a critical role in determining the rate of hepatic TG secretion in very low-density lipoprotein (VLDL) particles [66]. In addition, adipose tissue is a major site of extraction of plasma TG, with LPL the rate-limiting enzyme. Adipose tissue LPL is least active in the postprandial state, but even then there is significant removal of plasma TG. In fact, systemic plasma TG concentrations correlate inversely with adipose tissue TG clearance [67], suggesting a role for adipose tissue in "setting" the fasting plasma TG concentration. TG clearance in skeletal muscle does not relate in such a way to the plasma TG concentration [30].

The importance of white adipose tissue to whole-body amino acid metabolism is not entirely clear, although for some amino acids it may approach that of skeletal muscle, especially in obesity [68].

Adipose tissue also exerts major effects on energy metabolism through the secretion of a range of peptides and other factors (sometimes collectively termed adipokines or adipocytokines), some of which may act in a local paracrine manner, but some of which undoubtedly act as hormones signaling to the brain, skeletal muscle and other tissues. The best understood is the adipocyte-derived hormone leptin. Leptin deficiency in humans is characterized by widespread metabolic and physiologic disturbances, many of which are normalized on treatment with recombinant leptin [69]. Another adipocyte-derived peptide that seems important is adiponectin (also known as adipoQ or Acrp30). Adiponectin secretion decreases with increasing adipose tissue mass, contrary to the pattern with leptin and other adipokines [70]. Adiponectin has clear insulin-sensitizing effects in tissues other than adipose [71,72]. Although these aspects of adipose tissue function are not the subject of this chapter, they may well complement the better established functions of adipose tissue in energy metabolism. Secretory functions of adipose tissue have been extensively reviewed elsewhere [4,73,74]. This is further discussed in Chapter 9.

Postabsorptive metabolism in other tissues

The metabolism of brown adipose tissue (as seen in rodents) is different in many respects from that of white adipose tissue and, as its contribution to whole-body energy fluxes in adult humans is probably small, it will not be covered in this chapter. Nonetheless, measurement of regional heat production suggests that even in the absence of classic brown adipose tissue with the same histologic features as seen in rodents, there may be human fat depots that do have specialized thermogenetic actions. This regional heat production is inducible by cold exposure, but it is unclear how much of a role it plays in clinical obesity. It is arguable whether human adipose tissue depots should be considered as different shades of beige rather than strictly brown or white.

Additionally, the study of brown adipose tissue led to the elucidation of a potentially very important aspect of energy metabolism. Brown adipose tissue is specialized for the production of heat. This is achieved by the expression of a protein, uncoupling protein 1 (UCP-1) or thermogenin, in the inner mitochondrial membrane. UCP1 is a member of the mitochondrial proton transporter family. The proton gradient generated by the electron transport chain across the inner mitochondrial membrane is normally used for the synthesis of ATP. The effect of UCP1 is to instead discharge this gradient. Metabolic energy is therefore released as heat. Brown adipose tissue generates most of its heat by oxidation of fatty acids. A family of UCPs [75] have been discovered, related to UCP1. UCP2 is ubiquitously expressed, whereas UCP3 is expressed mainly in skeletal muscle. It remains uncertain whether these UCPs (2 and 3 especially) are involved in uncoupling of oxidative phosphorylation in tissues other than brown adipose tissue, although this has also been much debated [76–78]. UCP3, in particular, could potentially play an important role in energy metabolism because of its expression in skeletal muscle.

Postabsorptive liver metabolism in obesity shows some important changes. Of note, hepatic glucose output is increased [79]. The circulating concentrations of gluconenogenic precursors (glycerol, lactate, amino acids) are themselves increased in obesity. The other major change has already been mentioned: increased delivery of NEFA to the liver seems to produce both a fatty liver (discussed in greater detail in Chapter 16) and an increased hepatic production of VLDL. There are multiple steps regulating the number and size of VLDL particles, but the "mass action" of excess intrahepatocellular triglyceride coupled with increased NEFA influx into the liver from the circulation seems to be an irresistible drive to increase VLDL-TG [66,80,81].

Postprandial conditions

The postprandial period starts promptly with ingestion of a significant meal (and of course, due to the "cephalic phase," some changes may precede it). Its duration varies with the size of the meal, with the composition of the meal and with interactions between the contents of the meal. Isocaloric meals of hamburger versus baked potato with beans, or brown rice versus fruit juice show different postprandial characteristics. As the postprandial period ends, the subject gradually changes back towards a postaborptive metabolic state, the carbohydrate changes usually preceding the lipid changes.

It is not the intention of this chapter to discuss the differences in diets of obese and lean people, beyond suggesting that obese people may have genetic [82], or non-genetic reasons for eating a different diet (see Chapter 7).

The metabolic changes of the fasting/postprandial transition appear to be orchestrated almost entirely via insulin (see Fig. 10.1).

Whole-body postprandial metabolism

On a typical Western diet in which fat provides around 40% of energy, humans eat 200–300 g of carbohydrate and 70–100 g of fat (mainly TG) per day (approximate figures, for illustration only). If these are split between three main meals, a "typical" meal might contain around 80 g of carbohydrate and 30 g of fat.

The free glucose content of the body in the postabsorptive state is around 12 g. (The plasma glucose concentration is 5 mmol/L or about 0.9 g/L, and the extracellular fluid volume is about 20% of body weight or 13 L.) Therefore, at one meal we eat enough glucose to raise the plasma glucose concentration around eightfold. Likewise, if one compared the R_a of glucose in the fasting state, which depends upon hepatic glucose output [83], to the R_a of glucose after a meal, the R_a glucose would increase more than 10-fold after most meals. In normal people, however, the rise in plasma glucose concentration is no more than 60% of basal. These figures attest to homeostatic mechanisms that minimize the excursions of plasma glucose concentration. These mechanisms include rapid suppression of endogenous hepatic glucose production, together with increased glucose disposal into cells.

The many changes that occur after a typical meal have proven difficult to study in a reproducible manner and hence techniques have developed for studying isolated components of the postprandial state. Foremost amongst these is the "glucose clamp" approach suggested by Sherwin. This has provided a great deal of consistent information on skeletal muscle substrate utilization [84]. In this technique, glucose is infused intravenously, usually against a background of insulin infusion at a constant rate, to raise the plasma insulin concentration to some predetermined level (hyperinsulinemic clamp). The rate of glucose infusion is varied as necessary to keep the plasma glucose concentration, measured regularly at the bedside, constant within narrow limits: hence the plasma glucose concentration is "clamped." Under these conditions the rate of glucose disappearance from the plasma must equal the rate of glucose entry, which is known (as it is being infused). Any contribution from hepatic glucose release is usually small under these conditions, although it may be estimated by infusion of a labeled glucose tracer. The technique therefore provides a means for assessing whole-body glucose utilization at controlled plasma insulin concentrations, and thus gives a measure of whole-body insulin sensitivity: it is usually regarded as providing the "gold standard" assessment of this parameter [85,86].

Postprandially, indirect calorimetry shows an increase in REE with an increase in the whole-body RQ to above 0.9 (usually above 0.95). Similar changes are seen during a hyperinsulinemic glucose clamp. Whole-body rates of carbohydrate oxidation and lipid oxidation can be measured. It is usually found that under hyperinsulinemic conditions (post meal or hyperinsulinemic clamp) glucose oxidation increases and accounts for around 20–30% of the total glucose disposal rate [87,88, 89]. The remainder reflects "nonoxidative glucose disposal," sometimes called glucose storage, although anaerobic glycolysis is also included in this portion.

Postprandial lipid fluxes are also different from fasting values. Extracellular TG is confined to the plasma volume (in a normal individual, around 3 L at 1 mmol/L or 0.85 g/L, i.e. 2.5–3 g of extracellular TG). We eat enough TG in a typical meal to raise our plasma TG concentration at least 10-fold. This does not happen; a typical postprandial excursion in plasma TG concentration is more like 50–60% of the fasting concentration [90,91]. This must also imply the existence of co-ordinated mechanisms for regulating the delivery of endogenous TG to the circulation, and stimulating TG clearance. These have been much less studied than those responsible for glucose homeostasis, particularly the regulation of hepatic TG secretion in the postprandial period (because of the methodologic difficulties of such experiments), but it is clear that peripheral tissues are responsible for most of the increased TG clearance in the postprandial period. Obesity and high-fat meals each cause relative hypertriglyceridemia [92,93].

Muscle postprandial metabolism

After eating, skeletal muscle metabolism switches within a few minutes from the low carbohydrate uptake of fasting to a postprandial state of rapid glucose uptake, such that skeletal muscle is undoubtedly the major extrahepatic tissue involved in this co-ordinated regulation of glucose metabolism. The contribution of white adipose tissue is very small in comparison.

To study muscle behavior, the glucose clamp technique may be combined with selective catheterization of the venous drainage of a skeletal muscle bed (e.g. forearm or leg) (see Fig. 10.2). Making assumptions about the uniformity of the muscle mass, such studies suggest that the contribution of skeletal muscle in whole-body glucose disposal during hyperinsulinemia is a major one (70–85%) [87,94]. A corollary is that skeletal muscle is the tissue which predominantly "sets" the insulin sensitivity of glucose metabolism for the whole body [95].

In the postprandial state, the increased plasma glucose and insulin concentrations lead to increased glucose uptake by muscle, mainly via the insulin-regulatable glucose transporter GLUT4, and to increased glucose disposal within the muscle cell by co-ordinated regulation of the pathways of glycogen deposition, glycolysis and pyruvate oxidation. The glucose taken up from the plasma by muscle is either oxidized or stored as glycogen or released as lactate. Measurements made by selective venous catheterization suggest that around 25% [93,96,97] to 45% [28] of an oral glucose load (whether given as a pure glucose load or as part of a mixed meal) is disposed of by resting skeletal muscle

during the 4–6 hour postprandial period. Direct measurements of muscle glycogen deposition by ^{13}C-NMR spectroscopy show muscle glycogen content increasing by around 25%; net glycogen deposition in muscle during the 7 h following a mixed meal accounted for around 20% of that ingested [98].

Postprandially, fatty acid utilization by skeletal muscle decreases rapidly as glucose uptake and oxidation become the more important processes. It seems that muscle fatty acid utilization is actually regulated by the release of NEFA from adipose tissue, which is rapidly inhibited by insulin after a meal (see Figs 10.1,10.4). Also, rat studies indicate that insulin may regulate fatty acid uptake and esterification in the myocyte [99,100], suggesting there may also be direct control of muscle fatty acid uptake in the postprandial state. However, the physiologic significance of these latter findings remains uncertain in humans.

Among tissues that clear circulating triglyceride, skeletal muscle and adipose tissue play major roles postprandially [101]. The role of skeletal muscle appears to be very variable from person to person, and greatest in the highly endurance-trained individual, in whom TG clearance is very rapid [102]. It may be much less in the habitually sedentary person. The extraction of plasma TG fatty acids by muscle has been little explored. Although it may not occur at a high rate per unit mass of skeletal muscle, the bulk of skeletal muscle means that its contribution to whole-body plasma TG clearance may be substantial. The expression of skeletal muscle LPL is increased considerably by training [103] and training is also associated with a marked improvement in fat tolerance (i.e. the increase in plasma TG concentration following a fat load, also called "postprandial lipemia") [102,104,105]. It has been suggested that plasma TG fatty acids extracted by skeletal muscle serve mainly to replenish the intramuscular TG pool [106]. However, on the basis of a studies in rats, a model has been proposed in which fatty acids from TG mix locally at the capillaries with plasma NEFA, where they would lead to an increase in local NEFA concentration and hence NEFA uptake. This suggests that muscle does not distinguish between TG-derived NEFA and plasma NEFA [107].

Skeletal muscle LPL is suppressed by insulin [108], in contrast with adipose tissue, in which LPL is activated by insulin. This suggests that adipose tissue plays a more important role than skeletal muscle in clearance of plasma TG in the postprandial state. This may not be true for all subjects, because the suppression of skeletal muscle LPL by insulin is not very marked, and the bulk of skeletal muscle, especially in an athlete in whom muscle LPL is particularly active, may give it an equally or even more important role.

Adipose tissue postprandial metabolism

The uptake of glucose by white adipocytes has been extensively studied *in vitro*. Unfortunately, it seems clear that adipose tissue contributes relatively little (5–10%) to fasting whole-body glucose utilization, and in the postprandial period its contribution to glucose metabolism is dwarfed by that of skeletal muscle [109]. Adipocytes have a small store of glycogen, the concentration of which varies with feeding and fasting [110], but again, this cannot be a major contributor to whole-body carbohydrate economy. The role of glucose in adipocyte metabolism is twofold. First, glucose metabolism (mainly complete oxidation) seems to be a major route of ATP generation in white adipocytes [111]. Second, in the postprandial period, glycolysis provides glycerol-3-phosphate, which is needed for esterification of the fatty acids delivered to adipocytes from LPL in the capillaries. It might therefore be expected that adipose tissue glucose uptake would increase at this time, but the proportion of glucose metabolism diverted to glycerol-3-phosphate production, even after a high-fat meal, is only around 20% [112].

In sedentary people (in contrast to athletes), the role of adipose tissue appears to be larger than that of skeletal muscle in clearing circulating triglyceride-rich lipoproteins (compare Fig. 10.2 and Fig. 10.3). Partly this is the effect of varying body composition and partly due to insulin activating adipose tissue LPL. Adipose tissue also plays a key role in overall lipid homeostasis since a major and dramatic effect of meal ingestion is to suppress intra-adipocyte TG hydrolysis and thus the release of NEFA from adipose tissue The rate of supply of NEFA to the liver is a major determinant of hepatic TG secretion, and reduction in adipose tissue NEFA release is an important component of the suppression of hepatic TG secretion by insulin *in vivo* [66,80,81]. These considerations have led to the description of adipose tissue as a "buffer" for the daily influx of dietary fatty acids into the circulation [113]. As dietary fat enters the circulation, adipose tissue TG clearance is increased by insulin, and the release of NEFA is suppressed. By these means, postprandial excursions of "fatty acids" (TG and NEFA) are minimized, just as the liver and skeletal muscle "buffer" the daily influx of glucose.

As mentioned above, adipose tissue LPL is activated by insulin, and possibly by other hormones, including those released from the gut in response to feeding [114] (Fig. 10.5). Adipose tissue extraction of chylomicron-TG is avid, averaging around 30% of the arterial concentration in a single passage through the tissue [30] although this varies considerably from person to person. The quantitative role of adipose tissue in removal of plasma TG in the postprandial period has been estimated by a number of means. Marin et al. fed a meal containing 120 g of fat labeled with 14C-oleic acid [115]. After 24 hours, biopsies showed 60 g of this had been deposited in adipose tissue (in a group who had eaten a carbohydrate-rich breakfast), and the figure increased slowly over the next month. Romanski et al. performed similar studies and found that 24% (in men) to 35% (in women) of an oral fat load had been deposited in subcutaneous adipose tissue after 24 hours [116]. Arteriovenous difference studies suggest that in lean subjects about 35% of the fat load in a mixed meal is stored in adipose tissue over the subsequent 6 hours [89]. The magnitude of postprandial lipemia is inversely related to the LPL activity measured in plasma following injection of heparin, which releases LPL from its endothelial binding sites [117] although this does not distinguish between LPL released from different tissues. Defective activation of adipose tissue LPL is associated with increased postprandial lipemia [118].

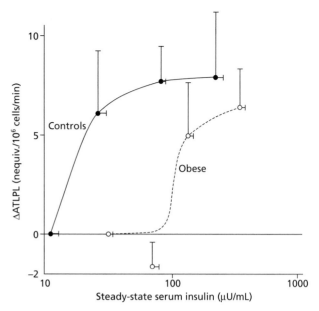

Figure 10.5 Insulin resistance of the activation of white adipose tissue lipoprotein lipase (LPL) in obesity. Dose–response curves were constructed by infusing insulin at different rates on different occasions for 6 h, and activation of adipose tissue LPL was measured as the difference in LPL activity in biopsies taken before and after insulin infusion. (Reproduced from Eckel [127] with permission.)

The fatty acids released by LPL can have different fates in different tissues. In skeletal muscle it appears that the fatty acids released by the action of LPL on plasma TG are quantitatively extracted by the muscle: no net "overspill" of fatty acids is seen during the postprandial period, for instance, when skeletal muscle LPL is active against chylomicron-TG [119]. The fate of these fatty acids is either esterification to replenish the intramuscular TG pool (ultimately a source for fatty acid oxidation) or direct oxidation. In adipose tissue, plasma TG extraction by LPL provides the source of fatty acids for deposition as intracellular TG, the ultimate energy store of the body. Teleologically, this process should be highly regulated, as the body's fat store is closely related to whole-body energy balance. It is not therefore surprising to find an additional level of control in adipose tissue. LPL-derived fatty acids in adipose tissue are not all taken up by adipocytes for esterification and storage. A proportion of these appear always to be released into the venous plasma in the form of NEFA [112,119]. So far as is known at present, this role of LPL in delivery of NEFA into the plasma is specific to white adipose tissue. However, regulation of the fate of LPL-derived fatty acids is a key process in the regulation of fat storage. In the fasted state there would seem little teleologic value in storage of plasma TG-derived fatty acids, when the adipocyte itself is liberating fatty acids at a high rate into the plasma. Accordingly, in that state there is almost complete release of LPL-derived fatty acids as NEFA into the plasma [112]. Adipose tissue LPL in the fasted state acts as a generator of plasma NEFA additional to the intracellular HSL. In the postprandial period, however, this changes markedly with much greater "capture" of

LPL-derived fatty acids for esterification within the adipocytes (although never complete in the relatively normal meals studied) [112,119,120].

Regulation of fat storage in white adipose tissue therefore primarily involves regulation of LPL, but the fine-tuning is provided by regulation of the pathway of fatty acid uptake and esterification in adipocytes. The regulation of this pathway is becoming clearer. First, it depends upon simultaneous suppression of HSL activity, generating a concentration gradient so that fatty acids flow into rather than out from adipocytes. It is stimulated by insulin [112] and by the acylation-stimulating protein (ASP). ASP is a potent stimulator of fatty acid esterification in adipocytes [121] and is produced locally within adipose tissue by the interaction of three components of the alternative complement pathway (D or adipsin, B and C3). These adipsin components are secreted from adipocytes, and their interaction is stimulated by the presence of chylomicrons [122,123]. Regulation of the fate of LPL-derived fatty acids in adipose tissue is of interest, not least because of the potentially adverse consequences of disturbed regulation of this pathway [124].

Adipose tissue metabolism is profoundly altered by obesity *per se*, and potentially by a previous history of obesity, but these possible influences are difficult to separate. Nevertheless, there are some very plausible mechanisms whereby particular characteristics of adipose tissue might predispose to obesity. It was previously considered that the number of fat cells is determined in infancy and invariant thereafter, suggesting that an overweight child may become an overweight adult because the capacity is there, whereas a lean child could not so easily become obese in adulthood. Attractive as this idea is, there is no evidence for it [125]; in fact, even octogenarians have adipocyte precursors that can differentiate into mature adipocytes [126].

Much attention has centered upon adipose tissue LPL as a cause for obesity. The idea that overexpression of LPL might provide a stimulus to fat storage has found some favor, not least because many studies show adipose tissue LPL activity to be increased in established obesity [127,128]. However, it is difficult to distinguish cause and effect. Because of the complex regulation of fat storage discussed above, it seems unlikely that overactivity of LPL in itself could cause excessive storage. Adipose tissue can regulate the amount of fat it stores independently of LPL capacity. For instance, in human LPL deficiency, adipocytes are normally fat filled [129] and in mice with adipose tissue-specific deficiency of LPL, adipose tissue lipid stores are maintained by upregulation of *de novo* lipogenesis [130]. The possibility that disturbed regulation of other components of the fat storage system [131] e.g. of the enzymes of fatty acid esterification or of ASP, could lead to excessive fat deposition has not been explored extensively, although it is known that ASP concentrations are increased in obese subjects [132].

Postprandial metabolism in other tissues
Perhaps the most important postprandial abnormality seen in the liver is the failure to suppress hepatic glucose output in obese,

insulin resistant subjects [79,133]. There may be well be a similar failure to suppress release of VLDL particles, but this has not been so thoroughly studied.

Exercise
Whole-body metabolism during exercise
During exercise, the metabolic flux in skeletal muscle may increase enormously and skeletal muscle metabolism dominates whole-body energy fluxes. During exercise, glucose metabolism changes dramatically.

During light exercise (25%, VO_{2max}) there is little mobilization of muscle glycogen, but glucose uptake, oxidation and conversion to lactate are stimulated. In this condition whole-body glucose turnover increases initially by about 50% and it seems likely that all this increase is directed to skeletal muscle [134].

During heavier exercise (e.g. 65%VO_{2max}) muscle glycogen breakdown is stimulated and glucosyl residues from this source are a major fuel for anaerobic and oxidative metabolism. Plasma glucose utilization is also increased and lactate may thus be recycled via hepatic gluconeogenesis. Whole-body glucose turnover increases to more than three times its resting value after 2 hours of exercise at this intensity, and again this is largely taken up by skeletal muscle [134]. Whole-body glucose oxidation measured by indirect calorimetry may increase by about 12-fold [134] and most of this must be accounted for by skeletal muscle; at 85% VO_{2max} glucose oxidation increases about 30-fold. Metabolic and physiologic adjustments bringing about this increased carbohydrate oxidation include increased cardiac output and muscle vasodilation, vastly increasing glucose delivery to working muscle and the co-ordinated regulation, via changes in intracellular Ca^{2+} and Pi concentrations, of contraction and of glycogenolysis and glycolysis [20,135]. During moderate or heavy exercise skeletal muscle is therefore by far the dominant tissue in glucose disposal in the body.

Muscle metabolism during exercise
During exercise, the O_2 consumption of skeletal muscle increases enormously; values of 350 mL of O_2/min per kilogram wet weight have been recorded [136] and under those conditions muscle oxygen uptake dominates that of the body.

Skeletal muscle is a major site of ATP turnover in the body, especially during exercise (Fig. 10.6). During a marathon run, the mass of ATP turned over in skeletal muscle alone is approximately equal to body mass [20]. Clearly, skeletal muscle has very efficient pathways for regeneration of ATP.

The main sources of free energy for ATP synthesis in skeletal muscle are anaerobic glycolysis and the complete oxidation of both carbohydrate and fatty acids. Amino acid oxidation also plays an important role, especially oxidation of the branched chain amino acids valine, leucine and isoleucine: in humans, these are largely completely oxidized within skeletal muscle. These substrates arise from the circulation (plasma glucose, NEFA, TG fatty acids and amino acids), from the intramuscular stores of glycogen and TG and from muscle protein. Typical

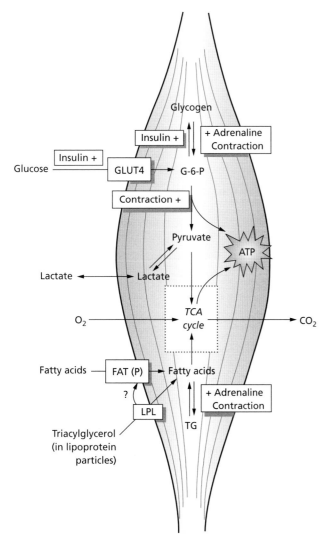

Figure 10.6 Major routes of ATP generation in skeletal muscle. Each arrow may represent more than one step in a pathway. Glucose uptake is mainly by the insulin-regulatable transporter GLUT4 in the fed state but GLUT1 may play an important role in the fasting state. The contribution of amino acids to oxidative metabolism is not shown for simplicity. "Contraction" refers to stimulation of muscle contraction, which is co-ordinated with metabolism via a number of intracellular mediators including intracellular Ca^{2+}. FAT(P) represents a possible fatty acid transporter; G-6-P, glucose-6-phosphate; LPL, lipoprotein lipase; TG, triacylglycerol; TCA cycle, tricarboxylic acid (Krebs) cycle. (Reproduced from Frayn [20]with permission.)

muscle contents of glycogen and of TG show considerable variability among muscles, nutritional states and individuals, but some representative figures are collated in Table 10.2.

The relative use of carbohydrate or lipid fuels is a function of the intensity and duration of exercise. The shorter the duration, the more intense the exercise and the less fit the subject, the greater the dependence on carbohydrate fuels, as rapid and greater usage of lipid fuel is a hallmark of the trained athlete.

The relative contributions of extramuscular and intramuscular sources of fuel have been the subject of much research, although there are many methodologic difficulties in such studies. Muscle biopsy techniques have clearly shown the utilization of muscle glycogen during exercise, and a reasonably consistent picture of glycogen depletion during exercise and repletion after refeeding has been built up [137]. Muscle glycogen deposition in the resting state after a meal has been confirmed by the technique of ^{13}C-nuclear magnetic resonance (NMR) spectroscopy [98].

Several biopsy studies have tried to clarify the contribution of intramuscular TG during exercise to the muscles energy needs. The results are not consistent, due in part to the fact that skeletal muscle TG concentrations are extremely variable even from site to site within a single muscle [138]. These studies mostly show the expected decline in muscle TG concentration during exercise [139,140] although one study using sequential biopsy suggested that muscle TG utilization was most pronounced during the postexercise period [141]. This postexercise decline has not been substantiated in other studies [140].

The contribution of plasma NEFA to oxidative metabolism can be estimated by the infusion of a labeled ^{13}C-NEFA tracer to measure [13]CO_2 production in expired air, whereas whole-body fat oxidation is measured by indirect calorimetry, and the difference is assumed to reflect oxidation of intramuscular TG fatty acids (after correcting for the incomplete recovery of the ^{13}C-label in expired air, "acetate recovery factor" [142]). However, this technique does not distinguish intramuscular TG fatty acids from those arising from plasma TG. Measurement of intramuscular TG (assumed to be intramyocellular lipid, IMCL) by magnetic resonance spectroscopy [143] has been used in muscle before and after exercise. Such measurements show the expected duration-dependent decline in IMCL with endurance exercise, although no change with high-intensity exercise [144]. This body of data suggests that intramuscular TG is, indeed, a significant source of fatty acids for oxidation during exercise [145].

Muscles clearly also increase their uptake from the circulation of glucose and lipid fuels during exercise. For glucose, exercise can increase uptake over 10-fold. The major point of regulation of increased glucose uptake is not entirely clear, but muscle vasodilation with increased glucose delivery may be an important factor. Furthermore, the amount of GLUT4 protein is a primary factor in determining the maximal rate of glucose transport into skeletal muscle. Under normal resting conditions, most of the GLUT4 molecules reside in membrane vesicles inside the muscle cells. In response to insulin or muscle contraction, GLUT4 translocates to the cell membrane, where it inserts to stimulate glucose transport. Plasma insulin concentrations do not change during light exercise.

However, rapid changes in GLUT4 mRNA and protein may occur in response to exercise. Increased GLUT4 expression may be mediated by the enzyme AMP-activated kinase, which is activated during exercise and has been demonstrated to increase GLUT 4 transcription [146–148].

Table 10.2 Typical glycogen and triacylglycerol (TG) contents of human skeletal muscle

	Units	Low-carbohydrate diet	Mixed diet	High-carbohydrate diet	Reference
Glycogen	g/kg wet weight	10	20	30–40	Bergström et al [179]
	kJ/kg wet weight	170	340	510–680	
Typical whole-body store*	MJ	4.25	8.5	15	
TG	mmol/kg wet weight	–	15 (range 1–100)	–	Collated**
	kJ/kg wet weight	–	450 (range 30–3000)	–	
Typical whole-body store*	MJ	–	11	–	

*Assumes 25 kg of muscle.
**Collated from a number of sources: range from Phillips et al. [180].

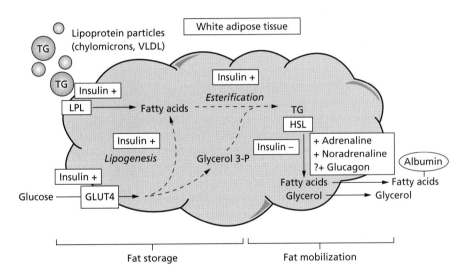

Figure 10.7 Major routes of fat deposition and mobilization in white adipose tissue. GLUT4, insulin-regulated glucose transporter; HSL, hormone-sensitive lipase; LPL, lipoprotein lipase; TG, triacylglycerol. (Reproduced from Frayn [20]with permission.)

During exercise, muscle NEFA utilization increases dramatically. Plasma NEFAs are the major fuel for exercise at low intensity (25% VO$_{2max}$) [134]. At greater intensities of exercise they are also important, but other fuel sources are more important for the first 2 hours or so. After that, these other sources (e.g. muscle glycogen) are depleted, and the ultra-endurance athlete utilizes almost entirely plasma NEFA as a fuel. Considering the size of the adipose tissue TG store, and greater ATP production per mole of oxygen from lipid compared to carbohydrate oxidation, this seems advantageous. For moderate-intensity exercise, trained subjects show rapid and extensive increases in lipid oxidation and the failure to make such changes is a hallmark of untrained (and obese) individuals.

It is generally considered that plasma TG fatty acids make only a small contribution to oxidative fuel metabolism during exercise. This seems to be true for exercise carried out in the fasting state, in which plasma TG is mainly present as very VLDL-TG. However, it is possible that the situation is different after a meal containing fat [2,149]. Chylomicron-TG is a better substrate for muscle LPL than is VLDL-TG [30] and there is some evidence for marked TG clearance from postprandial plasma by exercising muscle [149,150]. In addition, if the marked improvement of fat tolerance evident in highly trained subjects does indeed reflect improved TG clearance by skeletal muscle then this again suggests more than a modest contribution to muscle fatty acid delivery.

Adipose tissue during exercise
During exercise, there is a marked increase in NEFA delivery from adipose tissue [151,152] (Figure 10.7) and this is undoubtedly

mediated primarily by β-adrenergic stimulation [57]. In sustained high-intensity exercise, it may be reinforced by a slight fall in the plasma insulin concentration, and by secretion of both cortisol and growth hormone [153]. Despite these changes, the rate of NEFA delivery does not increase in proportion to the intensity of exercise [134]. It seems that adipose tissue perfusion during intense exercise may be inadequate to carry away all the fatty acids released in lipolysis [154]. Evidence for this comes from the sudden release of NEFA that is observed when exercise stops [134,153]; presumably a sudden relief of relative vasoconstriction allows "flushing out" of NEFA that have been trapped within the tissue.

Other

Exercise typically sees a reduced metabolic activity in visceral tissue as the available fuels and oxygen are funneled towards exercising muscle, for example NEFA uptake by the splanchnic bed being reduced by exercise [152]. Hepatic glucose output can increase by around 2–3-fold during exercise [83].

Impact of diets and energy imbalance

Effect of dietary manipulation on metabolic fuels

Under conditions of energy balance, whole-body RQ over 24 hours will mirror the ingested diet [148,155]. This metabolic "law" will mean that low-fat diets will inevitably reduce fat oxidation and low-carbohydrate diets will do the opposite.

It has long been recognized that obese people have an increased basal metabolic rate [156] (see Chapters 6 and 12). This seems to be a function of their greater lean body mass [157] and the basal metabolic rate of weight-stable people seems to change in proportion to their lean body mass [LBM]. Despite concerted searching there have been no changes identified in basal metabolic rate (corrected for LBM) in weight-stable obese patients (in the absence of recognized endocrine disease such as hypothyroidism). This clearly leaves open the possibilities that:
1. obesity is caused by increased energy intake
2. obesity is caused by decreased activity-associated energy expenditure (or other forms of energy expenditure such as thermoregulatory energy expenditure)
3. obesity is caused by excess weight gain during positive energy balance ("I will put on a stone in a couple of days if I am not careful")
4. obesity is caused by reduced weight loss during negative energy balance ("I've tried every diet and can't lose an ounce")
5. combinations of 1–4.
Possibilities 1 and 2 are discussed elsewhere (Chapters 6 and 12). I will briefly touch on possibilities 3 and 4.

Subjects who are weight-stable after losing weight usually are intermediate between those who have always been lean and those who have remained obese [158–161]. There are usually difficulties in being sure whether the "postobese" obese are similar to the "never obese" in terms of physical activity and body composition.

Overall studies of postobese subjects suggest that most of the abnormalities characteristic of obesity are mostly reversible by weight loss.

Weight-gaining states

In everyday life, most subjects are in approximate energy balance over the average week or month. However, there are few data as to how many days have significant positive energy balances (energy in exceeding energy out by >5%) and how many the converse. It is apparent that there is a general tendency for subjects to get heavier, less muscular and more adipose as they age over the decades of adult life (as discussed in Chapters 2 and 6). However, this is a gradual process and has not been studied in depth, although most believe that the change in body composition is a consequence of the gradual reduction in physical activity with aging.

In terms of the etiology of obesity, it seems easier to demonstrate differences between obesity-prone and obesity-resistant subjects during conditions of energy excess (or deficiency) compared to situations of energy balance. Thus subjects with personal or family history of obesity gain weight more rapidly than lean subjects.

Deliberate overfeeding studies show that deliberate overeating produces weight gain, the rate of gain varying between individuals [162,163]. In at least some people, excess calories from overeating can be diverted away from conversion to fat by increased energy expenditure [164]. Neumann in 1902 and Gulick in 1920 termed such disappative mechanisms "luxurkonsumption." However, there has been a prolonged and unresolved debate about the size of the effect and mechanisms that might be involved [163]. In some studies (reviewed by Tappy [162] and Joosen and Westerterp [165]) obesity-prone subjects (who have been selected either because they were currently or previously obese, or because they have a strong family history of obesity) gain weight more rapidly when overfed experimentally. The putative mechanisms for this include reduced nonexercise activity thermogenesis (NEAT) [166] and there may also be reduced diet-induced and cold-induced thermogenesis [162,165]. However, these studies are time-consuming and difficult to reproduce. No clear-cut changes in intermediary metabolism have been established to explain the changes in speed of weight gain with overfeeding whereas changes in food preference and NEAT have been demonstrated more convincingly.

Weight-losing states

Weight-losing states have traditionally been studied by underfeeding studies. There are solid data that negative energy balance induces weight maintaining counter-regulatory mechanisms. Reductions in basal metabolic rate are seen in both short-term [164,167] and longer-term studies [168]. Detailed studies of metabolic changes during short-term studies have been reported. They show both whole-body changes (e.g. whole-body energy expenditure decreased by 10% with 3 days of severe (−66%) underfeeding) and changes at the level of individual tissues

[169,170]. Perhaps the most famous underfeeding studies are the Minnesota Starvation Experiment [171] and Biosphere 2 [172] which demonstrate multiple behavioral, hormonal and metabolic changes in response to prolonged calorie restriction.

Differences in effectiveness of these "weight-maintaining" mechanisms might underlie some propensity to obesity. However, there is debate as to whether weight-maintaining mechanisms are triggered by "slow and steady" diets as currently recommended for overweight subjects or whether they only become apparent when body weight goes below a healthy norm. Of course, differences in either the threshold or the efficiency of weight-maintaining mechanisms could be crucial for successful obesity management. Garrow, reviewing his own clinical studies of controlled weight loss usually of obese inpatients under supervision, reported no evidence of "weight defence" which slowed the weight loss from the expected rate within a 3-week period.

Conversely, there are multiple possible mechanisms for differences in weight defence that could predispose to obesity [21]. For example, HSL has been suggested as having a role in susceptibility to obesity. Net fat deposition reflects the balance between two processes: fat mobilization and fat storage. If HSL activity is reduced, then there will be an increase in net fat deposition. This possibility was examined by measurement of HSL activity in adipose tissue biopsies in nonobese first-degree relatives of obese subjects [173]; it was found that maximal HSL activity was reduced by about 50% in the relatives, compared with control subjects with no immediate family history of obesity. In the more physiologic setting of responses *in vivo* to a mixed meal or to insulin infusion, there is evidence that in postobese women (formerly obese women who have reduced their weight to the normal range, and who are considered to be a model of the genetically "at risk") the ability of insulin to suppress plasma NEFA concentrations is enhanced [92,160]. Thus, the tendency towards net fat storage would again be enhanced.

Overall, partly because they are more difficult to undertake, over- and underfeeding studies have not clarified the changes seen in obesity to the same extent as has been achieved in weight-stable patients. The importance of differences between individuals in "weight maintenance" mechanisms as a cause for the development of obesity has not been established.

Metabolic inflexibility

As indicated above, there are multiple changes in metabolic behavior including fuel selection in obesity. However, the "denominator problem" makes it difficult to be sure whether these changes are adaptive or not, as discussed by Frayn [113,174]. Eckel has questioned whether the insulin resistance may be actually adaptive [175]. One aspect that seems unequivocally maladaptive is the metabolic inflexibility typical of obese patients (and also seen in insulin-resistant and glucose-intolerant subjects).

Table 10.3 Some examples of metabolic inflexibility seen in obesity.

Physiologic stimulus	Tissue	Normal response	Change in obesity	Consequence
Food/glucose	Pancreas	Good 1st phase, insulin response	Blunted and delayed	May lead to other delays
Food/glucose/insulin clamp	Muscle	Increase in glucose uptake, local RQ, switch to glucose oxidation & increase in glycogen storage	Blunted	Glucose intolerance
Food/glucose	Adipose tissue	Increase in local blood flow	Blunted	Uncertain
Food/glucose	Adipose tissue	Suppression of NEFA, release (HSL action)	Blunted and delayed	Excess lipid fuel availability in postprandial state – may drive dyslipidemia
Prolongation of fasting	Adipose tissue	Reduced leptin secretion and increase in lipolysis	Blunted	
Exercise	Whole body	Increase in VO_{2max}	Blunted	Reduced exercise capacity
Exercise	Muscle	Glucose uptake from circulation, switch to fatty acid oxidation	Blunted and delayed	Reduced exercise capacity

This key concept, introduced by Kelley [95,96], points out that in most aspects, obese subjects show slow, and often incomplete, responses to metabolic changes. Some examples are given in Table 10.3 and Figures 10.8 and 10.9.

Although it has been suggested that the interpretation of metabolic inflexibility needs to be "corrected" for defects in glycemic regulation, this does not detract from the central proposal that metabolic inflexibility has many features. Many of these features are clearly maladaptive and none appear adaptive. Some genes have been identified that may induce metabolic inflexibility but the most obvious causes in the general population are obesity and low physical fitness. The mechanisms causing metabolic inflexibility are currently being studied.

An important feature of metabolic inflexibility is that weight loss reverses (at least partially) all the elements that have been tested (see Fig. 10.10).

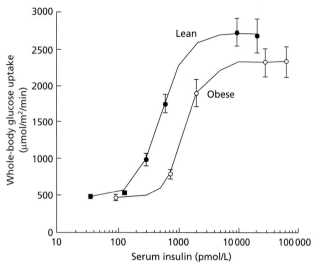

Figure 10.8 Insulin resistance of skeletal muscle glucose uptake in obesity. Glucose uptake was measured across the leg by femoral venous catheterization and measurement of blood flow, and insulin was infused at increasing rates to construct the dose–response curves. Plasma glucose concentrations were "clamped" at 5 mmol/L. There is a clear shift to the right of the dose–response curve of glucose uptake against serum insulin concentration in the obese group. (Reproduced from Laakso et al. [177] with permission.)

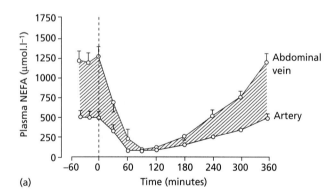

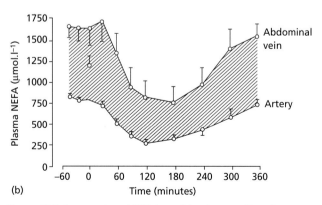

Figure 10.9 Concentrations of NEFA in arterial and venous effluent from adipose tissue, before and after a mixed meal given at time zero, in (a) lean and (b) obese subjects. Values are means (±SEM). (Data from Coppack et al. [80].)

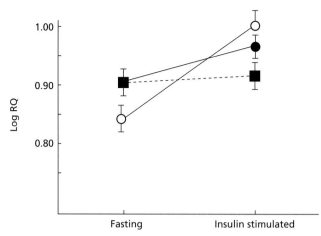

Figure 10.10 Illustration of the metabolic response in the leg (largely indicative of skeletal muscle response) to elevation of insulin levels at euglycemia in lean (○), obese (■), and obese maintained at plateau after substantial (approximately 15kg) weight loss (●). Values are means with their standard errors represented by vertical bars. The results show the complete metabolic inflexibility of the obese individual compared with lean healthy individuals, which is only very partially restored by weight loss. (Redrawn, with permission from the American Physiological Society, from Kelley 1999 et al. [178].)

Acknowledgments

This chapter was written drawing heavily on the excellent previous contributions to earlier editions of this book by my colleagues Lucinda Summers, Ellen Blaak and Keith Frayn. Whilst the mistakes are probably mine, the erudition mostly comes from their chapters which I have pirated. I am extremely grateful for their generosity in letting me use their work in this way. I am continuingly grateful to the Wellcome Trust for funding most of my own studies in this area.

References

1. Jones DA, Round JM. *Skeletal Muscle in Health and Disease. A Textbook of Muscle Physiology*. Manchester: Manchester University Press, 1990.
2. Henriksson J. Muscle fuel selection: effect of exercise and training. Proc Nutr Soc 1995;54:125–38.
3. Crandall DL, DiGirolamo M. Hemodynamic and metabolic correlates in adipose tissue: pathophysiologic considerations. FASEB J 1990;4:141–7.
4. Frayn KN, Karpe E, Fielding BA, Macdonald LA,Coppack SW. Integrative physiology of human adipose tissue. Int J Obes 2003; 27:875–88.
5. Hollenberg CH. Perspectives in adipose tissue physiology. Int J Obes 1990;14(suppl 3):135–52.
6. Johnson MA, Polgar J, Weightman D, Appleton D. Data on the distribution of fibre types in thirty-six human muscles. An autopsy study. J Neurol Sci 1973;18:111–29.
7. Bjorntorp P. Metabolic implications of body fat distribution. Diabetes Care 1991;14:1132–43.

8. Bjorntorp P. "Portal" adipose tissue as a generator of risk factors for cardiovascular disease and diabetes. Arteriosclerosis 1990; 10:493–6.

9. Kissebah AH, Krakower GR. Regional adiposity and morbidity. Physiol Rev 1994;74:761–811.

10. Banerji MA, Buckley MC, Chaiken RL, et al. Liver fat, serum triglycerides and visceral adipose tissue in insulin-sensitive and insulin-resistant black men with NIDDM. Int J Obes 1995;19:846–50.

11. Abate N, Garg A, Peshock RM, Stray-Gundersen J, Grundy SM. Relationships of generalized and regional adiposity to insulin sensitivity in men. J Clin Invest 1995;96:88–98.

12. Arner P. Impact of visceral fat. Int J Obes 1997;21(suppl 2):S20.

13. Couillard C, Bergeron N, Prud'homme D, et al. Gender difference in postprandial lipemia: importance of visceral adipose tissue accumulation. Arterioslcer Thromb Vasc Biol 1999;19:2448–55.

14. Arner P, Bülow J. Assessment of adipose tissue metabolism in man: comparison of Fick and microdialysis techniques. Clin Sci 1993;85:247–56.

15. Frayn KN, Coppack SW. Assessment of white adipose tissue metabolism by measurement of arteriovenous differences. Methods Mol Biol 2001;155:269–79.

16. Coppack SW, Jensen MD, Miles JM. In vivo regulation of lipolysis in humans. J Lipid Res 1994;35:177–93.

17. Opie LH, Walfish PG. Plasma free fatty acid concentrations in obesity. N Engl J Med 1963;268:757–60.

18. Flatt J-P. Role of the increased adipose tissue mass in the apparent insulin insensitivity of obesity. Am J Clin Nutr 1972;25:1189–92.

19. Björntorp P, Bergman H, Varnauskas E. Plasma free fatty acid turnover rate in obesity. Acta Med Scand 1969;185(4):351–6.

20. Frayn KN. *Metabolic Regulation: A Human Perspective*, 2nd edn. Oxford: Blackwell Publishing, 2003.

21. Astrup A, Buemann B, Christensen NJ, Toubro S. Failure to increase lipid oxidation in response to increasing dietary fat content in formerly obese women. Am J Physiol 1994;266:E592–E599.

22. Itani SI, Ruderman NB, Schmieder E, Boden G. Lipid-induced insulin resistance in human muscle is associated with changes in diacylglycerol, protein kinase C, and IkappaB-alpha. Diabetes 2002;51:2005–11.

23. Snyder WS. *Report of the Task Force on Reference Man*. Oxford: Pergamon Press for the International Commission on Radiological Protection,1975.

24. Spenst LF, Martin AD, Drinkwater DT. Muscle mass of competitive male athletes. J Sports Sci 1993;11:3–8.

25. Zurlo F, Larson K, Bogardus E, Ravussin E. Skeletal muscle metabolism is a major determinant of resting energy expenditure. J Clin Invest 1990;86:1423–7.

26. Acheson KJ., Schutz Y, Bessard T, Anantharaman K, Flatt J-P, Jequier E. Glycogen storage capacity and de novo lipogenesis during massive carbohydrate overfeeding in man. Am J Clin Nutr 1988;48:240–7.

27. Baltzan MA, Andres R, Cader G, ZierIer KL. Heterogeneity of forearm metabolism with special reference to free fatty acids. J Clin Invest 1962;41:116–25.

28. Jackson RA, Hamling JB, Sim BM, et al. Peripheral lactate and oxygen metabolism in man: the influence of oral glucose loading. Metabolism 1987;36:144–50.

29. Kiens B, Lithell H. Lipoprotein metabolism influenced by training-induced changes in human skeletal muscle. J Clin Invest 1989;83:558–64.

30. Potts JL, Fisher RM, Humphreys SM, et al. Peripheral triacylglycerol extraction in the fasting and post-prandial states. Clin Sci 1991;81:621–6.

31. Coppack SW, Persson M, Judd RL, Miles JM. Glycerol and nonesterified fatty acid metabolism in human muscle and adipose tissue in vivo. Am J Physiol 1999;276(2 Pt 1):E233–40.

32. Capaldo B, Napoli R, Di Marino L, Guida R, Pardo E, Sacca L. Role of insulin and free fatty acid (FFA) availability on regional FFA kinetics in the human forearm. J Clin Endocrinol Metab 1994;79:879–82.

33. Dagenais GR, Tancredi RG, ZierIer KL. Free fatty acid oxidation by forearm muscle at rest, and evidence for an intramuscular lipid pool in the human forearm. J Clin Invest 1976;58:421–31.

34. Sidossis LS, Coggan AR, Gastaldelli A, Wolfe RR. Pathway of free fatty acid oxidation in human subjects. Implications for tracer studies. J Clin Invest 1995;95:278–84.

35. Schrauwen P, Wagenmakers AJ, van Marken Lichtenbelt WD, Saris WH, Westerterp KR. Increase in fat oxidation on a high-fat diet is accompanied by an increase in triglyceride-derived fatty acid oxidation. Diabetes 2000;49:640–6.

36. Soop M, Bjorkman O, Cederblad G, Hagenfeldt L, Wahren J. Influence of carnitine supplementation on muscle substrate and carnitine metabolism during exercise. J Appl Physiol 1988;64:2394–9.

37. Glatz JE, Storch J. Unravelling the significance of cellular fatty acid-binding proteins. Curr Opin Lipidol 2001;12:267–74.

38. Randle PJ, Garland PB, Hales CN, Newsholme EA. The glucose fatty-acid cycle. Its role in insulin sensitivity and the metabolic disturbances of diabetes mellitus. Lancet 1963;1:785–9.

39. Piatti PM, Monti LD, Pacchioni M, Pontiroli AE, Pozza G. Forearm insulin- and non-insulin-mediated glucose uptake and muscle metabolism in man: role of free fatty acids and blood glucose levels. Metabolism 1991;40:926–33.

40. Roden M, Price TB, Perseghin G, et al. Mechanism of free fatty acidinduced insulin resistance in humans. J Clin Invest 1996;97:2859–65.

41. Roden M, Krssak M, Stingl H, et al. Rapid impairment of skeletal muscle glucose transport/ phosphorylation by free fatty acids in humans. Diabetes 1999;48:358–64.

42. Sidossis LS, Stuart EA, Shulman GI, Lopaschuk GD, Wolfe RR. Glucose plus insulin regulate fat oxidation by controlling the rate of fatty acid entry into the mitochondria. J Clin Invest 1996;98:2244–50.

43. Sidossis LS, Wolfe RR. Glucose and insulin-induced inhibition of fatty acid oxidation: the glucose-fatty acid cycle reversed. Am J Physiol 1996;270:E733–E738.

44. Zammit VA. The malonyl-CoA-long-chain acyl-CoA axis in the maintenance of mammalian cell function. Biochem J 1999;343:505–15.

45. Bergstrom J, Fürst P, Noree LO, Vinnars E. Intracellular free amino acid concentration in human muscle tissue. J Appl Physiol 1974;36:693–7.

46. Daniel PM, Pratt OE, Spargo E. The metabolic homoeostatic role of muscle and its function as a store of protein. Lancet 1977;ii:446–8.

47. Pond CM. An evolutionary and functional view of mammalian adipose tissue. Proc Nutr Soc. 1992;51(3):367–77.

48. Forouhi NG, Jenkinson G, Thomas EL, et al. Relation of triglyceride stores in skeletal muscle cells to central obesity and insulin sensitivity in European and South Asian men. Diabetologia 1999;42:932–5.

49. Savage DB, Petersen KF, Shulman GI. Disordered lipid metabolism and the pathogenesis of insulin resistance. Physiol Rev 2007;87: 507–20.

50. Bjorntorp P. Importance of fat as a support nutrient for energy: metabolism of athletes. J Sports Sci 1991;9:71–6.

51. Marin P, Hogh-Kristiansen I, Jansso, S, Krotkiewski M, Holm G, Bjorntorp P. Uptake of glucose carbon in muscle glycogen and adipose tissue triglycerides in vivo in humans. Am J Physiol 1992; 263:E473–E480.

52. Virtanen KA, Peltoniemi P, Marjamaki P, et al. Human adipose tissue glucose uptake determined using (18FI-fluoro-deoxy-glucose ([18F]FDG) and PET in combination with microdialysis. Diabetologia 2001;44:2171–9.

53. Horowitz JF, Coppack SW, Klein S. Whole-body and adipose tissue glucose metabolism in response to short-term fasting in lean and obese women. Am J Clin Nutr 2001;73:517–22.

54. Kissebah, AH, Alfarsi S, Adams PW, Wynn V. Role of insulin resistance in adipose tissue and liver in the pathogenesis of endogenous hypertriglyceridaemia in man. Diabetologia 1976;12:563–71.

55. Lillioja S, Foley J, Bogardus C, Mott D, Howard BV. Free fatty acid metabolism and obesity in man: in vivo and in vitro comparisons. Metabolism 1986;35:505–14.

56. Guo Z, Hensrud DO, Johnson CM, Jensen MD. Regional postprandial fatty acid metabolism in different obesity phenotypes. Diabetes 1999;48:1586–92.

57. Arner P, Kriegholm E, Engfeldt P, Bolinder J. Adrenergic regulation of lipolysis in situ at rest and during exercise. J Clin Invest 1990;85:893–8.

58. Samra JS, Clark ML, Humphreys SM, et al. Effects of morning rise in cortisol concentration on regulation of lipolysis in subcutaneous adipose tissue. Am J Physiol 1996;271:E996–E1002.

59. Cersosimo E, Danou E, Persson M, Miles JM. Effects of pulsatile delivery of basal growth hormone on lipolysis in humans. Am J Physiol 1996;271:E123–E126.

60. Samra JS, Clark ML, Humphreys SM, et al. Suppression of the nocturnal rise in growth hormone reduces subsequent lipolysis in subcutaneous adipose tissue. Eur J Clin Invest 1999;29:1045–52.

61. Osuga J, Ishibashi S, Oka T, et al. Targeted disruption of hormone-sensitive lipase results in male sterility and adipocyte hypertrophy, but not in obesity. Proc Nat Acad Sci USA 2000;97:787–92.

62. Wang SP, Laurin N, Himms-Hagen J, et al. The adipose tissue phenotype of hormone-sensitive lipase deficiency in mice. Obes Res 2001;9:119–28.

63. Okazaki H, Osuga J, Tamura Y, et al. Lipolysis in the absence of hormone-sensitive lipase: evidence for a common mechanism regulating distinct lipases. Diabetes 2002;51:3368–75.

64. Londos C, Gruia-Gray J, Brasaernle DL, et al. Perilipin: possible roles in structure and metabolism of intracellular neutral lipids in adipocytes and steroidogenic cells. Int J Obes 1996;20(suppl 3):S97-S101.

65. Clifford GM, Londos C, Kraemer EB, Vernon RG, Yeaman SJ. Translocation of hormone-sensitive lipase and perilipin upon lipolytic stimulation of rat adipocytes. J Biol Chem 2000;275,5011–15.

66. Malmstrom R, Packard CJ, Caslake M, et al. Effects of insulin and acipimox on VLDLl and VLDL2 apolipoprotein B production in normal subjects. Diabetes 1998;47:779–87.

67. Potts JL, Coppack SW, Fisher RM, et al. Impaired postprandial clearance of triacylglycerol-rich lipoproteins in adipose tissue in obese subjects. Am J Physiol 1995;268:E588–E594.

68. Patterson BW, Horowitz JF, Wu G, Watford M, Coppack SW, Klein S. Regional muscle and adipose tissue amino acid metabolism in lean and obese women. Am J Physiol Endocrinol Metab 2002;282:E931–6.

69. Farooqi IS, Matarese G, Lord GM, et al. Beneficial effects of leptin on obesity, T cell hyporesponsiveness, and neuroendocrine/ metabolic dysfunction of human congenital leptin deficiency. J Clin Invest 2002;110:1093–103.

70. Weyer C, Funahashi T, Tanaka S, et al. Hypoadiponectinemia in obesity and type 2 diabetes: close association with insulin resistance and hyperinsulinemia. J Clin Endocrinol Metab 2001;86: 1930–15.

71. Berg AH, Combs TP, Du X, Brownlee M, Scherer PE. The adipocyte-secreted protein Acrp30 enhances hepatic insulin action. Nat Med 2001;7:947–53.

72. Yamauchi T, Kamon J, Waki H, et al. The fat-derived hormone adiponectin reverses insulin resistance associated with both lipoatrophy and obesity. Nat Med 2001;7:941–6.

73. Frühbeck G, Gomez-Ambrosi J, Muruzabal EJ, Burrell MA. The adipocyte: a model for integration of endocrine and metabolic signaling in energy metabolism regulation. Am J Physiol 2001;280:E827–E847.

74. Mohamed-Ali V, Pinkney JH,Coppack SW. Adipose tissue as an endocrine and paracrine organ. Int J Obes 1998;22:1145–58.

75. Ricquier, D, Bouillaud E. The uncoupling protein homologues: UCPl, UCP2, UCP3, StUCP and AtUCP. Biochem J 2000;345:161–79.

76. Ricquier D, Bouillaud E. Mitochondrial uncoupling proteins: from mitochondria to the regulation of energy balance. J Physiol 2000;529:3–10.

77. Dulloo AG, Samec S. Uncoupling proteins: their roles in adaptive thermogenesis and substrate metabolism reconsidered. Br J Nutr 2001;86:123–39.

78. Hesselink MK, Greenhaff PL, Constantin-Teodosiu D, et al.Increased uncoupling protein 3 content does not affect mitochondrial function in human skeletal muscle in vivo. J Clin Invest 2003;111:479–86.

79. Gastaldelli A, Miyazaki Y, Pettiti M, et al. Separate contribution of diabetes, total fat mass, and fat topography to glucose production, gluconeogenesis, and glycogenolysis. J Clin Endocrinol Metab 2004;89:3914–21.

80. Coppack SW, Evans RD, Fisher RM, et al. Adipose tissue metabolism in obesity: lipase action in vivo before and after a mixed meal. Metabolism 1992;41:264–72.

81. Lewis GE, Uffelman KD, Szeto LW, Weller B, Steiner G. Interaction between free fatty acids and insulin in the acute control of very low density lipoprotein production in humans. J Clin Invest 1995;95:158–66.

82. Barsh GS, Farooqi IS, O'Rahilly S. Genetics of body weight regulation. Nature 2000;404:1.

83. Wahren J, Ekberg K. Splanchnic regulation of glucose production. Annu Rev Nutr 2007;27:329–45.

84. DeFronzo RA, Tobin J, Andres R. Glucose clamp technique: a method for quantifying insulin secretion and resistance. Am J Physiol 1979;237:E214–E223.

85. Kahn BB, Flier JS. Obesity and insulin resistance. J Clin Invest 2000;106:473–8l.

86. Laakso M, Edelman SV, Olefsky JM, Brechtel G, Wallace P, Baron AD. Kinetics of in vivo muscle insulin-mediated glucose uptake in human obesity. Diabetes 1990;39:965–74.

87. DeFronzo RA, Jacot E, Jequier E, et al. The effect ofinsulin on the disposal of intravenous glucose. Results from indirect calorimetry

and hepatic and femoral venous catheterization. Diabetes 1981;30: 1000–7.

88. Felber J-P, Acheson KJ, Tappy L. *From Obesity to Diabetes.* Chichester: John Wiley, 1993.

89. Clausen JO, Borch-Johnsen K, Ibsen H, et al. Insulin sensitivity index, acute insulin response, and glucose effectiveness in a population-based sample of 380 young healthy Caucasians. Analysis of the impact of gender, body fat, physical fitness, and lifestyle factors. J Clin Invest 1996;98:1195–209.

90. Coppack SW, Fisher RM, Gibbons GE, et al. Postprandial substrate deposition in human forearm and adipose tissues in vivo. Clin Sci 1990;79:339–48.

91. Summers LKM, Fielding BA, Herd SL, et al. Use of structured triacylglycerols containing predominantly stearic and oleic acids to probe early events in metabolic processing of dietary fat. J Lipid Res 1999;40:1890–8.

92. Raben A, Andersen HB, Christensen NJ, et al. Evidence for an abnormal postprandial response to a high-fat meal in women predisposed to obesity. Am J Physiol 1994;267:E549–E559.

93. Campbell PJ, Carlson MG, Nurjhan N. Fat metabolism in human obesity. *American Journal of Physiology.* Am J Physiol 1994;266: E600–E605.

94. Yki-Jarvinen H, Young AA, Lamkin C, Foley JE. Kinetics of glucose disposal in whole body and across the forearm in man. J Clin Invest 1987;79:1713–19.

95. Kelley DE, Mintun MA, Watkins SC, et al. The effect of non-insulin-dependent diabetes mellitus and obesity on glucose transport and phosphorylation in skeletal muscle. J Clin Invest 1996;97: 2705–13.

96. Kelley D, Mitrakou A, Marsh H, et al. Skeletal muscle glycolysis, oxidation, and storage of an oral glucose load. J Clin Invest 1988;81:1563–71.

97. Elia M, Folmer P, Schlatmann A, Goren A, Austin S. Carbohydrate, fat, and protein metabolism in muscle and in the whole body after mixed meal ingestion. Metabolism 1988;37:542–51.

98. Taylor R, Price TB, Katz LD, Shulman RG, Shulman GI. Direct measurement of change in muscle glycogen concentration after a mixed meal in normal subjects. Am J Physiol 1993;265:E224–E229.

99. Dyck DJ, Steinberg G, Bonen A. Insulin increases FA uptake and esterification but reduces lipid utilization in isolated contracting muscle. Am J Physiol 2001;281:E600–E607.

100. Luiken JJ, Koonen DP, Willems J, et al. Insulin stimulates long-chain fatty acid utilization by rat cardiac myocytes through cellular redistribution of FAT / CD36. Diabetes 2002;51:3113–19.

101. Binnert C, Pachiaudi C, Beylot M, et al. Influence of human obesity on the metabolic fate of dietary long- and medium-chain triacylglycerols. Am J Clin Nutr 1998;67:595–601.

102. Tsetsonis NV, Hardman AE, Mastana SS. Acute effects of exercise on postprandial lipemia: a comparative study in trained and untrained middle-aged women. Am J Clin Nutr 1997;65:525–33.

103. Seip RL, Angelopoulos TJ, Semenkovich EF. Exercise induces human lipoprotein lipase gene expression in skeletal muscle but not adipose tissue. Am J Physiol 1995;268:E229–E236.

104. Herd SL, Hardman AE, Boobis LH, Cairns CJ. The effect of 13 weeks of running training followed by 9 d of detraining on postprandial lipaemia. Br J Nutr 1998;80:57–66.

105. Malkova D, Evans RD, Frayn KN, et al. Prior exercise and postprandial substrate extraction across the human leg. Am J Physiol Endocrinol Metab 2000;279:El 020–El 028.

106. Oscai LB, Essig DA, Palmer WK. Lipase regulation of muscle triglyceride hydrolysis. J Appl Physiol 1990;69:1571–7.

107. Teusink B, Voshol PJ, Dahlmans VE, et al. Contribution of fatty acids released from lipolysis of plasma triglycerides to total plasma fatty acid flux and tissue-specific fatty acid uptake. Diabetes 2003;52:614–20.

108. Farese RV, Yost TJ, Eckel RH. Tissue-specific regulation of lipoprotein lipase activity by insulin/ glucose in normal-weight humans. Metabolism 1991;40:214–16.

109. Coppack SW, Fisher RM, Humphreys SM et al. Carbohydrate metabolism in insulin resistance: glucose uptake and lactate production by adipose and forearm tissues in vivo before and after a mixed meal. Clin Sci 1996;90:409–15.

110. Rigden DJ, Jellyman AE, Frayn KN, Coppack SW. Human adipose tissue glycogen levels and responses to carbohydrate feeding. Eur J Clin Nutr 1990;44:689–92.

111. Frayn KN,Humphreys SM, Coppack SW. Fuel selection in white adipose tissue. Proc Nutr Soc 1995;54:177–89.

112. Frayn KN, Shadid S, Hamlani R, et al. Regulation of fatty acid movement in human adipose tissue in the postabsorptive-to-postprandial transition. Am J Physiol 1994;266:E308–E317.

113. Frayn KN. Adipose tissue as a buffer for daily lipid flux. Diabetologia 2002;45:1201–10.

114. Oben J, Elliott R, Morgan L, Fletcher J, Marks V. The role of gut hormones in the adipose tissue metabolism of lean and genetically obese (ob/ob) mice. In: Ailhaud G, Guy-Grand B, Lafontan M, Ricquier D (eds) *Obesity in Europe 91.* Proceedings of the 3rd European Congress on Obesity. London: Libbey, 1992:269–72.

115. Marin P, Rebuffe-Scrive M, Bjorntorp P. Uptake of triglyceride fatty acids in adipose tissue in vivo in man. Eur J Clin Invest 1990;20:158–65.

116. Romanski SA, Nelson RM, Jensen MD. Meal fatty acid uptake in adipose tissue: gender effects in nonobese humans. Am J Physiol 2000;279:E455–E462.

117. Jeppesen J, Hollenbeck CB, Zhou MY, et al. Relation between insulin resistance, hyperinsulinemia, postheparin plasma lipoprotein lipase activity, and postprandial lipemia. Arterioslcer Thromb Vasc Biol 1995;15:320–4.

118. Katzel LI, Busby-Whitehead MJ, Rogus EM, Krauss RM, Goldberg AP. Reduced adipose tissue lipoprotein lipase responses, postprandial lipemia, and low high-density lipoprotein-2 subspecies levels in older athletes with silent myocardialischemia. Metabolism 1994; 43:190–8.

119. Evans K, Burdge G, Wootton SA, Clark ML, Frayn KN. Regulation of dietary fatty acid entrapment in subcutaneous adipose tissue and skeletal muscle. Diabetes 2002;51:2684–90.

120. Frayn KN, Coppack SW, Fielding BA, Humphreys SM. Coordinated regulation of hormone-sensitive lipase and lipoprotein lipase in human adipose tissue in vivo: implications for the control of fat storage and fat mobilization. Adv Enzyme Regul 1995;35: 163–78.

121. Sniderman AD, Cianflone K, Summers LKM, Fielding BA, Frayn KN. The acylation-stimulating protein pathway and regulation of postprandial metabolism. Proc Nutr Soc 1997;56:703–12.

122. Maslowska M, Scantlebury T, Germinario R, Cianflone K. Acute in vitro production of acylation stimulating protein in differentiated human adipocytes. J Lipid Res 1997;38:1–11.

123. Scantlebury T, Maslowska M, Cianflone K. Chylomicron-specific enhancement of acylation stimulating protein and precursor protein

C3 production in differentiated human adipocytes. J Biol Chem 1998;273:20903–9.

124. Sniderman AD, Cianflone K, Arner P, Summers LKM, Frayn KN. The adipocyte, fatty acid trapping and atherogenesis. Arterioslcer Thromb Vasc Biol 1998;18:147–51.

125. Ashwell M. Why do people get fat: is adipose tissue guilty? Proc Nutr Soc 1992;51353–5.

126. Hauner H, Entenmann G, Wabitsch M, et al. Promoting effect of glucocorticoids on the differentiation of human adipocyte precursor cells cultured in a chemically defined medium. J Clin Invest 1989;84:1663–70.

127. Eckel RH. Adipose tissue lipoprotein lipase. In: Borensztajn J (ed) *Lipoprotein Lipase*. Chicago: Evener, 1987:79–132.

128. Eckel RH. Lipoprotein lipase. A multifunctional enzyme relevant to common metabolic diseases. N Engl J Med 1989;320:1060–8.

129. Peeva E, Brun DL, Yen Murthy MR, et al. Adipose cell size and distribution in familial lipoprotein lipase deficiency. Int J Obes 1992;16:737–44.

130. Weinstock PH, Levak Frank S, Hudgins LE, et al. Lipoprotein lipase controls fatty acid entry into adipose tissue, but fat mass is preserved by endogenous synthesis in mice deficient in adipose tissue lipoprotein lipase. Proc Nat Acad Sci USA 1997;94:10261–6.

131. Kalant D, Phelis S, Fielding BA, et al. Increased postprandial fatty acid trapping in subcutaneous adipose tissue in obese women. J Lipid Res 2000;41:1963–8.

132. Cianflone K, Kalant D, Marliss EB, et al. Response of plasma ASP to a prolonged fast. Int J Obes 1995;19:604–9.

133. Gastaldelli A, Miyazaki Y, Pettiti M, et al. Metabolic effects of visceral fat accumulation in type 2 diabetes. J Clin Endocrinol Metab 2002;87(11):5098–103.

134. Romijn JA, Coyle EE, Sidossis LS, et al. Regulation of endogenous fat and carbohydrate metabolism in relation to exercise intensity and duration. Am J Physiol 1993;265:E380–E391.

135. Crowther GJ, Carey MF, Kemper WF, Conley KE. Control of glycolysis in contracting skeletal muscle. 1 Turning it on. Am J Physiol 2002;282:E67–E73.

136. Radegran G, Blomstrand E, Saltin B. Peak muscle perfusion and oxygen uptake in humans: importance of precise estimates of muscle mass. J Appl Physiol 1999;87:2375–80.

137. Coyle EF. Substrate utilization during exercise in active people. Am J Clin Nutr 1995;61(suppl):968S–979S.

138. Frayn KN. Skeletal muscle triacylglycerol in the rat: methods for sampling and measurement, and studies of biological variability. J Lipid Res 1980;21:139–44.

139. Carlson LA, Ekelund LG, Froberg SO. Concentration of triglycerides, phospholipids and glycogen in skeletal muscle and of free fatty acids and beta-hydroxybutyric acid in blood in man in response to exercise. Eur J Clin Invest 1971;1:248–54.

140. Kimber NE, Heigenhauser GJ, Spriet LL, Dyck DJ. Skeletal muscle fat and carbohydrate metabolism during recovery from glycogen-depleting exercise in humans. J Physiol 2003;548:919–27.

141. Kiens B, Richter EA. Utilization of skeletal muscle triacylglycerol during postexercise recovery in humans. Am J Physiol 1998;275:E332–E337.

142. Sidossis LS, Coggan AR, Gastaldelli A, Wolfe RR. A new correction factor for use in tracer estimations of plasma fatty acid oxidation. Am J Physiol 1995;269:E649–E656.

143. Boesch C, Slotboom J, Hoppeler H, Kreis R. In vivo determination of intra-myocellular lipids in human muscle by means oflocalized IH-MR-spectroscopy. Magn Res Med 1997;37:484–93.

144. Brechtel K, Niess AM, Machann J, et al. Utilisation of intramyocellular lipids (lMCLs) during exercise as assessed by proton magnetic resonance spectroscopy (1H-MRS). Hormone Metab Res 2001;33:63–6.

145. Watt MJ, Heigenhauser GJ, Spriet LL. Intramuscular triacylglycerol utilization in human skeletal muscle during exercise: is there a controversy? J Appl Physiol 2002;93:1185–95.

146. Rodnick KJ, Slot JW, Studelska DR, et al. Immunocytochemical and biochemical studies of GLVT4 in rat skeletal muscle. J Biol Chem 1992;267:6278–6285.

147. Ren JM, Semenkovich CE, Gulve EA, Gao J, Holloszy JO. Exercise induces rapid increases in GLVT4 expression, glucose transport capacity, and insulin-stimulated glycogen storage in muscle. J Biol Chem 1994;269:14396–401.

148. Dohm GL. Invited review: regulation of skeletal muscle GLUT-4 expression by exercise. J Appl Physiol 2002;93:782–7.

149. Griffiths AJ, Humphreys SM, Clark ML, Frayn KN. Forearm substrate utilization during exercise after a meal containing both fat and carbohydrate. Clin Sci 1994;86:169–75.

150. Ruys T, Sturgess I, Shaikh M, Watts GE, Nordestgaard BG, Lewis B. Effects of exercise and fat ingestion on high density lipoprotein production by peripheral tissues. Lancet 1989;ii:1119–22.

151. Bülow J. Physical activity and adipose tissue metabolism. Scand J Med Sci Sports 2004;14(2):72–3.

152. Enevoldsen LH, Simonsen L, Macdonald IA, Bülow J. The combined effects of exercise and food intake on adipose tissue and splanchnic metabolism. J Physiol 2004;561:871–82.

153. Hodgetts V, Coppack SW, Frayn KN, Hockaday TDR. Factors controlling fat mobilization from human subcutaneous adipose tissue during exercise. J Appl Physiol 1991;71:445–51.

154. Bülow J. Lipid mobilization and utilization. Med Sport Sci 1993;38:158–85.

155. Frayn KN. Indirect calorimetry. Metabolism 1988;37:1185.

156. Prentice AM, Black AE, Coward WA, et al. High levels of energy expenditure in obese women. BMJ 1986;292:983–7.

157. Hall KD. Body fat and fat-free mass inter-relationships: Forbes's theory revisited. Br J Nutr 2007;97:1059–63.

158. Friedman JE, Dohm GL, Leggett Frazier N, et al. Restoration of insulin responsiveness in skeletal muscle of morbidly obese patients after weight loss. Effect on muscle glucose transport and glucose transporter GLUT4. J Clin Invest 1992;89:701–5.

159. Simoneau JA, Veerkamp JH, Turcotte LP, Kelley DE. Markers of capacity to utilize fatty acids in human skeletal muscle: relation to insulin resistance and obesity and effects of weight loss. FASEB J 1999;13:2051–60.

160. Toubro S, Western P, Bülow J, et al. Insulin sensitivity in post-obese women. Clin Sci 1994;87:407–13.

161. Froidevaux E, Schutz Y, Christin L, Jequier E. Energy expenditure in obese women before and during weight loss, after refeeding, and in the weight-relapse period. Am J Clin Nutr 1993;57:35–42.

162. Tappy L. Metabolic consequences of overfeeding in humans. Curr Opin Clin Nutr Metab Care 2004;7:623–8.

163. Siervo M, Frühbeck G, Dixon A, et al. Efficiency of autoregulatory homeostatic responses to imposed caloric excess in lean men. Am J Physiol Endocrinol Metab 2008;294:E416–24.

164. Katzeff HL, O'Connell M, Horton ES, Danforth E Jr, Young JB, Landsberg L. Metabolic studies in human obesity during overnutrition and undernutrition: thermogenic and hormonal responses to norepinephrine. Metabolism 1986;35:166–75.

165. Joosen AM, Westerterp KR. Energy expenditure during overfeeding. Nutr Metab (Lond) 2006;3:25.

166. Levine JA, McCrady SK, Lanningham-Foster LM, Kane PH, Foster RC, Manohar CU. The role of free-living daily walking in human weight gain and obesity. Diabetes 2008;57:548–54.

167. Heymsfield SB, Harp JB, Reitman ML, et al. Why do obese patients not lose more weight when treated with low-calorie diets? A mechanistic perspective. Am J Clin Nutr 2007;85:346–54.

168. Leyton GB. Effects of slow starvation. Lancet 1946;2:73–79.

169. Jebb SA, Prentice AM, Goldberg GR, Murgatroyd PR, Black AE, Coward WA. Changes in macronutrient balance during over- and underfeeding assessed by 12-d continuous whole-body calorimetry. Am J Clin Nutr 1996;64:259–66.

170. Seevaratnam N, Bennett AJ, Webber J, Macdonald IA. The effects of underfeeding on whole-body carbohydrate partitioning, thermogenesis and uncoupling protein 3 expression in human skeletal muscle. Diabetes Obes Metab 2007;9:669–78.

171. Keys A, Brozek J, Henschel A, Mickelsen O, Taylor HL. *The Biology of Human Starvation*. Minneapolis, MN: University of Minnesota Press; 1950.

172. Walford RL, Mock D, Verdary R, MacCallum T Calorie restriction in biosphere 2: alterations in physiologic, hematologic, hormonal, and biochemical parameters in humans restricted for a 2-year period. J Gerontol A Biol Sci Med Sci 2002;57(6):B211–24.

173. Hellstrom L, Langin D, Reynisdottir S, Dauzats M, Arner P. Adipocyte lipolysis in normal weight subjects with obesity among first-degree relatives. Diabetologia 1996;39:921–8.

174. Frayn KN. Visceral fat and insulin resistance: causative or correlative? Br J Nutr 2000;83(suppl 1):S71-S77.

175. Eckel RH. Insulin resistance: an adaptation for weight maintenance. Lancet 1992;340:1452–3.

176. Chen YD, Golay A, Swislocki AL, Reaven GM. Resistance to insulin suppression of plasma free fatty acid concentrations and insulin stimulation of glucose uptake in noninsulin-dependent diabetes mellitus. J Clin Endocrinol Metab 1987;64:17–21.

177. Laakso M, Edelman SV, Brechtel G, Baron AD. Decreased effect of insulin to stimulate muscle blood flow in obese man. A novel mechanism for insulin resistance. J Clin Invest 1990;85:1844–52.

178. Kelley DE, Goodpaster B, Wing RR, Simoneau JA. Skeletal muscle fatty acid metabolism in association with insulin resistance, obesity, and weight loss. Am J Physiol 1999;277:E1130–41.

179. Bergstrom J, Hermansen E, Hultman E, Saltin B. Diet, muscle glycogen and physical performance. Acta Physiol Scand 1967; 71:140–50.

180. Phillips DI, Caddy S, Ilic V, Fielding BA, Frayn KN, Borthwick AC, Taylor R. Intramuscular triglyceride and muscle insulin sensitivity: evidence for a relationship in nondiabetic subjects. Metabolism 1996;45:947–50.

11 Eating Behavior

John E. Blundell,[1] Graham Finlayson[1] and Jason C.G. Halford[2]

[1] Institute of Psychological Sciences and Biopsychology Group, University of Leeds, Leeds, UK
[2] School of Psychology, University of Liverpool, Liverpool, UK

How eating behavior and appetite control contribute to an understanding of obesity

It is often asserted that obesity arises because of an imbalance in the management of the energy budget. In simple terms, a positive energy balance leads to a storage of energy (mainly as fat). The energy balance equation is often represented as a set of kitchen scales with energy intake on one side and energy expenditure on the other. The model suggests a simple mechanical operation in the effects on energy storage of changes in the provision and utilization of energy. This model is certainly false since the instrument that manages flows of body energy is not a simple mechanical device but a physiologically regulated system. Therefore, changes in either the intake or expenditure of energy do not have a simple additive or subtractive effect on the body's energy stores but are subject to physiologically regulated processes. This has many implications, one of the most important being that the system tolerates an energy surplus (positive energy balance) much more readily than it accepts an energy deficit. The system operates asymmetrically [1] although both surpluses and deficits are subject to physiologic adjustment [2].

Since eating behavior is obviously involved in the energy intake side of the equation, this asymmetry has implications for understanding how eating behavior, in the form of overconsumption, contributes to weight gain and how eating behavior can be adjusted to bring about weight loss (and weight maintenance). In understanding how eating behavior contributes to weight gain, one principal factor is that the overconsumption is largely "passive" [3] although there are definite mechanisms that are involved in this passive overconsumption. We can speak of drivers of overconsumption even though the process is conceived

to be passive, i.e. it happens without any deliberate attempt to overeat. In contrast, the achievement of an energy deficit through eating behavior will require a definite and positive intervention through a cognitively mediated process or through some coercive adjustment of the environment. Therefore, understanding eating behavior, and the processes responsible for its expression, can throw light on how eating (rather easily) contributes to weight gain, and how it can be adjusted (with considerable difficulty) to bring about weight loss and the prevention of weight regain.

The processes influencing eating behavior that allow overconsumption, and that create impediments for a reduction in energy intake, overlap. These processes involve the so-called energy homeostasis system and the hedonic system. Overconsumption is now widely regarded as arising from the strength and abundance of environmental stimuli (mainly foods) that cause a potent hedonic response which, in turn, overcomes the capacity of the homeostatic processes to inhibit food seeking and ingestion. The treatment of obesity through attempts to restrict eating behavior are resisted by a number of factors including: the willingness of people to relinquish a source of enjoyment in their lives (the hedonic response to eating), by difficulties in reversing the long-term rewarding effects of food on established eating habits, and by the opposing physiologic response to weight loss (decrease in leptin and increase in ghrelin, for example) (see also Rosenbaum et al. [4]). At the present time the treatment of obesity has not revealed a strategy capable of dealing with these forces on a scale required to curb the epidemic of obesity.

An examination of eating behavior can indicate possibilities for a deeper understanding of energy intake and how it can be controlled. Considering the human eating response, it is clear that we are not dealing with a uniform or homogeneous entity. There appears to be no unique pattern of eating, or form of energy intake, that will exclusively and inevitably lead to an excess of intake over expenditure. Nevertheless, some characteristics of the expression of appetite do render individuals vulnerable to overconsumption of food – these can be regarded as *risk factors*. Moreover, it is clear that, when considering the impact of the

Clinical Obesity in Adults and Children, 3rd edition. Edited by Peter G. Kopelman, Ian D. Caterson and William H. Dietz.
© 2010 Blackwell Publishing, ISBN: 978-1-4051-8226-3.

obesogenic environment on weight gain, there is enormous variability – some people are susceptible whilst others are resistant. Therefore we should not expect forms of eating behavior that create vulnerability to overconsumption to occur in all people. Any attempt to describe universal factors that link eating behavior with weight gain is likely to end in failure. Therefore the ideologic framework within which scientists conduct research on eating behavior is important in coming up with insights and solutions.

Conceptualization of the system controlling food intake behavior

It is now accepted that the control of appetite is based on a network of interactions forming part of a psychobiologic system. The system can be conceptualized on three levels (Fig. 11.1).

These are the levels of psychologic events (hunger perception, cravings, hedonic sensations) and behavioral operations (meals, snacks, energy and macronutrient intakes); the level of peripheral physiology and metabolic events; and the level of neurotransmitter and metabolic interactions in the brain [5]. Appetite reflects the synchronous operation of events and processes in the three levels. When appetite is disrupted, as in certain eating disorders, these three levels become desynchronized. Neural events trigger and guide behavior, but each act of behavior involves a response in the peripheral physiologic system; in turn, these physiologic events are translated into brain neurochemical activity. This brain activity represents the strength of motivation to eat and the willingness to refrain from feeding.

The lower part of the psychobiologic system (see Fig. 11.1) illustrates the appetite cascade which prompts us to consider the events which stimulate eating and which motivate organisms to

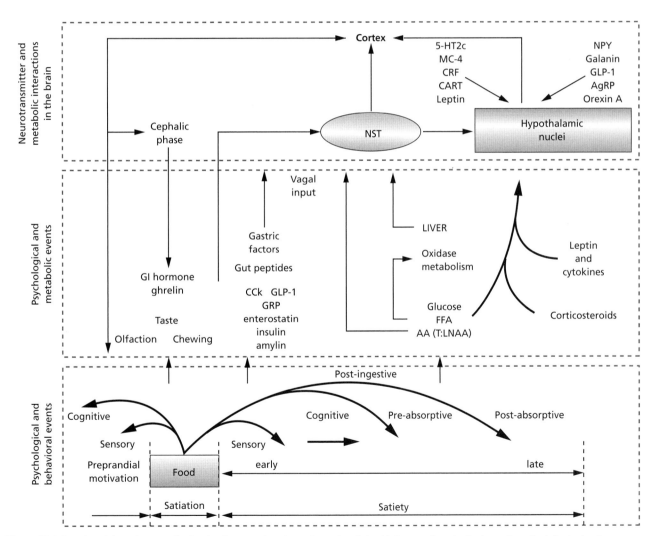

Figure 11.1 A version of the satiety cascade, showing the expression of appetite as the relationship between three levels of operations: the behavioral pattern, peripheral physiology and metabolism, and brain activity. PVN, paraventricular nucleus; NST, nucleus of the solitary tract; CCK, cholecystokinin; FFA, free fatty acids; T, tryptophan; LNAA, large neutral amino acids (see Blundell 1991 [5] for detailed diagram).

seek food. It also includes those behavioral actions which actually form the structure of eating, and those processes which follow the termination of eating and which are referred to as postingestive or postprandial events.

Even before food touches the mouth, physiologic signals are generated by the sight and smell of food. These events constitute the cephalic phase of appetite. Cephalic-phase responses are generated in many parts of the gastrointestinal tract; their function is to anticipate the ingestion of food. During and immediately after eating, afferent information provides the major control over appetite. It has been noted that "afferent information from ingested food acting in the mouth provides primarily positive feedback for eating; that from the stomach and small intestine is primarily negative feedback" [6].

It is useful here to distinguish between signals involved in appetite control. Traditionally, a distinction has been drawn between short-term and long-term regulation of appetite, but the connotation of episodic and tonic is more functionally appropriate [7]. Episodic signals are mainly inhibitory (but can be excitatory) and are usually generated by episodes of eating. These signals oscillate in accordance with the pattern of eating, and most are intimately associated with the signaling of satiety. Tonic signals arise from tissue stores – including adipose tissue – and exert a tonic pressure on the expression of appetite. These two sets of signals – one set responding sharply to changes in behavior and the other providing a slow modulation – are integrated within complex brain networks that control the overall expression of appetite.

Episodic signals and the satiety cascade

Important episodic signals are those physiologic events which are triggered as responses to the ingestion of food. These form the inhibitory processes which first of all stop eating and then prevent its reoccurrence and so are termed satiety signals. The types of signals involved in terminating a meal (satiation) and preventing further consumption (postmeal satiety) can be represented by the satiety cascade. The cascade demonstrates how *satiation*, the complex of processes which brings eating to a halt (cause meal termination), and *satiety*, those events which arise from food consumption which serve to suppress hunger (the urge to eat) and inhibit further eating, co-ordinate our eating behavior by controlling the size and frequency of eating episodes [8].

As the satiety cascade shows, the brain receives initial information about the amount of food ingested and its nutrient content through sensory input (sight, then taste and smell). Sensory as well as psychologic factors, along with past experience of consumption, are critical in initiating, sustaining and terminating intake as well as affecting food choice. However, from the first swallow, food enters the gastrointestinal (GI) tract. The GI tract is equipped with specialized chemo- and mechanoreceptors that monitor physiologic activity and pass information to the brain, mainly via the vagus nerve [9]. This afferent information constitutes one class of "satiety signals" and forms part of the preabsorptive control of appetite. It is usual to identify a postabsorptive

phase that arises when nutrients have undergone digestion and have crossed the intestinal wall to enter the circulation. These products, which accurately reflect the food consumed, may be metabolized in the peripheral tissues or organs or may enter the brain directly via the circulation. In either case, these products constitute a further class of metabolic satiety signals. Additionally, products of digestion and agents responsible for their metabolism may reach the brain and bind to specific chemoreceptors, influence neurotransmitter synthesis or alter some aspect of neuronal metabolism. In each case the brain is informed about some aspects of the metabolic state resulting from food consumption.

There is any number of components to the cascade which could be elaborated on. However, our focus is the key physiologic episodic and tonic signals critical to human appetite expression. As the cascade demonstrates, chemicals released by gastric stimuli or by food processing in the GI tract are critical to the development of within-meal satiation [10]. Many of these chemicals are peptide neurotransmitters, and many peripherally administered peptides produce changes in food consumption [11] and these will be described below.

Cholecystokinin (CCK)

Much recent research has confirmed the status of CCK as a hormone released in the proximal small intestine mediating meal termination (satiation) and possibly early-phase satiety. CCK will reduce meal size and also suppress hunger before the meal; these effects do not depend on the nausea that sometimes accompanies an IV infusion [12]. Food consumption (mainly protein and fat) stimulates the release of CCK (from duodenal mucosal cells) which in turn activates CCK-A type receptors in the pyloric region of the stomach. Fat in the form of free fatty acids (FFA) of carbon chain lengths C12 and above produce pronounced CCK releases [13,14]. This signal is transmitted via afferent fibers of the vagus nerve to the nucleus tractus solitarius (NTS) in the brainstem. From here the signal is relayed to the hypothalamic region where integration with other signals occurs.

Animal data suggest that endogenous CCK release mediates the preabsorptive satiating effect of intestinal fat infusions, and may in turn be critical in regulating the intake of fat [15]. As in rats, intestinal infusions of fat produce a reduction in food intake and promote satiety in humans [16]. In humans the satiety effect of fat infused directly into the duodenum can be blocked by the CCK-A receptor antagonist loxiglumide. Fat infusions significantly decrease both food intake and hunger in both male and female volunteers, effects that are reversed by the CCK-A antagonist [17]. High-fat breakfasts have been shown to produce both greater feelings of satiety (signified by reduced levels of hunger, desire to eat and prospective consumption) and elevated endogenous plasma CCK levels. Collectively, these studies support the theory that CCK plasma levels are a potent fat (or fatty acid)-stimulated endogenous satiety factor, whose effects on food intake and feeding behavior are mediated by CCK-A receptors. The CCK-A receptor antagonist loxiglumide blocks the effect of CCK-8 on appetite in humans [18], demonstrating that the appetite-suppressing effect of CCK-8 infusions, like that of duodenal fat, is mediated by CCK-A receptors. However, it should be noted that fat hydrolysis is essential for endogenous CCK release and for any subsequent effects on appetite [19,20].

It has also been shown that synthetic CCK-A type agonists suppress food intake in humans. This type of drug has been developed because of its potential as an anti-obesity agent, and it has been necessary to design the chemical structure in order to prolong the duration of action. In one example, the drug was administered by a nasal spray; when taken by mouth the drug was too rapidly metabolized in the stomach. This drug, ARL1718, caused a significant reduction in meal size and had a longer duration of action than observed after infusions of CCK itself [21]. A number of other CCK analogs/CCK-1 receptor agonists treatments have been developed, including most recently GW181771 (GlaxoSmithKline) and SR146131 (Sanofi-Aventis). However, development of at least one of these drugs was recently halted in clinical trials. Nonetheless, studies with such drugs, together with those on the peptide hormone itself, do suggest that CCK has the properties of a true satiation signal which contributes, under normal circumstances, to the termination of a meal. The action of CCK certainly acts in concert with other meal-related events, such as gastric distension, for example.

Glucagon-like peptide (GLP)-1
Glucagon-like peptide (GLP)-1 is an incretin hormone, released from the distal small intestine into the bloodstream in response to intestinal nutrients such as carbohydrate, fats, proteins and fiber, an effect associated with a decrease in appetite [13,22–26]. Rodent studies indicate that GLP-1 administration into the CNS reduces food intake and GLP-1 receptors are found in the brainstem, particularly in the NTS and the area postrema and key hypothalamic nuclei [27]. There are data suggesting that peripheral GLP-1 can also cross the blood–brain barrier and could act directly in other areas of the brain [28]. Thus, endogenous GLP-1 appears to be a key component of appetite regulation involving vagal afferent mechanisms, direct action on receptors in the brainstem and possibly in higher areas. However, the role of these central receptors in the action of peripherally administered GLP-1 remains to be determined.

Early studies demonstrated that in healthy men of normal weight, infusions of synthetic human GLP-1 [7–36] during the consumption of a fixed breakfast test meal enhanced ratings of fullness and satiety when compared to the placebo infusion [29]. During a later *ad libitum* lunch, food intake was also significantly reduced by the earlier GLP-1 infusion. Intravenous GLP-1 also dose dependently reduces spontaneous food intake and adjusts appetite in lean male volunteers. This marked reduction in food intake and enhancement in satiety is also observed in overweight/obese male patients with type 2 diabetes. In obese men, intravenous GLP-1 potently reduces food intake either during or post infusion [30] and, at lower subanorectic doses, slows gastric emptying. Reductions in intake and slowed gastric emptying are accompanied by decreased feelings of hunger, desire to eat and

prospective consumption, and a prolonged period of postmeal satiety. These data demonstrate that exogenous GLP-1 reduces food intake and enhances in satiety in humans, both lean and obese, a conclusion substantiated by a meta-analysis of the data from a number of GLP-1 infusion studies [31]. Subcutaneous injections of GLP-1 also induce weight loss in the obese [32]. Unfortunately, GLP-1 is normally rapidly inactivated by the enzyme dipeptidyl peptidase IV (DPP IV). Exendin-4, a naturally occurring GLP-1 agonist, is resistant to DPP IV and has been shown to reduce food intake in lean healthy humans [33]. Exenatide (Byetta; Amylin Pharmaceuticals, Eli Lilly) is a synthetic version of exendin-4 licensed for the treatment of type 2 diabetes and has been shown to produce moderate but sustained weight loss [34,35]. Other GLP-1 agonists under development include liraglutide from Novo Nordisk.

Peptide YY$_{3-36}$
Peptide YY$_{3-36}$ (PYY$_{3-36}$) is one of the two main endogenous forms of PYY. It is produced from the cleavage of PYY$_{1-36}$ (the other major form of PYY) by DPP IV. PYY is a 36 amino acid "hindgut" peptide released from endocrine cells in the distal small intestine and large intestine. This hormone is similar in structure to the orexigenic neuropeptide NPY (70% amino acid sequence identity), and in the past, peptide YY (PYY) has been regarded, like NPY, as a potent stimulator of food intake. However, a series of studies in rats, mice and one human study (all included in one paper) [36] demonstrated that peripheral PYY$_{3-36}$ administration reduces food intake and inhibits weight gain in rodents. These effects on intake and body weight are not observed in transgenic animals lacking NPY Y2 receptors (the NPY Y2 receptor knockout), thereby implicating these receptors in mediating the anorectic effects of PYY. PYY release in the distal intestine is triggered by a variety of nutrients, including fats (particularly FFA), some forms of fiber and bile acids [14,37–39]. In humans, endogenous PYY is released predominantly *after* rather than during a meal [36,40] and causes a decrease in gastric emptying (the so-called "ileal brake"). Thus, it is more associated with postmeal satiety. PYY (including PYY$_{3-36}$) can cross the blood–brain barrier via a nonsaturatable mechanism. Moreover, some of the effects of peripheral PYY$_{3-36}$ on food intake are either "independent of" or "dependent on" vagal afferents running from the periphery to the brain [41,42].

With regard to the effect of PYY on human appetite, Batterham et al. [36] demonstrated that in healthy humans a 90-minute PYY$_{3-36}$ infusion reduced hunger. Two hours after this infusion, at a buffet meal, food intake was also significantly reduced. In addition, in a further report, PYY infusions were made in both lean and obese subjects causing a 30% reduction in the size of a lunch offered after the infusion, and also decreasing the 24-hour energy intake by 23% in lean and by 16% in the obese subjects [40]. The feeling of hunger was also suppressed for over 3 hours following the PYY infusion, as well as plasma levels of ghrelin (see later). Moreover, the natural plasma levels of PYY were lower in the obese than in the lean subjects, and were inversely correlated with the Body Mass Index. The lower levels of PYY in the obese could mean a weaker satiety signaling through this hormone and therefore a greater possibility of overconsumption. All these findings are consistent, and together they make a coherent story concerning the role of PYY in appetite control and obesity.

The effects of PYY$_{3-36}$ on human food intake have been described in three other studies to date. However, as the authors noted, these effects required doses greater than the normal physiologic range of endogenous PYY and marked nausea was observed in one experiment [43–45]. Nonetheless, a PYY$_{3-36}$ nasal spray from Nastech Pharmaceuticals, AC162352 a synthetic version of human PYY$_{3-36}$ from Amylin Pharmaceuticals, and CJC-1681 from Conjuchem, and an Y2 agonist (TM30338 7TM Pharma) are currently in clinical development.

Amylin

Much recent research has also focused on amylin, a pancreatic rather than a GI hormone, which also has a potent effect on both food intake and body weight [46]. Amylin, a 37 amino acid peptide hormone, is co-secreted with insulin from pancreatic β-cells in response to blood glucose and other nutrient stimuli. Peripheral administration of amylin reduces food intake in mice and rats, and meal size in rats. Chronic or peripheral administration of amylin over a period of 5–10 days produces significant reductions in cumulative food intake, body weight and body mass of rats [47]. Amylin administration blocks the hyperphagic effects of NPY [48]. With regard to mechanism, the effect of amylin on gastric emptying may contribute to its effect on short-term appetite. However, vagotomy abolishes amylin's effect on gastric emptying but not its effect on food intake. The primary anorexic effects of amylin appear to be mediated by amylin receptors in the area postrema of the brainstem [49]. Here are located neurons which are co-responsive to both circulating glucose and amylin. Amylin can also cross the blood–brain barrier and is transported into brain regions such as the hypothalamus. Amylin receptors are located in the nucleus accumbens. Some authors have suggested that amylin entering the CNS may act like insulin and leptin as a signal of adiposity. This seems plausible as circulating levels of these hormones correlate with body weight [50]. Thus, amylin appears to be a component part of the appetite regulation system [51].

The effects of amylin on human food intake, food choice or appetite expression have yet to be fully assessed. However, pramlintide (a human amylin analog), given to replace deficits in endogenous amylin in diabetics, has been shown to reduce body weight in diabetic insulin-treated obese [52–54] and nondiabetic obese [55] subjects. In lean healthy volunteers pramlintide induces reductions in meal intake and duration, and reduces premeal appetite [56]. Similar effects of pramlintide on intake and eating behavior are reported in obese subjects (with and without type 2 diabetes) [57,58].

Satiety cascade peptides

In the overall control of the eating pattern, the sequential release and then deactivation of the peptides, described above, can

account for the evolving biologic profile of influence over the sense of hunger and the feeling of fullness [59]. The actions of these hormones therefore contribute to the termination of an eating episode (thereby controlling meal size) and subsequently influence the strength and duration of the suppression of eating after a meal. Individual variability in the release and maintenance of the levels of hormones (or the sensitivity of receptors) may determine whether some individuals are prone to snacking between meals or to other forms of opportunistic eating. The overall strength or weakness of the action of these peptides will help to determine whether individuals are resistant or susceptible to weight gain.

Tonic signals of appetite control
Role of leptin

One of the classic theories of appetite control has involved the notion of a so-called long-term regulation involving a signal which informs the brain about the state of adipose tissue stores. This idea has given rise to the notion of a lipostatic or ponderstatic mechanism [60]. Indeed, this is a specific example of a more general class of peripheral appetite (satiety) signals believed to circulate in the blood reflecting the state of depletion or repletion of energy reserves which directly modulate brain mechanisms. Such substances may include satietin, adipsin, tumor necrosis factor (TNF or cachectin – so named because it is believed to be responsible for cancer-induced anorexia), adiponectin and resistin together with other substances belonging to the family of neural active agents called cytokines.

In 1994 a landmark scientific event occurred with the discovery and identification of a mouse gene responsible for obesity. A mutation of this gene in the *ob/ob* mouse produces a phenotype characterized by the behavioral trait of hyperphagia and the morphologic trait of obesity. The gene controls the expression of a protein (the *ob* protein) by adipose tissue and this protein can be measured in the peripheral circulation. The identification and synthesis of the protein made it possible to evaluate the effects of experimental administration of the protein either peripherally or centrally [61]. Because the *ob* protein caused a reduction in food intake (as well as a possible increase in metabolic energy expenditure), it has been termed "leptin." There is some evidence that leptin interacts with NPY, one of the brain's most potent neurochemicals involved in appetite, and with the melanocortin system. Together, these and other neuromodulators are involved in a peripheral–central circuit which links an adipose tissue signal with central appetite mechanisms and metabolic activity (Fig. 11.2).

In this way the protein called leptin probably acts in a similar manner to insulin which has both central and peripheral actions; for some years it has been proposed that brain insulin represents a body weight signal with the capacity to control appetite.

At the present time the precise relationship between the leptin and weight regulation has not been determined. However, it is known that in animals and humans who are obese, the measured amount of leptin in the plasma is greater than in lean

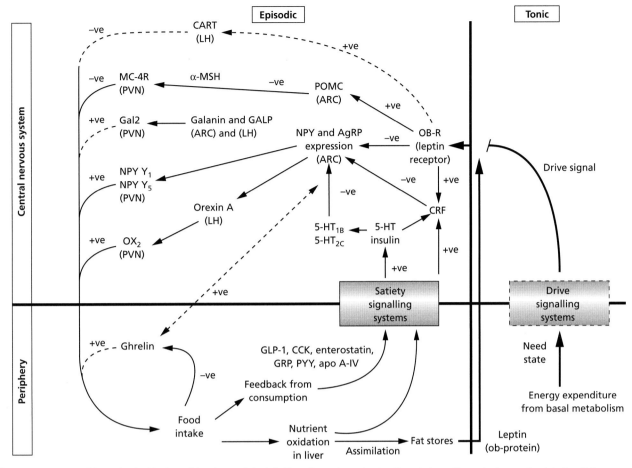

Figure 11.2 Neuromodulators involved in the peripheral–central circuit linking adipose tissue signals with central appetite mechanisms and metabolic activity.

counterparts. Indeed, there is always a very good correlation between the plasma levels of leptin and the degree of bodily fatness [62]. Therefore although leptin is perfectly positioned to serve as a signal from adipose tissue to the brain, high levels of the protein obviously do not prevent obesity or weight gain. Since the specific receptors for the protein (*ob* receptors) have been identified in the brain (together with the gene responsible for their expression) a defect in body weight regulation could reside at the level of the receptor itself. It is now known that a number of other molecules are linked in a chain to transmit the action of leptin in the brain. These molecules are also involved in the control of food intake, and in some cases a mutation in the gene controlling these molecules is known and is associated with the loss of appetite control and obesity. For example, the melanocortin concentrating hormone receptor 4 (MC4R) mutation leads to an excessive appetite and massive obesity in children, just like leptin deficiency (see below).

The prospects for leptin-based obesity treatments seem limited as most obese individuals are leptin insensitive rather than leptin deficient. Nonetheless, for individuals with leptin deficiency studies have shown that leptin treatment produces dramatic

weight loss, an effect associated with marked decreases in hunger [63–65]. The administration of exogenous leptin to humans with either an insufficiency or a specific deficit of endogenous leptin appears to strengthen within-meal satiation and postmeal satiety [65,66]. Under the right physiologic conditions, the effects of leptin on human appetite could be still exploited to treat obesity. Leptin insensitivity (characterized by high levels of circulating leptin) appears reversible with weight loss [67–69]. In such circumstances, part way through or after weight loss, exogenous leptin could be employed to suppress appetite, in the same way as in leptin-deficient individuals. However, this has yet to be robustly demonstrated.

Ghrelin and hunger drive
Ghrelin is found in both the gut and the brain, the gut being the major source of plasma ghrelin. The highest concentrations of ghrelin are found in the stomach, and then in the small intestine. Endogenous ghrelin levels appear responsive to nutritional status; for instance, human plasma ghrelin immunoreactivity increases during fasting and decreases after food intake. It is also found in hypothalamic nuclei critical to energy regulation [70]. Unlike the

other peripheral peptides described earlier, ghrelin stimulates rather than inhibits feeding behavior. Both peripheral and central infusions of ghrelin have been shown to stimulate food intake in rats and mice [71]. Decreased endogenous ghrelin levels are observed in genetically obese rats and mice, and in dietary-induced obese rats exposed to a high-fat diet [72]. The peripheral effects of ghrelin may be vagally mediated but a direct effect of circulating ghrelin on the CNS cannot be ruled out given that receptors are found for it on the arcuate nucleus outside the blood–brain barrier and that it can cross the blood–brain barrier also [73].

In lean humans, endogenous plasma ghrelin levels rise markedly before a meal [74] and are suppressed by food intake. However, initial studies suggested the obese appear to possess lower levels of endogenous ghrelin which are less responsive to food intake [75]. Dietary carbohydrate appears to suppress ghrelin in particular, but other nutrients such as fat (possibly FFAs) and fiber also have similar effects [39,76–81]. In lean healthy volunteers, ghrelin infusions or injections increase food intake, premeal hunger, palatability and prospective consumption, and increase gastric emptying, demonstrating a marked but short-term effect on human appetite [82–84]. Similarly, a ghrelin agonist, the growth hormone (GH) secretagog GH-related peptide (GHRP)-2, stimulates food intake in the obese [85].

It has been proposed that ghrelin, linked to the initiation of eating, acts as a compensatory hormone. This means that in obese people and in animals experimentally made fat, ghrelin levels would be reduced in an apparent attempt to restore a normal body weight status. Therefore ghrelin exhibits the characteristics of both an episodic and tonic signal in appetite control. From meal to meal the oscillations in the ghrelin profile act to initiate and to suppress hunger; over longer periods of time, some factor associated with fat mass applies a general modulation over the profile of ghrelin and therefore, in principle, over the experienced intensity of hunger. This means that when weight is lost, for example following a period of food restriction and weight loss, ghrelin levels would rise and therefore promote the feeling of hunger. This is likely to be one of the signals that make the loss of body weight so difficult to maintain and so ghrelin blockade may prove a useful anti-obesity treatment.

The drive to eat

For years the focus of investigations of appetite control has centered upon the termination of eating. This is because the termination of an eating episode – being the endpoint of a behavioral act – was perceived to be an unambiguous event around which empiric studies could be organized. Consequently, satiety came to be the concept which formed the basis for accounts of appetite.

However, some 50 years ago there was an equal emphasis on the excitatory or drive features of appetite. This was embodied in

Morgan's "central motive state" and in Stellar's location of this within the hypothalamus [86]. One major issue was to explain what gave animals (and humans) the energy and direction which motivated the seeking of food. These questions are just as relevant today but the lack of research has prevented much innovative thinking. In the light of knowledge about the physiology of energy homeostasis, and the utilization of different fuel sources in the body, it is possible to make some proposals. One source of the drive for food arises from the energy used to maintain physiologic integrity and behavioral adaptation. Consequently, there is a drive for food generated by energy expenditure. Over 60% of total energy expenditure is contributed by the resting metabolic rate (RMR). Consequently RMR provides a basis for drive and this resonates with the older concept of "needs translated into drives." In addition, through adaptation, it can be envisaged that other components of energy expenditure would contribute to the drive for food. The actual signals that help to transmit this energy need into behavior could be reflected in oxidative pathways of fuel utilization [87], abrupt changes in the availability of glucose in the blood [61] and eventually brain neurotransmitters such as NPY, which appears to be linked to metabolic processes. Leptin is also likely to play a role via this system.

In turn this drive to seek food, arising from a need generated by metabolic processing, is given direction through specific sensory systems associated with smell, but more particularly with taste. It is logical to propose that eating behavior will be directed to foods having obvious energy value. Of particular relevance to the current situation are the characteristics of sweetness and fattiness of foods. In general most humans possess a strong liking for the sweet taste of foods and for the fatty texture. Both of these commodities indicate foods which have beneficial (energy-yielding) properties.

Accordingly, appetite can be considered as a balance between excitatory and inhibitory processes. The excitatory processes arise from bodily energy needs and constitute a drive for food (which in humans is reflected in the subjective experience of hunger). The most obvious inhibitory processes arise from postingestive physiologic processing of the consumed food and these are reflected in the subjective sensation of fullness and a suppression of the feeling of hunger. However, the sensitivity of both the excitatory and inhibitory processes can be modulated by signals arising from the body's energy stores.

It should be noted that the drive system probably functions in order to ensure that energy intake at least matches energy expenditure. This has implications for the maintenance of obesity since total energy expenditure is proportional to body mass. This means that the drive for food may be strong in obese individuals in order to ensure that a greater volume of energy is ingested to match the raised level of expenditure. At the same time, whilst there is a process to prevent energy intake falling below expenditure, there does not seem to be a strong process to prevent intake rising above expenditure. Consequently, any intrinsic physiologic disturbance which leads to a rise in excitatory (drive) processes or a slight weakening of inhibitory (satiety) signals would allow consumption to drift upwards without generating a compensatory response. For some reason, a positive energy balance does not generate an error signal that demands correction. Consequently, the balance between the excitatory and inhibitory processes has implications for body weight regulation and the induction of obesity.

Homeostatic and hedonic processes of appetite control

A key issue in the study of appetite control is the relationship between "hedonic" (cognitive/emotional processes relating to reward) and "homeostatic" (metabolically regulated) drives arising from biologic needs (e.g. see Yeomans et al. [88]). Historically, hedonic processes have been viewed as a function of nutritional or caloric deficiency. In a state of depletion, the hedonic response (experienced as palatability or pleasure) to energy-providing foods is enhanced and when replete, the hedonic effect of these foods is reduced [89]. This view is compatible with the link between energy density and palatability [90]. However, the idea of reward as a consequence of the fulfillment of nutritional need is not sufficient to explain nonhomeostatic food intake (noncompensated patterns of overconsumption) and it is perhaps more useful to try and distinguish the neural substrates of homeostatic and hedonic systems and to assign them separate identities [91].

Separating homeostatic and hedonic systems

As discussed above, the homeostatic substrate comprises a network of neuropeptides and biogenic aminergic neurotransmitters which link peripheral and central components. This system has been well characterized [92] and involves insulin, leptin, NPY, AgRP, MSH, CART, GLP-1, orexins, ghrelins, PYY, and other peptides along with serotonin pathways and other aminergic systems. A biologic substrate mediating the reward processes of consumption is also being characterized and ostensibly involves glutamate, benzodiazepines, endocannabinoids, opioids and dopamine [93,94].

The implication of distinct neural substrates for homeostatic and hedonic systems is that processes of reward can operate free from biologic need, and the extent to which this occurs can be investigated. For example, pharmacologic evidence suggests that these circuits are somewhat separate. In obese subjects, administration of the serotonin drug D-fenfluramine suppressed the sensation of hunger but had no effect on the appreciation of the pleasantness of food [95]. Conversely, an opioid antagonist reduced the rated pleasantness of palatable foods but had no effect on hunger [96]. This double-dissociation concept indicates that hedonic processes are associated with a specific biologic substrate that can be pharmacologically dissected from the substrate mediating hunger [97]. This is supported by evidence from animal studies. In one study [98], saline (control), NPY or an opioid agonist (DAMGO) was injected into the paraventricular nucleus of rats. The rats could freely consume from standard chow and 10% sucrose solution. After injection of NPY, food intake was increased relative to saline, and the rats were found to consume approximately half their calories from the chow and half from the sucrose solution. Injection of DAMGO also stimulated intake, but in this condition 85% of calories came from the sucrose. Therefore, NPY and opioids may represent a demarcation between energy-driven versus reward-driven feeding.

Interaction of homeostatic and hedonic systems

Advances in our understanding of the molecular and neural mechanisms behind appetite regulation are revealing how the reward system can interact with homeostatic mechanisms. Information about nutritional need is relayed to the brain via tonic and episodic signals that are registered in the caudal brainstem and hypothalamic centers (including the arcuate nucleus, mediobasal, paraventricular and lateral hypothalamus) that comprise the homeostatic neural network. During homeostatic feeding, consumption of food leads to the downregulation of hunger signals and the upregulation of various satiety peptides by the hypothalamus, causing consumption to cease. However, when consumption is driven by hedonic processes, for example in response to highly palatable food, a different scenario is apparent. Erlanson-Albertsson [99] describes how with ingestion of high palatability food, taste sensing is different from that with low palatability food; sensory properties are registered before food is swallowed and these qualities therefore act as triggers through action on sensory receptors. These triggers are transmitted to the reward circuit, leading to the release or upregulation of reward mediators like dopamine, endocannabinoids, and endogenous opioids. The reward circuit has connections with appetite-controlling neurons in the hypothalamus that can increase the expression of hunger peptides such as NPY and orexins, while blunting the signaling of satiety peptides like insulin, leptin and cholecystokinin. Therefore when food is highly palatable, the drive to eat is maintained, with any subsequent overconsumption now mediated by hedonic stimulation rather than biologic need (see Fig. 11.3).

Hence although homeostatic and hedonic systems can be given separate identities [91], they are also to an extent inseparable, with neural cross-talk permitting functional interactions which may influence the organization of eating behavior. From this standpoint, the interaction of homeostatic and nonhomeostatic pathways in the neuroregulatory control of feeding may be more important than the two systems studied in isolation.

In a series of recent reviews, Berthoud [100–103] demonstrates how projections from the hypothalamus to the nucleus accumbens and other structures in the hedonic neural network modulate the motivation to feed via metabolic signals. Furthermore, direct and indirect projections from various corticolimbic systems to the hypothalamus may explain the ability of cognitive, emotional and hedonic processes – activated by relevant environmental cues and incentives – to over-ride the homeostatic regulatory circuits and drive up energy intake. For example, manipulation of the nucleus accumbens by GABA agonism was found to activate orexin and NPY neurons in the hypothalamus and deactivate POMC/CART

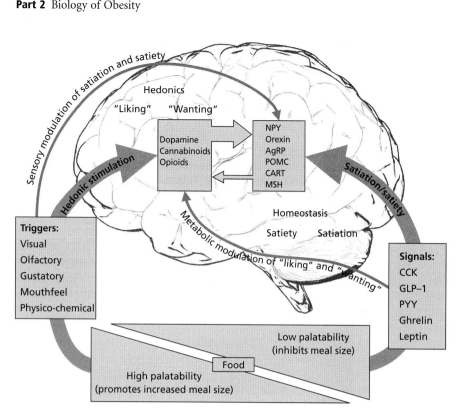

Figure 11.3 Model to explain overconsumption with high palatability food (see also Erlanson-Albertsson 2005 [99]). Exposure to highly palatable food causes an imbalance between hedonic and homeostatic processes. Sensory properties act as triggers causing the upregulation of reward mediators implicated in "liking" and "wanting." These triggers may also modulate homeostatic processes directly (e.g. Cornier et al 2007 [115]). The hedonic system connects with appetite-controlling neurons in the hypothalamus to over-ride homeostatic signaling in favor of continued eating. Defective or hyperactive metabolic signaling may also act directly to upregulate hedonic processes (e.g. Farooqi et al. 2007 [113]; Malik et al. 2008 [114]). Refer to Figs 11.1 and 11.2 for satiety mediators.

neurons [104]. Others have reported that high levels of endocannabinoids in the hypothalamus interfere with leptin signaling [105] while activation of CB1 receptors can prevent the hypothalamic melanocortin system from altering food intake [106]. Therefore, the hypothalamus may be a crucial point of convergence for hedonic and homeostatic interactions that determine eating behavior [107]. Metabolic signals may also act directly to modulate hedonic processing of food stimuli. For example, leptin, ghrelin and PYY can all act directly on neurons in the mesolimbic dopamine system, suggesting their influence on energy intake can depend in part on the modulation of the incentive value of foods [108–110].

Neuroimaging of homeostatic and hedonic interaction in humans

Advances in technology for imaging human brain activity provide the opportunity for researchers to experimentally investigate interactions between homeostatic and hedonic processes with increasing spatiotemporal acuity. In particular, improvements in functional magnetic resonance imaging (fMRI) have led to the localization of brain areas involved in the processing of rewarding stimuli. These "reward circuits" include the midbrain (ventral tegmental area), ventral striatum (nucleus accumbens and ventral pallidum), amygdala, hippocampus, orbitofrontal cortex (OFC), cingular and insular cortex [111–112].

Farooqi et al. [113] used fMRI to measure neural activation in response to visual food stimuli in two adolescent patients with congenital leptin deficiency. They found that subjective ratings of liking for the food stimuli correlated with activation in the nucleus accumbens in fed and fasted states, compared to a correlation in the fasted state only in the nonleptin-deficient controls. After treatment with leptin, the relationship between accumbens activation and liking for the foods in the experimental group was similar to control. These findings support previous evidence from the animal literature to suggest that leptin acts on homeostatic and hedonic circuits in the brain to dampen reward in addition to its role in enhancing satiety.

There is also evidence from fMRI to indicate a dual-process action for the gut peptide ghrelin. Malik et al. [114] administered ghrelin or saline intravenously between two 15-minute exposures to a series of food and nonfood images. Compared to control, ghrelin was associated with an increase in neural activity in the anterior insular, striatum, OFC and amygdala. Furthermore, activation in the OFC and amygdala, thought specifically to code the hedonic value of associated stimuli, was positively correlated with subjective ratings of hunger. Therefore, a known homeostatic metabolic signal may also promote eating via modulation of hedonic processes. The authors point out that ghrelin's action on hedonic circuits in the brain may be indirect via hypothalamic projections to the ventral tegmental area and amygdala, or directly through ghrelin receptors in these areas.

Another imaging study [115] measured responses to food stimuli of neutral or high hedonic value in lean subjects after 2 days of overfeeding by 30% or 0% (energy balance) relative to energy expenditure. In a state of energy balance, differences in neural activation were observed between foods of high hedonic value compared to neutral value foods including the visual cortices, premotor cortex, hippocampus and hypothalamus. On comparison with the energy balance state, overfeeding was associated with a reduction in activity in the hypothalamus and visual cortex. By demonstrating hypothalamic activity with manipulation of energy balance and the hedonic value of visual stimuli, the authors show that hedonic processes can influence homeostatic regulation but furthermore that energy balance status can modulate this interaction.

Liking versus wanting food

Food intake from the first anticipatory moments through to postingestive evaluation is regarded as a rewarding and satisfying experience. "Liking" and "wanting" are emerging constructs in a conceptual approach to food hedonics where separable processes of affect and motivation can be viewed as major influences on food intake. Liking and wanting achieve importance in light of the recognition of the contrast between homeostatic and hedonic processes that control eating [116].

The liking and wanting constructs stem from research exploring the neural basis of palatability and addictive behavior [117]. With principal focus on distinct dopamine and opioid function in the brain, the research suggests that processes of liking and wanting can be separately manipulated to produce patterns of behavior that are either exclusively affective or motivational (goal driven) in conjunction with a food stimulus. The proposal that food reward may comprise separable liking and wanting components has since attracted a great deal of attention and controversy among scientists concerned with human food intake and obesity. Many people would assume that liking and wanting are identical phenomena, both of which signify a positive attraction to food. The logical view is that liking and wanting co-vary in a natural two-way sequence. In behavioral terms, we assume that a change in liking will lead to proportional adjustments in wanting and, likewise, differences in wanting will predict changes in liking. Therefore, some researchers suggest that a clear behavioral distinction might not be possible. However, there are strong grounds for recognizing that liking and wanting can be clearly dissociated and have distinct identities. This means that they have much greater resolving potential for understanding the role of hedonics on eating and therefore on overconsumption.

Thus, the issue of liking versus wanting is concerned with the functional significance of these two distinguishable processes, operating within the hedonic domain, for overconsumption and weight regulation in humans. Liking and wanting are thought to reflect "core" processes that can operate without conscious awareness. This means that they have implicit components. However, their explicit counterparts express themselves subjectively in the form of hedonic feelings from the ingestion of a specific food (i.e. explicit liking) and thoughts relating to the intent or desire to consume a specific food (i.e. explicit wanting). Under normal circumstances, explicit liking ("I like this") is closely associated with explicit wanting ("I want this"). However,

there is evidence to suggest that wanting can be "irrational", i.e. when implicit wanting for a food is greater than explicit wanting, and not proportional to experienced or expected liking [118].

Liking and wanting appear to have separate and disproportionate roles in promoting overconsumption. In terms of liking, some individuals at risk of weight gain may experience an exaggerated hedonic response to palatable foods, so that foods are enjoyed more and therefore eaten in greater amounts for longer periods of time [119,120]. Conversely, susceptible individuals may have a diminished ability to experience pleasure from food and therefore consumption of palatable food is driven up to satisfy an optimum level of stimulation [121]. Processes of wanting may also bring about vulnerability to weight gain through disproportionate reactivity towards cues signaling the availability of food [122,123]. Moreover, a reduced ability to resist the motivation to eat when satiated may promote nonhomeostatic overconsumption [124]. A widely held notion is that wanting rather than liking may be the crucial process in maintaining an obese state. For example, research on chronic drug abusers indicates that repeated drug-taking behavior and strong motivation to obtain a "fix" can occur in the absence of any pleasant sensations during ingestion [125]. Moreover, food liking is often a rather stable characteristic within an individual and appears relatively uninfluenced by increasing weight status [126]. The implication is that liking may be important in establishing the motivational properties of food, but once these are retained it is the upregulation of implicit wanting in an obesogenic environment – insensitivity to homeostatic signals but susceptibility to external cues – that promotes overconsumption by influencing what and possibly how much is eaten from moment to moment.

As liking and wanting are theoretical constructs with separate identities, achieving an operational definition for experimental research is very important but could be difficult. Measures are required that not only reflect the existence of each process but permit dissociations to be detected by preventing the confounding of one process with the other. In research on rats and mice, liking is commonly operationalized by observing positive and negative behavioral reactions to the taste of food. These reactions are thought to be universal affective expressions because some of them can also be observed in primates and human infants [127]. They can be dissociated from the desire to eat and they often correspond to human subjective ratings of palatability [117]. However, in older children and adults, facial reactions to tastes are much less reliable, making them unsuitable as objective measures. In contrast to liking, wanting concerns the anticipatory or instrumental phase of reward-seeking behavior. Therefore, measures that reflect active engagement with the environment in pursuit of a known food can be said to contain at least an element of wanting. Importantly, wanting is not adequately captured by appetitive drive or the nonspecific desire for food in general. Wanting is thought to be the consequence of an active process of assigning value to perceptual events wherein sensory and cognitive inputs are transformed into desirable, attractive entities [128]. Therefore, wanting is likely to be modulated by sensory and/or cognitive influences which set it apart from other appetitive processes (e.g. needing). Wanting implies a direction, not just a force.

It should be noted that under normal circumstances, liking and wanting are assumed to co-vary, and in humans, few studies have been conducted to demonstrate that these processes can be differentiated. A convincing argument for the existence of two separate processes is that they can be influenced by distinct neural pathways in the brain.

Indeed, studies using fMRI are likely to offer new insights to the liking/wanting distinction. For example, Gottfried et al [129] induced selective sensory devaluation of peanut and vanilla food odors by consumption of peanut butter sandwiches or vanilla ice cream to satiety. They found that presentation of the devalued odor was associated with reduced activation in the amygdala and OFC compared to the nondevalued odor. However, they also observed increased activity in the striatum, insula and cingulate cortices in response to both odors when nondevalued compared to when they were devalued. These findings support behavioral data from our own laboratory where postingestive ratings of explicit liking were reduced for visual food stimuli regardless of their sensory properties, whereas an implicit measure of motivation using the same food stimuli revealed an increase in wanting for food items that contrasted with the food consumed [130]. These studies suggest there may be a neurologic explanation for why an uneaten food can increase in salience after consumption of food that is dissimilar in its sensory properties.

Phenotypes for appetite control

There exist many mechanisms through which an individual could gain weight and become obese. This diversity is reflected at the

level of analysis of genetics, central and peripheral physiology, and the behavioral and psychologic profile. It is also clear that a great number of environmental features can exploit intrinsic risk factors (Table 11.1) to induce susceptibility. In recent years, dietary features, such as high energy-dense foods, high-fat, high-carbohydrate, high-GI, high intake of sweet beverages, high-sucrose, high-fructose corn syrup and highly palatable foods, plus various combinations of these, have been proposed as causal agents provoking susceptibility to weight gain. Consequently, in studying susceptibility, the unfettered operation of a plethora of dietary variables could easily occlude the disclosure of key factors.

Therefore, in order to reduce the complexity of this nutritional environment and to allow nonnutrient-related features of susceptibility to be more easily identified, we have worked with individuals defined according to their habitual consumption of a particular type of diet. Such individuals have been called phenotypes. In principle, a number of behavioral phenotypes could be defined based on taste preferences, patterns of eating or motivational responses [131]. Because of the importance of dietary fat to energy balance and body weight regulation [132], researchers have paid attention to the habitual consumption of high-fat or low-fat foods. These have now been well defined and can be termed phenotypes [133]. The phenotype is defined by a particular pattern of behavior characterized by the selection of high-fat or low-fat food items.

High- and low-fat phenotypes: different routes to weight gain

High- (HF) and low-fat (LF) phenotypes are classified according to the type of diet habitually consumed, measured by a food frequency questionnaire (FFQ) and diary record, and with underreporters excluded. The records indicate that these groups habitually consume different types of foods and display different patterns of eating [134]. In principle, phenotypes can be identified independently of age or sex. However, in the first series of studies, the characteristics of young adult males have been examined. When subjected to energy and macronutrient challenges in order to evaluate the responses of the appetite control system, clear differences between the groups were demonstrated. Initially, HF displayed higher initial hunger levels, with a much sharper decline in hunger in response to meals or nutrient loads [135]. After eating, hunger recovered more rapidly in HF compared with LF. In addition, the size of a test meal consumed was closely related to the suppression of hunger in HF; in contrast, the appetite response system in LF appeared to be somewhat insensitive and damped.

This relationship between habitual fat intake and hunger is reminiscent of a previous finding. French et al [136] found that during 2 weeks of high-fat overfeeding to normal-weight subjects, which caused a significant gain in weight, subjects displayed a progressive increase in hunger and a decrease in fullness before a test meal. Taken together, these findings may indicate that eating a high-fat diet may facilitate feelings of hunger. A further feature of these behavior studies was that HF and LF differed in the

Table 11.1 Postulated interactions between behavioral risk factors and the obesogenic environment which generate a tendency for overconsumption

Biologic vulnerability (behavioral risk factor)	Environmental influence	Potential for overconsumption
Preference for fatty foods	Abundance of high fat (high energy-dense)	↑ Fat intake
Weak satiation (end of meal signals)	Large portion size	↑ Meal size
Hedonic responsiveness	Availability of highly palatable foods with specific sensory-nutrient combinations	↑ Amount eaten
Weak postingestive satiety	Easy accessibility to foods and presence of potent priming stimuli	↑ Frequency ↑ Frequency of eating ↑ Tendency to re-initiate eating

control over meal size when offered an unlimited range of either high-fat or high-carbohydrate foods. HF consumed a similar weight of food on both diets, and therefore took in a much higher amount of energy with the high-fat (high-energy dense) foods. In contrast, LF consumed a much smaller amount of the high-fat foods, and consequently took in a similar amount of energy on both diets. These findings suggest that signaling systems for meal termination (satiation) and postmeal inhibition of appetite (satiety) operate with differing strengths in HF and LF. This finding may not be surprising in view of the fact that the GI tract has become adapted to dealing with quite different dietary components, and this factor will have exerted a priming effect on specific satiety signals.

The existence of distinctive profiles of appetite control in HF and LF indicates different patterns of physiologic responses to food ingestion. The possibility of other physiologic differences was investigated using indirect calorimetry to measure basal metabolic rate (BMR), respiratory quotient (RQ) and dietary-induced thermogenic responses to specific fat and carbohydrate loads [137]. The results indicated that HF have a lower RQ than LF; this finding confirmed that fat oxidation was higher in HF, as would be expected due to the habitual high intake of fat-containing foods. However, an unexpected finding was the significantly higher BMR in HF than LF, together with different profiles of "thermogenic" responses to the high-fat and high-carbohydrate loads. A further important finding was that HF had higher plasma leptin levels than LF [138] despite having similar levels of body fat. However, the notion of individuals with different BMRs is consistent with the concept of "energy-sparing" and "energy-profligate" individuals which has been used to describe two distinct groups of women [139]. Interestingly, these two types of individuals are associated with different habitual intakes: the marginally nourished and the very well nourished. For years some researchers in the field of obesity research have maintained the idea that individuals exist who are capable of consuming prodigious amounts of food yet remaining lean. It is possible, therefore, that the HF and LF may constitute a useful investigative approach for examining the relationship between energy intake and energy utilization [140].

Resistant and susceptible phenotypes

In parallel with the characterization of individuals displaying different routes to weight gain with distinctive habitual diets – dietary phenotypes [140] – we can identify people who show differing degrees of responsiveness to an obesogenic diet. These groups of individuals can be termed susceptible or resistant phenotypes [119]. The principle is demonstrated in Figure 11.4 which shows the predicted Body Mass Index (BMI) response of a large number of people exposed to a restricted or obesogenic dietary environment [141]. People with diverse allelic profiles vary in their responsiveness to dietary conditions. When the dietary environment is restrictive, as in parts of sub-Saharan Africa, the genetic potential makes little difference. However, in an obesogenic environment that encourages overconsumption,

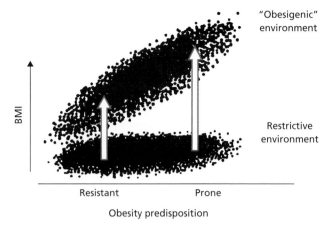

Figure 11.4 Potential effects of genetic background (obesity disposition) in individuals defined as resistant or prone, in a restrictive or obesogenic environment. (After Ravussin and Kozak 2004 [141].)

the genetic variability is more fully expressed and differences between susceptible (prone) and resistant individuals can be seen [142]. It should be noted that this situation mirrors that seen in outbred laboratory rats which, when subjected to high-fat diets, show marked differences in body weight response; some become obese whilst others remain lean [143]. Consequently the differences between lean and obese humans should not necessarily be attributed to varying attitudes towards weight and shape, or to the cognitive control of dieting. The differences may involve more fundamental psychobiologic processes.

In investigating susceptibility at the human level, we have identified changes in both homeostatic and hedonic processes of appetite control, as well as in the expression of physical activity. Careful examination of appetite responsiveness under controlled laboratory and free-living conditions has shown that susceptibility to weight gain on a high-fat diet is marked by a weak satiety response to dietary fat, a strong preference for high-fat food (particularly in the postprandial period), a moderate tendency to show "passive overconsumption" and a high score on the TFEQ factor Disinhibition – as well as low levels of leisure-time physical activity. Consequently, susceptibility is characterized by a cluster of variables including weak control over meal size and postmeal hunger and a strong attraction to highly palatable, high-fat foods. A qualitative analysis of the cognitions of susceptible phenotypes has revealed a strong emotional relationship with foods that is not displayed by the resistant phenotype. Coupled with a low level of physical activity energy expenditure, the susceptible phenotype displays an acquisitive and conservative psychobiologic profile, over which any deliberate control is difficult to achieve. The phenomenologic aspects of the susceptible individual suggest a "thrifty" pattern, and this type can therefore be regarded as the phenotypic expression of a thrifty genotype [144,145]. The term "thrifty phenotype" would be appropriate here, but this term has already been used with a slightly different connotation [146].

Postscript: individual variability – a key feature of eating behavior

The description of susceptible and resistant phenotypes (together with much other research not mentioned here) has drawn attention to the wide diversity in the pattern of the human eating response in the face of an obesogenic culture. Perhaps this should not be surprising given the great variability in the nutritional patterns that have been adopted by the human species in quite extreme ranges of climate and habitat. What are the implications of this diversity? One methodologic issue concerns the use of the statistical mean – or other measures of central tendency – to describe responses to interventions or treatments. Very often, the *mean* outcome fails to adequately reveal the true effect of the intervention or treatment (the weight loss response to enforced exercise is a good example). A truer reflection of the operation of the challenge is described by the diversity of responses which encourages a deeper examination of the internal processes responsible. In common language this means that one unique explanation cannot account for all outcomes.

This issue draws attention, once again, to the nomothetic and idiographic approaches to scientific explanation [147]. What should be the balance between seeking a common unifying principle and a regard for individual differences (quantitative and qualitative)? In the light of this question it may be an appropriate time for a shift in ideology in order to focus attention on individual variability, rather than on the mean value of any set of responses. The value of such a combined approach has recently been proposed [148]. Although the mean response is the statistical parameter associated with the elucidation of scientific principles, cause–effect relationships and other features normally seen as the objectives of scientific enquiry, the great diversity of the human eating response suggests that we are dealing with a phenomenon for which the "average" is often inappropriate. The identification of phenotypes – their behavioral expression and their underlying physiology and genetics – constitutes a partial step towards a recognition of the variability inherent in human eating.

References

1. Blundell JE. Food intake and appetite control: from energy intake to dietary patterns. Int J Obes 1995;19:2–3.
2. Stubbs RJ, Hughes DA, Johnstone AM, Horgan GW, King NA, Blundell JE. A decrease in physical activity affects appetite, energy, and nutrient balance in lean men feeding ad libitum. Am J Clin Nutr 2004;79:62–9.
3. Blundell JE, Tremblay A. Appetite control and energy (fuel) balance. Nutr Res Rev 1995;8:225–42.
4. Rosenbaum M, Murphy EM, Heymsfield SB, Matthews DE, Leibel RL. Low dose leptin administration reverses effects of sustained weight-reduction on energy expenditure and circulating concentrations of thyroid hormones. J Clin Endocrinol Metab 2002;87:2391–4.
5. Blundell JE. Pharmacological approaches to appetite suppression. Trends Pharmacol Sci 1991;12:147–57.
6. Smith GP, Greenberg D, Corp E, Gibbs J. Afferent information in the control of eating. In: Bray GA, Liss AR (eds) *Obesity: Towards a Molecular Approach*. New York: Alan R. Liss, 1990:63–79.
7. Halford JCG, Blundell JE. Differing roles for serotonin and leptin in appetite regulation. Ann Med 2000;32:222–32.
8. Blundell JE, Green S, Burley V. Carbohydrates and human appetite. Am J Clin Nutr 1994;59:728S–734S.
9. Mei N. Intestinal chemosensitivity. Physiol Rev 1985;65:211–37.
10. Read NW. Role of gastrointestinal factors in hunger and satiety in man. Proc Nutr Soc 1990;51:7–11.
11. Smith GP, Gibbs J. Peripheral physiological determinants of eating and body weight. In: Brownell KD, Fairburn CG (eds) *Eating Disorders and Obesity: A Comprehensive Handbook*. New York: Guilford Publications, 1995:8–12.
12. Greenough A, Cole G, Lewis J, Lockton JA, Blundell JE. Intranasal administration of a novel CCK agonist on appetite control in lean men. Int J Obes 1998;22(suppl):S16.
13. Feltrin KL, Little TJ, Meyer JH, et al. Effects of intraduodenal fatty acids on appetite, antropyloroduodenal motility, and plasma CCK and GLP-1 in humans vary with their chain length. Am J Physiol 2004;287:R524–R533.
14. Little TJ, Russo A, Meyer JH, et al. Free fatty acids have more potent effects on gastric emptying, gut hormones, and appetite than triacylglycerides. Gastroenterology 2007;133:1124–31.
15. Greenberg D, Smith GP, Gibbs J. Cholecystokinin and the satiating effect of fat. Gastroenterology 1992;102:1801–3.
16. Welch I, Saunders K, Read NW. Effect of ileal and intravenous infusions of fat emulsions on feeding and satiety in human volunteers. Gastroenterology 1985;89:1293–7.
17. Lieverse RJ, Jansen JBMJ, Masclee AAM, Rovati LC, Lamer CBHW. Effect of a low dose of intraduodenal fat on satiety in humans: studies using the type A cholecystokinin (CCK) receptor antagonist loxiglumide. Gut 1994;35:501–5.
18. Gutzwiller JP, Drewe J, Ketter S, et al. Interaction between CCK and a preload on food intake is mediated by CCK-A receptors in humans. Am J Physiol 2000;279:R189–195.
19. Hildebrand P, Petrig C, Buckhardt B, et al. Hydrolysis of dietary fat by pancreatic lipase stimulates cholecsytokinin releases. Gastroenterology 1998;114:123–9.
20. Degan L, Matzinger D, Drewe J, et al. Role of free fatty acids in regulating gastric emptying and gallbladder contraction. Digestion 2007;74(3–4):131–9.
21. Greenhough A, Cole G, Lewis J, Lockton A, Blundell J. Untangling the effects of hunger, anxiety, and nausea on energy intake during intravenous cholecystokinin octapeptide (CCK-8) infusion. Physiol Behav 1998;65:303–10.
22. Ranganath LR, Beety JM, Morgan LM, Wright W, Howland R, Marks V. Attenuated GLP-1 secretion in obesity: cause or consequence? Gut 1996;38:916–19.
23. Lavin JH, Wittert GA, Andrews J, et al. Interaction of insulin, glucagon-like peptide 1, gastric inhibitory polypeptide, and appetite in response to intraduodenal carbohydrate. Am J Clin Nutr 1998;68:591–8.
24. Frost GS, Brynes AE, Dhillo WS, Bloom SR, McBurney MI. The effects of fibre enrichment of pasta and fat content on gastric emptying, GLP-1, glucose, and insulin responses to a meal. Eur J Clin Nutr 2003;57:293–8.

25. Thomsen C, Storm H, Holst JJ, Hermansen K. Differential effects of saturated and monounsaturated fats on postprandial lipemia and glucagon-like peptide 1 responses in patients with type 2 diabetes. Am J Clin Nutr 2003;77:605–11.

26. Westerterp-Plantenga MS, Luscombe-Marsh N, Lejeyne MPGM, et al. Dietary protein, metabolism, and body-weight regulation: dose response effects. Int J Obes 2006;30(suppl 3):s16–s22.

27. Turton MD, Oshea D, Gunn I, Beak SA, Edwards CMB, Meeran K, et al. A role for glucagon like peptide 1 in the central regulation of feeding. Nature 1996;379:69–72.

28. Kastin AJ, Akerstrom V, Pan W. Interaction of glucagon-like petide-1 (GLP-1) with the blood-brain barrier. J Mol Neurosci 2002;18:7–14.

29. Flint A, Raben A, Astrup A, Holst J. Glucagon like peptide 1 promotes satiety and suppresses energy intake in humans. J Clin Invest 1998;101:515–20.

30. Näslund E, Gutniak M, Skogar S, Rössner S, Hellström PM. Glucagon-like peptide 1 increase the period of postprandial satiety and slows gastric emptying in obese men. Am J Clin Nutr 1998;68: 525–30.

31. Verdich A, Flint A, Gutwzwiller J, et al. A meta-analysis of the effects of glucagon-like peptide-1(7–36) amide on ad libitum energy intake in humans. J Clin Endocrinol Metab 2001;86:4382–9.

32. Näslund E, King N, Mansten S, Adner N, Holst JJ, Gutniak M. Prandial subcutaneous injections of glucagon like peptide 1 cause weight loss in obese human subjects. Br J Nutr 2004;91: 439–46.

33. Edwards CMB, Stanley SA, Davis R, Brynes AE, Frost GS, Seal LJ, et al. Exendin-4 reduces fasting and postprandial glucose and decreases energy intake in healthy volunteers. Am J Physiol 2001;291:E155–E161.

34. DeFronzo RA, Kim DD, Ratner RE, Fineman MS, Han J, Baron AD. Effects of extenatide (exendin-4) on glycemic control over 30 weeks in metformin-treated patients with type 2-diabetes. Diabetes Care 2005;28:1083–91.

35. Gallwitz B. Exenatide in type 2 diabetes: treatment effects in clinical studies and animal study data. Int J Clin Pract 2006;60(12):1654–61.

36. Batterham RL, Ffytche DH, Rosenthal JM, et al. PYY modulation of cortical and hypothalamic brain areas predicts feeding behavior in humans. Nature 2007;450:106–9.

37. Ongaa T, Zabieski R, Kato S. Multiple regulation of peptide YY in the digestive tract. Peptides 2002;23:279–90.

38. Feltrin KL, Patterson M, Ghetei MA, et al. Effect of fatty acid chain length on suppression of ghrelin and stimulation of PYY, GLP-2 and PP secretion in health men. Peptides 2006;27: 1638–43.

39. Weickert MO, Spranger J, Holst JJ, et al. Wheat-fibre-induced changes of postprandial peptide YY and ghrelin responses are not associated with acute alterations of satiety. Br J Nutr 2006;96: 795–8.

40. Batterham RL, Cohen MA, Ellis S, et al. Inhibition of food intake in obese subjects by peptide YY3–36. N Engl J Med 2003;349: 941–8.

41. Renshaw D, Batterham RL. Peptide YY: a potential therapy for obesity. Curr Drug Targets 2005;6:171–9.

42. Koda S, Dae Y, Murakami N, Shimbara T, Hanada T, Toshinai K, et al. The role of the vagal nerve in peripheral PYY3-36 induced feeding reduction in rats. Endocrinology 2005;146:2369–75.

43. Degan L, Oesch S, Casanva M, Graf S, Ketterer S, Drewe J, Beglinger C. Effect of peptide PYY3-36 on food intake in humans. Gastroenterology 2005;129:1430–6.

44. Sloth B, Holst JJ, Flint A, Gregersen NT, Astrup A. Effects of PYY1-36 and PYY3-36 on appetite, energy intake, energy expenditure, glucose and fat metabolism in obese and lean subjects. Am J Physiol 2007;292:E1062–E1066.

45. Sloth B, Davidsen L, Holst JJ, Flint A, Astrup A. Effect of subcutaneous injections of PYY1–36 and PYY3–36 on appetite, ad libitum energy intake, and plasma free fatty acid concentrations in obese males. Am J Physiol 2007;293:E604–E609.

46. Reda TK, Geliebter A, Pi-Sunyer FX. Amylin, food intake, and obesity. Obes Res 2002;10:1087–91.

47. Rushing PA, Hagan MM, Seeley RJ, et al. Inhibition of central amylin signaling increases food intake and body adiposity in rats. Endocrinology 2001;142:5035–8.

48. Morris MJ, Nguyen T. Does neuropeptide Y contribute to the anorectic action of amylin? Peptides 2001;22:541–6.

49. Lutz TA, Tschudy S, Mollet A, Geary N, Scharrer E. Dopamine D2 receptors mediate amylin's acute satiety effect. Am J.Physiol Regul Integr Comp Physiol 2001;280:R1697–R1703.

50. Rushing PA. Central amylin signalling and the regulation of energy homeostasis. Curr Pharmaceut Design 2003;9:819–25.

51. Lutz TA. Pancreatic amylin as a centrally acting satiating hormone. Curr Drug Targets 2005;6:181–9.

52. Hollander P, Maggs D, Ruggles JA, Fineman M, Shen L, Kolterman O, et al. Effect of pramlintide on weight in overweight and obese insulin treated type 2 diabetes patients. Obes Res 2004;12: 661–8.

53. Hollander P, Ratner R, Fineman M, Strobel S, Shen L, Maggs D, et al. Addition of pramlintide to insulin therapy lowers HbA(1c) in conjunction with weight loss in patients with type 2 diabetes approaching glycaemic targets. Diabetes Obes Metab 2003;5: 408–14.

54. Riddle M, Frias J, Zhang B, et al. Pramlintide improved glycemic control and reduced weight in patients with type 2 diabetes using basal insulin. Diabetes Care 2007;30:2794–9.

55. Aronne L, Fujioka K, Aroda V, et al. Progessive reduction in body weight after treatment with the amylin analog pramlintide in obesie subjects: a phase 2, randomized, placebo-controlled, dose-escalation study. J Clin Endocrinol Metab 2007;92:2977–83.

56. Chapman I, Parker N, Doran S, et al. Low-dose pramlintide reduced food intake and meal duration in healthy, normal weight subjects. Obesity 2007;15:1170–86.

57. Chapman I, Parker B, Doran S, Feinle-Bisset C, Wishart J, Strobel S, et al. Effect of pramlintide on satiety and food intake in obese subjects and subjects with type 2 diabetes. Diabetologia 2005;48: 838–48.

58. Smith SR, Blundell JE, Burns C, et al. Pramlintide treatment reduces 24-h caloric intake and meal-sizes and improves feeding control in obese subjects: a 6-wk translational research study. Am J Physiol 2007;293:E620–7.

59. Blundell JE, Naslund E. Invited commentary: glucagon like peptide-1, satiety and appetite control. Br J Nutr 1999;81:259–60.

60. Weigle, D. Appetite and the regulation of body composition. J Fed Am Soc Exper Biol 1994;8:302–10.

61. Campfield LS, Smith FJ, Guiswz Y, Devos R, Burn P. Recombinant mouse ob protein: evidence for a peripheral signal linking adiposity and central neural networks. Science 1995;269:546–9.

62. Maffei M, Halaas J, Ravussin E, et al. Leptin levels in human and rodent: measurement of plasma leptin and ob RNA in obese and weight reduced subjects. Nat Med 1995;1:1151–61.

63. Farooqi SF, Matarese G, Lord GM, Keogh JM, Lawrence E, Agwu C, et al. Beneficial effects of leptin on obesity, T cell hyporesponsiveness, and neuroendocrine/metabolic dysfunction of human congenital leptin deficiency. J Clin Invest 2002;110:1093–103.

64. Farooqi IS, Jebb SA, Langmack G, Lawrence E, Cheetham CH, Prentice AM, et al. Effects of recombinant leptin therapy in a child with congenital leptin deficiency. N Engl J Med 1999;341:879–84.

65. Williamson DA, Ravussin E, Wong M-L, DiPaoli A, Caglayan S, Ozata M, et al. Micro analysis of eating behavior of three leptin deficient adults treated with leptin therapy. Appetite 2005;45:75–80.

66. McDuffie JR, Riggs PA, Calis KA, et al. Effects of exogenous leptin on satiety and satiation in patients with lipodystrophy and leptin insufficiency. J Clin Endocrinol Metab 2004;89:4258–63.

67. Heini AF, Lara-Castro C, Kirk KA, Considine RV, Caro JF, Weinsier RL. Association of leptin and hunger-satiety ratings in obese women. Int J Obes 1998;22:1084–7.

68. Keim NL, Stern JS, Havel P. Relation between circulating leptin concentrations and appatite during a prolonged, moderate energy deficit in women. Am J Clin Nutr 1998;68:794–801.

69. Mars M, de Graf C, de Groot CPGM, van Rossum CTM, Kok FJ. Fasting leptin and appetite responses induced by a 4-day 65%-energy restricted diet. Int J Obes 2006;30:122–8.

70. Cummings DE. Ghrelin and short and long term regulations of appetite and body weight. Physiol Behav 2006;71:71–84.

71. Wren AM, Small CJ, Ward HL, et al. The novel hypothalamic peptide ghrelin stimulates food intake and growth hormone secretion. Endocrinology 2000;141:4325–8.

72. Ariyasu H, Takaya K, Hosoda H, et al. Delayed short-term secretory regulation of ghrelin in obese animals: evidenced by a specific RIA for the active form of ghrelin. Endocrinology 2002;143:3341–50.

73. Cummings DE. Ghrelin and short and long term regulations of appetite and body weight. Physiol Behav 2006;71:71–84.

74. Cummings DE, Purnell JQ, Frayo RS, Schmidova K, Wisse BE, Weigle DS. A preprandial rise in plasma ghrelin levels suggests a role in meal initiation in humans. Diabetes 2001;50:1714–19.

75. Tschöp M, Weyer C, Tataranni A, Devenarayan V, Ravussin E, Heiman ML. Circulating ghrelin levels are decreased in human obesity. Diabetes 2001;50:707–9.

76. Blom WAM, Stafleu A, de Graaf C, Kok FJ, Schaafsma G, Hendricks HFH. Ghrelin response to carbohydrate-enriched breakfast is related to insulin. Am J Clin Nutr 2005;81:367–75.

77. Feinle-Bisset C, Patterson M, Ghatei MA, Bloom SR, Horowitz M. Fat digestion is required for suppression of peptide YY and pancreatic polypeptide seactration by intraduodenal lipid. Am J Physiol 2005;289:E948–53.

78. Bowen J, Noakes M, Trenerry C, Clifton PM. Energy intake, ghrelin and cholecystokinin after difference carbohydrate and protein preloads in overweight men. J Clin Endocrinol Metab 2006;91(4):1477–83.

79. Erdmann J, Leibl M, Wagenpfeil S, Lippl F, Schusdziarra V. Ghrelin response to protein and carbohydrate meals in relation to food intake and glycerol levels in obese subjects. Regul Pept 2006;135(1–2):23–9.

80. Murray CD, Le Roux CW, Gouveia C, et al. The effect of different macronutrient infusions on appetite, ghrelin and peptide YY in parenterally fed patients. Clin Nutr 2006;25:626–33.

81. El Khoury DT, Obeid O, Azar ST, Hwalla N. Variations in postprandial ghrelin status following ingestion of high carbohydrate, high fat and high protein meals in males. Ann Nutr Metab 2006;50:260–9.

82. Wren AM, Small CJ, Ward HL, et al. The novel hypothalamic peptide ghrelin stimulates food intake and growth hormone secretion. Endocrinology 2000;141:4325–8.

83. Druce MR, Wren AM, Park AJ, et al. Ghrelin increases food intake in obese as well as lean subjects. Int J Obes 2005;29(9);1130–6.

84. Levin F, Edholm T, Schmidt PT, et al. Ghrelin stimulated gastric emptying and hunger in normal weight humans. J Clin Endocrinol Metab 2006;91(9):3296–302.

85. Laferrere B, Hart AB, Bowers CY. Obese subjects respond to the stimulatory effect of the ghrelin agonist growth hormone-releasing peptide-2 on food intake. Obesity 2006;14(6);1056–63.

86. Stellar E. The physiology of motivation. Psychol Rev 1954;61:5–22.

87. Friedman, MI, Rawson, NE. Fuel metabolism and appetite control. In: Fernstrom JD, Miller GD (eds) *Appetite and Body Weight Regulation*. Boca Raton, FL: CRC Press, 1994;63–76.

88. Yeomans MR, Blundell JE, Leshem M. Palatability: response to nutritional need or need-free stimulation of appetite? Br J Nutr 2004;92:S3–14.

89. Cabanac M. Maximization of pleasure, the answer to a conflict of motivations. C R Acad Sci III 1989;309:397–402.

90. Drewnowski A. Energy density, palatability, and satiety: implications for weight control. Nutr Rev 1998;56:347–53.

91. Blundell JE, Finlayson GS. Is susceptibility to weight gain characterised by homeostatic or hedonic risk factors for overconsumption? Physiol Behav 2004;82:21–5.

92. Schwartz MW, Woods SC, Porte D, Seeley RJ, Baskin DG. Central nervous system control of food intake. Nature 2000;404:661–71.

93. Saper CB, Chou CT, Elemquist JK. The need to feed: homeostatic and hedonic control of eating. Neuron 2002;36:199–211.

94. Flier JS. Obesity wars: molecular progress confronts and expanding epidemic. Cell 2004;116:337–50.

95. Blundell JE, Hill AJ. Nutrition, serotonin and appetite: case study in the evolution of a scientific idea. Appetite 1987;8:183–94.

96. Yeomans MR, Gray RW. Opioid peptides and the control of human ingestive behavior. Neurosci Biobehav Rev 2002;26:713–28.

97. Rogers PJ, Blundell JE. Mechanisms of diet selection: the translation of needs into behavior. Proc Nutr Soc 1991;50:65–70.

98. Giraudo SQ, Grace MK, Billington CJ, Levine AS. Differential effects of neuropeptides Y and the mu-agonist DAMGO on "palatability" vs. "energy". Brain Res 1999;10:160–3.

99. Erlanson-Albertsson C. How palatable food disrupts appetite regulation. Basic Clin Pharmacol Toxicol 2005;97:61–73.

100. Berthoud HR. Neural control of appetite: cross-talk between homeostatic and non-homeostatic systems. Appetite 2004;43:315–17.

101. Berthoud HR. Homeostatic and non-homeostatic pathways involved in the control of food intake and energy balance. Obesity 2006;14:S197–S200.

102. Berthoud HR. Interactions between the "cognitive" and "metabolic" brain in the control of food intake. Physiol Behav 2007;91:486–98.

103. Zheng H, Berthoud HR. Eating for pleasure or calories. Current Opinion in Pharmacology, Curr Opin Pharmacol 2008;7;607–12.

104. Zheng H, Corkern M, Stoyanova I, Patterson LM, Tian R, Berthoud HR. Peptides that regulate food intake: appetite-inducing accumbens manipulation activates hypothalamic orexin neurons and inhibits POMC neurons. Am J Physiol Regul Comp Physiol 2003;284; R1436–44.

105. di Marzo V, Goparaju SK, Wang L, et al. Leptin-regulated endocannabinoids are involved in maintaining food intake. Nature 2001;410:822–5.

106. Verty AN, Geller F, Dempfle A, et al. Ghrelin receptor gene: identification of several sequence variants in extremely obese children and adolescents, healthy normal-weight and underweight students, and children with short normal stature. J Clin Endocrinol Metab 2004;89:157–62.

107. Zheng H, Patterson LM, Berthoud HR. Orexin-signaling in the ventral tegmental area is required for high-fat appetite induced by opioid stimulation of the nucleus accumbens. J Neurosci 2007;27: 11075–82.

108. Fulton P, Pissios RP, Manchon L, et al. Leptin regulation of the mesoaccumbens dopamine pathway Neuron 2006;51:811–22.

109. Abizaid A, Liu ZW, Andrews ZB, et al. Ghrelin modulates the activity and synaptic input organization of midbrain dopamine neurons while promoting appetite. J Clin Invest 2006;116:3229–39.

110. Batterham RL, Cowley MA, Small CJ, et al. Gut hormone PYY3–36 physiologically inhibits food intake. Nature 2002;418:650–4.

111. McClure SM, York MK, Montague PR. The neural substrates of reward processing in humans: the modern role of fMRI. Neuroscientist 2004;10:260–8.

112. O'Doherty JP. Reward representations and reward-related learning in the human brain: insights from neuroimaging. Curr Opin Neurobiol 2004;14:769–76.

113. Farooqi IS, Bullmore E, Keogh J, Gillard J, O'Rahilly S, Fletcher PC. Leptin regulates striatal regions and human eating behavior. Science 2007;317:1355.

114. Malik S, McGlone F, Bedrossian D, Dagher A. Ghrelin modulates brain activity in areas that control appetitive behavior. Cell Metab 2008;7:400–9.

115. Cornier M-A, von Kaenel SS, Bessesen DH, Tregellas JR. Effects of overfeeding on the neuronal response to visual food cues. Am J Clin Nutr 2007;86:965–71.

116. Finlayson GS, King NA, Blundell JE. Liking vs. wanting food: importance for human appetite control and weight regulation. Neurosci Biobehav Rev 2007;31:987–1002.

117. Berridge KC. Food reward: brain substrates of wanting and liking. Neurosci Biobehav Rev 1996;20:1–25.

118. Berridge KC. Pleasure, unconscious affect and irrational desire. In: Manstead ASR, Frijda NH, Fischer AH (eds) *Feelings and Emotions: The Amsterdam Symposium*. Cambridge: Cambridge University Press, 2004:43–62.

119. Blundell JE, Stubbs RJ, Golding C, et al. Resistance and susceptibility to weight gain: individual variability in response to a high-fat diet. Physiol Behav 2005;86:614–22.

120. LeNoury JC, Lawton C, Blundell JE. Food choice and hedonic responses: differences between overweight and lean high fat phenotypes. Int J Obes 2002;26:S125.

121. Davis C, Fox J. Sensitivity to reward and body mass index (BMI): evidence of a non-linear relationship. Appetite 2008;50:43–9.

122. Saelens BE, Epstein LH. Reinforcing value of food in obese and non-obese women. Appetite 1996;27:41–50.

123. Tetley AC, Brunstrom JM, Griffiths P. Individual differences in food-cue reactivity. Appetite 2006;47:278.

124. Nasser JA, Geliebter A, Pi-Sunyer FX. Persistence of food reinforcement after a caloric preload in women is correlated with binge eating score and hunger in the fasted state. Appetite 2007; 44:329.

125. Lamb RJ, Preston KL, Schindler CW, et al. The reinforcing and subjective effects of morphine in post-addicts: a dose response study. J Pharmacol Exp Ther 1991;259:1165–73.

126. Cox DN, Perry L, Moore PB, Vallis L, Mela DJ. Sensory and hedonic associations with macronutrient and energy intakes of lean and obese consumers. Int J Obes 1999;23:403–10.

127. Berridge KC. Measuring hedonic impact in animals and infants: microstructure of affective taste reactivity patterns. Neurosci Biobehav Rev 2000;24:173–98.

128. Berridge KC, Robinson TE. Parsing reward. Trends Neurosci 2003;26:507–13.

129. Gottfried JA, O'Doherty J, Dolan RJ. Encoding predictive reward value in human amygdala and orbitofrontal cortex. Science 2003;301:1104–7.

130. Finlayson GS, King NA, Blundell JE. The role of implicit wanting in relation to explicit liking and wanting for food: implications for appetite control. Appetite 2008;50:120–7.

131. Drewnowski A. The behavioral phenotype in human obesity. In: Capaldi E (ed) *Why We Eat What We Eat: The Psychology of Eating*. Washington, DC: American Psychological Association, 1996: 291–308.

132. Blundell JE, Lawton CL, Cotton JR, Macdiarmid JI. Control of human appetite: implications for the intake of dietary fat. Annu Rev Nutr 1996;16:285–319.

133. Blundell JE, Cooling J. High-fat and low-fat (behavioral) phenotypes: biology or environment? Proc Nutr Soc 1999;58:1–5.

134. Macdiarmid JI, Cade JE, Hamilton KV, Blundell JE. High and low fat consumers, their macronutrient intake and body mass index: further analysis of the national diet and nutrition survey of British adults. Eur J Obes 1996;20:S48.

135. Cooling J, Blundell JE. High-fat and low-fat phenotypes: methodological issues concerning energy intake and expenditure. Int J Obes 1999;23:S91.

136. French SJ, Murray B, Rumsey RDE, Fadzlin R, Read NW. Adaptation to high-fat diets: effects on eating behavior and plasma cholecystokinin. Br J Nutr 1995;73:179–89.

137. Cooling J, Blundell JE. Differences in energy expenditure and substrate oxidation between habitual high fat and low fat consumers (phenotypes). Int J Obes 1998;22:612–18.

138. Cooling J, Barth J, Blundell J. The high-fat phenotype: is leptin involved in the adaptive response to a high fat (high energy) diet? Int J Obes 1998;22:1132–5.

139. Goldberg GR. From individual variation in energy intakes to variations in energy requirements and adaptations to them. Br J Nutr 1997;78:S81–S94.

140. Blundell JE, Cooling J. Routes to obesity: phenotypes, food choices and activity. Br J Nutr 2000;20:S33–38.

141. Ravussin E, Kozak LP. Energy homeostasis. In: Hofbauer KG, Keller U, Boss O (eds) *Pharmacotherapy of Obesity – Options and Alternatives*. Boca Raton, FL: CRC Press, 2004:488.

142. Ravussin E, Bogardus C. Energy balance and weight regulation: genetics versus environment. Br J Nutr 2000;83:S17–20.

143. Levine AS, Kotz CM, Gosnell BA. Sugars and fats: the neurobiology of preference. J Nutr 2003;133:S831–4.

144. Prentice AM. The emerging epidemic of obesity in developing countries. Int J Epidemiol 2006;35:93–9.

145. Speakman JR. A nonadaptive scenario explaining the genetic predisposition to obesity: the "predation release" hypothesis. Cell Metab 2007;6:5–12.

146. Hales CN, Barker DJ. The thrifty phenotype hypothesis. Br Med Bull 2001;60:5–20.

147. Allport GW. *Personality: A Psychological Interpretation*. New York: Holt, Rinehart and Winston, 1937.

148. Kaplan AS, Olmstead MP, Carter JC, Woodside D. Matching patient variables to treatment intensity. The continuum of care. Psychiatr Clin North Am 2001;24:281–92.

12 Energy Expenditure in Humans: The Influence of Activity, Diet and the Sympathetic Nervous System

Jose Lara, Moira A. Taylor and Ian A. Macdonald

School of Biomedical Sciences, University of Nottingham, Queen's Medical Centre, Nottingham, UK

The various chemical processes that underlie the functions of the body require the continuous provision of energy. In most cases, this energy is supplied by high-energy bonds within adenosine triphosphate (ATP). ATP availability is maintained by the utilization of the major fuels, glucose and fatty acids. Although in the short term some fuel utilization and ATP production can occur anaerobically (e.g. by the production of lactate from glucose), the capacity and duration of such provision are limited, and for all practical purposes only the oxidation of the fuels to carbon dioxide (CO_2) and water is of importance. Thus, the overall processes involved in the body's energy metabolism can be summarized by, first, the oxidation of fuels producing CO_2, water and ATP (with approximately 60% of the food energy being released as heat during the production of ATP) and second, the utilization of the ATP in the chemical processes of the body. Thus, the energy contained within the fuels (originally the food consumed) is first converted to ATP or lost as heat, and subsequently utilized in various metabolic processes (Fig. 12.1). This overall process is referred to as energy expenditure (EE), and represents the utilization of food energy to maintain the functions of the body. The close relationship between EE and the metabolic processes of the body explains why the term "metabolic rate" is used synonymously with EE.

History of the measurement of energy expenditure

Our understanding of EE and its measurement originated during the late 1800s and early 1900s when prominent scientists developed the concepts we now use when measuring EE and substrate metabolism. The mysteries of life lead to the proposition of obscure theories and doctrines that governed the medical sciences in the Middle Ages. The belief that a "vital force" or "vital heat" was responsible for the functioning of most living organisms characterized the theory of vitalism before the 1500s. During the next two centuries, the "phlogiston theory" supported the existence of a mysterious colorless, weightless "substance" (phlogiston) contained in all flammable materials and released when these were burned (e.g. dephlogistation) [1].

Pioneering work by two British scientists, Joseph Black and Joseph Priestley, lead to the discovery of CO_2 and oxygen (O_2), respectively [1]. However, it was Lavoisier's early experiments on O_2 combustion, and respiration and heat production in guinea pigs that replaced the "phlogiston theory" and formed the basis of the concept of EE [1,2].

Following the work of Lavoisier, Carl von Voit, a German physiologist, was among the first to develop an apparatus to measure CO_2 production in humans and animals. However, it was Max Rubner, a student of Voit, who improved Voit's apparatus and established the concepts of metabolic rate, and "specific dynamic action" (thermic effect of food) [3]. Table 12.1 lists some of the prominent physiologists contributing to the development of our understanding of energy metabolism.

Although new terminology has been introduced, the early concepts still remain. An example of this is the specific dynamic action of protein, now called thermic effect of food (TEF). Similarly, because of the difficulty in achieving the conditions required to measure basal metabolic rate (BMR), it is actually resting metabolic rate (RMR) that is commonly measured.

Some concepts have been surrounded by controversy. Neumann in 1902 [4] coined the term "Luxuskonsumption" to describe the capacity of some individuals to maintain a constant body weight at different levels of energy intake (EI). Others have been unable to confirm these findings [4]. A new term to describe this mechanism has been coined, adaptive thermogenesis, and its clinical significance is still debated.

Measuring RMR proved useful in the diagnosis of thyroid disorders characterized by altered energy metabolism. Early during

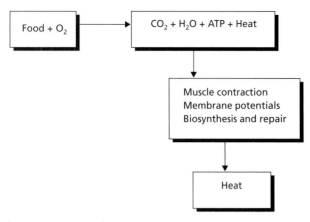

Figure 12.1 Summary of energy exchanges in the body.

the 19th century, the measurement of RMR became a routine test in most hospitals [1]. However, with advances in the development of techniques to measure thyroid hormones, measuring RMR was replaced by tests directed to hormone release.

During the early 1980s, indirect calorimetry (IC) became a fundamental tool in assessing the nutritional status of hospitalized patients [5]. During the same period, a renewed interest in measuring EE arose. Measuring EE was of interest to see whether low EE, in the context of low self-reported EI, might be a cause of obesity.

Methods of measuring energy expenditure

Calorimetric and noncalorimetric (direct and indirect) methods are available to assess EE under laboratory and free-living conditions. We will focus on those that for one or another reason have a wider use. Table 12.2 provides a list of methods used to assess EE in human subjects.

Calorimetric methods

Direct calorimetry (DC)
Because the measurement of EE implies measuring heat loss and heat production, DC remains the gold standard method. Heat loss can be measured accurately (0.1%), although this accuracy varies according to the routes of heat loss (e.g. evaporative heat 2–3%). However, the high cost of building and maintaining a calorimetric chamber impedes its widespread use. Indeed, only a few direct calorimetric chambers are available in the world. The technical aspects of DC and the different systems available are described in detail elsewhere [6,7].

Indirect calorimetry (IC)
Indirect calorimetry is more widely used to assess EE, which is estimated from the rates of respiratory gas exchange, i.e. O_2 consumption (VO_2) and CO_2 production (VCO_2). IC has the advantage of allowing an assessment of which fuel (i.e. carbohydrate or fat) is being used as a substrate for energy metabolism.

Table 12.1 Prominent contributors to EE developments and research

	Dates	Contributions/ area of work/ key experiments
Joseph Black	1728–1799	Discovered CO_2
Joseph Priestley	1733–1804	Discovered O_2
Antoine Lavoisier	1743–1794	Used a calorimeter to show respiration associated with heat production in guinea pigs
		Identified increased thermogenesis associated with food intake (later described as SDA (specific dynamic action), DIT, TEF)
Carl von Voit	1831–1908	Built a metabolic chamber to collect water and CO_2 in humans, probably the first open-circuit chamber
Nathan Zuntz	1847–1920	Developed an open-circuit calorimeter to measure VO_2 and VCO_2 – the first portable respirometer
Wilbur O. Atwater	1844–1907	Developed a respiration chamber for use in humans (the Atwater–Rosa calorimeter)
		Investigated EB in resting, active, fed and/or fasted humans
		Modified his respiration chamber to allow measurements of O_2
Max Rubner	1854–1908	Succeeded in measuring carbon and energy balance in a dog using his respiration chamber
		Attributed with developing the concept of basal metabolism
		Showed that different animal species produced the same amount of heat per unit of body surface area
		Described the specific dynamic action of food (SDA, now denoted TEF)
Graham Lusk	1866–1932	Showed that SDA (TEF) was not exclusive to proteins
Francis G. Benedict	1870–1957	Studied RMR in children and adults
		Report on metabolic standards
		Developed the most quoted equation to estimate BMR
		Developed a helmet for IC measurements, an early version of a ventilated hood
Max Kleiber	1893–1976	Found an exponential relationship between RMR and body mass in mammals leading to what we know as the Kleiber's law: $RMR = constant \times (body\ weight)^{0.75}$
		Provided the basis for the conclusion that total efficiency of energy utilization is independent of body size

There are two basic approaches towards IC, closed-circuit and open-circuit systems. In the closed-circuit system, the subject breathes from an O_2 reservoir and changes in the volume are used to calculate VO_2. In the open circuit, the more common of the two systems, the subject breathes ambient (room) air of a constant composition, and expires into a gas-sampling system. Studies comparing these approaches show that closed-circuit systems produce higher RMR values (5–10%) than open-circuit systems [8].

Table 12.2 Methods of measuring energy expenditure

Method	Accuracy	Advantages	Disadvantages	Complexity of use	Cost (£)
Direct calorimetry	++++	Very accurate Suitable for 24-hour or longer periods	Not widely available High maintenance costs	+++++	££££
Respiratory chamber	++++	Very accurate Suitable for 24-hour or longer periods	Not widely available	++++	££££
Ventilated hood systems	+++	Widely available in laboratory and clinical settings	Unsuitable for longer periods than a few hours	+++	£££
Douglas bag	+++	Can be used for outdoor measurements during PA	Interference with locomotive activity Limited sampling duration	+++	££
Portable calorimeters	+++	Availability of new smaller devices Useful for outdoor measurement of PAEE	Validation outside the sports science area is needed	+++	££
PA monitors	++	Used in large-scale studies Provides specific information on PA	Studies validating PA monitors against DLW are required	++	£
PA diaries	+	Most accessible method Used in a wide number of settings	Inaccurate Subject to bias/misreporting	+	£
HR monitors	+(+)	Satisfactory results in estimating EE at a group level	High variability at the individual level and in small groups	++	£
DLW	++++	Nonradioactive tracer Long-term estimation of TEE	Expensive (isotope and analytic equipment)	+++++	£££
Labeled bicarbonate	++++	Less expensive than DLW and provides EE estimations over shorter periods (e.g.12–24 h)	Subject to carbon fixation with variable recovery of labeled bicarbonate Invasive: IV infusion of labeled carbonate	++++	£££

++++ very high; +++ high; ++ moderate; +low.
££££ very high cost; £££ high cost; ££ moderate cost; £ low cost.

A disadvantage of IC is the need for a respiratory valve and a noseclip or facemask in exercising subjects or a ventilated hood in resting subjects, which limits the length of the measurement to only a few hours. A respiration chamber, usually the size of a small room (9–30 m^3), can be used for longer-term (e.g. 24 hours or longer) resting and exercising measurements. Some calorimeters have been designed to allow simultaneous IC and DC measurements, reporting an agreement of 1% between methods [9]. The lower complexity and expense of a respiratory chamber compared with DC has encouraged the use of this methodology.

Availability of a number of IC commercial devices using a ventilated hood has made the measurement of EE a common test in the field, clinical setting and laboratory. Early portable devices such as the Kofranyi–Michaelis respirometer [7] or the Oxylog offered the opportunity to measure the energy costs of physical activity (PAEE). A number of new and smaller computerized devices such as the K4b2 (Kosmed), Oxycon mobile (Jaeger) or VO$_{2000}$ (MedGraphics) are now popular in sports science.

Respiratory quotient (RQ)

Box 12.1 illustrates the major differences in VO$_2$ and energy release for the different macronutrients, showing the more than

Box 12.1 Summary of oxidation of the macronutrients. Adapted from [15]

Glucose
1 g glucose + 0.747 LO$_2$ = 0.747 LCO$_2$ + 0.6g H$_2$O + 15.15 kJ
RQ = 1.0
Energy content = 15 kJ/g
Energy release = 20.83 kJ/LO$_2$

Triglyceride
1 g fat + 2.023 LO$_2$ = 1.436 LCO$_2$ + 1.07g H$_2$O + 39.63 kJ
RQ = 0.71
Energy content = 39.63 kJ/g
Energy release = 19.59 kJ/LO$_2$

Protein
1 g protein + 1.031 LO$_2$ = 0.859 LCO$_2$ + 0.403g H$_2$0 + (urea, ammonia and creatinine) + 19.72 kJ
RQ = 0.833
Energy content = 19.72 kJ/g
Energy release = 19.13 kJ/LO$_2$

Table 12.3 Range of RQ values and interpretation

	RQ value	Related causes/factors
Physiologic range	0.70 to 1.0	
Glucose oxidation	1.0	High-CHO low-fat energy-sufficient diet
Fat oxidation	0.70	Underfeeding
		Low-carbohydrate high-fat energy-restricted diet
		Starvation
		Diabetes
Lipogenesis	>1.0	Overfeeding

twofold difference in energy released per gram of nutrient during the oxidation of fat compared with carbohydrate or protein, and that for a given EE a greater VO_2 is needed when using fat as a fuel compared to carbohydrate. The other major difference between the substrates is the CO_2/O_2 ratio – the RQ. The RQ value provides an indication of the principal substrate(s) being utilized. The standard RQ values for the main macronutrients are given in Box 12.1. These were obtained using conventional foods; however, RQ values may vary slightly for specific amino acids and fatty acids. The RQ value for alcohol, a common element of the diet contributing 5–10% of daily EI, is 0.67. The mean RQ for a standard Western diet is around 0.83–0.85. RQ values outside the physiologic range may be due to instrument or measurement error; however, a number of other factors may influence RQ [10] (Table 12.3).

High RQs indicating a low fat oxidation have been identified as a predictor of weight gain [11]. A study using a respiratory chamber has shown that muscle sympathetic nerve activity, a measure of sympathetic nervous outflow, is negatively associated ($r = -0.41$; $p = 0.01$) with RQ measured over 24 hours; regression analysis showed that sympathetic nerve activity, together with age and energy balance (EB, e.g. 24-hour EE minus EI) are independent determinants of 24-hour RQ [12]. In addition, there is evidence suggesting a familial resemblance in 24-hour RQ values independently of co-variates such as age, gender, and EB, recent preceding diet, and plasma variables such as free fatty acids (FFA) and insulin [13,14].

A more extensive account of the principles of IC in the measurement of EE can be found elsewhere [6,7,15,16].

Doubly labeled water (DLW) and the bicarbonate-urea methods

The traditional approaches of using direct or IC techniques to determine EE are able to detect minute-by-minute changes in EE but are of limited use in longer-term studies or for measuring free-living EE. This problem can be overcome by using the DLW method (using the nonradioactive isotopes deuterium and ^{18}O to assess mean daily EE (TEE) over a period of 10–14 days [17]. The DLW method is based on the principle that the metabolic processes of the body involve the incorporation of water in a number

of reactions. When such reactions occur the O_2 from the water can end up as CO_2 (and be lost from the body in expired air) whereas both the hydrogen and O_2 can end up in water and only be lost in sweat, urine and as respiratory water vapor. The rate of incorporation of water into these metabolic pathways is proportional to the rate of whole-body energy metabolism, so a measurement of the differential loss of O_2 and hydrogen labels from an initial, "doubly-labeled" loading dose provides an estimate of the body's rate of VCO_2, and thus VO_2, over the period of measurement [16]. The disadvantages of the DLW method are the availability and cost of the isotope, and the duration of the measurement. The method is unsuitable for detecting short-term differences in EE and is also unable to determine what fuel mix is being used. The former problem can be overcome with the "bicarbonate-urea" method [18], which produces valid estimates of TEE over a period of 2–3 days, involving the measurement of 14-carbon appearance in urinary urea. This method is relatively inexpensive, but does involve administering a radioactive substance (admittedly in very small amounts).

Noncalorimetric methods

Many researchers have attempted to use techniques such as heart rate monitoring (HR) and movement sensing to find cheaper and more feasible ways of measuring EE.

24-hour HR

There is a reasonably close relationship between HR and EE. Studies show a modest correlation between HR and VO_2 ($r = 0.68$), which improves ($r = 0.87$) after adjusting for age and fitness level; HR accounts for approximately 50% of the variability of VO_2 [19]. A recent study using HR to estimate PAEE in well-trained subjects with a predictive model including HR, gender, weight, age, and VO_{2max} showed a correlation coefficient of 0.91 between HR-predicted and IC-measured PAEE, explaining 83% of the variation in measured EE [20]. A predictive model without VO_{2max} still showed a high correlation ($r = 0.86$), explaining around 70% of the variation in measured EE.

A number of HR devices (usually in the form of a transmitter chest-strap and a watch-receiver) are commercially available. HR is usually monitored for approximately 16 hours (i.e. waking hours) during at least 3–4 days including weekdays and weekends in which work-related PA may vary. One of the approaches to estimate EE via HR monitoring is called the FLEX-HR method [21]. In this method, HR and VO_2 for each individual are simultaneously monitored while lying down, sitting, standing and doing exercise. The FLEX-HR is determined from the highest HR at rest and the lowest HR from light activity. RMR can be calculated from the VO_2 measured during resting or through a predictive equation. EE for values under this FLEX-HR threshold will be calculated as RMR; EE for HR values above the FLEX-HR threshold will be derived minute by minute from the VO_2 regression line obtained during exercise.

At low levels of EE (i.e. changes in posture at rest), HR rises more steeply than EE. HR is, furthermore, affected by factors other than PA such as emotional stress, high temperature and humidity, dehydration and illness in which changes in HR are unrelated to VO_2. The HR method is suitable for groups but its performance at the individual level can show great variation from the reference methods.

Accelerometry

Accelerometry [22] provides information on the amount, intensity, frequency and duration of most physical activities, an exception being swimming. Because triaxial monitors are designed to incorporate more planes of measurement (anteroposterior, mediolateral and vertical) than uniaxial (measuring acceleration in only one direction, usually vertical), these are probably more suitable to assess PA. A number of accelerometers have been developed, but only a few have been validated against EE calorimetric methods. The triaxial accelerometer, Tracmor (Philips Research, Eindhoven, The Netherlands), showed a correlation coefficient of 0.6–0.8 between EE from DLW and the activity counts [22].

The combination of HR and accelerometry has been used to estimate EE. The principle is to use a motion sensor as a back-up measure to confirm that elevations in HR are representative of response to PA. The preliminary studies showed the validity of this method in estimating EE [23]. A couple of devices are now available: the ActiReg that combines two pairs of motion sensors combined with HR monitoring, and the Intelligent Device for Energy Expenditure and Activity (IDEEA) that uses multiple sensors to assess body posture and body movement; validation against DLW is still pending.

Predictive equations

Information on RMR in conjunction with a multiplier for PA is essential to estimate energy requirements at a population level. Over 200 different predictive equations have been reported in the literature. However, the Harris–Benedict [24] and Schofield [25] equations remain the most commonly used when IC methodology is not available to estimate RMR. These formulae differ in terms of the inclusion of weight, height, age and sex.

The Schofield equations which were derived from a larger database, containing among other data those used by Harris and Benedict, were adopted by FAO/WHO/UNU in 1985. This database includes studies involving European and American individuals with most other groups being poorly represented. Therefore it is no surprise that overestimation of RMR in different populations has been reported [26].

Henry [26] has reported that Italian individuals, who had higher RMR than any of the other groups, comprise nearly 50% of the Schofield database. High RMRs among Italians might be related to the use of closed-circuit IC (see section on IC above), and to samples comprising young highly active subjects [26]. Therefore, a new database, "the Oxford database," excluding the Italian group and including RMR data from under-represented groups, has been used to derive new predictive equations (Table 12.4).

Components of energy expenditure

Whole-body EE can be separated into a number of components, with the major distinctions being between rest and activity (Fig. 12.2). The actual distribution of TEE between these two components obviously depends on the level of PA.

Resting EE
Fasting metabolic rate: BMR or RMR?

There is confusion and controversy about the usage of BMR and RMR. A simple search in PubMed for any of these terms gives very close results (BMR 6209, RMR 6370 items). The term "basal metabolism" was intended to differentiate between the energy expended under resting and active conditions. BMR is defined as "the daily rate of energy metabolism an individual needs in order to preserve the integrity of vital functions" [26]. Ideally, BMR should be measured under strictly standardized conditions. Subjects must be at complete rest (before and during the measurement, abstaining from significant muscle activity), in the postabsorptive state (fasting of at least 8–12 hours), under no emotional distress, wakeful, well nourished (e.g. weight-stable), free of disease or infection, and tested in a thermoneutral environment (22–26°C). However, in practice, it is very difficult to fulfill all these criteria; for example, measurements reported in the literature are often carried out at temperatures ranging from 9 to 15°C. BMR should not be confused with the sleeping metabolic rate which is approximately 10% lower than BMR. The fasting RMR, measured after an overnight fast and a period of at least 30 minutes supine rest, at a comfortable temperature, is a more appropriate assessment of someone's baseline level of metabolism. BMR is of little value when considering energy metabolism in relation to obesity, and is an expression which should not be used. The fasting RMR is slightly higher than BMR (approx. 10%), the reason for this being that it includes the thermic effect of arousal.

In most adult individuals the major component of TEE is RMR (65–75%) [27]. Mean day-to-day variability in the measurement of RMR using a ventilated hood is approximately 4% (range, 2–10%). Haugen et al [28] reported that RMR measured in the afternoon, after 4 hours fasting and 12 hours post exercise, was significantly greater (5%) than RMR measured in the morning (i.e. after 12 hours fasting and 12 hours post exercise). These results show a potential carry-over effect of the TEF and/or PA, increased afternoon RMR. In another study [29] the variability between repeated RMR measurements (assessed three times at 2-week intervals) was not explained by differences in prior nonexercise PA but by noncompliance with the protocol (e.g. fasting).

The main determinants of fasting RMR are body size and composition, in particular the size of the fat-free mass (FFM), the metabolically active tissue. Thus, the larger a person is, the greater their fasting RMR will be. Segal et al [30] showed in young men

Table 12.4 Prediction formulas for RMR

Author(s)	Formula*	Population in which formula was developed
Males		
Harris–Benedict	[66 + (13.8 × W) + (5 × H) − (6.8 × A) × 4.18]	Normal weight
Age category (yrs) (18–29)	[(63 × W) + 2896]	Normal weight, obese
(30–59)	[(48 × W) + 3653]	
(18–29)	[(63 × W) − (0.42 × H) + 2953]	
(30–59)	[(48 × W) − (0.11 × H) + 3670]	
Oxford equations		
Age category (yrs) (0–3)	[(0.255 × W) − 0.141]	
(3–10)	[(0.0937 × W) + 2.15]	
(10–18)	[(0.0769 × W) + 2.43]	
(18–30)	[(0.0669 × W) + 2.28]	
(30–60)	[(0.0592 × W) + 2.48]	
(60+)	[(0.0563 × W) + 2.15]	
(60–70)	[(0.0543 × W) + 2.37]	
(70+)	[(0.0573 × W) + 2.01]	
Females		
Harris–Benedict	[655 + (9.5 × W) + (1.9 × H) − (4.7 × A) × 4.18]	Normal weight
Age category (yrs) (18–29)	[(62 × W) + 2036]	Normal weight, obese
(30–59)	[(34 × W) + 3538]	
(18–29)	[(57 × W) + (11.84 × H) + 411]	
(30–59)	[(34 × W) + (0.06 × H) + 3530]	
Oxford equations		
Age category (yrs) (0–3)	[(0.246 × W) − 0.0965]	
(3–10)	[(0.0842 × W) + 2.12]	
(10–18)	[(0.0465 × W) + 3.18]	
(18–30)	[(0.0546 × W) + 2.33]	
(30–60)	[(0.0407 × W) + 2.90]	
(60+)	[(0.0424 × W) + 2.38]	
(60–70)	[(0.0429 × W) + 2.39]	
(70+)	[(0.0417 × W) + 2.41]	

*W, weight in kilograms; H, height in centimeters; A, age in years.
Harris–Benedict equations estimate RMR in kJ/24 h; Oxford equations in MJ/24 h.

(thus removing influences of age and gender) that when differences in FFM were taken into account by analysis of co-variance, there was no residual effect of fat mass, even though their subjects had a wide range of fat masses. Others [31] have reported that FFM accounts for up to 73% of the variation in 24-hour RMR while fat mass accounts for only 2%. Whilst size of FFM is the major determinant of fasting RMR, other variables also contribute to explain such variation. For example, it is known that RMR decreases with age at a rate of approximately 1–2% per decade in weight-stable subjects. Together, FFM, fat mass, age and sex account for approximately 80% of between-individuals variation in fasting RMR [32].

Some variation in the metabolic activity of the FFM does occur, as a consequence of differences in the composition of the FFM [33]. Small organs such as brain, heart, liver, and kidneys, contributing to approximately 5% of body weight, account for up to 70%

of RMR in adults. On the other hand, skeletal muscle comprises up to 50% of body weight but accounts for only 20–30% RMR.

Variations in RMR appear to be lower within families than between them, which indicates that RMR is to some extent genetically determined. In a study assessing familial dependence of RMR in American Indians [34], FFM, age and sex accounted for 83% of RMR variance; however, an additional 11% was accounted for by family membership.

Adrenoceptors have attracted substantial attention as possible genetic factors contributing to EE regulation. It was reported that a missense mutation in codon 64 of the gene for the β3-adrenoceptor with a replacement of tryptophan by arginine (Trp64Arg) may be implicated in obesity [35,36]. However, this was not confirmed by others [37]. Studies on the association between the Trp64Arg polymorphism and RMR also showed contradictory results [35,36,38].

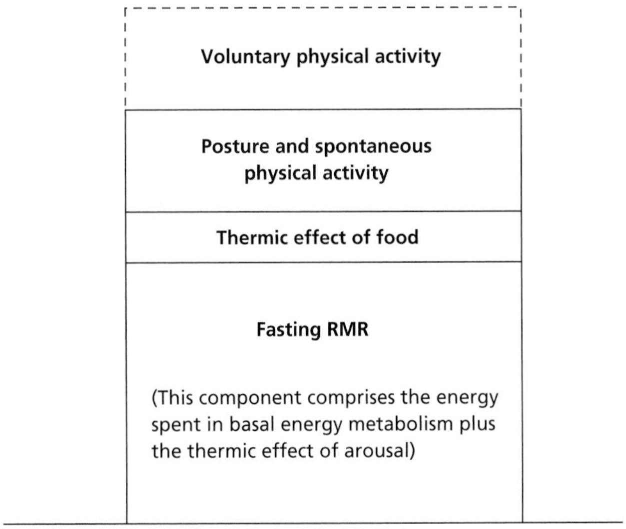

Figure 12.2 Components of TEE – the distribution represents a sedentary individual. Broken lines indicate that voluntary activity can be variable; a large amount of voluntary activity will increase TEE and reduce the proportional contribution of the other components.

Uncoupling proteins (UCPs) have also been investigated as factors controlling heat generation at the mitochondrial level which might affect EB, but the results were inconclusive [39]. Overall, in light of the emerging importance of gene polymorphisms in EE regulation, further investigations are required.

Other factors affecting RMR

Factors such as cold, stress, drugs, and hormonal changes can affect RMR. Growth in children involves numerous complex chemical processes which have a substantial energy cost. Protein synthesis and turnover alone account for approximately 25% of fasting RMR in healthy adults. The increased protein deposition during growth has an additional energy cost contributing to the elevated EE seen during growth spurts in children.

In many animal species (e.g. rats), chronic exposure to cold is associated with an increase in EE. During the early stages of cold exposure, EE increases due to shivering, but this is soon replaced by nonshivering mechanisms (nonshivering thermogenesis). Exposure of human beings to cold will produce an increase in EE due to shivering. Vigorous shivering can raise EE at least fourfold above baseline resting values. There is some controversy over the effects of cold exposure on nonshivering EE in humans. There is some evidence of increased thyroid hormone function and sleeping EE in nonobese women exposed to mild cold [40], which may represent a stimulation of nonshivering thermogenesis. In addition, 10 days of continued exposure to mild/moderate cold was associated with a 10–15% increase in fasting RMR [41]. This effect was small compared to the effect seen in cold-adapted rodents, and was only observed in those subjects demonstrating

adaptation to cold by a lowering of the core temperature threshold needed to elicit a shivering response.

It is known that thyroid hormone administration for several days increases RMR. Hyperthyroid patients have a higher RMR due to increased blood T_3 level and may attain 180% of the standard value [42]. There is no general agreement about the mechanism of thyroid hormone effect, but increases in the Na, K-ATPase activity in various tissues and in the protein turnover rate are likely contributors.

RMR varies over the menstrual cycle, probably due to changes in sex hormones. It may on average be 8% higher during the luteal phase of the menstrual cycle [43], while use of oral contraceptives may increase RMR by 5% [44].

Food ingestion: TEF

The consumption of food is associated with an increase in EE and VO_2. This was first observed over 200 years ago by Lavoisier, and since then has been described by a number of terms. Max Rubner called it specific dynamic action of protein. However, more appropriate terms for this process are the thermic effect of food (TEF) and diet-induced thermogenesis (DIT). Thermogenesis literally means heat production, and so can be equated with EE. However, it is generally used to represent conditions in which EE is stimulated above baseline. The term TEF defines the increase in EE after a single meal, while DIT describes the long-term (24-hour or longer) effect of dietary intake.

Diet-induced thermogenesis can be reduced during periods of underfeeding or when consuming a high-fat diet, and increased during overfeeding, especially with a high-carbohydrate intake. TEF for carbohydrates is approximately 5–10% of the energy ingested while for fat and protein it represents 3–5% and 20–30%, respectively [1,3]. Total TEF is approximately 7–9% of energy consumed after mixed meals of 400–1200 kcal in nonobese and obese subjects. The peak in TEF occurs between 60 and 180 minutes in most individuals, but it is delayed in obese and older people [45].

Potential influencing factors in TEF include the following.

Meal size

A major problem when trying to draw conclusions about possible differences in TEF after different-sized meals is the duration of the responses. Large meals (in excess of 4 MJ) can stimulate EE for several hours, making it very difficult to determine the total response. Reed and Hill [45] measured TEF for 6 hours after consumption of moderate-to-large meals with different composition and reported that at 3 hours 57% of TEF had been expended, at 4 hours 77%, and at 5 hours 91%. Calorimetric chamber studies measuring 24-hour EE show that at 5 hours after a meal, EE has not completely returned to baseline values [46].

There is some evidence that small meals produce smaller overall TEF than large meals, but in many cases the conclusions may not be reliable because of inappropriate study designs. For example, Tai et al [47] compared TEF over a 5-hour period to a single 3.1 MJ meal or to six 0.52 MJ meals eaten at 30-minute intervals. Overall, TEF over the 5 hours was less with the six meals, but this is likely to be in part due to the intermittent nature of the measurements, and the failure to measure the total response to the multiple small meals. Similarly, Vaz et al. [48] found a smaller TEF over 2 hours to three 1.05 MJ meals consumed in the first 60 minutes, compared to a single 3.15 MJ meal at the start of the 2 hours. However, neither response was maximal by 2 hours and measurements of EE were only made for 10–12 minutes in every 30. Thus, it would be unsafe to conclude that for the same total EI, a series of small meals is associated with a smaller TEF than a single large meal.

Meal frequency

We recently found that an irregular meal frequency led to a lower postprandial EE over 1–3 hours after a test meal, compared with a regular meal frequency in lean [49] and obese women [50]. Whilst a comprehensive feeding study is required to investigate the mechanism of this effect, it may have some practical significance as Western populations are increasingly moving away from regular meals, perhaps because of the wider availability of ready-prepared meals at home and greater opportunity to eat more meals outside the home.

It appears that meal type affects TEF, with solid food producing a greater response than homogenized liquids with the same nutrient content [51]. This has been attributed to the solid food being more palatable, producing a hedonistic response that increases the activation of the sympathetic nervous system (SNS). However, whilst we have confirmed this effect of solid food (compared with a liquid test meal), we did not find an accompanying enhancement of the plasma noradrenaline response (an index of the SNS) to the test meal [52].

An oral component of TEF has also been suggested. Some studies report lower TEF (40%) over 6 hours after tube feeding than after oral ingestion of isoenergetic meals by normal-weight subjects [53], an effect not observed in obese subjects. It is suggested that this may be a mechanism of adaptive thermogenesis.

Meal composition

It is widely believed that TEF is greater when consuming a high-carbohydrate meal than after an isoenergetic high-fat meal. This is partly based on the demonstrations that administration of glucose (either orally or intravenously) stimulates EE by the equivalent of 7–10% of the amount of glucose stored [54] but triglyceride infusion only produces an EE increase equivalent to 2% of the fat stored [55]. However, these effects are not always apparent when food is ingested, as Kinabo and Durnin [56] found no difference in TEF over 5 hours when meals with 70% carbohydrate or 65% fat were compared.

The types of carbohydrate and fat ingested may also have significant effects on TEF. Oral ingestion of fructose produces a greater TEF than the same amount of glucose [57]; it is less clear whether similar effects occur with nutrient mixtures (test meals). Meals containing saturated fat appear to produce a lower TEF than meals containing medium-chain triglyceride [58]. It has

been shown that substitution of 6 g visible fat by fish oil for a 3-week period was accompanied by an increase in fasting EE and fat oxidation [59]. Further work is needed to establish the effect of diet composition on EE.

Other nutritional factors

Recently much attention has been focused on the flavanol content of foods and their possible influence on EE. Tea consumption can promote fat oxidation and increase 24-hour EE [60,61]. These promoting effects are related not only to caffeine content but also to other constituents such as polyphenols, which have a synergistic effect on thermogenesis. Polyphenols may increase the turnover of noradrenaline, explaining the synergistic impact of these components on EE.

Insulin resistance

Several studies have now reported [62] a decreased thermic response to glucose ingestion in insulin-resistant and diabetic obese subjects compared with young noninsulin-resistant subjects. This is associated with a reduced rate of glucose uptake.

DIT: effects on TEE

With normal diets, eaten in sufficient quantities to satisfy energy requirements, the overall stimulation of EE is equal to 8–10% of EI [63]. Thus, an individual with a fasting RMR of 4 kJ/min, remaining supine and fasting for 24 hours, would use 5.76 MJ of energy. In order to maintain EB, the individual would require an equivalent to 110% of this (6.34 MJ) because of the amount of energy expended in DIT. Thus, it should be obvious that a low total EI will be associated with a lower DIT, and thus smaller TEE. This contributes to the reduction in EE seen with negative EB. However, the adaptation to excess EI is controversial. It was reported that an excessive total EI can lead to increased DIT and TEE [64], especially if consisting of excessive carbohydrate. This implies that the weight gain is lower than expected according to the raised EI. On the other hand, other investigations failed to confirm this phenomenon [65,66]. It was suggested that there is a threshold in cumulative overfeeding which could trigger the facultative thermogenesis to maintain EB. However, this is unlikely to occur with the modest degrees of overeating which are likely to contribute to the development of obesity.

Physical activity (PA)
PA level

The majority of the population is now so sedentary that PA only accounts for approximately 30% of TEE. This has undoubtedly contributed to the increased prevalence of obesity in recent years, and low levels of PA are also an independent risk factor for cardiovascular disease. Thus, increased levels of PA are important for promoting health, and as part of the lifestyle strategy needed to reduce the risk of obesity. This section will focus on the latter, considering the levels of EE associated with different types of PA, and also assessing the potential effects of regular PA on RMR and weight control.

Table 12.5 Energy costs of physical activities

Activity	kJ/min
Sleeping	4.5
Sitting	5.0
Standing	6.0
Brisk walking (6.4 km/h)	30.0
Running (8 km/h)	43.0
Cycling (l6 km/h)	30.0
Swimming (25 rn/min)	28.0

Values are estimations for a nonobese 70 kg individual.

At the simplest level, activity-related EE can be defined as any situation which raises EE above resting levels. Thus, maintaining an upright posture requires a higher EE (20–50%) than when seated. Any type of activity which is weight bearing (e.g. walking, running, climbing) requires an EE which is proportional to body weight and speed of movement. By contrast, activities such as swimming, rowing and to some extent cycling are less affected by body weight. Table 12.5 shows approximate EE for standard activities, although the actual value for any individual is dependent on his/her body weight and how the exercise is performed. One of the effects of learning and performing an activity regularly is that it may improve the effectiveness (or efficiency) of movements, so that a slightly lower EE is needed for the same activity. However, this effect is fairly modest and is unlikely to alter the EE by more than a few percent.

Types of PA

The simplest distinction which can be made is to separate the types of activity into those involving aerobic metabolic pathways and those requiring anaerobic mechanisms of energy release. The latter are of short duration, high-intensity types of activity such as sprinting (e.g. running for a bus) or running up the stairs. These types of activity have very high rates of EE (over 100 kJ/min) but can only be sustained for a few seconds. In addition, because the immediate energy release is anaerobic (usually with production of lactate) it takes several minutes to recover from the metabolic disturbances produced. Anaerobic PA is of little value in weight loss, although it may be of value in developing and maintaining muscle mass.

Aerobic PA is of much greater importance for TEE and the prevention and treatment of obesity. When describing an individual's capacity for aerobic activity, the term maximal VO_2 (VO_{2max}) is widely used. This is usually expressed as mL O_2/kg body weight (or FFM)/min, and describes the maximum rate an individual can sustain for at least 1 minute. Sedentary individuals have low VO_{2max} with values ranging from 30 to 40 mL/kg/min; highly active subjects can exceed 60 mL/kg/min. When one considers that a nonobese individual would have a fasting RMR of approximately 75 J/kg/min (equivalent to 3.8 mL O_2/kg/min), if

their VO_{2max} was 35 mL/kg/min, they would be exhausted when increasing EE by less than tenfold above resting.

PA at a large proportion of VO_{2max} (above 70%) cannot be maintained for long periods of time, except in physically highly trained subjects. However, provided someone becomes accustomed to being active, lower intensities of effort (40–60% VO_{2max}) can be sustained for up to several hours. Under these conditions, PA can make a substantial contribution to TEE, especially if the person's VO_{2max} is reasonably high.

The term nonexercise activity thermogenesis (NEAT) has been introduced to define the EE of all physical activities other than volitional sporting-like exercise, i.e. occupation-related (working, going to school) and leisure-related activities (dancing, playing the guitar, walking while shopping) [67]. There is now evidence suggesting that orexin, one of the body's neurochemical signals for vigilance and wakefulness, is associated with NEAT. Orexin-deficient animals suffer from sleep disorders and are obese, while orexin injected into the hypothalamus in rats increases NEAT in a dose-dependent fashion [68]. In addition, low orexin levels in cerebrospinal fluid are associated with abdominal fat in obese subjects [69].

Fuel utilization during activity

High-intensity activity requires a continuous supply of carbohydrate to the exercising muscles; lower-intensity exercise (e.g. below 50% VO_{2max}) can be sustained through the oxidation of fat [70]. Thus, if increased PA is to be used as part of a lifestyle strategy to prevent or treat obesity, it is usually of benefit to use lower-intensity activities which maximize the rates of fat oxidation. It has been suggested that obese individuals may have an altered fiber type profile within their skeletal muscles, such that they have a reduced capacity for oxidizing fat [71], but this is a controversial topic which has not been confirmed by subsequent studies. It is clear that increasing the level of habitual PA (training) can improve fat utilization at a given exercise intensity, but as most obese individuals are physically inactive, obesity will reduce the level of fat utilization during activity.

Effects of PA on RMR

There has been substantial debate as to whether the level of PA, or training, can affect RMR. It is well established that prolonged, high-intensity exercise can elevate RMR for several hours but it is less clear whether regular exercise training, or increased habitual PA, has a similar effect. Cross-sectional studies [72] show no relationship between VO_{2max} and RMR (per kg FFM); interestingly the subjects with the lowest VO_{2max} had the highest body fat content. In an intervention study the same authors [73] found no effect of 12-week increased PA, which increased VO_{2max} by 10%, on RMR of young men. However, the trained subjects in this study showed small reductions in body fat, indicative of a slight negative EB over the study period. Normally, negative EB is associated with a reduction in RMR, but the exercise-trained subjects did not show such a reduction. By contrast, Poehlman et al. [74] found a weak but significant relationship between RMR and VO_{2max} in nonobese young women ($r = 0.54$), even when controlling for body composition ($r = 0.38$).

PA, EB and body weight

One argument against the use of increased PA as a means of regulating EB is that it will stimulate EI. However, many studies show that when subjects change from a sedentary lifestyle to moderate PA levels, there is no increase in EI. The study by Broeder et al. [73] provides an example of this, where 1 hour of exercise, 4 days/week for 12 weeks was not accompanied by any increase in voluntary FI. Obviously, very high PA levels need to be accompanied by an appropriate EI, with a high-carbohydrate diet being of particular importance when high-intensity exercise is performed.

Increasing PA as an adjunct to dietary modification for weight loss in obesity would result in greater negative EB and body fat loss. However, of greater importance is that the combination of diet and exercise produces a greater loss of body fat (but not FFM) than diet alone [75]. Furthermore, Racette et al. [76] showed that increasing PA level improved the ability of obese subjects to comply with a dietary restriction program.

In addition, PA is widely recommended to prevent and treat obesity-related complications such as type 2 diabetes and coronary heart disease (CHD).

Increasing PA favorably influences several markers of vascular risk such as high-density lipoprotein (HDL) cholesterol, serum triglyceride concentration and both low-density lipoprotein (LDL) and HDL particle sizes. PA, furthermore, increases insulin sensitivity and reduces the risk of type 2 diabetes. These beneficial effects are modest and variable; however, they are important in reducing the morbidity and mortality from CHD on a population level, and specifically important in patients with atherogenic dyslipidemia.

Mechanisms and sites of thermogenesis and the sympathetic nervous system

There are numerous thermogenic mechanisms, including substrate cycling, mitochondrial uncoupling in brown adipose tissue and increased sodium pump activity, the details of which are beyond the scope of this chapter. However, it is worthwhile considering which tissues and organs may be important sites of thermogenesis (i.e. increased resting EE) in adult humans, and what role the SNS may have in regulating their metabolic activity.

Thermogenic stimuli

It has been known for over 70 years that the catecholamines noradrenaline and adrenaline can stimulate RMR in humans [77]. The plasma adrenaline threshold for stimulating EE is just above normal resting concentrations [78], with mild stimuli such as postural change and mental arithmetic being capable of raising the concentrations above this threshold. Maximal stimulation of EE (25–30% above resting) occurs when adrenaline

concentrations rise to 5–10-fold above basal. It was originally thought that catecholamine-induced thermogenesis was due to a stimulation of lipolysis in adipose tissue and increased fat oxidation [79] but it is now clear that at steady state there is a generalized stimulation of metabolism with increased fat and carbohydrate oxidation and little change in RQ. In association with this, it is clear that many tissues of the body are involved in the thermogenic response to catecholamines, with skeletal muscle and the viscera being particularly important [80].

It is possible that some of the nutrient-induced thermogenesis discussed earlier is due to a stimulatory effect of catecholamines, as in some circumstances the β-adrenoceptor antagonist propranolol can reduce the thermogenic response to glucose [81] and food [82]. However, it is of interest that not all nutrients produce thermogenic responses in the same tissues or organs. Intravenous infusion of amino acids increases whole-body EE by 19%, with half of the effect occurring in the splanchnic tissues [83]. By contrast, the stimulation of EE due to oral ingestion of fructose or glucose has no effect on the splanchnic tissues [84].

The SNS

Since the demonstration by Landsberg and Young [85] of reduction in SNS activity during fasting in rats, there has been great interest in the possibility that altered sympathoadrenal control of metabolism and thermogenesis may contribute to the development of obesity. Furthermore, sympathomimetics which stimulate EE are viewed as of potential therapeutic value for obese individuals. However, review of the literature on the assessment of sympathoadrenal activity in the obese yields conflicting information, with similar numbers of studies showing reduced, unchanged or increased SNS activity in obese compared to lean subjects [86]. Interestingly, this review provided clearer evidence of reduced adrenal medullary activity in the obese, and the implications of this for EE deserve further attention. An extension to this review [87] revealed an altered relationship between an index of SNS activity (muscle sympathetic nerve activity) and resting EE in Pima Indians, indicating that the development of obesity in this group may be associated with a defective SNS influence on metabolism.

Whilst there is some evidence of a link between SNS activation and TEF, especially in younger but not older subjects [88], the administration of a β-adrenoceptor antagonist does not always reduce TEF [89]. However, we have observed an effect of diet composition on fasting plasma noradrenaline concentrations (an index of SNS activity) and the responses to meal ingestion, such that high-sucrose diets and test meals produce larger responses than high starch or high fat [90]. In addition, the high-sucrose diet was associated with greater 24-hour EE than the other two diets. Thus, further studies are needed to examine the influence of diet composition on any SNS effect on EE.

Some caution is needed when considering the possible use of sympathomimetics to stimulate EE in the obese, because undesirable cardiovascular effects may occur. It is clear that catecholamine stimulation of EE in humans is mediated by β-adrenoceptors, with some debate as to the dominant receptor subtype (β$_2$ or β$_3$). However, the concern is that any generalized activation of the SNS or release of adrenaline from the adrenal medulla has the potential of producing stimulation of the heart (β$_1$-adrenoceptors) or of increasing blood pressure due to α-adrenoceptor effects causing arterial vasoconstriction. Thus, any pharmacologic approach needs to be selective for effects on EE, in order that undesirable side-effects are avoided.

Obesity and energy expenditure

Obesity can only develop as a consequence of a prolonged period of positive EB; therefore a reduction in EE can theoretically contribute to weight gain. For many years there was a widely held view that very low RMRs may be a cause of obesity. However, it is now clear that such low RMRs only occur in severe hypothyroidism, and that this is a negligible cause of obesity. The advent of the DLW method has shown that the obese do not have reduced TEE compared to nonobese subjects. In fact, because the obese are larger, with a greater FFM than the nonobese, they usually have a greater TEE [91]. This higher TEE is usually accompanied, in weight-stable obese subjects, by a fasting RMR per kg/FFM similar to nonobese subjects.

Table 12.6 compares the body composition of a nonobese 70 kg individual and a 100 kg obese person. The difference in total body fat (26.6 kg) is equivalent to 1037 MJ of stored energy. If the nonobese person's TEE was 10 MJ/day, with a positive EB of +10% of this (1 MJ/day), it would take at least 3 years to increase body weight and fat content to those of the 100 kg person. In reality, most cases of obesity probably develop over a longer period of time with a smaller daily positive EB. Prospective studies in the Pima Indians (a group with high prevalence of obesity) have shown that in adults a low 24-hour EE is associated with a high weight gain over the next 2 years [90]. Similar observations have been made in infants [93] and children [94]; however, on average the low 24-hour EE only explains 40% of the weight gain. Subsequent observations on the Pima Indians

showed that in males (but not females), weight gain was associated with a lower EE associated with spontaneous PA [95].

Thus, a low 24-hour EE, due at least in part to low PA, is a risk factor for weight gain and the development of obesity. The weight-stable obese do not have a low EE, if anything it is elevated, but PA makes a smaller contribution to TEE than in the nonobese. Whilst there is evidence of reduced TEF responses to meals in the obese, this is probably secondary to their insulin resistance and possibly the insulating effect of the adipose tissue [96]. Weight reduction to nonobese values is almost always associated with a normalization of these reduced TEF responses [97,98].

Table 12.6 Body composition and body energy content

	Nonobese	Obese
Weight (kg)	70	100
Fat mass (kg)	8.4	35
Fat % body weight	12	35
Fat energy (MJ)	327	1365
FFM (kg)	61.6	65
Glycogen (kg)	1	1
CHO energy (MJ)	16	16
Protein (kg)	15	16
Protein energy (MJ)	255	272
Total energy (MJ)	598	1653
Fat energy as % total	55	83

References

1. Kleiber M. *The Fire of Life: An Introduction to Animal Energetics.* Huntington: Krieger, 1975.
2. Prentice AM. Le Symposium Lavoisier. Proc Nutr Soc 1995;54:1–8.
3. Lusk G. *The elements of the science of nutrition.* Philadelphia: Saunders, 1928.
4. Forbes GB. Energy intake and body weight: a reexamination of two "classic" studies. Am J Clin Nutr 1984;39:349–50.
5. Kinney JM. Indirect calorimetry in malnutrition: nutritional assessment or therapeutic reference? J Parenteral Enteral Nutr 1987;11: 90S–94S.
6. Webb P. *Human Calorimeters.* New York: Praeger, 1985.
7. Maclean JA, Tobin G. *Animal and Human Calorimetry.* New York: Cambridge University Press, 1987.
8. Clark HD, Hoffer LJ. Reappraisal of the resting metabolic rate of normal young men. Am J Clin Nutr 1991;53:21–6.
9. Dauncey MJ, Murgatroyd PR, Cole TJ. A human calorimeter for the direct and indirect measurement of 24-h energy expenditure. Br J Nutr 1978;39:557–66.
10. Schutz Y, Ravussin E. Respiratory quotients lower than 0.70 in ketogenic diets. Am J Clin Nutr 1980;33:1317–19.
11. Zurlo F, Lillioja S, Esposito-Del Puente A, et al. Low ratio of fat to carbohydrate oxidation as predictor of weight gain: study of 24-h RQ. Am J Physiol 1990;259:E650–E657.
12. Snitker S, Tataranni PA, Ravussin E. Respiratory quotient is inversely associated with muscle sympathetic nerve activity. J Clin Endocrinol Metab 1998;83:3977–9.
13. Toubro S, Sørensen TI, Hindsberger C, et al. Twenty-four-hour respiratory quotient: the role of diet and familial resemblance. J Clin Endocrinol Metab 1998;83:2758–64.
14. Jacobson P, Rankinen T, Tremblay A, et al. Resting metabolic rate and respiratory quotient: results from a genome-wide scan in the Quebec Family Study. Am J Clin Nutr 2006;84:1527–33.
15. Frayn KN, Macdonald IA. Assessment of substrate and energy metabolism in vivo. In: Draznin B, Pizza R (eds) *Clinical Research in Diabetes and Obesity,* vol1. Totowa, NJ: Humana Press, 1997:101 –24.
16. Murgatroyd PR, Shetty PS, Prentice AM. Techniques for the measurement of human energy expenditure: a practical guide. Int J Obes 1993;17:549–68.
17. Prentice AM. Applications of the doubly labelled water (^{2}H$_2$^{18}O) method in free-living adults. Proc Nutr Soc 1988;47:259–68.

18. Elia M, Jones MG, Jennings G, et al. Estimating energy expenditure from the specific activity of urine urea during lengthy subcutaneous NaH^{14}C0$_3$ infusion. Am J Physiol 1995;269:E172–E182.

19. Strath SJ, Swartz AM, Bassett DR Jr, et al. Evaluation of heart rate as a method for assessing moderate intensity physical activity. Med Sci Sports Exerc 2000;32:S465–S470.

20. Keytel LR, Goedecke JH, Noakes TD, et al. Prediction of energy expenditure from heart rate monitoring during submaximal exercise. J Sports Sci 2005;23:289–97.

21. Spurr G, Prentice A, Murgatroyd P, et al. Energy expenditure from minute-by-minute heart-rate recording: comparison with indirect calorimetry. Am J Clin Nutr 1988;48:552–9.

22. Plasqui G, Westerterp KR. Physical activity assessment with accelerometers: an evaluation against doubly labeled water. Obesity 2007;15:2371–9.

23. Rennie K, Rowsell T, Jebb S, et al. A combined heart rate and movement sensor: proof of concept and preliminary testing study. Eur J Clin Nutr 2000;54:409–14.

24. Harris J, Benedict F. A biometric study of basal metabolism in man. (Publication no. 279). Washington, DC: Carnegie Institute, 1919.

25. Schofield WN. Predicting basal metabolic rate, new standard and review of previous work. Hum Nutr Clin Nutr 1985;39c:5–41.

26. Henry CJ. Basal metabolic rate studies in humans: measurement and development of new equations. Pub Health Nutr 2005;8:1133–52.

27. Ravussin E, Lillioja S, Anderson TE, et al. Determinants of 24-hour energy expenditure in man. Methods and results using a respiratory chamber. J Clin Invest 1986;78:1568–78.

28. Haugen HA, Melanson EL, Tran ZV, et al. Variability of measured resting metabolic rate. Am J Clin Nutr 2003;78:1141–4.

29. Adriaens MP, Schoffelen PF, Westerterp K. Intra-individual variation of basal metabolic rate and the influence of daily habitual physical activity before testing. Br J Nutr 2003;90:419–23.

30. Segal KR, Lacayanga I, Dunaif A, et al. Impact of body fat mass and percent fat on metabolic rate and thermogenesis in men. Am J Physiol 1989;256:E573–E579.

31. Nelson KM, Weinsier RL, Long CL, et al. Prediction of resting energy expenditure from fat-free mass and fat mass. Am J Clin Nutr 1992;56:848–56.

32. Rising R, Harper LT, Fontvieille AM, et al. Determinants of total daily energy expenditure: variability in physical activity. Am J Clin Nutr 1994;59:800–4.

33. Elia M. Organ and tissue contribution to metabolic rate. In: Kinney JM, Tucker HN (eds) *Energy Metabolism: Tissue Determinants and Cellular Corollaries.* New York: Raven Press, 1992:61–79.

34. Bogardus C, Lillioja S, Ravussin E, et al. Familial dependence of the resting metabolic rate. N Engl J Med 1986;315:96–100.

35. Clement K, Ruiz J, Cassard-Doulcier A, et al. Additive effect of A → G (−3826) variant of the uncoupling protein gene and the Trp64Arg mutation of the beta 3-adrenergic receptor gene on weight gain in morbid obesity. Int J Obes 1996;20:1062–6.

36. Clement K, Vaisse C, Manning BSJ, et al. Genetic variation in the β3-adrenergic receptor and an increased capacity to gain weight in patients with morbid obesity. N Engl J Med 1995;333:352–4.

37. Gagnon J, Mauriege P, Roy S, et al. The Trp64Arg mutation of the beta3 adrenergic receptor gene has no effect on obesity phenotypes in the Quebec Family Study and Swedish Obese Subjects Cohorts. J Clin Invest 1996;98:2086–93.

38. Sipilainen R, Uusitupa M, Heikkinen S, et al. Polymorphism of the β3-adrenergic receptor gene affects basal metabolic rate in obese Finns. Diabetes 1997;46:77–80.

39. Ricquier D, Bouillaud F. Mitochondrial uncoupling proteins: from mitochondria to the regulation of energy balance. J Physiol 2000;529:3–10.

40. Lean MEJ, Murgatroyd PR, Rothnie I, et al. Metabolic and thyroid responses to mild cold are abnormal in obese and diabetic women. Clin Endocrinol 1988;28:665–73.

41. Bruck K, Baum E, Schwennicke HP. Cold-adaptive modifications in man induced by repeated short-term cold exposures and during a 10-day and night cold exposure. Pflugers Arch 1976;363:125–33.

42. Randin J, Schutz Y, Scazziga B, et al. Unaltered glucose-induced thermogenesis in Graves' disease. Am J Clin Nutr 1986;43:738–44.

43. Bisdee JT, James WP, Shaw MA. Changes in energy expenditure during the menstrual cycle. Br J Nutr 1989;61:187–99.

44. Diffey B, Piers LS, Soares MJ, et al. The effect of oral contraceptive agents on the basal metabolic rate of young women. Br J Nutr 1997;77:853–62.

45. Reed GW, Hill JO. Measuring the thermic effect of food. Am J Clin Nutr 1996;63:164–9.

46. Westerterp KR. Diet induced thermogenesis. Nutr Metab 2004;1:5.

47. Tai MM, Carsillo P, Pi-Sunyer FX. Meal size and frequency: effect on the thermic effect of food. Am J Clin Nutr 1991;54:783–7.

48. Vaz M, Tuner A, Kingwell B, et al. Postprandial sympathoadrenal activity: its relation to metabolic and cardiovascular events and to changes in meal frequency. Clin Sci 1995;89:349–57.

49. Farshchi H, Taylor MA, Macdonald IA. Decreased thermic effect of food after an irregular compared with a regular meal pattern in healthy lean women. Int J Obes 2004;28:653–60.

50. Farshchi HR, Taylor MA, Macdonald IA. Beneficial metabolic effects of regular meal frequency on dietary thermogenesis, insulin sensitivity, and fasting lipid profiles in healthy obese women. Am J Clin Nutr 2005;81:16–24.

51. LeBlanc J, Brondel I. Role of palatability on meal-induced thermogenesis in human subjects. Am J Physiol 1985;248:E333–E336.

52. Habas ME, Macdonald IA. Metabolic and cardiovascular responses to a liquid and solid test meal. Br J Nutr 1998;79:241–7.

53. Garrel DR, de Jonge L. Intragastric vs oral feeding: effect on the thermogenic response to feeding in lean and obese subjects. Am J Clin Nutr 1994;59:971–4.

54. Thiebaud D, Schutz Y, Acheson K, et al. Energy cost of glucose storage in human subjects during glucose-insulin infusions. Am J Physiol 1983;244:E216–E221.

55. Thiebaud D, Acheson K, Schutz Y, et al. Stimulation of thermogenesis in men after combined glucose, long-chain triglyceride infusion. Am J Clin Nutr 1983;37:603–11.

56. Kinabo JL, Durnin JVGA. Thermic effect of food in man: effect of meal composition and energy content. Br J Nutr 1990;64:37–44.

57. Tappy L, Randin JP, Felber JP, et al. Comparison of thermogenic effect of fructose and glucose in normal humans. Am J Physiol 1986;250:E718–E724.

58. Scalfi L, Coltorti A, Contaldo F. Post-prandial thermogenesis in lean and obese subjects after meals supplemented with medium-chain and long-chain triglycerides. Am J Clin Nutr 1991;53:1130–3.

59. Couet C, Delarue J, Ritz P, et al. Effect of dietary fish oil on body fat mass and basal fat oxidation in healthy adults. Int J Obes 1997;21:637–43.

60. Dulloo AG, Duret C, Rohrer D, et al. Efficacy of a green tea extract rich in catechin polyphenols and caffeine in increasing 24-h energy expenditure and fat oxidation in humans. Am J Clin Nutr 1999;70: 1040–5.

61. Rumpler W, Seale J, Clevidence B, et al. Oolong tea increases metabolic rate and fat oxidation in men. J Nutr 2001;131:2848–52.

62. Golay A, Schutz Y, Meyer HU, et al. Glucose – induced thermogenesis in nondiabetic and diabetic obese subjects. Diabetes 1982;31:1023–8.

63. Schutz Y, Bessard T, Jequier E. Diet-induced thermogenesis measured over a whole day in obese and nonobese women. Am J Clin Nutr 1984;40:542–52.

64. Webb P, Annis JF. Adaptation to overeating in lean and overweight men and women. Hum Nutr Clin Nutr 1983;37:117–31.

65. Norgan NG, Durnin JV. The effect of 6 weeks of overfeeding on the body weight, body composition, and energy metabolism of young men. Am J Clin Nutr 1980;33:978–88.

66. Siervo M, Fruhbeck G, Dixon A, et al. Efficiency of autoregulating homeostatic responses to imposed caloric excess in lean men. Am J Physiol Endocrinol Metab 2008;294:E416–E424.

67. Levine JA. Nonexercise activity thermogenesis – liberating the life-force. J Intern Med 2007;262:273–87.

68. Kiwaki K, Kotz CM, Wang C, et al. Orexin A (hypocretin 1) injected into hypothalamic paraventricular nucleus and spontaneous physical activity in rats. Am J Physiol Endocrinol Metab 2004;286:E551–E559.

69. Kok SW, Overeem S, Visscher TL, et al. Hypocretin deficiency in narcoleptic humans is associated with abdominal obesity. Obes Res 2003;11:1147–54.

70. Astrand PO, Rodahl K. *Textbook of Work Physiology*, 2nd edn. New York: McGraw-Hill, 1977.

71. Wade AJ, Marbut MM, Round JM. Muscle fibre type and aetiology of obesity. Lancet 1990;335:805–8.

72. Broeder CE, Burrhus KA, Svanevik LS, et al. The effects of aerobic fitness on resting metabolic rate. Am J Clin Nutr 1992;55:795–801.

73. Broeder CE, Burrhus KA, Svanevik LS, et al. The effects of either high-intensity resistance or endurance training on resting metabolic rate. Am J Clin Nutr 1992;55:802–10.

74. Poehlman ET, Viers HF, Detzer M. Influence of physical activity and dietary restraint on resting energy expenditure in young, non-obese females. Can J Physiol Pharmacol 1991;69:320–6.

75. Kempen KPG, Saris WHM, Westerterp KR. Energy balance during an 8-wk energy-restricted diet with and without exercise in obese women. Am J Clin Nutr 1995;62:722–9.

76. Racette SB, Schoeller DA, Kushner RF, et al. Exercise enhances dietary compliances during moderate energy restriction in obese women. Am J Clin Nutr 1995;62:345–9.

77. Cori CF, Buchwald KW. Effect of continuous injection of epinephnine on the carbohydrate metabolism, basal metabolism and vascular system of normal man. Am J Physiol 1930;95:71–8.

78. Macdonald IA, Bennett T, Fellows IW. Catecholamines and the control of metabolism in man. Clin Sci 1985;68:613–19.

79. Steinberg D, Nestel PI, Buskirk ER, et al. Calorigenic effect of norepinephrine correlated with plasma free fatty acid turnover and oxidation. J Clin Invest 1964;43:167–76.

80. Webber J, Macdonald IA. Metabolic actions of catecholamines in man. Baillière's Clin Endocrinol Metab 1993;7:393–413.

81. Acheson KJ, Jequier E, Wahren J. Influence of f~-adrenergic blockade on glucose induced thermogenesis in man. J Clin Invest 1983;72: 893–902.

82. Astrup A, Christensen NJ, Simonsen L, et al. Effects of nutrient intake on sympathoadrenal activity and thermogenic mechanisms. J Neurosci Methods 1990;34:187–92.

83. Aksnes AK, Brundin T, Hjeltnes N, et al. Metabolic, thermal and circulatory effects of intravenous infusion of amino acids in tetraplegic patients. Clin Physiol 1995;15:377–96.

84. Brundin T, Wahren J. Whole body and splanchnic oxygen consumption and blood flow after oral ingestion of fructose or glucose. Am J Physiol 1993;264:E504–E513.

85. Landsberg L, Young JB. Fasting, feeding and the regulation of the sympathetic nervous system. N Engl J Med 1978;298:1295–301.

86. Young JB, Macdonald IA. Sympathoadrenal activity in human obesity: heterogeneity of findings since 1980. Int J Obes 1992;16: 959–67.

87. Macdonald IA. Advances in our understanding of the role of the sympathetic nervous system in obesity. Int J Obes 1995;19:S2–S7.

88. Schwartz RS, Jaeger LF, Veith RC. The thermic effect of feeding in older men: the importance of the sympathetic nervous system. Metabolism 1990;39:733–7.

89. Nacht CA, Christin L, Temler E, et al. Thermic effect of food: possible implication of parasympathetic nervous system. Am J Physiol 1987;253:E481–E488.

90. Raben A, Macdonald IA, Astrup A. Replacement of dietary fat by sucrose or starch: effects on 14 days' ad libitum energy intake, energy expenditure and body weight in formerly obese and non-obese subjects. Int J Obes 1997;21:846–59.

91. Welle S, Forbes GB, Start M, et al. Energy expenditure under free-living conditions in normal weight and overweight women. Am J Clin Nutr 1992;55:14–21.

92. Ravussin E, Lillioja S, Knowler WC, et al. Reduced rate of energy expenditure as a risk factor for body weight gain. N Engl J Med 1988;318:467–72.

93. Roberts SB, Savage J, Coward WA, et al. Energy expenditure and intake in infants born to lean and overweight mothers. N Engl J Med 1988;318:461–6.

94. Griffiths M, Payne PR, Stunkard AJ, et al. Metabolic rate and physical development in children at risk of obesity. Lancet 1990;336:76–7.

95. Zurlo F, Ferraro R, Fontvieile AM, et al. Spontaneous physical activity and obesity: cross-sectional and longitudinal studies in Pima Indians. Am J Physiol 1992;263:E296–E300.

96. Brundin T, Thörne A, Wahren J. Heat leakage across the abdominal wall and meal-induced thermogenesis in normal-weight and obese subjects. Metabolism 1992;41:49–55.

97. Bukkens SGF, McNeill G, Smith JS, et al. Postprandial thermogenesis in post-obese women and weight matched controls. Int J Obes 1991;15:147–54.

98. Tataranni PA, Mingrone G, Greco AV, et al. Glucose-induced thermogenesis in post-obese women who have undergone biliopancreatic diversion. Am J Clin Nutr 1994;60:320–6.

3 Obesity and Disease

13 Obesity and Dyslipidemia: Importance of Body Fat Distribution

André Tchernof[1] and Jean-Pierre Després[2]

[1] Endocrinology and Genomics, Laval University, Quebec, Canada
[2] Quebec Heart Institute, Laval University, Quebec, Canada

Overview of lipid and lipoprotein metabolism

Cholesterol and triglycerides are hydrophobic compounds which are transported in the blood by lipoproteins. On the basis of their density and composition, four major subclasses of lipoproteins have been identified: chylomicrons, very low-density lipoproteins (VLDL), low-density lipoproteins (LDL) and high density lipoproteins (HDL) (Fig. 13.1).

Chylomicrons are the largest, most buoyant lipoproteins and contain mostly triglycerides. The protein constituents of these particles are apolipoprotein (Apo) E and C (II and III) as well as intestine-synthesized Apo B48, which are responsible for lipoprotein catabolism and structural integrity. Chylomicrons are synthesized in the intestine shortly after a meal and represent the form by which most of the dietary fatty acids are transported in the plasma in the form of triglycerides. Endothelial lipoprotein lipase (LPL) is responsible for the hydrolysis of triglycerides contained within chylomicrons [1]. The resulting chylomicron remnants are taken up by remnant receptors in the liver including the LDL receptor and LDL receptor-related protein (LRP) through an Apo E-dependent process [2]. VLDLs are synthesized by the liver and contain Apo B-100, E and C. VLDL synthesis rates rely mainly on the availability of neutral lipids from either *de novo* lipogenesis, hepatocyte cytoplasmic triglyceride stores, fatty acids derived from lipoproteins taken up by the liver (mainly chylomicron remnants) or plasma free fatty acids (FFA). The relative contribution of each of these sources varies according to the nutritional, hormonal and metabolic status of the patient [3]. In the fasting state, most triglycerides are contained within VLDL particles. Intermediate-density lipoproteins (IDLs) and LDLs are the catabolic products of VLDLs, resulting from the hydrolysis of the triglyceride content of VLDL particles by both LPL and hepatic lipase [1]. LDL particles are the main carriers of cholesterol in the blood. Apo B-100 synthesized in the liver is their main protein constituent, and only one molecule of Apo B is found per LDL particle. IDL and LDL are taken up by the liver through binding of Apo B and E to the LDL receptor. The formation of HDL particles results from the hydrolysis of VLDL to LDL, a process during which excess surface components aggregate to form nascent HDL particles (see Fig. 13.1). The major apolipoproteins of HDL particles are Apo A-I and Apo A-II. According to the concept of reverse cholesterol transport [4], HDL particles promote the net movement of cholesterol from extrahepatic tissues back to the liver [5].

Dyslipidemic states and the risk of coronary heart disease

Coronary heart disease (CHD) is recognized as a major cause of mortality and morbidity in affluent societies. In this regard, scientific evidence supporting the notion that high plasma cholesterol and LDL-cholesterol concentrations are associated with an increased risk of CHD is unequivocal[6–8]. Epidemiologic studies have established that each 1% increase in LDL-cholesterol leads to a 1–2% increase in coronary artery disease mortality rate [9]. Accordingly, interventions aimed at plasma LDL-cholesterol reduction have been shown to decrease coronary artery disease events significantly [10–15]. However, measuring LDL-cholesterol levels, along with traditional CHD risk factors such as cigarette smoking, hypertension, diabetes and family history of cardiovascular disease (CVD), only allows the identification of approximately 50% of the population that will eventually develop

Clinical Obesity in Adults and Children, 3rd edition. Edited by Peter G. Kopelman, Ian D. Caterson and William H. Dietz.
© 2010 Blackwell Publishing, ISBN: 978-1-4051-8226-3.

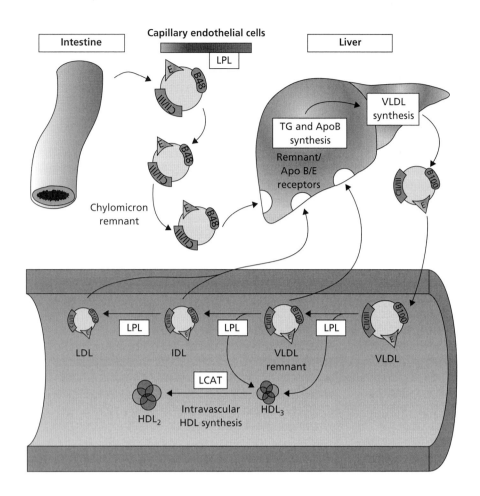

Figure 13.1 Overview of lipoprotein metabolism and lipid transport. Dietary fatty acids are incorporated in the form of triglycerides into chylomicrons in the intestine. Endothelial lipoprotein lipase (LPL) is responsible for the hydrolysis of triglycerides contained in chylomicrons. The resulting chylomicron remnants are taken up by the remnant receptors in the liver. VLDL particles containing Apo B-100 are synthesized by the liver. These particles are submitted to the catabolic activity of endothelial LPL in the circulation, leading to the formation of VLDL remnants, IDL and LDL particles, which are progressively depleted in triglycerides and enriched in cholesterol. VLDL remnants are taken up by the remnant receptors in the liver, whereas IDL and LDL bind to the Apo B/E receptor (LDL receptor). HDL particles are generated by aggregation of excess surface components resulting from the hydrolysis of Apo B-containing particles by LPL. The cholesterol ester content of HDL is also increased during this process (HDL$_2$ subfraction).

the disease [16]. For instance, a study from Genest and colleagues [17] has shown that there is considerable overlap in plasma cholesterol concentrations among subjects with and without CHD, as almost 50% of patients with the disease had rather "normal" plasma cholesterol levels [17]. Accordingly, Sniderman and Silberberg [18] have suggested that although mean plasma cholesterol levels may be higher in patients with CHD compared to healthy subjects, the overlap of cholesterol values in these two groups of individuals is such that the ability of cholesterol alone to discriminate subjects at risk for CHD is relatively weak [18,19].

With respect to cholesterol lowering, although the reduction in coronary heart disease event rate has been clearly established in clinical trials, a significant number of treated patients still develop a first or a recurrent event [7,10,14]. Consequently, beyond traditional risk factors and LDL-cholesterol levels, a collection of nontraditional risk factors has emerged including prothrombotic factors and proinflammatory markers, as well as measures reflecting lipoprotein heterogeneity such as apolipoprotein B levels, triglyceride concentrations, and small, dense LDL particles. This was well illustrated in the large myocardial infarction case versus control INTERHEART study, which reported that almost 90% of all cases could be explained by the following modifiable factors: the Apo B/Apo A1 ratio, smoking,

hypertension, diabetes, abdominal obesity, psychosocial factors, consumption of fruits, vegetables and alcohol, and regular physical activity [20]. These results clearly emphasize that a lower number of myocardial infarction cases remained unexplained once new and important risk factors are considered.

Apolipoprotein concentrations could reflect the concentrations of lipoproteins which protect against or promote premature atherosclerosis, and thereby provide clinically relevant information. As mentioned, the ratio of Apo B over Apo A-I has been shown to be a strong predictor of CHD risk in several studies [19–23]. Patients with elevated LDL-Apo B, but with LDL-cholesterol values within the normal range, are generally characterized by an elevated number of small, dense LDL particles, which have been shown in several studies to be associated with an increased risk of cardiovascular disease [24]. The presence of these atherogenic LDL particles most likely arises from an increased flow of triglycerides from triglyceride-rich lipoproteins to LDLs through the action of the cholesteryl ester transfer protein (CETP). Such transfer, which contributes to deplete LDL particles in cholesterol ester and increase their triglyceride content, is amplified in hypertriglyceridemic states [24]. LDL heterogeneity reflecting differences in LDL particle composition and density is now recognized as an important factor which contributes to the link between dyslipidemic states and the risk of coronary heart disease.

Epidemiologic studies have also clearly established that a low plasma HDL-cholesterol concentration is a very potent and independent risk factor for coronary heart disease [25,26]. The levels of Apo A-I, the main protein component of HDL, are also reduced in patients with coronary heart disease [27]. Despite the fact that HDL-cholesterol has long been recognized as an independent risk factor, HDL particles are also heterogeneous in size and composition [5,28]. As for LDL, the presence of hypertriglyceridemia also appears to be a major factor modulating HDL metabolism [5]. There is a well-established negative relationship between plasma HDL-cholesterol level and triglyceride concentrations [29–32] and patients characterized by high plasma triglyceride levels frequently have low HDL-cholesterol as well as small HDL particles. Among mechanisms explaining this association, small HDL particles, which are the product of intravascular lipolysis of triglyceride-enriched HDL, could be cleared more rapidly, are stable or are more prone to shed Apo A-I than large HDL particles [5]. Thus, although the contribution of plasma triglyceride level itself as a risk factor for CHD remains equivocal (several studies have shown that high plasma triglyceride levels were no longer a risk factor for CHD after statistical adjustment for HDL-C concentration [33]) triglyceride enrichment of HDL particles plays a significant role in modulating HDL metabolism.

The clinical importance of HDL particle composition and size remains to be established. Nevertheless, knowledge about lipid and lipoprotein metabolism has considerably evolved in recent years and future studies are likely to further refine cardiovascular disease risk prediction through the measurement of additional lipid lipoprotein-related variables. Clinicians now need to go beyond simple plasma cholesterol level measurements in CHD risk assessment.

Obesity and dyslipidemia: importance of visceral adipose tissue

Obesity is commonly associated with chronic diseases such as hypertension, type 2 diabetes and cardiovascular disease [34–38]. Excess body fatness has also been frequently associated with dyslipidemic states and with alterations in other cardiovascular disease risk factors [38–41]. Some prospective studies have found that obesity was a significant predictor of cardiovascular disease-related mortality, although this association appears to be of lower magnitude than the relationships of cardiovascular disease mortality to well-known risk factors such as smoking, hypertension and dyslipidemia [38,42–44]. This section describes how the morphologic heterogeneity of obesity, more specifically regional body fat distribution, accounts for the most important part of the association between obesity and the related metabolic complications.

In 1947, Jean Vague [45] was the first to describe the sex-related difference in body fat distribution and to foresee its

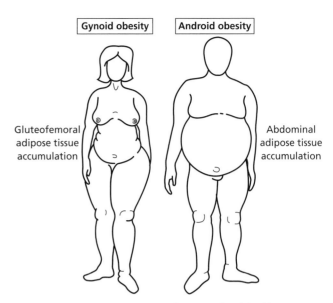

Figure 13.2 Android and gynoid types of obesity as first defined by Vague [45], with preferential accumulation of adipose tissue in the abdominal and gluteofemoral region, respectively. The android pattern of adipose tissue distribution is more closely associated with the metabolic complications of obesity.

correlation with the complications of obesity. He defined the accumulation of upper body fat mostly found in men as *android* obesity, this type of obesity being more frequently associated with diabetes, hypertension and cardiovascular disease. He also referred to *gynoid* obesity to describe a condition where body fat was preferentially accumulated in the gluteal-femoral region. He suggested that this pattern of fat distribution, mostly found in women, was not associated with the expected complications of obesity [45,46] (Fig. 13.2). Several prospective studies which have used the ratio of waist and hip circumferences (the widely used waist-to-hip ratio, WHR) have now confirmed that the android type of obesity, now referred to as abdominal obesity, is more closely associated with a cluster of metabolic complications such as dyslipidemias, hyperinsulinemia and a higher risk of diabetes and cardiovascular diseases, rather than an excess of total body fatness *per se* [47–53].

Age and sex differences in visceral adipose tissue accumulation

As mentioned above, the most widely used measurement of body fat distribution has been the WHR. The rationale for using this index is that the higher the accumulation of abdominal fat, the higher the ratio of waist-to-hip circumferences. However, this measurement does not distinguish the amount of adipose tissue located in the abdominal cavity (the intra-abdominal or visceral adipose tissue) from the subcutaneous abdominal adipose tissue. With the development of imaging techniques such as computed tomography (CT) and magnetic resonance (MRI), it has become possible to accurately quantify the amount of fat located in the

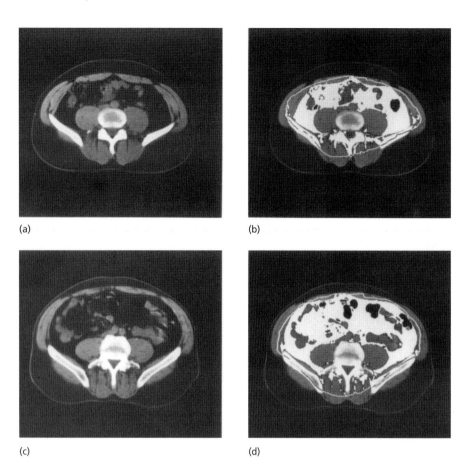

(a)

(b)

(c)

(d)

Figure 13.3 (a,b) Cross-sectional abdominal adipose tissue area measured by CT at the L4–L5 vertebrae level in a young man and a middle-aged man with comparable levels of total body fat in kg. (c,d) The visceral cavity was delineated with a graph pen and adipose tissue was highlighted with an attenuation range of -190 to -30 Hounsfield units.

various body compartments, including the abdominal cavity [54–56]. On the basis of differences in the density of tissues, adipose tissue can be distinguished from bone and muscle, and the size of the visceral and subcutaneous adipose tissue compartments can be reliably estimated by measuring areas of the corresponding tissues on a single scan at the abdominal level, usually at the L4–L5 vertebrae [54–57] (Fig. 13.3).

Starting in the late 1980s, studies were published creating an increasingly large body of knowledge regarding correlates of abdominal-visceral obesity in various populations and physiologic conditions. These studies have indicated that age and sex are important correlates of visceral adipose tissue accumulation. Using computed tomography methodology, Lemieux and colleagues have noted that for any given body fat mass value, men have significantly higher amounts of visceral adipose tissue compared to premenopausal women [58] (Fig. 13.4). Whether such a sex difference in visceral adipose tissue accumulation could account for the well-known difference in cardiovascular risk factors between men and women has also been examined in a cross-sectional comparison of subgroups of men and women who were individually matched for the level of visceral adipose tissue. This procedure largely eliminated most of the differences in glucose tolerance and plasma lipoprotein levels, including concentrations of Apo B and triglycerides [59]. In the latter study,

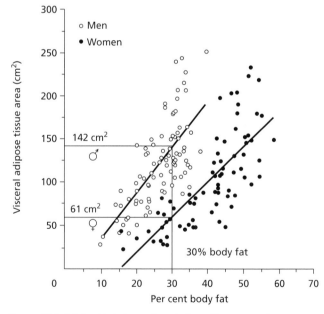

Figure 13.4 Relationship between visceral adipose tissue area and percentage body fat in men (open circles) and women (closed circles) (r = 0.71, p < 0.0001 in men and r = 0.76, p < 0.0001 in women). At 30% body fat, regression equations predict a 142 cm² vs 61 cm² visceral fat accumulation in men and women respectively. (Adapted from Lemieux et al. [58].)

plasma HDL-C concentrations remained higher in women than in men, even after controlling for sex differences in visceral adiposity [59]. Accordingly, androgens and estrogens have been shown to modulate hepatic lipase activity levels directly, contributing to the well-known sex difference in HDL-cholesterol levels [60]. Moreover, the association between the androgenicity marker sex hormone-binding globulin (SHBG) and HDL-cholesterol levels or hepatic lipase activity was found to be independent of interindividual differences in visceral adipose tissue accumulation [61–63].

Additional studies have been performed on visceral fat accumulation and the sex difference in LDL particle size, as men usually have smaller LDL particles than women [64]. When comparing subgroups of men and women with similarly elevated triglyceride concentrations (>2 mmol/L) and visceral adipose tissue areas (>100 cm^2), LDL particle size remained significantly lower in men than in women. These results suggest that despite being strong predictors of LDL size [65], plasma triglyceride levels and visceral adipose tissue area could not entirely explain sex-related differences in LDL size [64]. Genome-wide association and heritability studies have now confirmed a very strong genetic component to the small, dense LDL phenotype [66,67] which could mask the contribution of visceral fat to sex differences in LDL size. In summary, visceral adipose tissue accumulation, along with other hormonal and genetic factors, is a significant contributor to sex-related differences in several metabolic parameters.

The prevalence of obesity increases with age [68] and total body fat mass as well as visceral adipose tissue accumulations are significant positive correlates of age [69–72]. The cardiovascular disease risk profile also generally deteriorates with age, and the concomitant increase in visceral adipose tissue was one of the important factors associated with the development of a more atherogenic metabolic profile [73,74]. However, other age-related processes that are independent of the variation in total adiposity and visceral adipose tissue deposition also contribute to the alterations in plasma lipid and lipoprotein concentrations as well as in insulin sensitivity [73,74]. Nevertheless, a substantial proportion of age and sex differences in the metabolic risk profile predictive of the risk of type 2 diabetes and cardiovascular disease could still be attributed to concomitant variations in visceral adipose tissue accumulation.

The metabolic alterations of visceral obesity

Abdominal obesity is now recognized as a critical correlate of several metabolic complications found in obesity [38,75–77]. As an example to show the relative importance of obesity and visceral adipose tissue accumulation as correlates of metabolic alterations, we used a simple approach in which we compared two subgroups of obese men matched for total body fat mass but with either low or high levels of visceral adipose tissue measured by computed tomography [77,78]. These two groups were then compared to lean controls identified on the basis of a Body Mass Index (BMI) below 25 kg/m^2 (Fig. 13.5). As shown in panels A–E,

only men with high levels of visceral adipose tissue displayed significantly higher plasma triglyceride and apolipoprotein B levels, lower HDL-C concentrations as well as reduced HDL$_2$-C/HDL$_3$-C and HDL-C/total cholesterol ratios compared to the two other subgroups. Plasma total and LDL-cholesterol levels are often within the normal range in subjects with visceral obesity, as shown in panels F and G. We also observed that obese men with high levels of visceral adipose tissue were also characterized by significantly higher fasting plasma insulin concentrations and by higher insulinemic and glycemic responses to a standard oral glucose load, suggesting a link between visceral fat accumulation and insulin resistance (panels H–J) [77,79]. Similar results were obtained when these analyses were conducted in women (not shown).

Additional evidence shows that visceral fat accumulation is a strong correlate of plasma glucose and insulin homeostasis alterations found in obesity. For example, when comparing equally obese women who had either normal or altered insulin sensitivity, the major feature of insulin-resistant women was an increased visceral fat accumulation measured by computed tomography [80]. Other studies have now emphasized the importance of visceral fat accumulation in the association between obesity and risk factors for type 2 diabetes. Specifically, in both men and women, visceral adipose tissue accumulation has been positively associated with fasting insulin and C-peptide levels, as well as with the insulin response to an oral glucose challenge [77,79]. These associations appeared to be independent from concomitant variations in total body fat mass [76,78]. The negative correlation between CT-measured visceral fat accumulation and glucose disposal assessed with the hyperinsulinemic-euglycemic clamp technique is also a well-established phenomenon [16,74,81–86]. In addition, prospective studies have shown that visceral obesity is associated with an increased risk of developing type 2 diabetes [87,88]. Thus, individuals with visceral obesity are frequently characterized by both hyperinsulinemia and insulin resistance.

Measures of the proinflammatory/prothrombotic component of the metabolic syndrome are also closely correlated with the presence of excess body fatness and abdominal obesity. The acute-phase reactant C-reactive protein (CRP) is a sensitive marker of inflammation [89]. Circulating levels of this protein are generally low in patients without acute illness but using high-sensitivity assays, it has been possible to investigate the relationship between previously considered normal plasma CRP levels and cardiovascular disease [90]. Several studies have now demonstrated that elevated high-sensitivity CRP levels are independently associated with an increased risk for cardiovascular disease mortality and morbidity, as well as with acute coronary events in both men and women [91–95]. Elevated CRP levels are also correlated with body weight and BMI as well as insulin resistance [41,96–98]. In a sample of 159 men, Lemieux et al. [99] found that, among subjects with a high body fat mass, those with excess visceral adiposity had the highest CRP levels [99].

The nature of the relationship between CRP and adiposity has not been clearly established. However, other adipose

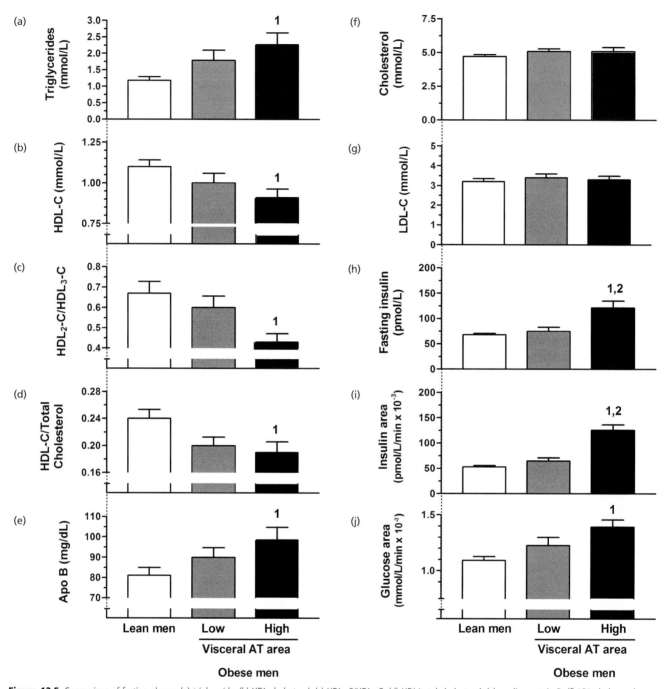

Figure 13.5 Comparison of fasting plasma (a) triglyceride; (b) HDL-cholesterol; (c) HDL$_2$-C/HDL$_3$-C; (d) HDL/total cholesterol; (e) apolipoprotein B; (f) LDL cholesterol; (g) total cholesterol; (h) fasting insulin; (i) insulinemic; and (j) glycemic responses to a 75 g oral glucose load (areas under the curves) among a subgroup of lean men and two subgroups of obese men with the same amount of total fat but with either low or high levels of visceral adipose tissue (AT). 1, Significantly different from lean controls; 2, significantly different from obese men with low levels of visceral adipose tissue, $p < 0.05$. (Adapted from Pouliot et al. [77].)

tissue-secreted proinflammatory cytokines such as interleukin-6 (IL-6), IL-1β or TNF-α may stimulate CRP production in obesity [96,97,100]. Accordingly, plasma levels of CRP and IL-6 are increased in obese subjects [101,102] and reduced by substantial weight loss [102–104]. The hemostatic and fibrinolytic systems may also be affected in obese patients as these patients tend to have higher fibrinogen, factor VII, factor VIII, von Willebrand factor and plasminogen activator inhibitor levels compared to nonobese individuals. A close association has generally been observed between abdominal obesity and disturbances in plasminogen activator inhibitor, fibrinogen, factor VIII and von Willebrand factor, while less consistent results have been found for factor VII [105–107]. Finally, adiponectin, an adipose tissue cytokine with insulin-sensitizing anti-inflammatory effects, has been shown to be decreased in visceral obese individuals [108,109].

Abdominal obesity and cardiovascular disease outcome

Convincing evidence that abdominal obesity is associated with cardiovascular disease is now available. CT-measured visceral fat accumulation was a significant and independent predictor of all-cause mortality in a small study by Kuk and colleagues [110]. In addition, results from the Nurses' Health Study examining the 8-year incidence of coronary heart disease among more than 44,000 women who were disease free at baseline revealed that within each tertile of BMI, a larger waist circumference was associated with an increased disease risk [111]. Similar conclusions were obtained in the INTERHEART case–control study, which included more than 27,000 individuals from several countries [112]. In each BMI category, subjects with the highest WHR were those with the highest risk of myocardial infarction.

This independent association between abdominal or visceral obesity and cardiovascular disease or mortality is likely accounted for by the risk associated with the clustering metabolic abnormalities of visceral obesity. The Quebec Cardiovascular Study examined this issue in a prospective design. In 1985, the cardiovascular disease risk profile of a random sample of 2443 middle-aged men living in the metropolitan area of Quebec City was evaluated [113]. This evaluation included the measurement of fasting plasma lipid and lipoprotein levels. After exclusion of men who showed clinical signs of ischemic heart disease (IHD) (exertion angina, coronary insufficiency, nonfatal myocardial infarction, and coronary death) and of men with triglyceride concentrations above 4.5 mmol/L, the incidence of IHD over 5 years was studied in a sample of 2103 men initially free from IHD. Over the 5-year follow-up, 114 men developed clinical signs of ischemic heart disease.

When comparing the risk profiles of these 114 men to the 1989 men who remained healthy over the 5-year follow-up, it was found that men who eventually developed IHD had an elevated systolic blood pressure and a much higher prevalence of diabetes [114]. Significant differences were also found in the plasma lipoprotein and lipid profile between men with IHD and men who remained healthy. Plasma total cholesterol and triglyceride levels were significantly higher in men who developed IHD compared to those who remained event free. The mean Apo B concentration was also 12% higher in men who developed IHD. In concordance with previous prospective data, plasma HDL-C concentrations were lower and the cholesterol/HDL-C ratio was substantially higher (by 16%) in men who developed IHD compared to men who remained healthy over the 5-year follow-up [114]. An elevated Apo B concentration was also found in 42% of men who developed IHD and appeared as the best predictor of disease in multiple regression analyses [115]. Fasting insulin levels were measured in a nested case–control substudy of the same cohort excluding diabetic patients. Fasting plasma insulin concentration was found to be an independent predictor of IHD risk even after control for other risk variables, including plasma lipid and lipoprotein concentrations [116]. Stratified analyses showed that the combination of both hyperinsulinemia and elevated Apo B levels was associated with more than a 10-fold increase in IHD risk [116].

Small, dense LDL particles have been reported to be more prevalent in coronary heart disease patients than in healthy controls [117–125] and there is evidence suggesting that these particles have atherogenic properties, which could be mediated by an increased filtration rate in the endothelial space of the artery wall [126,127], an increased susceptibility to oxidation [128–130], a reduced affinity for the LDL receptor leading to longer residence time in circulation [131] and an increased capacity to bind to intimal proteoglycans [132]. In the Quebec Cardiovascular Study, small LDL particles were, indeed, predictive of a significant increase in the risk of ischemic heart disease over the 5-year follow-up [133]. This association was later confirmed within the large-scale, population-based, prospective design of this cohort [134]. As the predominance of small, dense LDL particles is closely associated with the hypertriglyceridemic-low HDL-cholesterol dyslipidemic state of visceral obesity [65,135,136], our results provide further support to the notion that small, dense LDL particles represent another component of the dyslipidemic profile of visceral obesity which increases cardiovascular disease risk.

The contribution of the inflammation marker CRP to the 5-year risk of developing ischemic heart disease was also examined within the Quebec Cardiovascular Study design [137,138]. Results reported by Pirro et al. [137] indicated that CRP levels predicted the short-term risk for IHD (<2 years), but not the long-term risk. Moreover, the risk associated with high CRP levels was independent of other known risk factors only in younger men (≤55 years). These results suggest that disease prediction by elevated CRP may be especially relevant for younger middle-aged men and in the case of events occurring early after the evaluation [137].

Thus, results from the Quebec Cardiovascular Study clearly show that nontraditional risk factors generally associated with abdominal obesity are also strong predictors of the disease outcome. Most interestingly, we found that the use of a particular combination of nontraditional risk factors, namely elevated insulin and apolipoprotein B levels and dense LDL particles, predicted a more than 20-fold increase in ischemic heart disease risk compared to those not showing this atherogenic triad of metabolic abnormalities [139]. The strength of the relationship between nontraditional risk factors and ischemic heart disease risk was not significantly affected by adjustment for traditional risk factors. Once again, these results emphasize the ability of typical features of the insulin-resistant/dyslipidemic state of visceral obesity to identify individuals at risk for cardiovascular disease [139].

The metabolic syndrome and global cardiometabolic risk

In 1988, Reaven was the first to suggest the term "insulin resistance syndrome" (or syndrome X) to describe a cluster of metabolic abnormalities including: hypoalphalipoproteinemia, hypertriglyceridemia, hyperinsulinemia and increased blood pressure [140]. Several organizations have since provided guidelines to identify obese individuals characterized by such a pattern of risk factors [8,141–144]. Among others, experts from the American National Cholesterol Education Program (Adult Treatment Panel III) issued a new designation for the syndrome, called "metabolic syndrome," which included abdominal obesity, atherogenic dyslipidemia, raised blood pressure, insulin resistance with or without glucose intolerance, and a prothrombotic/proinflammatory state. To screen for the presence of the metabolic syndrome, the ATPIII panel recommended that the simultaneous occurrence of three or more of the following components:
- abdominal obesity (as defined by a waist circumference greater than 102 cm in men and 88 cm in women)
- elevated plasma triglyceride levels (greater than or equal to 1.69 mmol/L)
- low HDL-cholesterol (below 1.04 mmol/L in men and 1.29 mmol/L in women)
- high blood pressure (greater than or equal to 130/85 mmHg)
- elevated fasting plasma glucose (greater than or equal to 6.1 mmol/L)[8].

Other components of the metabolic syndrome, such as insulin resistance, the proinflammatory state, and the prothrombotic state, were not included in the clinical variables to identify individuals affected by the metabolic syndrome as they cannot be used in routine clinical evaluation at the present time [8]. Quite consistently, visceral adipose tissue accumulation was found to be a critical determinant of the metabolic syndrome identified using the ATPIII panel criteria [145,146]. The International Diabetes Federation (IDF) organized a consensus committee to revise the original World Health Organization guidelines [143] in an attempt to align these recommendations to those of the ATP III panel [147]. Recognizing that the most prevalent form of the metabolic syndrome was found in patients with elevated waist circumference, this measure was recommended as an obligatory criterion to identify individuals likely to have the syndrome. Thus, under the IDF guidelines, diagnosis of the metabolic syndrome requires the necessary presence of an elevated waist circumference combined with two of the four additional clinical criteria of NCEP-ATP III [147].

As an additional screening tool to identify patients with the metabolic syndrome, we have proposed that the simultaneous presence of an increased waist circumference and elevated triglyceride levels could help efficiently identify those characterized by the clustering metabolic abnormalities of abdominal obesity [148]. The rationale for using these variables was that waist circumference, a reliable predictor of visceral adipose tissue accumulation [149], and triglyceride levels would each predict specific components of the previously described atherogenic triad [139],

namely elevated insulin and Apo B and the presence of dense LDL particles [148]. In the initial studies using cutoffs of 90 cm and 2.0 mmol/L for waist circumference and triglyceride levels respectively, as many as 84% of the male subjects with elevated waist and triglyceride levels were characterized by the atherogenic triad of risk factors whereas less than 10% of the subjects with low waist and triglyceride levels had these risk factors [148,150]. A large number of studies have now examined the association of hypertriglyceridemic waist with features of the metabolic syndrome, type 2 diabetes or cardiovascular disease, reinforcing the notion that this specific phenotype is a useful clinical tool in the identification of obese individuals at the highest risk of disease (reviewed in Lemieux et al [151]).

As discussed in the previous sections of this chapter, the presence of metabolic syndrome features is predictive of an increased relative cardiovascular disease risk. However, the absolute risk of cardiovascular disease is also strongly influenced by the presence or absence of traditional risk factors. At the present time, global risk assessment algorithms are still lacking to help quantify diabetes and cardiovascular disease risk resulting from the presence of both classic risk factors and abdominal obesity- or insulin resistance-related metabolic markers [152]. The term "cardiometabolic risk" [152] has been proposed and also used by the American Diabetes Association [153] and the American Heart Association [154] to describe the overall risk of developing type 2 diabetes and cardiovascular disease [152]. Cardiometabolic risk encompasses the global risk of cardiovascular disease and type 2 diabetes associated with traditional risk factors while also taking into consideration the potential additional contribution of abdominal obesity and/or insulin resistance to global disease risk. Thus, to properly evaluate cardiovascular risk, physicians must first consider traditional CVD risk factors. Whether the presence of clinical criteria for the metabolic syndrome increases the risk of CVD beyond that of traditional risk factors remains uncertain. Resolving this issue has now become crucial for the optimal assessment of global CVD risk [152].

Fat depot-specific characteristics and their link with predictors of disease outcome

The morphology and physiologic characteristics of adipose tissue differ from one fat depot to another. A very large number of studies have compared an extremely wide variety of parameters in visceral versus subcutaneous fat depots. Specific features of the visceral adipose tissue depots have been shown to be closely related or even lead to metabolic alterations. This section will provide an overview of how the biologic nature of visceral adipose tissue may explain the link between visceral obesity and the metabolic disturbances generally associated with this condition.

Adipocyte size
The mature adipocyte population of a given fat depot varies in cell size according to the volume of the triglyceride droplet

located in each cell. Sex, adiposity level, nutritional status and anatomic location have all been shown to modulate fat cell size [155–159]. In both sexes, omental and subcutaneous adipocytes become larger with obesity, but adipocyte size reaches a plateau in massively obese subjects [156,159]. In normal-weight to obese women, omental adipocytes are 20–30% smaller than subcutaneous adipocytes over most of the spectrum of adiposity values [156,159]. Omental and subcutaneous adipocytes only reach a similar size at markedly elevated BMI values in women (>45 kg/m²) [156,159]. In men, omental and subcutaneous adipocytes have similar cell sizes through most of the adiposity range. In addition, maximal adipocyte size is lower in men (approximately 120 μm) than in women (approximately 140 μm) [155]. Studies assessing differences between small and large adipocytes from the same adipose tissue depot of a given individual showed that lipolysis, lipid synthesis and glucose uptake [155,160,161], as well as gene expression [162], were strongly influenced by adipocyte size. Thus, fat cell size is a critical determinant of adipocyte function [155] and sex-, depot- and adiposity-related differences in this parameter likely play a critical role in the link between visceral obesity and metabolic alterations.

Adipocyte metabolism

The response of adipose cells to lipolytic agonists is different in the visceral and subcutaneous compartments [156,159,163–165], one of the main determinants of these regional differences being adipocyte size [155,156,159]. Larger adipocytes in a given adipose tissue depot appear to have increased lipid synthesis, increased lipolysis and, therefore increased fatty acid flux across the cell membrane [166]. Lower basal lipolysis is found in the omental compared to the subcutaneous depot in women, consistent with the difference in adipocyte size [159,163,165]. Thus, in women and possibly in very lean men, visceral adipose tissue is not believed, at least in the basal condition, to be a major contributor to the pool of circulating free fatty acids [167]. However, compared to the subcutaneous adipose tissue depot, lipolysis in omental fat was found to be more responsive to β-adrenergic agonist stimulation [159,163,165] and less to insulin suppression [168,169]. In men, lipolytic activity is higher than that observed in women, although no regional difference is observed in isoproterenol-stimulated lipolysis [156,159]. In absolute terms, however, more free fatty acids are released into the portal circulation by visceral adipose tissues in men [167]. Compared to women, this may increase the impact of omental adipose tissue on hepatic metabolism and subsequently contribute to the development of a diabetogenic and atherogenic metabolic profile [156].

Triglyceride accumulation in adipose tissue depots relies mainly on the hydrolysis of triglyceride-rich lipoproteins by LPL and on triglyceride synthesis inside the adipocyte. The regional differences in the rate of these processes are also tightly associated with adipocyte size. Some studies including both sexes failed to find differences in omental versus subcutaneous LPL activity [170,171]. However, higher LPL activity in subcutaneous adipose tissue was observed in studies including mostly women

[159,169,172] and the opposite was observed in studies that included mostly men [156,172,173]. Thus, we propose that regional differences in LPL activity are sex specific and likely reflect the propensity of each compartment to accumulate lipids in each sex. Concordant with these observations, triglyceride synthesis in women is reduced in omental compared to subcutaneous adipose tissue [163,174] whereas no regional difference is observed in men [163].

The mechanisms underlying the relationship between adipocyte function and the metabolic abnormalities of visceral obesity have been extensively studied. Hepatic VLDL synthesis is a central factor in the dyslipidemic state of abdominal obesity [3,175]. In fact, the hypertriglyceridemic state of this condition is primarily due to VLDL overproduction, particularly large VLDL particles [176,177], while the concomitant low HDL-cholesterol levels and predominance of small, dense LDL particles appear to be consequences of high triglyceride levels [3,5,175]. Availability of fatty acids in the liver is recognized as the primary determinant of reduced Apo B degradation and VLDL overproduction [3]. Thus an increased fatty acid flux from visceral adipose tissue to the liver could potentially explain abdominal obesity-related hypertriglyceridemia [178]. The high concentrations of triglyceride-rich lipoproteins found in visceral obesity could then favor increased lipid transfer by the cholesterol ester transfer protein (CETP) between VLDL particles and LDL as well as HDL particles. HDL particles then become relatively depleted in cholesterol esters and enriched in triglycerides. Triglycerides can also be transferred to LDL by CETP and this phenomenon also reduces the cholesterol-to-triglyceride ratio in LDL particles. Since hepatic triglyceride lipase (HL) activity has been reported to be increased in visceral obesity [179,180], triglyceride-rich HDL and LDL particles are then submitted to hydrolysis by this enzyme, generating on the one hand small, dense LDL and HDL particles and, as a consequence, reduced HDL cholesterol levels, especially in the HDL$_2$ subfraction.

With respect to insulin resistance, excess FFA release from adipose tissue may be associated with reduced hepatic insulin extraction [181,182], which could partly contribute to the hyperinsulinemic state of this condition [39,178]. It may also be associated with increased hepatic gluconeogenesis, leading to elevated hepatic glucose production, which could contribute to the deterioration of glucose tolerance [180,183]. Current literature suggests that excess systemic FFA release is involved in skeletal muscle insulin resistance through inhibition of insulin signaling and glucose transport, as well as inhibition of glycogen synthase, pyruvate dehydrogenase and hexokinase [184–187]. Several papers have now emphasized that increased muscle lipid content is closely associated with insulin resistance [83,188] and this phenomenon would result from a state of "metabolic inflexibility," that is, a reduced capacity to switch from fatty acid oxidation in the fasting state to glucose oxidation and glycogen synthesis in the postprandial state [189].

Insulin resistance and dyslipidemia can also be observed in rare genetic forms of lipodystrophies in humans or in a number of murine models of fat storage deficiency [190]. These models paradoxically show that lack of adequate lipid storage, much like excess lipid storage, is associated with metabolic disturbances. For example, selective disruption of the key adipose tissue adipogenic transcription factor PPARγ2 in mice leads to phenotypes of insulin resistance, with or without lipodystrophy [191,192]. Together with several other studies, such findings led to the suggestion that metabolic alterations may arise from reduced adipose tissue expandability when facing caloric excess and "spillover" of lipids to other tissues such as the liver and muscle [190,193–195]. According to this concept, adipose tissue stores, especially the peripheral subcutaneous compartments, are viewed as lipid-buffering tissues that help maintain the homeostasis of daily lipid fluxes [193]. Consistent with the postulated negative impact of excess lipid flux in ectopic sites, overexpression of LPL in the liver or skeletal muscle LPL causes insulin resistance specific to the tissue overexpressing LPL. These results suggest that added fatty acid burden in a given tissue is causative of insulin resistance [196]. The lipid-storing function of adipose tissue and its expandability have since emerged as major determinants of dyslipidemia and insulin resistance in obesity, and also as targets for therapeutic intervention. Stimulation of fat cell hyperplasia with compounds such as PPARγ agonists thiazolidinediones, generates small, insulin-sensitive adipocytes in subcutaneous compartments and leads to improvements of the metabolic profile, especially in prediabetic subjects [197,198].

To study the relative capacity of each abdominal fat compartment to store excess lipids through fat cell hypertrophy and hyperplasia, we examined a sample of women in whom we performed measures of abdominal adipose tissue areas by CT and also obtained omental and subcutaneous adipose tissue samples by surgery to characterize adipocyte size and adipogenic gene expression [199]. We observed a marked difference in, on the one

hand, the regressions of omental and subcutaneous adipocyte size to total body fat mass and on the other, the regressions of adipose tissue areas and total body fat mass (Fig. 13.6). The fact that the regression slopes of subcutaneous and omental fat cell size were parallel showed that obese women have proportionately larger adipocytes in both fat compartments compared to lean women. Conversely, the fact that the regression of subcutaneous adipose tissue area was much steeper than that of visceral adipose tissue area with total body fat mass suggests that subcutaneous fat is hyperplasic in obese women. Thus, in women, hyperplasia is predominant in the subcutaneous fat depot, whereas fat cell hypertrophy is observed both in the omental and subcutaneous compartments (see Fig. 13.6) [199].

Considering that adipocyte number and anatomic localization are major determinants of metabolic consequences related to obesity [166], we suggest that a higher storage capacity of the subcutaneous compartment through fat cell hyperplasia such as that seen in women could theoretically decrease the reliance on the visceral and other ectopic lipid storage compartments, and thereby exert a protective metabolic role when facing energy excess.

Adipokines

Adipose tissue is known to produce a number of cytokines, or adipokines, and many other factors involved in the regulation of numerous biologic processes [200]. Adipokines are secreted by adipocytes or preadipocytes but also, especially in obesity, by macrophages invading the tissue [200]. Visceral and subcutaneous adipose tissues often do not uniformly contribute to the secretion of these factors [201–204] and the literature also suggests that, much like adipocyte metabolism, adipocyte size has a critical influence on their secretory patterns [205].

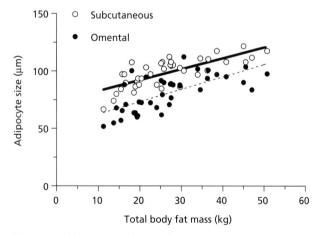 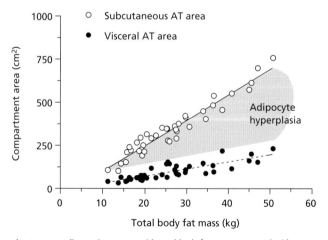

Figure 13.6 (a) Regressions of mean adipocyte size in omental and subcutaneous adipose tissue in relation to total body fat mass. (b) Regressions of adipose tissue areas of abdominal subcutaneous and visceral fat depots in relation to total fat body mass. Given the parallel regressions of subcutaneous and omental adipocyte size versus fat mass, the steeper regression of subcutaneous adipose tissue area with total body fat mass compared with visceral adipose tissue area suggests predominant adipocyte hyperplasia in subcutaneous fat in this sample of women. These analyses were performed in a sample of 40 women undergoing abdominal hysterectomies (age: 47 ± 5 years; BMI 27.9 ± 5.3 kg/m²). (Adapted from Drolet et al. [199].)

Blood levels of adiponectin, a cytokine with insulin-sensitizing and anti-inflammatory properties, are inversely related to adiposity levels [206]. The decrease in adiponectin concentration with obesity is believed to have negative consequences on whole-body glucose homeostasis [206]. Visceral adipose tissue accumulation is an independent predictor of circulating adiponectin levels [108,109]. Omental adipose tissue adiponectin secretion also seems to be a critical determinant of circulating adiponectin levels. Indeed, omental adipocyte adiponectin secretion is significantly reduced in obesity, while subcutaneous adipocyte adiponectin secretion is maintained in abdominally obese women [201,207].

Interleukin-6, a proinflammatory cytokine, is positively associated with obesity and especially with visceral fat accumulation [102,208]. IL-6 is also tightly linked to CRP production and other markers of cardiovascular disease [209]. Adipose tissue generates up to a third of total IL-6 production, suggesting a significant systemic impact [209]. Moreover, local production and accumulation of this cytokine modulate lipid homeostasis directly in adipose tissue [205,209,210]. For example, elevated plasma IL-6 is associated with increased omental fat cell β-adrenergic lipolytic responsiveness [211] and β-adrenergic-dependent lipolysis is increased by high levels of IL-6 [212]. Moreover, LPL activity is reduced by half in subcutaneous and omental adipose tissue depots exposed to chronic IL-6 treatment [212,213]. Although the metabolism of both adipose tissue depots is affected by IL-6, the local impact of the cytokine may be more pronounced in visceral fat since this tissue releases 2–3 times more IL-6 than subcutaneous fat [210]. Thus, increased secretion of IL-6 in obesity could alter lipid metabolism of visceral adipose tissue and possibly increase FFA release rates from this depot [209].

Tumor necrosis factor α (TNF-α) is a proinflammatory cytokine secreted by immune cells such as macrophages [209]. Obesity is associated with increased circulating and adipose tissue TNF-α [203]. This increase has been mainly attributed to macrophage infiltration in adipose tissue and increased secretion by adipocytes [205,214]. Chronically elevated TNF-α levels tend to reduce fat mass through lipolysis induction, impairment of insulin-induced lipogenesis and reduced glucose uptake [215,216]. TNF-α may also contribute to skeletal muscle insulin resistance through induction of nitric oxide production in that tissue [217]. TNF-α is positively correlated with visceral fat accumulation [218,219]. However, its role in adipose tissue distribution remains unclear. Studies measuring regional expression differences in TNF-α and its receptor failed to find consistent results [202,215] and the alteration of fat disposal by this cytokine seems to be greater in subcutaneous adipose tissue [215]. Taken together with the fact that hypertrophic adipocytes may secrete high amounts of TNF-α [205], it may be hypothesized that TNF-α could contribute to reduce fat accumulation in subcutaneous adipose tissue and drive the lipid overflow to the visceral and ectopic fat compartments.

Mature adipocytes also secrete significant amounts of plasminogen activator inhibitor-1 (PAI-1) [220]. The release of this cytokine by omental adipose tissue is higher compared to that of subcutaneous adipose tissue and this regional difference is even more pronounced in obese individuals [204,221,222]. Positive correlations have been observed between plasma PAI-1 levels and measures of visceral obesity [223]. Thus, part of the prothrombotic state of visceral obesity may be explained by impaired fibrinolysis due to PAI-1 secretion by intra-abdominal adipocytes [220]. This may represent another mechanism linking visceral obesity to cardiovascular disease [220].

In summary, the physiologic and metabolic nature of visceral and subcutaneous adipose tissues provides interesting clues to decipher the complex association between visceral fat accumulation and clustering metabolic abnormalities (Fig. 13.7). Visceral adipocyte lipolysis responds more to β-adrenergic agonists and less to its suppression by insulin. Even if visceral fat is not a major contributor to whole-body FFA production, its altered lipolytic responsiveness, amplified by the release of FFA directly in the portal vein of abdominally obese individuals, may play a significant role. As previously described, visceral adipocytes and other cells contained in the visceral fat depots have a distinct secretory pattern of pro- and anti-inflammatory adipokines compared to cells located in subcutaneous compartments. The greater proinflammatory and prothrombotic potential of visceral fat may alter local and systemic metabolism by affecting lipid synthesis, lipolysis, insulin sensitivity and fibrinolysis. Moreover, in abdominally obese individuals, visceral fat has lower adiponectin secretion rates, which could also contribute to inflammation and insulin resistance. The proinflammatory-prothrombotic adipokine profile, together with altered lipolysis and subcutaneous adipogenesis, may contribute to the metabolic alterations observed in abdominally obese individuals, and subsequently increase the risk of type 2 diabetes and cardiovascular disease.

Therapeutic implications

As reviewed in this chapter, visceral obesity is a feature of a dysfunctional adipose tissue phenotype referred to as ectopic fat disposition. Excess visceral and ectopic fat is associated with a cluster of metabolic abnormalities contributing to increase the risk of type 2 diabetes and ischemic heart disease. The proper identification of patients with visceral obesity has important public health implications. The use of CT represents a precise and reliable procedure to identify viscerally obese patients. However, this expensive methodology is not readily available to most clinicians. Moreover, depending on how the procedure is performed, a significant amount of radiation can be associated with this test [224]. Several studies have used the WHR as a measurement of abdominal obesity and until recently, this variable had been considered as a relevant tool in the assessment of abdominal fat accumulation [225]. We and others have suggested that the waist circumference by itself is a better correlate of visceral adipose tissue accumulation than the WHR or other anthropometric measures [149,226,227]. As mentioned earlier, the combined use

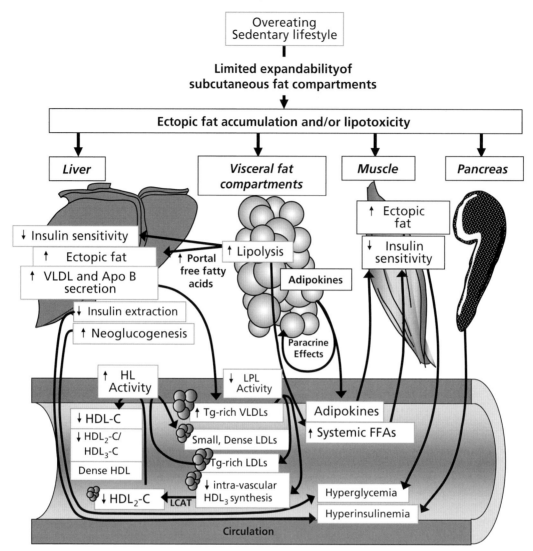

Figure 13.7 Complex metabolic interactions that presumably occur in the insulin-resistant, dyslipidemic, proinflammatory and prothrombotic state of visceral obesity. Increased food intake and a sedentary lifestyle lead to excess accumulation of fat in the visceral compartments as well as ectopic fat deposition. As a result, the liver is exposed to high concentrations of free fatty acids (FFA) generated by the highly lipolytic activity of the enlarged visceral adipose tissue mass and poor inhibition of lipolysis by insulin. This phenomenon stimulates VLDL synthesis and secretion as well as gluconeogenesis in the liver and inhibits hepatic extraction of insulin. The activity of lipoprotein lipase (LPL) is low, which leads to increased plasma concentrations of triglycerides (TG). The increased hepatic lipase (HL) activity contributes to the formation of small, dense LDL particles from TG-enriched LDL particles. It also leads to decreased HDL cholesterol concentrations, HDL_2-C/HDL_3-C and HDL size. Adipose tissue releases cytokines which may modulate adipose tissue metabolism via paracrine effects, exert direct effects on the vascular endothelium and atherogenic plaque, or interfere with insulin signaling in the muscle, thereby contributing to insulin resistance. Reduced insulin extraction and increased gluconeogenesis in the liver contribute to alterations in plasma glucose-insulin homeostasis.

of waist circumference and fasting plasma triglyceride levels contributes to a rapid and inexpensive identification of individuals with excess visceral/ectopic fat [151].

As discussed, excess visceral adipose tissue accumulation plays a significant role in the pathophysiology of a number of clustering abnormalities. Accordingly, weight loss therapy leading to a reduction in visceral adipose tissue mass has been suggested to be associated with improvements in several aspects of the metabolic risk profile [103,104,228–230]. A critical review of weight loss

studies suggested that the visceral adipose tissue compartment may be preferentially mobilized in response to a negative energy balance [231]. Thus, it appears that interventions producing a significant mobilization of visceral adipose tissue may contribute to alleviate some of the abnormalities leading to type 2 diabetes and cardiovascular disease.

When considering weight reduction, however, the clinician is confronted with crucial questions: which mode of intervention should be chosen, how much weight loss will be required to obtain significant health benefits, and how the relapse most often observed in the postweight loss period should be addressed. Solutions to these problems and questions remain very important. Lifestyle intervention studies revealed that counseling patients with the aim of reducing weight, total intake of fat and saturated fat, while increasing fiber intake and physical activity, significantly reduced the risk of developing type 2 diabetes [232]. Most interestingly, changes in the diabetes incidence rates were largely dependent upon the participant's compliance with clinical recommendations. This highly effective lifestyle intervention was found to be even more effective than metformin therapy alone [233].

These results clearly emphasize the fact that if high-risk patients with abdominal obesity and glucose intolerance are offered support by additional health professionals to reshape their nutritional and physical activity habits, such behavioral modifications have a high potential for health improvements. Although the latter studies were not designed to evaluate the respective contributions of exercise, caloric restriction and weight loss on health outcomes, the inclusion of an exercise prescription likely played a significant role in the results achieved and in contributing to the long-term maintenance of a reduced body weight. In this regard, physical activity may represent an interesting adjunct to weight reduction interventions since it has been shown to have beneficial effects on carbohydrate and lipid metabolism irrespective of the magnitude of weight loss achieved [234]. Regarding the amount of weight loss required to obtain health-related benefits, studies tend to suggest that body weight normalization is not necessary to achieve substantial metabolic benefits [235]. The question of whether it is necessary to reach low levels of visceral adipose tissue to induce favorable metabolic changes was examined in a weight loss protocol in postmenopausal women [229]. Interestingly, results did not support the notion of reaching a given threshold (below $110\,cm^2$ in that study) of visceral adipose tissue area in order to improve the risk profile. Moreover, a moderate visceral fat loss yielded similar metabolic improvement compared to more substantial losses in a study conducted in obese postmenopausal women [229]. These results suggest that moderate weight loss, specifically in the abdominal region, may represent an effective strategy for risk management in abdominal obesity. Keeping realistic expectations and objectives regarding weight loss, focusing on maintenance of a reduced body weight and adding a significant amount of exercise may help to reduce the risk of relapse.

Conclusion

Excess visceral adipose tissue accumulation appears to represent a central component of the clustering metabolic abnormalities leading to an increased risk of type 2 diabetes and cardiovascular disease. When present, this condition is associated, in both men and women, with insulin resistance, compensatory hyperinsulinemia, glucose intolerance, a dyslipidemic state including high plasma triglycerides, low HDL-C, an increased cholesterol/HDL-C ratio, hyperapolipoprotein B and an increased proportion of small, dense LDL particles as well as with a prothrombotic and proinflammatory profile. This cluster of metabolic abnormalities clearly increases the risk of type 2 diabetes and cardiovascular disease. It is, therefore, clinically relevant to identify and treat these high-risk patients who are characterized by an excess of visceral and ectopic fat. On the basis of its high prevalence in affluent societies, it is proposed that visceral obesity and the concomitant development of the metabolic syndrome will likely represent the most prevalent cause of type 2 diabetes and coronary heart disease in the coming years. Concerted efforts to prevent and treat this condition are needed.

References

1. Shepherd J, Packard CJ. Lipoprotein metabolism. In: Fruchart JC, Shepherd J (eds) *Human Plasma Lipoproteins*. Berlin: De Gruyter, 1989:55–78.
2. Mahley RW, Ji ZS. Remnant lipoprotein metabolism: key pathways involving cell-surface heparan sulfate proteoglycans and apolipoprotein E. J Lipid Res 1999;40(1):1–16.
3. Lewis GF. Fatty acid regulation of very low density lipoprotein production. Curr Opin Lipidol 1997;8:146–53.
4. Reichl D, Miller NE. Pathophysiology of reverse cholesterol transport. Insights from inherited disorders of lipoprotein metabolism. Arteriosclerosis 1989;9(6):785–97.
5. Lamarche B, Rashid S, Lewis GF. HDL metabolism in hypertriglyceridemic states: an overview. Clin Chim Acta 1999;286:145–61.
6. Gotto AM, LaRosa JC, Hunninghake D, et al. The cholesterol facts: a summary of the evidence relating dietary fats, serum cholesterol and coronary heart disease. Circulation 1990;81(5):1721–33.
7. Kwiterovich PO Jr. Clinical relevance of the biochemical, metabolic, and genetic factors that influence low-density lipoprotein heterogeneity. Am J Cardiol 2002;90(8A):30i–47i.
8. Adult Treatment Panel III. Third Report of the National Cholesterol Education Program (NCEP) Expert Panel on Detection, Evaluation, and Treatment of High Blood Cholesterol in Adults (Adult Treatment Panel III) final report. Circulation 2002;106(25):3143–421.
9. Kwiterovich PO Jr. State-of-the-art update and review: clinical trials of lipid-lowering agents. Am J Cardiol 1998;82(12A):3U–17U.
10. Josan K, Majumdar SR, McAlister FA. The efficacy and safety of intensive statin therapy: a meta-analysis of randomized trials. CMAJ 2008;178(5):576–84.
11. Kearney PM, Blackwell L, Collins R, et al. Efficacy of cholesterol-lowering therapy in 18,686 people with diabetes in 14 randomised trials of statins: a meta-analysis. Lancet 2008;371(9607):117–25.
12. O'Regan C, Wu P, Arora P, Perri D, Mills EJ. Statin therapy in stroke prevention: a meta-analysis involving 121,000 patients. Am J Med 2008;121(1):24–33.
13. Levantesi G, Scarano M, Marfisi R, et al. Meta-analysis of effect of statin treatment on risk of sudden death. Am J Cardiol 2007;100(11):1644–50.
14. Afilalo J, Duque G, Steele R, Jukema JW, de Craen AJ, Eisenberg MJ. Statins for secondary prevention in elderly patients: a hierarchical bayesian meta-analysis. J Am Coll Cardiol 2008;51(1):37–45.

15. Henyan NN, Riche DM, East HE, Gann PN. Impact of statins on risk of stroke: a meta-analysis. Ann Pharmacother 2007;41(12): 1937–45.

16. Wilson PW, Castelli WP, Kannel WB. Coronary risk prediction in adults (the Framingham Heart Study). Am J Cardiol 1987;59(14): 91G–4G.

17. Genest JJ, McNamara JR, Salem DN, Schaefer EJ. Prevalence of risk factors in men with premature coronary heart disease. Am J Cardiol 1991;67:1185–9.

18. Sniderman AD, Silberberg J. Is it time to measure apolipoprotein B? Arteriosclerosis 1990;10:665–7.

19. Sniderman A, Shapiro S, Marpole D, Skinner B, Teng B, Kwiterovich PO Jr. Association of coronary atherosclerosis with hyperapo-betalipoproteinemia [increased protein but normal cholesterol levels in human plasma low density (b) lipoproteins]. Proc Natl Acad Sci USA 1980;77(1):604–8.

20. Yusuf S, Hawken S, Ounpuu S, et al. Effect of potentially modifiable risk factors associated with myocardial infarction in 52 countries (the INTERHEART study): case-control study. Lancet 2004;364 (9438):937–52.

21. Walldius G, Aastveit AH, Jungner I. Stroke mortality and the apoB/apoA-I ratio: results of the AMORIS prospective study. J Intern Med 2006;259(3):259–66.

22. Walldius G, Jungner I, Holme I, Aastveit AH, Kolar W, Steiner E. High apolipoprotein B, low apolipoprotein A-I, and improvement in the prediction of fatal myocardial infarction (AMORIS study): a prospective study. Lancet 2001;358(9298):2026–33.

23. Sniderman AD, Holme I, Aastveit A, Furberg C, Walldius G, Jungner I. Relation of age, the apolipoprotein B/apolipoprotein A-I ratio, and the risk of fatal myocardial infarction and implications for the primary prevention of cardiovascular disease. Am J Cardiol 2007;100(2):217–21.

24. Lamarche B, Lemieux I, Després JP. The small, dense LDL phenotype and the risk of coronary heart disease: epidemiology, pathophysiology and therapeutic aspects. Diabetes Metab 1999;25(3): 199–211.

25. Gordon DJ, Rifkind BM. High-density lipoprotein – the clinical implications of recent studies. N Engl J Med 1989;321(19): 1311–16.

26. Després JP, Lemieux I, Dagenais GR, Cantin B, Lamarche B. HDL-cholesterol as a marker of coronary heart disease risk: the Quebec Cardiovascular Study. Atherosclerosis 2000;153(2):263–72.

27. Rader DJ, Hoeg JM, Brewer HM. Quantification of plasma apolipoproteins in the primary and secondary prevention of coronary artery disease. Ann Intern Med 1994;120:1012–25.

28. Rader DJ. High-density lipoproteins and atherosclerosis. Am J Cardiol 2002;90(8A):62i–70i.

29. Gordon T, Castelli WP, Hjortland MC, Kannel WB, Dawber TR. High density lipoprotein as a protective factor against coronary heart disease: the Framingham Study. Am J Med 1977;62:707–14.

30. Davis CE, Gordon D, LaRosa JC, Wood PD, Halperin M. Correlation of plasma high density lipoprotein cholesterol levels with other plasma lipid and lipoprotein concentrations. Circulation 1980;62(suppl IV):IV24–IV30.

31. Albrink MJ, Krauss RM, Lindgren FT, von der Groeben VD, Wood PD. Intercorrelation among high density lipoprotein, obesity, and triglycerides in a normal population. Lipids 1980;15:668–78.

32. Petersson B, Trell E, Hood B. Premature death and associated risk factors in urban middle-aged men. Am J Med 1984;77:418–26.

33. Austin MA. Plasma triglyceride and coronary heart disease. Arterisocler Thromb 1991;11:2–14.

34. Sims EAH, Berchtold P. Obesity and hypertension: mechanisms and implications for management. JAMA 1982;247:49–52.

35. NIH Consensus Conference. Lowering blood cholesterol to prevent heart disease. JAMA 1985;253(14):2080–6.

36. Bray GA. Complications of obesity. Ann Intern Med 1985;103: 1052–62.

37. Garrison RJ, Kannel WB, Stokes III J, Castelli WP. Incidence and precursors of hypertension in young adults: the Framingham off-spring study. Prev Med 1987;16:235–51.

38. Kissebah AH, Freedman DS, Peiris AN. Health risks of obesity. Med Clin North Am 1989;73:111–38.

39. Després JP. Obesity and lipid metabolism: relevance of body fat distribution. Curr Opin Lipidol 1991;2:5–15.

40. Després JP. Dyslipidaemia and obesity. Baillières Clin Endocrinol Metab 1994;8(3):629–60.

41. Ford ES. Body mass index, diabetes, and C-reactive protein among U.S. adults. Diabetes Care 1999;22:1971–7.

42. Barrett-Connor E. Obesity, atherosclerosis, and coronary artery disease. Ann Intern Med 1985;103:1010–19.

43. Manson JE, Willet WC, Stampfer MJ, et al. Body weight and mortality among women. N Engl J Med 1995;333:677–85.

44. Bray GA, Davidson MB, Drenick EJ. Obesity: a serious symptom. Ann Intern Med 1972;77(5):797–805.

45. Vague J. La différenciation sexuelle, facteur déterminant des formes de l'obésité. Presse Med 1947;30:339–40.

46. Vague J. The degree of masculine differentiation of obesities: a factor determining predisposition to diabetes, atherosclerosis, gout and uric calculous disease. Am J Clin Nutr 1956;4(1):20–34.

47. Kissebah AH, Vydelingum N, Murray R, et al. Relation of body fat distribution to metabolic complications of obesity. J Clin Endocrinol Metab 1982;54(2):254–60.

48. Björntorp P. Hazards in subgroups of human obesity. Eur J Clin Invest 1984;14:239–41.

49. Larsson B, Svardsudd K, Welin L, Wilhemsen L, Björntorp P, Tibblin G. Abdominal adipose tissue distribution, obesity and risk of cardiovascular disease and death: 13-year follow-up of participants in the study of men born in 1913. BMJ 1984;288:1401–4.

50. Lapidus L, Bengtsson C, Larsson B, Pennert K, Rybo E, Sjöström L. Distribution of adipose tissue and risk of cardiovascular disease and death: a 12 year follow up of participants in the population study of women in Gothenburg, Sweden. BMJ 1984;289:1261–3.

51. Donahue RP, Abbot RD, Bloom E, Reed DM, Yano K. Central obesity and coronary heart disease in men. Lancet 1987;1:821–4.

52. Ohlson LO, Larsson B, Svardsudd K, et al. The influence of body fat distribution on the incidence of diabetes mellitus 13.5 years of follow-up of the participants in the study of men born in 1913. Diabetes 1985;34:1055–8.

53. Ducimetière P, Richard J, Cambien F. The pattern of subcutaneous fat distribution in middle-aged men and the risk of coronary heart disease: the Paris prospective study. Int J Obes 1986;10:229–40.

54. Sjöström L, Kvist H, Cederblad A, Tylen U. Determination of total adipose tissue and body fat in women by computed tomography, 40K, and tritium. Am J Physiol 1986;250:E736–E745.

55. Després JP, Prud'homme D, Pouliot MC, Tremblay A, Bouchard C. Estimation of deep abdominal adipose-tissue accumulation from simple anthropometric measurements in men. Am J Clin Nutr 1991;54(3):471–7.

56. Ferland M, Després JP, Tremblay A, et al. Assessment of adipose tissue distribution by computed axial tomography in obese women: association with body density and anthropometric measurements. Br J Nutr 1989;61:139–48.

57. Kuk JL, Church TS, Blair SN, Ross R. Does measurement site for visceral and abdominal subcutaneous adipose tissue alter associations with the metabolic syndrome? Diabetes Care 2006;29(3):679–84.

58. Lemieux S, Prud'homme D, Bouchard C, Tremblay A, Després JP. Sex differences in the relation of visceral adipose tissue accumulation to total body fatness. Am J Clin Nutr 1993;58(4):463–7.

59. Lemieux S, Després JP, Moorjani S, et al. Are gender differences in cardiovascular disease risk factors explained by the level of visceral adipose tissue? Diabetologia 1994;37(8):757–64.

60. Tikkanen MJ, Nikkilä EA. Regulation of hepatic lipase and serum lipoproteins by sex steroids. Am Heart J 1987;113:562–7.

61. Desmeules A, Couillard C, Tchernof A, et al. Post-heparin lipolytic enzyme activities, sex hormones and sex hormone-binding globulin (SHBG) in men and women: the HERITAGE Family Study. Atherosclerosis 2003;171:343–50.

62. Tchernof A, Toth MJ, Poehlman ET. Sex hormone-binding globulin levels in middle-aged premenopausal women: association with visceral obesity and metabolic profile. Diabetes Care 1999;22 (11):1875–81.

63. Tchernof A, Labrie F, Bélanger A, et al. Relationships between endogenous steroid hormone, sex hormone-binding globulin and lipoprotein levels in men: contribution of visceral obesity, insulin levels and other metabolic variables. Atherosclerosis 1997;133: 235–44.

64. Lemieux I, Pascot A, Lamarche B, et al. Is the gender difference in LDL size explained by the metabolic complications of visceral obesity? Eur J Clin Invest 2002;32(12):909–17.

65. Tchernof A, Lamarche B, Prud'homme D, et al. The dense LDL phenotype: association with plasma lipoprotein levels, visceral obesity, and hyperinsulinemia in men. Diabetes Care 1996;19(6): 629–37.

66. Bossé Y, Pérusse L, Després JP, et al. Evidence for a major quantitative trait locus on chromosome 17q21 affecting low-density lipoprotein peak particle diameter. Circulation 2003;107(18):2361–8.

67. Bossé Y, Vohl MC, Després JP, et al. Heritability of LDL peak particle diameter in the Quebec Family Study. Genet Epidemiol 2003;25(4):375–81.

68. Reeder BA, Angel A, Ledoux M, Rabkin SW, Young TK, Sweet LE. Obesity and its relation to cardiovascular disease risk factors in Canadian adults. Canadian Heart Health Surveys Research Group. CMAJ 1992;146(11):2009–19.

69. Enzi G, Gasparo M, Biondetti PR, Fiore D, Semisa M, Zurlo F. Subcutaneous and visceral fat distribution according to sex, age and overweight, evaluated by computed tomography. Am J Clin Nutr 1986;44:739–46.

70. Kotani K, Tokunaga K, Fujioka S, et al. Sexual dimorphism of age-related changes in whole-body fat distribution in the obese. Int J Obes 1994;18:207–12.

71. Schwartz RS, Shuman WP, Bradbury VL, et al. Body fat distribution in healthy young and older men. J Gerontol 1990;45(6):M181–M185.

72. Seidell JC, Oosterlee A, Deurenberg P, Hautvast JGA, Ruijs JHJ. Abdominal fat depots measured with computed tomography: effects of degree of obesity, sex, and age. Eur J Clin Nutr 1988;42: 805–15.

73. Lemieux S, Prud'homme D, Moorjani S, et al. Do elevated levels of abdominal visceral adipose tissue contribute to age-related differences in plasma lipoprotein concentrations in men? Atherosclerosis 1995;118:155–64.

74. DeNino WF, Tchernof A, Dionne IJ, et al. Contribution of abdominal adiposity to age-related differences in insulin sensitivity and plasma lipids in healthy nonobese women. Diabetes Care 2001;24(5): 925–32.

75. Kissebah AH, Krakower GR. Regional adiposity and morbidity. Physiol Rev 1994;74(4):761–811.

76. Wajchenberg BL. Subcutaneous and visceral adipose tissue: their relation to the metabolic syndrome. Endocr Rev 2000;21(6):697–738.

77. Pouliot MC, Després JP, Nadeau A, et al. Visceral obesity in men: associations with glucose tolerance, plasma insulin, and lipoprotein levels. Diabetes 1992;41:826–34.

78. Lemieux S, Després JP. Metabolic complications of visceral obesity: contribution to the aetiology of type 2 diabetes and implications for prevention and treatment. Diabetes Metab 1994;20(4):375–93.

79. Després JP, Nadeau A, Tremblay A, et al. Role of deep abdominal fat in the association between regional adipose tissue distribution and glucose tolerance in obese women. Diabetes 1989;38:304–9.

80. Brochu M, Tchernof A, Sites CK, Eltabbakh GH, Sims EAH, Poehlman ET. What are the physical characteristics associated with a normal metabolic profile despite a high level of obesity in postmenopausal women? J Clin Endocrinol Metab 2001;86(3):1020–5.

81. Dvorak R, DeNino WF, Ades PA, Poehlman ET. Phenotypic characteristics associated with insulin resistance in metabolically obese but normal-weight young women. Diabetes 1999;48:2210–14.

82. Brochu M, Starling RD, Tchernof A, Matthews DE, Poehlman ET. Visceral adipose tissue as an independent correlate of glucose disposal in older postmenopausal women. J Clin Endocrinol Metab 2000;85:2378–84.

83. Goodpaster BH, Thaete FL, Simoneau JA, Kelley DE. Subcutaneous abdominal fat and thigh muscle composition predict insulin sensitivity independently of visceral fat. Diabetes 1997;46:1579–85.

84. Bonora E, del Prato S, Bonadonna RC, et al. Total body fat content and fat topography are associated differently with in vivo glucose metabolism in nonobese and obese nondiabetic women. Diabetes 1992;41:1151–9.

85. Rendell M, Hulthen UL, Tornquist C, Groop L, Mattiasson I. Relationship between abdominal fat compartments and glucose and lipid metabolism in early postmenopausal women. J Clin Endocrinol Metab 2001;86(2):744–9.

86. Sites CK, Calles-Escandon J, Brochu M, Butterfield M, Ashikaga T, Poehlman ET. Relation of regional fat distribution to insulin sensitivity in postmenopausal women. Fertil Steril 2000;73(1):61–5.

87. Bergstrom RW, Newell-Morris LL, Leonetti DL, Shuman WP, Wahl PW, Fujimoto WY. Association of elevated fasting C-peptide level and increased intra-abdominal fat distribution with development of NIDDM in Japanese-American men. Diabetes 1990;39:104–11.

88. Boyko EJ, Fujimoto WY, Leonetti DL, Newell-Morris L. Visceral adiposity and risk of type 2 diabetes: a prospective study among Japanese Americans. Diabetes Care 2000;23(4):465–71.

89. Gabay C, Kushner I. Acute-phase proteins and other systemic responses to inflammation. N Engl J Med 1999;340(6):448–54.

90. Ross R. Atherosclerosis – an inflammatory disease. N Engl J Med 1999;340(2):115–26.

91. Koenig W, Sund M, Fröhlich M, et al. C-reactive, a sensitive marker of inflammation, predicts future risk of coronary heart disease in initially healthy middle-aged men. Results from the MONICA (Monitoring Trends and Determinants in Cardiovascular Disease) Augsburg Cohort Study, 1984 to 1992. Circulation 1999;99:237–42.

92. Ridker PM, Hennekens CH, Buring JE, Rifai N. C-reactive protein and other markers of inflammation in the prediction of cardiovascular disease in women. N Engl J Med 2000;342:836–43.

93. Ridker PM, Cushman M, Stampfer MJ, Tracy RP, Hennekens CH. Inflammation, aspirin, and the risk of cardiovascular disease in apparently healthy men. N Engl J Med 1997;336:973–9.

94. Ridker PM, Glynn RJ, Hennekens CH. C-reactive protein adds to the predictive value of total and HDL cholesterol in determining risk of first myocardial infarction. Circulation 1998;97:2007–11.

95. Thompson SG, Kienast J, Pyke SDM, Haverkate F, van de Loo JCW. Hemostatic factors and the risk of myocardial infarction or sudden death in patients with angina pectoris. N Engl J Med 2000;332:635–41.

96. Visser M, Bouter LM, McQuillan GM, Wener MH, Harris TB. Elevated C-reactive protein levels in overweight and obese adults. JAMA 1999;282:2131–5.

97. Yudkin JS, Stehouwer CDA, Emeis JJ, Coppack SW. C-reactive protein in healthy subjects: associations with obesity, insulin resistance, and endothelial dysfunction. A potential role for cytokines originating from adipose tissue? Arterioscler Thromb Vasc Biol 1999;19:972–8.

98. Hak AE, Stehouwer CDA, Bots ML, et al. Associations of C-reactive protein with measures of obesity, insulin resistance, and subclinical atherosclerosis in healthy, middle-aged women. Arterioscler Thromb Vasc Biol 1999;19:1986–91.

99. Lemieux I, Pascot A, Prud'homme D, et al. Elevated C-reactive protein: another component of the atherothrombotic profile of abdominal obesity. Circulation 2001;21:961–7.

100. Yudkin JS, Kumari M, Humphries SE, Mohamed-Ali V. Inflammation, obesity, stress and coronary heart disease: is interleukin-6 the link? Atherosclerosis 2000;148:209–14.

101. Hotamisligil GS. Molecular mechanisms of insulin resistance and the role of the adipocyte. Int J Obes 2000;24 (suppl 4):S23–S27.

102. Bastard JP, Jardel C, Bruckert E, et al. Elevated levels of interleukin 6 are reduced in serum and subcutaneous adipose tissue of obese women after weight loss. J Clin Endocrinol Metab 2000;85(9):3338–42.

103. Tchernof A, Nolan A, Sites CK, Ades PA, Poehlman ET. Weight loss reduces C-reactive protein levels in obese postmenopausal women. Circulation 2002;105:564–9.

104. Heilbronn LK, Noakes M, Clifton PM. Energy restriction and weight loss on very-low-fat diets reduce C-reactive protein concentrations in obese, healthy women. Arterioscler Thromb Vasc Biol 2001;21:968–70.

105. Juhan-Vague I, Alessi MC, Vague P. Increased plasma plasminogen activator inhibitor 1 levels. A possible link between insulin resistance and atherothrombosis. Diabetologia 1991;34(7):457–62.

106. Vague P, Juhan-Vague I, Chabert V, Alessi MC, Atlan C. Fat distribution and plasminogen activator inhibitor activity in nondiabetic obese women. Metabolism 1989;38(9):913–15.

107. Mertens I, van Gaal LF. Obesity, haemostasis and the fibrinolytic system. Obes Rev 2002;3(2):85–101.

108. Cnop M, Havel PJ, Utzschneider KM, et al. Relationship of adiponectin to body fat distribution, insulin sensitivity and plasma lipoproteins: evidence for independent roles of age and sex. Diabetologia 2003;46:459–69.

109. Park KG, Park KS, Kim M-J, et al. Relationship between serum adiponectin and leptin concentrations and body fat distribution. Diabetes Res Clin Pract 2004;63:135–42.

110. Kuk JL, Katzmarzyk PT, Nichaman MZ, Church TS, Blair SN, Ross R. Visceral fat is an independent predictor of all-cause mortality in men. Obesity 2006;14(2):336–41.

111. Rexrode KM, Carey VJ, Hennekens CH, et al. Abdominal adiposity and coronary heart disease in women. JAMA 1998;280(21):1843–8.

112. Yusuf S, Hawken S, Ôunpuu S, et al. Obesity and the risk of myocardial infarction in 27 000 participants from 52 countries: a case-control study. Lancet 2005;366:1640–9.

113. Dagenais GR, Robitaille NM, Lupien PJ, et al. First coronary heart disease event rates in relation to major risk factors: Québec Cardiovascular Study. Can J Cardiol 1990;6:274–80.

114. Lamarche B, Després JP, Moorjani S, Cantin B, Dagenais GR, Lupien PJ. Prevalence of dyslipidemic phenotypes in ischemic heart disease: prospective results form the Quebec Cardiovascular Study. Am J Cardiol 1995;75:1189–95.

115. Lamarche B, Moorjani S, Lupien PJ, Cantin B, Dagenais GR, Després JP. Apolipoprotein A-I and B levels and the risk of ischemic heart disease during a five-year follow-up of men in the Québec Cardiovascular Study. Circulation 1996;94:273–8.

116. Després JP, Lamarche B, Mauriège P, et al. Hyperinsulinemia as an independent risk factor for ischemic heart disease. N Engl J Med 1996;334:952–7.

117. Fisher WR. Heterogeneity of plasma low density lipoproteins manifestations of the physiologic phenomenon in man. Metabolism. 1983;32:283–91.

118. Crouse JR, Parks JS, Schey HM. Studies of low density lipoprotein molecular weight in human beings with coronary artery disease. J Lipid Res 1985;26:566–74.

119. Austin MA, Breslow JL, Hennekens CH, Buring JE, Willet WC, Krauss RM. Low-density lipoprotein subclass patterns and risk of myocardial infarction. JAMA 1988;260:1917–21.

120. Griffin BA, Caslake MJ, Yip B, Tait GW, Packard CJ, Shepherd J. Rapid isolation of low density lipoprotein (LDL) subfractions from plasma by density gradient ultracentrifugation. Atherosclerosis 1990;83:59–67.

121. Tornvall P, Karpe F, Carlson LA, Hamsten A. Relationships of low density lipoprotein subfractions to angiophauically defined coronary artery disease in young survivors of myocardial infarction. Atherosclerosis 1991;90:67–80.

122. Campos H, Genest JJ, Blijlevens E, et al. Low density lipoprotein particle size and coronary artery disease. Arterisocler Thromb 1992;12:187–95.

123. Coresh J, Kwiterovich PO Jr, Smith HH, Bachorik PS. Association of plasma triglyceride concentration and LDL particle diameter, density, and chemical composition with premature coronary artery disease in men and women. J Lipid Res 1993;34:1687–97.

124. Jaakkola O, Solakivi T, Tertov VV, Orekhov AN, Miettinen TA, Nikkari T. Characteristics of low-density lipoprotein subfractions from patients with coronary artery disease. Coron Artery Dis 1993;4:379–85.

125. Griffin BA, Freeman DJ, Tait GW, et al. Role of plasma triglyceride in the regulation of plasma low density lipoprotein (LDL) subfractions: relative contribution of small dense LDL to coronary heart disease risk. Atherosclerosis 1994;106:241–53.

126. Rajman I, Maxwell S, Cramb R, Kendall M. Particle size: the key to the atherogenic lipoprotein? Q J Med 1994;87(12):709–20.

127. Packard CJ. Plasma triglycerides, LDL heterogeneity and atherogenesis. Ther Exp 1994;85:1–6.

128. Dejager S, Bruckert E, Chapman MJ. Dense low density lipoprotein subspecies with diminished oxidative resistance predominate in combined hyperlipidemia. J Lipid Res 1993;34(2):295–308.

129. de Graaf J, Hendriks JCM, Demacker PNM, Stalenhoef AF. Identification of multiple dense LDL subfractions with enhanced susceptibility to in vitro oxidation among hypertriglyceridemic subjects. Normalization after clofibrate treatment. Arterisocler Thromb 1993;13(5):712–19.

130. Chait A, Brazg RL, Tribble DL, Krauss RM. Susceptibility of small, dense, low-density lipoproteins to oxidative modification in subjects with the atherogenic lipoprotein phenotype, pattern B. Am J Med 1993;94(4):350–6.

131. Silliman K, Shore V, Forte TM. Hypertriglyceridemia during late pregnancy is associated with the formation of small dense low-density lipoproteins and the presence of large buoyant high-density lipoproteins. Metabolism 1994;43(8):1035–41.

132. La Belle M, Krauss RM. Differences in carbohydrate content of low density lipoproteins associated with low density lipoprotein subclass patterns. J Lipid Res 1990;31:1577–88.

133. Lamarche B, Tchernof A, Moorjani S, et al. Small, dense low-density lipoprotein particles as a predictor of the risk of ischemic heart disease in men. Prospective results from the Québec Cardiovascular Study. Circulation 1997;95(1):69–75.

134. Lamarche B, St Pierre AC, Ruel IL, Cantin B, Dagenais GR, Després JP. A prospective, population-based study of low density lipoprotein particle size as a risk factor for ischemic heart disease in men. Can J Cardiol 2001;17(8):859–65.

135. Katzel LI, Krauss RM, Goldberg AP. Relations of plasma TG and HDL-C concentrations to body composition and plasma insulin levels are altered in men with small LDL particles. Arterisocler Thromb 1994;14:1121–8.

136. Campos H, Bailey SM, Gussak LS, Siles X, Ordovas JM, Schaefer EJ. Relations of body habitus, fitness level, and cardiovascular risk factors including lipoproteins in a rural and urban Costa Rican population. Arterisocler Thromb 1991;11(4):1077–88.

137. Pirro M, Bergeron J, Dagenais GR, et al. Age and duration of follow-up as modulators of the risk for ischemic heart disease associated with high plasma C-reactive protein levels in men. Arch Intern Med 2001;161(20):2474–80.

138. St Pierre AC, Bergeron J, Pirro M, et al. Effect of plasma C-reactive protein levels in modulating the risk of coronary heart disease associated with small, dense, low-density lipoproteins in men (The Quebec Cardiovascular Study). Am J Cardiol 2003;91(5):555–8.

139. Lamarche B, Tchernof A, Mauriège P, et al. Fasting insulin and apolipoprotein B levels and low-density lipoprotein particle size as risk factors for ischemic heart disease. JAMA 1998;279(24):1955–61.

140. Reaven GM. Role of insulin resistance in human disease. Diabetes 1988;37:1595–607.

141. National Institutes of Health. Clinical Guidelines on the Identification, Evaluation, and Treatment of Overweight and Obesity in Adults – The Evidence Report. National Institutes of Health. Obes Res 1998;6(suppl 2):51S–209S.

142. National Heart Lung Association. *Practical Guide to the Identification, Evaluation, and Treatment of Overweight and Obesity in Adults.* Publication No. 00–4084. Bethesda, MD: National Institutes of Health. 2000.

143. World Health Organization. *Obesity: Preventing and Managing the Global Epidemic.* WHO Technical Report Series 894. Geneva: World Health Organization, 2000.

144. Grundy SM, Brewer HB Jr, Cleeman JI, Smith SC Jr, Lenfant C. Definition of metabolic syndrome: report of the National Heart, Lung, and Blood Institute/American Heart Association conference on scientific issues related to definition. Circulation 2004;109(3):433–8.

145. Carr DB, Utzschneider KM, Hull RL, et al. Intra-abdominal fat is a major determinant of the National Cholesterol Education Program Adult Treatment Panel III criteria for the metabolic syndrome. Diabetes 2004;53(8):2087–94.

146. Goodpaster BH, Krishnaswami S, Harris TB, et al. Obesity, regional body fat distribution, and the metabolic syndrome in older men and women. Arch Intern Med 2005;165(7):777–83.

147. Alberti KG, Zimmet P, Shaw J. Metabolic syndrome – a new worldwide definition. A Consensus Statement from the International Diabetes Federation. Diabet Med 2006;23(5):469–80.

148. Lemieux I, Pascot A, Couillard C, et al. Hypertriglyceridemic waist. A marker of the atherogenic metabolic triad (hyperinsulinemia; hyperapolipoprotein B; small, dense LDL) in men? Circulation 2000;102:179–84.

149. Pouliot MC, Després JP, Lemieux S, et al. Waist circumference and abdominal sagittal diameter: best simple anthropometric indexes of abdominal visceral adipose tissue accumulation and related cardiovascular risk in men and women. Am J Cardiol 1994;73:460–8.

150. Mauriège P, Després JP, Moorjani S, et al. Abdominal and femoral adipose tissue lipolysis and cardiovascular disease risk factors in men. Eur J Clin Invest 1993;23(11):729–40.

151. Lemieux I, Poirier P, Bergeron J, et al. Hypertriglyceridemic waist: a useful screening phenotype in preventive cardiology? Can J Cardiol 2007;23(suppl B):23B–31B.

152. Després JP, Lemieux I. Abdominal obesity and metabolic syndrome. Nature 2006;444(7121):881–7.

153. Beckley ET. New ADA initiative moves beyond "metabolic syndrome". DOC News 2006;3(7):1–19.

154. Eckel RH, Kahn R, Robertson RM, Rizza RA. Preventing cardiovascular disease and diabetes: a call to action from the American Diabetes Association and the American Heart Association. Circulation 2006;113(25):2943–6.

155. Farnier C, Krier S, Blache M, et al. Adipocyte functions are modulated by cell size change: potential involvement of an integrin/ERK signalling pathway. Int J Obes 2003;27:1178–86.

156. Boivin A, Brochu G, Marceau S, Marceau P, Hould FS, Tchernof A. Regional differences in adipose tissue metabolism in obese men. Metabolism 2007;56(4):533–40.

157. Fried SK, Kral JG. Sex differences in regional distribution of fat cell size and lipoprotein lipase activity in morbidly obese patients. Int J Obes 1987;11:129–40.

158. Salans LB, Cushman SW, Weismann RE. Studies of human adipose tissue. Adipose cell size and number in nonobese and obese patients. J Clin Invest 1973;52(4):929–41.

159. Tchernof A, Bélanger C, Morisset AS, et al. Regional differences in adipose tissue metabolism in women: minor effect of obesity and body fat distribution. Diabetes 2006;55(5):1353–60.

160. Zinder O, Shapiro B. Effect of cell size on epinephrine- and ACTH-induced fatty acid release from isolated fat cells. J Lipid Res 1971;12(1):91–5.

161. Franck N, Stenkula KG, Ost A, Lindstrom T, Stralfors P, Nystrom FH. Insulin-induced GLUT4 translocation to the plasma membrane is blunted in large compared with small primary fat cells isolated from the same individual. Diabetologia 2007;50(8):1716–22.

162. Jernas M, Palming J, Sjoholm K, et al. Separation of human adipocytes by size: hypertrophic fat cells display distinct gene expression. FASEB J 2006;20(9):1540–2.

163. Edens NK, Fried SK, Kral JG, Hirsch J, Leibel RL. In vitro lipid synthesis in human adipose tissue from three abdominal sites. Am J Physiol 1993;265(3 Pt1):E374–E379.

164. Reynisdottir S, Dauzats M, Thörne A, Langin D. Comparison of hormone-sensitive lipase activity in visceral and subcutaneous human adipose tissue. J Clin Endocrinol Metab 1997;82(12):4162–6.

165. Richelsen B, Pedersen SB, Moller-Pedersen T, Bak JF. Regional differences in triglyceride breakdown in human adipose tissue: effects of catecholamines, insulin, and prostaglandin E$_2$. Metabolism 1991; 40:990–6.

166. Smith J, Al-Amri M, Dorairaj P, Sniderman A. The adipocyte life cycle hypothesis. Clin Sci 2006;110:1–9.

167. Nielsen S, Guo Z, Johnson M, Hensrud DD, Jensen MD. Splanchnic lipolysis in human obesity. J Clin Invest 2004;113(11):1582–8.

168. Zierath JR, Livingston JN, Thorne A, et al. Regional difference in insulin inhibition of non-esterified fatty acid release from human adipocytes: relation to insulin receptor phosphorylation and intracellular signalling through the insulin receptor substrate-1 pathway. Diabetologia 1998;41(11):1343–54.

169. Mauriège P, Marette A, Atgie C, et al. Regional variation in adipose tissue metabolism of severely obese premenopausal women. J Lipid Res 1995;36(4):672–84.

170. Fried SK, Russell CD, Grauso NL, Brolin RE. Lipoprotein lipase regulation by insulin and glucocorticoid in subcutaneous and omental adipose tissue of obese men and women. J Clin Invest 1993;92:2191–8.

171. Panarotto D, Poisson J, Devroede G, Maheux P. Lipoprotein lipase steady-state mRNA levels are lower in human omental versus subcutaneous abdominal adipose tissue. Metabolism 2000;49(9):1224–7.

172. Rebuffé-Scrive M, Andersson B, Olbe L, Björntorp P. Metabolism of adipose tissue in intraabdominal depots of nonobese men and women. Metabolism 1989;38(5):453–8.

173. Mårin P, Andersson B, Ottosson M, et al. The morphology and metabolism of intraabdominal adipose tissue in men. Metabolism 1992;41(11):1242–8.

174. Maslowska MH, Sniderman AD, MacLean LD, Cianflone K. Regional differences in triacylglycerol synthesis in adipose tissue and in cultured preadipocytes. J Lipid Res 1993;34(2):219–28.

175. Lewis GF, Carpentier A, Adeli K, Giacca A. Disordered fat storage and mobilization in the pathogenesis of insulin resistance and type 2 diabetes. Endocr Rev 2002;23(2):201–29.

176. Adiels M, Borén J, Caslake MJSP, et al. Overproduction of VLDL1 driven by hyperglycemia is a dominant feature of diabetic dyslipidemia. Arterioscler Thromb Vasc Biol 2005;25:1697–703.

177. Adiels M, Taskinen MR, Packard C, et al. Overproduction of large VLDL particles is driven by increased liver fat content in man. Diabetologia 2006;49:755–65.

178. Björntorp P. "Portal" adipose tissue as a generator of risk factors for cardiovascular disease and diabetes. Arteriosclerosis 1990;10:493–6.

179. Després JP, Ferland M, Moorjani S, et al. Role of hepatic-triglyceride lipase activity in the association between intra-abdominal fat and plasma HDL-cholesterol in obese women. Arteriosclerosis 1989;9(4):485–92.

180. Després JP, Marette A. Relation of components of insulin resistance syndrome to coronary disease risk. Curr Opin Lipidol 1994;5(4):274–89.

181. Hennes M, Shrago E, Kissebah AH. Receptor and postreceptor effects of FFA on hepatocyte insulin dynamics. Int J Obes 1990;14:831–41.

182. Svedberg J, Björntorp P, Smith V, Lonnroth P. FFA inhibition of insulin binding, degradation, and action in isolated hepatocytes. Diabetes 1990;39:570–4.

183. Björntorp P. Metabolic abnormalities in visceral obesity. Ann Med 1992;24(1):3–5.

184. Kelley DE, Mokan M, Simoneau JA, Mandarino LJ. Interaction between glucose and free fatty acid metabolism in human skeletal muscle. J Clin Invest 1993;92(1):91–8.

185. Griffin ME, Marcucci MJ, Cline GW, et al. Free fatty acid-induced insulin resistance is associated with activation of protein kinase C theta and alterations in the insulin signaling cascade. Diabetes 1999;48(6):1270–4.

186. Thompson AL, Cooney GJ. Acyl-CoA inhibition of hexokinase in rat and human skeletal muscle is a potential mechanism of lipid-induced insulin resistance. Diabetes 2000;49(11):1761–5.

187. Boden G, Chen X, Ruiz J, White JV, Rossetti L. Mechanisms of fatty acid-induced inhibition of glucose uptake. J Clin Invest 1994;93(6):2438–46.

188. Goodpaster BH, Kelley DE. Skeletal muscle triglyceride: marker or mediator of obesity-induced insulin resistance in type 2 diabetes mellitus? Curr Diabet Rep 2002;2(3):216–22.

189. Kelley DE, Mandarino LJ. Fuel selection in human skeletal muscle in insulin resistance. A reexamination. Diabetes 2000;49:677–83.

190. Gray SL, Vidal-Puig AJ. Adipose tissue expandability in the maintenance of metabolic homeostasis. Nutr Rev 2007;65(6 Pt 2):S7–S12.

191. Medina-Gomez G, Virtue S, Lelliott C, et al. The link between nutritional status and insulin sensitivity is dependent on the adipocyte-specific peroxisome proliferator-activated receptor-gamma2 isoform. Diabetes 2005;54(6):1706–16.

192. Zhang J, Fu M, Cui T, et al. Selective disruption of PPARgamma 2 impairs the development of adipose tissue and insulin sensitivity. Proc Natl Acad Sci USA 2004;101(29):10703–8.

193. Frayn KN. Adipose tissue as a buffer for daily lipid flux. Diabetologia 2002;45(9):1201–10.

194. Nadler ST, Attie AD. Please pass the chips: genomic insights into obesity and diabetes. J Nutr 2001;131:2078–81.

195. Reitman ML, Mason MM, Moitra J, et al. Transgenic mice lacking white fat: models for understanding human lipoatrophic diabetes. Ann NY Acad Sci 1999;892:289–96.

196. Kim JK, Fillmore JJ, Chen Y, et al. Tissue-specific overexpression of lipoprotein lipase causes tissue-specific insulin resistance. Proc Natl Acad Sci USA 2001;98(13):7522–7.

197. Furnsinn C, Waldhausl W. Thiazolidinediones: metabolic actions in vitro. Diabetologia 2002;45(9):1211–23.

198. Giannini S, Serio M, Galli A. Pleiotropic effects of thiazolidinediones: taking a look beyond antidiabetic activity. J Endocrinol Invest 2004;27(10):982–91.

199. Drolet R, Richard C, Sniderman AD, et al. Hypertrophy and hyperplasia of abdominal adipose tissues in women. Int J Obes 2008;32:283–91.

200. Trayhurn P, Wood IS. Signalling role of adipose tissue: adipokines and inflammation in obesity. Biochem Soc Trans 2005;33(Pt 5):1078–81.

201. Drolet R, Bélanger C, Fortier M, et al. Fat depot-specific impact of visceral obesity on adipocyte adiponectin release in women. Obesity 2009;17(3):424–30.

202. Hube F, Birgel M, Lee YM, Hauner H. Expression pattern of tumour necrosis factor receptors in subcutaneous and omental human adipose tissue: role of obesity and non-insulin-dependent diabetes mellitus. Eur J Clin Invest 1999;29(8):672–8.

203. Hotamisligil GS, Arner P, Caro JF, Atkinson RL, Spiegelman BM. Increased adipose tissue expression of tumor necrosis factor-alpha in human obesity and insulin resistance. J Clin Invest 1995;95(5):2409–15.

204. He G, Pedersen SB, Bruun JM, Lihn AS, Jensen PF, Richelsen B. Differences in plasminogen activator inhibitor 1 in subcutaneous versus omental adipose tissue in non-obese and obese subjects. Horm Metab Res 2003;35(3):178–82.

205. Skurk T, Alberti-Huber C, Herder C, Hauner H. Relationship between adipocyte size and adipokine expression and secretion. J Clin Endocrinol Metab 2007;92(3):1023–33.

206. Whitehead JP, Richards AA, Hickman IJ, Macdonald GA, Prins JB. Adiponectin – a key adipokine in the metabolic syndrome. Diabetes Obes Metab 2006;8(3):264–80.

207. Motoshima H, Wu X, Sinha MK, et al. Differential regulation of adiponectine secretion from cultured human omental and subcutaneous adipocytes: effects of insulin and rosiglitazone. J Clin Endocrinol Metab 2002;87:5662–7.

208. Fenkci S, Rota S, Sabir N, Sermez Y, Guclu A, Akdag B. Relationship of serum interleukin-6 and tumor necrosis factor alpha levels with abdominal fat distribution evaluated by ultrasonography in overweight or obese postmenopausal women. J Invest Med 2006;54(8):455–60.

209. Wisse BE. The inflammatory syndrome: the role of adipose tissue cytokines in metabolic disorders linked to obesity. J Am Soc Nephrol 2004;15(11):2792–800.

210. Fried SK, Bunkin DA, Greenberg AS. Omental and subcutaneous adipose tissues of obese subjects release interleukin-6: depot difference and regulation by glucocorticoid. J Clin Endocrinol Metab 1998;83(3):847–50.

211. Morisset AS, Huot C, Légaré D, Tchernof A. Circulating IL-6 concentrations and abdominal adipocyte isoproterenol-stimulated lipolysis in women. Obesity 2008;16(7):1487–92.

212. Trujillo ME, Sullivan S, Harten I, Schneider SH, Greenberg AS, Fried SK. Interleukin-6 regulates human adipose tissue lipid metabolism and leptin production in vitro. J Clin Endocrinol Metab 2004;89(11):5577–82.

213. Greenberg AS, Nordan RP, McIntosh J, Calvo JC, Scow RO, Jablons D. Interleukin 6 reduces lipoprotein lipase activity in adipose tissue of mice in vivo and in 3T3-L1 adipocytes: a possible role for interleukin 6 in cancer cachexia. Cancer Res 1992;52:4113–16.

214. Weisberg SP, McCann D, Desai M, Rosenbaum M, Leibel RL, Ferrante AW Jr. Obesity is associated with macrophage accumulation in adipose tissue. J Clin Invest 2003;112(12):1796–808.

215. Good M, Newell FM, Haupt LM, Whitehead JP, Hutley LJ, Prins JB. TNF and TNF receptor expression and insulin sensitivity in human omental and subcutaneous adipose tissue – influence of BMI and adipose distribution. Diab Vasc Dis Res 2006;3(1): 26–33.

216. Grunfeld C, Feingold KR. The metabolic effects of tumor necrosis factor and other cytokines. Biotherapy 1991;3(2):143–58.

217. Perreault M, Marette A. Targeted disruption of inducible nitric oxide synthase protects against obesity-linked insulin resistance in muscle. Nat Med 2001;7(10):1138–43.

218. Park HS, Park JY, Yu R. Relationship of obesity and visceral adiposity with serum concentrations of CRP, TNF-alpha and IL-6. Diabetes Res Clin Pract 2005;69(1):29–35.

219. Tsigos C, Kyrou I, Chala E, et al. Circulating tumor necrosis factor alpha concentrations are higher in abdominal versus peripheral obesity. Metabolism 1999;48(10):1332–5.

220. Alessi MC, Juhan-Vague I. PAI-1 and the metabolic syndrome: links, causes, and consequences. Arterioscler Thromb Vasc Biol 2006;26(10):2200–7.

221. Gottschling-Zeller H, Birgel M, Rohrig K, Hauner H. Effect of tumor necrosis factor alpha and transforming growth factor beta 1 on plasminogen activator inhibitor-1 secretion from subcutaneous and omental human fat cells in suspension culture. Metabolism 2000;49(5):666–71.

222. Alessi MC, Peiretti F, Morange P, Henry M, Nalbone G, Juhan-Vague I. Production of plasminogen activator inhibitor 1 by human adipose tissue: possible link between visceral fat accumulation and vascular disease. Diabetes 1997;46(5):860–7.

223. Kockx M, Leenen R, Seidell J, Princen HM, Kooistra T. Relationship between visceral fat and PAI-1 in overweight men and women before and after weight loss. Thromb Haemost 1999;82(5):1490–6.

224. Brenner DJ, Hall EJ. Computed tomography – an increasing source of radiation exposure. N Engl J Med 2007;357(22):2277–84.

225. Kissebah AH, Peiris AN. Biology of regional body fat distribution. Relationship to non-insulin-dependent diabetes mellitus. Diabet Metab Rev 1989;5:83–109.

226. Rankinen T, Kim SY, Pérusse L, Després JP, Bouchard C. The prediction of abdominal visceral fat level from body composition and anthropometry: ROC analysis. Int J Obes 1999;23(8):801–9.

227. Chan DC, Watts GF, Barrett PH, Burke V. Waist circumference, waist-to-hip ratio and body mass index as predictors of adipose tissue compartments in men. Q J Med 2003;96(6):441–7.

228. Kreisberg RA, Oberman A. Medical management of hyperlipidemia/dyslipidemia. J Clin Endocrinol Metab 2003;88(6):2445–61.

229. Brochu M, Tchernof A, Turner AN, Ades PA, Poehlman ET. Is there a threshold of visceral fat loss that improves the metabolic profile in obese postmenopausal women? Metabolism 2003;52(5):599–604.

230. Després JP, Lamarche B. Effects of diet and physical activity on adiposity and body fat distribution: implications for the prevention of cardiovascular disease. Nutr Res Rev 1993;6:137–59.

231. Smith SR, Zachwieja JJ. Visceral adipose tissue: a critical review of intervention strategies. Int J Obes 1999;23:329–35.

232. Tuomilehto J, Lindstrom J, Eriksson JG, et al. Prevention of type 2 diabetes mellitus by changes in lifestyle among subjects with impaired glucose tolerance. N Engl J Med 2001;344(18):1343–50.

233. Knowler WC, Barrett-Connor E, Fowler SE, et al. Reduction in the incidence of type 2 diabetes with lifestyle intervention or metformin. N Engl J Med 2002;346(6):393–403.

234. Lamarche B, Després JP, Pouliot MC, et al. Is body fat loss a determinant factor in the improvement of carbohydrate and lipid metabolism following aerobic exercise training in obese women? Metabolism 1992;41(11):1249–56.

235. Poirier P, Després JP. Waist circumference, visceral obesity, and cardiovascular risk. J Cardiopulm Rehabil 2003;23(3):161–9.

14 Obesity Insulin Resistance and Gut Hormones

Joseph Proietto

Department of Medicine, University of Melbourne, Melbourne, Australia

Insulin resistance

There is now little doubt that a significant cause of insulin resistance is excess fat. To understand obesity-induced insulin resistance, it is necessary to have knowledge of how insulin signals. Briefly, when insulin binds to its receptor, a conformational change in the receptor activates the intrinsic tyrosine kinase located in the β chain. The initial target of the tyrosine kinase is its companion β chain. Cross tyrosine phosphorylation of the β chains more powerfully activates the tyrosine kinase which then activates its primary downstream target, one of a family of proteins called insulin receptor substrates (IRS) 1–4. The most important IRS in peripheral tissues is IRS-1 while in the liver and pancreatic β cell it is IRS-2 [1]. Insulin phosphorylates multiple tyrosine residues on IRS proteins. Tyrosine-phosphorylated IRS proteins attract several downstream proteins that contain SH2 domains in their structures, including PI-3 kinase, and Grb2, which in turn mediate the metabolic and growth effects of insulin respectively. PI-3 kinase phosphorylates P(4,5)P2 to P(3,4,5)P3 which activates PDK and in turn it activates both Akt (PKB) and PKC ζ. In muscle and adipose tissues, these mediate an increase in glucose transport by translocating the glucose transporter GLUT4 from an intracellular compartment to the cell surface. They also stimulate glycogen synthesis and have antilipolytic activity. The Grb2 pathway mediates the growth effects of insulin via activation of the MAP kinase pathway.

In the previous edition of this book some mechanisms of obesity-induced insulin resistance were reviewed. In particular, the effects of free fatty acids (FFA) and obesity-induced changes in cytokine levels were highlighted. Briefly, it was shown that free fatty acids cause peripheral insulin resistance by overproduction of long-chain acyl-CoA secondary to the oversupply of FFAs, which in turn activate protein kinase θ [2], that serine-phosphorylates and thus impairs the action of IRS-1. Long-chain acyl-CoA may also increase the production of ceramide [3] which inhibits Akt (PKB) [4]. Finally, long-chain acyl-CoAs inhibit hexokinase, the enzyme involved in the first step in glucose metabolism [5].

Free fatty acids also cause hepatic insulin resistance by stimulating gluconeogenesis [6] by several proposed mechanisms including upregulation of fructose 1,6 bisphosphatase [7], elevation of acetyl-CoA, citrate, NADH or ATP [8,9] and accumulation of PKC δ [8]. Recently, transgenic mice overexpressing fructose 1,6 bisphosphatase in the liver were produced and showed that despite an increase in gluconeogenesis from glycerol, there was no measurable increase in endogenous glucose production [10], suggesting that fat-induced increase in FBPase on its own is not sufficient to explain enhanced EGP and that other fat-induced mechanisms must contribute.

In the previous edition of this book, the role of tumor necrosis factor (TNF)-α, resistin, interleukin 6 (IL-6), adiponectin and leptin in modulating insulin action was discussed. Since the publication of the last edition, the following has been discovered about these adipokines.

TNF-α

Diet-induced obesity is associated with an upregulation of protein tyrosine phosphatase 1B (PTP1B), a negative regulator of insulin signaling. Perhaps the most significant advance in knowledge relative to TNF-α is the finding that this cytokine can upregulate PTP1B [11]. This phosphatase dephosphorylates (and hence inhibits) the insulin receptor, leading to insulin resistance.

Resistin

In rodents, resistin is secreted mainly from adipocytes while in humans, monocytes and macrophages are the main source [12]. Fat feeding increases resistin levels, resulting in hepatic insulin resistance [13]. In mice, resistin deficiency improves glucose

Clinical Obesity in Adults and Children, 3rd edition. Edited by Peter G. Kopelman, Ian D. Caterson and William H. Dietz.
© 2010 Blackwell Publishing, ISBN: 978-1-4051-8226-3.

tolerance and insulin sensitivity by enhancing Akt phosphorylation in muscle and liver and decreasing suppressor of cytokine signalling-3 (SOCS-3) levels [14]. Infusion of resistin into the brain resulted in elevated endogenous glucose production associated with an increased hepatic expression of SOCS-3, IL-6 and TNF-α [15].

Adiponectin

As mentioned in the last edition of this book, low levels of adiponectin in obese subjects may contribute to the insulin resistance seen in obesity. More recent work has shown that mice in which the adiponectin gene has been deleted demonstrate differential insulin resistance in various tissues. Adiponectin knockout (KO) mice demonstrate hepatic but not peripheral insulin resistance [16]. Interestingly, these mice are also unresponsive to the insulin-sensitizing effects of PPARγ agonists, suggesting that the glitazones partly enhance insulin sensitivity by upregulating adiponectin expression [16]. This is inconsistent with evidence from human studies showing that the PPARγ agonists (glitazones) predominantly improve peripheral insulin action with only a minor beneficial effect on hepatic insulin resistance [17]. It is possible that there is a species difference in the actions of adiponectin.

Novel obesity-related mechanisms for insulin resistance
Retinol binding protein 4

A surprising outcome of deletion of the insulin-responsive glucose transporter (GLUT4) in individual tissues was that mice with deletion specifically in adipocytes developed muscle insulin resistance [18]. Investigating this surprising phenotype, Qin et al. identified genes that were differentially expressed between GLUT4-deficient and normal adipocytes [19]. A surprising finding was that GLUT4-deficient adipocytes overexpressed retinol binding protein 4 (RBP-4) 2.3-fold [19]. Retinol binding protein was previously known only as a transporter of vitamin A. In a subsequent series of elegant experiments, it was shown that circulating levels of RBP-4 are elevated in obese mouse models, including the melanocortin 4 receptor (MC4R) KO, leptin deficient (ob/ob) and high fat fed mice [19]. In addition, serum RBP-4 levels were elevated 1.9-fold in obese human subjects. Modulation of RBP-4 levels, by genetic manipulation, RBP-4 infusion or infusion of a compound that reduces RBP-4 level, resulted in changes in insulin sensitivity, suggesting that elevated RBP-4 can cause insulin resistance. Of interest is that the PPARγ agonist, the thiazolidenedione rosiglitazone which is known to improve insulin resistance, normalized RBP-4 in the GLUT4 KO mice.

Mitochondrial dysfunction and oxidative stress

Mitochondrial dysfunction as a cause of insulin resistance has been proposed for some time [20–22]. In addition, it was shown that excess fat availability resulted in a decrease in the expression of transcriptional regulators such as PGC1α required for mitochondrial production and in the expression of genes coding for proteins in the electron transport chain [23]. To further

investigate possible mechanisms involved in the development of mitochondrial dysfunction, Bonnard et al. [24] fed mice a high-fat, high-sucrose diet for a prolonged period of time. This resulted in mitochondrial dysfunction. The diet-induced high-fat fed insulin-resistant mice had an increase in reactive oxygen species (ROS) production in skeletal muscle. Antioxidant treatment decreased muscle ROS production and restored mitochondrial integrity, suggesting that the high ROS induced by the diet was the cause of the mitochondrial dysfunction, which in turn led to insulin resistance. These studies were repeated *in vitro* and confirmed that glucose or lipid-induced reactive oxygen species production caused mitochondrial dysfunction.

Thus, it appears that mitochondrial alterations in obese type 2 diabetic subjects do not precede the onset of insulin resistance, but rather are the result of reactive oxygen species production in muscle as a result of fat overfeeding. The authors proposed that excess nutrient supply results in the uncoupling of mitochondrial oxidative phosphorylation, leading to overproduction of free oxygen radicals. These in turn are postulated to suppress expression of PGC1α and other regulators of mitochondrial biogenesis, thus reducing mitochondrial biogenesis. This reduces fatty acid oxidation, leading to the excess accumulation of intracellular fat and subsequent insulin resistance [24].

However, this view of the role of mitochondrial dysfunction as a cause of insulin resistance has recently been challenged. It has been proposed that rather than insulin resistance being linked to a reduction in fatty acid β oxidation, and the subsequent accumulation of intracellular fat, the cause is mitochondrial overload and an increase in incomplete FFA oxidation coupled with reduced fat oxidation in the liver [25].

Blood flow abnormalities leading to insulin resistance

It has been proposed that part of insulin's action to stimulate glucose uptake in muscle tissues is to open what have been called nutrient capillaries [26]. It follows that any abnormality in this effect of insulin could contribute to what is perceived as insulin resistance. Insulin appears to have antagonistic effects to both vasodilate (mediated by nitric oxide) and vasoconstrict (mediated by endothelin-1) resistance arterioles [27]. It has been proposed that localized excess fat deposited around arterioles may lead to impaired insulin-stimulated nitric oxide synthesis, resulting in unopposed constriction caused by endothelin-1 [28]. It has been further suggested that this is a consequence of increased production of TNF-α from excess localized fat surrounding the vessel [28]. Another, possibly related mechanism may be the reduced expression of eNOS as was demonstrated in resistance arterioles of obese Zucker rats [29].

Abnormal fatty acid re-esterification as the cause of insulin resistance in central obesity

In a recent study it has been proposed that an abnormality in fatty acid re-esterification in women with central obesity is a possible cause of insulin resistance in central obesity [30]. The authors compared women with and without abdominal obesity. They performed euglycemic clamps at an insulin infusion rate of 40 mU/m^2/min and assessed glucose disposal, endogenous glucose production and lipolysis. They found that centrally obese women demonstrated peripheral and hepatic insulin resistance. Using the ratio of the rate of appearance of glycerol (as a measure of lipolysis) and the level of circulating free fatty acids (Ra$_{gly}$/FFA), they were able to estimate the rate of re-esterification of free fatty acids to triglyceride. Obese women had a marked reduction in the rate of FFA re-esterification, and fatty acid re-esterification was significantly related to abdominal circumference and peripheral and hepatic insulin resistance independent of total body fat [30]. The inability to re-esterify FFA results in higher FFA levels which then induce widespread insulin resistance.

Obesity and gut hormones

The center of weight control is the hypothalamus. There are several available reviews of its role [31,32]. While the hypothalamus determines the desire to eat or the sensation of fullness, its net state is in turn determined by the balance of the actions of circulating signals. These signals, as might be expected, are derived from relevant tissues including fat tissue (leptin, adiponectin, TNF-α and other cytokines) and the gut. Not surprisingly, the gut and its extension, the pancreas, which receive and respond to ingested energy, are a rich source of signals to the hypothalamus. This section of the chapter will review current knowledge of the gut signals that can regulate food intake.

Several gut peptides have been described that influence food intake. These come from different areas of the gastrointestinal tract and can be subdivided several ways. If subdivided functionally, they are:
• short-term satiety peptides (CCK)
• long-term feeding signals (PYY, GLP-1, PP, amylin, insulin, neuromedin B, oxyntomodulin)
• feeding stimulator (ghrelin).
If subdivided anatomically, they are:
• stomach (ghrelin)
• duodenum (CCK, GIP)
• pancreas (PP, amylin, insulin)
• ileum (GLP-1, oxyntomodulin, PYY)
• colon (GLP-1, oxyntomodulin, PYY).
Before discussing hormonal signals it is important to state that there is evidence that gastric distension *per se* can terminate a meal, although a large volume of food is required for this to occur [33,34]. To achieve this function the stomach has well-characterized stretch receptors [35,36].

General gut hormones
Ghrelin
Ghrelin is a 28 amino acid protein that stimulates both food intake and growth hormone release [37]. It has been shown to stimulate food intake in rodents [38] and man [39]. It is produced in the stomach and the brain, although the major component of the circulating hormone is stomach derived. When ghrelin is administered peripherally it stimulates food intake and activates neurons in the arcuate nucleus of the hypothalamus that express neuropeptide Y (NPY) [40,41]. The growth hormone secretagog receptor 1a (GHS-R1a) is expressed at a high level in the hypothalamus consistent with a role in ghrelin's food intake-stimulating effects.

Unlike leptin, plasma ghrelin levels vary significantly during the day, rising prior to meals and falling rapidly after meals [42]. Of interest, ghrelin levels are higher following weight loss [42], a mechanism contributing to weight regain after weight loss. Ghrelin has been shown to stimulate insulin-induced glucose uptake in adipocytes [43] and insulin secretion [44]. It is possible therefore that the rise in ghrelin that occurs following weight loss not only contributes to weight regain but may also contribute to the metabolic benefits on glucose tolerance seen with weight loss.

Cholecystokinin (CCK)
Cholecystokinin is produced predominantly by the I cells of the duodenal and jejunal mucosa. Other sites of production so far described include the brain and the nerves supplying the gut. The CCK parent hormone is cleaved by endoproteolytic enzymes into at least six peptides including CCK8, CCK22, CCK33 and CCK58. Of these, it appears that CCK58 is the major circulating form in both rats [45] and humans [46]. CCK is secreted in response to the presence of food (in particular fat and protein) in the gut. It has a multitude of effects, including stimulation of pancreatic secretion, contraction of the gallbladder and, of relevance to this discussion, the induction of satiety. If injected just before a meal, CCK reduces the size of the meal [47]; however, the effect is short-lived.

There are two CCK receptors: CCK1R (CCK-A), mainly expressed in the gastrointestinal system, and CCK2R (CCK-B), which is predominantly found in the brain. The satiating effects of CCK are mediated by both central and peripheral actions of the hormone. CCK1R receptors are expressed in the vagus nerve, and subdiaphragmatic vagotomy reduces the satiating effect of peripherally administered CCK [48], showing the peripheral action of CCK. Injection of CCK directly into selected brain nuclei decreases food intake [49]. Of interest is the fact that CCK also slows gastric emptying, thus contributing to the gastric distension that occurs after feeding. As mentioned above, there is evidence that distension *per se* inhibits food intake. CCK and gastric distension may have additive effects [50].

Because of its short duration of action, CCK may not be a good target for the treatment of obesity. When CCK is repeatedly administered peripherally to rats it reduces meal size but this does not lead to weight loss as the rats simply increase the number of meals [51], a testament to the highly complex regulatory mechanism that controls body weight. Recently it has been demonstrated that CCK release following a meal is reduced following weight loss [52] (Fig. 14.1), demonstrating that CCK takes part in the multifaceted adaptation to voluntary weight loss.

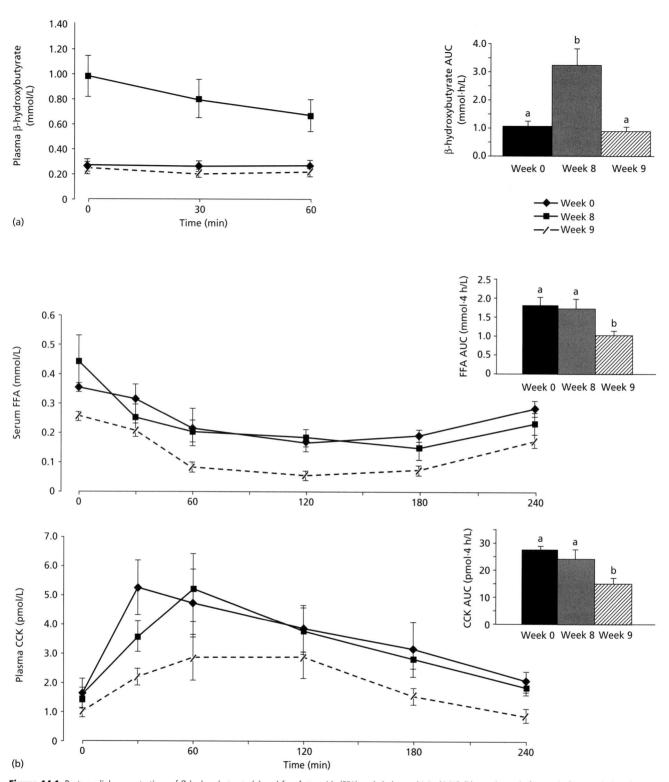

Figure 14.1 Postprandial concentrations of β-hydroxybutyrate (a) and free fatty acids (FFA) and cholecystokinin (CCK) (b) are shown before and after weight loss (error bars indicate SEM; n = 12). The bar graphs depict the cumulative postprandial responses (area under the curve) of the metabolites. (Reproduced with permission from Chearskul et al. [52].).

Gastric inhibitory polypeptide (GIP)

Glucose-dependent insulinotropic polypeptide or gastric inhibitory polypeptide (GIP) is a 42 amino acid hormone produced in the proximal small bowel in K cells. It is known as one of the two incretin hormones (with GLP-1) and is a major inducer of postprandial insulin secretion [53]. Like GLP-1, it is degraded by dipeptidyl peptidase-IV (DPP-IV). GIP acts through a G-coupled receptor, generating cAMP as the intracellular signal. As expected, this receptor is expressed in pancreatic β cells but it is also expressed in adipocytes [54] and osteoblasts [55]. It was the deletion of the receptor in mice that uncovered the actions of GIP on fat and bone metabolism. GIP has the effect of encouraging nutrient storage by stimulating glucose uptake and activation of lipoprotein lipase in adipocytes [56]. This is the reason why GIP receptor KO mice are resistant to the weight gain associated with a high-fat diet [56]. Thus, it has been proposed that GIP can be seen as a direct link between overnutrition and obesity since the stimulation of GIP is nutrient dependent. GIP is not the only factor acting in this manner, since insulin is also stimulated by nutrients and encourages energy storage by activating glucose uptake and lipoprotein lipase. The effect of GIP on bone is to encourage bone formation after food intake [57].

Glucagon-like peptide-1 (GLP-1)

The physiology of glucagon-like peptide-1 has recently been thoroughly reviewed [58]. There are many examples in biology of a single gene giving rise to multiple bio-active proteins and peptides. In endocrinology, pro-opiomelanocortin (POMC) is the typical example. Proglucagon is another, giving rise to GLP-1, glucagon, GLP-2, glicentin, and oxyntomodulin (Fig. 14.2). The same proglucagon gene is expressed in the pancreatic α cells and in the intestine so the different hormones produced in these tissues are

the result of differential processing of proglucagon mRNA [59]. In the gut, processing results in the formation of glicentin (1–69) which includes oxyntomodulin (33–69) and GLP-1 (72–108), intervening peptide 2 (111–123) and GLP-2 (126–160). It was found that a truncated fragment of GLP-1 (78–107) was a powerful stimulator of insulin secretion while the full-length hormone (72–108) was inactive [60]. The majority of GLP-1 secreted from the gut in humans is the amidated version [61].

There is some evidence that there is a very low level of basal GLP-1 secretion but clearly most GLP-1 is secreted in response to food arriving in the distal gut. In addition, the response is proportional to the size of the meal. Strangely, GLP-1 secretion is quite rapid, possibly before the food has had a chance to arrive in the distal small bowel, which may be explained by several mechanisms including the existence of some L cells in more proximal areas of the small bowel and a direct effect of GIP to stimulate GLP-1 secretion via the vagus nerve [62].

The receptor for GLP-1 is G-coupled and is expressed in pancreatic islets, brain, heart, kidney, and gastrointestinal tract. GLP-1 has multiple functions including:
- stimulation of insulin secretion (but only in the presence of elevated glucose)
- suppression of glucagon secretion
- inhibition of gastrointestinal secretion and motility
- inhibition of food intake [63,64].

Both GLP-1 [65] and its receptor [66] are expressed in the brain. The receptor is particularly expressed in key food-regulating centers such as the arcuate nucleus and other hypothalamic areas [66]. Nutrients infused into the ileum stimulate GLP-1 release [67] and induce satiety [68], suggesting that peripherally produced GLP-1 may have a physiologic role in modulating satiety. Indeed, infusion of GLP-1 dose-dependently enhances

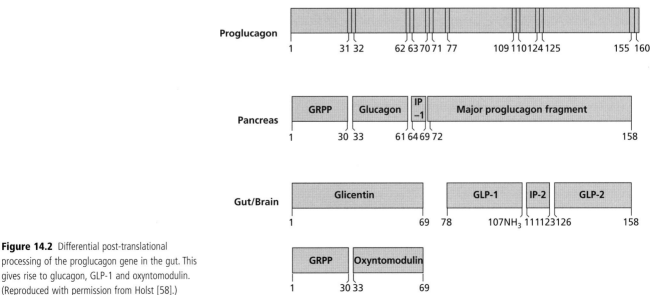

Figure 14.2 Differential post-translational processing of the proglucagon gene in the gut. This gives rise to glucagon, GLP-1 and oxyntomodulin. (Reproduced with permission from Holst [58].)

satiety and reduces food intake [69,70]. An analog of GLP-1 developed for the treatment of type 2 diabetes (Exendin 4) when administered daily resulted in mild but steady and progressive weight loss [71]. The mechanism for GLP-1 mediated weight loss is not clear. Is it acting via the vagus nerve or by a direct action on the brain? It could possibly be a combination of both.

Peptide YY (PYY)

Peptide YY is a 36 amino acid peptide secreted from the L cells into the distal gut. Its secretion is stimulated by food. Two forms of PYY are found in the circulation: PYY1–36 and PYY3–36 [72]. Dipeptidyl peptidase IV, the same enzyme that degrades GLP-1, also cleaves off the first two N terminal amino acids to form PYY3–36, the active form of the hormone. Thus while DPP-IV inactivates GLP-1, it activates PYY.

Peptide YY, NPY and pancreatic polypeptide (PP) (see below) belong to the same family and share a high degree of homology (67% with NPY). PYY acts predominantly through the Y2-R receptor and has been shown to inhibit food intake in both humans and rodents. Y2 receptors are found in the arcuate nucleus of the hypothalamus. In addition, they are also expressed in the vagal nodose ganglion. Infusion of PYY3–36 reduces NPY mRNA in the arcuate nucleus. Although it had been suggested that this action arose via activation of POMC neurons, a direct suppressive effect on NPY neurons is now considered more likely [73]. Indeed, PYY3–36 appears to inhibit POMC neurons, leading to the suggestion that it temporarily reduces the role of arcuate nuclear cells, thus increasing the influence of other circuits [73].

Infusion of PYY3–36 into humans [74] and rodents [75] results in a sustained reduction in appetite and food intake. PYY3–36 possibly acts two ways to mediate these effects. Direct injection of the hormone into the arcuate nucleus suppressed food intake and NPY neuronal firing [75], suggesting a direct effect of the hormone in the brain. However, rat studies suggest that there is a major role for the vagus nerve in PYY3–36's action. Abdominal vagotomy abolished the anorectic effect of peripherally administered PYY3–36 and the activation of arcuate nucleus neurons [76]. Y2-R receptors are synthesized in the nodose ganglion and transported along vagal fibers to the nerve endings. There is also evidence that this action of the vagus nerve is mediated via the solitary tract [76]. It is important to note that the weight loss effects of PYY3–36 administration into rodents has been questioned [77].

Oxyntomodulin

The term "oxyntomodulin" was first applied in 1981 to a bioactive form of enteroglucagon that increased cAMP in the fundus of the rat stomach [78]. It was shown to have some activity as an incretin hormone when it was demonstrated to stimulate insulin secretion from perfused rat pancreas [79]. In addition, it inhibits pentagastrin-stimulated acid secretion [80]. Indeed, most of the initial work was directed towards its action in the gut. However, in 2001 oxyntomodulin was shown to inhibit food intake in the rat when it was injected into the the brain of 24-hour fasted animals [81]. It also increases energy expenditure since the weight loss in oxyntomodulin-treated rats is greater than pair fed controls [82].

This hormone is made in the L cells of the gut in the same cells that also make GLP-1 and PYY. With them, it is secreted following a meal. There is evidence that DPP-IV degrades the hormone [83]. Oxyntomodulin has been shown to suppress appetite and reduce food intake in humans without inducing nausea [84]. It is possible that it signals through the GLP-1 receptor since it was unable to suppress food intake in GLP-1R KO mice [85]. However, there are some differential physiologic effects of these two related hormones, Compared to GLP-1, oxyntomodulin causes less nausea and has a weaker incretin effect but a more potent effect on food intake and energy expenditure [86]. More work is required to clarify this issue.

Bombesin-like peptides (gastrin-releasing peptide (GRP), neuromedin B (NMB))

Bombesin, originally discovered in amphibians, is a 14 amino acid peptide which suppresses feeding, induces hypothermia and hyperglycemia and induces grooming [87,88]. While intraventricular administration reduces food intake, it has been shown that the main effect of peripheral bombesin on food intake may be mediated neurally since neurally disconnecting the gut from the brain blocks its effect [89]. However, bombesin is not expressed in mammals. Instead, mammals express two bombesin-like compounds: gastrin-releasing peptide (GRP) (27 amino acids) and neuromedin B (NMB) (10 amino acids). GRP18–27 is known as neuromedin C. GRP was first isolated in 1979 and shown to have potent gastrin-secreting effects [90]. It is expressed widely in the gastrointestinal tract and brain. It was subsequently found to reduce meal size in rats although it was not as potent as bombesin itself [91]. Two separate and distinct receptors have been identified for GRP and neuromedin B although they share a high degree of homology. Interestingly, bombesin binds equally well to both receptors. The distribution of these receptors in the brain is also different, with the GRP receptor more highly expressed than the neuromedin B receptor in all areas of the hypothalamus [92]. Both receptors are involved in inhibition of feeding [93]. The order of potency for the suppression of feeding is bombesin > GRP > neuromedin B. The physiologic role of bombesin-like proteins in mammals remains unclear.

The pancreas

Embryologically the pancreas is an extension of the gut. The islets of Langerhans are the source of several peptides that can influence food intake in response to meals. These include pancreatic polypeptide, amylin and insulin.

Pancreatic polypeptide

As mentioned previously, pancreatic polypeptide (PP) is a member of a family of peptides that includes PYY and NPY. PP has 36 amino acids and is made in specific cells found in the islets of Langerhans. It is secreted in a biphasic manner and in proportion to the amount of food ingested and the level remains elevated for approximately 6 hours postprandially [94]. CCK, hypoglycemia and exercise also stimulate its secretion, the latter two mediated by the sympathetic nervous system [95]. Transgenic mice overexpressing PP in the pancreas developed a lean phenotype and demonstrated reduced gastric emptying [96].

It is interesting that while peripherally administered PP reduces food intake, when PP is administered directly into the brain it stimulates food intake [97]. Centrally, PP acts by binding to the Y4 receptor found in hypothalamic orexin-expressing neurons. Deletion of the Y4 receptor in mice resulted in reduced food intake and a lean phenotype [98]. Infusion of PP into humans reduced food intake by 25% over the next 24 hours [99]. It is believed that PP acts on the area postrema, a region of the brainstem that is outside the blood–brain barrier and is close to both the nucleus of the solitary tract and the dorsal motor nucleus of the vagus nerve [100,101]. Low levels of PP are found in obese children with the Prader–Willi syndrome [102] while they are elevated in patients with anorexia nervosa [103].

Amylin

Amylin, also known as islet amyloid polypeptide (IAPP), was isolated independently by two groups in 1987 [104,105]. It is a 37 amino acid protein produced by the pancreatic β cells and co-secreted with insulin. Since it was found in amyloid-like fibrils around β cells, it was originally thought to contribute to the pathogenesis of type 2 diabetes. However, it was soon realized that amylin is part of a larger family of calcitonin gene-related peptides. Subsequent work clarified the different roles of amylin. It is now known to suppress food intake, gastric emptying, glucagon secretion and digestive enzyme secretion, leading to the suggestion that its overall role is to limit the entry of nutrients into the circulation [106].

The role of amylin in inhibiting food intake has been reviewed [107]. Briefly, it appears to have both short- and long-term effects on reducing food intake by reducing meal size via its satiating effect [108] but also possibly by reducing the number of meals [109]. A physiologic role for amylin's satiating effect was questioned when it was realized that the minimal dose of exogenous amylin that led to a reduction in feeding produced twice the levels that are normally seen postprandially. However, the most powerful evidence that amylin has a physiologic role in food intake comes from studies showing that an antagonist of amylin increases food intake in rats [110]. Amylin's effect on reducing food intake is mediated via receptors located in the area postrema in the hindbrain [110].

Recently, it has been shown that amylin may restore leptin responsiveness in fat-fed rats, a model of diet-induced leptin insensitivity [111]. Amylin improved leptin signaling (measured by assessing level of leptin-induced STAT3 phosphorylation) in the ventromedial nucleus of the hypothalamus (but not the arcuate nucleus) and in the area postrema. Interestingly, neither PYY3–36 nor a GLP-1 analog induced an enhancement of leptin signaling [111].

Insulin

More has been written about insulin than about any other hormone. Most of the studies deal with its metabolic effects, which will not be covered here. When insulin is prescribed to patients with poorly controlled type 2 diabetes, it nearly always leads to weight gain. The exact mechanism for this is not known, but some proposed causes include a reduction in glycosuria, increased food intake in patients who see that their sugars are lower and the lipogenic effect of insulin on fat cells. In fact, like amylin, when administered into the brain, insulin suppresses feeding.

Insulin is known to enter the brain slowly and, like leptin, could possibly transmit a signal indicating the level of adiposity, since the amount of insulin secreted is generally proportional to the level of adiposity [112]. Insulin receptors have been found in many areas of the brain, including the arcuate nucleus. Deletion of brain insulin receptors leads to an increased food intake and an obese phenotype [113]. Woods et al [112] suggest that insulin levels correlate better with visceral fat (higher in men) while leptin levels correlate better with subcutaneous fat (higher in women). It is of interest therefore that insulin seems to act more powerfully in the male brain while leptin works better in the female brain [114].

Gut hormone changes after weight loss, including bariatric surgery

There appear not to be differences in the levels or secretion profiles of the various gut hormones in obesity [115,116]. However, it is well known that both insulin and leptin are elevated in proportion to the amount of fat in the body and that ghrelin is lower in obese subjects. These differences in hormone levels are likely to be the result rather than the cause of obesity. Apart from elevated ghrelin levels in Prader–Willi syndrome [117,118], no differences in gut hormone levels, that could lead to obesity, have so far been reported in nonsyndromic obesity.

However, when a stably obese individual loses weight, the secretion of hormones is altered. When discussing this, the mode of weight loss may be important. Thus caloric restriction, gastric banding and bypass procedures need to be discussed separately. Weight loss achieved with caloric restriction is associated with changes in several circulating hormones that appear to be part of a co-ordinated response to defend body weight. Thus it has been shown that the levels of inhibitors of food intake fall, including leptin, CCK, insulin [52] and PYY [115], while two hormones known to increase food intake rise, including ghrelin [42] and adiponectin [119]. There is evidence that these changes in hunger-controlling hormones lead to a measurable increase in hunger and a desire to eat [120], possibly contributing to weight regain after weight loss.

The changes in hormones that occur with weight loss induced with adjustable gastric banding need further study, but appear to

Table 14.1 Summary of changes in gut hormones associated with different ways of achieving weight loss

Hormone	Mode of weight loss		
	Caloric restriction	**Gastric banding**	**Gastric bypass**
Ghrelin	Increase[1]	No change[3]	No change[7]
CCK	Decrease[2]	NA	NA
Insulin	Decrease[2]	No change[3]	Decrease basal Increase postprandial[5]
PP	NA	No change[3]	NA
PYY	Decrease[4]	NA	Increase[6]
GIP	No change[5]	No change[3]	Increase[5]
GLP-1	No change[5]	No change[3]	Increase[5]

NA, no data available.
[1]Cummings et al. 2002 [42]. [2]Chearskul et al. 2008 [52]. [3]Shak et al. 2008 [124]. [4]Pfluger et al. 2007 [115]. [5]Laferrere et al. 2008 [123]. [6]Morinigo et al. 2006 [122]. [7]Korner et al. 2005 [121].

be similar to caloric restriction (Table 14.1). In contrast, when gastric bypass surgery is undertaken, the anatomic change delivers partially digested food to the lower gut which appears to trigger a substantially different response, including a failure of ghrelin to rise [121] and an increase in PYY [122], GIP and GLP-1 [123], which contribute to a reduction in hunger and an increase in satiety following surgery, despite the occurrence of weight loss [112], no doubt contributing to the long-term success of this procedure (Fig. 14.3).

Potential role of gut hormones in the treatment of obesity

Patients who have surgery for the treatment of obesity do not require pharmacotherapy to maintain weight loss. However, if indeed the adaptive changes that occur in gut hormones and the fat-derived adipokines (leptin and adiponectin) are the main reason for the failure to maintain weight loss, it follows that after weight loss, replacement of one or more of these reduced satiety signals may assist with long-term weight maintenance. Thus inhibitors of ghrelin and agonists of oxyntomodulin, PP, amylin, PYY and GLP-1 may have therapeutic potential.

Ghrelin inhibitors

Ghrelin could theoretically be used to treat several conditions associated with anorexia. Short-term studies in humans have reported increased food intake following ghrelin infusions in patients who were anorectic because of cancer [125], chronic obstructive pulmonary disease [126] and renal dialysis [127]. So far there are no published human studies on ghrelin inhibition to reduce food intake. One study in rats has shown that the inhibitor [D-Lys]-GHRP-6 reduced food intake in both obese (fa/fa) and lean (Fa/fa) rats [128].

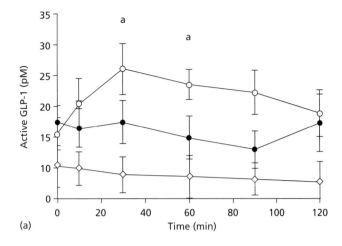

(a)

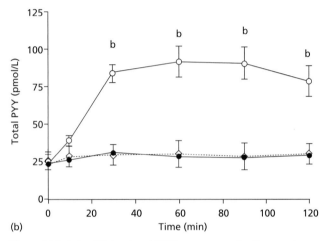

(b)

Figure 14.3 Active GLP-1 and total PYY in response to a liquid test meal. Active GLP-1 (a) and total PYY (b) circulating concentrations over the course of the test in obese subjects before (*black circles*, n = 9) and 6 weeks after (*open circles*, n = 9) RYGBP and in obese subjects matched with the experimental group for the BMI attained 6 weeks after surgery (*open diamonds*, n = 6). Data are expressed as mean (± SEM). (a) p < 0.05 and (b) p < 0.01 values are indicated for comparison relative to baseline (Bonferroni). (Reproduced with permission from Morinigo et al. [122].)From Morinigo R, et al. *J Clin Endocrinol and Metab* 91: 1735–40 2006 with permission).

GLP-1 agonists

Glucagon-like peptide-1 agonism has been a therapeutic target for the treatment of diabetes because of the multiple actions of GLP-1 that are beneficial to the maintenance of normal glucose levels, such as stimulation of insulin release, inhibition of glucagon secretion, slowing of gastric emptying and reduction in food intake. However, this has proven to be a difficult problem because of the very short half-life of the native hormone. Eventually three ways of overcoming the problem of half-life were arrived at. The first was the finding of a stable analog from the saliva of a reptile from the deserts of North America, the Gila monster (*Heloderma suspectum*), called extendin 4 and now marketed as exenatide (Byetta). This hormone is administered by injection and has been shown to lower blood glucose and to modestly reduce body weight in patients with type 2

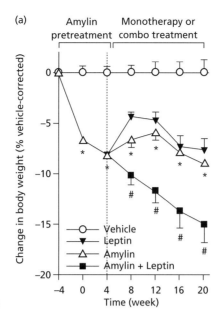 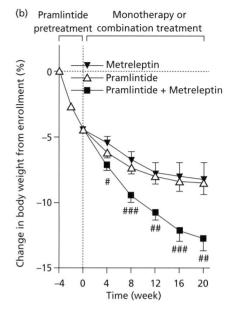

Figure 14.4 Weight loss effect of combined amylin and leptin agonism in DIO rats and overweight/obese humans. (a) Change in body weight for DIO rats pretreated for 14 days with amylin and then maintained on amylin (*open triangles*) or switched to either leptin monotherapy (*filled inverted triangles*) or amylin + leptin combination therapy (*filled squares*) for an additional 28 d. (b) Change in body weight for 93 evaluable human subjects pretreated with pramlintide for 4 weeks and then treated with pramlintide (*open triangles*), metreleptin (*filled inverted triangles*) or pramlintide + metreleptin combination (*filled squares*). Mean ± SE (a) and LS mean ± SE (b): *, $p < 0.05$ vs vehicle controls; #, $p < 0.01$; ##, $p < 0.01$; ###, $p < 0.001$ vs monotherapies. (Reproduced with permission from Roth et al. [111].)

diabetes [129]. Its main side-effect is mild nausea. The second approach has been to inhibit DPP-4, the enzyme responsible for the degradation of GLP-1 and GIP. These agents are marketed as sitagliptin and vildagliptin and have been shown to lower blood glucose [130]. Interestingly, they do not lower body weight and while this may be due to a lower level of GLP-1 activity than is achieved with exenatide, another possible reason may be that less PYY3–36 is made. As mentioned above, DPP-4 is the enzyme that produces the active hormone PYY3–36 from PYY1–36. The third approach has been to attach a fatty acid molecule to the native GLP-1 [131]. This compound has undergone clinical trials.

Oxyntomodulin, another product of the glucagon gene, degraded by DPP-4, is thought to act via the GLP-1 receptor. However, some of its actions are different to GLP-1 and it appears to cause less nausea, possibly giving it therapeutic advantage as a weight loss therapy. Studies in humans have shown that preprandial subcutaneous injection of oxyntomodulin reduces body weight [127] and increases energy expenditure [132]. More studies are required.

Amylin agonists

Pramlintide, an analog of human amylin, is administered by subcutaneous injection and is now clinically available. It has been shown that when added to insulin, it improves glucose control in patients with type 2 diabetes [133]. Of particular interest is its potential to enhance the action of leptin [111] (Fig. 14.4). Since leptin is one of those hormones that falls dramatically following weight loss and given that most obese subjects have leptin insensitivity, a combination of leptin and pramlintide could be a promising post weight loss therapy to assist with weight maintenance.

PYY agonists

Intravenous administration of PYY3–36 was shown to inhibit food intake [75] and therefore hope rose that it could be effective as a weight loss agent. However, a more recent study in which PYY3–36 was administered intranasally showed that the higher dose (600 μgm tid) was not tolerated due to nausea and vomiting while the lower dose (200 μgm tid) was not effective when compared to placebo [134].

Pancreatic polypeptide

Intravenous infusion of PP into humans has been reported to reduce appetite and to decrease energy intake up to 24 hours after the termination of the infusion [99]. Longer term studies are required to determine if PP has therapeutic potential.

Conclusion

Gut hormones offer some hope for the development of new therapeutics for the treatment of obesity. The main obstacles are the issues of nausea, duration of action and the need for parenteral administration. The future may also lie in combinations of hormones.

References

1. White MF, Kahn CR. The insulin signaling system. J Biol Chem 1994;269:1–4
2. Griffin ME, Marcucci MJ, Cline GW, et al. Free fatty acid-induced insulin resistance is associated with activation of protein kinase C

theta and alterations in the insulin signaling cascade. Diabetes 1999;48:1270–4.

3. Schmitz-Peiffer C, Craig DL, Biden TJ. Ceramide generation is sufficient to account for the inhibition of the insulin-stimulated PKB pathway in C2C12 skeletal muscle cells pretreated with palmitate. J Biol Chem 1999;274:24202–10.

4. Zhou H, Summers SA, Birnbaum MJ, Pittman RN. Inhibition of Akt kinase by cell-permeable ceramide and its implications for ceramide-induced apoptosis. J Biol Chem 1998;273:16568–75.

5. Thompson AL, Cooney GJ. Acyl-CoA inhibition of hexokinase in rat and human skeletal muscle is a potential mechanism of lipid-induced insulin resistance. Diabetes 2000;49:1761–5.

6. Andrikopoulos S, Proietto J. The biochemical basis of increased hepatic glucose production in a mouse model of type 2 (non-insulin-dependent) diabetes mellitus. Diabetologia 1995;38:1389–96.

7. Song S, Andrikopoulos S, Filippis C, Thorburn AW, Khan D, Proietto J. Mechanism of fat-induced hepatic gluconeogenesis: effect of metformin. Am J Physiol Endocrinol Metab 2001;281:E275–82.

8. Lam TK, Yoshii H, Haber CA, et al. Free fatty acid-induced hepatic insulin resistance: a potential role for protein kinase C-delta. Am J Physiol Endocrinol Metab 2002;283:E682–91.

9. Lam TK, van de Werve G, Giacca A. Free fatty acids increase basal hepatic glucose production and induce hepatic insulin resistance at different sites. Am J Physiol Endocrinol Metab 2003;284:E281–90.

10. Lamont BJ, Visinoni S, Fam BC, et al. Expression of human fructose-1,6-bisphosphatase in the liver of transgenic mice results in increased glycerol gluconeogenesis. Endocrinology 2006;147:2764–72.

11. Zabolotny JM, Kim Y-B, Welsh LA, Kershaw EE, Neel BG, Kahn B. Protein tyrosine phosphatase 1B (PTP1B) expression is induced by inflammation in vivo. J Biol Chem 2008;14:1–27.

12. Patel L, Buckels AC, Kinghorn IJ, et al. Resistin is expressed in human macrophages and directly regulated by PPAR gamma activators. Biochem Biophys Res Commun 2003;300:472–6.

13. Muse ED, Obici S, Bhanot S, et al. Role of resistin in diet-induced hepatic insulin resistance. J Clin Invest 2004;114:232–9.

14. Qui Y, Nie Z, Lee YS, et al. Loss of resistin improves glucose homeostasis in leptin deficiency. Diabetes 2006;55:3083–90.

15. Muse ED, Lam TKT, Scherer PE, Rossetti L. Hypothalamic resistin induces hepatic insulin resistance. J. Clin Invest 2007;117:1670–8.

16. Nawrocki AR, Rajala MW, Tomas E, et al. Mice lacking adiponectin show decreased hepatic insulin sensitivity and reduced responsiveness to peroxisome proliferator-activated receptor gamma agonists. J Biol Chem 2006;281:2654–60.

17. Inzucchi SE, Maggs DG, Spollett GR, et al. Efficacy and metabolic effects of metformin and troglitazone in type II diabetes mellitus. N Engl J Med 1998;338:867–72.

18. Abel ED, Peroni O, Kim JK, et al. Adipose-selective targeting of the GLUT4 gene impairs insulin action in muscle and liver. Nature 2001;409:729–33.

19. Qin Y, Graham TE, Mody N, et al. Serum retinol binding protein 4 contributes to insulin resistance in obesity and type 2 diabetes. Nature 2005;436:356–62.

20. Simoneau JA, Kelley DE. Altered glycolytic and oxidative capacities of skeletal muscle contribute to insulin resistance in NIDDM. J Appl Physiol 1997;83:166–71.

21. Kelley DE, He J, Menshikova EV, Ritov VB. Dysfunction of mitochondria in human skeletal muscle of type 2 diabetes. Diabetes 2002;51:2944–50.

22. Lowell BB, Shulman GI. Mitochondrial dysfunction and type 2 diabetes. Science 2005;307:384–7.

23. Sparks LM, Xie H, Koza RA, et al. A high fat diet co-ordinately downregulates genes required for mitochondrial oxidative phosphorylation in skeletal muscle. Diabetes 2005;54:1926–33.

24. Bonnard C, Durand A, Peyrol S, et al. Mitochondrial dysfunction results from oxidative stress in the skeletal muscle of diet-induced insulin resistant mice. J Clin Invest 2008;118:789–800.

25. Koves TR, Ussher JR, Noland RC, et al. Mitochondrial overload and incomplete fatty acid oxidation contribute to skeletal muscle insulin resistance. Cell Metab 2008;7:45–56.

26. Clark MG, Wallis MG, Barrett EJ, et al. Blood flow and muscle metabolism: a focus on insulin action. Am J Physiol Endocrinol Metab 2003;284:E241–E258.

27. Cardillo C, Nambi SS, Kilcoyne CM, et al. Insulin stimulates both endothelin and nitric oxide activity in the human forearm. Circulation 1999;100:820–5.

28. Yudkin JS, Eringa E, Stehouwer CD. "Vasocrine" signalling from perivascular fat: a mechanism linking insulin resistance to vascular disease. Lancet 2005;365:1817–20.

29. Eringa EC, Stehouwer CDA, Roos MH, Westerhof N, Sipkema P. Selective resistance to vasoactive effects of insulin in muscle resistance arteries of obese Zucker (fa/fa) rats. Am J Physiol Endocrinol Metab 2007;293:E1134–E1139.

30. Yeckel CW, Dziura J, DiPietro L. Abdominal obesity in older women: potential role for disrupted fatty acid re-esterification in insulin resistance. J Clin Endocrinol Metab 2008;93(4):1285–91.

31. Shimizu H, Inoue K, Mori M. The leptin-dependent and -independent melanocortin signaling system: regulation of feeding and energy expenditure. J Endocrinol 2007;197:1–9.

32. Cota D, Proulx K, Seeley RJ. The role of CNS fuel sensing in energy and glucose regulation. Gastroenterology 2007;132:2158–68.

33. Smith GP. *Satiation: From Gut to Brain*. New York: Oxford University Press, 1998.

34. Powley TL, Phillips RJ. Gastric satiation is volumetric, intestinal satiation is nutritive. Physiol Behav 2004;82:69–74.

35. Berthoud HR, Powley TL. Vagal afferent innervation of the rat fundic stomach: morphological characterization of the gastric tension receptor. J Comp Neurol 1992;319:261–76.

36. Phillips RJ, Powley TL. Tension and stretch receptors in gastrointestinal smooth muscles: re-evaluating vagal mechanoreceptor electrophysiology. Brain Res Rev 2000;34:1–26.

37. Wren AM, Small CJ, Ward HL, et al. The novel hypothalamic peptide ghrelin stimulates food intake and growth hormone secretion. Endocrinology 2000;141:4325–8.

38. Tschöp M, Smiley DL, Heiman ML. Ghrelin induces adiposity in rodents. Nature 2000;407:908–13.

39. Wren AM, Seal LJ, Cohen MA, et al. Ghrelin enhances appetite and increases food intake in humans. J Clin Endocrinol Metab 2001;86:5992–5.

40. Wang L, Saint-Pierre DH, Taché Y. Peripheral ghrelin selectively increases Fos expression in neuropeptide Y-synthesizing neurons in mouse hypothalamic arcuate nucleus. Neurosci Lett 2002;325:47–51.

41. Traebert M, Riediger T, Whitebread S, Scharrer E, Schmid HA. Ghrelin acts on leptin-responsive neurones in the rat arcuate nucleus. J Neuroendocrinol 2002;14:580–6.

42. Cummings DE, Weigle DS, Frayo RS, et al. Plasma ghrelin levels after diet-induced weight loss or gastric bypass surgery. N Engl J Med 2002;346:1623–30.

43. Patel AD, Stanley SA, Murphy KG, et al. Ghrelin stimulates insulin-induced glucose uptake in adipocytes. Regul Pept 2006;134:17–22.

44. Lee HM, Wang G, Englander EW, Kojima M, Greeley GH Jr. Ghrelin, a new gastrointestinal endocrine peptide that stimulates insulin secretion: enteric distribution, ontogeny, influence of endocrine, and dietary manipulations. Endocrinology 2002;143:185–90.

45. Reeve JR Jr, Green GM, Chew P, Eysselein VE, Keire DA. CCK-58 is the only detectable endocrine form of cholecystokinin in rat. Am J Physiol Gastrointest Liver Physiol 2003;285:G255–G265.

46. Eysselein VE, Eberlein GA, Schaeffer M, et al. Characterization of the major form of cholecystokinin in human intestine: CCK-58. Am J Physiol Gastrointest Liver Physiol 1990;258:G253–G260.

47. Gibbs J, Young RC, Smith GP. Cholecystokinin elicits satiety in rats with open gastric fistulas. Nature 193;245:323–5.

48. Smith GP, Jerome C, Cushin BJ, Eterno R, Simansky KJ. Abdominal vagotomy blocks the satiety effect of cholecystokinin in the rat. Science 1981;213:1036–7.

49. Blevins JE, Stanley BG, Reidelberger RD. Brain regions where cholecystokinin suppresses feeding in rats. Brain Res 2000;860:1–10.

50. Kissileff HR, Carretta JC, Geliebter A, Pi-Sunyer FX. Cholecystokinin and stomach distension combine to reduce food intake in humans. Am J Physiol Regul Integr Comp Physiol 2003;285:R992–R998.

51. West DB, Fey D, Woods SC. Cholecystokinin persistently suppresses meal size but not food intake in free feeding rats. Am J Physiol 1984;246:R776–R787.

52. Chearskul S, Delbridge E, Shulkes A, Proietto J, Kriketos A. Effect of weight loss and ketosis on postprandial cholecystokinin and free fatty acid concentrations. Am J Clin Nutr 2008;87:1238–46.

53. Dupre J, Ross SA, Watson D, Brown JC. Stimulation of insulin secretion by gastric inhibitory polypeptide in man. J Clin Endocrinol Metab 1973;37:826–8.

54. Yip RG, Boylan MO, Kieffer TJ, Wolfe MM. Functional GIP receptors are present on adipocytes. Endocrinology 1998;139:4004–7.

55. Bollag RJ, Zhong Q, Phillips P, et al. Osteoblast-derived cells express functional glucose-dependent insulinotropic peptide receptors. Endocrinology 2000;141:1228–35.

56. Miyawaki K, Yamada Y, Ban N, et al. Inhibition of gastric inhibitory polypeptide signaling prevents obesity. Nat Med 2002;8:738–42.

57. Tsukiyama K, Yamada Y, Yamada C, et al. Gastric inhibitory polypeptide as an endogenous factor promoting new bone formation after food ingestion. Mol Endocrinol 2006;20:1644–51.

58. Holst JJ. The physiology of glucagon-like peptide 1. Physiol Rev 2007;87:1409–39.

59. Mojsov S, Heinrich G, Wilson IB, Ravazzola M, Orci L, Habener JF. Preproglucagon gene expression in pancreas and intestine diversifies at the level of post-translational processing. J Biol Chem 1986;261:11880–9.

60. Holst JJ, Orskov C, Nielsen OV, Schwartz TW. Truncated glucagon-like peptide I, an insulin-releasing hormone from the distal gut. FEBS Lett 1987;211:169–74.

61. Orskov C, Rabenhøj L, Wettergren A, Kofod H, Holst JJ. Tissue and plasma concentrations of amidated and glycine-extended glucagon-like peptide I in humans. Diabetes 1994;43:535–9.

62. Rocca AS, Brubaker PL. Role of the vagus nerve in mediating proximal nutrient-induced glucagon-like peptide-1 secretion. Endocrinology 1999;140:1687–94.

63. Tang-Christensen M, Larsen PJ, Göke R, et al. Central administration of GLP-1-(7–36) amide inhibits food and water intake in rats. Am J Physiol 1996;271:R848–56.

64. Turton MD, O'Shea D, Gunn I, et al. A role for glucagon-like peptide-1 in the central regulation of feeding. Nature 1996;379:69–72.

65. Jin SL, Han VK, Simmons JG, Towle AC, Lauder JM, Lund PK. Distribution of glucagonlike peptide I (GLP-I), glucagon, and glicentin in the rat brain: an immunocytochemical study. J Comp Neurol 1988;271:519–32.

66. Göke R, Larsen PJ, Mikkelsen JD, Sheikh SP. Distribution of GLP-1 binding sites in the rat brain: evidence that exendin-4 is a ligand of brain GLP-1 binding sites. Eur J Neurosci 1995;7:2294–300.

67. Layer P, Holst JJ, Grandt D, Goebell H. Ileal release of glucagon-like peptide-1 (GLP-1). Association with inhibition of gastric acid secretion in humans. Dig Dis Sci 1995;40:1074–82.

68. Read N, French S, Cunningham K. The role of the gut in regulating food intake in man. Nutr Rev 1994;52:1–10.

69. Flint A, Raben A, Astrup A, Holst JJ. Glucagon-like peptide 1 promotes satiety and suppresses energy intake in humans. J Clin Invest 1998;101:515–20.

70. Verdich C, Flint A, Gutzwiller JP, et al. A meta-analysis of the effect of glucagon-like peptide-1 (7–36) amide on ad libitum energy intake in humans. J Clin Endocrinol Metab 2001;86:4382–9.

71. Blonde L, Klein EJ, Han J, et al. Interim analysis of the effects of exenatide treatment on A1C, weight and cardiovascular risk factors over 82 weeks in 314 overweight patients with type 2 diabetes. Diabetes Obes Metab 2006;8:436–47.

72. Eberlein GA, Eysselein VE, Schaeffer M, et al. A new molecular form of PYY: structural characterization of human PYY(3–36) and PYY(1–36). Peptides 1989;10:797–803.

73. Acuna-Goycolea C, van den Pol AN. Peptide YY(3–36) inhibits both anorexigenic proopiomelanocortin and orexigenic neuropeptide Y neurons: implications for hypothalamic regulation of energy homeostasis. J Neurosci 2005;25:10510–19.

74. Batterham RL, Cohen MA, Ellis SM, et al. Inhibition of food intake in obese subjects by peptide YY3–36. N Engl J Med 2003;349:941–8.

75. Batterham RL, Cowley MA, Small CJ, et al. Gut hormone PYY(3–36) physiologically inhibits food intake. Nature 2002;418:650–4.

76. Koda S, Date Y, Murakami N, et al. The role of the vagal nerve in peripheral PYY3–36-induced feeding reduction in rats. Endocrinology 2005;146:2369–75.

77. Tschöp M, Castañeda TR, Joost HG, et al. Physiology: does gut hormone PYY3–36 decrease food intake in rodents? Nature 2004;430(6996):1.

78. Bataille D, Gespach C, Tatemoto K, et al. Bioactive enteroglucagon (oxyntomodulin): present knowledge on its chemical structure and its biological activities. Peptides 1981;2(suppl 2):41–4.

79. Jarrousse C, Bataille D, Jeanrenaud B. A pure enteroglucagon, oxyntomodulin (glucagon 37), stimulates insulin release in perfused rat pancreas. Endocrinology 1984;115:102–5.

80. Schjoldager BT, Baldissera FG, Mortensen PE, Holst JJ, Christiansen J. Oxyntomodulin: a potential hormone from the distal gut. Pharmacokinetics and effects on gastric acid and insulin secretion in man. Eur J Clin Invest 1988;18:499–503.

81. Dakin CL, Gunn I, Small CJ, et al. Oxyntomodulin inhibits food intake in the rat. Endocrinology 2001;142:4244–50.

82. Dakin CL, Small CJ, Park AJ, Seth A, Ghatei MA, Bloom SR. Repeated ICV administration of oxyntomodulin causes a greater reduction in body weight gain than in pair-fed rats. Am J Physiol Endocrinol Metab 2002;283:E1173–7.

83. Zhu L, Tamvakopoulos C, Xie D, et al. The role of dipeptidyl peptidase IV in the cleavage of glucagon family peptides: in vivo metabolism of pituitary adenylate cyclase activating polypeptide-(1–38). J Biol Chem 2003;278:22418–23.

84. Cohen MA, Ellis SM, Le Roux CW, et al. Oxyntomodulin suppresses appetite and reduces food intake in humans. J Clin Endocrinol Metab 2003;88:4696–701.

85. Baggio LL, Huang Q, Brown TJ, Drucker DJ. Oxyntomodulin and glucagon-like peptide-1 differentially regulate murine food intake and energy expenditure. Gastroenterology 2004;127:546–58.

86. Chaudhri OB, Wynne K, Bloom SR. Can gut hormones control appetite and prevent obesity? Diabetes Care 2008;31(suppl 2):S284–9.

87. Kulkosky PJ, Gibbs J, Smith GP. Feeding suppression and grooming repeatedly elicited by intraventricular bombesin. Brain Res 1982;242: 194–6.

88. Flynn FW. Bombesin-like peptides in the regulation of ingestive behavior. Ann NY Acad Sci 1994;739:120–34.

89. Stuckey JA, Gibbs J, Smith GP. Neural disconnection of gut from brain blocks bombesin-induced satiety. Peptides 1985;6:1249–52.

90. McDonald TJ, Jörnvall H, Nilsson G, et al. Characterization of a gastrin releasing peptide from porcine non-antral gastric tissue. BBRC 1979;90:227–33.

91. Stein LJ, Woods SC. Gastrin releasing peptide reduces meal size in rats. Peptides 1982;3:833–5.

92. Battey J, Wada E. Two distinct receptor subtypes for mammalian bombesin-like peptides. Trends Neurosci 1991;14:524–8.

93. Ladenheim EE, Wirth KE, Moran TH. Receptor subtype mediation of feeding suppression by bombesin-like peptides. Pharmacol Biochem Behav 1996;54:705–11.

94. Adrian TE, Bloom SR, Bryant MG, Polak JM, Heitz PH, Barnes AJ. Distribution and release of human pancreatic polypeptide. Gut 1976;17:940–4.

95. Havel PJ, Parry SJ, Curry DL, Stern JS, Akpan JO, Gingerich RL. Autonomic nervous system mediation of the pancreatic polypeptide response to insulin-induced hypoglycemia in conscious rats. Endocrinology 1992;130:2225–9.

96. Ueno N, Inui A, Iwamoto M, et al. Decreased food intake and body weight in pancreatic polypeptide-overexpressing mice. Gastroenterology 1999;117:1427–32.

97. Clark JT, Kalra PS, Crowley WR, Kalra SP. Neuropeptide Y and human pancreatic polypeptide stimulate feeding behavior in rats. Endocrinology 1984;115:427–9.

98. Sainsbury A, Schwarzer C, Couzens M, et al. Y4 receptor knockout rescues fertility in ob/ob mice. Genes Dev 2002;16:1077–88.

99. Batterham RL, Le Roux CW, Cohen MA, et al. Pancreatic polypeptide reduces appetite and food intake in humans. J Clin Endocrinol Metab 2003;88:3989–92.

100. Whitcomb DC, Puccio AM, Vigna SR, Taylor IL, Hoffman GE. Distribution of pancreatic polypeptide receptors in the rat brain. Brain Res 1997;760:137–49.

101. Kojima S, Ueno N, Asakawa A, et al. A role for pancreatic polypeptide in feeding and body weight regulation. Peptides 2007;28: 459–63.

102. Zipf WB, O'Dorisio TM, Cataland S, Sotos J. Blunted pancreatic polypeptide responses in children with obesity of Prader-Willi syndrome. J Clin Endocrinol Metab 1981;52:1264–6.

103. Fujimoto S, Inui A, Kiyota N, et al. Increased cholecystokinin and pancreatic polypeptide responses to a fat-rich meal in patients with restrictive but not bulimic anorexia nervosa. Biol Psychiatr 1997;41:1068–70.

104. Cooper GJ, Willis AC, Clark A, Turner RC, Sim RB, Reid KB. Purification and characterization of a peptide from amyloid-rich pancreases of type 2 diabetic patients. Proc Natl Acad Sci USA 1987;84:8628–32.

105. Westermark P, Wernstedt C, Wilander E, Hayden DW, O'Brien TD, Johnson KH. Amyloid fibrils in human insulinoma and islets of Langerhans of the diabetic cat are derived from a neuropeptide-like protein also present in normal islet cells. Proc Natl Acad Sci USA 1987;84:3881–5.

106. Young A, Denaro M. Roles of amylin in diabetes and in regulation of nutrient load. Nutrition 1998;14:524–7.

107. Lutz TA. Amylinergic control of food intake. Physiol Behav 2006;89: 465–71.

108. Lutz TA, Geary N, Szabady MM, del Prete E, Scharrer E. Amylin decreases meal size in rats. Physiol Behav 1995;58(6):1197–202.

109. Arnelo U, Permert J, Adrian TE, Larsson J, Westermark P, Reidelberger RD. Chronic infusion of islet amyloid polypeptide causes anorexia in rats. Am J Physiol 1996;271:R1654–9.

110. Mollet A, Gilg S, Riediger T, Lutz TA. Infusion of the amylin antagonist AC 187 into the area postrema increases food intake in rats. Physiol Behav 2004;81:149–55.

111. Roth JD, Roland BL, Cole RL, et al. Leptin responsiveness restored by amylin agonism in diet-induced obesity: evidence from nonclinical and clinical studies. Proc Natl Acad Sci USA 2008;105:7257–62.

112. Woods SC, Lutz TA, Geary N, Langhans W. Pancreatic signals controlling food intake; insulin, glucagon and amylin. Philos Trans R Soc Lond B Biol Sci 2006;361:1219–35.

113. Brüning JC, Gautam D, Burks DJ, et al. Role of brain insulin receptor in control of body weight and reproduction. Science 2000;289:2122–5.

114. Clegg DJ, Riedy CA, Smith KA, Benoit SC, Woods SC. Differential sensitivity to central leptin and insulin in male and female rats. Diabetes 2003;52:682–7.

115. Pfluger PT, Kampe J, Castaneda TR, et al. Effect of human body weight changes on circulating levels of peptide YY and peptide YY3–36. J Clin Endocrinol Metab 2007;92:583–8.

116. Rubio IG, Castro G, Zanini AC, Medeiros-Neto G. Oral ingestion of a hydrolyzed gelatin meal in subjects with normal weight and in obese patients: postprandial effect on circulating gut peptides, glucose and insulin. Eat Weight Disord 2008;13:48–53.

117. Haqq AM, Farooqi IS, O'Rahilly S, et al. Serum ghrelin levels are inversely correlated with body mass index, age, and insulin concentrations in normal children and are markedly increased in Prader-Willi syndrome. J Clin Endocrinol Metab 2003;88:174–8.

118. Feigerlová E, Diene G, Conte-Auriol F, et al. Hyperghrelinemia precedes obesity in Prader-Willi syndrome. J Clin Endocrinol Metab 2008;93(7):2800–5.

119. Turyn J, Korczynska J, Presler M, Stelmanska E, Goyke E, Swierczynski J. Up-regulation of rat adipose tissue adiponectin gene expression by long-term but not by short-term food restriction. Mol Cell Biochem 2008;312:185–91.

120. Keim NL, Stern JS, Havel PJ. Relation between circulating leptin concentrations and appetite during a prolonged, moderate energy deficit in women. Am J Clin Nutr 1998;68:794–801.

121. Korner J, Bessler M, Cirilo LJ, et al. Effects of Roux-en-Y gastric bypass surgery on fasting and postprandial concentrations of

plasma ghrelin, peptide YY, and insulin. J Clin Endocrinol Metab 2005;90:359–65.

122. Morínigo R, Moizé V, Musri M, et al. Glucagon-like peptide-1, peptide YY, hunger, and satiety after gastric bypass surgery in morbidly obese subjects. J Clin Endocrinol Metab 2006;91:1735–40.

123. Laferrère B, Teixeira J, McGinty J, et al. Effect of weight loss by gastric bypass surgery versus hypocaloric diet on glucose and incretin levels in patients with type 2 diabetes. J Clin Endocrinol Metab 2008;93(7):2479–85.

124. Shak JR, Roper J, Perez-Perez GI, et al. The effect of laparoscopic gastric banding surgery on plasma levels of appetite-control, insulinotropic, and digestive hormones. Obes Surg 2008;18(9):1089–96.

125. Neary NM, Small CJ, Wren AM, et al. Ghrelin increases energy intake in cancer patients with impaired appetite: acute, randomized, placebo-controlled trial. J Clin Endocrinol Metab 2004;89:2832–6.

126. Nagaya N, Itoh T, Murakami S, et al. Treatment of cachexia with ghrelin in patients with COPD. Chest 2005;128:1187–93.

127. Wynne K, Park AJ, Small CJ, et al. Subcutaneous oxyntomodulin reduces body weight in overweight and obese subjects: a double-blind, randomized, controlled trial. Diabetes 2005;54:2390–5.

128. Beck B, Richy S, Stricker-Krongrad A. Feeding response to ghrelin agonist and antagonist in lean and obese Zucker rats. Life Sci 2004;76:473–8.

129. DeFronzo RA, Ratner RE, Han J, Kim DD, Fineman MS, Baron AD. Effects of exenatide (exendin-4) on glycemic control and weight over 30 weeks in metformin-treated patients with type 2 diabetes. Diabetes Care 2005;28:1092–100.

130. Aschner P, Kipnes MS, Lunceford JK, Sanchez M, Mickel C, Williams-Herman DE. Sitagliptin Study 021 Group. Effect of the dipeptidyl peptidase-4 inhibitor sitagliptin as monotherapy on glycemic control in patients with type 2 diabetes. Diabetes Care 2006;29:2632–7.

131. Degn KB, Juhl CB, Sturis J, et al. One week's treatment with the long-acting glucagon-like peptide 1 derivative liraglutide (NN2211) markedly improves 24-h glycemia and alpha- and beta-cell function and reduces endogenous glucose release in patients with type 2 diabetes. Diabetes 2004;53:1187–94.

132. Wynne K, Park AJ, Small CJ, et al. Oxyntomodulin increases energy expenditure in addition to decreasing energy intake in overweight and obese humans: a randomised controlled trial. Int J Obes 2006; 30:1729–36.

133. Riddle M, Frias J, Zhang B, et al. Pramlintide improved glycemic control and reduced weight in patients with type 2 diabetes using basal insulin. Diabetes Care 2007;30:2794–9.

134. Gantz I, Erondu N, Mallick M, et al. Efficacy and safety of intranasal peptide YY3–36 for weight reduction in obese adults. J Clin Endocrinol Metab 2007;92:1754–7.

15 Obesity as an Endocrine Disease

Yuji Matsuzawa

Department of Internal Medicine and Molecular Science, Osaka University Graduate School,
Sumitomo Hospital, Osaka, Japan

Classifications of obesity with respect to morbidity

Developed countries provide an increasing number of opportunities for overeating and decreased physical activity, with obesity closely correlated to this overnutritional state and health problems as a typical consequence. Obesity has become a main target for medical research in the field of preventive medicine.

Obesity-related diseases that range from type 2 diabetes mellitus, hyperlipidemia, hypertension, fatty liver, hyperuricemia, atherosclerotic diseases, sleep apnea, cardiac or respiratory dysfunction, orthopedic diseases and menstrual disorder to cancers are reviewed in other chapters in this book. Studies on the morbidity of obesity have indicated that the overall extent of body fat accumulation is not necessarily the major determinant of the occurrence of these diseases; body fat distribution, particularly intra-abdominal visceral fat accumulation plays an important role in the development of a variety of diseases.

Until this concept was established, several classifications of obesity were proposed in order to distinguish the possible mechanisms of its morbidity. In 1947, Vague first reported that the incidence of metabolic complications among equally obese subjects may differ depending on their physique [1]. He differentiated between android obesity, in which adipose tissue is likely to accumulate in the abdomen, and gynoid obesity, in which adipose tissue accumulation occurs in the femoral region. He showed that morbidity is higher in the android type compared to the gynoid type. Kissebah simplified the indicators for adipose tissue distribution by applying waist-to-hip circumference ratio (WHR) and defined those with higher WHR as upper body segment obesity and those with lower WHR as lower body segment obesity [2].

He reported abnormalities in glucose metabolism more frequently in upper body segment obesity than in lower body segment obesity and revealed that upper body segment obesity is a high-risk group for metabolic disorders. Bjorntorp gave the name "abdominal obesity" or "central obesity" to subjects with high WHR and confirmed the higher incidence of type 2 diabetes mellitus, hyperlipidemia and ischemic heart disease in this group compared to the peripheral obesity group [3].

High WHR as an expression of upper body or abdominal obesity has provided a practical index for predicting risks associated with fat accumulation. However, the concept of "waist" originally included both subcutaneous and intra-abdominal visceral fat: discrimination of these two types of abdominal adipose tissue is necessary to analyze the relationship between fat distribution and morbidity of obesity. At present, computed tomography (CT) is the most useful method for measuring fat volume and fat distribution and enabling the analysis of intra-abdominal visceral fat [4]. Metabolic disorders such as glucose intolerance or hyperlipidemia occur more frequently in visceral fat obesity than in subcutaneous obesity. In addition to metabolic disorders, visceral fat accumulation is closely correlated with cardiovascular disorders [5].

The entity of visceral fat obesity corresponds to the terms upper body segment obesity, central or abdominal obesity.

Pathophysiology of visceral fat obesity

Metabolic and cardiovascular disorders in visceral fat obesity

A number of clinical studies have demonstrated the contribution of visceral fat accumulation to the development of metabolic disorders including glucose intolerance and hyperlipidemia. Our studies have demonstrated that visceral fat area/subcutaneous fat area (V/S) at the umbilical level (determined by CT scan) correlates significantly with the glucose area under the curve after an oral glucose tolerance test (OGTT), plasma triglyceride and cholesterol levels in obese subjects [6]. Visceral fat accumulation is

Clinical Obesity in Adults and Children, 3rd edition. Edited by Peter G. Kopelman, Ian D. Caterson and William H. Dietz.
© 2010 Blackwell Publishing, ISBN: 978-1-4051-8226-3.

associated not only with quantitative changes in serum lipids and lipoproteins but also qualitative changes in lipoproteins. An example is small, dense low-density lipoprotein (LDL) particles related to triglyceride-high density lipoprotein (HDL) dyslipidemic state found in visceral fat obesity [7].

Insulin resistance, or hyperinsulinemic state, in visceral obesity may be one of the key abnormalities for these metabolic disorders, at least for glucose intolerance. Previous reports have shown that hyperinsulinemia is present in visceral fat obesity. Studies on tissue glucose uptake performed by Kissebah and the steady-state plasma glucose method performed by our group clearly demonstrate that visceral fat obesity has greater insulin resistance than subcutaneous fat obesity [8].

Visceral fat accumulation has been shown to have causative effects on circulatory disorders in addition to metabolic disorders, as already mentioned. There is a close correlation between systolic and diastolic blood pressure and V/S in premenopausal female subjects. We have demonstrated a close correlation between V/S and the diastolic dimension index or stroke index in obese subjects, which reflected the prevalence of hypervolemic state or impaired cardiac function in visceral obesity.

We have also demonstrated that sleep apnea syndrome occurs more frequently in visceral fat obesity than in subcutaneous obesity [9]. Previously it was assumed that neck adiposity was the major causative factor.

Visceral fat obesity can be characterized as high-risk obesity with multiple complications including insulin resistance, disorders of lipid and glucose metabolism, hypertension, cardiac dysfunction and sleep apnea syndrome (Fig. 15.1).

Significance of visceral fat accumulation in nonobese subjects

Obesity is conventionally defined by a relationship between body weight and height for an individual. Body Mass Index (BMI) most commonly defines obesity (weight in kg/height in m²),

although cutoff points of obesity are different in Western and Asian countries. Analysis of adipose tissues by CT scan, however, indicates that there is a substantial variation in visceral fat volume even among subjects with normal body weight. The visceral fat area correlates significantly with fasting plasma glucose, serum triglyceride and cholesterol in normal weight subjects. Visceral fat area also correlates with blood pressure. It is noted that the V/S ratio has no significant correlation with these markers, which is different from the case in obese subjects [10]. These data suggest that subcutaneous fat may have a protective role against the ill effects of visceral fat accumulation in obese subjects. The detrimental influence of visceral adiposity is more clearly demonstrated in subjects with normal body weight, since these individuals generally have less subcutaneous fat is than their more obese peers.

These results confirm that visceral fat accumulation is related to the development of both metabolic and cardiovascular disorders even in nonobese subjects. Thus, the disease entity "visceral fat syndrome" is proposed as a disorder frequently accompanied by glucose intolerance, lipid disorders and hypertension irrespective of absolute body weight [11].

Visceral fat syndrome and metabolic syndrome

In recent years, a pathologic state with clustering of multiple risk and visceral fat accumulation has been recognized as the highly atherogenic syndrome, identified as "syndrome X" by Reaven [12] or the "deadly quartet" by Kaplan [13]. More recently, the term "metabolic syndrome" has been applied. In the consensus on the definition of the metabolic syndrome from the International Diabetes Federation (IDF) and National Cholesterol Education Program (NCEP), the crucialrole of intra-abdominal visceral fat in the development of multiple risks and cardiovascular diseases has been recognized [14]. Previous epidemiologic studies suggested that WHR is a significant predictor for coronary artery disease independent of BMI. Furthermore, several studies

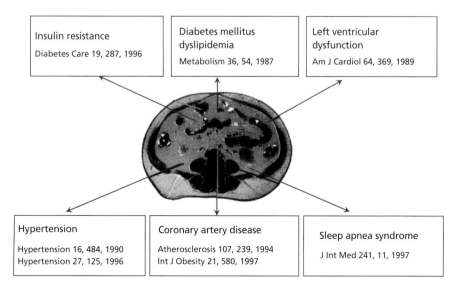

Figure 15.1 Visceral fat accumulation is related to a variety of diseases, such as insulin resistance, diabetes mellitus, dyslipidemia, hypertension, coronary artery disease, cardiac dysfunction and sleep apnea syndrome.

have shown that visceral adiposity determined by CT scan is related to coronary artery disease (CAD). For example, according to our study on the correlation between fat distribution and CAD in nonobese subjects, visceral fat area was found to be increased twofold compared to control subjects without CAD, while comparisons between BMI and subcutaneous fat area showed no difference. Thirty eight percent of nonobese CAD subjects had greater visceral fat area over two standard deviations (SD) of the mean visceral fat area of non-CAD control subjects [15].

These results, together with previous reports, confirm that visceral fat accumulation plays a key role in both metabolic disorders and cardiovascular disease in the metabolic syndrome/visceral fat syndrome.

Important questions arise from the association: why does visceral fat accumulation cause a variety of metabolic and circulatory disorders, and why is this syndrome so atherogenic? In order to answer these questions, we have investigated the functions of adipose tissue, a tissue which has traditionally been regarded as a passive store of excess energy in the form of triglyceride.

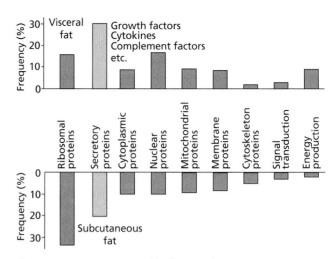

Figure 15.2 Gene expression profile of human adipose tissue.

Molecular mechanism of visceral fat syndrome

Adipose tissue as an endocrine organ

In recent years, biologic characterization of adipose tissue has been extensively investigated. For example, we have analyzed the gene expression profile of visceral fat and subcutaneous fat. We initiated a systemic analysis of active genes by constructing a 3'-directed cDNA library, in which the mRNA population is faithfully reflected. Out of approximately 1000 independent clones, 60% of the whole genes have already been identified as known human genes through searching the non-ST division of the GeneBank. The remaining 40% are composed of novel and unidentified genes. The most surprising finding from this project was that adipose tissue frequently and abundantly expressed the genes encoding secretory proteins, most of which were important bio-active substances [16]. We named these adipose tissue-derived bioactive substances adipocytokines. Figure 15.2 shows the distribution of the gene groups classified by their functions or subcellular localization, showing that the proportion of genes encoding secretory proteins comprises about 20% and 30% of the whole genes expressed in subcutaneous fat and visceral fat, respectively.

Thus, adipose tissue seems to be an endocrine organ that can affect the function of other body organs, through the secretion of various adipocytokines. This includes the vascular system. Adipocytokines include heparin-binding epidermal growth factor-like growth factor (HB-EGF), leptin, tumor necrosis factor-α (TNF-α), plasminogen activator inhibitor type 1 (PAI-1) and angiotensinogen [17,18]. The expression and plasma levels of these adipocytokines increase with visceral fat accumulation and are implicated in insulin resistance and atherosclerosis.

HB-EGF is a potent stimulator of smooth muscle cell proliferation and increased secretion from accumulated adipose tissue

may induce intimal thickening of vascular walls. TNF-α is a typical cytokine that plays a major role in inflammatory cellular phenomena. Since Hotamisligil first reported that adipose tissue secretes this cytokine, it has been recognized as one of the candidate molecules inducing insulin resistance [17]. It has been shown that adipose TNF-α mRNA and plasma TNF-α protein are increased in most animal models as well as human obesity, and associated with insulin resistance. Neutralizing TNF-α in blood from obese rats with a soluble TNF-α receptor-immunoglobulin G fusion protein markedly improves insulin resistance. These results support the hypothesis that higher production of TNF-α in accumulated adipose tissue may be causative for obesity-associated insulin resistance. In addition to TNF-α, IL-1β, IL-6 macrophage migration factor, nerve growth factor and haptoglobin have been shown to be secreted from adipose tissue and linked to inflammation and the inflammatory response. The elevated production of these inflammation-related adipocytokines is considered important in the development of disease linked to obesity, particularly type 2 diabetes and cardiovascular disease. Adipose tissue is involved in extensive cross-talk with other organs and multiple metabolic systems through the various adipocytokines.

PAI-1, an inhibitor of fibrinolysis, has been shown to be produced abundantly in accumulated visceral adipose tissue in experimental models using ventromedial hypothalamus (VMH)-lesioned rats. Plasma levels of PAI-1 and visceral adiposity determined by CT are correlated in humans, suggesting that increased plasma levels of PAI-1 might be an important additional mechanism of vascular disease in visceral obesity (Fig. 15.3) [18].

Adiponectin and its clinical significance

When my laboratory started a comprehensive analysis of expressed genes in human adipose tissue, 40% of expressed genes in adipose tissue were unknown – novel genes. The gene expressed most abundantly in adipose tissue was a novel gene, which

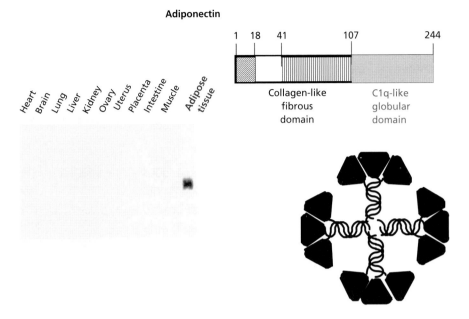

Figure 15.3 Tissue distribution of adiponectin mRNA expression and adiponectin structure.

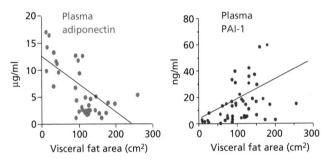

Figure 15.4 Correlation between visceral adiposity and adiponectin or PAI-1.

we named adipose most abundant gene transcript-1 (apM-1) [19]. The molecule encoded by apM-1 possesses a signal peptide, collagen-like motif and globular domain, and has notable homology with collagen X, VIII and complement factor C1q. We applied the term "collagen-like protein adiponectin" (Fig. 15.4) [20].

The mouse homolog of adiponectin has been cloned as AdipoQ or ACRP30. My laboratory established a method for the measurement of plasma adiponectin levels in humans using an enzyme-linked immunosorbent assay. The concentration of adiponectin in human plasma is extremely high – up to 5–10 μg/mL. Plasma concentrations are negatively correlated with BMI, whereas leptin increases with BMI [21]. The negative correlation of adiponectin levels and visceral adiposity is stronger than between adiponectin levels and subcutaneous adiposity, in contrast to the profile of PAI-1 levels which correlates positively with visceral adiposity (see Fig. 15.4) [22].

The mechanism by which plasma levels are reduced in individuals with visceral fat accumulation is not yet clarified. Co-culture with visceral fat inhibits adiponectin secretion from subcutaneous adipocytes. This finding suggests that inhibiting factors for adiponectin synthesis or secretion are re-secreted from visceral adipose tissue. TNF-α is reported to be a strong inhibitor of adiponectin promoter activity. One mechanism to explain the negative correlation between visceral adiposity and adiponectin levels may be increased secretion of TNF-α from accumulated visceral fat [23].

Plasma adiponectin concentrations are lower in people who have type 2 diabetes mellitus than in BMI-matched controls [24]. The plasma adiponectinconcentrations have been shown to correlate strongly with insulin sensitivity, which suggests that low plasma concentrations are associated with insulin resistance. In a study of Pima Indians, individuals with high levels of adiponectin were less likely than those with low concentrations to develop type 2 diabetes. High adiponectin concentration is, therefore, a notable protective factor against the development of type 2 diabetes [25,26].

Studies on knockout, adiponectin[-/-] mice support the human observations [27]. The knockout mice show no specific phenotype when they are fed a normal diet but a high-sucrose and high-fat diet induces marked elevation of plasma glucose and insulin levels. Notably insulin resistance, estimated by an insulin tolerance test during the high-sucrose, high-fat diet, also develops in the knockout mice. The supplementation of adiponectin by adenovirus transfection clearly improved this insulin resistance [27]. Adiponectin has been shown to exert its actions on muscle fatty acid oxidation and insulin sensitivity by activation of AMP-activated protein kinase [28].

Plasma levels of adiponectin are also decreased in hypertensive humans, despite the presence of insulin resistance. Endothelium-dependent vasoreactivity is impaired in people with hypoadiponectinemia, which could be a contributing factors to hypertension in visceral obesity [29].

Importantly, plasma concentrations of adiponectin are lower in people with coronary heart disease than in controls, even when BMI and age are matched [30]. A Kaplan–Meier analysis in Italian individuals with renal insufficiency demonstrated that those with high adiponectin concentrations experienced a delay in death from cardiovascular causes compared to other groups [31]. A case–control study performed in Japan demonstrated that the group with plasma levels less than $4\,\mu g/mL$ had increased risk of CAD and multiple metabolic risk factors, which suggests that hypoadiponectinemia is a key factor in the metabolic syndrome [32]. A prospective study also confirmed that high adiponectin concentrations are associated with reduced risk of acute myocardial infarction in men [33]. A genetically induced syndrome of hypoadiponectinemia caused by a missense mutation has been reported. The mutant rodents exhibit the clinical phenotype of the metabolic syndrome [34]. These clinical associations strongly suggest that hypoadiponectinemia is an important risk factor for cardiovascular disease.

Adiponectin as a potent anti-inflammatory adipocytokine

As previously mentioned, adiponectin has multiple functions in the prevention of metabolic and cardiovascular diseases. More recently, adiponectin has been shown to prevent liver fibrosis [35] and some kinds of cancer including endometrial, breast and colon cancer [36,37]. Besides these well-characterized biologic functions, recent evidence supports a strong anti-inflammatory function.

My laboratory reported that adiponectin suppresses the production of the potent proinflammatory cytokine TNF-α in macrophages [38]. Treatment of cultured macrophages with adiponectin significantly inhibits their phagocytic activity and their lipopolysaccharide-induced production of TNF-α. Suppression of phagocytosis by adiponectin is mediated by one of the complement C1q receptors, C1qRp; this function is completely abrogated by the addition of an anti-C1qRp monoclonal antibody. Such observations suggest that adiponectin is an important regulator of immune and inflammatory systems through an inhibitory involvement to suppress inflammatory responses [39].

In the development process of atherosclerosis, macrophages play a crucial role in plaque formation. Adiponectin attenuates cholesteryl ester accumulation in macrophages The adiponectin-treated macrophages contain fewer lipid droplets stained by oil red O. Adiponectin suppresses the expression of the class A macrophage scavenger receptor (MSR) at both mRNA and protein levels measured by Northern and immunoblot analyses without affecting the expression of CD36 [40]. Adiponectin inhibits TNF-α induced mRNA expression of monocyte adhesion molecules without affecting the interaction between TNF-α and its receptors in human aortic endothelial cells [39]. Additionally, adiponectin suppresses TNF-α induced IκB-α phosphorylation and subsequent NF-κB activation without affecting other TNF-α mediated signals, including Jun N-terminal kinase, p38 kinase and Akt kinase [41]. This inhibitory effect of adiponectin is accompanied by cAMP accumulation and is blocked by either adenylate cyclase inhibitor or protein kinase A (PKA) inhibitor [36]. These observations suggest that plasma adiponectin modulates the inflammatory response of both macrophages and endothelial cells through cross talk between cAMP-PKA and NF-κB signaling pathways [41]. Anti-inflammatory function of adiponectin may result in the prevention of atherogenic cell phenomena such as monocyte adhesion to endothelial cells, differentiation of monocytes to macrophages and foam cell formation [21].

Current studies have shown that adiponectin also induces various anti-inflammatory cytokines, such as interleukin-10 (IL-10) or IL-1 receptor antagonists [42]. Acute coronary syndrome, accompanied by sudden-onset severe chest pain and characteristic ECG changes, is considered an important prognostic marker of outcome for coronary artery disease: the vulnerability of atheromatous plaque is the important determinant of plaque rupture. In this process, matrix metalloproteinase (MMP) secreted by macrophages may play an important part in plaque vulnerability. Tissue inhibitor of metalloproteinase (TIMP) may protect against plaque rapture by inhibition of MMP activity. Adiponectin increases the expression of mRNA and protein production of TIMP in macrophages. Prior to the induction of TIMP formation and secretion, adiponectin is shown to induce IL-10 synthesis in macrophages, suggesting that adiponectin induces TIMP formation and secretion via induction of IL-10 synthesis in an autocrine manner in macrophages. It may also inhibit MMP activity [42].

These functions may potentially prevent acute coronary syndrome. A possible mechanism of prevention of atherosclerosis and acute coronary syndrome by adiponectin is shown in Figure 15.5.

C-reactive protein (CRP) is a characteristic marker of inflammation and elevation of high-sensitive CRP is considered a risk factor for atherosclerosis [43]. A number of studies have shown

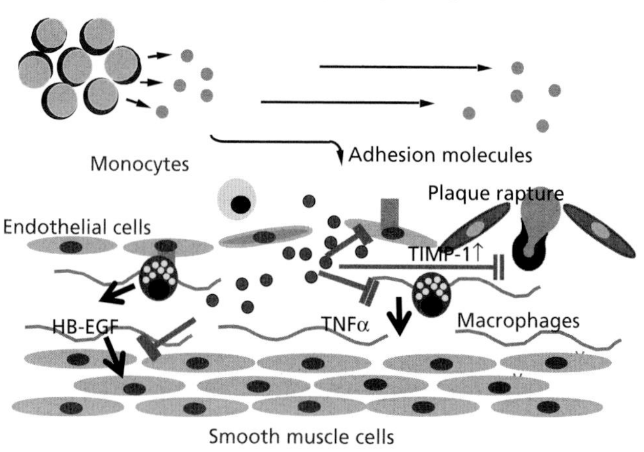

Mechanism of anti-atherogenicity of adiponectin

Figure 15.5 The mechanism of prevention of atherosclerosis and plaque rapture by adiponectin.

that there is a reciprocal association of adiponectin and CRP in plasma in healthy subjects and in subjects with a variety of diseases including type 2 diabetes, metabolic syndrome and end-stage kidney disease. The mechanism of this reciprocal association of CRP and adiponectin remains to be clarified. My laboratory detected the expression of adiponectin mRNA in human adipose tissue and demonstrated a significant inverse correlation between CRP and adiponectin mRNA. In addition, the CRP mRNA level of white adipose tissue in adiponectin-deficient mice is higher than that of wild-type mice. The reciprocal association of adiponectin and CRP levels in both human plasma and adipose tissue might participate in the development of atherosclerosis via an inflammatory response [44].

Increased influx of free fatty acids (FFA) and glycerol from accumulated visceral fat to the liver

Visceral fat is characterized by enhanced lipolysis and augmented plasma FFA flux to the portal circulation and into the liver. Insulin resistance has been shown to be exacerbated by an increased supply of FFA to peripheral tissue and the liver. *In vitro* studies have demonstrated that palmitate exposure causes a dose-dependent reduction in cell surface insulin receptor binding of isolated hepatocytes. It is associated with a proportionally diminished receptor-mediated internalization and decreased intracellular and total receptor-mediated insulin degradation [45]. This phenomenon may contribute to reduced hepatic insulin extraction and peripheral hyperinsulinemia.

Increased FFA influx in the liver from accumulated visceral fat is the process of lipoprotein secretion. Recent studies indicate that microsomal triglyceride transfer protein (MTP) plays a key role in lipoprotein assembly of apolipoprotein B and lipids to form very low-density lipoprotein (VLDL) in the liver [46]. This process is considered to be a limiting factor for VLDL secretion from the liver to plasma. My group has reported that FFA enhances mRNA expression of MTP in the liver. This suggests that increased FFA influx to the liver from visceral fat contributes to increased VLDL formation and secretion resulting in hyperlipidemia [47].

In contrast to the observation for FFA metabolism, there have been few investigations of the fate of glycerol, another metabolite of triglyceride lipolysis. During the Body Map Project, my group identified an adipose tissue-specific water channel named aquaporin adipose, or aquaporin 7 which has been found to play an important role in membrane transport of glycerol [48]. Messenger RNA of aquaporin adipose responds to feeding and fasting; fasting remarkably enhances its expression while feeding suppresses it [49]. This regulation causes increased glycerol release from adipose tissue during fasting in order to supply glycerol from visceral fat to the liver to maintain hepatic glucose production. Insulin has a major role in the suppression of aquaporin mRNA on feeding [50]. However, mRNA expression of aquaporin adipose in visceral fat is enhanced in obese model animals such as the db/db mouse and feeding-induced suppression does not occur. This results in an increase of portal glycerol

influx to the liver during feeding [51]. It can be speculated that the physiologic role of aquaporin adipose is to maintain blood glucose levels by glycerol transport and prevent hypoglycemia during fasting. However, in visceral obesity, suppression by insulin during feeding is impaired and excess glycerol influx to the liver may contribute to hyperglycemia, especially postprandially.

Factors inducing visceral fat accumulation

Sex hormones may be a factor in determining body fat distribution. Visceral fat accumulation is more predominant in men than in women when comparisons are made between age-matched subjects with comparable BMI [52]. Previous studies have shown that there is a negative correlation between plasma levels of sex hormone-binding globulin (SHBG) and WHR in females [53]. This suggests that testosterone is an important determinant of visceral adiposity in females. In contrast, low testosterone levels in males correlate with visceral adiposity.

Aging is also an important factor in the accumulation of visceral fat. A close linear correlation between age and visceral fat volume was demonstrated in male subjects in a cross-sectional study of 1557 obese subjects of varying ages [52]. Although this correlation was also present in female obese subjects, the slope became much steeper after the menopause, compatible with that seen in men.

Among dietary factors, high sucrose intake is a candidate for promoting visceral fat accumulation. High sucrose loading is known to cause an increase of mesenteric fat in both human and animal models [54].

Physical exercise has been suggested to prevent and reduce visceral fat accumulation. My laboratory analyzed fat distribution in Japanese Sumo wrestlers in order to investigate the effects of physical exercise on visceral adiposity. Sumo wrestlers eat a high-energy diet (7000–10000 kcal daily) to gain weight, but at the same time they perform strenuous physical training. Although they show marked obesity and have markedly high waist circumference, the average V/S ratio is 0.25 in young Sumo wrestlers which is comparable to subcutaneous obesity. Their glucose and lipid levels are within normal values. A typical CT image of abdominal fat in Sumo wrestlers is shown in Figure 15.6 with little intra-abdominal visceral fat and developed muscularity and increased subcutaneous fat [10,11]. The incidence of diabetes mellitus increases in retired wrestlers who do not continue to take physical exercise.

Physical exercise is not only useful in preventing visceral fat accumulation, but also in reducing visceral adiposity. It is noteworthy that subcutaneous adiposity is rather insensitive and not so markedly altered by physical activity. Genetic factors for visceral adiposity might be present since visceral obesity sometimes clusters in the same family. A nonconservative missense mutation in the β3-adrenergic receptor gene has been suggested as a candidate for the genetic factor of visceral obesity [55].

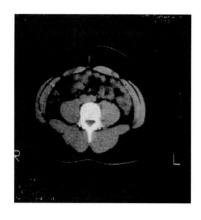

	Sumo wrestlers	Control
BMI (kg/m2)	36 ± 6	23 ± 4
TC (mg/dL)	160 ± 29	189 ± 17
TG (mg/dL)	105 ± 13	79 ± 44
FPG (mg/dL)	95 ± 21	92 ± 5
V/S	0.25 ± 0.13	

Figure 15.6 Metabolic profiles in young Sumo wrestlers. (Reproduced with permission from Matsuzawa Y, Fujioka S, Tokunaga K, Tarui S. Classification of obesity with respect to morbidity. Proc Soc Exp Biol Med 1992;200(2):197–201.)

Conclusion

Adipocytes secrete various adipocytokines to control cell function of other organs. Production and secretion of adipocytokines are dynamically regulated mainly by nutritional circumstance. Lifestyle factors, such as overeating and physical inactivity, induce visceral fat accumulation. Oversecretion of adipocytokines, such as PAI-1 or TNF-α, and hyposecretion of adipocytokines, such as adiponectin, may be factors in the development of lifestyle-related diseases, including type 2 diabetes mellitus, hyperlipidemia, hypertension and atherosclerosis. These, in turn, constitute the so-called metabolic syndrome. The reduction of visceral fat is an essential preventive measure for the metabolic syndrome and the resulting cardiovascular disease. The regulation of key adipocytokines including adiponectin provide potential therapeutic tools for the treatment of overweight and obesity.

References

1. Vague J. La differentiation sexuelle, facteur determinant des formes de l'obesite. Press Med 1947;55:388–40.
2. Kissebah AH, Vydelingum N, Murray, R, et al. Relation of body fat distribution to metabolic complications of obesity. J Clin Endocrinol Metab 1982;54:254–60.
3. Bjorntorp P. Regional patterns of fat distribution. Ann Intern Med 1985;103:994–5.
4. Tokunaga K, Matsuzawa Y, Ishikawa K, et al. Novel technique for the determination of body fat by computed tomography. Int J Obes 1983;7:437–45.
5. Matsuzawa Y, Fujioka S, Tokunaga K, et al. A novel classification: visceral fat obesity and subcutaneous fat obesity. In: Berry EM, Blondheim SH (eds) *Recent Advances in Obesity Research V*. London: John Libbey, 1987:92–6.
6. Fujioka S, Matsuzawa Y, Tokunaga K, et al. Contribution of inra-abdominal fat accumulation to the impairment of glucose and lipid metabolism. Metabolism 1987;36:54–9.
7. Depres JP. Obesity and lipid metabolism: relevance of body fat distribution. Curr Opin Lipidol 1991;2:5–15.
8. Evans DJ, Muller RA, Kissebah P. Relationship between skeletal muscle insulin resistance, insulin-mediated glucose disposal and insulin binding: effect of obesity and body fat topography. J Clin Invest 1984;74:1515–25.
9. Shinohara E, Kihara S, Yamashita S. Visceral fat accumulation as an important factor for obstructive sleep apnea syndrome in obese subjects. J Intern Med 1997;241:11–18.
10. Matsuzawa Y, Fujioka S, Tokunaga K, et al. Classification of obesity with respect to morbidity. Proc Soc Exp Biol Med 1992;200:197–201.
11. Matsuzawa Y. Pathophysiology and molecular mechanism of visceral fat syndrome: the Japanese case. Diabetes Metab Rev 1997;13:3–13.
12. Reaven GM. Role of insulin resistance in human disease. Diabetes 1988;37:1595–607.
13. Kaplan NM. The deadly quartet. Arch Intern Med 1989;149:1514–20.
14. Alberti KG, Zimmet P, Shaw J. Metabolic syndrome – a new worldwide definition. A consensus statement from the International Diabetes Federation. Diabet Med 2006;23:1385–6.
15. Nakamura T, Tokunaga K, Shimomura I, et al. Contribution of visceral fat accumulation to the development of coronary artery disease in non-obese men. Atherosclerosis 1994;107:239–46.
16. Maeda K, Okubo K, Shimomura I, et al. Analysis of expression profile of genes in the human adipose tissue. Gene 1997;190:227–35.
17. Uysal KT, Wiesblock SM, Mario MW, et al. Protection from obesity-induced insulin risistance in mice lacking TNF-alpha function. Nature 1997;389:610–14.
18. Shimomura I, Funahashi T, Takahashi M, et al. Enhanced expression of PAI-1 in visceral fat: possible contribution to vascular disease in obesity. Nature Med 1997;2:1–5.
19. Maeda K, Okubo K, Shimomura I, Funahashi T, et al. cDNA cloning and expression of a novel adipose specific collagen-like factor, apM1 (adipose most abundant gene transcript 1). Biochem Biophys Res Commun 1996;22:286–9.
20. Matsuzawa Y. Adiponectin: identification, physiology and clinical relevance and vascular disease. Atherosclerosis 2005;6(Suppl):7–14.
21. Arita Y, Kihara S, Ouchi Y, et al. Paradoxical decrease of an adipose-specific protein, adiponectin in obesity. Biochem Biophys Res Commun 1999;257:79–83.
22. Matsuzawa Y, Funahashi T, Kihara S, et al. Adiponectin and metabolic syndrome. Arterioscler Thromb Vasc Biol 2004;24:29–33.

23. Matsuzawa Y. Therapy insight: adipocytokines in metabolic syndrome and related cardiovascular disease. Nature Clin Prac Cardiovasc Med 2006;3:35–42.

24. Hotta K, Funahashi T, Tanaka S, et al. Circulating concentrations of the adipocyte-specific protein, adiponectin, are decreased in the patient with reduced insulin sensitivity during progression of type-2 diabetes in rhesus monkeys. Diabetes 2001;50:1126–33.

25. Weyer C, Funahashi T, Tanaka S, et al. Hypoadiponectinemia in obesity and type 2 diabetes: evidence for a role of insulin resistance and/or hyperinsulinemia. J Clin Endocrinol Metab 2001;86:1930–5.

26. Lindsay RS, Funahashi T, Hanson RI, et al. Adiponectin protects against development of type 2 diabetes in the Pima Indian population. Lancet 2002;360:57–8.

27. Maeda N, Shimomura I, Kishida K, et al. Diet-induced insulin resistance in mice lacking adiponectin/ACRP30. Nat Med 2002;8:731–7.

28. Ruderman NB, Saha AK, Kragen EW. Minireview: malonyl CoA, AMP-activated protein kinase, and adiposity. Endocrinology 2003;144:5166–71.

29. Ouchi N, Ohnishi M, Kihara S, et al. Association of hypoadiponectinemia with impaired vasoreactivity. Hypertension 2003;42:231–4.

30. Ouchi N, Kihara S, Arita Y. Novel modulator for endothelial adhesion molecules: adipocyte-derived plasma protein, adiponectin. Circulation 1999;100:2473–6.

31. Zoccali C, Mallamaci F, Tripepi G, et al. Adiponectin, the most abundant adipocyte-derived protein, is functionally related to metabolic risk factors and predicts cardiovascular outcomes in end stage renal disease. J Am Soc Nephrol 2002;13:134–41.

32. Kumada M, Kihara S, Sumitsuji S, et al. Association of hypo-adiponectinemia with coronary artery disease. Arterioscler Thromb Vasc Biol 2003;23:85–9.

33. Piscon T, Girman CJ, Hotamisligil G, et al. Plasma adiponectin levels and risk of myocardial infarction in men. JAMA 2005;291:1730–7.

34. Ohashi K, Ouchi N, Kihara S, et al. Adiponectin I164T mutation is associated with the metabolic syndrome and coronary artery disease. J Am Coll Cardiol 2004;43:1195–200.

35. Kamada Y, Tamura S, Kiso S, et al. Enhanced carbon tetrachloride-induced liver fibrosis in mice lacking adiponectin. Gastroenterology 2003;125(6):1796–807.

36. Miyoshi Y, Funahashi T, Kihara S, et al. Association of serum adiponectin levels with breast cancer risk. Clin Cancer Res 2003;9:5699–704.

37. Petridou E, Manzoros C, Dessypris N, et al. Plasma adiponectin concentration in relation to endometrial cancer: a case-control study. J Clin Endocrinol Metab 2003;88:993–7.

38. Yokota T, Oritani K, Takahashi I, et al. Adiponectin, a new member of the family of soluble defence collagens, negatively regulates the growth of monocytic progenitors and the functions of macrophages. Blood 1999;96:1727–32.

39. Ouchi N, Kihara S, Arita Y, et al. Adiponectin, adipocyte-derivede plasma protein, inhibits endothelial NF-κB signaling through cAMP-dependent pathway. Circulation 2000;102:1296–301.

40. Ouchi N, Kihara S, Arita Y, et al. Adipocyte-derived plasma protein, adiponecin, suppresses lipid accumulation and class A scavenger receptor expression in human monocyte-derived macrophages. Circulation 2001;103:1057–63.

41. Ouchi N, Kobayashi H, Kihara S, et al. Adiponectin stimulates angiogenesis by promote cross-talk between AMP-activated protein kinase and Akt signaling in endothelial cells. J Biol Chem 2004;279:1304–9.

42. Kumada M, Kihara S, Ouchi N, et al. Adiponectin specifically increased tissue inhibitor of metalloproteinase-1 through interleukin-10 expression in human macrophages. Circulation 2004;109:2046–9.

43. Ridker PM, Glynn RJ, Hennekens CH. C-reactive protein adds to predictive value of total and HDL cholesterol in determining risk of first myocardial infarction. Circulation 1998;97:2007–11.

44. Ouchi N, Kihara S, Funahashi T, et al. Reciprocal association of C-reactive protein with adiponectin in blood stream and adipose tissue. Circulation 2003;107:671–4.

45. Hennes MMI, Shargo E, Kissebah AH. Mechanism of free fatty acid effects on hepatocytes insulin receptor binding and processing. Obes Res 1993;1:18–28.

46. Watterau JR, Zilversmit DM. Purification and characterization of microsomal triglyceride and cholesterol ester transfer protein from bovine liver microsomes. Chem Phys Lipid 1985;38:205–22.

47. Kuriyama H, Yamashita S, Shimomura I, et al. Enhanced expression of hepatic acylcoA synthetase and microsomal triglyceride transfer protein mRNAs in the obese and hypertriglyceridemic rats with visceral fat accumulations. Hepatology 1998;2:557–62.

48. Kishida K, Kuriama H, Funahashi T, et al. Aquaporin adipose, a putative glycerol channel in adipocytes. J Biol Chem 2000;275:20896–902.

49. Maeda N, Funahashi T, Hibuse T, et al. Adaptation to fasting by glycerol transport through aquaporin 7 in adipose tissue. Proc Natl Acad Sci USA 2004;101:17801–6.

50. Kishida K, Shimomura I, Kondo H, et al. Genomic structure and insulin-mediated repression of the aquaporin adipose, adipose-specific glycerol channel. J Biol Chem 2001;276:36251–60.

51. Kuriyama H, Shimomura I, Kishida K, et al. Coordinated regulation of fat-specific glycerol channes, aquaporin adipose and aquaporin 9. Diabetes 2002;51:2915–21.

52. Kotani K, Tokunaga K, Fujioka S, et al. Sexual dimorphism of age-related changes in whole body fa distribution in the obese. Int J Obes 1994;18:207–12.

53. Evans DJ, Barth JH, Burke CW. Body fat topography in women with androgen excess. Int J Obes 1988;12:157–62.

54. Keno Y, Matsuzawa Y, Tokunaga K, et al. High sucrose diet increases visceral fat accumulation in VMH-lesioned obese rats. Int J Obes 1991;15:205–11.

55. Clemens K, Vaisse C, Manning BSJ, et al. Genetic variation in the β3-adrenergic receptor and increased capacity to gain weight in patients with morbid obesity. N Engl J Med 1995;333:352–4.

16 Metabolic Syndrome, Diabetes and Nonalcoholic Steatohepatitis

Ioannis Kyrou,[1,2] **John Willy Haukeland,**[1,3] **Neeraj Bhala**[1,4] **and Sudhesh Kumar**

[1] WISDEM, University Hospital Coventry and Warwickshire, Clinical Sciences Research Institute, Warwick Medical School, University of Warwick, Coventry, UK
[2] Endocrinology, Metabolism and Diabetes Unit, Evgenidion Hospital, Athens University Medical School, Athens, Greece
[3] Faculty Division, Aker University Hospital, University of Oslo, Oslo, Norway
[4] Clinical Trial Service Unit and Epidemiological Studies Unit (CTSU), Nuffield Department of Clinical Medicine, University of Oxford, Oxford, UK

Introduction

Obesity is the most frequent metabolic disease globally, with rapidly increasing prevalence in both adults and children. The escalating epidemic of obesity poses a major threat to public health and has reached critical proportions over the past two decades. Current estimations classify 1.2–1.5 billion people as overweight and almost 400–500 million as clinically obese, with Body Mass Index (BMI) exceeding 25 kg/m^2 and 30 kg/m^2, respectively [1]. Weight gain and particularly visceral fat accumulation are associated with increased risk for developing a wide range of co-morbidities that primarily include insulin resistance, type 2 diabetes mellitus, atherosclerosis, hypertension, dyslipidemia and liver disorders [2,3]. The term "metabolic syndrome" describes a clinical entity characterized by the synchronous presentation of obesity, insulin resistance, hypertension and dyslipidemia [4]. Although not included in the diagnostic criteria of the metabolic syndrome, nonalcoholic fatty liver disease (NAFLD) is now increasingly regarded as one of its manifestations, since it is pathogenetically linked to obesity and insulin resistance [5]. NAFLD represents a broad spectrum of hepatic abnormalities, extending from simple steatosis to nonalcoholic steatohepatitis (NASH), and has become one of the most common chronic liver disorders worldwide. NASH is the most severe form of NAFLD and can progress to cirrhosis, liver failure and more rarely hepatocellular cancer [6]. As advances in the treatment of cardiovascular risk factors and acute coronary syndromes are offering improved cardioprotection to obese and diabetic patients, reduced early cardiovascular mortality in these populations is expected to increase the incidence of complications which were previously underestimated, such as NAFLD and NASH-related cirrhosis.

Pathogenesis of type 2 diabetes

Type 2 diabetes is the prevalent form of diabetes, comprising 80–90% of diagnosed cases. The pathogenesis of type 2 diabetes is typically a complex and progressive process that reflects multifactorial effects of various genes and environmental factors. Monogenic forms of diabetes have been identified, but are uncommon, attributed to a number of rare gene mutations that cause distinct defects associated with either insulin resistance or impaired insulin secretion. This chapter will focus on the most common form of diabetes which is related to the presence of obesity and develops over a period of time as the result of insulin resistance combined with impaired insulin secretion.

Epidemiologic associations between diabetes and obesity

Type 2 diabetes prevalence has increased dramatically over the past two decades in developed and developing countries,

Clinical Obesity in Adults and Children, 3rd edition. Edited by Peter G. Kopelman, Ian D. Caterson and William H. Dietz.

following closely the concurrent epidemic spread of obesity. Globally, 220–250 million adults are estimated to have diabetes and this number is expected to rise rapidly to 350–380 million by 2025. Depending on age, ethnicity and gender, 50–90% of type 2 diabetic patients exhibit BMI values over 25 kg/m². Obesity and diabetes are now characterized as twin epidemics and even as the epidemic of "diabesity" [7,8].

The recent type 2 diabetes epidemic has been disproportionately affecting non-Caucasian populations (e.g. Hispanic, South Asian, Pacific and Indian Ocean populations, as well as Native American, Canadian and Australian Aboriginal communities), coinciding with high prevalence rates of obesity [9]. These identified ethnic variations are primarily explained by increased genetic susceptibility in combination with a rapid transition from traditional to Westernized lifestyle patterns (sedentary behaviors, smoking and diets rich in energy-dense foods, carbohydrates and saturated fats) and by early malnutrition effects on intrauterine and infantile growth [10–12].

Type 2 diabetes in the pediatric population constitutes another relatively new development in the epidemiology of the disease. Although type 1 diabetes accounts for the majority of diabetes cases in young people, glucose intolerance and overt type 2 diabetes incidence are steadily increasing among children and adolescents [13]. This novel trend is attributed to the alarming problem of childhood obesity globally and will be further discussed in the chapter concerning the consequences of childhood obesity.

Evidence from large-scale population studies suggests that the duration and degree of weight gain in adult life are powerful predictors of type 2 diabetes and that obesity constitutes the most important independent risk factor for the disease (Fig. 16.1)

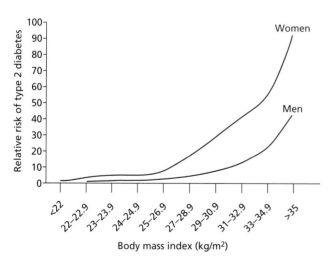

Figure 16.1 Body Mass Index (BMI) and age-adjusted relative risk of type 2 diabetes in adults. The relative risk for diabetes begins to increase at BMI values that are considered within the healthy weight range, 22 kg/m² for women and 24 kg/m² for men. Severe obesity (BMI over 35 kg/m²) is associated with an extremely high relative risk in both women and men, approximately 90 and 40, respectively. (Data based on [15] and [16].)

[14–16]. Notably, the relative risk for diabetes in adults appears to increase at BMI values that are considered within the healthy weight range, 22 kg/m² for women and 24 kg/m² for men, and rises exponentially as BMI progresses in the overweight (25–30 kg/m²) and obese (>30 kg/m²) range. Severe obesity (BMI over 35 kg/m²) is associated with an extremely high relative risk for diabetes in both women and men, approximately 90 and 40, respectively [15,16]. Furthermore, the documented incidence of type 2 diabetes in nonobese populations is low and clinical studies have proven that even moderate sustained weight loss has a significant impact on diabetes prevention [17].

Cross-sectional and prospective studies that included assessments of fat distribution have shown a powerful correlation between central obesity and type 2 diabetes, above and beyond the impact of BMI, confirming the initial reports from Vague, who first described this association more than half a century ago [18–20]. Central fat distribution is now a well-established independent risk factor for diabetes and correlates positively with the presence of insulin resistance and hyperinsulinemia. Accordingly, anthropometric indices of central obesity, such as waist circumference and waist-to-height ratio (an index that takes body height into account, WHtR), are proposed as better risk indicators for glucose intolerance and type 2 diabetes compared to BMI [21].

Natural history of progression to type 2 diabetes

Insulin resistance is necessary but not sufficient for the development of type 2 diabetes. Pancreatic adaptation to insulin resistance, through increased β cell mass and enhanced insulin secretion, prevents the onset of marked hyperglycemia and glucose intolerance. Normoglycemia is maintained for as long as the β cells increase insulin secretion appropriately to compensate for reduced insulin sensitivity. β Cell decompensation and secretory dysfunction is an essential step in the natural history of progression to type 2 diabetes. Thus, the pathogenesis of the disease represents an imbalance characterized by progressive insulin resistance and relatively inadequate insulin secretion [22].

Insulin sensitivity exhibits a nonlinear relationship with insulin secretion which is described by a hyperbolic curve (Fig. 16.2) [23]. Obese patients with insulin resistance and adequate compensatory β cell function typically move upward on this curve, by increasing insulin secretion, and maintain normal glucose tolerance (NGT). Conversely, obese patients who develop impaired glucose tolerance (IGT) and type 2 diabetes deviate and fall off this curve because of β cell failure concomitant with deteriorating insulin sensitivity [24]. Notably, these patients still secrete more insulin compared to lean individuals, but the degree of relative hyperinsulinemia is not sufficient to offset the underlying insulin resistance. The deterioration of insulin sensitivity begins several years before the onset of diabetes, worsens over time and may stabilize after a point. It is considered that IGT corresponds to the near maximum insulin resistance state. β Cell dysfunction progresses concurrently with insulin resistance and is already significantly impaired before the conversion from NGT to IGT. Patients with IGT are estimated to have a loss of β cell function

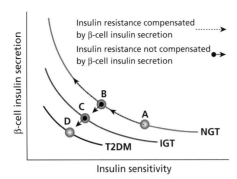

NGT criteria
FPG <100 mg/dL (5.6 mmol/l)
2-hr PG <140 mg/dL (7.8 mmol/l)
IFG criteria
FPG ≥100 mg/dL and <126 mg/dL (7.0 mmol/l)
IGT criteria
2-hr PG ≥140 mg/dL and <200 mg/dL
T2DM criteria
FPG ≥126 mg/dL
2-hr PG ≥200 mg/dL (11.1 mmol/l)
DM symptoms and random PG ≥200 mg/dL

Figure 16.2 Hyperbolic relationship between insulin secretion and insulin sensitivity and the criteria for the diagnosis of diabetes. Obese insulin-resistant patients who do not progress to diabetes increase appropriately the β cell insulin secretion (upward movement on the curve from point A to point B) and maintain normal glucose tolerance (NGT). Conversely, obese patients that progress to impaired glucose tolerance (IGT) and type 2 diabetes (T2DM) deviate and fall off this curve because of β cell failure to compensate for decreasing insulin sensitivity (falling off the curve from point B to point C for IGT and to point D for T2DM). IFG, impaired fasting glucose; FPG, fasting plasma glucose levels after at least 8 hours without caloric intake; 2-h PG, plasma glucose levels 2 hours after an oral glucose load containing the equivalent of 75 g anhydrous glucose dissolved in water; Random PG, plasma glucose levels measured without regard to the interval since the last meal.

that reaches 60–80%, initially reflected as elevated postprandial plasma glucose levels [25]. Further decline in β cell function leads to overt type 2 diabetes and fasting hyperglycemia.

Insulin resistance state and type 2 diabetes

Insulin resistance is defined as a state characterized by decreased peripheral tissue sensitivity to the actions of insulin, leading to increased insulin secretion and hyperinsulinemia. Decreased insulin sensitivity at the cellular level indicates that stimulation of signaling pathways via the insulin receptor requires higher insulin concentrations than those required in healthy individuals. Glucose homeostasis can be severely affected in insulin-resistant states due to reduced biologic effectiveness of insulin to promote glucose utilization and suppress hepatic glucose production.

Insulin resistance is a natural consequence of aging and can also appear under physiologic conditions, such as puberty and pregnancy. Temporary fluctuations in insulin sensitivity are frequent in normal daily life and depend on multiple factors (e.g. variations in food intake, physical activity and hormonal secretion rhythms). Thus, insulin resistance is not a disease in itself but rather a description of a physiologic state. However, obesity-related insulin resistance develops as a prolonged and progressive pathophysiologic state that may lead to type 2 diabetes in predisposed individuals. Adipose tissue accumulation, especially visceral, induces metabolic and hormonal changes, which gradually cause significant defects in the insulin signal transduction pathway and manifest as various degrees of insulin resistance in adipose tissue, liver and skeletal muscle [22,23,26]. The causes of these defects will be discussed in the following sections of this chapter about the role of adipose tissue in insulin resistance. Decreased insulin sensitivity in obese patients induces persistent stimulation of insulin secretion and leads to chronic hyperinsulinemia, which in turn contributes to further weight gain. Thus, in the course of obesity, fat accumulation promotes insulin resistance combined with increased insulin secretion and vice versa, forming

co-existing vicious cycles that steadily progress within each insulin-resistant tissue (Fig. 16.3).

Adipose tissue insulin resistance plays a critical role in initiating and perpetuating these vicious cycles. Thus, adipocytes regulate glycemia in type 2 diabetes, despite the fact that adipose tissue glucose uptake accounts for less than 5% of the total glucose disposal. In normal conditions, insulin-mediated inhibition of the hormone-sensitive lipase in adipocytes attenuates free fatty acid (FFA) release from fat depots into the circulation. This effect causes decreased FFA plasma concentrations which promote muscle glucose uptake and inhibition of hepatic glucose production. Conversely, type 2 diabetes is characterized by persistently increased FFA efflux from insulin-resistant adipocytes, due to uninhibited lipolysis. Chronic elevations of circulating FFA levels reduce peripheral glucose utilization, increase the rate of hepatic glucose production and promote the establishment of generalized insulin resistance, in concert with hormonal and cytokine effects induced by the expanded adipose tissue (see Fig. 16.3) [27,28].

Hepatic insulin resistance is the primary defect accounting for fasting hyperglycemia in type 2 diabetes. In the liver, insulin activates enzymes that promote glycogenesis and suppresses those involved in gluconeogenesis, thus regulating the rate of hepatic glucose production. Fasting is associated with stimulated hepatic gluconeogenesis and glycogenolysis due to low circulating insulin levels. In normal conditions, fasting hepatic glucose production matches precisely the basal glucose utilization and is created by equal gluconeogenesis and glycogenolysis rates. Type 2 diabetes, despite the presence of hyperinsulinemia, is characterized by markedly increased fasting glucose production in the liver due to hepatic insulin resistance [22]. This increase is caused predominantly by accelerated glucose synthesis via the gluconeogenic pathway and exhibits a positive linear correlation with the severity of fasting hyperglycemia [29].

Insulin resistance in skeletal muscle contributes significantly to postprandial hyperglycemia in type 2 diabetes. Skeletal muscle

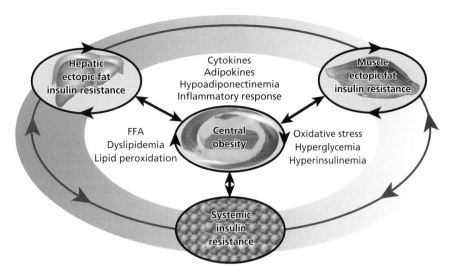

Figure 16.3 Schematic representation of the primary sites of insulin resistance. Weight gain causes adipose tissue accumulation and ectopic fat deposition in the liver and skeletal muscle. In the course of obesity, particularly when fat is accumulated centrally, various degrees of insulin resistance develop gradually in all these tissues, due to an adverse profile of circulating adipokines and free fatty acids (FFA), in combination with proinflammatory and oxidative stress responses. In response, β cell insulin secretion is stimulated, causing chronic hyperinsulinemia that, in turn, favors further weight gain. Thus, obesity promotes decreased insulin sensitivity combined with increased insulin secretion and vice versa, forming co-existing vicious cycles which steadily progress within each insulin-resistant tissue and feed back to each other at the systemic level. This state of obesity-related insulin resistance may lead to type 2 diabetes in genetically predisposed individuals.

accounts for most of the glucose disposal after meal ingestion in healthy individuals. Type 2 diabetic patients exhibit impaired insulin-stimulated glucose uptake in skeletal muscle, which is reduced and delayed in proportion to the underlying degree of decreased insulin sensitivity [22,30]. This underutilization of glucose following food intake is superimposed on increased hepatic glucose production rates, dictating the magnitude and, to an extent, the duration of postprandial elevations in plasma glucose levels.

Impaired insulin secretion and type 2 diabetes pathogenesis

Normal insulin secretion is the *sine qua non* for the preservation of glucose homeostasis. β Cell secretory function is pulsatile, characterized by multiple rapid pulses that are superimposed on slower (ultradian) oscillations. Rapid pulses occur every 8–15 minutes and have small amplitudes, while ultradian oscillations occur every 80–150 minutes and exhibit larger amplitudes. Ultradian pulses are amplified postprandially, are tightly coupled to oscillations in plasma glucose levels (insulin–glucose feedback loop) and appear unrelated to neural stimuli and the counter-regulatory hormones. Circadian variations in insulin secretion are also present, with more potent postprandial responses after breakfast, probably because of reduced β cell sensitivity to glucose during the evening and at night [31].

Approximately half of the total daily insulin secretion occurs in response to meals. After meal ingestion, a rapid insulin secretory response is induced and insulin secretion peaks within an hour. Insulin release in response to an intravenous glucose load is distinctively biphasic, with an early rapid phase within the first 10 minutes which is followed by a depression and then by a slower and more prolonged second secretory phase. This first-phase response plays a significant physiologic role by acutely mobilizing the target tissues, particularly the liver through the portal circulation, to handle the glucose challenge. Oral glucose loads do not produce such a clear biphasic response due to the more gradually induced increase in plasma glucose levels [32]. However, glucose ingestion elicits a much greater insulin release than the intravenous administration of a comparable glucose load, because of vagal nerve stimulation (cephalic phase insulin response) and secretion of gut-derived hormones that enhance glucose-stimulated insulin secretion (incretins) [33].

The number and mass of β cells in the pancreas determine the amount of insulin secretion. The pancreatic β cell population reflects a dynamic balance between neogenesis, replication and apoptotic processes in the islets of Langerhans [34]. Increased pancreatic β cell mass is a crucial compensatory mechanism against insulin resistance in the periphery.

Insulin secretion in IGT is characterized by decreased and delayed first-phase response to glucose loads and by abnormalities in the rhythm of both rapid and ultradian pulses. In type 2 diabetes the first-phase insulin secretion is almost absent and the second phase is also reduced. Additionally, the pulsatile pattern of insulin secretion is markedly impaired, with short and irregular rapid pulses and with ultradian oscillations that are decreased in amplitude and less synchronized with oscillations in plasma glucose levels [31,35]. As a result, type 2 diabetic patients secrete most of the total daily insulin under basal conditions. Furthermore, the mass of functional β cells in IGT and type 2 diabetes fails to match the degree of underlying insulin resistance and

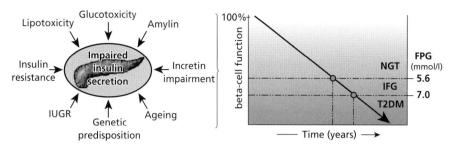

Figure 16.4 Factors causing impaired insulin secretion and schematic representation of the relationship between progressive β cell failure and the development of glucose intolerance and type 2 diabetes. β Cell function deteriorates for years before the onset of glucose intolerance and type 2 diabetes and is already significantly impaired at the time of diagnosis. NGT, normal glucose tolerance; IFG, impaired fasting glucose; IUGR, intrauterine growth restriction; T2DM, type 2 diabetes; FPG, fasting plasma glucose levels after at least 8 hours without caloric intake.

long-standing disease is associated with a further progressive decline in β cell mass (Fig 16.4) [24,34].

These insulin secretion defects are essential for the progression to IGT and type 2 diabetes and develop gradually for years before the onset of overt hyperglycemia, representing the cumulative result of multiple factors (see Fig 16.4) [22]. Some of these factors, such as genetic predisposition and aging, are intrinsic to the individual and cannot be modified. Thus, specific interest is focused on factors related to the insulin-resistant state in obesity, which cause acquired β cell defects that can be, at least partially, restored with weight loss and tight glycemic control.

Glucotoxicity leads to abnormal insulin secretion, depending on the degree and, more importantly, the duration of hyperglycemia. *In vitro*, prolonged β cell exposure to high glucose concentrations causes glucose desensitization, impairs insulin gene transcription and induces apoptosis. In animal studies restoration of normoglycemia alone, by pharmacologically inducing renal glucosuria, was sufficient to improve insulin secretion [22]. Human studies evaluating the rate of insulin secretion also support the role of glucotoxicity, showing that reduced glucose sensitivity is a predominant defect in IGT patients [36,37]. Notably, *in vitro* and *in vivo* studies have reported that hyperglycemia can potentiate insulin secretion responses provided that time is allowed for the β cells to recover between glucose challenges. All these data indicate that chronic hyperglycemia, despite increasing the absolute insulin secretion, exerts toxic effects in the pancreas primarily by impairing β cell glucose sensitivity.

Lipotoxicity is another factor proposed to induce β cell dysfunction. Toxic effects of FFA in the pancreas appear to depend decisively on the degree of FFA exposure and on genetic predisposition for type 2 diabetes. Short-term β cell exposure to physiologic increases in FFA has been shown to stimulate insulin secretion. Conversely, prolonged β cell exposure to high FFA concentrations increases the islet triglyceride content, impairs glucose-stimulated insulin secretion and promotes apoptosis. It is suggested that, under these conditions, FFA oxidation is enhanced and intracellular metabolites, such as citrate and ceramide, accumulate. Elevated citrate levels inhibit glycolysis which is essential for glucose-stimulated insulin secretion. Additionally,

elevated ceramide levels increase nitric oxide synthesis, which subsequently induces the expression of proinflammatory cytokines and leads to apoptosis [22,38]. Human studies have also shown that sustained physiologic increases in FFA plasma levels can impair β cell insulin secretion, but mostly in the presence of genetic predisposition (family history of type 2 diabetes) [39]. Furthermore, in nondiabetic subjects with strong family history of type 2 diabetes, pharmacologic inhibition of lipolysis significantly improved insulin secretion, highlighting the role of lipotoxicity in genetically predisposed individuals [40].

The incretin effect (the ratio between the integrated insulin response to an oral glucose load and to an isoglycemic intravenous glucose infusion) is distinctively decreased in type 2 diabetes, due to incretin deficiency and/or incretin resistance [41,42]. Glucose-dependent insulinotropic polypeptide (GIP, formerly referred as gastric inhibitory polypeptide) and glucagon-like peptide-1 (GLP-1) are released from neuroendocrine cells of the small intestine (K and L cells, respectively) and represent the main incretins, accounting for more than 90% of the incretin effect. GLP-1 and GIP rapidly stimulate insulin secretion and exhibit potential β cell preserving properties. Incretin secretion occurs in response to intraluminal carbohydrates, is proportional to the ingested glucose load and depends upon the absorption of glucose across the intestinal mucosa. Their secretion is not stimulated by plasma glucose levels, but the incretin effects on β cell secretion are largely glucose dependent and proportional to the increase in circulating glucose. GLP-1 meal-induced secretion is decreased in patients with IGT and deteriorates more with the progression to type 2 diabetes; however, its insulinotropic activity is preserved [43]. Conversely, GIP secretion remains normal in type 2 diabetes, but exhibits diminished bioactivity on β cells, indicating resistance to its action [44].

Amylin (islet amyloid polypeptide, IAPP) is suggested to promote β cell failure in type 2 diabetes. β Cells synthesize amylin, which is co-secreted with insulin. Thus, amylin secretion is increased together with insulin secretion in the presence of insulin resistance. Amylin is rather insoluble and has a strong tendency to self-aggregate and form fibrils, which are the main constituent of amyloid deposits in the pancreas. Islet amyloid deposits are frequently identified in type 2 diabetic patients and were proposed as a potential cause of β cell dysfunction. However, this hypothesis has recently been challenged and it is now proposed that amylin toxicity on β cells derives from its ability to form membrane permeant oligomers. These toxic intracellular oligomers, rather than the extracellular amyloid, are considered to induce β cell defects, especially in the presence of elevated plasma FFA levels [45].

Intrauterine growth restriction (IUGR) and perinatal nutrient restriction are also associated with β cell defects. Epigenetic, structural and functional adaptive responses to prenatal and postnatal malnutrition have been shown to cause reduced β cell mass and decreased insulin secretory capacity early in the development of the endocrine pancreas. This adverse early-life programming may became detrimental later in life and lead to type 2 diabetes during periods of increased insulin demand, especially since low birth weight is also a risk factor for obesity and insulin resistance [46].

Adipose tissue and the links to insulin resistance and metabolic syndrome

Obesity, the endocrine function of adipose tissue and adipokine secretion

Traditionally, adipose tissue has been regarded as a passive energy depot with a role limited to storing transient energy surpluses until they can be retrieved later through lipolysis. The discovery that adipocytes synthesize and secrete a broad spectrum of novel hormones, cytokines and factors has radically changed this view. This provides new insights into the function of adipose tissue, which is now considered a highly active and complex endocrine organ. The endocrine functions of adipocytes reflect their metabolic status and relay this information to other organs and tissues and to the central nervous system [47]. Furthermore, adipocytes express a wide variety of receptors that enable them to respond to different stimuli which either originate from adjacent cells or are transported via the systemic circulation (Fig. 16.5). Thus, adipose tissue becomes the center of a multileveled reciprocal network with a key role in regulating metabolic homeostasis. Defects of this dynamic cross-talk predispose to fat accumulation and are implicated in the pathogenesis of obesity and its related complications [48].

The adipose tissue exhibits a characteristic adapting capacity to grow in size. Pronounced weight gain induces substantial adipose tissue remodeling with marked changes in the local cellularity. Obesity is characterized by increases in both the number (hyperplasia) and mass (hypertrophy) of the adipocytes, attributed to preadipocytes being stimulated to proliferate and differentiate (adipogenesis) and to small adipocytes being filled with lipid droplets (lipogenesis), respectively. Notably, hypertrophy of adipocytes initially precedes adipogenesis and has been shown to plateau after reaching a maximum size for each adipocyte. In contrast, hyperplasia-adipogenesis continues to progress in

relation to weight gain and subsequently the number of large adipocytes in fat depots rises proportionally to BMI (see Fig. 16.5) [49]. Enlarged adipocytes tend to more insulin resistant and lipolytic compared to small adipocytes and their overall secretory function promotes metabolic dysregulation [50]. The hypertrophic and hyperplastic growth of adipose tissue is also accompanied by increased local vascularization and stromal cell proliferation [51]. Furthermore, circulating mononuclear cells transmigrate from the bloodstream into the expanding adipose tissue and augment the number of resident macrophages [52].

Increasing attention is currently focused on a novel family of adipose-derived proteins, collectively termed adipokines or adipocytokines [53]. The main members of this group include leptin, adiponectin, resistin, visfatin, tumor necrosis factor-α (TNF-α) and interleukin-6 (IL-6) (Fig. 16.6). Adipokine expression and secretion are markedly altered in obesity and strongly correlate with the manifestations of the metabolic syndrome [54]. Notably, most of the adipokines that exert deleterious effects on metabolism are more potently expressed in visceral adipose tissue. This translates into higher visceral than subcutaneous adipokine secretion in the obese state and supports the association between visceral fat accumulation and increased risk for metabolic complications [55,56].

Leptin represents the prototypical adipokine and is responsible for the revived research interest in adipose tissue biology [57]. The plasma concentration of this hormone is proportional to the total fat mass and strongly correlates to BMI [58]. Specific cell membrane receptors (LEPR) directly mediate the actions of leptin, which primarily acts to suppress appetite and enhance energy expenditure at the hypothalamic level [59]. Extensive investigation of the leptin effects exposed a wide range of biologic functions, so that this hormone is now regarded as a multipotent endocrine mediator, interacting with all the major endocrine axes. It is also intriguing that leptin structurally belongs to the type I cytokine superfamily and exhibits proinflammatory properties [60].

Equally significant is the identification of adiponectin (Acrp30, apM1, AdipoQ, GBP28), an adipokine with unique properties, since it appears to play a protective physiologic role [61]. Adiponectin is secreted by adipocytes and exerts its actions via distinct receptors, AdipoR1 and AdipoR2, mainly expressed in skeletal muscle and the liver, respectively. Improved insulin sensitivity is the most recognized beneficial effect of adiponectin, as it stimulates glucose uptake in skeletal muscle, inhibits glucose production in the liver and also induces fatty acid oxidation in both these tissues [62]. Additionally, adiponectin mediates antiatherogenic and anti-inflammatory functions. In contrast to other adipokines, adiponectin is characterized by markedly reduced synthesis in the obese state, particularly in visceral fat depots, and, hence, by decreased circulating concentrations (hypoadiponectinemia). Plasma adiponectin levels correlate inversely with cardiometabolic complications [63,64].

Resistin and visfatin are newer members of the adipokine family with more uncertainty regarding their precise actions.

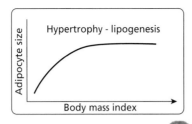

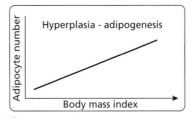

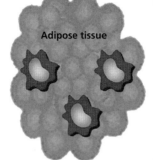

Figure 16.5 Schematic representation of the endocrine and signaling role of adipose tissue. Adipocytes secrete a broad spectrum of hormones, cytokines and factors with potent autocrine, paracrine and endocrine effects. Furthermore, they express a plethora of receptors that receive various signals from adjacent cells and the periphery. In addition to adipocytes which constitute the primary local cell population, adipose tissue also contains other cell types, such as preadipocytes, stromal cells and macrophages. The endocrine significance of adipose tissue is amplified as the body fat mass increases.

Hypertrophy-lipogenesis of adipocytes initially precedes adipogenesis and has been shown to plateau after reaching a maximum size for each adipocyte. Hyperplasia-adipogenesis continues to progress in relation to weight gain and subsequently the number of large adipocytes in fat depots rises proportionally to BMI. TSH, thyroid stimulating hormone; T3, tri-iodothyronine; PPAR-γ, peroxisome proliferator-activated receptor-γ; HDL, high-density lipoprotein; LDL, low-density lipoprotein; VLDL, very-low-density lipoprotein.

Resistin (adipocyte-specific secretory factor, ADSF, FIZZ3) is upregulated in obese individuals and has been described as causing insulin resistance in rodent models and inducing proinflammatory effects [65]. In humans, however, the exact mode of resistin production and its involvement in glucose regulation pathways remain to be elucidated. Uncertainty also exists regarding the role of visfatin, which is expressed by adipocytes and was originally identified as a growth factor for early B lymphocytes (pre-B cell colony enhancing factor, PBEF). Visfatin has been reported as an insulin-mimetic adipokine secreted from visceral adipose tissue. However, subsequent studies on visfatin have failed to confirm the original findings and more research is needed to establish its clinical relevance and mechanisms of action [66].

Finally, the adipokine family includes two of the major proinflammatory cytokines, TNF-α and IL-6, which are also secreted by adipocytes (see Fig. 16.6). Apart from their well-known immune effects, these cytokines can cause metabolic disturbances with detrimental consequences. TNF-α is implicated in the development of insulin resistance by disrupting the tyrosine phosphorylation of the insulin receptor substrates (IRS) 1 and 2, thus blocking the insulin signal transduction pathway [67]. IL-6 promotes hyperglycemia, dyslipidemia and atherogenesis [68,69].

Both cytokines exhibit elevated plasma levels in obesity, with a large fraction of IL-6 and most of the TNF-α secretion originating from the amplified population of resident macrophages in fat depots [52,70–72]. Increased circulating concentrations of TNF-α and IL-6 contribute to the pathophysiology of obesity by triggering pathogenetic pathways in multiple tissues that lead to manifestations of the metabolic syndrome (insulin resistance, dyslipidemia, hypertension, hypercoagulability, enhanced acute-phase response and liver dysfunction).

Obesity as a chronic inflammatory state

Another novel viewpoint concerning the complex function of adipose tissue in obesity is the association of its expansion with the development of a low-grade chronic inflammatory state [73]. The proinflammatory nature of adipose tissue is heightened proportionally to the increased fat mass and shows consistently strong correlations with visceral adipose tissue accumulation and BMI [74]. Obesity has been shown to induce an unremitting proinflammatory response, which continues to evolve for as long as the weight gain is maintained (Fig. 16.7). Recent evidence links this prolonged activation of inflammatory signaling pathways to the pathogenesis of both type 2 diabetes and atherosclerosis [75,76].

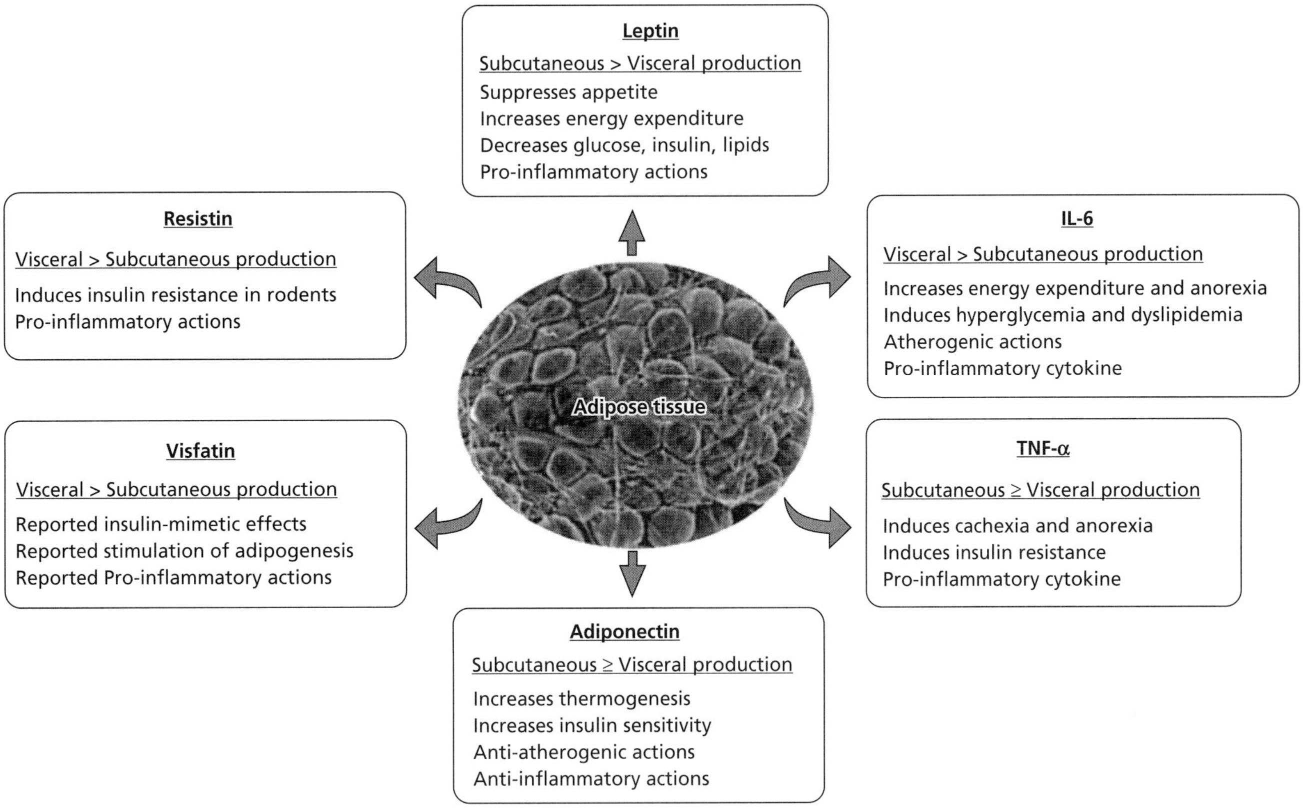

Figure 16.6 Schematic representation of the major adipokines secreted by adipose tissue. Most of the adipokines are secreted into the plasma proportionally to the adipose tissue mass and exert deleterious metabolic and proinflammatory effects. Adiponectin plays a protective role in metabolic homeostasis and exhibits decreased secretion in obesity, particularly in visceral fat depots. TNF-α, tumor necrosis factor-α: IL-6, interleukin-6.

The obesity-related inflammatory state is characterized by failure to properly resolve due to an adversely altered adipose tissue milieu. The underlying molecular interplay ultimately forms a vicious cycle between preadipocytes, enlarged adipocytes and macrophages inside each fat depot. As lipogenesis and adipogenesis progress, adipose-derived adipokines and chemokines, such as monocyte chemotactic protein-1 (MCP-1) and interleukin 8 (IL-8), are increasingly released into the systemic circulation (see Fig. 16.7a). Thus, mononuclear cells are recruited from the bloodstream and transmigrate into the expanding adipose tissue, where they are activated and function as resident macrophages [52,77]. In turn, these macrophages secrete locally cytokines (e.g. TNF-α, IL-6, IL-1β) which further stimulate the proinflammatory adipocyte secretion, suppress the expression of adiponectin and promote insulin resistance in enlarged adipocytes [78]. It is important to note that, unlike this continuous feedback loop generated inside the accumulated fat, conventional inflammatory responses are typically programmed to quickly subside once the original stimulus/threat is contained. Thus, at usual inflammatory sites, such as local infections and injuries, cytokines are secreted transiently by the recruited immune cells in order to avoid prolonged macrophage responses which would have destructive consequences (see Fig. 16.7b) [79]. It becomes apparent that sustained fat accumulation initiates a subclinical inflammatory response, which is perpetuated locally because of ongoing reciprocal interactions between the increasing populations of adipocytes and macrophages. Progressively this leads to a chronic, low-grade, generalized inflammatory state mediated by the persistent adipokine secretion of either adipocyte or macrophage origin [80]. Constantly increased circulating adipokine and cytokine concentrations induce potent adverse metabolic effects on other tissues and organs (e.g. liver, skeletal muscle, endothelium), contributing to the overall deterioration of metabolic homeostasis [73,81,82].

Central obesity and the significance of fat distribution

It is recognized that regional adiposity plays an equally significant, if not greater, role in the development of obesity-related metabolic complications [18]. In 1947, Jean Vague described the existence of two distinct clinical types of obesity in relation to fat distribution and reported that the degree of upper body adiposity is a factor determining type 2 diabetes predisposition [19]. Central obesity (visceral, abdominal, android, upper body or apple-shaped obesity) is characterized by fat accumulation intra-abdominally and subcutaneously around the abdomen, and is associated with increased risk for metabolic and cardiovascular

(a) Progressive weight gain

(b) Typical inflammatory response

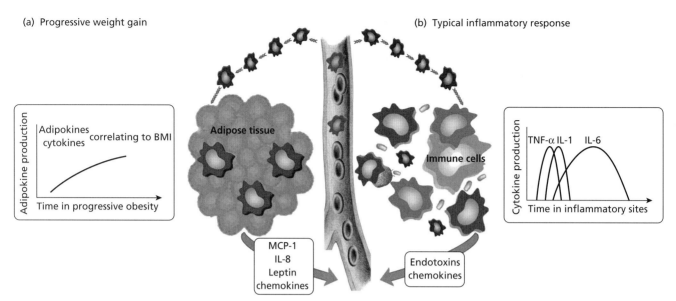

Figure 16.7 Schematic representation of the chronic proinflammatory state related to obesity versus the conventional immune response at inflammatory sites. (a) Progressive weight gain causes an unremitting secretion of proinflammatory adipokines, cytokines and chemokines from fat depots into the circulation, which strongly correlates with BMI. Subsequently, mononuclear cells transmigrate from the bloodstream into the expanding adipose tissue and increase the local population of resident macrophages, which becomes the major source of cytokine secretion from adipose tissue. A vicious cycle is formed inside fat depots, where adipocytes release FFA and adipokines that stimulate macrophages to secrete cytokines and vice versa. The end result is a chronic low-grade inflammatory state which is perpetuated for as long as the weight gain is maintained. (b) Immune responses at inflammatory sites (e.g. local infections, injuries) are usually time-restricted and subside once the original stimulus-threat is contained. The main inflammatory cytokines, TNF-α, IL-1 and IL-6 are secreted by the recruited immune cells transiently in order to avoid prolonged macrophage responses that would have destructive consequences. MCP-1, monocyte chemotactic protein-1; IL-8, interleukin 8.

diseases, independent of BMI. Conversely, in gluteofemoral obesity (peripheral, gynoid, lower body or pear-shaped obesity) the fat is stored predominantly in the subcutaneous regions of hips, thighs and lower trunk and, to some extent, appears to be protective against metabolic complications [83].

Waist circumference, measured in the horizontal plane midway between the superior iliac crest and the lower margin of the last rib, correlates positively with abdominal fat mass (subcutaneous and intra-abdominal) and provides a simple and reliable assessment of central obesity [84]. The waist-to-hip circumference ratio (WHR) may also be used to define central obesity, but it is a weaker marker of abdominal fat content and does not appear to have greater prognostic value compared to waist circumference alone [20,85]. The waist circumference cut-off points for the diagnosis of central obesity are still a matter of debate. Different thresholds must be used according to gender and ethnicity due to significant variations in susceptibility to central adiposity, as will be discussed in the following section on the metabolic syndrome.

Several hypotheses have been proposed to explain the correlation of central fat distribution with high cardiometabolic risk. Visceral adipose tissue is more lipolytic in obesity, probably due to increased catecholamine-induced lipolysis and decreased insulin-mediated inhibition of the hormone-sensitive lipase. Thus, central obesity is associated with a greater flux of FFA into the portal circulation with potential lipotoxic effects on several metabolic pathways, primarily in the liver and skeletal muscle [74,86]. Additionally, in the obese state, visceral fat is characterized by markedly upregulated secretion of adipokines, downregulated secretion of adiponectin and enhanced activation of inflammatory pathways [55,56]. Neuroendocrine abnormalities, including dysregulation of the hypothalamic-pituitary-adrenal axis, are also related to visceral adiposity and appear implicated in its adverse consequences [87,88]. These mechanisms may act in concert during weight gain and are considered crucial steps in the pathogenic process that links central obesity to cardiometabolic complications.

Metabolic syndrome: diagnostic criteria and the significance of central obesity

Obesity, type 2 diabetes, hypertension and dyslipidemia, all independent risk factors for cardiovascular disease (CVD), exhibit a marked tendency to cluster together. Two decades ago, Reaven proposed the term "syndrome X" in order to illustrate such a constellation of metabolic abnormalities revolving around insulin resistance and to emphasize its correlation with high morbidity and mortality rates due to CVD [4]. Since then, the term "metabolic syndrome" has been adopted to better describe this clustering of powerful CVD risk factors, which is estimated to affect approximately 20–25% of the adult population in Western societies [89,90]. Although there is continuing controversy about whether it constitutes a distinct pathophysiologic entity, a number of international medical bodies propose that the metabolic syndrome should be clearly defined, based on standardized criteria, in order to help both research and clinical practice [90–93].

Until recently the diagnostic criteria varied significantly between different metabolic syndrome definitions, resulting in confusion and limiting the comparability between studies. To address this issue, the International Diabetes Federation (IDF) issued a consensus statement in 2005 and proposed a new worldwide metabolic syndrome definition which is easy to enforce, since it is based on the evaluation of simple anthropometric and plasma measurements (waist circumference, blood pressure and plasma levels of triglycerides, high-density lipoprotein cholesterol and fasting glucose) [92]. According to this definition, central obesity becomes a prerequisite for the diagnosis of the metabolic syndrome. Establishing the presence of insulin resistance with an oral glucose tolerance test is no longer necessary and is replaced as a criterion by the assessment of fasting glucose (Table 16.1). Another problem addressed was the applicability of the criteria to various ethnic groups, especially regarding obesity. It is well documented that individuals of specific ethnic origin, regardless of the country of residence, are more prone to central obesity and more susceptible to its complications [94–97]. Given that Asian populations exhibit an amplified risk of morbidity at lower adiposity levels, rigorous cut-off points are being proposed for the management of these patients, considering clinical interventions for BMI values that exceed $23 \, kg/m^2$ and confirming obesity with a BMI threshold as low as $25 \, kg/m^2$ [96,98]. Accordingly, the IDF consensus defines central obesity in adult men and nonpregnant women based on ethnicity-specific values of waist circumference (see Table 16.1). These values were incorporated as initial guidelines and epidemiologic studies are expected to provide more comprehensive data that will supplement the current knowledge and offer new insights concerning additional populations (e.g. South and Central Americans, sub-Saharan Africans, Eastern Mediterranean and Middle East populations).

To date, the new IDF definition of the metabolic syndrome has helped significantly to set uniformly accepted diagnostic criteria worldwide and emphasize the significance of central obesity; it can be generally regarded as a valuable tool in forming and evaluating strategies for diagnosis and treatment [92,99]. However, it should be noted that, in order to more accurately predict increased risk of heart disease or type 2 diabetes, additional risk factors, such as age, smoking and cholesterol plasma levels, must also be assessed [100,101].

Nonalcoholic fatty liver disease

The recent progress in our understanding of the pathways regulating metabolic homeostasis has shed new light on the cross-talk between liver and adipose tissue. Derangements of glucose and lipid metabolism, such as those involved in obesity and type 2

Table 16.1 Criteria for the diagnosis of the metabolic syndrome according to the International Diabetes Federation definition [92]

I. Central obesity: defined according to ethnicity specific values of waist circumference

Ethnic group	Men	Women	Until more specific data are available:
Europids	≥94 cm	≥80 cm	Sub-Saharan Africans, Eastern
South Asians	≥90 cm	≥80 cm	Mediterranean Middle East (Arab)
Chinese	≥90 cm	≥80 cm	populations: use European data
Japanese	≥85 cm	≥90 cm	Ethnic South and Central Americans: use South Asian recommendations

II. Plus any two of the following factors:

A. ↑ TG levels: ≥150 mg/dL (1.7 mmol/L)
  or
  specific treatment for this lipid abnormality

B. ↓ HDL-c levels: males ≤40 mg/dL (1.03 mmol/L), females ≤50 mg/dL (1.29 mmol/L)
  or
  specific treatment for this lipid abnormality

C. ↑ Blood pressure: systolic BP ≥130 mm Hg
  or
  diastolic BP ≥85 mm Hg
  or
  treatment of previously diagnosed hypertension

D. ↑ FPG: ≥100 mg/dL (5.6 mmol/L)
  or
  previously diagnosed type 2 diabetes

TG, triglycerides; HDL-c, high-density lipoprotein cholesterol; BP, blood pressure; FPG, fasting plasma glucose.

diabetes, combined with ectopic fat accumulation in the liver can impair hepatic function and lead to manifestations that may progress from asymptomatic steatosis to cirrhosis and terminal liver failure.

Definition of NAFLD and NASH

In 1980 the term "nonalcoholic steatohepatitis (NASH)" was introduced by Ludwig et al. to describe a previously unnamed nonalcohol-related liver disease with histologic features that resembled those of alcoholic hepatitis [102]. The term "nonalcoholic fatty liver disease (NAFLD)" is now applied to describe the entire spectrum of these hepatic abnormalities, which extends from simple fatty liver infiltration (steatosis) to steatohepatitis and fibrosis. The hallmark of NAFLD is steatosis, typically regarded as a triglyceride content exceeding 5–10% of the total liver weight [103]. The identified steatosis represents ectopic deposition of fat in the liver and is usually macrovesicular with a large singular intracellular fat droplet displacing the nucleus [104].

Nonalcoholic steatohepatitis is defined as the most severe histologic form of NAFLD, types 3 and 4 as proposed by Matteoni et al., characterized by distinctive features of inflammation, hepatocyte injury (ballooning degeneration) and varying degrees of fibrosis in addition to steatosis (Table 16.2) [105,106]. Histologic distinction between NASH and alcoholic hepatitis may not be feasible, highlighting the importance of a detailed alcohol consumption history.

Epidemiology of NAFLD

Nonalcoholic fatty liver disease has become one of the most common causes of chronic liver disease globally, characterized by high prevalence rates and distribution patterns that follow the trends of weight gain and diabetes in developed and developing countries. Additionally, as both obese and diabetic populations are expected to continue to grow rapidly, with earlier onset and longer duration of the underlying metabolic derangements,

NAFLD prevalence and disease burden are predicted to steadily increase worldwide in the next decades [107–109].

The prevalence of NAFLD in the general population varies according to the modality used for diagnosis, with a consensus figure of 20–30% for several developed countries and more moderate estimations in the 10–15% range [109–114]. The corresponding prevalence of NASH is estimated to reach approximately 2–3% [115,116]. Contrary to the initial reports that implied female predominance, NAFLD appears to be more common in males. The disease is reported to peak during the fourth decade of life in men and after the fifth decade in women [109,110].

Prevalence data for NAFLD in cohorts of obese and diabetic patients document an overwhelming presence of the disease, indicating potential pathogenetic relations. According to these data, almost 75% of the patients with clinical obesity or type 2 diabetes develop steatosis. NASH can be diagnosed in 10–20% of these obese individuals, especially if the fat is accumulated centrally [108–109]. NAFLD prevalence rises with increasing BMI and reaches 90–95% in bariatric surgery patients, who usually suffer from morbid obesity (BMI exceeding $40\,kg/m^2$) and other manifestations of the metabolic syndrome [117–119].

Table 16.2 Nonalcoholic fatty liver disease (NAFLD) histologic classification as proposed by Matteoni et al. [105]. Nonalcoholic steatohepatitis (NASH) is defined as the most severe form of NAFLD (types 3 and 4 of NAFLD)

Type 1	Type 2	Type 3 – NASH	Type 4 – NASH
Steatosis	Steatosis	Steatosis	Steatosis
No inflammation	Mild inflammation	Inflammation	Inflammation
No other hepatocyte injury findings	No other hepatocyte injury findings	Ballooning degeneration	Ballooning degeneration
No fibrosis	No fibrosis	No fibrosis	Fibrosis and/or Mallory bodies
Considered stable & nonprogressive	Considered of benign prognosis	Progressive to cirrhosis	Progressive to cirrhosis

Natural history of NAFLD and the risk for cirrhosis and hepatocellular carcinoma

Data concerning the natural history of NAFLD are based primarily on studies with relatively small cohorts of selected patients [120–123]. However, it is now evident that NAFLD is not always benign, as previously perceived, and can potentially cause severe liver complications (Fig. 16.8). Indeed, according to a

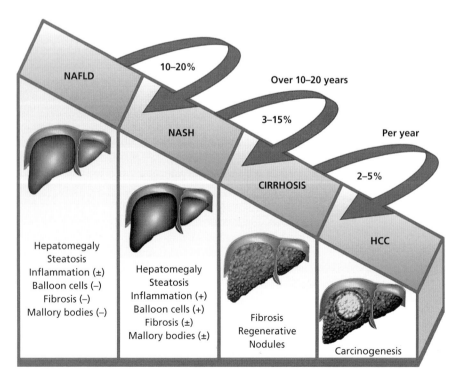

NAFLD

10–20%

Over 10–20 years

NASH

3–15%

Per year

CIRRHOSIS

2–5%

HCC

Hepatomegaly
Steatosis
Inflammation (±)
Balloon cells (–)
Fibrosis (–)
Mallory bodies (–)

Hepatomegaly
Steatosis
Inflammation (+)
Balloon cells (+)
Fibrosis (±)
Mallory bodies (±)

Fibrosis
Regenerative
Nodules

Carcinogenesis

Figure 16.8 Schematic representation of the natural history of nonalcoholic fatty liver disease (NAFLD). NASH, non-alcoholic steatohepatitis; HCC, hepatocellular carcinoma.

population-based cohort study, mortality among community-diagnosed NAFLD patients was higher than in the general population. Liver disease was the third leading cause of death in this group, compared to the 13th leading cause in the general population, although the absolute risk was low [120].

Long-term prognosis of NAFLD depends crucially on the histologic stage. Simple steatosis is typically benign and stable (1–2% risk of developing clinical evidence of cirrhosis over 15–20 years) [124,125]. Conversely, patients with NASH are at increased risk for developing cirrhosis, end-stage liver failure and hepatocellular carcinoma (HCC) (see Fig. 16.8). Advancement of NASH to cirrhosis ranges between 3% and 15% over 10–20 years and has a particularly poor prognosis, since almost a third of these cirrhotic patients will require a liver transplant or die from hepatic associated complications [126–128]. HCC is estimated to develop in patients with NASH-related cirrhosis at an annual rate of 2–5%, with data suggesting that chronic hyperinsulinemia may directly promote hepatic carcinogenesis [129,130].

The severity of NAFLD tends to increase with age, although regression is also possible over time. Signs of regression should be evaluated with caution, particularly in older patients. The progression of fibrosis can be silent and is often associated with normalization of plasma aminotransferases and abated histologic features of steatosis and inflammation. Loss of the characteristic histology is frequently consistent with the transition of NASH to a "burned-out" state, typically recognized as cryptogenic cirrhosis, which correlates with high HCC risk and is a common indication for liver transplantation [131,132]. Indeed, this transition seems to explain the pathogenesis in many patients with cryptogenic cirrhosis, most of whom are older than NASH patients,

but otherwise exhibit the same risk factors (obesity, insulin resistance and/or diabetes) [133].

Ethnic variations characterize both the prevalence and the natural history of NAFLD, suggesting that genetic predisposition plays a role in the pathogenesis of the disease [109,110,134]. Published data show that Asian and Hispanic populations are more prone to steatosis and may develop more severe forms of NASH, while African-Americans are reported to exhibit the disease less frequently than would be predicted by the corresponding obesity and diabetes trends [135–137]. Notably in regions like India, where obesity rates remain lower compared to Western societies, the prevalence of NAFLD in the general population still reaches 20–30% [138,139]. Interestingly, these differences are in complete accord with the aforementioned predisposition of certain ethnic groups to central obesity, insulin resistance and type 2 diabetes.

NAFLD pathogenesis and the relation to obesity and diabetes

Nonalcoholic fatty liver disease can be classified into primary and secondary types depending on the underlying cause. Primary NAFLD is associated with the metabolic syndrome components, while the category of secondary disease includes a diverse variety of causes (Table 16.3) [106]. Although this classification is rather arbitrary, it emphasizes the fact that NAFLD is predominantly associated with the presence of obesity, insulin resistance and their related metabolic complications [140,141]. Notably, many of the secondary causes may in fact exacerbate cases of undiagnosed primary NAFLD, indicating significant overlap in this classification.

Table 16.3 Nonalcoholic fatty liver disease (NAFLD) classification into primary and secondary types based on the underlying cause

PRIMARY

Metabolic Syndrome Components
Obesity (particularly central)
Insulin resistance – type 2 diabetes
Hypertriglyceridemia
Low HDL cholesterol
Hypertension

SECONDARY

Nutrition	Metabolic-genetic	Drugs	Toxins	Other
Starvation	A-& hypobetalipoproteinemia	Amiodarone	Organic solvents	Hepatitis C virus
Rapid weight loss	Lipodystrophy	Methotrexate	Phosphorus	Human
Total parenteral nutrition	Hypothalamic conditions	Tamoxifen	Petrochemicals	immunodeficiency virus
Intestinal bypass surgery	Hypopituitarism	Corticosteroids	Toxic mushrooms	Inflammatory bowel
	Acute fatty liver of pregnancy	Valproic acid	*Bacillus cereus* toxins	disease
	Reyes syndrome	Isoniazid		Small bowel
	Weber–Christian syndrome	Antiretroviral therapy		diverticulosis & bacterial overgrowth

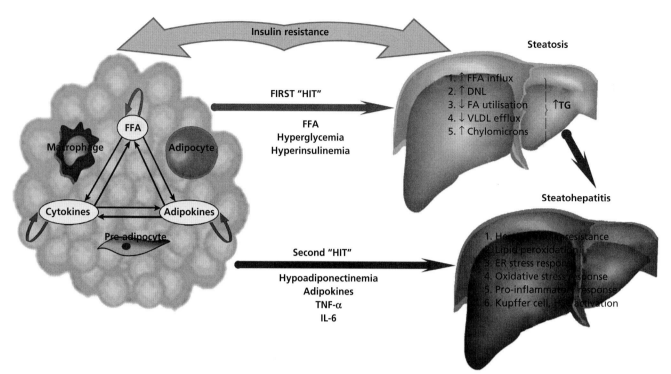

Figure 16.9 Schematic representation of the "two hit" model in the pathogenesis of nonalcoholic fatty liver disease (NAFLD). The first "hit" induces steatosis and enhances the susceptibility of the liver to the second "hit." Steatosis results primarily from an amplified hepatic free fatty acid (FFA) influx due to increased release of FFA from insulin-resistant fat depots (reduced insulin inhibition of lipolysis). In the liver this FFA influx is combined with increased *de novo* lipogenesis (DNL), impaired fatty acid oxidation and suppressed VLDL efflux, which are caused by the underlying hyperinsulinemia, hyperglycemia and hepatic insulin resistance. Dietary fat may also contribute to the total hepatic triglyceride (TG) content through the delivery of chylomicrons from the intestines. The second "hit" causes progression to steatohepatitis (NASH) and is promoted by elevated plasma levels of TNF-α and IL-6, hyperleptinemia and hypoadiponectinemia. Circulating adipokines in obesity, in combination with steatosis, induce hepatic insulin resistance, hepatic lipid peroxidation, oxidative stress responses, endoplasmic reticulum (ER) stress responses and activation of Kupffer and hepatic stellate cells (HSC). The end result is the development of a chronic proinflammatory state in the steatotic liver, characterized by hepatic cell injury, inflammation, apoptosis and fibrosis.

The tight association between obesity, insulin resistance and NAFLD has been supported by strong epidemiologic data. Furthermore, nondiabetic patients with either simple steatosis or steatohepatitis have been shown to be insulin resistant in numerous studies, utilizing various methods to demonstrate glucose intolerance [142–146]. Obesity-related insulin resistance is now considered the cornerstone in the pathogenesis of NAFLD [147,148]. Whether insulin resistance can originate first from the liver, caused independently by the increased hepatocyte triglyceride content, is a matter of debate: most data suggest that adipose tissue represents the primary site triggering the subsequent cascade. Day et al. have proposed the "two-hit" model in order to describe the chain of events leading from obesity to steatosis and NASH [148–150]. According to this model, the first "hit" facilitates the development of steatosis and enhances the susceptibility of the liver to the second "hit" which is considered responsible for the progression to hepatic injury, inflammation and fibrosis (Fig. 16.9).

The first "hit" is directly related to the presence of insulin resistance. Reduced insulin sensitivity causes decreased inhibition of lipolysis and decreased glucose uptake in adipocytes; concomitantly it increases lipogenesis and decreases the inhibition of gluconeogenesis in the liver. The increased and sustained FFA release from insulin-resistant fat depots enhances the hepatic FFA influx, which is considered the primary contributing factor in the development of steatosis (see Fig. 16.9). Notably, central obesity, due to high rates of visceral lipolysis, induces markedly increased delivery of FFA directly to the liver via the portal circulation [151]. The triglyceride content of hepatocytes is further augmented due to stimulated *de novo* lipogenesis, impaired hepatic fatty acid oxidation and decreased VLDL efflux, which are caused by the underlying hyperinsulinemia, hyperglycemia and hepatic insulin resistance [152,153]. Dietary triglycerides, transported from the intestines to the liver via chylomicrons, may also contribute to steatosis. The extent of steatosis correlates with the degree of insulin resistance and reflects the risk for development of NASH and NASH-related cirrhosis [149].

The second "hit" facilitates the progression from steatosis to steatohepatitis. NASH results from a vicious cycle in the steatotic liver, which involves increasing hepatic insulin resistance and lipid peroxidation, in combination with proinflammatory, oxidative stress and endoplasmic reticulum stress responses (see Fig. 16.9). All these processes are triggered and supported by the circulating adipokines and are amplified locally by detrimental pathways activated in hepatocytes. Thus, increased TNF-α and IL-6 plasma levels, hyperleptinemia and hypoadiponectinemia promote a chain of adverse effects in the liver that leads to cell injury, mitochondrial dysfunction, inflammation, apoptosis and fibrosis, especially in the presence of steatosis [150,154]. Furthermore, circulating adipokines and the steatosis itself stimulate the local secretion of proinflammatory cytokines (e.g. TNF-α, IL-6, IL-1β) by hepatocytes. Kupffer and hepatic stellate cells are also activated and more inflammatory cells transmigrate from the circulation to the liver [155,156]. It becomes evident that NASH progressively develops a chronic proinflammatory hepatic state that bears resemblance to the inflammatory state of adipose tissue in obesity. The exact molecular mechanisms implicated in these interactions are the subject of intense research, aiming to identify critical steps which could be modulated in order to offer specific therapeutic approaches for NASH.

Diagnosis of NAFLD

A definitive diagnosis of NAFLD requires exclusion of alcohol abuse and histologic confirmation, although performing a liver biopsy in all the patients with suspected steatosis is not practical. The precise level of daily ethanol intake that conclusively distinguishes nonalcoholic from alcoholic disease is not known. The National Institutes of Health Clinical Research Network on NAFLD has reached a consensus which defines that the maximum allowed alcohol intake level for NAFLD diagnosis is 140 g ethanol/week (two standard drinks/day) for men and 70 g ethanol/week (one standard drink/day) for women [108]. Detailed information concerning past alcohol habits should also be obtained, since the overall lifetime consumption appears to be significant.

In the usual clinical setting, NAFLD can be diagnosed with relative confidence in patients having no history of alcohol abuse, metabolic co-morbidities and abnormal laboratory or imaging findings suggesting liver disease. The initial assessment must also include a detailed medical history, evaluation for metabolic syndrome and testing for human immunodeficiency virus, hepatitis B and C infection, serum ferritin, ceruloplasmin, autoantibodies, and α1-antitrypsin [157,158]. The key points for the diagnosis of NAFLD are summarized in Table 16.4.

The need to perform a liver biopsy to establish the diagnosis is still debated due to the risk of complications and limitations associated with sampling and interpretation errors. Nevertheless, histologic assessment is considered important in managing patients with high clinical suspicion for NASH, since the underlying type and stage of NAFLD determine the prognosis and are crucial variables in forming the therapeutic strategy. Clinical and laboratory predictors of underlying severity have been reported, in order to support a justified selection of the NAFLD patients who would benefit most from a biopsy [159], but conflicting data exist about their accuracy to predict more advanced histology.

Adult obesity and implications for the treatment of type 2 diabetes, metabolic syndrome and NAFLD

Effective treatment of obesity represents a primary objective in the therapeutic approach to obese patients with associated metabolic diseases, such as type 2 diabetes, metabolic syndrome and NAFLD, since reduction of the excessive body weight can mitigate all the associated risks. The currently available treatment options will be discussed in detail in the following chapters about the management of adult obesity. The key message for clinicians providing care to these patients is that early and aggressive weight loss interventions should always complement the treatment of co-existing complications and that this approach is essential for a favorable long-term outcome.

After the initial evaluation, a structured plan of action must be formulated in co-operation with each patient in order to set precise and realistic goals for steady weight reduction and to establish optimal adherence. Lifestyle modification, including appropriate diet and exercise, is the initial step and must be keenly encouraged. Pharmacotherapy for tackling obesity in these patients should be initiated early in the treatment plan, in addition to other agents prescribed for diabetes, hypertension and dyslipidemia. Failure to achieve or maintain weight loss with lifestyle interventions and antiobesity drugs is an indication for bariatric surgery, which should be promptly considered as the next step in the weight management strategy [160]. Following the proposed guidelines, surgical interventions in morbidly obese patients with metabolic complications can effectively treat not

Table 16.4 Key points in the diagnostic process for nonalcoholic fatty liver disease (NAFLD)

Definite diagnosis	Symptoms and signs	Laboratory	Imaging
Alcohol	Asymptomatic	↑ ALT, AST	Ultrasonography
Men <2 standard	(50–100%)	Usually ALT, AST <2–4 x upper	Computed tomography
drinks/day	Fatigue (0–70%)	normal	Magnetic resonance
Women <1 standard	RUQ pain (0–50%)	Usually ALT > AST	imaging
drink/day	Hepatomegaly	↑ ALP, GGT	Magnetic resonance
	Splenomegaly (rare)	↑ IgA (about 25%)	spectroscopy
Liver biopsy	Palmar erythema (rare)	Hyperglycemia (about 30–35%)	Reliable for diagnosis
Histologic confirmation		Hyperlipidemia (about 20–30%)	Not reliable for staging
& staging			

RUQ, Right upper quadrant: AST, aspartate transaminase; ALT, alanine transaminase; GGT, γ-glutamyl transpeptidase; ALP, alkaline phosphatase; IgA, immunoglobulin A.

only obesity but also the entire metabolic syndrome spectrum, and thus significantly decrease the overall long-term mortality [161,162].

In the presence of diagnosed type 2 diabetes the treatment strategy is principally determined by the primary goal of tight glycemic control. Although useful as adjunct treatment, the available weight loss medications cannot be recommended as primary therapy for diabetes due to low compliance and sustainability and potential adverse side-effects which often restrict their use in clinical practice. Thus, at the time of diagnosis antidiabetic agents should be initiated together with lifestyle interventions to manage hyperglycemia. The American Diabetes Association (ADA) and the European Association for the Study of Diabetes (EASD) have issued a consensus algorithm for the initiation and adjustment of therapy in type 2 diabetes, recently updated regarding the use of peroxisome proliferator-activated receptor-γ agonists (PPARγ agonists, thiazolidinediones, glitazones) [163,164]. According to this consensus, the HbA$_{1c}$ (A1C) target level for each individual patient should be as close to the nondiabetic range (A1C: 6%) as possible without significant risk of hypoglycemia and an A1C value greater or equal to 7% should prompt actions to initiate or change therapy until A1C levels lower than 7% are achieved.

Adopting regimens not favoring weight gain and not enhancing hyperinsulinemia should be generally preferred for the treatment of type 2 diabetes, but not at the expense of hyperglycemia. Metformin is a valuable option because it is associated with weight stability or modest weight loss, does not cause hypoglycemia as monotherapy and is inexpensive. Unless not tolerated due to gastrointestinal side-effects or contraindicated due to impaired renal function (increased risk of lactic acidosis), metformin is recommended as the initial pharmacologic treatment to manage hyperglycemia [163]. Additionally required therapy (oral agent or insulin) should be added on top of metformin. Sulfonylureas and glinides, which both stimulate the endogenous insulin secretion, as well as glitazones and insulin therapy, are options that may promote weight gain. It must be noted that pioglitazone and rosiglitazone have also been associated with fluid retention and increased risk for congestive heart failure, while particularly the latter appears to increase the risk of myocardial ischemic events [164,165]. Initiation and intensification of insulin therapy should be combined with metformin and considered as a treatment option at an early stage.

The identification of incretin defects in type 2 diabetes has prompted new treatment approaches, leading to the development of novel classes of antidiabetic agents. Exogenous administration of GLP-1 and GIP cannot be used for treatment, since both peptides exhibit extremely short plasma half-lives (2 minutes for GLP-1 and 5–7 minutes for GIP) due to rapid proteolytic degradation into biologically inactive metabolites by the enzyme dipeptidyl peptidase-4 (DPP-4) [166]. Incretin-based treatments currently include incretin mimetics and DPP-4 inhibitors. Incretin mimetics (e.g. exenatide, liraglutide) are injectable GLP-1 analogs with prolonged half-life in the circulation, aiming to compensate for GLP-1 deficiency. DPP-4 inhibitors (gliptins, e.g.

sitagliptin, vildagliptin) are administered orally and aim to potentiate the endogenous incretin effect by inhibiting the degradation of the secreted GLP-1. Both approaches are effective in improving glycemic control by enhancing insulin secretion and preserving β cell mass. Furthermore incretin mimetics promote weight loss, while DPP-4 inhibitors are considered weight-neutral agents [167].

Treatment strategies for patients with metabolic syndrome should follow the proposed guidelines for treating obesity, dyslipidemia, hypertension and type 2 diabetes, according to the components that are present in each case. It must be emphasized that prompt recognition is pivotal in the management of any independent cardiometabolic risk factor, which should be treated in the context of the individual patient, even when the concept of the metabolic syndrome is not taken into account [100,101]. However, applying the new IDF metabolic syndrome criteria in regular clinical practice is expected to motivate physicians and patients for early and more aggressive weight loss interventions, since precise assessment of central obesity becomes a prerequisite for both diagnosis and follow-up care [92,99].

Specific treatment guidelines for NAFLD are lacking because of the limited number of large randomized clinical trials in the literature. Thus, the proposed therapeutic strategies for optimal care of NAFLD patients rely on effectively treating each co-existing component of the metabolic syndrome, focusing particularly on weight loss. The associated risk of CVD dictates this approach, which concurrently helps to prevent and reverse hepatic abnormalities. Restricted alcohol consumption and even abstinence should be recommended after the diagnosis of NAFLD in order to avoid additional stress to the liver. Given the different prognosis according to the underlying histologic stage, the cases of simple steatosis can be followed in a primary care setting, whereas NASH requires rigorous and long-term follow-up combined with more aggressive interventions [158,168].

Insulin-sensitizing agents appear to have a valid role in NAFLD treatment, even in the absence of overt type 2 diabetes [169,170]. Their application in nondiabetic NAFLD patients who exhibit glucose intolerance is encouraging, but larger and more prolonged studies are required before these agents can be incorporated into guideline treatment recommendations. Metformin has initially yielded contradictory results regarding long-term improvement in biochemical and histologic features of NAFLD. Recent data are more supportive of the effects of metformin in reducing steatosis, hepatic cellular injury and inflammation [171,172]. Studies with pioglitazone and rosiglitazone have also provided promising evidence about their efficacy in NAFLD [173,174]. Glitazones offer an attractive therapeutic option in these patients, due to the combination of insulin-sensitizing and anti-inflammatory effects, but their long-term safety and benefits need further validation with increased vigilance regarding the associated risk of weight gain and heart failure [164,165,175].

Liver transplantation represents the last option in the treatment of NASH-related cirrhosis and HCC. Based on current prevalence trends of NASH, the number of patients reaching this terminal stage is predicted to rise significantly in the forthcoming decades. Notably, many of these patients are also expected to be poor candidates for transplantation due to severe co-morbidities. Post-transplantation recurrence of steatosis and NASH is an additional problem, related to inadequate treatment of underlying risk factors and to the required immunosuppressive therapy [176]. Thus, prevention and early intervention are regarded as vital in NASH patients.

The treatment of obesity-related metabolic diseases poses a challenge in modern clinical practice and requires a co-ordinated approach, aiming to control every co-existing complication and achieve lifelong weight management. Specific interventions directly tackling pathogenetic mechanisms (e.g. the use of anti-inflammatory and cytoprotective agents) are expected to provide more therapeutic options for the entire spectrum of the metabolic syndrome in the future.

Acknowledgments

Fellowship support from the European Foundation for the Study of Diabetes Albert Renold Fellowship for Young Scientists for I. Kyrou is gratefully appreciated.

References

1. James WP. The epidemiology of obesity: the size of the problem. J Intern Med 2008;263(4):336–52.
2. Kopelman P. Health risks associated with overweight and obesity. Obes Rev 2007;8(suppl 1): 13–17.
3. Bray GA. Medical consequences of obesity. J Clin Endocrinol Metab 2004;89(6):2583–9.
4. Reaven GM. Banting lecture 1988. Role of insulin resistance in human disease. Diabetes 1988;37(12):1595–607.
5. Abdelmalek MF, Diehl AM. Nonalcoholic fatty liver disease as a complication of insulin resistance. Med Clin North Am 2007;91(6): 1125–49.
6. Day CP. Non-alcoholic steatohepatitis (NASH): where are we now and where are we going? Gut 2002;50(5):585–8.
7. Smyth S, Heron A. Diabetes and obesity: the twin epidemics. Nat Med 2006;12(1):75–80.
8. Astrup A, Finer N. Redefining type 2 diabetes: "diabesity" or "obesity dependent diabetes mellitus"? Obes Rev 2000;1(2):57–9.
9. Zimmet P, Alberti KG, Shaw J. Global and societal implications of the diabetes epidemic. Nature 2001;13;414(6865):782–7.
10. Adeghate E, Schattner P, Dunn E. An update on the etiology and epidemiology of diabetes mellitus. Ann NY Acad Sci 2006; 1084:1–29.
11. Junien C, Nathanielsz P. Report on the IASO Stock Conference 2006: early and lifelong environmental epigenomic programming of metabolic syndrome, obesity and type II diabetes. Obes Rev 2007;8(6):487–502.
12. Yoon KH, Lee JH, Kim JW, et al. Epidemic obesity and type 2 diabetes in Asia. Lancet 2006;368(9548):1681–8.
13. Alberti G, Zimmet P, Shaw J, et al. Type 2 diabetes in the young: the evolving epidemic: the international diabetes federation consensus workshop. Diabetes Care 2004;27(7):1798–811.
14. Wannamethee SG, Shaper AG. Weight change and duration of overweight and obesity in the incidence of type 2 diabetes. Diabetes Care 1999;22:1266–72.
15. Colditz GA, Willett WC, Rotnitzky A, et al. Weight gain as a risk factor for clinical diabetes mellitus in women. Ann Intern Med 1995;1;122(7):481–6.
16. Chan JM, Rimm EB, Colditz GA, et al. Obesity, fat distribution, and weight gain as risk factors for clinical diabetes in men. Diabetes Care 1994;17(9):961–9.
17. van Gaal LF, Mertens I, Ballaux D. What is the relationship between risk factor reduction and degree of weight loss? Eur Heart J 2005;7(suppl):L21–L26.
18. Pi-Sunyer FX. The epidemiology of central fat distribution in relation to disease. Nutr Rev 2004;62(7 Pt 2):S120–6.
19. Vague J. The degree of masculine differentiation of obesities: a factor determining predisposition to diabetes, atherosclerosis, gout, and uric calculous disease. Am J Clin Nutr 1956;4(1):20–34.
20. Klein S, Allison DB, Heymsfield SB, et al. Waist circumference and cardiometabolic risk: a consensus statement from shaping America's health: Association for Weight Management and Obesity Prevention; NAASO, the Obesity Society; the American Society for Nutrition; and the American Diabetes Association. Diabetes Care 2007;30(6):1647–52.
21. Schneider HJ, Glaesmer H, Klotsche J, et al. Accuracy of anthropometric indicators of obesity to predict cardiovascular risk. J Clin Endocrinol Metab 2007;92(2):589–94.
22. DeFronzo RA. Pathogenesis of type 2 diabetes mellitus. Med Clin North Am 2004;88(4):787–835.
23. Kahn SE, Hull RL, Utzschneider KM. Mechanisms linking obesity to insulin resistance and type 2 diabetes. Nature 2006;444(7121): 840–6.
24. Kahn SE. The importance of beta-cell failure in the development and progression of type 2 diabetes. J Clin Endocrinol Metab 2001;86(9):4047–58.
25. Gastaldelli A, Ferrannini E, Miyazaki Y, et al. Beta-cell dysfunction and glucose intolerance: results from the San Antonio metabolism (SAM) study. Diabetologia 2004;47(1):31–9.
26. Guilherme A, Virbasius JV, Puri V, et al. Adipocyte dysfunctions linking obesity to insulin resistance and type 2 diabetes. Nat Rev Mol Cell Biol 2008;9(5):367–77.
27. Bays H, Mandarino L, DeFronzo RA. Role of the adipocyte, free fatty acids, and ectopic fat in pathogenesis of type 2 diabetes mellitus: peroxisomal proliferator-activated receptor agonists provide a rational therapeutic approach. J Clin Endocrinol Metab 2004;89(2): 463–78.
28. Boden G. Effects of free fatty acids (FFA) on glucose metabolism: significance for insulin resistance and type 2 diabetes. Exp Clin Endocrinol Diabetes 2003;111(3):121–4.
29. DeFronzo RA, Ferrannini E, Simonson DC. Fasting hyperglycemia in non-insulin-dependent diabetes mellitus: contributions of excessive hepatic glucose production and impaired tissue glucose uptake. Metabolism 1989;38(4):387–95.
30. Shulman GI, Rothman DL, Jue T, et al. Quantitation of muscle glycogen synthesis in normal subjects and subjects with non-insulin-dependent diabetes by 13C nuclear magnetic resonance spectroscopy. N Engl J Med 1990; 322(4):223–8.
31. Pørksen N, Hollingdal M, Juhl C, et al. Pulsatile insulin secretion: detection, regulation, and role in diabetes. Diabetes 2002;51(suppl 1):S245–54.

32. Caumo A, Luzi L. First-phase insulin secretion: does it exist in real life? Considerations on shape and function. Am J Physiol Endocrinol Metab 2004;287(3):E371–85.

33. Creutzfeldt W, Nauck M. Gut hormones and diabetes mellitus. Diabetes Metab Rev 1992;8(2):149–77.

34. Bonner-Weir S. Beta-cell turnover: its assessment and implications. Diabetes 2001;50(suppl 1):S20–4.

35. Polonsky KS. Dynamics of insulin secretion in obesity and diabetes. Int J Obes 2000;24(suppl 2):S29–31.

36. Ferrannini E, Gastaldelli A, Miyazaki Y, et al. Predominant role of reduced beta-cell sensitivity to glucose over insulin resistance in impaired glucose tolerance. Diabetologia 2003;46(9):1211–19.

37. Ferrannini E, Gastaldelli A, Miyazaki Y, et al. Beta-cell function in subjects spanning the range from normal glucose tolerance to overt diabetes: a new analysis. J Clin Endocrinol Metab 2005;90(1):493–500.

38. McGarry JD. Banting lecture 2001: dysregulation of fatty acid metabolism in the etiology of type 2 diabetes. Diabetes 2002;51(1):7–18.

39. Kashyap S, Belfort R, Gastaldelli A, et al. A sustained increase in plasma free fatty acids impairs insulin secretion in nondiabetic subjects genetically predisposed to develop type 2 diabetes. Diabetes 2003;52(10):2461–74.

40. Cusi K, Kashyap S, Gastaldelli A, et al. Effects on insulin secretion and insulin action of a 48-h reduction of plasma free fatty acids with acipimox in nondiabetic subjects genetically predisposed to type 2 diabetes. Am J Physiol Endocrinol Metab 2007;292(6):E1775–81.

41. Vilsbøll T, Holst JJ. Incretins, insulin secretion and type 2 diabetes mellitus. Diabetologia 2004;47(3):357–66.

42. Baggio LL, Drucker DJ. Biology of incretins: GLP-1 and GIP. Gastroenterology 2007;132(6):2131–57.

43. Holst JJ. The physiology of glucagon-like peptide 1. Physiol Rev 2007;87(4):1409–39.

44. Nauck MA, Baller B, Meier JJ. Gastric inhibitory polypeptide and glucagon-like peptide-1 in the pathogenesis of type 2 diabetes. Diabetes 2004;53(suppl 3):S190–6.

45. Haataja L, Gurlo T, Huang CJ, et al. Islet amyloid in type 2 diabetes, and the toxic oligomer hypothesis. Endocr Rev 2008;29(3):303–16.

46. McMillen IC, Robinson JS. Developmental origins of the metabolic syndrome: prediction, plasticity, and programming. Physiol Rev 2005;85(2):571–633.

47. Kershaw E, Flier JS. Adipose tissue as an endocrine organ. J Clin Endocrinol Metab 2004;89(6):2548–56.

48. Flier JS. Obesity wars: molecular progress confronts an expanding epidemic. Cell 2004; 116(2):337–50.

49. Björntorp P. Size, number and function of adipose tissue cells in human obesity. Horm Metab Res 1974;4:77–83.

50. Le Lay S, Krief S, Farnier C, et al. Cholesterol, a cell size-dependent signal that regulates glucose metabolism and gene expression in adipocytes. J Biol Chem 2001;276(20):16904–10.

51. Hausman DB, DiGirolamo M, Bartness TJ, et al. The biology of white adipocyte proliferation. Obes Rev 2001;2(4):239–54.

52. Weisberg SP, McCann D, Desai M, et al. Obesity is associated with macrophage accumulation in adipose tissue. J Clin Invest 2003; 112(12):1796–808.

53. Trayhurn P, Wood IS. Adipokines: inflammation and the pleiotropic role of white adipose tissue. Br J Nutr 2004;92(3):347–55.

54. Matsuzawa Y. The metabolic syndrome and adipocytokines. FEBS Lett 2006;580(12):2917–21.

55. Montague CT, O'Rahilly S. The perils of portliness: causes and consequences of visceral adiposity. Diabetes 2000;49(6):883–8.

56. Yang X, Smith U. Adipose tissue distribution and risk of metabolic disease: does thiazolidinedione-induced adipose tissue redistribution provide a clue to the answer? Diabetologia 2007;50(6):1127–39.

57. Zhang Y, Proenca R, Maffei M, et al. Positional cloning of the mouse obese gene and its human homologue. Nature 1994;372(6505):425–32.

58. Considine RV, Sinha MK, Heiman ML, et al. Serum immunoreactive-leptin concentrations in normal-weight and obese humans. N Engl J Med 1996;334(5):292–5.

59. Ahima RS. Central actions of adipocyte hormones. Trends Endocrinol Metab 2005;16(7):307–13.

60. Wauters M, Considine RV, van Gaal LF. Human leptin: from an adipocyte hormone to an endocrine mediator. Eur J Endocrinol 2000;143(3):293–311.

61. Ahima RS. Metabolic actions of adipocyte hormones: focus on adiponectin. Obesity (Silver Spring) 2006;14(suppl 1):9S-15S.

62. Kadowaki T, Yamauchi T, Kubota N, et al. Adiponectin and adiponectin receptors in insulin resistance, diabetes, and the metabolic syndrome. J Clin Invest 2006;116(7):1784–92.

63. Fisher FM, McTernan PG, Valsamakis G, et al. Differences in adiponectin protein expression: effect of fat depots and type 2 diabetic status. Horm Metab Res 2002;34(11–12):650–4.

64. Funahashi T, Matsuzawa Y. Hypoadiponectinemia: a common basis for diseases associated with overnutrition. Curr Atheroscler Rep 2006;8(5):433–8.

65. McTernan PG, Kusminski CM, Kumar S. Resistin. Curr Opin Lipidol 2006;17(2):170–5.

66. Pilz S, Mangge H, Obermayer-Pietsch B, et al. Visfatin/pre-B-cell colony-enhancing factor: a protein with various suggested functions. J Endocrinol Invest 2007;30(2):138–44.

67. Hotamisligil GS, Shargill NS, Spiegelman BM. Adipose expression of tumor necrosis factor-alpha: direct role in obesity-linked insulin resistance. Science 1993;259(5091):87–91.

68. Tsigos C, Papanicolaou DA, Kyrou I, et al. Dose-dependent effects of recombinant human interleukin-6 on glucose regulation. J Clin Endocrinol Metab 1997;82:4167–70.

69. Hoene M, Weigert C. The role of interleukin-6 in insulin resistance, body fat distribution and energy balance. Obes Rev 2008;9(1):20–9.

70. Coppack SW. Pro-inflammatory cytokines and adipose tissue. Proc Nutr Soc 2001;60(3):349–56.

71. Tsigos C, Kyrou I, Chala E, et al. Circulating tumor necrosis factor alpha concentrations are higher in abdominal versus peripheral obesity. Metabolism 1999;48(10):1332–5.

72. Maachi M, Piéroni L, Bruckert E, et al. Systemic low-grade inflammation is related to both circulating and adipose tissue TNFalpha, leptin and IL-6 levels in obese women. Int J Obes 2004;28(8):993–7.

73. Hotamisligil GS. Inflammation and metabolic disorders. Nature 2006;444(7121):860–7.

74. Weiss R. Fat distribution and storage: how much, where, and how? Eur J Endocrinol 2007;157(suppl 1):S39–45.

75. Shoelson SE, Lee J, Goldfine AB. Inflammation and insulin resistance. J Clin Invest 2006;116(7):1793–801.

76. Libby P. Inflammation in atherosclerosis. Nature 2002;420(6917): 868–74.

77. Xu H, Barnes GT, Yang Q, et al. Chronic inflammation in fat plays a crucial role in the development of obesity-related insulin resistance. J Clin Invest 2003;112(12):1821–30.

78. Wellen KE, Hotamisligil GS. Obesity-induced inflammatory changes in adipose tissue. J Clin Invest 2003;112(12):1785–8.

79. Chrousos GP. The hypothalamic-pituitary-adrenal axis and immune-mediated inflammation. N Engl J Med 1995;332:1351–62.

80. Tilg H, Moschen AR. Adipocytokines: mediators linking adipose tissue, inflammation and immunity. Nat Rev Immunol 2006;6(10): 772–83.

81. Yudkin JS. Inflammation, obesity, and the metabolic syndrome. Horm Metab Res 2007;39(10):707–9.

82. Lehrke M, Lazar MA. Inflamed about obesity. Nat Med 2004;10(2):126–7.

83. Snijder MB, Zimmet PZ, Visser M, et al. Independent and opposite associations of waist and hip circumferences with diabetes, hypertension and dyslipidemia: the AusDiab Study. Int J Obes 2004;28(3): 402–9.

84. Janssen I, Heymsfield SB, Allison DB, et al. Body mass index and waist circumference independently contribute to the prediction of nonabdominal, abdominal subcutaneous, and visceral fat. Am J Clin Nutr 2002;75(4):683–8.

85. Chan DC, Watts GF, Barrett PH, et al. Waist circumference, waist-to-hip ratio and body mass index as predictors of adipose tissue compartments in men. Q J Med 2003;96(6):441–7.

86. Björntorp P. "Portal" adipose tissue as a generator of risk factors for cardiovascular disease and diabetes. Arteriosclerosis 1990;10(4): 493–6.

87. Björntorp P, Rosmond R. Neuroendocrine abnormalities in visceral obesity. Int J Obes 2000;24(suppl 2):S80–5.

88. Kyrou I, Chrousos GP, Tsigos C. Stress, visceral obesity, and metabolic complications. Ann NY Acad Sci 2006;1083:77–110.

89. Pi-Sunyer X. The metabolic syndrome: how to approach differing definitions. Med Clin North Am 2007;91(6):1025–40.

90. Kahn R, Buse J, Ferrannini E, et al. The metabolic syndrome: time for a critical appraisal: joint statement from the American Diabetes Association and the European Association for the Study of Diabetes. Diabetes Care 2005;28(9):2289–304.

91. Alberti, KG, Zimmet PZ. Definition, diagnosis and classification of diabetes mellitus and its complications. Part 1: diagnosis and classification of diabetes mellitus provisional report of a WHO consultation. Diabet Med 1998;15:539–53.

92. Alberti KG, Zimmet PZ, Shaw J. The metabolic syndrome – a new worldwide definition. Lancet 2005;366:1059–62.

93. Expert Panel on Detection, Evaluation, and Treatment of High Blood Cholesterol in Adults. Executive Summary of The Third Report of The National Cholesterol Education Program (NCEP) Expert Panel on Detection, Evaluation, And Treatment of High Blood Cholesterol In Adults (Adult Treatment Panel III). JAMA 2001;285:2486–97.

94. James WP. Assessing obesity: are ethnic differences in body mass index and waist classification criteria justified? Obes Rev 2005;6(3):179–81.

95. James WP, Rigby N, Leach R. Obesity and the metabolic syndrome: the stress on society. Ann NY Acad Sci 2006;1083:1–10.

96. WHO Expert Consultation. Appropriate body-mass index for Asian populations and its implications for policy and intervention strategies. Lancet 2004;363:157–63.

97. Barnett AH, Dixon AN, Bellary S, et al. Type 2 diabetes and cardiovascular risk in the UK south Asian community. Diabetologia 2006;49(10):2234–46.

98. Huxley R, Barzi F, Stolk R, et al. Ethnic comparisons of obesity in the Asia-Pacific region: protocol for a collaborative overview of cross-sectional studies. Obes Rev 2005;6(3):193–8.

99. Grundy SM. Metabolic syndrome: a multiplex cardiovascular risk factor. J Clin Endocrinol Metab 2007;92(2):399–404.

100. Reaven GM. The metabolic syndrome: requiescat in pace. Clin Chem 2005;51(6):931–8.

101. Sattar N. Why metabolic syndrome criteria have not made prime time: a view from the clinic. Int J Obes 2008;32(suppl 2): S30–4.

102. Ludwig J, Viggiano TR, McGill DB, et al. Nonalcoholic steatohepatitis: Mayo Clinic experiences with a hitherto unnamed disease. Mayo Clin Proc 1980;55(7):434–8.

103. Yeh MM, Brunt EM. Pathology of nonalcoholic fatty liver disease. Am J Clin Pathol 2007;128(5):837–47.

104. Brunt EM. Nonalcoholic steatohepatitis. Semin Liver Dis 2004; 24(1):3–20.

105. Matteoni CA, Younossi ZM, Gramlich T, et al. Nonalcoholic fatty liver disease: a spectrum of clinical and pathological severity. Gastroenterology 1999;116(6):1413–19.

106. Angulo P. Nonalcoholic fatty liver disease. N Engl J Med 2002;346(16):1221–31.

107. Angulo P. GI epidemiology: nonalcoholic fatty liver disease. Aliment Pharmacol Ther 2007;25(8):883–9.

108. Farrell GC, Larter CZ. Nonalcoholic fatty liver disease: from steatosis to cirrhosis. Hepatology 2006;43(2 suppl 1):S99–S112.

109. Clark JM. The epidemiology of nonalcoholic fatty liver disease in adults. J Clin Gastroenterol 2006;4(3 suppl 1):S5–10.

110. Browning JD, Szczepaniak LS, Dobbins R, et al. Prevalence of hepatic steatosis in an urban population in the United States: impact of ethnicity. Hepatology 2004;40(6):1387–95.

111. Clark JM, Brancati FL, Diehl AM. The prevalence and etiology of elevated aminotransferase levels in the United States. Am J Gastroenterol 2003;98(5):960–7.

112. Jimba S, Nakagami T, Takahashi M, et al. Prevalence of nonalcoholic fatty liver disease and its association with impaired glucose metabolism in Japanese adults. Diabet Med 2005;22(9): 1141–5.

113. Bellentani S, Tiribelli C, Saccoccio G, et al. Prevalence of chronic liver disease in the general population of northern Italy: the Dionysos Study. Hepatology 1994;20(6):1442–9.

114. Bedogni G, Miglioli L, Masutti F, et al. Prevalence of and risk factors for nonalcoholic fatty liver disease: the Dionysos nutrition and liver study. Hepatology 2005;42(1):44–52.

115. Clark JM, Brancati FL, Diehl AM. Nonalcoholic fatty liver disease. Gastroenterology 2002;122(6):1649–57.

116. Neuschwander-Tetri BA, Caldwell SH. Nonalcoholic steatohepatitis: summary of an AASLD Single Topic Conference. Hepatology 2003;37(5):1202–19.

117. Machado M, Marques-Vidal P, Cortez-Pinto H. Hepatic histology in obese patients undergoing bariatric surgery. J Hepatol 2006;45(4): 600–6.

118. Gholam PM, Kotler DP, Flancbaum LJ. Liver pathology in morbidly obese patients undergoing Roux-en-Y gastric bypass surgery. Obes Surg 2002;12:49–51.

119. Beymer C, Kowdley KV, Larson A, et al. Prevalence and predictors of asymptomatic liver disease in patients undergoing gastric bypass surgery. Arch Surg 2003;138(11):1240–4.

120. Adams LA, Lymp JF, St Sauver J, et al. The natural history of nonalcoholic fatty liver disease: a population-based cohort study. Gastroenterology 2005;129(1):113–21.

121. Adams LA, Sanderson S, Lindor KD, et al. The histological course of nonalcoholic fatty liver disease: a longitudinal study of 103 patients with sequential liver biopsies. J Hepatol 2005;42(1): 132–8.

122. Ekstedt M, Franzén LE, Mathiesen UL, et al. Long-term follow-up of patients with NAFLD and elevated liver enzymes. Hepatology 2006;44(4):865–73.

123. Bedogni G, Miglioli L, Masutti F, et al. Incidence and natural course of fatty liver in the general population: the Dionysos study. Hepatology 2007;46(5):1387–91.

124. Dam-Larsen S, Franzmann M, Andersen IB, et al. Long term prognosis of fatty liver: risk of chronic liver disease and death. Gut 2004;53(5):750–5.

125. Day CP. Natural history of NAFLD: remarkably benign in the absence of cirrhosis. Gastroenterology 2005;129(1):375–8.

126. Falck-Ytter Y, Younossi ZM, Marchesini G, et al. Clinical features and natural history of nonalcoholic steatosis syndromes. Semin Liver Dis 2001;21(1):17–26.

127. Ratziu V, Poynard T. Assessing the outcome of nonalcoholic steatohepatitis? It's time to get serious. Hepatology 2006;44(4):802–5.

128. Haukeland JW, Lorgen I, Schreiner LT, et al. Incidence rates and causes of cirrhosis in a Norwegian population. Scand J Gastroenterol 2007;12:1–8.

129. Ong JP, Younossi ZM. Epidemiology and natural history of NAFLD and NASH. Clin Liver Dis 2007;11(1):1–16.

130. Bugianesi E. Steatosis, the metabolic syndrome and cancer. Aliment Pharmacol Ther 2005;22(suppl 2):40–3.

131. Bugianesi E, Leone N, Vanni E, et al. Expanding the natural history of nonalcoholic steatohepatitis: from cryptogenic cirrhosis to hepatocellular carcinoma. Gastroenterology 2002;123(1):134–40.

132. Maheshwari A, Thuluvath PJ. Cryptogenic cirrhosis and NAFLD: are they related? Am J Gastroenterol 2006;101(3):664–8.

133. Poonawala A, Nair SP, Thuluvath PJ. Prevalence of obesity and diabetes in patients with cryptogenic cirrhosis: a case-control study. Hepatology 2000;32(4 Pt 1):689–92.

134. Day CP. Genes or environment to determine alcoholic liver disease and non-alcoholic fatty liver disease. Liver Int 2006;26(9):1021–8.

135. Weston SR, Leyden W, Murphy R, et al. Racial and ethnic distribution of nonalcoholic fatty liver in persons with newly diagnosed chronic liver disease. Hepatology 2005;41(2):372–9.

136. Chitturi S, Farrell GC, Hashimoto E, et al. Non-alcoholic fatty liver disease in the Asia-Pacific region: definitions and overview of proposed guidelines. J Gastroenterol Hepatol 2007;22(6):778–87.

137. Caldwell SH, Harris DM, Patrie JT, et al. Is NASH underdiagnosed among African Americans? Am J Gastroenterol 2002;97(6):1496–500.

138. Singh SP, Nayak S, Swain M, et al. Prevalence of nonalcoholic fatty liver disease in coastal eastern India: a preliminary ultrasonographic survey. Trop Gastroenterol 2004;25(2):76–9.

139. Sanyal AJ. Nonalcoholic fatty liver disease in the Indian subcontinent: a medical consequence of globalization? Indian J Gastroenterol 2001;20(6):215–16.

140. Marchesini G, Bugianesi E, Forlani G, et al. Nonalcoholic fatty liver, steatohepatitis, and the metabolic syndrome. Hepatology 2003;37(4): 917–23.

141. Kotronen A, Yki-Järvinen H. Fatty liver: a novel component of the metabolic syndrome. Arterioscler Thromb Vasc Biol 2008;28(1): 27–38.

142. Bugianesi E, Gastaldelli A, Vanni E, et al. Insulin resistance in non-diabetic patients with non-alcoholic fatty liver disease: sites and mechanisms. Diabetologia 2005;48(4):634–42.

143. Pagano G, Pacini G, Musso G, et al. Nonalcoholic steatohepatitis, insulin resistance, and metabolic syndrome: further evidence for an etiologic association. Hepatology 2002;35(2):367–72.

144. Chitturi S, Abeygunasekera S, Farrell GC, et al. NASH and insulin resistance: insulin hypersecretion and specific association with the insulin resistance syndrome. Hepatology 2002;35(2):373–9.

145. Haukeland JW, Konopski Z, Linnestad P, et al. Abnormal glucose tolerance is a predictor of steatohepatitis and fibrosis in patients with non-alcoholic fatty liver disease. Scand J Gastroenterol 2005;40(12):1469–77.

146. Sanyal AJ, Campbell-Sargent C, Mirshahi F, et al. Nonalcoholic steatohepatitis: association of insulin resistance and mitochondrial abnormalities. Gastroenterology 2001;120(5):1183–92.

147. Qureshi K, Abrams GA. Metabolic liver disease of obesity and role of adipose tissue in the pathogenesis of nonalcoholic fatty liver disease. World J Gastroenterol 2007;13(26):3540–53.

148. Day CP, James OF. Steatohepatitis: a tale of two "hits"? Gastroenterology 1998;114(4):842–5.

149. Day CP. Pathogenesis of steatohepatitis. Best Pract Res Clin Gastroenterol 2002;16(5):663–78.

150. Day CP. From fat to inflammation. Gastroenterology 2006;130(1): 207–10.

151. Nielsen S, Guo Z, Johnson CM, et al. Splanchnic lipolysis in human obesity. J Clin Invest 2004;113(11):1582–8.

152. Parekh S, Anania FA. Abnormal lipid and glucose metabolism in obesity: implications for nonalcoholic fatty liver disease. Gastroenterology 2007;132(6):2191–207.

153. McCullough AJ. Pathophysiology of nonalcoholic steatohepatitis. J Clin Gastroenterol 2006;40(3 suppl 1):S17–29.

154. Haukeland JW, Damas JK, Konopski Z, et al. Systemic inflammation in nonalcoholic fatty liver disease is characterized by elevated levels of CCL2. J Hepatol 2006;44(6):1167–74.

155. Tomita K, Tamiya G, Ando S, et al. Tumour necrosis factor alpha signalling through activation of Kupffer cells plays an essential role in liver fibrosis of non-alcoholic steatohepatitis in mice. Gut 2006;55(3):415–24.

156. Ikejima K, Okumura K, Kon K, et al. Role of adipocytokines in hepatic fibrogenesis. J Gastroenterol Hepatol 2007; 22(suppl 1):S87–92.

157. Adams LA, Talwalkar JA. Diagnostic evaluation of nonalcoholic fatty liver disease. J Clin Gastroenterol 2006;40(3 suppl 1):S34–8.

158. Day CP. Non-alcoholic fatty liver disease: current concepts and management strategies. Clin Med 2006;6(1):19–25.

159. Angulo P, Keach JC, Batts KP, et al. Independent predictors of liver fibrosis in patients with nonalcoholic steatohepatitis. Hepatology 1999;30(6):1356–62.

160. Tsigos C, Hainer V, Basdevant A, et al. Management of obesity in adults: European clinical practice guidelines. Obes Facts 2008;1:106–16.

161. Fried M, Hainer V, Basdevant A. Interdisciplinary European guidelines for surgery for severe (morbid) obesity. Obes Surg 2007;17(2): 260–70.

162. Sjöström L, Narbro K, Sjöström CD, et al. Effects of bariatric surgery on mortality in Swedish obese subjects. N Engl J Med 2007;357(8):741–52.

163. Nathan DM, Buse JB, Davidson MB, et al. Management of hyperglycemia in type 2 diabetes: a consensus algorithm for the initiation and adjustment of therapy: a consensus statement from the American Diabetes Association and the European Association for the Study of Diabetes. Diabetes Care 2006;29(8):1963–72.

164. Nathan DM, Buse JB, Davidson MB, et al. Management of hyperglycemia in type 2 diabetes: a consensus algorithm for the initiation and adjustment of therapy: update regarding thiazolidinediones: a consensus statement from the American Diabetes Association and the European Association for the Study of Diabetes. Diabetes Care 2008;31(1):173–5.

165. Home PD, Pocock SJ, Beck-Nielsen H, et al. Rosiglitazone evaluated for cardiovascular outcomes – an interim analysis. N Engl J Med 2007;357(1):28–38.

166. Baggio LL, Drucker DJ. Biology of incretins: GLP-1 and GIP. Gastroenterology 2007;132(6):2131–57.

167. Amori RE, Lau J, Pittas AG. Efficacy and safety of incretin therapy in type 2 diabetes: systematic review and meta-analysis. JAMA 2007;298(2):194–206.

168. Younossi ZM. Current management of non-alcoholic fatty liver disease and non-alcoholic steatohepatitis. Aliment Pharmacol Ther 2008;28(1):2–12.

169. Khashab M, Chalasani N. Use of insulin sensitizers in NASH. Endocrinol Metab Clin North Am 2007;36(4):1067–87.

170. Angelico F, Burattin M, Alessandri C, et al. Drugs improving insulin resistance for non-alcoholic fatty liver disease and/or non-alcoholic steatohepatitis. Cochrane Database Syst Rev 24;(1), CD005166, 2007.

171. Marchesini G, Brizi M, Bianchi G, et al. Metformin in non-alcoholic steatohepatitis. Lancet 2001;358(9285):893–4.

172. Bugianesi E, Gentilcore E, Manini R, et al. A randomized controlled trial of metformin versus vitamin E or prescriptive diet in nonalcoholic fatty liver disease. Am J Gastroenterol 2005;100(5):1082–90.

173. Belfort R, Harrison SA, Brown K, et al. A placebo-controlled trial of pioglitazone in subjects with nonalcoholic steatohepatitis. N Engl J Med 2006;355(22):2297–307.

174. McCullough AJ. Thiazolidinediones for nonalcoholic steatohepatitis – promising but not ready for prime time. N Engl J Med 2006; 355(22):2361–3.

175. Henriksen JH, Ring-Larsen H. Rosiglitazone: possible complications and treatment of non-alcoholic steatohepatitis (NASH). J Hepatol 2008;48(1):174–6.

176. Angulo P. Nonalcoholic fatty liver disease and liver transplantation. Liver Transpl 2006;12(4):523–34.

17 Cardiovascular Consequences of Obesity

Ian Wilcox

Sydney Medical School, University of Sydney, Sydney, Australia; Department of Cardiology, Royal Prince Alfred Hospital, Sydney, Australia

Introduction

Obesity is a well-recognized cardiovascular risk factor which exerts effects on the heart and circulation, both directly and also by its association with other known risk factors such as hypertension or diabetes [1]. Impaired cardiovascular fitness is also common in obese subjects and is an adverse factor which appears to predict increased mortality from cardiovascular disease independently of the degree of obesity and thus both "fitness" and "fatness" are important independent and modifiable risk factors for heart disease [2] which is clearly of major importance to both obese individuals and to the health of the community as a whole.

In the past, the effects of obesity on respiratory function have been considered separately from the cardiovascular effects despite the known importance of heart–lung interactions on pathophysiology in the obese. In this chapter we will explore the interaction between obesity, heart and lung disease in an attempt to understand the cardiorespiratory consequences of obesity better.

Obesity, especially upper body obesity, is linked with snoring, obstructive sleep apnea (OSA) and also cardiovascular disease and thus has important influences on cardiorespiratory function, while both awake and asleep [3]. The term "syndrome Z" has been used to describe the frequent association between components of the metabolic syndrome, including type 2 diabetes, and OSA (Box 17.1). This relationship is an important confounder of the relationship between obesity and its cardiovascular consequences. A report from the International Taskforce on Epidemiology and Prevention recently strongly recommended that health professionals working in type 2 diabetes and sleep-disordered breathing consider this possible relationship [4]. Although not explicitly stated, the statement should also apply to those health professionals working in obesity and those in cardiovascular

disease. We will explore the protean ways in which the cardiorespiratory consequences of obesity are affected by the presence of co-existent obstructive sleep apnea, present in a substantial proportion of the obese.

Physical fitness and obesity as predictors of mortality risk in obesity

Lack of physical fitness due to a sedentary lifestyle is believed to be a predictor of increased mortality risk. A series of reports from a longitudinal study of a population which were predominantly white US male college graduates (Aerobics Center Longitudinal Study) showed that performance on a maximal treadmill test indicated that those individuals in the lowest quartile of fitness had an increased mortality risk independent of their degree of obesity. These findings were confirmed by the Lipid Research Study [2] which used data from 7589 subjects (2506 women, 2860 men) aged 30–75 examined in eight US centers between 1972 and 1976 and followed until 1988. The subjects had a mean age of approximately 46 years and Body Mass Index (BMI) of 27.4 for males and 24.9 for women, and potentially there was a bias in favor of including healthy subjects; 12% of subjects were obese (BMI $\geq$30), while 33% of women and 50% of men were overweight (BMI 25–29.9 kg/m^2). The adjusted mortality hazard ratio for fit-fat women was 1.3 compared to 1.30 for unfit-not fat

> ### Box 17.1 Components of a proposed "syndrome Z" (Wilcox et al. [3])
>
> - Obstructive sleep apnea
> - Hypertension
> - Increased sympathetic nerve activity
> - Central (visceral) obesity
> - Insulin resistance
> - Atherogenic dyslipidemia

Clinical Obesity in Adults and Children, 3rd edition. Edited by Peter G. Kopelman, Ian D. Caterson and William H. Dietz.
© 2010 Blackwell Publishing, ISBN: 978-1-4051-8226-3.

women and 1.57 for unfit-fat women. The values for men were 1.44, 1.25 and 1.49 respectively with no significant interaction between fitness or fatness in men or women.

Physical fitness does not completely ameliorate the health hazard of obesity [1,2]. Therefore, it appears that both fatness and fitness are potentially modifiable risk factors for mortality [5].

Obesity and sudden death

Obesity increases the risk of sudden death [6]. A variety of mechanisms have been suggested which include increased sympathetic nerve activity, prolongation of the QT interval and structural heart disease such as coronary artery disease and cardiomyopathy.

The US Nurses' Health Study is a prospective study of a cohort of 121,701 nurses aged 30–55 years who completed a questionnaire about their medical history, coronary heart disease (CHD) risk factors, lifestyle and menopausal status at entry in 1976 and have been followed up at 2-year intervals by mail. In this cohort, the risk of sudden death increased with age and was associated with at least one known coronary disease risk factor in most instances, of which smoking, hypertension and diabetes conferred a 2.5–4-fold increase in risk of sudden death. Obesity and a family history of myocardial infarction before the age of 60 years each conferred a moderate (1.6-fold) increase in risk. These data showed that, as in men, the risk of sudden death was associated with risk factors for coronary disease, including obesity, and as expected, most deaths (88%) were classified as arrhythmic [7,8]. Given that other vascular risk factors are common in the obese, the total risk of sudden death in obese women is likely to be substantially increased. Although coronary heart disease is the underlying factor responsible for sudden death in most instances, other diseases such as cardiomyopathy are also common in the obese.

Increased sympathetic nerve activity promotes cardiac arrhythmias and has been shown to be increased in obesity in normotensive [9] and hypertensive subjects, whereas weight reduction tends to normalize these changes. The degree of sympathetic nerve overactivity during sleep and while awake is further increased by co-existent obstructive sleep apnea which occurs in a significant proportion of the obese [10].

The long QT syndrome is a genetically diverse inherited disorder of cardiac myocyte ion channels, which leads to prolonged ventricular repolarization and predisposes individuals to a characteristic type of ventricular tachycardia (torsades de pointes) and sudden death [11]. In susceptible individuals, changes in autonomic nerve activity (sympathetic overactivity) and electrolyte disturbances can prolong the duration of ventricular repolarization to a critical degree, causing serious, and potentially fatal, cardiac arrhythmias.

The use of diuretics and laxatives is well known to cause electrolyte changes, particularly hypokalemia and hypomagnesemia, which prolong ventricular repolarization, lengthen the QT interval on the surface ECG and increase the risk of ventricular tachycardia/fibrillation, especially in those with the long QT syndrome [11]. Treatment of obesity with ultra low-energy diets has been reported in some but not all studies to be associated with a risk of sudden death, and changes in electrolytes caused by these types of diets may be the mechanism responsible, especially in susceptible subjects.

In a study of both obese and nonobese women with a normal QT interval corrected for heart rate (QTc) at rest, Corbi and colleagues [12] compared free fatty acid (FFA) and catecholamine levels in women separated by the presence and pattern of obesity and examined the effects of weight loss of of approximately 12 kg. Obese women were subdivided into either peripheral (waist:hip ratio (WHR) ≤0.85) or central (WHR >0.85) fat distributions and showed that there was a positive relationship between obesity, free fatty acid levels, QTc and plasma catecholamines including both adrenaline and noradrenaline. Weight reduction over 12 months of the same magnitude in both groups of obese women reduced QTc and FFA, and both noradrenaline and adrenaline levels were significantly higher in women with central obesity. These findings suggest that weight reduction may reduce the risk of sudden death in the obese by reducing sympathetic nerve activity and its effects on ventricular repolarization.

It is likely that the changes in sympathetic nerve activity and QTc on obese subjects, particularly those with abdominal obesity, are most important in the subgroup with an inherited ion channel disorder. Although patients in this study had a normal QT interval at rest, this group can be assumed to contain some subjects with ion channel abnormalities in whom these changes are potentially very important.

Dietary fat and fatty acid content have been linked to risk of coronary heart disease and sudden death in the population in general and may also be important in the obese. While the traditional view of the "diet–heart" hypothesis focused on the importance of unsaturated fat intake, a number of studies have demonstrated that dietary intake of n-3 polyunsaturated fatty acids (PUFA) may be an important factor in sudden death in those with or without known coronary heart disease. Of special interest has been the long chain n-3 PUFA, mainly derived from seafood, and intermediate chain n-3 PUFA, derived from canola oil and walnuts in Western diets, neither of which are synthesized by humans and are therefore essential fatty acids. Leaf and colleagues proposed a cellular mechanism to explain the link between dietary intake of fat and risk of sudden death based on observations from a number of animal and human studies which suggest that n-3 PUFA reduce the risk of ventricular fibrillation, and therefore sudden death, by stabilizing myocyte ion channels [13].

Taken together, these findings suggest that the diet of obese subjects is likely to affect their health in a number of ways. Given that obesity is associated with an increased risk of sudden death, consideration should be given to measures such as improving physical fitness and increasing the dietary intake of intermediate and long chain essential polyunsaturated fatty acids, which may reduce the risk of sudden death without necessarily leading to loss of adipose tissue. Finally, the health benefits of weight reduction using caloric restriction may also be adversely affected by the composition of the diet used to achieve it.

Sudden death in the obese may be due to obstructive sleep apnea, particularly when sudden death occurs during sleep. Habitual snoring is a useful marker of OSA in that approximately one-third of heavy snorers have OSA and is a relatively simple addition to epidemiologic studies of the health consequences of snoring. It should be stressed that it remains to be shown that snoring without OSA is benign. In a study of unexpected sudden death in Finland [14], a history of heavy snoring, obtained from relatives *post mortem*, was an independent risk factor for sudden death, particularly between midnight and 6 am when these subjects were presumably asleep. In a retrospective study of patients with documented OSA who died suddenly during follow-up [15], the presence of severe OSA (Apnea/Hypopnea Index (AHI) >30/h) conferred an increased risk of sudden death with a hazard ratio for early morning sudden death of 2.6:1. The cause of sudden death clearly includes primary cardiac arrhythmias, including slow (sinus arrest or high-grade atrioventricular block) or fast rhythms (ventricular tachycardia or ventricular fibrillation) and acute myocardial infarction with secondary cardiac arrhythmias or pump failure. The Sleep Heart Health Study examined the relationship between OSA and cardiac arrhythmias prospectively in a large cohort of apparently healthy subjects. In this study the presence of OSA was an independent predictor of complex ventricular arrhythmias including ventricular tachycardia [16]. This does not exclude bradycardia, known to be important in sudden death in other settings, as an important mechanism of sudden death in OSA.

There are clearly multiple pathophysiological mechanisms by which obesity can lead to sudden death. These data provide us with further evidence of the importance of prevention of obesity in children and adults and the impetus to treat it once established. The major new diagnostic question in the obese subject is whether or not OSA co-exists which can be screened for using the Berlin Questionnaire and others and tested for in the home (ambulatory) or laboratory-based settings.

Obesity and vascular disease

Obesity has been suspected for many years to confer an increased risk of morbidity and mortality due to coronary artery and peripheral vascular diseases. However, differences in how obesity is defined and measured as well as methodologic problems have made proving the validity of this apparent relationship more difficult. As discussed earlier, obesity often occurs in a cluster with established metabolic vascular risk factors and lack of physical fitness, making it more difficult to establish whether the presence and pattern of obesity is an *independent* vascular risk factor.

A number of studies have reported that predominantly abdominal fat distribution may be at least as important as BMI as a determinant of cardiac risk. The Gothenburg study reported by

Larsson and co-workers [17] demonstrated that in men, abdominal fat distribution was a risk factor for coronary heart disease but this was not statistically significant once smoking, blood pressure and total cholesterol levels were adjusted for.

A prospective study of a cohort of middle-aged Finnish men followed for 11 years [18], which used two indices of abdominal obesity (waist measurement and WHR) and reported coronary events defined using MONICA criteria, showed the risk of coronary events in men with a WHR of 0.91 was increased almost threefold. The study confirmed that the WHR was more powerful and consistent than BMI in predicting risk of future coronary heart disease events. In this study, smoking and poor fitness, not only more common in the obese but, as in other studies, independent risk factors for coronary disease, augmented the risk of coronary heart disease and increased the potential benefits of identifying and modifying all these risk factors in the obese.

The effects of obesity, and particularly fat distribution, on coronary heart disease risk have also been shown to occur in both men and women. In an 8-year follow-up of the US Nurses' Health Study, Rexrode and co-workers [19] reported that the waist circumference and WHR were strongly and independently associated with an increased age-adjusted risk of coronary heart disease among women. The adverse effects of abdominal fat distribution were also seen in relatively lean women (BMI <25 kg/m^2). For example, after adjusting for BMI and other cardiac risk factors, women with a WHR of 0.88 or higher had a relative risk of coronary heart disease of 3.25, as compared with those with a ratio below 0.72 (Fig. 17.1).

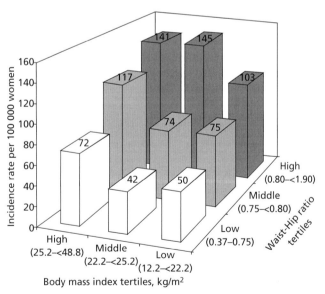

Figure 17.1 Age-adjusted incidence rates for coronary heart disease according to body mass index and WHR tertiles. Numbers at the top of each bar indicate incidence. At each level of obesity, risk of coronary heart disease was significantly increased by an abdominal fat distribution. (Reproduced with permission from Rexrode et al. [19].)

Detection of coronary artery calcification using X-rays has been used as a marker of atherosclerotic coronary artery disease in the past but although highly specific, it lacked sensitivity. The advent of high-resolution, 64- and 128-slice CT scanners has increased the sensitivity of this noninvasive method of detecting coronary disease without apparent loss in specificity. In a study of 1160 asymptomatic men, Arad and co-workers compared anthropomorphic, metabolic and insulin resistance measurements with coronary calcium scores derived from electron beam CT examinations, and showed that coronary calcium scores were positively and independently correlated with visceral obesity, glucose levels and insulin resistance [20]. The relationship between visceral obesity and coronary calcification as a measure of coronary heart disease was present whether subjects had elevated blood glucose levels or not.

A critical question in those at risk of vascular disease is the mode of presentation. Calcification is a marker of relatively stable plaques and therefore, while it identifies those with risk factors who actually have developed vascular disease, these are not necessarily those at highest risk and therefore most likely to benefit from interventions. The development of acute coronary syndromes in patients with vascular disease identifies a group of patients with a markedly increased temporal risk of adverse outcomes. The spectrum of presentations of acute coronary syndromes includes sudden death, acute myocardial infarction with either ST elevation or depression and unstable angina. Acute rupture of an atherosclerotic plaque is well known to be responsible for the clinical manifestations of acute coronary syndromes in most patients and while this is usually a single lesion, multiple unstable plaques can occur in some patients. It is also clear that subclinical plaque rupture can occur. Identifying the factors responsible for the development of acute phases in the course of otherwise stable disease has been the subject of intensive investigation.

Inflammation is increasingly understood to be an important factor in the pathophysiology of atherosclerosis and in the development of acute vascular syndromes [21]. Elevated inflammatory markers such as C-reactive protein and cytokines have been shown to occur both in acute vascular syndromes but also in those at future risk of developing acute vascular events [21,22].

Interleukin (IL)-6 is a cytokine which is produced in response to several factors, including infection, IL-1 and interferon-γ. Tumor necrosis factor (TNF-α) has pleiotropic effects on cellular and humoral immunity in response to infection, inflammation and tissue injury, while IL-6 is a central mediator of the acute-phase response and a primary determinant of production of C-reactive protein by the liver.

The Physicians' Health Study was a randomized, double-blind, placebo-controlled trial of the effectiveness of aspirin and β-carotene in the primary prevention of cardiovascular disease and cancer in 22,071 US male physicians aged 40–84 years with no prior history of myocardial infarction, stroke, transient ischemic attack or cancer. As part of this study a prospective, nested, case–control study of IL-6 as a potential marker for future myocardial infarction among participants was performed and this showed that IL-6 levels at baseline appeared to identify men at future risk of acute myocardial infarction [21].

Adipose tissue is now well recognized to be a source of inflammatory mediators and increased production of TNF-α and interleukin-6 and release of these mediators may play a significant role in promoting the development of atherosclerosis and its complications [23–4].

The effect of obesity on the risk of developing atherosclerosis and its acute and chronic complications is compounded by the apparent prothrombotic effects of obesity. This may mean that the consequences of plaque rupture are likely to be more adverse than in lean subjects. The identification of adipose tissue as a source of inflammatory mediators with production of proinflammatory cytokines such as TNF-α, interleukins, including interleukin 6, and also C-reactive protein provides a conceptual framework linking obesity, insulin resistance and atherosclerosis [17–23].

Cholesterol lowering has been shown to reduce the risk of future vascular events and in obese subjects, relatively modest weight loss achieved by diet and drugs [24] or a combination of the two is associated with significant changes in lipid levels which, if sustained, would have major beneficial effects on future risk of vascular events.

Drugs such as statins appear to have pleiotropic effects which include stabilization, or "passivization", of potentially vulnerable atherosclerotic plaques. Inflammatory markers such as C-reactive protein have been shown to be reduced during statin treatment and may be a marker of risk reduction.

Obstructive sleep apnea is increasingly accepted as a confounding factor in the relationship between obesity, inflammation and cardiovascular risk [25]. In a Japanese study of 30 men with OSA and 14 obese controls (mean BMI 27.7 kg/m^2), levels of C-reactive protein and IL-6 produced from peripheral blood monocytes were significantly higher in obese subjects with OSA than controls and fell after a month's treatment of OSA using nasal continuous positive airway pressure (CPAP) [26], an effect independent of the effects of obesity. These findings were extended recently by Jelic and co-workers [27] who showed that OSA promotes inflammation and oxidative stress and reduces availability of nitric oxide and repair capacity in vascular endothelial cells *in vivo*. They also found that treatment with nasal CPAP reversed these adverse alterations in endothelial function.

Our understanding of the relationship between obesity and risk of coronary heart disease has advanced substantially in recent years. Evidence that obesity, especially abdominal obesity, is related to increased risk of atherosclerotic vascular disease has become increasingly convincing. Advances in our understanding of the key role inflammation plays in the development and course of atherosclerosis have allowed us to examine the potential mechanisms by which obesity may contribute to this process, and perhaps provide clinicians with better measures to assess the risk reduction conferred by modification of obesity and other factors, such as smoking and physical inactivity, which are commonly clustered with it.

Obesity and hypertension

Obesity is associated with increased blood pressure levels in both normotensive and hypertensive children and adults in a large number of studies. In lean subjects, elevated blood pressure levels are a more accurate reflection of increased peripheral resistance, whereas in the obese, increased resting cardiac output due to the increased metabolic demands of adipose tissue means blood pressure measurements will tend to overestimate the increase in peripheral resistance. While the mechanisms by which obesity leads to hypertension are not completely understood, studies have shown that weight reduction can lower blood pressure and some of its effects on the heart and circulation.

The relationship between obesity and hypertension and cardiovascular risk in adults has varied somewhat between studies. Some suggest that there may be a stronger relationship between blood pressure and future risk of cardiovascular disease in lean rather than obese subjects. In a study of over 1 million Swedish men having military preconscription health assessments, there was no evidence that this was the case [28] (Silvenoinen et al 2008) with the greatest risk of hypertension and future CVD being in the obese rather than lean subjects.

Obesity in childhood has increased dramatically since the 1960s in the US and similar trends have been noted in other countries. In children, obesity increases the risk of hypertension approximately threefold across all levels of BMI with no threshold of effect. Interventional studies have shown that blood pressure reduction can be achieved, as in adults [29]. Whereas hypertension in pediatric practice was formerly considered more likely in children with genetic hypertension and those with renal disease, this pattern has changed and obesity-related hypertension has assumed much more importance.

The diagnosis of hypertension in adults is relatively straightforward but in children, blood pressure values have to be adjusted for age, gender and height, making accurate diagnosis more difficult than in adults. The significance of borderline elevated blood pressure in children is potentially more important since it appears to be a precursor of hypertension in adulthood. Unlike in adults, it has been reported that the early pattern in childhood has been that of systolic rather than diastolic hypertension. The use of an appropriate blood pressure cuff size is relatively more important than in adults. The recommended cuff size is one with a bladder width that is approximately 40% of the arm circumference midway between the olecranon and the acromion process [29].

The pathophysiology of hypertension in obesity-hypertension in children and adults remains to be fully elucidated. Characteristically such patients have increased sympathetic nerve activity, increased insulin levels and increased activity of the renin-angiotensin-aldosterone system. Obesity-hypertension is one of the salt-sensitive variants of essential hypertension. While there is clearly a strong association between obesity-hypertension, sodium sensitivity and insulin resistance, there is no simple relationship which integrates these observations into an explanation of why blood pressure is increased in these patients.

Activation of the sympathetic nervous system occurs early in the course of obesity and is involved in many of its chronic manifestations, including the cardiovascular complications of hypertension, left ventricular hypertrophy, congestive heart (CHF) failure and arrhythmias. Recent research interest has focused on the role of leptin, produced in adipocytes, on regulation of the sympathetic nervous system in obesity.

Leptin is a 16 kDa peptide produced mainly in adipose tissue and has been conceived to play a regulatory role ("adipostat") in determining fat mass by inhibiting food intake through reducing appetite, probably in the hypothalamus, and by increasing thermogenesis via increased sympathetic nerve activity. However, many of the results of studies in animal and human subjects have been contradictory.

In a study by Eikelis and co-workers [30], adrenaline secretion and leptin levels were measured in a range of healthy obese subjects with a wide variety of leptin levels, normal-weight healthy subjects and patients with heart failure (high noradrenaline levels), essential hypertension (high noradrenaline levels), pure autonomic failure (low noradrenaline levels) and healthy elderly subjects (reduced adrenaline levels). Leptin levels were not low in the two models of high sympathetic tone (heart failure and hypertension); in fact, elevated leptin levels found in heart failure were due to reduced renal clearance. Plasma leptin levels were normal in autonomic failure and in the elderly. The concept that leptin directly stimulates sympathetic efferent activity appears simplistic and further studies are needed to clarify the relationship between total fat mass, fat distribution and the autonomic nervous system in obesity.

Short-term weight loss reduces blood pressure substantially in adults [31–35]. Typically there is a fall in both weight and blood pressure associated with a natriuresis, which is most marked in the acute phase and increases gradually thereafter.

In a study of 26 obese Japanese women with a mean age of 50 years and a BMI of 34 kg/m^2 [36] an average weight loss of 9 kg reduced mean blood pressure by 11 mmHg. In this study, the fall in BP did not correlate with weight or BMI but did correlate with reduced intra-abdominal obesity as measured by CT scan. These results do not exclude the possibility that weight and adiposity expressed as BMI are important but do suggest that fat distribution is a more important factor than obesity alone in affecting blood pressure.

End-stage renal disease and congestive heart failure are major consequences of chronic essential hypertension. When hypertension and diabetes are both present, as they commonly are in obesity, the risk of end-stage renal disease is substantially increased. Obesity has a number of effects on renal function which promote an increase in blood pressure, including increasing renal tubular sodium reabsorption, impairing pressure natriuresis, intravascular volume expansion (due to activation of the sympathetic nervous system and renin-angiotensin system) and by physical compression of the kidneys, particularly when visceral obesity is present [37]. Early functional changes of micro-albuminemia and expression of growth- and/or fibrosis-promoting factors precede major histologic changes in the kidney [1]. It is believed that chronic obesity promotes gradual loss of nephron numbers and function.

In animal studies, a relationship can be shown between caloric intake and renal disease, with excess intake promoting and restriction protecting against glomerular injury. However, long-term studies of the effects of caloric restriction or weight reduction in human subjects are lacking [1,37].

Prevention of end-stage renal disease is a major objective of treatment in hypertension [1,37]. In the obese, treatment goals in hypertension should include not only weight reduction and good blood pressure control but also correction of the associated metabolic abnormalities to try to prevent further renal injury and consequent irreversible nephron loss.

Obesity, hypertension and patterns of cardiac hypertrophy

Obesity, when predominantly central in distribution, is characteristically associated with a number of cardiac structural changes, which include right and left ventricular (LV) dilation and hypertrophy, left atrial dilation and fatty infiltration of the conducting system. Peripheral obesity appears not to be associated with hypertension or structural changes in the heart and circulation.

The effect of obesity on blood pressure begins early in the course of this disorder. Hypertension occurs commonly in obese children and adults of all ages but daytime hypertension is not a prerequisite for the presence of LV hypertrophy in obese subjects and this observation, along with an apparent increase in cardiomyopathy and heart failure in obese subjects, led to the notion of the "cardiomyopathy of obesity" [8]. An additional factor contributing adversely to the severity of LV hypertrophy and systolic dysfunction in obese patients is co-existent obstructive sleep apnea [10]. Remodeling of the heart occurs in response to *chronic* changes in distending pressure in systole, diastole or both. This is distinct from the changes in cardiac function, which occur in response to an *acute* load. At a cellular level this process is due to hypertrophy of cardiac myocytes in a configuration which depends on the type of load the heart is responding to (Figs 17.2, 17.3).

Isolated pressure overload of the left ventricle, such as occurs in hypertension in the absence of obesity, produces a pattern of hypertrophy in which the left ventricle remodels with a symmetric increase in wall thickness, a reduction in end-systolic diameter but no increase in diastolic diameter or concentric hypertrophy. At a cellular level this pattern of hypertrophy results from addition of new myofibrils in a parallel format. This change in geometry has the effect of reducing LV systolic wall stress and therefore is an adaptation which reduces the LV work in response to this pressure overload (see Fig. 17.2).

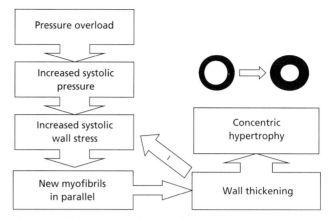

Figure 17.2 Pattern of ventricular remodeling: response to pressure overload. In this setting the pressure overload occurs in systole leading to increased systolic wall stress. (Adapted from Grossman et al. [60].)

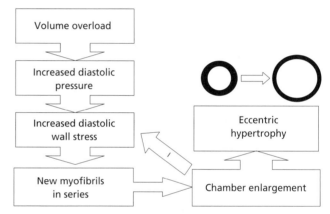

Figure 17.3 Pattern of ventricular remodeling: response to volume. In this setting the pressure overload occurs in diastole, resulting in increased diastolic wall stress to which the heart responds by "eccentric" hypertrophy. (Adapted from Grossman et al. [60].)

Volume overload of the left ventricle occurs typically in mitral or aortic regurgitation when the ventricle has to generate a greater stroke volume, because of valvular regurgitation, in order to maintain net forward stroke volume and hence cardiac output. Therefore the overload of the ventricle occurs in diastole, causing increased diastolic wall stress. The heart responds to this stress by adding new sarcomeres in series. Dilation of the ventricle in response to this chronic volume overload increases diastolic wall stress but typically end-systolic diameter and volume are unchanged. Left ventricular wall mass increases to a greater degree despite apparently more modest increases in wall thickness (see Fig. 17.3).

Obesity has been associated with eccentric ventricular hypertrophy in which both the diameter and wall thickness of the left ventricle are increased at all levels of blood pressure. The apparently different effects of obesity and hypertension on LV geometry led to the concept of the "dimorphic" effects of obesity and hypertension on LV hypertrophy and systolic function. Thus, lean hypertensives are expected to have concentric hypertrophy, centrally obese but normotensives will have eccentric hypertrophy, and those with both obesity and hypertension have an unfavorable combination of both volume and pressure overload or systolic and diastolic pressure overload. This results in dilation and dysfunction and potentially earlier heart failure in the course of the disease. However, the relationship between central obesity and LV hypertrophy is not as simple as first thought and many obese subjects have concentric hypertrophy even if they are normotensive.

Obstructive sleep apnea is another key confounder of the relationship between obesity and systemic hypertension. Acute and chronic hypoxia can be associated with LV hypertrophy and OSA is the most common disease process which causes hypoxia in subjects without lung disease. A recent substudy from the Sleep Heart Health Study has significantly enhanced our understanding of the relationship between LV mass and geometry in obstructive sleep apnea. A large subgroup had echocardiograms performed at baseline and the presence and pattern of LV hypertrophy was compared with the severity of sleep-disordered breathing (either AHI or SaO_2). There was a clear-cut "dose-dependent" relationship between the severity of OSA and LV hypertrophy, particularly eccentric hypertrophy, and worsening LV systolic function [39] (Fig. 17.4).

The importance of LV hypertrophy lies in its value as an adverse prognostic factor in hypertension. In hypertensive subjects, echocardiographically measured LV mass is a more powerful prognostic factor than systolic or diastolic blood pressure [40,41]. Antihypertensive drugs vary in their effects on regression of ventricular hypertrophy, and regression of cardiac and vascular hypertrophy is considered to be an important goal in treating hypertension.

Studies of the effect of weight reduction have provided evidence supporting the notion that obesity causes both hypertension and LV hypertrophy [31,32]. The effects of weight reduction (average of 8 kg) on LV hypertrophy were examined by MacMahon and co-workers in a population of young obese, predominantly male subjects (mean age 42 years and BMI of 33 kg/m²) [33]. Obesity, expressed as BMI, was independently associated with systolic and diastolic blood pressure and LV mass. Following weight reduction, blood pressure fell by an average of 13/14 (sys/dias) mmHg and echocardiographic LV mass by 20%; the effects of weight reduction on LV mass were reported to be statistically independent of effects on blood pressure.

In clinical practice, interventions to reduce weight typically involve a combination of increased physical exercise and potentially fitness, as well as weight loss with variable effects on fat mass and distribution in individual subjects. While assessing the relative impacts of these different factors on blood pressure and cardiac structure may be a relevant research question, in practice they are usually combined, and therefore the total benefit which this approach can achieve is more clinically relevant. Exercise itself has effects on cardiac structure, which vary with the type and intensity of the exercise program undertaken.

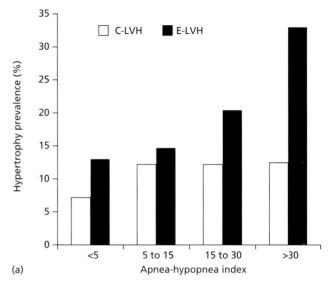

(a)

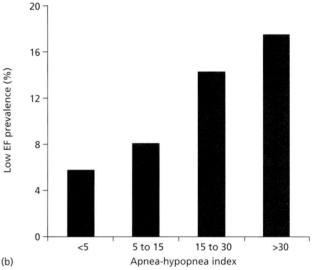

(b)

Figure 17.4 Sleep Heart Health Study and patterns of LV hypertension and systolic function in sleep apnea. (a) Association of OSA with concentric (C) or eccentric (E) hypertrophy. (b) OSA severity and systolic function. (Reproduced with permission from Chami et al. [39].)

Hinderliter and colleagues [42] studied the effect of either improved fitness through regular aerobic exercise or exercise plus a behavioral weight reduction program. This was a randomized controlled study of 82 overweight or obese men and women (mean BMI 31 kg/m²) who were sedentary and included normotensive and hypertensive subjects and normal-weight controls. Patients with hypertension had no drug treatment for at least 6 weeks. Over 6 months, blood pressure fell (6/7 mmHg in weight management group and ¾ mmHg in aerobic exercise group) and both groups had significant reductions in LV septal and posterior wall thickness, but not indexed LV mass, compared to controls. While previous studies have shown that weight reduction promotes ventricular remodeling in the obese, this study showed that regular aerobic exercise had beneficial effect on ventricular remodeling whether weight loss occurred or not.

There is increasing evidence that factors other than blood pressure itself lead to LV hypertrophy. Only approximately 50% of hypertensive subjects have LV hypertrophy, suggesting there may be genetic and other factors which determine the hypertrophic response to a given blood pressure load in an individual. The results of a number of studies in animals and human subjects have suggested that increased sympathetic nerve activity leads to LV hypertrophy and a study, which separately examined the role of cardiac sympathetic nerve activity, showed that the degree to which this was increased was a major determinant of LV hypertrophy [43].

Thus, obese subjects who appear to have increased sympathetic nerve activity independently of the presence of hypertension would be more likely to have increased LV mass, regardless of geometric changes, provided this involved cardiac as well as peripheral sympathetic nerve activity (measured using microneurographic techniques).

Obstructive sleep apnea is another cause of increased sympathetic nerve activity which increases substantially during apneic episodes and, persists during the early waking hours. This is reduced by effective treatment with nasal CPAP [44].

Obesity and stroke

Obesity is well recognized to be a risk factor for coronary artery disease, as described earlier. However, the relationship between obesity and stroke has been less clear-cut. Established stroke risk factors such as hypertension, LV hypertrophy, diabetes and hypercholesterolemia are common in the obese and these factors have been considered to explain the increased risk of stroke in obese subjects. As in other vascular consequences of obesity, obstructive sleep apnea is a potential confounder of this association given that it is common in the obese and in patients with stroke or transient ischemic attacks [45].

In a prospective study from the Physicians' Health Study, Kurth and co-workers examined the relationship between increasing adiposity, expressed as BMI, and self-reported stroke over a period of 12.5 years in the 21,414 participating US physicians [46]. The study population was relatively healthy and while 38% were overweight, only 6% were obese. There was little change in BMI during the course of the study. For each 1 unit increase in BMI, total, ischemic, and hemorrhagic stroke risk increased by 6%. Adjustment for the presence of hypertension, diabetes and hypercholesterolemia, attenuated risk of stroke in total and ischemic stroke but not hemorrhagic stroke but it remained significant at a relative risk of 4% per 1 unit increase in BMI. Therefore, obesity confers a significant risk of stroke which is independent of other known risk factors of hypertension and diabetes. There is no equivalent study in women; published studies have shown variable and inconclusive results.

The mechanism by which obesity might mediate an increased risk of stroke independent of associated hypertension or diabetes remains to be established but elevated inflammatory markers, cytokines and prothrombotic factors in obese subjects are all factors which may be involved in increasing the risk of acute vascular disease, including ischemic stroke, in the obese.

A series of recent studies have shown an important relationship between obesity, obstructive sleep apnea and atrial fibrillation. Atrial fibrillation is a major independent risk factor for stroke. Data from the Framingham Study and others have shown that obesity is an independent risk factor for atrial fibrillation and this, along with the relationship between obesity and hypertension, at least partly explains the increased risk of stroke in the obese. A retrospective study of 3542 Ohmstead County residents [47] showed that in subjects aged <65, BMI and OSA were both independent predictors of incident atrial fibrillation.

Obesity and congestive heart failure

Congestive heart failure is a major cause of morbidity and mortality whether manifested as predominantly systolic or diastolic heart failure. Given the ominous prognosis of this condition, prevention of this disorder is now considered to be a major medical health issue. The cardiac response to obesity is characterized by LV dilation and hypertrophy, which are known precursors of congestive heart failure. The progression from risk factor to heart failure has been shown clearly in systemic hypertension [48,49] in which pressure overload leads to concentric hypertrophy with early diastolic and late systolic dysfunction.

As in other disease processes linked with obesity, heart failure is complicated by co-existent risk factors which include not only hypertension and diabetes but also sleep apnea. Patients with severe congestive heart failure are often cachectic and this has the potential to complicate our understanding of a possible link between increasing adiposity and congestive heart failure. Therefore it is important to distinguish between obesity as a possible factor leading to heart failure and the effects of established heart failure on body metabolism and composition.

Obesity has been identified as a risk factor for heart failure in extremely obese patients and, more recently, this relationship has been shown to hold for patients with less severe obesity. Kenchaiah and co-workers followed 5881 subjects in the Framingham Heart Study for a mean of 14 years [50]. They excluded underweight subjects (BMI <18.5 kg/m^2) and used BMI to define overweight (BMI 25–29.9 kg/m^2) and obesity (BMI ≥30 kg/m^2). Presentation with an initial episode of heart failure was classified by a panel of three experienced cardiologists using criteria previously used as part of the study. Peripheral edema, common in obese subjects without heart failure, was only a minor criterion in the definition of heart failure in this study, and only included if not attributable to another non cardiac cause. Only 16% of the subjects were obese; half of the men and one-third of the women were overweight, whereas extreme obesity (BMI ≥40) was rare (only eight men). After adjustment for known heart failure risk factors, mainly hypertension and diabetes, both of which increased with increasing BMI, there was an incremental increase in risk of developing heart failure of approximately 5% for women and 7% for men for each increase of BMI by $1\,kg/m^2$. Compared with normal-weight women, overweight women had a 50% increase in CHF risk and obese women a doubling of risk. In men, being overweight was associated with a 20% increase and obesity a 90% increase in risk of CHF. There did not appear to be a threshold of effect of obesity on the risk of developing CHF in men or women (Fig 17.5). Based on these findings, obesity could be attributed as the cause of CHF in approximately 11% of men and 14% of women. The prospective nature of the study, demonstration of a progressive, stepwise increase in risk with increasing BMI and the temporal relationship between documentation of obesity and the subsequent development of heart failure are clearly strengths of this study.

The "obesity paradox" in congestive heart failure lies in the observation that while obesity is a risk factor for the development of heart failure, among patients with heart failure, those with a higher BMI have a better prognosis. Another factor which complicates our understanding of the relationship between adiposity and heart failure is obstructive sleep apnea. As previously discussed, snoring and sleep apnea occur commonly in obese subjects and when such patients have a dilated cardiomyopathy or LV systolic dysfunction from other processes such as coronary heart disease, the combination is an adverse one [38,39,51,52].

As a consequence of the development of congestive heart failure some patients develop periodic breathing and central apneas (Cheyne–Stokes respiration) during sleep and such patients are typically normal or underweight, have worse systolic function, typically quite severe (LV ejection fraction <20%), and have a worse prognosis than those with or without obstructive sleep apnea.

Exercise capacity or "fitness" is a prognostic factor in patients with heart failure and independent of LV systolic function. Patients with a lower maximal exercise capacity (often measured as maximal oxygen uptake or VO_{2max}), have a worse prognosis. While cachexia is a recognized adverse prognostic factor in patients with heart failure, this relationship persists even among patients who are not cachectic [53].

Therefore, even in patients with established systolic heart failure, physical fitness and fatness remain important prognostic factors, as they are in the obese with apparently normal cardiac function. Given the major burden imposed by congestive heart failure on patients, their families and the community in general, physicians must increasingly understand the importance of intervening to prevent the development of heart failure and obesity needs to be understood in this context.

Effects of obesity on intra-abdominal pressure

Abdominal pressure can be measured in various ways and intravesical and rectal pressures correlate well with directly measured

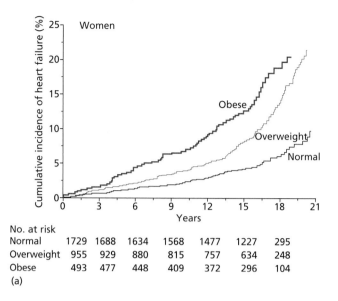

(a)

No. at risk							
Normal	1729	1688	1634	1568	1477	1227	295
Overweight	955	929	880	815	757	634	248
Obese	493	477	448	409	372	296	104

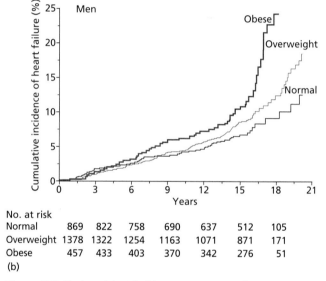

(b)

No. at risk							
Normal	869	822	758	690	637	512	105
Overweight	1378	1322	1254	1163	1071	871	171
Obese	457	433	403	370	342	276	51

Figure 17.5 Obesity and the risk of future congestive heart failure. Obesity was associated with an increased risk of heart failure in both men and women without evidence of a threshold effect. (Reproduced with permission from Kenchaiah et al. [50].)

intra-abdominal pressure. Increasing abdominal obesity increases not only intra-abdominal pressure but also intrathoracic pressure, central venous, pulmonary arterial and pulmonary venous pressure.

The effects of obesity on intra-abdominal pressure may be an important factor contributing to the cardiac, respiratory and other consequences of obesity. Raised intra-abdominal pressure is likely to be another factor causing breathlessness in the obese and, for example, partly explains why obese subjects commonly develop marked increases in dyspnea with postural changes, such as stooping or bending or lying down in the prone or supine position.

Studies in dogs have shown that increasing intra-abdominal pressure, using an implanted balloon progressively inflated to a pressure of 25 mmHg, resulted in elevated systolic and diastolic blood pressure in the systemic circulation. This returned to baseline values 2 weeks after balloon deflation [54]. These changes in blood pressure occurred without changes in renin, aldosterone, natriuretic peptides or catecholamines, suggesting that intra-abdominal pressure affects blood pressure by other means and may be an independent factor contributing to elevated blood pressures common in many, but not all, obese subjects.

Elevated abdominal and thoracic pressure result in increased cerebral venous pressure and therefore increased intracranial pressure. This may partly explain the association of obesity with increased intracranial pressure in pseudotumor cerebri [55].

Obesity, sleep-disordered breathing and cardiorespiratory disease

Obesity is associated with cardiovascular disease including systemic hypertension, pulmonary hypertension, atherosclerosis and congestive heart failure. Understanding the pathophysiological basis of this relationship is potentially confounded by emerging knowledge of the importance of the link between obesity, particularly central or upper body obesity, and sleep-disordered breathing, including sleep apnea and hypercapneic respiratory failure.

Obesity is strongly linked with obstructive sleep apnea as defined by obstructed breathing efforts, typically associated with snoring, and either partial (50% reduction in breathing amplitude – hypopnea) or complete apnea for 10 seconds or more [10]. An AHI of >5/h has been used to define "sleep apnea" and when associated with symptoms of tiredness or sleepiness is known as the "sleep apnea syndrome." Only a minority of patients with sleep apnea have symptoms of sleepiness and not all patients who are obese and who may snore have sleep apnea [56].

The definition of sleep apnea based on these respiratory parameters has been empirical and, almost certainly, overly simplistic. In making comparisons between the cardiovascular and respiratory consequences of sleep-disordered breathing, it becomes clear that the cardiovascular consequences of OSA are much more serious than the respiratory consequences, mainly hypercapneic respiratory failure with/without associated lung disease ("overlap syndrome").

The prevalence of OSA increases with age and obesity. Epidemiologic studies have shown that OSA (AHI ≥5/h) affects up to 24% of men and 12% of women between the ages of 30 and 65, and the "OSA syndrome" affects 4% of men and 2% of women in this age range. Among the morbidly obese the proportion with OSA rises to approximately 50%. It is important to note that obesity is less clearly related to OSA in older patients. Data from the Sleep Heart Health Study [56] showed that OSA in older people (age >60 years) was poorly predicted by higher BMI, neck circumference, WHR and self-reported breathing pauses. The reason for the differences in the sleep-disordered breathing risk factors by age was not clear. However, it is clear that OSA is a significant factor, which interacts with obesity and its cardiorespiratory consequences.

Obstructive sleep apnea is now established as a risk factor for daytime hypertension based on animal and human studies which include cross-sectional and prospective epidemiologic studies and treatment trials using nasal CPAP. Human studies have shown that nasal CPAP eliminates the nocturnal blood pressure changes and lowers daytime blood pressure independently of other factors such as obesity itself and antihypertensive drugs. The mechanism by which OSA causes hypertension is not fully known but increased peripheral sympathetic nerve activity has been shown to be present night and day and to be reduced by CPAP treatment [44,57]. There is also evidence that β-blockers are more effective antihypertensive drugs in OSA [58], providing additional support for the notion that the sympathetic nervous system is critically important for the development of systemic hypertension in OSA.

Sleep apnea and pulmonary hypertension

Pulmonary hypertension is associated with OSA, occurring in 20–40% of patients; while this is typically mild to moderate in severity, it can be severe. The prevalence of pulmonary hypertension in OSA is increased by increasing obesity and by the presence of parenchymal lung disease such as chronic obstructive pulmonary disease.

Evidence in favor of a causal relationship includes observation of pulmonary hypertension in animals exposed to repetitive hypoxia, regression of pulmonary hypertension in children with OSA due to enlarged tonsils, and some studies of the effect of treatment of OSA with nasal CPAP [59].

Given what is known about the relationship between increasing obesity and OSA, 50% of morbidly obese subjects would be expected to have OSA and 25% of these would be expected to have pulmonary hypertension.

Conclusion

Obesity has a plethora of effects on the heart, circulation, respiratory function and sleep, which combine to reduce quality and length of life. In considering the cardiovascular effects of obesity and given the physiological importance of these heart–lung interactions, it is clearly important to understand the respiratory effects of obesity. In addition, increasing recognition of snoring and sleep apnea among obese subjects, especially those with abdominal or visceral fat distributions, presents an opportunity to advance our understanding of the circadian health consequences of obesity and offers new opportunities to intervene. The fact that many different cardiovascular risk factors "cluster" together in obese subjects enables these to be identified more readily and, more importantly, modified.

References

1. Eckel RH, Barouch WW, Ershow AG. Report of the National Heart, Lung, and Blood Institute-National Institute of Diabetes and Digestive and Kidney Diseases Working Group on the Pathophysiology of Obesity-Associated Cardiovascular Disease. Circulation 2002;1(5):2923–8.

2. Stevens J, Cai J, Evenson KR, et al. Fitness and fatness as predictors of mortality from all causes and from cardiovascular disease in men and women in the Lipid Research Clinics Study. Am J Epidemiol 2002;156(9):832–41.

3. Wilcox I, McNamara SG, Collins FL, et al. Syndrome Z: the interaction of sleep apnea, vascular risk factors and heart disease. Thorax 1998;53(suppl 3):25S-28.

4. Shaw JE, Punjabi NM, Wilding JP, et al Sleep-disordered breathing and type 2 diabetes. A report from the International Diabetes Federation Taskforce on Epidemiology and Prevention. Diabetes Res Clin Pract. 2008;81:2–12.

5. Poirier P, Giles TD, Bray GA, et al. Obesity and cardiovascular disease: pathophysiology, evaluation, and effect of weight loss. Circulation 2006;113:898–918.

6. Messerli FH, Nunez BD, Ventura HO, et al. Overweight and sudden death: increased ventricular ectopy in cardiomyopathy of obesity. Arch Intern Med 1987;147:1725–8.

7. Albert CM, Chae CU, Grodstein F, et al. Prospective study of sudden cardiac death among women in the United States. Circulation 2003;107(16):2096–101.

8. Alpert MA. Obesity cardiomyopathy: pathophysiology and evolution of the clinical syndrome. Am J Med Sci 2001;321:225–36.

9. Grassi G, Seravalle G, Cattaneo BM, et al. Sympathetic activation in obese normotensive subjects. Hypertension 1995;25(4):560–3.

10. Grunstein R, Wilcox I, Yang TS, et al. Snoring and sleep apnea in men: interaction with central obesity and hypertension. Int J Obes 1993;17:503–40.

11. Schwartz PJ, Priori SG, Napolitano C. The long QT syndrome. In: Zipes DP, Jalife J (eds) *Cardiac Electrophysiology: From Cell to Bedside.* PhiladelphiaL Saunders 2000:597–615.

12. Corbi GM, Carbone S, Ziccardi P, et al. FFAs and QT intervals in obese women with visceral adiposity: effects of sustained weight loss over 1 year. J Clin Endocrinol Metab 2002;87(5):2080–3.

13. Leaf A, Kang JX, Xaio J-F, et al. Clinical prevention of sudden cardiac death by n-3 polyunsaturated fatty acids and mechanism of prevention of arrhythmias by n-3 fish oils. Circulation 2003;107(21):2646–52.

14. Seppala T, Partinen M, Penttilä A, et al. Sudden death and sleeping history among Finnish men. J Intern Med 1991;229(1):23–8.

15. Gami AS, Howard DE, Olson EJ, et al. Day-Night pattern of sudden death in obstructive sleep apnea. N Engl J Med 2005;352:1206–14.

16. Mehra R, Benjamin EJ, Shahar E, et al. Association of nocturnal arrhythmias with sleep-disordered breathing: The Sleep Heart Health Study. Am J Respir Crit Care Med. 2006;173:910–16.

17. Larsson B, Svärdsudd K, Welin L, et al. Abdominal adipose tissue distribution, obesity, and risk of cardiovascular disease and death: 13 year follow up of participants in the study of men born in 1913. BMJ 1984;289:1257–61.

18. Lakka HM, Lakka TA, Tuomilehto J, et al. Abdominal obesity is associated with increased risk of acute coronary events in men. Eur Heart J 2002;23:706–13.

19. Rexrode KM, Carey VJ, Hennekens CH, et al. Abdominal adiposity and coronary heart disease in women. JAMA 1998;280(21):1843–8.

20. Arad Y, Newstein D, Cadet F, et al. Association of multiple risk factors and insulin resistance with increased prevalence of asymptomatic coronary artery disease by an electron-beam computed tomographic study. Arterioscler Thromb Vasc Biol 2001;21(12):2051–8.

21. Rader DJ. Inflammatory markers of coronary risk. N Engl J Med 2000;343(16):1179–82.

22. Ridker PM, Rifai N, Stampfer MJ, et al. Plasma concentration of interleukin-6 and the risk of future myocardial infarction among apparently healthy men. Circulation 2000;101(15):1767–72.

23. Loskutoff DJ, Samad F. The adipocyte and hemostatic balance in obesity : studies of PAI-1. Arterioscler Thromb Vasc Biol 1998;18(1):1–6.

24. Marks SJ, Chin S, Strauss BJ. The metabolic effects of preferential reduction of visceral adipose tissue in abdominally obese men. Int J Obes 1998;22(9):893–8.

25. Lattimore JD, Celermajer DS, Wilcox I. Obstructive sleep apnea and cardiovascular disease. J Am Coll Cardiol 2003;41(9):1429–37.

26. Yokoe T, Minoguchi K, Matsuo H, et al. Elevated levels of C-reactive protein and interleukin-6 in patients with obstructive sleep apnea syndrome are decreased by nasal continuous positive airway pressure. Circulation 2003;107(8):1129–34.

27. Jelic S, Padeletti M, Kawut SM, et al. Inflammation, oxidative stress, and repair capacity of the vascular endothelium in obstructive sleep apnea. Circulation. 2008; 29;117(17):2270–8.

28. Silventoinen K, Magnusson PKE, Neovius M, et al. Does Obesity Modify the Effect of Blood Pressure on the Risk of Cardiovascular Disease?: A Population-Based Cohort Study of More Than One Million Swedish Men. Circulation, Oct 2008;118:1637–1642.

29. Sorof J, Daniels S. Obesity hypertension in children: a problem of epidemic proportions. Hypertension 2002;40(4):441–7.

30. Eikelis N, Schlaich M, Aggarwal A, et al. Interactions between leptin and the human sympathetic nervous system. Hypertension 2003; 41(5):1072–9.

31. Dahl LK, Silver L, Christie RW. The role of salt in the fall of blood pressure accompanying reduction in obesity. N Engl J Med 1958;258:1186–92.

32. Tuck ML, Sowers J, Dornfeld L, et al. The effect of weight reduction on blood pressure, plasma renin activity, and plasma aldosterone levels on obese patients. N Engl J Med 1981;304:930–3.

33. MacMahon SW, Wilcken DE, Macdonald GJ. The effect of weight reduction on left ventricular mass. N Engl J Med 1986;314(6):334–43.

34. Rocchini AP, Key J, Bondie D, et al. The effect of weight loss on the sensitivity of blood pressure to sodium in obese adolescents. N Engl J Med 1989;321(9):580–5.

35. Kotchen JM, Cox-Ganser J, Wright CJ, et al. Gender differences in obesity-related cardiovascular disease risk factors among participants in a weight loss programme. Int J Obes 1993;17(3):145–51.

36. Kanai H, Tokunaga K, Fujioka S, et al. Decrease in intra-abdominal visceral fat may reduce blood pressure in obese hypertensive women. Hypertension 1996;27:125:129.

37. Hall JE, Jones DW, Kuo JJ, et al. Impact of the obesity epidemic on hypertension and renal disease. Curr Hypertens Rep 2003;5(5):386–92.

38. Wilcox I, McNamara SG, Wessendorf T, et al. Prognosis and sleep disordered breathing in heart failure. Thorax 1998;53(suppl 3):33S–36.

39. Chami HA, Devereux RB, Gottdiener JS, et al. Left Ventricular Morphology and Systolic Function in Sleep-Disordered Breathing. Circulation. 2008;117:2599–260.

40. Levy D, Garrison RJ, Savage DD, et al. Prognostic implications of echocardiographically determined left ventricular mass in the Framingham Heart study. N Engl J Med 1990;322:1561–6.

41. Levy D, Salomon M, D'Agostino RB, et al. Prognostic implications of baseline echocardiographic features and their serial changes in subjects with left ventricular hypertrophy. Circulation 1994;90: 1786–93.

42. Hinderliter A, Sherwood A, Gullette EC, et al. Reduction of left ventricular hypertrophy after exercise and weight loss in overweight patients with mild hypertension. Arch Intern Med 2002;162(12): 1333–9.

43. Schlaich MP, Kaye DM, Lambert E, et al. Relation between cardiac sympathetic activity and hypertensive left ventricular hypertrophy. Circulation 2003;108(5):560–5.

44. Hedner JA, Darpö B, Ejnell H, et al. Reduction in sympathetic activity after long-term CPAP treatment in sleep apnea: cardiovascular implications. Eur Respir J 1995;8(2):222–9.

45. Harbison JA, Gibson GJ. Snoring, sleep apnea and stroke: chicken or scrambled egg? Q J Med 2000;93(10):647–54.

46. Kurth T, Gaziano JM, Berger K, et al. Body Mass Index and the risk of stroke in men. Arch Intern Med 2002;162(22):2557–62.

47. Gami AS, Hodge DO, Herges RM, et al. Obstructive sleep apnea, obesity, and the risk of incident atrial fibrillation. J Am Coll Cardiol 2007;49(5):565–71.

48. Levy D, Larson MG, Vasan RS, et al. The progression from hypertension to congestive heart failure. JAMA 1996;275(20):1557–62.

49. Lloyd-Jones DM, Larson MG, Leip EP, et al. Lifetime risk for developing congestive heart failure: the Framingham Heart Study. Circulation 2002;106(24):3068–72.

50. Kenchaiah S, Evans JC, Levy D, et al. Obesity and the risk of heart failure. N Engl J Med 2002;347(5):305–13.

51. Malone S, Liu PP, Holloway R, et al. Obstructive sleep apnea in patients with dilated cardiomyopathy: effects of continuous positive airway pressure. Lancet 1991;338:1480–4.

52. Kaneko Y, Floras JS, Usui K, et al. Cardiovascular effects of continuous positive airway pressure in patients with heart failure and obstructive sleep apnea. N Engl J Med 2003;348(13):1233–41.

53. Davos CH, Doehner W, Rauchhaus M, et al. Body mass and survival in patients with chronic heart failure without cachexia: the importance of obesity. J Cardiac Fail 2003;9(1):29–35.

54. Bloomfield G, Sugerman H, Blocher CR, et al. Chronically increased intra-abdominal pressure produces systemic hypertension in dogs. Int J Obes 2003;24(7):819–24.

55. Sugerman H, DeMaria E, Felton WL 3rd, et al. Increased intra-abdominal pressure and cardiac filling pressure in obesity-associated pseudotumor cerebri. Neurology 1997;49(2):507–11.

56. Young T, Shahar E, Nieto FJ, et al. Predictors of sleep-disordered breathing in community-dwelling adults: the Sleep Heart Health Study. Arch Intern Med 2002;162(8):893–900.

57. Narkiewicz K, van de Borne PJ, Cooley RL, et al. Sympathetic activity in obese subjects with and without obstructive sleep apnea. Circulation 1998;98(8):772–6.

58. Kraiczi H, Hedner J, Peker J, et al. Comparison of atenolol, amlodipine, enalapril, hydrochlorothiazide, and losartan for antihypertensive treatment in patients with obstructive sleep apnea. Am J Respir Crit Care Med 2000;161(5):1423–8.

59. Lattimore JD, Wilcox I, Adams MR, et al. Treatment of obstructive sleep apnea leads to enhanced pulmonary vascular nitric oxide release. Int J Cardiol 2007;126(2):229–33.

60. Grossman W, Carabello BA. *Ventricular Wall Stress and the Development of Cardiac Hypertrophy and Failure*. New York: Raven Press, 1993.

18 Adult Obesity: Fertility

Renato Pasquali, Alessandra Gambineri, Valentina Vicennati and Uberto Pagotto

Division of Endocrinology, Department of Internal Medicine, S. Orsola-Malpighi Hospital, University Alma Mater Studiorum of Bologna, Italy

Introduction

The effect of adiposity is manifest in nearly every aspect of female reproductive life and in several aspects of male reproduction. The worldwide epidemic of obesity has considerable responsibility for the increasing rates of infertility problems in both sexes.

This is particularly relevant for women, since there is consistent evidence that early-onset obesity, particularly during adolescence, may predispose to infertility later in life by affecting spontaneous ovulation and increasing the likelihood of the development of hyperandrogenic states, particularly the polycystic ovary syndrome (PCOS). Moreover, in adult women, obesity may act adversely by interfering with assisted reproductive technology (ART) efficiency and outcomes, increasing miscarriages and early pregnancy loss, and worsening the physiologic process and delivery in pregnancy.

In men, obesity may reduce androgen concentrations in proportion to excess body fat and, in massively obese individuals, may impair spermatogenesis. Additional adverse effects of male obesity are represented by erectile dysfunction and poor semen quality.

Infertility can be reversed by weight loss in both sexes, which emphasizes the need for its careful investigation and recognition, together with related pathophysiologic aspects in the presence of obesity. In turn, physicians involved in human fertility, such as obstetricians and gynecologists, should be aware that the treatment of obesity may improve fertility, particularly after ART, and pregnancy outcomes.

The worldwide epidemic of obesity

We are facing a worldwide public health emergency due to the increasing epidemic of obesity and related disorders [1]. Recent estimates show that the increasing prevalence of obesity is recognized worldwide, with few exceptions. The International Obesity Task Force estimates that at least 1.1 billion adults are currently overweight, including 312 million who are obese, and that with the new Asian Body Mass Index (BMI) criteria, the number is even higher [2]. Most importantly, there is emerging evidence that overweight is increasing not only in adults but in children too [2].

The price of obesity is represented by a long list of co-morbidities and social, psychologic and demographic problems. Obese women have similar co-morbidities to men, particularly type 2 diabetes mellitus (T2DM) and cardiovascular diseases [3]. On the other hand, they also have some specific problems, including fertility-related disorders [4,5]. Obesity affects every aspect of reproduction in both males and females. Undoubtedly, social and cultural factors must be considered while estimating these effects, particularly in women. Fertility and reproduction unfortunately have a well-defined biologic time interval, particularly in women, which is shorter than life expectation, at least in industrialized and developed countries. This can undoubtedly expose women to a greater impact of negative environmental and biologic factors and events, such as obesity, T2DM and hypertension. Although there are very few studies on this topic, it is possible that this may also apply to men.

Box 18.1

- The price of obesity is represented by a long list of co-morbidities including fertility-related disorders.

Clinical Obesity in Adults and Children, 3rd edition. Edited by Peter G. Kopelman, Ian D. Caterson and William H. Dietz.

Obesity and infertility in women

Obesity may affect infertility and reproduction in women in different ways: (i) by affecting spontaneous ovulation, (ii) by interfering with ART efficiency and outcomes, and (iii) by worsening the physiologic process and delivery in pregnancy.

Epidemiologic evidence that obesity is associated with menstrual and ovulatory disorders

The association between obesity and alterations of the reproductive functions in women was recognized a long time ago [6,7] and has been confirmed more recently [8].

The relationship between excess body fat and reproductive disorders appears to be stronger for early-onset obesity particularly during adolescence [9]. There are several epidemiologic studies which suggest that changes in body weight or body composition are critical factors regulating pubertal development in young women, and the discovery of leptin provided critical evidence for an endocrine regulation of puberty and the fertile reproductive system, particularly in females [10]. Menarche generally occurs at a younger age in obese girls than in normal-weight counterparts [9] and there is evidence that in adolescent and young women the age of onset of obesity and of menstrual irregularities and oligoanovulation is significantly correlated [9.11]. Although many multiparous women are obese, there is nonetheless evidence that obesity may also affect fertility rates in women within the fertile age range. The Nurses' Health Study [12] reported that the risk of ovulatory infertility increased in women with increasing BMI values. Several other cross-sectional and prospective studies have produced similar findings [4]. In a recent observational study performed in the United Kingdom, the authors found that lifestyle (smoking, alcohol and coffee consumption) and BMI had a significant and cumulative dose-dependent and weight-dependent negative impact on fecundity [13].

The abdominal pattern of fat distribution may have a specific impact on ovulation and fertility. In one study examining a large group of nulliparous healthy women who presented for artificial insemination due to infertility of their partners, Zaadstra and co-workers [14] found that abdominal fatness was more negatively associated with a decreasing chance of conception than total body fat.

The paradigm of PCOS: independent effects of obesity on fertility and reproduction

Although they are not included in the current diagnostic criteria of PCOS [15,16], it has nonetheless been widely recognized that insulin resistance and hyperinsulinemia, as well as obesity and the metabolic syndrome, affect most PCOS women [17–19].

The prevalence of obesity in PCOS women appears to be much larger than expected in the general population. Although the cause of this association remains unknown, a recent comprehensive review by Ehrmann [18] reported an estimated prevalence

rate for more than 30% of cases and, in some series, a percentage as high as 75%.

Mechanisms by which obesity influences the pathophysiology and clinical expression of PCOS are complex and not completely understood [20,21]. However, obesity is believed to play a distinct pathophysiologic role in the development of hyperandrogenism in women with PCOS [17,21]. Several factors are relevant to understanding the complex pathophysiologic network relating obesity with PCOS. They include insulin, the insulin–growth factor system, the opioid system, estrogens and several adipokines, particularly leptin, which have been extensively reviewed in recent articles to which interested readers can refer [19–22].

The phenotype of PCOS largely depends on the presence of obesity [17,20]. Androgen abnormalities are usually more pronounced, despite lower luteinizing hormone (LH) concentrations with respect to normal-weight PCOS women. This is particularly evident in those with central fat distribution, which characterizes more than 60% of PCOS women, even if they have normal BMI values. In addition, a higher proportion of obese PCOS women complain of hirsutism and menstrual disorders in comparison to normal-weight women. Chronic oligoanovulation is likely to be more pronounced in obese women with PCOS, although longitudinal studies on this specific topic have not been performed.

The relative contribution of the long list of metabolic derangements in influencing ovulation and fertility in PCOS women has been discussed [20,21,23]. Other than ovulatory dysfunctions, obese PCOS women are characterized by blunted responsiveness to pharmacologic treatments to induce ovulation, recurrent miscarriages, more frequent early pregnancy loss and a reduced incidence of pregnancy. Finally, from recent studies performed in PCOS women conceiving after ART, there is evidence that those with obesity had higher gonadotropin requirements during stimulation, fewer oocytes, a higher abortion rate and a lower livebirth rate than their nonobese counterpart [20,23]. Therefore, a decreased efficiency of the different treatments for anovulation and infertility may be expected in obese PCOS women.

Obesity and ART outcomes

Obesity can impair the outcome of ART. It is reported that raising BMI by one unit decreases the odds for pregnancy by 0.84 in *in vitro* fertilization (IVF) and that each reduction of BMI by one unit after lifestyle intervention increases the chance of pregnancy by 1.19 [24].

Obesity-related alterations to steroid metabolism and altered secretion and action of insulin and several adipokines may influence follicle growth, embryo development and implantation in natural conception or following ART [23–26]. Higher gonadotropin requirements in obese women undergoing controlled ovarian hyperstimulation for ART are necessary, which suggests some exogenous gonadotropin resistance [27], particularly when associated with PCOS [28].

Longer periods of ovarian stimulation, higher cancellation rates and higher incidence of follicular asynchrony have been found in obese patients undergoing controlled ovarian hyperstimulation (COH) and IVF [24,29]. Different studies have shown that decreased periovulatory human chorionic gonadotropin (HCG) concentrations and an inverse correlation between HCG levels and BMI are associated with diminished fertilization rates [30] and that lower peak estradiol concentrations (HCG day) noted in obese women undergoing COH for IVF was associated with an impaired cycle outcome [31].

Reduced oocyte retrieval in overweight and obese women has been reported [27], mainly due to their poorer ovarian response: this is additionally associated with PCOS [24].

Oocyte quality may be impaired as a result of obesity, which implies lower fertilization rates [27], although similar data have not been reported by others [24]. Whether poorer embryo quality may be associated with obesity is unclear, since positive and negative reports have been published [24,28,29]. Finally, a lower incidence of embryo transfer and lower mean number of transferred embryos have been observed in linear association with increasing BMI in some but not all studies [24].

Discrepancies in the current literature regarding reproductive outcome in obese patients may be due to the different cut-off points used to define obesity, and/or the inclusion of a combination of overweight and obese patients in some study populations, the type of obesity considered, and the individual endocrine and metabolic pattern of each woman, which is likely to vary among subjects within the same BMI group. In a recent meta-analysis performed by Maheshwari et al. [32] aimed at assessing the effects of obesity on the outcome of ART, the authors found that, compared with women with a BMI of 25 or less, women with a BMI >25 have a lower chance of pregnancy following IVF (odds ratio (OR) 0.71), require higher doses of gonadotropins (weighted mean differences: 210.08) and have an increased miscarriage rate (OR 1.31). By contrast, they found no evidence of the effect of BMI on livebirth, cycle cancellation, oocyte recovery and ovarian hyperstimulation syndrome. However, they suggest that further studies with clear entry criteria and uniform reporting of outcomes are needed to investigate the true impact of weight on the outcome of ART.

The oocyte donation model has still not definitively established an hypothesis related to the impact of obesity but recent studies are suggestive [24]. Since the impact of obesity on extraovarian factors and its influence on ART outcome are critical issues [33], continuing studies are required.

Obesity and pregnancy outcome

Most reports show decreased livebirth rates in obese patients with spontaneous pregnancies or pregnancies following ART. It has been suggested that obesity and associated hormonal alterations may affect the function of the corpus luteum and trophoblast function, early embryo development and endometrial receptivity [24,32]. Implantation seems additionally to be detrimentally affected by obesity, although this is still disputed by some [27]. Furthermore, the question as to whether obese women have lower pregnancy rates following ovulation induction or ART is still unresolved [24]. Nevertheless, Wang et al [34] showed that

---

Box 18.2

- The relationship between excess body fat and reproductive disorders appears to be stronger for early-onset obesity, particularly during adolescence.
- Hyperandrogenic states, particularly PCOS, are commonly associated with obesity.
- Obesity can impair the outcome of ART. Obesity is also associated with lower pregnancy rates following ovulation induction or ART and increases risk for miscarriages.
- The negative impact of obesity can also be extended to fetal malformation.

---

the probability of achieving at least one pregnancy during ART treatment was reduced by almost 30% in women with a BMI of 30–35, and by 50% in those with a BMI greater than 35.

Miscarriages may occur more frequently in obese women not only following conceptions achieved through ART [27,28,34]. Although no consensus exists, it is commonly accepted that only those women with a BMI greater than 30 should be considered at high risk [35]. The discrepancies in findings between certain studies may be related to the lack of differentiation according to fat distribution pattern [36].

Obesity is associated with a higher risk of obstetric causes of maternal death and of anesthesia-related deaths [37]. Obese women present higher rates of complications in pregnancy, mainly in the third trimester, such as hypertension, pre-eclampsia, gestational diabetes, thromboembolism, urinary tract infection, fetal macrosomia, preterm labor and delivery, sudden and unexplained intrauterine death, operative vaginal deliveries, shoulder dystocia, cesarean section delivery, and anesthetic and surgical complications [4,24,35,37–39].

The negative impact of obesity can also be extended to fetal malformations, such as defects of the central nervous system (neural tube defects), great vessels, ventral wall and intestine [4,37]. Apart from congenital anomalies, children of obese mothers run a higher risk of intrauterine fetal death, head trauma, shoulder dystocia, brachial plexus lesions, fractures of the clavicle, meconium aspiration, fetal distress and increased risk of death within the first year [4,29].

Obesity and infertility in men

In men, obesity may affect fertility by altering the hormonal milieu and by reducing spermatogenesis. In addition, obesity in men may be associated with erectile dysfunction (ED). These topics will be addressed in the following sections.

Male obesity as a hypoandrogenic state

In the obese male, total and free testosterone blood concentration levels progressively decrease with increasing body weight, and this reduction is associated with a progressive decrease of sex hormone-binding globulin (SHBG) concentrations. Androstenedione and dihydrotestosterone circulating levels are usually normal or slightly reduced. Changes in testosterone metabolism through 5α-reductase activity may also occur in obesity, although this is still questionable [40]. Abdominal fat distribution may have a further negative effect on testosterone levels in men [40,41].

Factors responsible for altered androgen status in male obesity

Gonadotropin levels are usually normal or slightly reduced in obese men, as are their responses following gonadotropin-releasing hormone stimulation (GnRH) [42]. This specifically occurs in obese men with high BMI values, probably due to impaired secretion of GnRH at the hypothalamic level [43]. The absence of classic clinical signs of hypogonadism can be explained by the fact that the testosterone free fraction is only 2% of total testosterone, and that obesity predominantly affects circulating bound testosterone, due to the concurrent decrease of SHBG production, as a result of hepatic synthesis inhibition by excessive circulating insulin [44]. However, as demonstrated in women, insulin may also stimulate testosterone production *in vivo* in men [40]. Therefore, reduced testosterone in male obesity is due to a balance between inhibiting and stimulating processes.

Estrogen production rates in male obesity are increased in proportion to body weight [45]. It has been suggested that hypotestosteronemia in obese men may in some way result from negative feedback, inhibiting the regulation of estrogen upon gonadotropin secretion [40]. Alternatively, higher aromatase activity has been hypothesized, based on the reversal of reduced testosterone levels after administration of an aromatase inhibitor, testolactone [40].

As occurs in endogenous hypercortisolism which is invariably associated with inhibition of the hypothalamic-pituitary-gonadal axis [40], recent data support the concept that reduced testosterone in obese males may partly depend on hyperactivity of the hypothalamic-pituitary-adrenal axis [46].

Leptin receptors are widely expressed in the human testes [47]. Long-term exposure of human fat cells to testosterone inhibits leptin expression *in vitro* [47] and in male rodent cultured Leydig cells, leptin receptors have been shown to negatively influence gonadotropin hormone- and HCG-stimulated androgen production, by mechanisms probably involving the 17,20 lyase activity [48]. Hypogonadal men show lowered leptin levels, which are restored to normal by testosterone replacement therapy [49]. Studies in obese men have shown a significantly negative relationship between leptin levels and basal and HCG-stimulated testosterone levels [50]. This supports the theory that excess circulating leptin contributes to the decreased testosterone levels in obese men.

Effect of obesity on reproduction in men

Despite the important impact of obesity on steroidogenesis, the impact of obesity on fertility in men has been much less investigated than in women. Epidemiologic association studies are lacking. Spermatogenesis and fertility may, however, be reduced in subjects with massive obesity [51]. On the other hand, there is evidence for an emerging subfertility condition in male obesity. This may be due to multiple factors. As previously reported, this may be partly explained by the hypotestosteronemic state, which represents a true functional state of hypogonadotropic hypogonadism. In these conditions, oligospermia may also occur [40].

An underestimated problem is ED, which is common in obese men and tends to increase with increasing BMI values. In the Massachusetts Male Aging Study [52] which was performed in a large cohort of men aged 40–70 years, the overall prevalence of ED was 17%, but it increased to 45% in subjects with BMI values greater than 30. In the Health Professionals Follow-up Study, it was found that men with a BMI higher than 28.7 had a 30% higher risk for ED than those with a normal BMI (<25) [53]. Although there are no formal studies of the prevalence of ED in obesity, it is anticipated to be high [54,55]. Interestingly, ED can be reversed through weight loss [56]. Since ED represents an indirect but very common cause of infertility in men, this must be taken into consideration in the clinical setting. This is further emphasized by the strong association between ED and T2DM and recent findings demonstrating that ED also represents a risk factor for cardiovascular diseases [57].

Several studies have suggested that the quality of semen has declined over the last few decades [58]. Since the onset of these alterations appears to be recent, changes in lifestyle or environmental factors have been postulated. Particular attention has been paid to environmental pollutants. Among these disruptors, persistent organochlorines, used as pesticides or industrial chemicals, have been considered. Many organochlorines have hormone-disrupting properties and are therefore suspected candidates for determining poorer fertility [59]. A potential link between these environmental disruptors and obesity was recently investigated in a Danish study [60], showing that men with poor semen quality

---

Box 18.3

- In males, obesity decreases testosterone level in proportion to increasing body fat.
- In massively obese patients, hypogonadotropic hypogonadism and hypospermatogenesis may also occur.

Box 18.4

- Obese patients may have a higher prevalence of erectile dysfunction, which can be recovered after weight loss.
- Poor semen quality may be associated with obesity in men.

were three times more likely to be obese than men with normal semen quality. An additional finding was that there was even a significant negative correlation between semen quality parameters and BMI among men with the best semen quality. More research is needed in this area, particularly in young individuals.

References

1. Haslan DW, James WPT. Obesity. Lancet 2005;366:1197–209.

2. James WPT, Rigby N, Leach R. The obesity epidemic, metabolic syndrome and future preventive strategies. Eur J Cardiovasc Prev Rehabil 2004;11:3–8.

3. Ford ES. Prevalence of the metabolic syndrome in US population. Endocrinol Metab Clin North Am 2004;33:333–50.

4. Linnè Y. Effects of obesity on women's reproduction and complications during pregnancy. Obes Rev 2004;5:137–43.

5. Pasquali R, Pelusi C, Genghini S, Cacciari M, Gambineri A. Obesity and reproductive disorders in women. Hum Reprod Update 2003; 9:359–72.

6. Rogers J, Mitchell GW. The relation of obesity to menstrual disturbances. N Engl J Med 1952;247:53–6.

7. Hartz AJ, Barboriak PN, Wong A, Katayama KP, Rimm AA. The association of obesity with infertility and related menstrual abnormalities in women. Int J Obes 1979;3:57–77.

8. Norman RJ, Clark AM. Obesity and reproductive disorders: a review. Reprod Fertil Dev 1998;10:55–63.

9. Pelusi C, Pasquali R. Polycystic ovary syndrome in adolescents. Pathophysiology and treatment implication. Treat Endocrinol 2003; 2:215–30.

10. Farooqi IS, Jebb SA, Langmack G. Effects of recombinant leptin therapy in a child with congenital leptin deficiency. N Engl J Med 1999;341:879–84.

11. Lake JK, Power C, Cole TJ. Women's reproductive health: the role of body mass index in early and adult life. Int J Obes 1997;21: 432–8.

12. Rich-Edwards JA, Goldman MB, Willet WC, et al. Adolescent body mass index and infertility caused by ovulatory dysfunction. Am J Obstet Gynecol 1994;71:171–7.

13. Hassan MA, Killick SR. Negative lifestyle is associated with a significant reduction in fecundity. Fertil Steril 2004;81:384–92.

14. Zaadstra BM, Seidell JC, van Noord PA, et al. Fat and female fecundity: prospective study of effect of body fat distribution on conception rates. BMJ 1993;306:484–7.

15. Zawadski JK, Dunaif A. Diagnostic criteria for polycystic ovary syndrome;towards a rational approach. In: Dunaif A, Givens JR, Haseltine F (eds) *Polycystic Ovary Syndrome*. Boston: Blackwell Scientific, 1992:377–84.

16. Rotterdam ESHRE/ASRM-Sponsored PCOS Consensus Workshop Group. Revised 2003 consensus on diagnostic criteria and long-term health risks related to polycystic ovary syndrome (PCOS). Hum Reprod 2004;19:41–7.

17. Gambineri A, Pelusi C, Vicennati V, Pagotto U, Pasquali R. Obesity and the polycystic ovary syndrome. Int J Obes 2002;26:883–96.

18. Ehrmann DA. Polycystic ovary syndrome. N Engl J Med 2005;352:1223–36.

19. Pasquali R, Gambineri A. PCOS: a multifaceted disease from adolescence to adult age. Ann NY Acad Sci 2006;1092:158–74.

20. Pasquali R, Gambineri A, Pagotto U. The impact of obesity on reproduction in women with polycystic ovary syndrome Br J Obstet Gynecol 2006;113:1148–59.

21. Barber TM, McCarthy MI, Wass JAH, Franks S. Obesity and polycystic ovary syndrome. Clin Endocrinol 2006;65:137–45.

22. Poretsky L, Cataldo NA, Rosenwaks Z, Giudice LC. The insulin-related ovarian regulatory system in health and disease. Endocrinol Rev 1999;20:535–82.

23. Andersen AN, Goossens V, Gianaroli L, Felberbaum R, de Mouzon J, Nygren KG. Assisted reproductive technology in Europe, 2003. Results generated from European registers by ESHRE. Hum Reprod 2007;22:1513–25.

24. Bellver J, Busso C, Pellicer A, Remohí J, Simón C. Obesity and assisted reproductive technology outcomes. Reprod Biomed Online 2006;12:562–8.

25. Budak E, Fernández Sánchez M, et al. Interactions of the hormones leptin, ghrelin, adiponectin, resistin and PYY3–36 with the reproductive system. Fertil Steril 2006;85:1563–81.

26. Mitchell M, Armstrong DT, Robker RL, Norman RJ. Adipokines: implications for female fertility and obesity. Reproduction 2005;130: 583–97.

27. Fedorcsák P, Dale PO, Storeng R, et al. Impact of overweight on assisted reproduction treatment. Hum Reprod 2004;11:2523–8.

28. Mulders AG, Laven JS, Eijkemans MJ, et al. Patient predictors for outcome of gonadotropin ovulation induction in women with normogonadotropic anovulatory infertility: a meta-analysis. Hum Reprod Update 2003;9:429–49.

29. van Swieten E, Leew-Harmsen L, Badings E, et al. Obesity and clomiphene challenge test as predictors of outcomes of in vitro fertilization and intracytoplasmatic sperm injection. Gynecol Obstet Invest 2005;170:541–548

30. Carrell DT, Jones KP, Peterson CM, et al. Body mass index is inversely related to intrafollicular HCG concentrations, embryo quality and IVF outcomes. Reprod Biomed Online 2001; 3:109–11

31. Nichols J, Crane M, Higdon H III, et al. Extremes of body mass index reduce in vitro fertilization pregnancy rates. Fertil Steril 2003;79:645–657.

32. Maheshwari A, Stofberg L, Bhattacharya S. Effect of overweight and obesity on assisted reproductive technology – a systematic review. Hum Reprod Update 2007;13:433–444.

33. Levens ED, Skarulis MC. Assessing the role of endometrial alteration among obese patients undergoing assisted reproduction. Fertil Steril 2008;89(6):1606–8.

34. Wang J, Davies M, Norman R. Body mass and probability of pregnancy during assisted reproduction treatment: retrospective study. BMJ 2000;321:1320–1.

35. Public Affairs Committee of the Teratology Society. Teratology Public Affairs Committee position paper: maternal obesity and pregnancy. Birth Defect Res 2006;76:73–7.

36. Winter E, Wang J, Davies M, et al. Early pregnancy loss following assisted reproductive technology treatment. Hum Reprod 2002;17: 3220–3.

37. Hall F, Neubert A. Obesity and pregnancy. Obstet Gynaecol Sur 2005;4:253–60.

38. Kabiru W, Raynor D. Obstetric outcome associated with increase in BMI category during pregnancy. Am J Obstet Gynecol 2004;191: 928–32.

39. Ramsay JE, Greer I, Sattar N. Obesity and reproduction. BMJ 2006;333:1159–62.

40. Pasquali R. Androgens and obesity: fact and perspectives. Fertil Steril 2006;85:1319–40.

41. Wajchenberg BL. Subcutaneous and visceral adipose tissue: their relation to the metabolic syndrome. Endocrinol Rev 2000;21:697–738.

42. Kokkoris P, Pi-Sunyer FX. Obesity and endocrine diseases. Endocrinol Metab Clin North Am 2003;32:895–914.

43. Vermeulen A, Kaufman JM, Deslypere JP, Thomas G. Attenuated luteinizing hormone (LH) pulse amplitude but normal LH pulse frequency, and its relation to plasma androgens in hypogonadism of obese men. J Clin Endocrinol Metab 1993;76:1140–6.

44. Plymate SR, Matej LA, Jones RE, Friedl KE. Inhibition of sex hormone-binding globulin production in the human hepatoma (Hep G2) cell line by insulin and prolactin. J Clin Endocrinol Metab 1988;67:460–4.

45. Longcope C, Kato T, Horton R. Conversion of blood androgens to estrogens in normal adult men and women. J Clin Invest 1969;48:2191–201.

46. Vicennati V, Ceroni L, Genghini S, Patton L, Pagotto U, Pasquali R. Sex difference in the relationship between the hypothalamic-pituitary-adrenal (HPA) axis and sex hormones in obesity. Obes Res 2006;14:235–43.

47. Moschos S, Chan JL, Mantzoros CS. Leptin and reproduction: a review. Fertil Steril 2002;77:433–44.

48. Caprio M, Isidori AM, Carta AR, Moretti C, Dufau ML, Fabbri A. Expression of functional leptin receptors in rodent Leydig cells. Endocrinology 1999;140:4939–47.

49. Jockenhövel F, Blum WF, Vogel E, et al. Testosterone substitution normalizes elevated serum leptin levels in hypogonadal men. J Clin Endocrinol Metab 1997;82:2510–13.

50. Isidori AM, Caprio M, Strollo F, et al. Leptin and androgens in male obesity: evidence for leptin contribution to reduced androgen levels. J Clin Endocrinol Metab 1999;84:3673–80.

51. Strain GW, Zumoff B, Kream J, et al. Mild hypogonadotropic hypogonadism in obese men. Metabolism 1982;31:871–5.

52. Feldman HA, Goldstein I, Hatzichristou DG, Krane RJ, McKinlay JB. Impotence and its medical and psychosocial correlates: results of the Massachusetts Male Aging Study. J Urol 1994;151:54–61.

53. Bacon CG, Mittleman MA, Kawachi I, Giovannucci E, Glasser DB, Rimm EB. Sexual function in men older than 50 years of age: results from the Health Professionals Follow-up Study. Ann Intern Med 2003;139:161–8.

54. Chung Ws, Sohn JH, Park YY. Is obesity an underlying factor in erectile dysfunction? Eur Urol 1999;36:68–70.

55. Shiri R, Koskimäki J, Hakama M, et al. Effect of lifestyle factors on incidence of erectile dysfunction. Int J Impot Res 2004;16:389–94.

56. Esposito K, Giugliano F, di Palo C, et al. Effect of lifestyle changes on erectile dysfunction in obese men: a randomized controlled trial. JAMA 2004;291:2978–84.

57. Russell ST, Khandheria BK, Nehra A. Erectile dysfunction and cardiovascular disease. Mayo Clin Proc 2004;79:782–94.

58. Micic D, Cubrilo KM. Obesity and male reproductive function. Obes Metab 2006;2:13–27.

59. Magnusdottir EV, Thorsteinsson T, Thorsteinsdottir S, Heimisdottir M, Olafsdottir K. Persistent organochlorines, sedentary occupation, obesity and human male subfertility. Hum Reprod 2005;20:208–15.

60. Jensen TK, Andersson AM, Jørgensen N, et al. Body mass index in relation to semen quality and reproductive hormones among 1558 Danish men. Fertil Steril 2004;82:863–70.

19 Obstructive Sleep Apnea

Brendon J. Yee and Ronald R. Grunstein

Department of Respiratory and Sleep Medicine, Royal Prince Alfred Hospital, Sydney, Australia; Woolcock Institute of Medical Research, University of Sydney, Sydney, Australia

Pathogenesis

The physiology of sleep

To sleep physiologists, humans exist in three states: wakefulness, nonrapid eye movement (NREM) sleep and rapid eye movement (REM or dreaming) sleep. There are marked differences between these three states in many aspects of physiology. Sleep has profound effects on breathing and these effects are usually greatest during REM sleep. Sleep can amplify the effects of drugs such as alcohol and opiates on breathing.

In normal subjects, sleep is associated with a fall in minute ventilation, primarily due to a drop in tidal volume. As a result, there is a small rise in arterial blood carbon dioxide tension ($PaCO_2$) and a small fall in arterial blood oxygen tension (PaO_2). During NREM sleep, the hypoxic drive to breathe is reduced and the ventilatory response to hypercapnia is diminished. This depression of chemosensitivity is greatest during REM sleep. Sleep is also associated with a reduction in tone of the upper airway dilator muscles, with a resulting increase in resistance to airflow. REM sleep is characterized by postural muscle atonia, with bursts of eye movements and associated peripheral muscle twitches (phasic REM). Phasic REM is associated with marked breathing irregularity. The loss of postural muscle tone during REM sleep leaves us largely reliant on the diaphragm (a nonpostural muscle) for maintaining ventilation. An individual with abnormal diaphragm function, either due to neuromuscular disease or to mechanical disadvantage (kyphoscoliosis, lung disease or obesity), will have impaired breathing in sleep, particularly during REM sleep. Someone with a combination of these factors, such as an obese patient with lung disease, will be at even greater risk of developing sleep-related respiratory failure.

Clinical Obesity in Adults and Children, 3rd edition. Edited by Peter G. Kopelman, Ian D. Caterson and William H. Dietz.
© 2010 Blackwell Publishing, ISBN: 978-1-4051-8226-3.

Definitions in sleep-disordered breathing

Sleep-disordered breathing is defined by the loss of a normal pattern of breathing during sleep and ranges from snoring through to profound nocturnal hypoventilation and respiratory failure during sleep. Intermittent snoring, with no associated sleep fragmentation (so-called "simple snoring"), is common and generally not considered part of the spectrum of sleep-disordered breathing. On the other hand, heavy snoring can result in arousals from sleep with accompanying sleep disruption [1] and should be considered part of the disease state.

Obstructive sleep apnea (OSA) is characterized by repetitive episodes of complete cessation of airflow (apnea) during sleep due to collapse of the upper airway, generally at the level of the pharynx [2]. During an apnea, continued respiratory efforts occur against the closed airway (Table 19.1), with resulting hypoxemia, until the apnea is terminated by arousal from sleep with restoration of upper airway patency. Typically, after a few deep breaths, this cycle is repeated, often hundreds of times through the night (Fig. 19.1). The recurrent arousals cause sleep fragmentation resulting in daytime sleepiness [3].

Significant upper airway obstruction can occur in the absence of complete collapse of the upper airway. Increased airway resistance can produce a measurable reduction in airflow (hypopnea) with the same consequences (hypoxemia and arousal) as an apnea. Even very minor increases in airway resistance (without detectable reductions in airflow) can produce recurrent arousals and excessive daytime sleepiness: the "upper airway resistance syndrome" [1].

Patients with impaired daytime respiratory function, whatever the cause, will have abnormal breathing, and will often develop impaired gas exchange, during sleep. These patients may have prolonged periods of hypoxemia lasting minutes, usually due to reduced ventilation (hypoventilation) although worsening ventilation-perfusion mismatch may also contribute. Hypercapnia also develops during sleep due to hypoventilation. These prolonged episodes of sleep-related hypercapnic hypoxia can lead to a "resetting" of chemoreceptors with subsequent blunted daytime chemosensitivity and the development or worsening of daytime hypercapnic respiratory failure. In addition, the prolonged exposure to hypoxemia and hypercapnia may lead to pulmonary hypertension and right-sided heart failure – "cor pulmonale." Patients with these severe forms of respiratory failure in sleep include those with many types of chronic lung disease, respiratory muscle failure due to neuromuscular disorders and, importantly, the obesity hypoventilation syndrome (OHS) (see below).

Central apnea refers to cessation of airflow with no detectable respiratory effort (in contrast to obstructive apneas where

breathing efforts are often vigorous). There is some confusion surrounding this term as it has been used to describe the patterns of breathing in patients in whom hypoventilation is the predominant pathology. This pattern of breathing that tends to occur in patients with awake hypercapnia and reduced respiratory drive should be differentiated from the "true" central apneas that classically occur as part of the periodic breathing seen in patients with cardiac failure [4] (also called Cheyne–Stokes breathing). In this breathing pattern, ventilation waxes and wanes from hyperventilation to central apnea. Periodic breathing can also occur in patients with neurologic disease due to strokes or rarely as an idiopathic form. Sporadic central apneas may also occur in patients with severe OSA and usually disappear when the OSA is treated. The etiology of central apnea in the patient with cardiac failure is complex, involving interplay between circulation time, brisk chemoreceptor drive and upper airway narrowing [4].

Pathogenesis of OSA: general

Upper airway collapse occurs when the negative (or suction) pressure applied to the upper airway during inspiration is greater than the dilating forces applied by the upper airway muscles such as genioglossus [2,5]. Collapse of the upper airway usually occurs in the retropalatal or retroglossal area and most patients have more than one site of collapse. Less frequently, upper airway collapse can occur at the epiglottis or glottis [4]. The determinants of the site of collapse in individual patients are unclear. Any factors which reduce airway size, decrease airway muscle tone, increase upper airway compliance or lead to the generation of a greater inspiratory pressure will predispose to the development of OSA [5]. Muscle tone and suction pressure are influenced by sleep stage and the relative respiratory drive to the diaphragm versus that to the upper airway dilator muscles.

Table 19.1 Definitions in sleep-disordered breathing

Term	Definition
Apnea	Complete cessation of airflow for at least 10 seconds
Hypopnea	Reduction in airflow for at least 10 seconds, ending with an arousal or associated with oxygen desaturation of at least 3%
Obstructive event	Continued respiratory effort occurs despite reduced airflow as above
Central event	Respiratory effort is absent, with absent airflow
Periodic breathing (Cheyne–Stokes respiration)	Respiration that waxes and wanes, alternating between hyperventilation and central apnea – seen in patients with heart failure or neurologic disease
Hypoventilation	An abnormal rise in PaCO$_2$ during sleep, usually associated with oxygen desaturation, with or without discrete respiratory events
Apnea-Hypopnea Index (AHI) (Respiratory Disturbance Index (RDI))	Number of apneic and hypopneic episodes per hour of sleep; >5 is usually considered abnormal

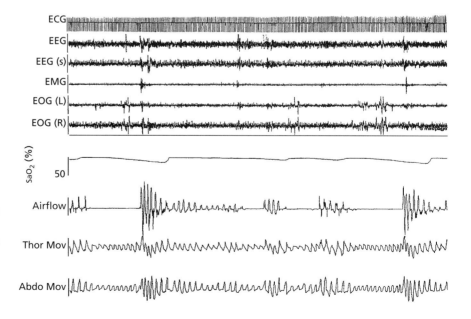

Figure 19.1 Five-minute tracing of a patient with typical severe obstructive sleep apnea. The upper traces show the variables used for sleep staging (ECG, electrocardiogram; EEG, electroencephalogram; EMG, electromyogram; EOG, electro-oculogram) and indicate this patient is in REM sleep. The apneas are indicated by intermittent cessation of airflow (Airflow, nasal airflow) and are obstructive in nature, as continued respiratory effort is seen when airflow is absent (Thor Mov, thoracic movement or effort; Abdo Mov, abdominal movement or effort). Repetitive falls in oxygen saturation (SaO$_2$) are seen following each apnea.

Several studies have shown that the pharyngeal airway is smaller in patients with OSA than normal subjects [6,7]. When the airway size is reduced, a greater suction pressure is required during inspiration. In the awake state, patients with OSA have increased upper airway dilator muscle activity that normalizes airflow resistance despite the anatomically smaller airway [8,9]. This compensatory increased upper airway muscle activity is lost during sleep, particularly in the genioglossus [2], resulting in airway closure. However, although the increased waking genioglossus activity is seen in some patients with OSA [9], some patients have similar genioglossus muscle activity values to control subjects. Compensatory muscle activity may be increased in other muscle groups or other mechanisms may be important in such patients.

Patients with OSA may also have defects in the sensory mechanisms that normally protect the upper airway from closure [10]. However, it is difficult to determine whether identified defects in sensory control (based on both clinical and histopathologic changes) in patients with OSA have a role in the genesis of OSA or are due to chronic airway vibration from snoring.

Pathogenesis of OSA: the role of obesity

Obesity is one of the strongest risk factors for OSA and there are a number of ways in which obesity can reduce upper airway size and therefore predispose the upper airway to collapse. External neck circumference is increased in patients with OSA and this measurement may explain some of the link between obesity and sleep apnea [11,12]. Neck circumference is an index of neck fat deposition, particularly in the lateral pharyngeal fat pads, and this fat deposition may lead to airway narrowing and OSA [13]. Imaging studies have shown that these fat pads are increased in size in obese patients with OSA [14]. However, excess fat deposition around the airway is not a universal finding in obese OSA patients [15] and well-matched controls are often difficult to obtain. Other studies have shown that obese sleep apnea patients have larger tongues [16] and smaller upper airway volumes [6] than nonobese patients. Obesity may predispose to OSA by increasing the size of upper airway soft tissue structures, although the cause of this increased size is unknown. There may be soft tissue edema from the repeated vibration of snoring and apnea. Human upper airway pathologic studies have been described infrequently in sleep apnea, though in one report more fat and muscle were observed in the uvula of sleep apnea patients [17,18].

A case–control study examining the upper airway using a sophisticated volumetric analysis MRI scan found that OSA patients had a larger volume of soft tissue surrounding the upper airway compared with controls. Controls were matched in terms of sex, age, ethnicity, craniofacial size and visceral neck fat. The authors concluded that OSA is associated with a significantly larger tongue, lateral pharyngeal walls, and total soft tissue. In a multivariable logistic regression the volume of the tongue and lateral walls was shown to independently increase the risk of sleep apnea [19].

Apart from upper airway narrowing, fat deposition in the chest and abdomen contributes to OSA. In morbidly obese patients, neck size is a better predictor of sleep apnea than other body anthropomorphic measures [20]. However, in a wide weight range of sleep apnea clinic patients, we observed that waist measurement provided similar or better statistical correlations with sleep apnea [21]. Abdominal obesity may reduce lung volumes particularly in the supine posture and so reduce upper airway size. Lung volume directly influences upper airway size during respiration. Thoracic inspiratory activity produces caudal traction on the trachea, increasing pharyngeal cross-sectional area [22]. This effect may be reduced in obese patients as impaired respiratory muscle force has been noted in these patients [23]. Cephalad movement of the trachea, as would occur with a decrease in lung volume, decreases upper airway size and increases pharyngeal resistance [24]. Passive inflation of the lung producing an increase in end-expiratory lung volume increases the size of the retropalatal airway [25].

It is likely that obesity promotes sleep apnea through a variety of mechanisms. In some patients, subcutaneous neck or peripharyngeal fat may be the critical "load" that tips the balance in favor of upper airway closure in sleep. In other patients, abdominal fat loading may be important. As yet there are no data on how weight loss relates to changes in upper airway fat.

In addition, more speculatively, the central obesity–sleep apnea link may be related to abnormal upper airway muscle function. Obesity is associated with changes in relative muscle fiber composition in skeletal muscle [26]. Some studies of sleep apnea patients before and after weight loss have shown changes in upper airway function rather than structure [27], supporting a hypothesis of abnormal upper airway muscle function in obese patients with sleep apnea.

Obesity hypoventilation syndrome

The majority of patients with OSA have normal arterial carbon dioxide ($PaCO_2$) tensions when awake. The term OHS describes those patients with obesity and daytime hypercapnia (and usually hypoxemia) in the absence of lung or neuromuscular disease. This association between obesity, hypersomnolence and hypercapnia was recognized for many years and was labeled "Pickwickian syndrome" (in honor of Joe, the fat boy, in Dickens' *Pickwick Papers*). However, the pathogenesis of the condition was poorly understood and the link with OSA not recognized. Early theories were that obesity produced a load to breathing, which together with depressed chemosensitivity produced OHS. The recognition that sleep apnea was present in these patients and that relief of upper airway obstruction by tracheostomy effectively treated the respiratory failure altered our understanding of OHS. Upper airway obstruction is a crucial factor in the pathogenesis of OHS [5]. However, most patients with OSA do not have hypercapnia when awake and so upper airway obstruction alone is not enough to produce OHS. In addition, the majority of patients with obesity and eucapnia have normal resting ventilation and occlusion pressures and normal or increased responses to hypoxia and

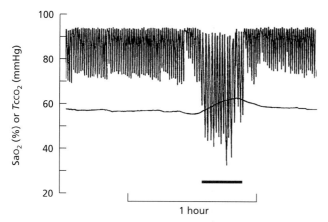

Figure 19.2 Two-hour oximetry recording, with transcutaneous (tc) CO_2 monitoring in a patient with severe OSA and OHS. The black bar indicates a period of REM sleep. There are repetitive arterial oxygen desaturations, with profound hypoxemia in REM sleep, associated with a marked rise in $tcCO_2$ indicating hypoventilation.

hypercapnia. The prevalence of OHS in the obese population is unknown, but it is probably underdiagnosed. A study found that 31% of obese patients (BMI >35 kg/m^2) admitted to medical wards had OHS [28].

There are no longitudinal studies on the development of OHS but almost certainly OHS starts out as heavy snoring, and then OSA and sleep-induced respiratory abnormalities occur before the development of daytime respiratory failure. During an apneic period, $PaCO_2$ rises acutely and PaO_2 falls (Fig. 19.2). When the apnea is terminated by an arousal, ventilation increases and oxygen and carbon dioxide levels can return to normal. If arousal responses *or* ventilatory responses to hypoxia or hypercapnia are depressed, the apneic periods will be longer, the degree of blood gas derangement greater and the normalization of blood gases in the period following arousal compromised [5]. In those patients able to compensate for the loss of ventilation during apneic periods by increased ventilation between events, overall eucapnia will be maintained. In contrast, if the compensatory mechanisms are poor, then overall ventilation will be reduced during sleep with the development of persistent hypercapnia and hypoxia during sleep. This will result in resetting of the chemoreceptors [29] and progression to daytime CO_2 retention. Sleep fragmentation as a result of repetitive arousals will also depress arousal responses. Arousal responses can be further impaired in patients prescribed sedatives/hypnotics to improve "insomnia," opiate analgesics to ease musculoskeletal pain or by consumption of alcohol. The term "Pickwickian syndrome" should be replaced by OHS or OSA with awake hypercapnic respiratory failure, which better describes the syndrome within the spectrum of sleep-disordered breathing.

It is likely that the development of OHS is multifactorial, with the key elements a combination of obesity (increased upper airway loading and reduced lung volumes), OSA, poor

chemoreceptor function (particularly defective arousal responses to hypoxia) and possibly alcohol consumption (reducing upper airway tone and arousal responses to asphyxia) [5]. Assessment of chemoreceptor function in this patient group is made difficult as prolonged exposure to hypoxia and hypercapnia will alter ventilatory responses, but studies in other diseases have shown familial clustering in the level of chemosensitivity, suggesting a genetic component [30]. It is important to stress that awake hypercapnia can occur in obese patients in the absence of any smoking history or lung or muscle disease [31].

More recently, leptin has been implicated in sleep-disordered breathing in obese subjects. In obese, leptin-deficient mice with OHS, leptin replacement resulted in an increase in minute ventilation (awake and asleep) and increased chemosensitivity to carbon dioxide during sleep [31]. These changes were independent of food intake, weight and CO_2 production. Patients with OSA have higher leptin levels than subjects with similar obesity without OSA [32]. Leptin levels fell significantly in a group of 22 patients with OSA after 4 days of treatment with continuous positive airway pressure (CPAP) [33], possibly due to reduced sympathetic activity. OSA may well be a confounder in some of the hormonal associations observed in central obesity and is possibly associated with resistance to the weight-reducing effects of leptin. In this context, hyperleptinemia and accelerated weight gain appear closely associated with worsening of sleep apnea [34]. Also, higher circulatory leptin levels were associated with hypoventilation in obesity. Interestingly higher leptin levels also fall with compliant noninvasive positive pressure ventilation (NIPPV) use independent of weight loss in OHS patients [35]. In human obesity, leptin "resistance" is common and leptin may act as a respiratory stimulant so that deficiency or resistance to the effects of leptin may promote OHS [36].

Epidemiology

Epidemiology in the general community

Studies examining prevalence in the area of sleep-disordered breathing have largely concentrated on self-reported estimates of snoring and daytime sleepiness. These symptoms are commonly reported in the general community, including obese subjects, and sleepiness may have many causes (Table 19.2). In addition, snoring may be underestimated if history from a bed partner is unavailable. Therefore questionnaire estimates of OSA are difficult to interpret and of limited usefulness.

The Wisconsin Sleep Cohort Study [37] is the largest reported prevalence study in which sleep studies were performed. This group found an apnea index of >5 events/h in 9% of female and 24% of male middle-aged public servants. The "OSA syndrome" (daytime sleepiness and an apnea index of >5/h) was found in 2% of women and 4% of men. An apnea index of >15 events/h was found in 4% of women and 9% of men. Our group has found a similar prevalence of OSA in an Australian rural community using home monitoring of breathing [37]. Population studies

Table 19.2 Sleepiness in the obese patient

Cause	Reason
Inadequate amounts of sleep	Lifestyle (especially shift work and commercial drivers)
	Insomnia
Drugs (causing sleepiness/disrupting sleep)	Hypnotics
	Alcohol
	Drug abuse
Disorders disrupting sleep	OSA
	PLMS
Primary brain disorders	Narcolepsy
	IHS

OSA, obstructive sleep apnea; PLMS, periodic leg movement disorder; IHS, idiopathic hypersomnolence.

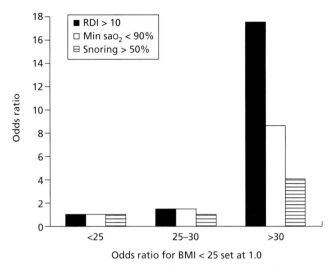

Figure 19.3 Obesity (measured by BMI) is an important predictor of OSA in the Busselton Sleep Survey. With the odds ratio for BMI <25 set at 1.0, a BMI >30 increased the odds ratio of either OSA (Respiratory Disturbance Index, RDI >10), desaturation during the night (min SaO$_2$ <90%) or heavy snoring (snoring for more than 50% of the night) by 4–18 times, depending on the variable.

show the prevalence of OSA with daytime sleepiness is approximately 3–7% for adult males and 2–5% for adult females in the general population [38].

Even where sleep studies are performed, estimates of prevalence are made difficult by the varying definitions of OSA used. In the past, researchers have used an apnea index of >5 events/h to define OSA. However, given that hypopneas and even increased upper airway resistance can produce the OSA syndrome, that definition is probably inadequate. Other measurements such as arousal index or changes in heart rate and blood pressure through the night may be important. In addition, more recent work (see later) has suggested that an apnea index as low as 1–5 events/h may influence the development of hypertension [38].

Epidemiology in the obese population

Multiple investigations have consistently shown that obesity, particularly central obesity, is strongly associated with sleep-disordered breathing in adults [36,37]. Measurements of central obesity such as waist or neck measurements are closely linked to OSA in sleep clinic populations and this association remains tight in the general population, although not as strong as in sleep clinic cohorts. In the Busselton Sleep Survey [38] there was a strong effect of BMI in increasing the risk of sleep-disordered breathing in the community (Fig. 19.3) [39].

There are limited data on the prevalence of sleep apnea in the obese population. The Swedish Obese Subjects study, which examined 3034 subjects with BMI >35, found that over 50% of obese men reported habitual loud snoring [40] as compared to 15% in age-matched nonobese subjects. Similarly, 33% of men and 12% of women in this study reported a history of frequent witnessed apneas. Questionnaires tend to underestimate the prevalence of OSA. The exact prevalence of the spectrum of sleep-breathing disorders in the obese is unknown, but it is clear that OSA and related conditions occur in a very high proportion of obese subjects.

Longitudinal studies have demonstrated a strong association between weight gain and the development of sleep-disordered breathing. The Wisconsin group prospectively evaluated 690 randomly selected local residents twice at 4-year intervals for the presence of sleep-disordered breathing [41]. They found that weight gain of 10% predicted an approximate 32% increase in the Apnea-Hypopnea Index (AHI) and similarly, weight loss of 10% predicted a 26% fall in the AHI. Therefore, even relatively small changes in baseline weight have a powerful impact on the degree of sleep-disordered breathing.

Epidemiology: other risk factors for OSA
Age
The prevalence of OSA increases with age. Some of this association may be due to increased central fat deposition with age, but other factors such as changes in tissue elasticity and ventilatory control and cardiopulmonary and neurologic co-morbidity may be important. Data from the community-based Sleep Heart Health Study have shown that disease prevalence increases steadily with age and reaches a plateau after the age of 60 years [42]. OSA in older adults may be distinct from OSA in middle-aged adults as there is conflicting evidence that OSA is associated with increased adverse effects in elderly OSA patients [43].

Gender
In the middle-aged population, the risk of OSA is three to four times greater in males than in females [44]. However, the prevalence of OSA increases in women after the menopause, suggesting a protective role for female hormones or an OSA-promoting role for male hormones. These effects may be due to hormonal influences on ventilatory control and mechanical behavior of the upper

airway [45] or on patterns of body fat deposition. The redistribution of fat from peripheral to central sites that occur with menopause may lead to increased prevalence of sleep apnea due to upper airway mass loading. Alternatively, the change in hormonal status may affect the arousal of ventilatory responses to blood gas changes during sleep. Finally, after menopause, the female airway may be more "collapsible" due to changes in upper airway mechanical properties from lowered female hormone levels.

A number of large epidemiologic studies have indicated that female hormone replacement therapy in menopause may protect against OSA [46,47]. However, clinical trials of estrogen administration in menopausal OSA have been disappointing [48]. Furthermore, despite only limited controlled data, exogenous androgen therapy in men and women may promote or worsen OSA [48].

Familial, genetic and maxillofacial factors

Familial clustering of OSA has been noted, independent of age and obesity. This association is probably due to similarities in facial structure affecting upper airway dynamics during sleep. Certain maxillofacial appearances such as class II malocclusion and retroposed mandible are strongly linked to OSA in nonobese subjects [49]. In obese patients, certain familial maxillofacial structures will further increase the likelihood of OSA. Static cephalometrics, CT and MRI have shown a number of skeletal and soft tissue structural differences between individuals with and without OSA during wakefulness. Features such as retrognathia, tonsillar hypertrophy, enlarged tongue or soft palate, inferiorly positioned hyoid bone, decreased posterior airway space, maxillary and mandibular retroposition can all narrow upper airway dimensions and promote OSA [50].

Some congenital conditions are linked to OSA. The Pierre–Robin sequence is strongly associated with OSA due to mandibular shortening. Patients with Down syndrome are predisposed to OSA due to oropharyngeal crowding and obesity. Nearly two-thirds of patients with Marfan syndrome have OSA [51], despite a thin body habitus, due to abnormal compliance of upper airway tissue.

Any condition causing narrowing of the upper airway, such as tonsillar and adenoid hypertrophy, macroglossia and high arched palates, will predispose to the development of OSA. Nasal obstruction is also a significant risk factor for OSA [52]. Again, the presence of these abnormalities will interact with obesity to produce a greater risk for OSA [53].

Co-morbid conditions

Many endocrine abnormalities are associated with an increased prevalence of OSA. Hypothyroidism reduces chemosensitivity and promotes airway narrowing by upper airway myopathy and myxedematous infiltration [54]. More than 50% of patients with acromegaly have OSA, and an increased prevalence of central sleep apnea has been seen associated with increased disease activity (as assessed by biochemical markers) [55]. Cushing disease is also associated with OSA [56].

Cardiac failure (whatever the cause) is associated with a high incidence of sleep-disordered breathing. In a study of 450 patients with cardiac failure referred to a sleep laboratory (either with sleep symptoms or persistent dyspnea), 72% had more than 10 apneas-hypopneas per hour [57]. Patients had OSA or central sleep apnea (Cheyne–Stokes respiration), with OSA more common in those patients with BMI >35 kg/m^2.

Cerebrovascular disease is associated with the presence of sleep-disordered breathing. One report examined patients in both the acute and convalescent stages of a first-ever stroke (hemorrhagic or ischemic) [58]. In the acute phase, 71% of patients had an AHI greater than 10, with an AHI >30 in 28%. Cheyne–Stokes breathing was seen in 26%. In the convalescent phase (3 months later), the overall AHI and the amount of Cheyne–Stokes breathing had fallen, but the obstructive apnea index was unchanged. Some patients had persistent central apneas following their stroke.

Clinical aspects

Symptoms and signs of sleep-disordered breathing

History and physical examination have fairly poor sensitivity and specificity for the detection of sleep-disordered breathing [59]. The typical symptoms associated with OSA are heavy snoring and excessive daytime sleepiness (EDS). The reporting of witnessed apneas is a relatively specific symptom but is also relatively insensitive. Other symptoms are listed in Box 19.1. Nocturnal symptoms include those related to the breathing disorder such as choking and gasping, nocturia and nocturnal gastroesophageal reflux. Daytime symptoms are related to the effects of sleep fragmentation and include morning headaches, fatigue, poor memory and concentration, alteration in mood and impotence [3]. Importantly, the arousal responses to upper airway narrowing during sleep can be so brisk that some patients (particularly women) can present with insomnia, restless sleep or anxiety [60].

These symptoms emphasize the importance of obtaining a confirmatory history from the spouse, bed partner and other family members. Few people are aware that they snore or stop

---

Box 19.1 Symptoms of sleep-disordered breathing

Snoring
Daytime sleepiness
Disrupted sleep
Choking or gasping during sleep
Dry throat/mouth in morning
Morning headaches
Nocturia
Heartburn
Poor memory/concentration
Fatigue
Impotence
Altered mood/irritability

breathing during sleep. The initial consultation is often precipitated by the bed partner's concerns about snoring and apnea. Excessive sleepiness may be recognized by the patient, but may be under-reported if patients are unaware that their sleepiness is abnormal or are afraid of the potential consequences of EDS (such as loss of driving license or work).

Examination of the upper airway may be important. Obvious pharyngeal crowding and tonsillar enlargement suggest upper airway obstruction [61]. The vibration of soft tissues due to heavy snoring can lead to a reddened and edematous uvula and soft palate. Systemic hypertension is commonly associated with OSA. Detailed cephalometric measurements, as predictors for OSA, seem to be more useful in the nonobese population [59].

Diagnosis of sleep-disordered breathing

The "gold standard" approach to the investigation of sleep-disordered breathing is an overnight in-laboratory sleep study (polysomnography, PSG). Sleep stage, sleep architecture and arousals from sleep are monitored during a full sleep study by two EEG channels, two electro-oculogram (EOG) channels and one electromyogram (EMG) channel. Breathing during sleep is usually monitored qualitatively with a measure of airflow at the nose/mouth, usually two measures of respiratory effort, such as diaphragm EMG and chest wall and abdominal movement, and oxygen saturation. Other variables measured include ECG, leg EMG, transcutaneous CO_2, body position and snoring. A sleep study should be scored manually and, as a minimum, the report should include the total amount of sleep and proportions of different sleep stages, the number of respiratory events seen (apneas and hypopneas per hour in both REM and non-REM sleep), the degree of oxygen desaturation recorded, the number of EEG arousals and the presence or absence of periodic leg movements. Definitions of events are not standard across all sleep laboratories and different methods for measuring airflow and other respiratory variables have differing sensitivities.

In the area of sleep-disordered breathing, the definitions of normal and abnormal sleep are under constant revision. In general, an AHI of less than 5 events/hour would be considered normal, with an AHI of greater than 15 events/hour considered to represent at least moderate disease. An AHI of 5–15 events/hour would be considered mild disease but there is significant individual variability in the symptoms related to this mild degree of OSA. If a patient is symptomatic, then a trial of treatment is warranted. However, more recent studies have suggested that an AHI between one and five may significantly increase the risk of developing hypertension, regardless of symptoms [44].

Although PSG is considered the best available test for the diagnosis of OSA, patients with OSA can have significant night-to-night variability in the severity of their disease, with the potential for a false-negative study (Box 19.2). A negative PSG with high clinical suspicion warrants further review and often even a repeat sleep study.

The expense and inconvenience of PSG have led to a search for alternative tools for the diagnosis of OSA. Overnight oximetry

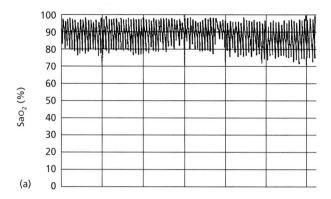

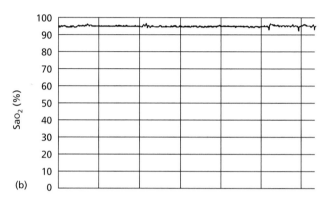

Figure 19.4 (a) One-hour oximetry recording during sleep in a patient with severe OSA, showing typical repetitive arterial oxygen desaturations. (b) One-hour oximetry recording during sleep in the same patient during treatment with nasal CPAP, with desaturations abolished and SaO_2 maintained above 90%.

Box 19.2 Reasons for false-negative sleep studies

Poor sleep efficiency (laboratory effect)
Little or no REM sleep seen
Usual sedatives or alcohol not taken
Patient not sleeping in usual position (especially supine)
Occurrence of "subcriterion events"
Night-to-night variability in the severity of OSA (significant in milder disease)

---

can detect repetitive oxygen desaturations seen in OSA (Fig. 19.4) and can be diagnostic in some patients [62]. However, not all apneic events produce significant desaturation and so a normal oximetry study does not exclude OSA. Similarly limited, portable or "at-home" systems have had some success in the diagnosis of OSA but again do not necessarily exclude the diagnosis if negative. Currently they are probably most useful in patients in whom the clinical suspicion is high or who cannot readily be studied in a laboratory, such as the immobile or medically unstable patient.

Consequences of sleep-disordered breathing
Psychosocial effects

Excessive daytime sleepiness is characteristic of sleep apnea. However, sleepiness and fatigue are commonly reported symptoms in the general community, particularly in the obese population. The sleepiness seen in patients with OSA is predominantly related to repetitive arousal and sleep fragmentation, but a direct effect of hypoxemia is possible [63]. However, OSA is characterized by a range of EDS and there is a relatively poor correlation between markers of severity of OSA, such as AHI, and daytime sleepiness. It seems likely that people vary in their susceptibility to the effects of sleep fragmentation and sleep deprivation. There are no simple tests to accurately quantify daytime sleepiness. Sleepiness may lead to both impaired work performance and driving [64]. Patients with untreated OSA form an important risk group for motor vehicle accidents. Driving performance on various simulators is impaired in patients with OSA [65]. Treatment with nasal CPAP dramatically improves daytime sleepiness and driving simulator performance [65,66,67].

Many studies have found that OSA patients perform poorly on psychometric tests compared to controls. Sleep apnea leads to defects in executive function and working memory in both adults and children [68]. There is a variable degree of improvement in cognitive function with nasal CPAP [63]. The detrimental effects of OSA have other social implications, with data from the Swedish Obese Subjects study showing that, in equally obese men and women, OSA is associated with impaired work performance, increased sick leave and a higher divorce rate [39].

Cardiovascular effects
Acute effects

The acute cardiovascular effects seen during obstructive events have been well characterized, with marked changes in both systemic and pulmonary arterial blood pressure. As an obstructive apnea progresses, there are increasing swings in pleural pressure, worsening hypoxemia, bradycardia (vagally mediated) and increased sympathetic nerve activity. As the apnea is terminated by arousal, with increased ventilation, heart rate increases and both systolic and diastolic blood pressure increase markedly (Fig. 19.5), often by more than 100 mmHg. These profound hemodynamic fluctuations are largely due to surges in sympathetic nerve activity resulting from the combination of blood gas derangement, large swings in intrathoracic pressure and arousals. Patients with OSA have increased sympathetic activity through the night, with persistence of this increased activity into wakefulness [69]. In addition, these patients have a potent pressor response to hypoxia compared to normal subjects [70], possibly due to repetitive nocturnal hypoxia. Studies using an elegant canine model of OSA have shown that sustained hypertension develops after 1–3 months of OSA [71]. Studies in rats have found that intermittent hypoxia induces a persistent increase in diurnal blood pressure, mediated through renal sympathetic nerve activity and the renin-angiotensin system [72].

Chronic effects: hypertension

Sleep apnea is a common finding among patients in hypertension clinics and similarly, many patients with OSA have hypertension

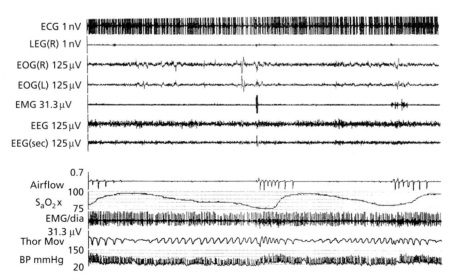

Figure 19.5 Five-minute tracing of a patient with typical severe obstructive sleep apnea. The upper traces show the variables used for sleep staging (ECG, electrocardiogram; Leg, leg electromyogram; EOG, electro-oculogram; EMG, submental electromyogram; EEG, electroencephalogram) and indicate this patient is in REM sleep. The apneas are indicated by intermittent cessation of airflow (Autoflowm nasal airflow) and are obstructive in nature, as continued respiratory effort is seen when airflow is absent (Thor Res, thoracic movement or effort; EMG/dia, diaphragm electromyogram). Repetitive falls in oxygen saturation (SaO_2) are seen following each apnea. The lowest trace is a noninvasive recording of blood pressure (BP) showing an increase in both systolic (>50 mmHg) and diastolic blood pressure (>25 mmHg) at the end of an apnea.

[73,74]. A cross-sectional study of 1400 patients referred for a sleep study showed that the degree of OSA was an independent predictor of morning blood pressure [21]. Left ventricular hypertrophy (as assessed by echocardiography), an important outcome of hypertension, was shown to be increased in normotensive patients with OSA compared to matched controls without OSA [75]. Studies of blood pressure as measured by intrarterial monitoring, automated daytime blood pressure readings or 24-hour ambulatory blood pressure have demonstrated a fall in blood pressure levels after CPAP treatment [76]. Despite these studies, a causal link between OSA hypertension has been disputed due to the presence of important confounders such as obesity and age. However, published data from two large epidemiologic studies have provided stronger evidence that OSA is an independent risk factor for hypertension, regardless of obesity. Data from the Sleep Heart Health Study, a large cross-sectional community based study with more than 6000 subjects, found that AHI and percentage of sleep time with an oxygen saturation below 90% were significantly associated with systemic hypertension, independent of anthropomorphic variables such as BMI, waist/hip ratio and neck circumference [77]. Similarly, prospective data from the Wisconsin Sleep Cohort Study [41], which followed more than 700 subjects for 4–8 years, have found a dose–response association between sleep-disordered breathing and hypertension, independent of measures of obesity. In this study, an AHI <4.9 events/hour had an odds ratio for hypertension at follow-up of 1.42, with an odds ratio of 2.03 and 2.89 for an AHI of 5.0–14.9 and >15 respectively. Therefore it is likely that the acute nocturnal surges in blood pressure in response to chemoreflex-mediated hypoxic stimulation of sympathetic activity lead to chronic hypertension [78]. A number of mechanisms have been postulated for this process including enhanced vasoconstriction and endothelial dysfunction [79,80]. Further support for an independent effect of OSA on blood pressure has been provided by studies showing that effective nasal CPAP reduces blood pressure compared with subtherapeutic CPAP [81,82]. These two studies were included in a recent meta-analysis of 12 placebo-controlled randomized trials (572 patients), which showed a statistically significant pooled reduction in mean blood pressure of 1.69 mmHg with CPAP treatment in OSA. Although this was only a modest reduction in blood pressure, most of the trials included normotensive individuals [83].

Chronic effects: cardiovascular disease and mortality

As with hypertension, cause and effect relationships between OSA and other cardiovascular endpoints are difficult to establish. A number of groups have reported an increased risk of myocardial infarction and stroke in sleep apnea [84,85]. Two recent observational cohorts have shown moderate to severe OSA to be a risk factor for stroke and with serial PSG measurements, pre-existng OSA may be a risk factor for incident stroke (and mortality) [86,87]. Potential mechanism of atherosclerosis include endothelial dysfunction and a vascular inflammatory response from hypoxia. C-reactive protein level (CRP) (an index of the presence of systemic inflammation and probably atherogenesis) is elevated in OSA [88]. Effective CPAP therapy was associated with a reduction in CRP in a population with severe OSA [89].

A number of proatherogenic factors have been shown to be promoted by untreated OSA [90]. Data from the Sleep Heart Health Study have demonstrated a relationship between AHI and prevalent cardiovascular disease (as defined by various manifestations of ischemic heart disease, heart failure and stroke) [91]. The odds ratios were fairly modest and surprisingly there did not appear to be a dose–response ratio above an AHI of 10. However, a criticism of this study is the mean age of the group (65 years). Prior work has suggested that the effects of OSA on cardiovascular disease, including mortality, are most marked in those patients under 50 years. A prospective study of more than 1600 patients found that age, BMI, hypertension and apnea index were independent predictors of death [92]. He et al. [93] observed an increased cumulative mortality in untreated patients with an apnea index >20 compared to AI <20, again most marked in patients under 50 years. Treatment with CPAP or tracheostomy reduced the mortality.

Snoring is a strong risk factor for sleep-related strokes while sleep apnea symptoms (snoring plus reported apneas or EDS) increase the risk of cerebral infarction, with an odds ratio of 8.0. Mechanisms other than increased blood pressure and sympathetic activity may be involved. Tests of platelet aggregation increased overnight in a group of patients with OSA compared to decreasing overnight in control subjects [94]. Treatment with CPAP decreased the night-time level of platelet aggregability and reversed the overnight rise seen before treatment. Other studies of vascular responsiveness have demonstrated impaired vasodilation in patients with OSA, both with and without hypertension [95]. These findings have implications in analysis of data linking obesity and cardiac disease.

Peker et al. did a 7-year follow-up study of 182 middle-aged men. They concluded that the risk for cardiovascular disease is increased fivefold in middle-aged men with OSA and that effective treatment decreases the risk to one-tenth of that in untreated men [96]. In the longest prospective cohort study (10 years), Marin and colleagues showed a higher risk of fatal and nonfatal cardiovascular events in men with severe OSA who were noncompliant with CPAP compared to healthy controls, snorers and treated patients with OSA (e.g. CPAP). Although there was potential bias with confounding variables at baseline, this is the best study to demonstrate the potential mortality associated with untreated severe OSA [97]. More difficult still is the issue of treating patients with OSA who do not have significant sleepiness, with the aim of preventing the effects of sleep-disordered breathing on cardiovascular outcomes [98].

Chronic effects: pulmonary hypertension and lung disease

Obstructive apneas can produce pulmonary hypertension acutely, largely due to hypoxic pulmonary vasoconstriction although hypercapnia may also play a role. A number of studies have found a relationship between OSA and the development of daytime pulmonary hypertension (PHT), with the prevalence of PHT ranging from 10% to 70% in patients presenting with OSA [99–101]. Some of these studies have included patients with lung disease, particularly chronic obstructive pulmonary disease (COPD), as well as OSA, possibly confounding the results. However, there are several studies that carefully excluded patients with any lung disease and these studies have found PHT in 10–40% of patients with OSA [102]. It seems likely that individual variation in the response of the pulmonary vasculature to hypoxia accounts for the development of PHT in some patients with OSA. Sleep-disordered breathing should therefore be excluded in any patient who has PHT. There are very limited data on the effects of CPAP treatment of OSA on PHT. However, a randomized cross-over study with sham and therapeutic CPAP demonstrated that CPAP reduced PHT in OSA, particularly in patients with higher PHT at baseline [103].

The "overlap syndrome" describes those patients with both OSA and lung disease, particularly COPD. The combination of these diseases results in a greater degree of pulmonary hypertension and blood gas abnormality than expected for each disease alone. In general, patients with COPD develop daytime hypercapnia only when their lung function falls below 30% of their predicted. However, patients with only moderate COPD (lung function >40% predicted) can develop significant awake hypercapnic hypoxic respiratory failure if they have co-existent OSA. The hypercapnia is due to hypoventilation secondary to changes in ventilatory control and can be partly or fully reversed with effective treatment of the sleep apnea.

Chronic effects: endocrine abnormalities

Impaired growth hormone (GH) secretion in adults can lead to central obesity and reduced bone and muscle mass; patients with obesity have low levels of GH. Men with OSA have a defect in both GH and testosterone secretion [104,105] that can be reversed with CPAP treatment, independent of any weight change. The low GH levels in OSA patients may be additive to the already low levels of obesity, but it remains unknown whether the changes in GH and testosterone in OSA result in any measurable changes in body composition or body fat distribution.

Numerous cross-sectional studies have consistently found a link between the presence and severity of OSA with glucose intolerance, insulin resistance and diabetes mellitus. In a group of patients with a high likelihood of OSA, based on questionnaire data, plasma insulin levels were found to be increased in both men and women, independent of obesity [18]. Ip et al. studied 250 consecutive subjects from a sleep clinic without known diabetes mellitus. They essentially found that obesity but also sleep apnea severity and minimum oxygen saturation were independent determinants of insulin resistance [106]. In another study of 150 mildly obese subjects sleep-disordered breathing was independently associated with glucose intolerance and insulin resistance [107]. Despite cross-sectional studies, only a few longitudinal studies have been reported with mainly subjective markers of OSA used. Finally interventional studies with CPAP have been

conflicting. Although several studies have demonstrated improvements in insulin sensitivity and HbA1c with CPAP in both nondiabetic and diabetic OSA subjects independent of any changes in weight, other recent reports, including two randomized controlled studies with larger sample sizes, showed no change in insulin sensitivity or HbA1c levels after 3 months of therapeutic versus sham CPAP in both diabetics and nondiabetics. Although negative, there were potential confounding factors, such as relatively low compliance of CPAP use suggesting insufficently treated OSA. Potential mechanisms linking OSA and insulin dysregulation include chronic intermittent hypoxia, sleep loss (due to sleep fragmentation), increased sympathetic activity, dysregulation of the hypothalamic-pituitary axis, generation of reactive oxygen species, activation of inflammatory pathways and possible changes in visceral fat in OSA with CPAP [108,109].

Treatment

The approach to any treatment should be tailored to suit the individual patient and in sleep-disordered breathing will be determined primarily by the severity of symptoms and the severity of the OSA. A secondary consideration is the presence or absence of cardiovascular risk factors. The question as to whether patients should be treated for this reason alone, regardless of symptoms, remains unanswered and this area is made more difficult by the fact that compliance with the most successful form of treatment available (CPAP) is related to the relief of symptoms. However, patient denial, either conscious or not, may produce an "asymptomatic" patient and if possible family input should be sought when a patient with a highly positive study denies symptoms. Patient occupation may also influence the decision to treat, particularly given data regarding motor vehicle accidents and OSA and the fact that sleep deprivation, common in commercial drivers, may act synergistically with even mild OSA to increase daytime sleepiness.

Weight loss

Weight loss is an important part of any treatment regime where the disease is related to obesity. Weight loss, either by caloric restriction [110–115] (Table 19.3) or bariatric surgery [116–119] (Table 19.4), significantly reduces the severity of OSA. Even moderate weight loss (10%) can decrease the AHI and improve daytime alertness. Longitudinal data on 690 subjects, followed over 8 years with sleep studies, showed that a 10% weight gain predicted an increase in the AHI of around 32% and a 10% weight loss predicted a decrease of 26% in the AHI [91,120]. In two controlled studies, 10–15% reduction in body weight lead to an approximately 50% reduction in OSA (AHI) in moderate obese males.

Short-term effects of weight loss

Several small clinical studies have evaluated the short-terms effects of varying degrees of weigh loss in patients with OSA. The

Table 19.3 Effects of dietary weight change on severity of OSA

Study	Baseline	Follow-up	Comment
Smith et al. (1985) [110]	AHI: 55 Weight: 106 kg	AHI: 29 Weight: 97 kg	Dietary means (15 patients)
Pasquali et al. (1990) [111]	AHI: 67	AHI: 33	Mean weight loss: 19 kg (23 patients)
Schwartz et al. (1990) [112]	AHI: 83	AHI: 32	Dietary means (13 patients)
Suratt et al. (1992) [113]	AHI: 90 BMI: 54 kg/m^2	AHI: 62 BMI: 46 kg/m^2	Very low-calorie diet (8 patients) 6/8 patients improved
Sampol et al. (1998) [114]			
Group I (67 patients)	AHI: 52 BMI: 32	AHI: 44 BMI: 26	Weight loss of >10% by dietary means in each group (follow-up time 11 months): cure in 34 patients in group II
Group II (34 patients)	AHI: 44 BMI: 33	AHI: 3 BMI: 27	At long-term follow-up (94 months) in group II, AHI increased to 40 from 24 in 6 patients with no change in weight
Kansanenen et al. (1998) [115]	AHI: 31	AHI: 19	Very low-calorie diet (15 patients). Mean weight loss 9 kg

Table 19.4 Effects of surgical weight change on severity of OSA

Study	Baseline	Follow-up	Comment
Harman et al. (1982) [116]	AHI: 78	AHI: 1.4	Jejuno-ileal bypass Mean weight loss 108 kg
Pillar et al. (1994) [117]	AHI: 40 BMI: 45	AHI: 11 BMI: 33	Gastric bypass/gastroplasty (14 patients) Initial results at 4/12
		AHI: 24 BMI: 35	Same group at follow-up at 7 years: note nonsignificant change in weight, but significantly worse OSA
Sugerman et al. (1992) [118]	AHI: 64	AHI: 26	Gastric bypass/gastroplasty (40 patients) Mean weight loss 57 kg
Charuzi et al. (1985) [119]	AHI: 89	AHI: 8	Gastric bypass (13 patients) Mean weight change 73%

majority of these studies all demonstrated that weight loss was associated with an improvement in OSA. These studies are, however, uncontrolled with varying degrees of obesity at baseline. Smith et al demonstrated not only a reduction in OSA with weight loss but also a reduction in pharyngeal critical closing

pressure, which indicated a reduction in upper airway collapsibility [110].

Several case series of significant weight loss through surgical procedures have been published. Although there was an improvement in OSA with dramatic weight loss, the amount of weight loss did not always correlate with the amount of improvement in OSA.

Recently a pharmacotherapy (sibutramine)-assisted weight loss study in obese men with moderate to severe OSA over 6 months was published. This study showed that weight loss of approximately 10% was associated with a reduction of AHI by approximately 30% and a reduction in subjective symptoms of OSA without a change in blood pressure [121].

Long-terms effects of weight loss

Detailed long-term studies of weight loss are lacking. In a group of 313 patients with BMI >35 kg/m^2 assessed by questionnaire 1 year after bariatric surgery, there were marked improvements in habitual snoring (82% preoperatively to 14% at follow-up), observed sleep apnea (33% to 2%) and daytime sleepiness (39% to 4%) [122]. This group had lost an average of 48% of their excess weight. However, the effects of weight loss on OSA are variable, and many patients have significant residual disease that warrants further treatment. In addition, there have been reports of OSA recurring despite maintenance of weight loss [103,106]. For these reasons, patients should be reassessed after weight loss progress.

With bariatric surgery being more frequently used for obesity, a recent meta-analysis showed dramatic improvements of OSA in the majority of patients after surgery, with an average reduction in AHI of 33.9 events/hour and OSA resolution in 85.7% [123].

Other general measures

Alcohol and sedatives such as benzodiazepines should be avoided in patients with sleep-disordered breathing. These drugs can reduce pharyngeal muscle tone and depress arousal responses, resulting in more and longer apneas during sleep. Similarly, sleep deprivation can impair upper airway muscle tone and increase arousal thresholds, increasing any tendency to OSA. Smoking cessation can reduce self-reported snoring, possibly by effects of smoke on airway inflammation, and should be encouraged (as always).

Body position may influence the frequency of apnea and hypopneas in 50–60% of patients [124]. AHI increases the in supine position and is lower in an elevated position (30–60°) and lateral position [125]. Some patients have predominantly positional apnea (related to the supine posture) and attempts to avoid this position during sleep may help reduce the severity of OSA. However, positional therapy may not be effective in the obese patient but be considered in patients with OSA who have at least twice the number of respiratory events in the supine compared to the lateral position and have an AHI <10 events/hour. Nasal obstruction will worsen any tendency to snoring and OSA and should be treated (usually pharmacologically); there is little evidence that nasal surgery is of any use in the treatment of OSA. The effects of external nasal dilator strips on snoring are variable, with some studies reporting success [126]. These strips have no effect on OSA.

Devices

Continuous positive airway pressure (CPAP)

The application of nasal CPAP for the treatment of OSA was first described by Sullivan et al. in 1981 and revolutionized the field of sleep-disordered breathing [127]. Nasal CPAP is the most effective treatment available for OSA. A CPAP machine works by delivering positive pressure to the upper airway via a nose (or face) mask, thus providing a pneumatic splint that prevents upper airway closure. The pressure is usually generated by an electromechanical blower that delivers airflow through wide-bore tubing to a nasal mask with a fixed expiratory resistance. Adjusting the airflow allows different pressures to be delivered at the nares. The optimal pressure required to prevent upper airway closure is determined by a sleep study. The required pressure can vary between 4 and 20 cmH$_2$O. Many patients show a rebound phenomenon during these treatment nights, with markedly increased amounts of REM and slow-wave sleep.

Treatment with nasal CPAP normalizes sleep architecture (see Fig. 19.4), decreases upper airway edema and significantly improves daytime sleepiness both subjectively and objectively [128]. Studies have shown that CPAP improves daytime alertness, cognitive function, mood and quality of life in patients with OSA of all degrees of severity, from mild (including "upper airway resistance syndrome") through to severe [129–133]. These studies include carefully controlled trials with either placebo tablets or subtherapeutic CPAP [134]. A recent study by Weaver et al. showed a dose–response relationship with CPAP. Normal levels of subjective and objective sleepiness, memory, and daily functioning have been achieved with more than 4.6, more than 6, and more than 7.5 hours of CPAP per night, respectively [135]. There is also evidence that treatment with CPAP reduces the incidence of actual and near miss traffic accidents in patients with OSA [136]. As discussed previously, CPAP treatment reverses many of the adverse effects of OSA on blood pressure, pulmonary hypertension, various hormonal levels, including leptin, and mortality. CPAP does not cure OSA. When treatment with CPAP is stopped, OSA recurs and symptoms return. However, regular use of CPAP may lead to a reduction in the underlying severity of OSA as assessed by sleep studies performed after a period of treatment. This reduction in severity is probably due to the effects of CPAP in reducing upper airway edema and treating sleep deprivation. Barnes et al. reported in a randomized cross-over study of CPAP versus a placebo tablet in mild OSA that CPAP failed to improve measures of objective or subjective sleepiness, and that placebo effect may account for some of the treatment responses previously reported [137].

The main problem limiting the efficacy of CPAP has been long-term compliance [138]. Various reports of compliance indicate that 40–70% of patients have difficulties with compliance [139]. On the whole, those centers that provide more intensive initial (within the first few weeks of treatment) assistance to patients have better long-term compliance; compliance with treatment in this initial period predicts long-term compliance. In addition, those patients who have the greatest symptomatic improvement with CPAP are, not surprisingly, the more compliant. The CPAP machine and mask are fairly cumbersome and inconvenient. Side-effects related to the patient–mask interface are the most common and, although often minor, have a major impact on patient tolerance and use of the treatment. Poorly fitting masks can cause skin irritation and even ulceration. More importantly, poor mask fit can result in air leak either around the mask or through the mouth. Due to the high airflow generated by the CPAP machine, leaks can produce major effects on the mouth and nose, with dryness of the mouth and nasal congestion and rhinorrhea. These problems can be effectively treated either by improving mask fit, providing a chin-strap to prevent mouth opening or humidifying and warming the air with humidifiers built into the circuit. The technology of mask and machine is constantly improving, with machines available now that ramp pressure up slowly at sleep onset and continuously adjust the required pressure through the night. These modifications may improve compliance in some patients. Those patients who require higher pressures or have milder disease are less likely to be compliant. Obese patients with OSA generally require higher pressures than patients who are not obese. Recently a study on the use of group cognitive behavioral therapy versus standard education for CPAP showed that behavioral therapy increased CPAP usage by 2.9 hours over the first month of treatment [140]. Despite these problems, CPAP remains highly effective for the treatment of all symptoms related to all degrees of OSA and should not be abandoned without intensive attempts to improve an individual's tolerance and compliance.

Newer generations of CPAP devices providing automatic adjustments of positive airway pressure are widely available. The algorithmis employed by these devices are not well known and are variable between various devices [141]. Auto-adjusting devices are generally just as effective as conventional fixed CPAP in OSA outcomes. There is also evidence that auto-adjusting devices are associated with lower mean pressures than conventional CPAP but this has not been shown to be associated with more significant compliance rates [142].

Mandibular advancement devices

Mandibular advancement devices (MAD) are intraoral orthodontic devices designed to displace the mandible anteriorly, increasing the anteroposterior diameter of the upper airway and so reducing upper airway closure and collapse when worn at night. These devices are effective at reducing snoring, assessed both objectively and subjectively [143]. The effects of these devices in OSA are less clear. Randomized controlled studies using an inactive acrylic dental plate as a placebo have confirmed the efficacy of MAD for improving OSA measured by PSG.

However, success rates depend on PSG definitions of OSA. Essentially, approximately 65% of patients achieve a 50% or greater reduction of AHI with MAD. Approximately 35–40% achieve a complete response (defined as a AHI <5 events/h) [144]. MAD have also been shown to reduce both subjective and objective measures of daytime sleepiness (including simulated driving performances). There is also evidence that MAD have a modest reduction in blood pressure (2–4 mmHg) after 1 and 3 month periods [145,146].

In comparison to CPAP, MAD are less effacious for improving PSG indices of OSA. In CPAP versus MAD cross-over studies, CPAP resulted in a greater improvement in AHI and oxyhemoglobin saturation. In a RCT comparing CPAP and MAD, sleepiness, health-related quality of life and AHI were more likely to be improved with CPAP. However, both treatments were similarly effective in reducing diastolic blood pressure compared to baseline values [147]. Despite various physiologic and PSG parameters associated with better MAD outcomes, it is not possible to predict with certainty which patients will respond to MAD in a clinical setting. These devices require careful orthodontic attention to ensure that adequate anterior displacement of the mandible is achieved. The efficacy of these devices is likely to be reduced in the more obese patients as skeletal factors and maxillofacial abnormalities are less important in the genesis of upper airway obstruction in this group. In general, these devices tend to be less effective in those patients with more severe OSA. However, if a patient is intolerant of CPAP, it may be worthwhile trialing a MAD. There are few data available on compliance but self-reported data suggest a pooled compliance rate of 77% at 1 year [148]. Short-term side-effects are generally minor and are related to excessive salivation, jaw and tooth discomfort, and occasional joint discomfort. Fortunately serious complications are not common, but occlusal changes may occur.

The American Academy of Sleep Medicine has revised its clinical practice guidelines for the treatment of snoring and OSA with oral appliances. MAD are now indicated for mild to moderate OSA in patients who prefer oral appliances to CPAP, who do not respond to CPAP, who are not suitable for treatment with CPAP, or in whom treatment attempts with CPAP are unsuccessful. CPAP should be considered before oral appliances in severe OSA and those in whom urgent treatment is required to treat severe symptoms (e.g. sleepiness) or significant co-morbidities (e.g. cardiovascular). MAD patients require sufficient teeth to retain the device. Caution is needed for those with periodontal disease or temporomandibular disease [143].

Surgery
Tracheostomy
Prior to the advent of CPAP, tracheostomy was the only effective treatment for OSA [149]. This operation is invasive, with significant morbidity, particularly in obese subjects, and is only partly effective in treating OHS. It should be reserved for those patients with very severe OSA who are completely intolerant of any other treatment. However, tracheostomy may be used as a temporary

measure for airway protection in patients with severe OSA with either morbid obesity or significant craniofacial anomalies that pose a high risk for airway compromise in the perioperative period. With skilful surgery and close follow-up, tracheostomy may be a "last-resort" therapeutic option in some patients.

Uvulopalatopharyngoplasty (UPPP) and other upper airway surgery
Surgery aims to alleviate anatomic sites of obstruction in the naso-, oro- and hypopharynx. Unfortunately, surgical success for OSA is often unpredictable and less effective than CPAP. Surgical success depends on appropriate patient selection, types of surgery and experience of surgical teams. Success rates have varied between 50% and 90% in improving OSA by greater than 50% [150].

Uvulopalatopharyngoplasty was originally described in Japan in the 1950s for the treatment of heavy snoring and involves a careful surgical removal of the uvula and part of the soft palate (with or without tonsillectomy). The operation was introduced to the US for the treatment of OSA in the early 1980s and was greeted with some enthusiasm. However, the efficacy of UPPP in the treatment of OSA is limited [151]. When treatment success is defined as a reduction in AHI of only 50%, a successful result is seen in less than 50% of patients. There are no preoperative tests that satisfactorily predict the response to surgery. There is a significant morbidity and even mortality. Excessive removal of palatal tissue can lead to velopharyngeal incompetence with nasal regurgitation and speech changes. Subsequent use of CPAP may be more difficult following UPPP. Not surprisingly, many studies report particularly poor results in obese patients. Current guidelines state that the efficacy of UPPP is variable and that it should only be considered after nonsurgical therapies have failed [149].

Modifications of the UPPP have been introduced where either a surgical laser is used to resect the palate (laser-assisted uvulopalatoplasty, LAUP) or high-frequency radio waves ("somnoplasty") are used in an attempt to stiffen palatal tissue. The treatment response is variable and unpredictable. Ryan and Love studied 44 patients at baseline and 3 months after LAUP and reported worsening of OSA (AHI increased by more than 100%) in 30% of their patient group, with a very poor relationship between subjective and objective measures of efficacy [152]. There is clearly a "placebo" effect in snoring surgery that has been demonstrated in other forms of surgical intervention. A randomized controlled study comparing temperature-controlled radiofrequency ablation to the tongue base and palate (TCRFTA) with CPAP and sham CPAP (ineffective CPAP) showed that treatment with TCRFTA and CPAP improved quality of life scores and sleepiness in mild to moderate OSA [153].

More complex maxillo-acial surgery, usually performed in two phases, has been used with some success in the treatment of OSA. The first phase involves a UPPP in combination with genioglossus advancement, via a mandibular osteotomy, and hyoid myotomy. The Stanford group has reported overall success rates of around 60% with this procedure, but with less success in those patients with more severe disease (>60 events per hour and desaturation to 70%) and in the morbidly obese [154]. The second phase involves bimaxillary advancement, which was reported to be as successful as CPAP in treating a group of patients with severe OSA (AHI 68/h) and a mean BMI of 31 kg/m² [155]. In contrast, Bettega et al. found that phase I surgery was generally ineffective in OSA, with successful results in only 22% of patients [156]. In their study, phase II surgery was successful in 75% of patients, but morbidity was significant. These complex surgical procedures are highly specialized and not widely available. Other surgical procedures including mandibular osteotomy with genioglossus advancement, hyoid myotomy suspension and distraction osteogenesis have been associated with surgical success in highly selected patients [150].

Pharmacologic treatment

There are no placebo-controlled studies showing constant efficacy of any medication in OSA or OHS [157]. Obviously, weight-lowering drugs will be of benefit through weight loss but no drug has been found that alters the collapsibility of the upper airway during sleep. Studies looking at agents such as medroxyprogesterone, protriptyline and SSRIs as a primary therapy for OSA have been disappointing. Although mirtazapine initially looked promising for OSA, a recent randomized placebo-controlled study showed negative effects of mirtazepine such as weight gain and a potential for worsening OSA [158]. A systematic review concluded that current data do not support the use of drugs as an alternative to CPAP in OSA [159].

Two randomized, double-blind placebo-controlled trials have shown that modafinil (nonamphetamine wakefulness promoter) may be useful as an adjunct therapy for OSA patients who are still sleepy despite CPAP use. Modafinil does not seem to affect sleep-disordered breathing (i.e. AHI) but improves measures of sleepiness compared to placebo [160,161].

Management of OSA with daytime respiratory failure (including OHS)

There are no current guidelines for the management of OHS. Oxygen therapy without PAP is usually inadequate as it does not improve upper airway obstruction or nocturnal hypoventilation. Respiratory stimulants have been trialled in small studies with very limited success. Obviously weight loss (including bariatric surgery) will be an important aspect of therapy but studies are limited. Patients should be managed in a specialist sleep and respiratory failure center and, depending on the chronicity and severity of their condition, many are best managed with a brief period of hospitalization. There is a wide range in the degree of hypercapnic hypoxic respiratory failure associated with the combination of OSA and obesity, and the management of these patients should be individualized.

Patients may come to medical attention with acute-on-chronic respiratory failure due to a superimposed condition such as a respiratory tract infection or even postanesthetic for an unrelated surgical procedure. In these decompensated patients, oxygen therapy alone should be used with caution and with very close monitoring of hypercapnia and, as the main pathology in these patients is impaired respiratory drive, sedatives or hypnotics should be avoided. Treatments available for these decompensated patients, and for those patients with severe chronic respiratory failure due to OHS, were very high CPAP pressures, CPAP plus added oxygen or NIPPV or, for the most unwell or obtunded patients, a short period of intubation and mechanical ventilation [162,163].

NIPPV can deliver either volume-cycled ventilation or positive pressure ventilation to the upper airway via nose- or facemask, effectively providing mechanical ventilation without the need for intubation. These devices can provide support to the patient's spontaneous respiratory efforts or deliver a set number of breaths as a back-up if the patient's inspiratory efforts are inadequate to trigger the machine. These devices are extremely effective in the treatment of both acute and chronic respiratory failure due to hypoventilation related to obesity and OSA [164,165] and are well tolerated by the patient (Fig. 19.6).

When the acutely unwell patient has been stabilized, sleep studies can be performed to determine whether home use of

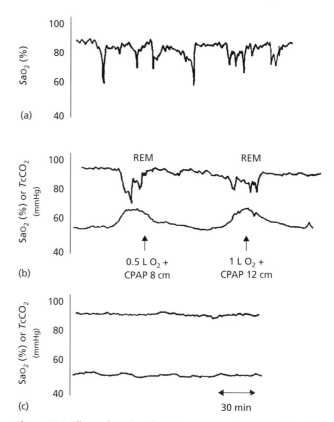

Figure 19.6 Efficacy of nasal ventilation in a patient with OHS. Recordings of oxygen saturation (SaO_2, %) show marked falls in oxygen level during sleep (a). Addition of CPAP and low-flow oxygen (0.5 L = 0.5 L/min of supplemental oxygen; 1 L = 1 L/min) results in normal oxygen saturation in NREM sleep but persisting hypoxemia in REM sleep (b). Use of nasal ventilation, either pressure support or volume cycled, will prevent oxygen desaturation in REM sleep (c) and prevent rises in transcutaneous CO_2 ($tcCO_2$) levels.

NIPPV is required, at what pressures and whether added oxygen is needed. A similar approach is used in the treatment of patients with chronic severe OHS. After a period of treatment with NIPPV (months), some of these patients can be treated with CPAP alone. A specialist sleep unit with expertise in the long-term management of sleep-related respiratory failure best manages these patients. Clinical consensus suggests NIPPV should be used in decompensated (e.g. impaired consciousness) OHS patients [166].

More commonly, patients with OHS or in stable hypercapnic respiratory failure without decompensation will present to sleep clinics. Most studies with stable OHS should undergo a CPAP titration (plus or minus oxygen) study with reasonable success but NIPPV may be required. A recent study showed that both CPAP and NIPPV will have similar outcomes at 3 months but patients were excluded if they failed an initial CPAP titration study (persisting marked hypoxemia with CPAP) [167]. Predictors of CPAP failure include greater degrees of obesity, significant restrictive physiology, severity of hypoxemia during PSG and higher $PaCO_2$ levels during wakefulness [168].

In summary, CPAP is effective in the majority of patients with stable OHS; however, NIPPV may be required in patients who fail CPAP, those with decompensated hypercapnic respiratory failure or those with predominat hypoventilation without upper airway obstruction (e.g. OSA) [169].

Conclusion

Obesity can produce a measurable reduction in lung function and is very strongly associated with breathing disorders in sleep such as obstructive sleep apnea (OSA) and hypoventilation. Moderate to severe degrees of obesity can lead to a restrictive abnormality in lung function due to the mechanical effects of central body fat. Obese subjects may have reduced lung volumes and an increased work of breathing. Central fat deposition is also linked to upper airway collapsibility in sleep and epidemiologic data have identified obesity as a crucial risk factor in the development of OSA. Sleep-disordered breathing has a number of clinical consequences, including excess cardiovascular morbidity. The combination of obesity-induced reduced pulmonary function and sleep-disordered breathing can lead to progressive respiratory failure during sleep, finally resulting in awake hypercapnic respiratory failure (OHS, central hypoventilation). This respiratory failure can occur without any intrinsic lung disease. Weight reduction can improve lung function and reduce the severity of sleep apnea and OHS. Treatment of sleep-breathing disorders has been advanced greatly by the use of positive airway pressure devices and OHS can be reversed with the use of these devices.

References

1. Guilleminault C, Stoohs R, Clerk A, Simmons J, Labanowski M. From obstructive sleep apnea syndrome to upper airway resistance syndrome: consistency of daytime sleepiness. Sleep 1992;15(6 suppl):S13–16.
2. Remmers JE, deGroot WJ, Sauerland EK, Anch AM. Pathogenesis of upper airway occlusion during sleep. J Appl Physiol 1978;44(6): 931–8.
3. McNamara SG, Grunstein RR, Sullivan CE. Obstructive sleep apnea. Thorax 1993;48(7):754–64.
4. Rubinstein I, Bradley TD, Zamel N, Hoffstein V. Glottic and cervical tracheal narrowing in patients with obstructive sleep apnea. J Appl Physiol 1989;67(6):2427–31.
5. Sullivan CE GR, Marrone O, Berthon-Jones M. Sleep apnea – pathophysiology: upper airway and control of breathing. In: Guilleminault CPM (ed) *Obstructive Sleep Apnea Syndrome: Clinical Research and Treatment*. New York: Raven Press, 1990.
6. Fleetham JA. Upper airway imaging in relation to obstructive sleep apnea. Clin Chest Med 1992;13(3):399–416.
7. Schwab RJ, Gefter WB, Hoffman EA, Gupta KB, Pack AI. Dynamic upper airway imaging during awake respiration in normal subjects and patients with sleep disordered breathing. Am Rev Respir Dis 1993;148(5):1385–400.
8. Horner RL, Innes JA, Murphy K, Guz A. Evidence for reflex upper airway dilator muscle activation by sudden negative airway pressure in man. J Physiol 1991;436:15–29.
9. Mezzanotte WS, Tangel DJ, White DP. Waking genioglossal electromyogram in sleep apnea patients versus normal controls (a neuromuscular compensatory mechanism). J Clin Invest 1992;89(5):1571–9.
10. Larsson H, Carlsson-Nordlander B, Lindblad LE, Norbeck O, Svanborg E. Temperature thresholds in the oropharynx of patients with obstructive sleep apnea syndrome. Am Rev Respir Dis 1992;146(5 Pt 1):1246–9.
11. Katz I, Stradling J, Slutsky AS, Zamel N, Hoffstein V. Do patients with obstructive sleep apnea have thick necks? Am Rev Respir Dis 1990;141(5 Pt 1):1228–31.
12. Davies RJ, Stradling JR. The relationship between neck circumference, radiographic pharyngeal anatomy, and the obstructive sleep apnea syndrome. Eur Respir J 1990;3(5):509–14.
13. Koenig JS, Thach BT. Effects of mass loading on the upper airway. J Appl Physiol 1988;64(6):2294–9.
14. Brown IG, Zamel N, Hoffstein V. Pharyngeal cross-sectional area in normal men and women. J Appl Physiol 1986;61:890.
15. Ciscar MA, Juan G, Martinez V. Magnetic resonance imaging of the pharynx in OSA patients and healthy subjects. Eur Respir J 2001;1(1):1–8.
16. Miles PG, Vig PS, Weyant RJ. Craniofacial structure and obstructive sleep apnea syndrome – a qualitative analysis and meta-analysis of the literature. Am J Orthod Dentofac Orthop 1996;109:163.
17. Do KL, Ferreyra H, Healy JF, Davidson TM. Does tongue size differ between patients with and without sleep-disordered breathing? Laryngoscope 2000;110:1552–5.
18. Schwab RJ, Gupta KB, Gefter WB, Metzger LJ, Hoffman EA, Pack AI. Upper airway and soft tissue anatomy in normal subjects and patients with sleep-disordered breathing. Significance of the lateral pharyngeal walls. Am J Respir Crit Care Med 1995;152(5 Pt 1): 1673–89.
19. Schwab RJ, Pasirstein M, Pierson R, Mackley A. Identification of upper airway anatomic risk factors for obstructive sleep apnea with volumetric magnetic resonance imaging. Am J Respir Crit Care Med 2003;168;522–30.

20. Grunstein RR, Stenlof K, Hedner J, Sjostrom L. Impact of obstructive sleep apnea and sleepiness on metabolic and cardiovascular risk factors in the Swedish Obese Subjects (SOS) Study. Int J Obes 1995;19(6):410–18.

21. Grunstein R, Wilcox I, Yang TS, Gould Y, Hedner J. Snoring and sleep apnea in men: association with central obesity and hypertension. Int J Obes 1993;17(9):533–40.

22. van de Graaff WB. Thoracic influence on upper airway patency. J Appl Physiol 1988;65(5):2124–31.

23. Lopata M, Onal E. Mass loading, sleep apnea, and the pathogenesis of obesity hypoventilation. Am Rev Respir Dis 1982;126(4):640–5.

24. Series F, Cormier Y, Desmeules M. Influence of passive changes of lung volume on upper airways. J Appl Physiol 1990;68(5):2159–64.

25. Begle RL, Badr S, Skatrud JB, Dempsey JA. Effect of lung inflation on pulmonary resistance during NREM sleep. Am Rev Respir Dis 1990;141(4 Pt 1):854–60.

26. Wade AJ, Marbut MM, Round JM. Muscle fibre type and aetiology of obesity. Lancet 1990;335(8693):805–8.

27. Rubinstein I, Colapinto N, Rotstein LE, Brown IG, Hoffstein V. Improvement in upper airway function after weight loss in patients with obstructive sleep apnea. Am Rev Respir Dis 1988;138(5):1192–5.

28. Nobar S, Burkart KM, Zwillich CW. Hypoventilation among obese patients: a common and under-diagnosed problem. Am J Respir Crit Care Med 2000;161:A890.

29. Berthon-Jones M, Sullivan CE. Time course of change in ventilatory response to CO_2 with long-term CPAP therapy for obstructive sleep apnea. Am Rev Respir Dis 1987;135(1):144–7.

30. Fleetham JA, Arnup ME, Anthonisen NR. Familial aspects of ventilatory control in patients with chronic obstructive pulmonary disease. Am Rev Respir Dis 1984;129(1):3–7

31. Leech JA, Onal E, Baer P, Lopata M. Determinants of hypercapnia in occlusive sleep apnea syndrome. Chest 1987;92(5):807–13.

32. O'Donnell C P, Schaub CD, Haines AS, et al. Leptin prevents respiratory depression in obesity. Am J Respir Crit Care Med 1999;159(5 Pt 1):1477–84.

33. Phillips BG, Kato M, Narkiewicz K, Choe I, Somers VK. Increases in leptin levels, sympathetic drive, and weight gain in obstructive sleep apnea. Am J Physiol Heart Circ Physiol 2000;279(1):H234–7.

34. Chin K, Shimizu K, Nakamura T, et al. Changes in intra-abdominal visceral fat and serum leptin levels in patients with obstructive sleep apnea syndrome following nasal continuous positive airway pressure therapy. Circulation 1999;100(7):706–12.

35. Yee BJ, Cheung J, Phipps P, Banerjee D, Piper AJ, Grunstein RR. Treatment of obesity hyponventilation syndrome and serum leptin. Respiration 2006;73:209–12

36. Phipps PR, Starritt E, Caterson I, Grunstein RR. Association of serum leptin with hypoventilation in human obesity. Thorax 2002;57:75–6.

37. Young T, Palta M, Dempsey J, Skatrud J, Weber S, Badr S. The occurrence of sleep-disordered breathing among middle-aged adults. N Engl J Med 1993;328(17):1230–5.

38. Bearpark H, Elliott L, Grunstein R, et al. Snoring and sleep apnea. A population study in Australian men. Am J Respir Crit Care Med 1995;151(5):1459–65.

39. Punjabi NM. The epidemiology of adult obstructive sleep apnea. Proc Am Thorac Soc 2008;5:136–43.

40. Grunstein RR, Stenlof K, Hedner JA, Sjostrom L. Impact of self-reported sleep-breathing disturbances on psychosocial performance in the Swedish Obese Subjects (SOS) Study. Sleep 1995;18(8):635–43.

41. Peppard PE, Young T, Palta M, Skatrud J. Prospective study of the association between sleep-disordered breathing and hypertension. N Engl J Med 2000;342(19):1378–84.

42. Young T, Shahar E, Nieto FJ, et al. Predictors of sleep-disordered breathing in community-dwelling adults: the Sleep Heart Health Study. Arch Intern Med 2002;162:893–900.

43. Launois SH, Pepin JL, Levy P. Sleep apnea in elderly: a specific entity? Sleep Med Rev 2007;131:1702–9.

44. Redline S, Kump K, Tishler PV, Browner I, Ferrette V. Gender differences in sleep disordered breathing in a community-based sample. Am J Respir Crit Care Med 1994;149(3 Pt 1):722–6.

45. Brooks LJ, Strohl KP. Size and mechanical properties of the pharynx in healthy men and women. Am Rev Respir Dis 1992;146(6):1394–7.

46. Bixler E, Vgontzas A, Lin H, ten Have T, Rein J. Prevalence of sleep-disordered breathing in women. Am J Respir Crit Care Med 2001;163:608–13.

47. Shahar E, Redline S, Young T, Boland L, Baldwin C. Hormone replacment therapy and sleep-disordered breathing. Am J Respir Crit Care Med 2003;167:1186–92.

48. Cistulli P, Barnes DJ, Grunstein RR, Sullivan CE. Effect of short-term hormone replacement in the treatment of obstructive sleep apnea in postmenopausal women. Thorax 1994;49:699–702.

49. Nelson S, Hans M. Contribution of craniofacial risk factors in increasing apneic activity among obese and nonobese habitual snorers. Chest 1997;111(1):154–62.

50. Cistulli PA. Cranialfacial abnormalities in obstructive sleep apnea: implications for treatment. Respirology 1996;1:167–74.

51. Cistulli PA, Sullivan CE. Sleep apnea in Marfan's syndrome. Increased upper airway collapsibility during sleep. Chest 1995;108(3):631–5.

52. Lofaso F, Coste A, d'Ortho MP, et al. Nasal obstruction as a risk factor for sleep apnea syndrome. Eur Respir J 2000;16(4):639–43.

53. Ferguson KA, Ono T, Lowe AA, Ryan CF, Fleetham JA. The relationship between obesity and craniofacial structure in obstructive sleep apnea. Chest 1995;108(2):375–81.

54. Grunstein RR, Sullivan CE. Sleep apnea and hypothyroidism: mechanisms and management. Am J Med 1988;85(6):775–9.

55. Grunstein RR, Ho KY, Sullivan CE. Sleep apnea in acromegaly. Ann Intern Med 1991;115(7):527–32.

56. Rosenow F, McCarthey V, Caruso AC. Sleep apnea in endocrine diseses. J Sleep Res 1998;7(1):3–11.

57. Sin DD, Fitzgerald F, Parker JD, Newton G, Floras JS, Bradley TD. Risk factors for central and obstructive sleep apnea in 450 men and women with congestive heart failure. Am J Respir Crit Care Med 1999;160(4):1101–6.

58. Parra O, Arboix A, Bechich S, et al. Time course of sleep-related breathing disorders in first-ever stroke or transient ischemic attack. Am J Respir Crit Care Med 2000;161(2 Pt 1):375–80.

59. Redline S, Strohl KP. Recognition and consequences of obstructive sleep apnea hypopnea syndrome. Clin Chest Med 1998;19(1):1–19.

60. Ambrogetti A, Olson LG, Saunders NA. Differences in the symptoms of men and women with obstructive sleep apnea. Aust NZ J Med 1991;21(6):863–6.

61. Hoffstein V, Szalai JP. Predictive value of clinical features in diagnosing obstructive sleep apnea. Sleep 1993;16(2):118–22.

62. Gyulay S, Olson LG, Hensley MJ, King MT, Allen KM, Saunders NA. A comparison of clinical assessment and home oiximetry in the diagnosis of obstructive sleep apnea. Am Rev Respir Dis 1993;147(1):50–3.

63. Montplaisir J, Bedard MA, Richer F, Rouleau I. Neurobehavioral manifestations in obstructive sleep apnea syndrome before and after treatment with continuous positive airway pressure. Sleep 1992;15(6 suppl):S17–19.

64. Findley LJ, Fabrizio MJ, Knight H, Norcross BB, LaForte AJ, Suratt PM. Driving simulator performance in patients with sleep apnea. Am Rev Respir Dis 1989;140(2):529–30.

65. Juniper M, Hack MA, George CF, Davies RJ, Stradling JR. Steering simulation performance in patients with obstructive sleep apnea and matched control subjects. Eur Respir J 2000;15(3):590–5.

66. Findley L, Smith C, Hooper J, Dineen M, Suratt PM. Treatment with nasal CPAP decreases automobile accidents in patients with sleep apnea. Am J Respir Crit Care Med 2000;161(3 Pt 1):857–9.

67. George CF, Boudreau AC, Smiley A. Effects of nasal CPAP on simulated driving performance in patients with obstructive sleep apnea. Thorax 1997;52(7):648–53.

68. Beebe DW, Gozal D. Obstructive sleep apnea and the prefrontal cortex: towards a comprehensive model linking nocturnal upper airway. obstruction to daytime cognitive and behavioural deficits. J Sleep Res 2002;11:1–16.

69. Carlson JT, Hedner J, Elam M, Ejnell H, Sellgren J, Wallin BG. Augmented resting sympathetic activity in awake patients with obstructive sleep apnea. Chest 1993;103(6):1763–8.

70. Hedner JA, Wilcox I, Laks L, Grunstein RR, Sullivan CE. A specific and potent pressor effect of hypoxia in patients with sleep apnea. Am Rev Respir Dis 1992;146(5 Pt 1):1240–5.

71. Brooks D, Horner RL, Kozar LF, Render-Teixeira CL, Phillipson EA. Obstructive sleep apnea as a cause of systemic hypertension. Evidence from a canine model. J Clin Invest 1997;99(1):106–9.

72. Fletcher EC, Bao G, Li R. Renin activity and blood pressure in response to chronic episodic hypoxia. Hypertension 1999;34(2):309–14.

73. Worsnop CJ, Naughton MT, Barter CE, Morgan TO, Anderson AI, Pierce RJ. The prevalence of obstructive sleep apnea in hypertensives. Am J Respir Crit Care Med 1998;157(1):111–15.

74. Stradling JR, Crosby JH. Predictors and prevalence of obstructive sleep apnea and snoring in 1001 middle aged men. Thorax 1991;46(2):85–90.

75. Hedner J, Ejnell H, Caidahl K. Left ventricular hypertrophy independent of hypertension in patients with obstructive sleep apnea. J Hypertens 1990;8(10):941–6.

76. Working Group on OSA and Hypertension. Obstructive sleep apnea and blood pressure elevation: what is the relationship? Blood Press 1993;2(3):166–82.

77. Nieto FJ, Young TB, Lind BK, et al. Association of sleep-disordered breathing, sleep apnea, and hypertension in a large community-based study. Sleep Heart Health Study. JAMA 2000;283(14):1829–36.

78. Somers VK, Mark AL, Zavala DC, Abbound FM. Contrasting effects of hypoxia and hypercapnia on ventilation and sympathetic activity in humans. J Appl Physiol 1989;67:2095–100.

79. Kato M, Roberts-Thompson P, Philips BG, Haynes WG. Impairment of endothelium-dependent vasodilation of resistance vessels in aptients with obstructive sleep apnea. Circulation 2000;102:2607–10.

80. Wolk R, Kara T, Somers VK. Sleep-disordered breathing and cardiovascular disease. Circulation 2003;108:9–12.

81. Becker HF, Jerrentrup A, Ploch T, Grote L, Penzel T. Effects of nasal continuous positive airway pressure treatment on blood pressure in patients with obstructive sleep apnea. Circulation 2003;107:68–73.

82. Pepperell JC, Ramdassingh-Dow S, Crosthwaite N, Mullins R. Ambulatory blood pressure after therapeutic and subtherapeutic nasal continuous positive airway pressure for obstructive sleep apnea: a randomised parallel trial. Lancet 2002;359:204–10.

83. Haentjens P, van Meerhaeghe A, Moscariello A, et al. The impact of continous positive airway pressure on blood pressure in patients with obstructive sleep apnea syndrome: evidence from a meta-analysis of placebo-controlled randomized trials. Arch Intern Med 2007;167:757–64.

84. Hung J, Whitford EG, Parsons RW, Hillman DR. Association of sleep apnea with myocardial infarction in men. Lancet 1990;336(8710):261–4.

85. Palomaki H, Partinen M, Erkinjuntti T, Kaste M. Snoring, sleep apnea syndrome, and stroke. Neurology 1992;42(7 suppl 6):75–81; discussion 82.

86. Arzt M, Young T, Finn L, Skatrud JB, Bradley TD. Association of sleep-disordered breathing and the occurance of stroke. Am J Respir Crit Care Med 2005;172:1447–51.

87. Yaggi HK, Concato J, Kernan WN, Lichtman JH, Brass LM, Mohsenin V. Obstructive sleep apnea as a risk factor for stroke and death. N Engl J Med 2005;353:2034–41.

88. Shamsuzzamam AS, Winnicki M, Lanfranchi P, Wolk R, Kara T. Elevated C-reactive protein in patients with obstructive sleep apnea. Circulation 2002;105:2462–4.

89. Yokoe T, Minoguchi K, Matsuo H, et al. Elevated levels of C-reactive protein and interleukin-6 in patients with obstructive sleep apnea syndrome are decreased by nasal continuous positive airway pressure. Circulation 2003;107:1129–34.

90. Dyugovskaya L, Lavie P, Lavie L. Increased adhesion molecules expression and production of reactive oxygen species in leukocytes of sleep. Am J Respir Crit Care Med 2002;165:934–9.

91. Shahar E, Whitney CW, Redline S, et al. Sleep-disordered breathing and cardiovascular disease: cross sectional results of the Sleep Heart Health Study. Am J Respir Crit Care Med 2001;163:19–25.

92. Lavie P, Herer P, Peled R, et al. Mortality in sleep apnea patients: a multivariate analysis of risk factors. Sleep 1995;18(3):149–57.

93. He J, Kryger MH, Zorick FJ, Conway W, Roth T. Mortality and apnea index in obstructive sleep apnea. Experience in 385 male patients. Chest 1988;94(1):9–14.

94. Sanner BM, Konermann M, Tepel M, Groetz J, Mummenhoff C, Zidek W. Platelet function in patients with obstructive sleep apnea syndrome. Eur Respir J 2000;16(4):648–52.

95. Carlson JT, Rangemark C, Hedner JA. Attenuated endothelium-dependent vascular relaxation in patients with sleep apnea. J Hypertens 1996;14(5):577–84.

96. Peker Y, Hedner J, Norum J, Kraiczi H, Carlson J. Increased incidence of cardiovascular disease in middle-aged men with obstructive sleep apnea: a 7-year follow up. Am J Respir Crit Care Med 2002;165:1395–9.

97. Marin JM, Carrizo SJ, Vicente E, Agusti AG. Long-term cardiovascular outcomes in men with obstructive sleep apnea-hypopnea

syndrome with or without treatment with continuous positive airway pressure: an observational study. Lancet 2005;365:1046–53.

98. Hedner J. Editorial. Am J Respir Crit Care Med 2001;163:5–6.

99. Weitzenblum E, Krieger J, Apprill M, et al. Daytime pulmonary hypertension in patients with obstructive sleep apnea syndrome. Am Rev Respir Dis 1988;138(2):345–9.

100. Sajkov D, Cowie RJ, Thornton AT, Espinoza HA, McEvoy RD. Pulmonary hypertension and hypoxemia in obstructive sleep apnea syndrome. Am J Respir Crit Care Med 1994;149(2 Pt 1):416–22.

101. Sajkov D, Wang T, Saunders NA, Bune AJ, Neill AM, Douglas Mcevoy R. Daytime pulmonary hemodynamics in patients with obstructive sleep apnea without lung disease. Am J Respir Crit Care Med 1999;159(5 Pt 1):1518–26.

102. Bady E, Achkar A, Pascal S, Orvoen-Frija E, Laaban JP. Pulmonary arterial hypertension in patients with sleep apnea syndrome. Thorax 2000;55(11):934–9.

103. Arias MA, Garcia-Rio F, Alonso-Fernandez A, Martinez I, Villamor J. Pulmonary hypertension in obstructive sleep apnea: effects of continous positive airway pressure: a randomised, controlled crossover study. Eur Heart J 2006;27:1106–13.

104. Grunstein RR, Handelsman DJ, Lawrence SJ, Blackwell C, Caterson ID, Sullivan CE. Neuroendocrine dysfunction in sleep apnea: reversal by continuous positive airways pressure therapy. J Clin Endocrinol Metab 1989;68(2):352–8.

105. Grunstein RR, Handelsman DJ, Stewart DA, Sullivan CE. Growth hormone secretion is increased by nasal CPAP treatment of sleep apnea. Am Rev Respir Dis 1993;147:A686.

106. Ip MS, Lam B, Ng MN, Lam WK, Tsang KW, Lam KS. Obstructive sleep apnea is independently associated with insulin resistacne. Am J Respir Crit Care Med 2002;165:670–6.

107. Punjabi NM, Sorkin JD, Katzel LI, Goldberg AP, Schwartz AR, Smoth PL. Sleep-disordered breathing and insulin resistance in middle-aged and overweight men. Am J Respir Crit Care Med 2002;165:677–82.

108. Tasali E, Ip MSM. Obstructive sleep apnea and metabolic syndrome. Proc Am Thorac Soc 2008;5:202–17.

109. Trennell MI, Ward JA, Yee BJ, et al. Influence of constant positive airway pressure on lipid storage, muscle metabolism and insulin action in obese patients with severe obstructive sleep apnea. Diabetes Obes Metab 2007;9:679–87.

110. Smith PL, Gold AR, Meyers DA, Haponik EF, Bleecker ER. Weight loss in mildly to moderately obese patients with obstructive sleep apnea. Ann Intern Med 1985;103(6 Pt 1):850–5.

111. Pasquali R, Colella P, Cirignotta F. Treatment of obese patients with obstructive sleep apnea syndrome: effect of weight loss and interference otorhinolaryngoiatric pathology. Int J Obes 1990;14:207–17.

112. Schwartz AR, Gold AR, Schubert N. Effect of weight loss on upper airway collapsibility in obstructive sleep apnea. Am Rev Respir Dis 1991;144:494–8.

113. Suratt PM, McTier RF, Findley LJ, Pohl SL, Wilhoit SC. Effect of very-low-calorie diets with weight loss on obstructive sleep apnea. Am J Clin Nutr 1992;56(1 suppl):182S–184S.

114. Sampol G, Munoz X, Sagales MT. Long term efficacy of dietary weight loss in sleep apnea/hypopnoea syndrome. Eur Respir J 1998;12:1156–9.

115. Kansanen M, Vanninen E, Tuunainen A. The effect of very low-calorie diet-induced weight loss on the severity of obstructive sleep apnea and autonomic nervous function in obese patients with obstructive sleep apnea syndrome. Clin Physiol 1998;18:377–85.

116. Harman EM, Wynne JW, Block AJ. The effect of weight loss on sleep disordered breathing and oxygen desaturation in morbidly obese men. Chest 1982;82:291–4.

117. Pillar G, Peled R, Lavie P. Recurrence of sleep apnea without concomitant weight increase 7.5 years after weight reduction surgery. Chest 1994;106(6):1702–4.

118. Sugerman HJ, Fairman RP, Sood RK. Long-term effects of gastric surgery for treating respiratory insufficiency of obesity. Am J Clin Nutr 1992;55:597S–601S.

119. Charuzi I, Ovnat A, Peiser J. The effect of surgical weight reduction on sleep quality in obese-related sleep apnea syndrome. Surgery 1985;97:535–8.

120. Peppard PE, Young T, Palta M, Dempsey J, Skatrud J. Longitudinal study of moderate weight change and sleep-disordered breathing. JAMA 2000;284(23):3015–21.

121. Yee BJ, Phillips CL, Banerjee D, Caterson I, Hedner JA, Grunstein RR. The effect of sibutramine-assisted weight loss in men with obstructive sleep apnea. Int J Obes 2007;312:161–8.

122. Dixon JB, Schachter LM, O'Brien PE. Sleep disturbance and obesity: changes following surgically induced weight loss. Arch Intern Med 2001;161(1):102–6.

123. Buchwald HA, Avidor Y, Braunwald E, et al. Bariatric surgery: a systemic review and meta-analysis. JAMA 2004;292:1724–37.

124. Cartwright RD. Effect of sleep position on sleep apnea severity. Sleep 1984;7:110–14.

125. McEvoy RD, Sharp DJ, Thornton AT. The effects of posture on obstructive sleep apnea. Am Rev Respir Dis 1986;133:662–6.

126. Pevernagie D, Hamans E, van Cauwenberge P, Pauwels R. External nasal dilation reduces snoring in chronic rhinitis patients: a randomized controlled trial. Eur Respir J 2000;15(6):996–1000.

127. Sullivan CE, Issa FG, Berthon-Jones M, Eves L. Reversal of obstructive sleep apnea by continuous positive airway pressure applied through the nares. Lancet 1981;1(8225):862–5.

128. Sullivan CE, Grunstein RR. Continuous positive airway pressure in sleep disordered breathing. In: Kryger MH, Dement WC, Roth TP (eds) *Principles and Practice of Sleep Medicine*. Philadelphia: WB Saunders, 1994: 559–70.

129. Engleman HM, Kingshott RN, Wraith PK, Mackay TW, Deary IJ, Douglas NJ. Randomized placebo-controlled crossover trial of continuous positive airway pressure for mild sleep apnea/hypopnea syndrome. Am J Respir Crit Care Med 1999;159(2):461–7.

130. Engleman HM, Martin SE, Kingshott RN, Mackay TW, Deary IJ, Douglas NJ. Randomised placebo controlled trial of daytime function after continuous positive airway pressure (CPAP) therapy for the sleep apnea/hypopnoea syndrome. Thorax 1998;53(5):341–5.

131. Jenkinson C, Stradling J, Petersen S. Comparison of three measures of quality of life outcome in the evaluation of continuous positive airways pressure therapy for sleep apnea. J Sleep Res 1997;6(3):199–204.

132. Ballester E, Badia JR, Hernandez L, et al. Evidence of the effectiveness of continuous positive airway pressure in the treatment of sleep apnea/hypopnea syndrome. Am J Respir Crit Care Med 1999;159(2):495–501.

133. Engleman HM, Martin SE, Deary IJ, Douglas NJ. Effect of continuous positive airway pressure treatment on daytime function in sleep apnea/hypopnoea syndrome. Lancet 1994;343(8897):572–5.

134. Jenkinson C, Davies RJ, Mullins R, Stradling JR. Comparison of therapeutic and subtherapeutic nasal continuous positive airway

pressure for obstructive sleep apnea: a randomised prospective par-allel trial. Lancet 1999;353(9170):2100–5.

135. Weaver TE, Maislin G, Dinges DF, et al. Relationship between hours of CPAP use and achieving normal levels of sleepiness and daily functioning. Sleep 2007;30:711–19.

136. Krieger J, Meslier N, Lebrun T, et al. Accidents in obstructive sleep apnea patients treated with nasal continuous positive airway pres-sure: a prospective study. The Working Group ANTADIR, Paris and CRESGE, Lille, France. Association Nationale de Traitement a Domicile des Insuffisants Respiratoires. Chest 1997;112(6): 1561–6.

137. Barnes M, Houston D, Worsnop CJ, et al. A randomised controlled trial of continuous positive airway pressure in mild obstructive sleep apnea. Am J Respir Crit Care Med 2002;165:773–80.

138. Grunstein RR. Sleep-related breathing disorders. 5. Nasal continu-ous positive airway pressure treatment for obstructive sleep apnea. Thorax 1995;50(10):1106–13.

139. Krieger J. Long-term compliance with nasal continuous positive airway pressure (CPAP) in obstructive sleep apnea patients and nonapneic snorers. Sleep 1992;15(6 suppl):S42–6.

140. Richards D, Bartlett DJ, Wong K, Malouff J, Grunstein RR. Increased adherence to CPAP with a group cognitive behavioural treatment intervention: a randomized trial. Sleep 2007;30:635–40.

141. Farre R, Montserrat JM, Rigau J, Trepat X. Response of automatic continuous positive airway pressure devices to different sleep breathing patterns: a bench study. Am J Respir Crit Care Med 2002;166:469.

142. Littner M, Hirshkowitz M, Davila D, Anderson WM, Kushida CA. Practice parameters for the use of auto-titrating continuous positive airway pressure devices for titrating pressures and treating adult patients with obstructive sleep panea syndrome: an American Academy of Sleep Medicine report. Sleep 2002;25:143.

143. Kushida CA, Morgenthaler TI, Littner MR, et al. Practice parame-ters for the treatment of snoring and obstrutive sleep apnea with orla appliances: an update for 2005. Sleep 2006;29:240–3.

144. Ng AT, Gotsopoulos H, Qian J, Cistulli PA. Effect of oral appliance therapy on upper airway collapsibility in obstructive sleep apnea. Am J Respir Crit Care Med 2003;168:238–41.

145. Barnes M, McEvoy RD, Banks S, et al. Efficacy of postitive airway pressure and oral appliances in mild to moderate obstrutive sleep apnea. Am J Respir Crit Care Med 2004;170:656–64.

146. Gotsopoulos H, Kelly JJ, Cistulli PA. Oral appliance therapy reduces blood pressure in obstructive sleep apnea: a randomized, controlled trial. Sleep 2004;27:934–41.

147. Lam B, Sam K, Mok WY, et al. Randomised study of three non-surgical treatments in mild to moderate obstructive sleep apnea. Thorax 2007;62:354–9.

148. Fergusson KA, Cartwright R, Rogers R, Schmidt-Nowara W. Oral appliances for snoring and obstructive sleep apnea: a review. Sleep 2006;29:244–62.

149. Standards of Practice Committee for the American Sleep Disorders Association. Practice parameters for the treatment of obstructive sleep apnea in adults: the efficacy of surgical modifications of the upper airway. Report of the American Sleep Disorders Association. Sleep 1996;19(2):152–5.

150. Won CHJ, Li KK, Guilleminault C. Surgical treatment of obstruc-tive sleep apnea. Proc Am Thorac Soc 2008;5:193–9.

151. Rodenstein DO. Assessment of uvulopalatopharyngoplasty for the treatment of sleep apnea syndrome. Sleep 1992;15(6 suppl):S56–62.

152. Ryan CF, Love LL. Unpredictable results of laser assisted uvu-lopalatoplasty in the treatment of obstructive sleep apnea. Thorax 2000;55(5):399–404.

153. Woodson T, Stewart D, Wraver E, Javaheri S. A randomised trial of temperature-controlled radiofrequency ablation, continuous posi-tive airway pressure and placebo for obstructive sleep apnea. Oto-tolaryngology 2002;128:848–61.

154. Powell NB, Riley RW, Robinson A. Surgical management of obstructive sleep apnea syndrome. Clin Chest Med 1998;19(1): 77–86.

155. Riley RW, Powell NB, Guilleminault C. Obstructive sleep apnea syndrome: a review of 306 consecutively treated surgical patients. Otolaryngol Head Neck Surg 1993;108(2):117–25.

156. Bettega G, Pepin JL, Veale D, Deschaux C, Raphael B, Levy P. Obstructive sleep apnea syndrome. Fifty-one consecutive patients treated by maxillofacial surgery. Am J Respir Crit Care Med 2000;162(2 Pt 1):641–9.

157. Hedner J, Grote L. Pharmacological therapy in sleep apnea. In: McNicholas WT, Phillipson EA (eds) *Breathing Disorders in Sleep*. London: WB Saunders, 2002: 149–56.

158. Marshall NS, Yee BJ, Desai AV, et al. Two randomised placebo-con-trolled trials to evaluate the efficacy and tolerability of mirtazapine for the treatment of obstructive sleep apnea. Sleep 2008;1:824–31.

159. Smith I, Lasserson T, Wright J. Drug treatments for obstructive sleep apnea. Cochrane Database of Systematic Reviews 2002;4.

160. Pack AI, Black JE, Schwartz JR. Modafinil as adjunct therapyv for daytime sleepiness in obstructive sleep panea. Am J Respir Crit Care Med 2001;164:1675–81.

161. Kingshott RN, Vennelle M, Coleman EL. Randomized, double-blind, placebo-controlled crossover trial of modafinil in the treat-ment of residual excessive sleeepiness in the sleep apnea/hypopnea syndrome. Am J Respir Crit Care Med 2001;163:918–23.

162. Piper AJ, Sullivan CE. Effects of long-term nocturnal nasal ventila-tion on spontaneous breathing during sleep in neuromuscular and chest wall disorders. Eur Respir J 1996;9(7):1515–22.

163. Sullivan CE, Berthon-Jones M, Issa FG. Remission of severe obesity-hypoventilation syndrome after short-term treatment during sleep with nasal continuous positive airway pressure. Am Rev Respir Dis 1983;128(1):177–81.

164. Piper AJ, Sullivan CE. Effects of short-term NIPPV in the treatment of patients with severe obstructive sleep apnea and hypercapnia. Chest 1994;105(2):434–40.

165. Piper AJ, Laks L, Sullivan CE. Effectiveness of short-term NIPPV in the management of patients with severe OSA and REM hypoventila-tion. Sleep 1993;16(8 suppl):S115–16; discussion S116–17.

166. Perez de Llano LA, Golpe R, Ortiz Piquer M, et al. Short term and long term effects of nasal intermittent positive pressure ventilation in patients with obesity hypoventilation syndorme. Chest 2005;128:587–94.

167. Piper AJ, Wang D, Yee BJ, Barnes DJ, Grunstein RR. Randomised trial of CPAP vs bilevel support in the treatment of obesity hypov-entilation syndrome without severe nocturnal desaturation. Thorax 2008;63:395–401.

168. Banerjee D, Yee BJ, Piper AJ, Zwilich CW, Grunstein RR. Obesity hypoventilation syndrome: hypoxemia during continous positive airway pressure. Chest 2007;131:1678–84.

169. Mokhlesi B, Kryger MH, Grunstein RR. Assessment and manage-ment of patients with obesity hypoventilation syndrome. Proc Am Thorac Soc 2008;5:218–25.

4 Management of Adult Obesity

20 An Overview of Obesity Management

Peter G. Kopelman[1] and Ian D. Caterson[2]

[1] St George's Hospital, University of London, London, UK
[2] Institute of Obesity Nutrition and Exercise, University of Sydney, Sydney, Australia

Introduction

Obesity management is perceived as a challenge: it requires considerable time, usually in a busy practice, skills with which a therapist may not have been trained and a feeling that successful outcome is unlikely. Such a situation tends to make many health professionals unprepared to become involved in obesity management.

There are reasons for the perceived lack of success that include lack of training, few long-term maintenance programs, little understanding of the pathophysiology of weight control and often a prejudice about obesity ("all it takes is self-control and will-power"). In addition, few health professionals have been taught about nutrition and physical activity or realistic weight loss goals. Obesity treatment is frequently instituted without the benefit of an integrated lifestyle management program.

Modern obesity treatment programs aim to improve health and well-being and this needs to be emphasized. Obesity treatment by health professionals should be for health benefit and not as a response to the dictates of fashion. Not all those who seek weight loss treatment require it. It is important for the therapist to recognize this and to let such individuals know when they do *not* need to lose weight. While most will accept such advice, in some cases it may be necessary to refer for specific counseling or therapy for an eating disorder.

Obesity therapy today is based on clinical assessment and the assessment of associated medical risks (such as metabolic and locomotor disease). For some patients general advice on eating and activity may be all that is required. For others, in need of therapy for health reasons, it is advisable to include a lifestyle program and, when necessary, to consider adjunctive therapy. Treatment requires sufficient consultation time and, once

Clinical Obesity in Adults and Children, 3rd edition. Edited by Peter G. Kopelman, Ian D. Caterson and William H. Dietz.
© 2010 Blackwell Publishing, ISBN: 978-1-4051-8226-3.

adequate weight loss (or other goal) has been achieved, an ongoing weight maintenance program. The need for long-term follow-up cannot be stressed too firmly: successful long-term weight maintenance depends on continuing follow-up [1,2]. This chapter summarizes such an approach to weight management.

How much weight loss?

There are few long-term studies of intentional weight loss and its effect on mortality. Some studies are currently under way and other larger studies are planned. It appears that intentional weight loss in women results in a reduction of mortality in the first 2 years, and that this reduction is particularly explained by cancer deaths [3]. Moreover, after 9 years of follow-up, self-reported intentional weight loss is associated with lower mortality rates whereas unintentional weight loss is associated with higher mortality rates [4]. There are also improvements in medical risk factors and complications from other diseases.

Many individuals have unrealistic expectations about weight loss and set themselves, or their patients, unachievable weight loss goals. It is not necessary to reach the "ideal" or "healthy" weight because health benefits can be obtained from firstly maintaining weight (not gaining more) and, secondly, from losing a moderate amount of weight, around 5–10% of presenting weight. This amount of weight loss produces reduction in risk and increased health benefits [5–8]. A list of potential benefits is given in Box 20.1.

Recent studies confirm that mild to moderate weight loss can be achieved by lifestyle intervention and maintained for up to 4 years. There have been several major trials on diabetes prevention in Scandinavia, China and the US [9,10]. The Diabetes Prevention Program study from the US studied the effects of placebo, metformin and a reasonably intensive lifestyle intervention in diabetes prevention. At the end of 4 years there was a 58% reduction in the incidence of diabetes. This was produced by a maintained mean weight loss of 4.6 kg. These benefits are sustained provided that subjects maintain their lowered weight and

Box 20.1 Health benefits of moderate weight loss (5–10% of presenting body weight)

Mortality
    20% decrease in overall
    30% decrease in diabetes related deaths
    40% decrease in cancer related deaths
Blood pressure
    10 mmHg decrease
Lipids
    15% decrease in cholesterol
    Reductions in other lipids
Diabetes
    Better blood glucose control

Box 20.2 Possible goals of obesity management

These will be individual and need to be negotiated with each patient.
Body weight
    Loss (5–10% of body weight)
    Possible maintenance of current weight (especially in the older patient)
Waist reduction
? Change in body composition
Metabolic disease
    Better control and/or fewer medications
    Diabetes
    Dyslipidemia
    Hypertension
Mechanical disease
    Better control, less intensive therapy
    OSA
    Arthritis
Activity
    Control of mechanical disease
    More able, less short of breath
    Less restriction
    Feeling of well-being
Fewer medications overall
Quality of life, well being and psychosocial functioning
Fertility (important for IVF programs)
Individual goals
    "The special dress"
    Occupational reasons, etc.

continue to be physically active. The other studies, with in general less intensive lifestyle interventions, produced similar results. A seemingly small weight loss of a few kilograms may have major benefits. Initial patient management should be a moderate weight loss of 5–10%. If successful then later treatment can set a new target for further weight loss.

Because of the difficulties in understanding appropriate and necessary weight loss, and in the absence of training and experience of weight management, many organizations and health departments have produced (and occasionally update) best practice guidelines. Examples of such guidelines are those of the Scottish Intercollegiate Guidelines Network [5], the NIH [6], the Royal College of Physicians of London (2003) [11], the National Health and Medical Research Council of Australia, 2003 [12], and Healthy Weight, Healthy Lives – toolkit for developing local strategies (2008) [13].

Such guidelines, with their evidence-based approach, highlight areas of difficulty. For example, the Body Mass Index (BMI) cut-off points for obesity, which were derived from largely Caucasian (indeed US) data, are probably inappropriate for other ethnic groups. Some organizations (including the WHO) and countries have suggested lower BMI cut-points for those from Asia and possibly higher values for those of Pacific Islands descent [14,15]. A further problem with such guidelines is their potential rigidity. It is essential to realize that with increasing risk factors or disease, or possibly with those of Asian origin, treatment needs to be instituted or intensified at the earliest stage and/or lower BMI level.

Aims of obesity treatment

With this in mind, what are the aims of obesity treatment? A 5–10% weight loss is one. However, weight loss should not be the sole objective for obesity treatment. Additional aims are to reduce risk to health and complications from associated disease that may

be present. Secondly, treatment is not just for the short term, but rather for a lifetime. A list of possible aims is given in Box 20.2. If weight loss cannot be achieved, an aim of no additional weight gain may be practical, achievable and of benefit. In some patients who find weight loss difficult due to mechanical complications (such as osteo-arthritis), or emotional or psychologic factors, prevention of further weight gain may be more appropriate than actual weight loss.

All such goals should be negotiated with the patient and documented. When the goals are achieved the patient must be congratulated and given credit for their success. New goals (which may include further loss or weight maintenance) should then be negotiated.

Overall, weight loss should be approached incrementally with new weight loss goals being set when the original target has been reached. It is likely that goals for older patients (>65 years) will be different from those who are young. There is a suggestion that although a population becomes heavier with age, the risk from obesity does not increase proportionately.

Assessment of the overweight and obese patient

General

For most health professionals, patients will be seen in a consulting room. Necessary equipment includes weighing scales that measure to 200 kg or more, large blood pressure cuffs, a long tape measure for waist circumference, and larger width chairs. A list of the requirements which are appropriate for a clinic treating obese individuals is given in Box 20.3.

Specific weight history

There are a number of specific factors which should be sought and a brief list is given in Box 20.4. The history of weight gain should be obtained to elucidate possible causative factors and to determine the patient's insight and understanding of the factors underlying their weight gain. Such questions might include, "At what stage did you gain weight, do you know of specific reasons for your weight gain, can you describe your eating patterns and what activity do you do?" It is helpful to decide whether childhood-onset obesity is due to a particular life event or a specific

syndrome. These latter are rare and may be identified by the length of history and specific associated clinical features. Specific single gene disorders are associated with the early onset of massive obesity, usually a strong family history and often characteristic clinical features such as hypogonadism.

A number of diseases may be associated with weight gain, though uncommonly with massive obesity, and clinical features of these should be sought. The diseases include endocrine diseases (hypothyroidism, acromegaly, Cushing syndrome, and diabetes), various types of arthritis or injury that may be associated with immobility, and cardiac disease which may also reduce activity. There are particular drugs that are associated with weight gain and a history of the use of such drugs should be obtained. Examples of such drugs are given in Box 20.5.

Physical examination and investigations

A detailed physical examination should always be performed. Weight and height should be measured and BMI calculated. (BMI

Box 20.3 Essential elements for an appropriate setting for the management of overweight and obesity

Trained staff directly involved in the running of the weight loss program. These staff (medical, nursing and other healthcare professionals) should have attended courses on the management of obesity and must be provided with an opportunity to continue their education.

A printed program for weight management that includes clearly outlined dietary advice, behavioral modification techniques, physical exercise and strategies for long-term lifestyle change. Such a program may include a family and/or group approach.

Suitable equipment, in particular accurate and regularly calibrated weighing scales and stadiometer.

Specified weight loss goals with energy deficits being achieved through moderating food intake and increasing physical expenditure.

Documentation of individual patients' health risks. This will include BMI, waist circumference, blood pressure, blood lipids, cigarette smoking and other co-morbid conditions.

A clearly defined follow-up procedure which involves collaboration between the different settings of care, provides regular monitoring and documentation of progress and includes details of criteria for judging the success of weight loss. This will allow a weight loss program to be properly supported, medical conditions to be monitored and problems or issues to be addressed at the earliest opportunity.

Box 20.4 Points that should be elucidated in any clinical history taken from a patient prior to obesity management

Medical history
  Risk factors
  Presence of established complications of obesity – remember to ask about snoring, sleep and daytime somnolence

Body weight history
  When was weight gained – puberty, stopping sport, employment, marriage, pregnancies, etc.
  Previous treatment(s) for obesity (including successes and failures)
  Family history of obesity, and related diseases and risk factors – type 2 diabetes, hypertension, premature coronary heart disease

Diet history
  Eating pattern and amount (compared to friends)
  Hunger
  Stress or emotional eating, binges
  Alcohol intake

Regular physical activity pattern

Relevant social history
  Cigarette smoking and cessation (did they gain weight then?)

Drug history
  Antipsychotics
  Antidepressants
  Steroids
  Anticonvulsants
  Lithium
  β-blockers

Reproductive history
  Irregular periods
  Polycystic ovary syndrome

Box 20.5 Drug treatment which may be associated with weight gain

Antipsychotic (olanapine, clozapine, risperidone)

Antidepressants (tricyclic antidepressants)

Lithium

Antiepileptic drugs (valproate, carbamazepine, gabapentin)

Diabetic medications (insulin, sulfonylureas, thiazolidinediones)

Steroid hormones (glucocorticoids, possibly oral contraceptives)

β-blockers

Antihistamines

Table 20.1 Classification of overweight and obesity in adults according to BMI and the cut-points of abdominal circumference (waist)

A. BMI values

Classification	BMI (kg/m^2)*	Risk of co-morbidities**
Underweight	<18.5	Low (but risk of other clinical problems increased)
Normal range	18.5–24.9	Average
Preobese	25.0–29.9	Mildly increased
Obese	**≥30.0**	
Class I	30.0–34.9	Moderate
Class II	35.0–39.9	Severe
Class III	≥40.0	Very severe

B. Abdominal circumference at which risk increases

	Risk increased	Substantial increase
Men	94 cm (OR 2.2)	102 cm (OR 4.6)
Women	80 cm (OR 1.6)	88 cm (OR 2.6)
Asian men	90 cm	
Asian women	80 cm	

OR, odds ratio, which is the increase in risk associated with this situation, compared to a lower waist circumference.

The values are those suggested by the WHO [25].

cut-off points are shown in Table 20.1.) It is worth recording the distribution of fat tissue by measuring the waist circumference. (The waist measurement is taken as the narrowest circumference midway between the lower border of the ribs and the upper border of the iliac crest.) Examination of the skin is important. Thin, atrophic skin (together with abdominal adiposity and relatively thinner extremities) is a feature of excess use or secretion of glucocorticoids; acanthosis nigricans (pigmented, "velvety" skin creases especially in the axillae or around the neck) is associated with insulin resistance; hirsutism in women may indicate the polycystic ovary syndrome or simply obesity *per se*. A neck circumference of >43 cm indicates the likelihood of obstructive sleep apnea (OSA) and the pharynx should be examined to exclude evidence of obstruction from tonsils, other causes of narrowing and for redness and edema of the uvula. Note should be taken of blood pressure and cardiovascular function.

Some investigations are useful but care should be taken to choose those appropriate for the individual. In addition to assessing for risk factors (see below), it may be useful to measure plasma thyroid-stimulating hormone (TSH) and testosterone; the latter is often low, particularly in men with OSA, while it may be elevated in obese women. Liver transaminases (alanine and aspartate) may be elevated, particularly in those with abdominal adiposity and/or the metabolic syndrome. This may reflect associated nonalcoholic fatty liver disease (NAFLD). Often, in the early stages of weight loss, these liver enzymes rise, but usually settle as weight stabilizes. The measurement of serum leptin is not recommended as a routine, but may be required in patients with extreme early-onset obesity. Although the rare leptin deficiency syndrome can be treated, the serial measurement of leptin in simple or spontaneous obesity may prove to be an useful marker of fat loss.

Assessment of risk

An initial risk measure is the presence of abdominal adiposity. The WHO has suggested the measures shown in Table 20.1 but for those of Asian origin, these measures may be 90 cm or greater in males and 80 cm or greater in females (the exact measurements are being decided at a recent WHO conference (December 2008)) [17].

As well as the presence of hypertension, assessment must be made of the presence of cardiac disease and of diabetes. OSA (as determined by sleep history, examination of the pharynx and neck circumference) is an added risk. Dyslipidemia (classically hypertriglyceridemia with low HDL cholesterol (<1 mmol/L)) and elevated LDL cholesterol (>3.5 mmol/L)) confers additional risk. Cigarette smoking is a major risk factor.

These risks may need to be quantified by specific investigations such as an exercise ECG or sleep studies.

Assessment of motivation to lose weight

Not all patients are prepared to lose weight. Sometimes it may be advisable to assess the patient's readiness and motivation by direct questioning or using the Stages of Change model. It may be necessary to suggest that rather than embarking on an intensive program at the current time, the patient should return at a later stage for reassessment and review, when they are prepared and motivated to lose weight.

Obesity management programs

The therapies and degree of intensity of any weight loss program should be based on an assessment of the degree of adiposity (anthropometry) and the presence or absence of medical risk factors. A suggested approach is outlined in Table 20.2. Mild to moderate "uncomplicated" overweight and obesity may require

Table 20.2 Practical approach to obesity treatment – clinical assessment and rational management outline

BMI	Risk rating	General advice	Eating	Activity	Lifestyle program	Obesity drugs	VLCDs	Surgery
18.5–24.9	Low	Use						
	High		Use	Use				
25–29.9	Low				Use			
	High				Use	Consider*		
30–34.9	Low				Use	Consider/use		
	High				Use	Use		
35–39.9	Low				Use	Use		
	High				Use	Use	Consider	Consider
40+	High				Use	Use	Use	Consider

Risk rating:

Low = waist <102 cm in men and <88 cm in women and no risk factors present.

High = waist greater than the above measures, or the presence of risk factors.

Risk factors:

Type 2 diabetes/impaired glucose tolerance, Hypertension, coronary heart disease, dyslipidemia, OSA.

*Pharmacotherapy should be considered at a BMI >27 in the presence of disease when there has been no weight loss in 12 weeks of a lifestyle program.

Pharmacotherapy might be considered earlier in those with greater BMI or with more risk factors and diseases.

advice with a specific eating and physical activity program. Greater degrees of obesity and risk, or the presence of disease, require more intensive lifestyle interventions, the use of pharmacotherapy, possibly very low-calorie/energy diets (meal replacements) or surgery. While all these aspects of obesity treatment are considered in detail in other chapters, it is worthwhile briefly reviewing each modality.

It also needs to be underlined that any weight program must provide a weight maintenance component. This is the most time-consuming component, but regular and long-term follow-up visits and intervention are part of the management of any chronic disorder.

The components of a weight management program are:
- general advice
- eating (diet intervention)
- physical activity
- behavior modification
- lifestyle program
- maintenance program – monitoring and longer term follow-up.

In addition, it may be necessary to consider adjunctive therapies for some patients.

General advice

General advice should be given in all circumstances and will include aspects of eating, physical activity and behavior modification. However, for most individuals with increased adiposity and/or medical risk, an additional planned program of intervention is necessary. Such a program usually involves a number of visits (10–12 over a period of 3–6 months) with specific tasks for each one. If weight loss is insufficient during this time, then consideration should be given to drug treatment or other therapies.

Eating (diet intervention)

While energy (calorie) restriction produces good weight loss, some individuals may find this irksome and impossible to maintain. For such patients, a low-fat eating plan may prove effective; such plans may be maintained for several years [18–20]. Fat intake can be reduced to less than 40 g per day (or lower for women) with the remainder of the diet being *ad libitum*. Greater losses may be obtained by additionally reducing energy intake. Men may also need to reduce energy intake by limiting their alcohol intake.

The major discussion of diet and obesity is in Chapter 21.

Physical Activity (exercise program)

Emphasis should be placed on increasing total daily activity to between 60 and 90 minutes each day [21,22]. While exercise and fitness are important, the initial emphasis should be on increasing the activities of daily living, in particular more walking. A formal written exercise prescription has been shown to increase effectiveness in general practice [23]. Giving patients the opportunity to use or purchase a pedometer and then setting the number of steps they need do in a day may prove an effective method of increasing activity. For patients with arthritis or other disabilities, hydrotherapy (exercising in water) may be a way of initiating movement and this type of activity can assist weight loss. A more detailed discussion appears in Chapter 23.

Behavior modification

This therapy is important and central to any weight loss program (see Chapter 22). There are many components to behavior modification, but a simple one is the use of a food and exercise diary. This allows habit recognition and change. All subjects, but most particularly those who are overweight or obese, under-report food intake and over-report the activity they undertake. A diary provides an important starting point for discussion and suggests possible interventions. Additional behavioral therapies include discussion about habits, change and alternative ways of approaching situations. Other techniques involve stress management, improving self-esteem and occasionally more specific counseling or psychiatric intervention.

Lifestyle program

Programs for lifestyle change usually have a number of initial intensive visits (10 or 12, for example) and then, depending on the patient's response, further visits may be scheduled or, in addition, drugs or other treatment initiated (see Chapters 24, 25). When goals are reached then the visits are extended. Such a lifestyle program should involve a range of health professionals (dietitians, physiotherapists, nurses, psychologists). Good results (and satisfaction for the treatment group) are usually obtained by the involvement of multidisciplinary teams.

Because of this partial abrogation of obesity treatment by health professionals and because of community perceptions, many organizations and groups have been established to "fill the gap." Some commercial groups use conventional therapy (e.g. Weight Watchers or programs used in some gyms), while others rely on alternative or natural therapies and still others use "magic" treatments which sound plausible but really have no scientific basis nor effectiveness. Examples of the latter would be total body wrapping, some herbal concoctions and bulking agents. Few have been tested rigorously, many are costly but the very existence of such programs and therapies shows that many individuals desire to lose weight but need to be guided into the correct approach and be provided with effective therapy.

Maintenance program

This is an essential part of any weight loss program and the most neglected. Follow-up programs are essential and effective [2].

Monitoring and longer term follow-up

Patients involved in an obesity treatment program require the following:
• monitoring of weight (ideally monthly – no more than two monthly)
• monitoring of pulse rate and blood pressure
• monitoring of obesity-related risks and diseases (e.g. dyslipidemia, type 2 diabetes).
The treatment plan should be recorded for each patient and incorporated into local audit data recording systems.
As weight loss progresses adjustments of medications for obesity-related or obesity-responsive diseases and risks taken by the patient may be necessary. For example, the dose of an oral hypoglycemic agent may need to be reduced as insulin sensitivity increases with weight loss.

Audit and outcome measures

Table 20.3 lists the process measures that may be used to judge the success or otherwise of an obesity management program. Ultimately, the success of antiobesity drugs must be judged by a reduction in outcome measures that include myocardial infarction, cerebrovascular accidents, physical disability and death.

Adjunctive therapies

Adjunctive therapies or more intensive treatments (discussed in Chapters 24, 25) should be considered for those patients at medical risk from their obesity when primary interventions have failed to achieve adequate weight loss after a sustained period of time (not less than 12 weeks). Such patients may include those with a BMI of:
• >35
• >25 with two or more risks
• >30, or <35 and who have been treated with a lifestyle program for 12 weeks without reaching goals (this is particularly important if they have risk factors)
• >27 who have not lost weight on a lifestyle program after 24 weeks, especially with risk factor(s).
For patients of Asian background, at particular risk of medical complications, it may be important to consider this type of adjunctive therapy earlier or at lower BMIs.

Low calorie/energy diets

Milk provides most of the essential macro- and micronutrients. A diet based on 1220 mL (2 pints) of milk is effective in inducing substantial weight loss. It may be used for several weeks as essentially the only form of food for 3–4 days each week.

Commercially produced very low-calorie diets (VLCDs) may also be effective. They contain between 400 and 800 kcal per day,

Table 20.3 Process measures to judge the success of antiobesity treatment

Measures	Immediate benefits	Longer term benefits
Physical measures	Weight loss	Reduced breathlessness
	Reduction in waist circumference	Decreased sleep apnea
		Reduced angina
	Improvement in co-morbidities	Reduced blood pressure
Metabolic measures	Decreased fasting blood glucose & plasma insulin	Reduction in doses of concomitant medications
	Improvement in fasting lipid profile	
	Decreased HbA1c (if diabetic)	
Functional measures	Increased mobility	Reduced time away from work
	Decreased symptoms	Improved involvement in social activities
	Increased well-being and mood	
	Increased health-related quality of life	Decreased number of consultations with health professionals

usually as protein, with added necessary vitamins and minerals. Such diets can be commenced after a period on a lifestyle program. There should be a definite protocol for their use which includes behavior modification. The initial lifestyle program is necessary to provide a base therapy to which a patient may return after the most "drastic" VLCD. It is important not to prescribe VLCDs for patients with liver or renal disease. However, with appropriate treatment modifications and precautions, they can be used for diabetic patients, even if treated with insulin. Insulin and sulfonylurea doses may need to be reduced substantially during the VLCD treatment program. Once treatment is completed, a maintenance program is essential. Subsequent weight regain may suggest a period of retreatment with VLCDs.

Pharmacotherapy

This treatment may prove effective as an adjunct to lifestyle intervention in selected patients: a detailed discussion appears in Chapter 24. The newer drugs available (worldwide) are orlistat (Xenical) and sibutramine (Reductil, Meridia). Rimonabant has now been withdrawn following advice from the European Medicines Agency (2008). Orlistat is additionally available from retail pharmacies ("over the counter") in North America, Australia and Europe.

Selection of patients for pharmacotherapy

It is important that doctors who prescribe such drugs are fully familiar with either the primary literature or an authoritative summary.

The criteria applied to the use of an antiobesity drug are similar to those applied to the treatment of other relapsing disorders. It is important to avoid offering antiobesity drug therapy to patients who are seeking a "quick fix" for their weight problem. The initiation of drug treatment will depend on the clinician's judgment about the risks to an individual from continuing obesity.

Obesity surgery

This is the most effective, but most drastic, form of treatment available for obesity. The Swedish Obese Study [24] has shown that with appropriate follow-up a substantial weight loss can be maintained for at least 10 years. Some surgical procedures are designed to reduce intake or absorption but more recent procedures such as gastric banding (laparoscopic) or stapling and gastric bypass have fewer side-effects and excellent results. Both an experienced surgical team and a dedicated long-term follow-up team are required. This treatment is discussed more fully in Chapter 25.

References

1. Bjorvell H, Rossner S. Long-term effects of commonly available weight reducing programmes in Sweden. Int J Obes 1987;11:67–71.
2. Bjorvell H, Rossner S. A ten-year follow-up of weight change in severely obese subjects treated in a combined behavioural modification programme. Int J Obes 1992;16:623–5.
3. Williamson DF, Pamuk E, Thun M, et al. Prospective study of intentional weight loss and mortality in never-smoking overweight US white women aged 40–64 years. American Journal of Epidemiology Am J Epidemiol 1995;141:1128–41.
4. Gregg EW, Gerzoff RB, Thompson TJ, Williamson DF. 2003 Intentional Weight Loss and Death in Overweight and Obese U.S. Adults 35 Years of Age and Older. Ann Int Med 2003:138;383–389.
5. Scottish Intercollegiate Guidelines Network (SIGN) *Obesity in Scotland: A National Clinical Guideline Recommended for Use in Scotland.* Glasgow: Scottish Intercollegiate Guidelines Network, 1996.
6. National Institutes of Health (NIH) Clinical Guidelines on the identification, evaluation, and treatment of overweight and obesity in adults. The Evidence Report. National Institutes of Health. Obes Res 1998;6(suppl 2(3)): 51S–209S.
7. Vidal, J. The Metabolic Challenge of Obesity. Int J Obesity 2002:26; S25–S28.
8. National Institute of Health and Clinical Excellence. Obesity: the prevention, identification, assessment and management of overweight and obesity in adults and children. NICE Clinical Guideline 43 December 2006 www.nice.org.uk/nicemedia/pdf/ CG43NICEGuideline.pdf
9. Tuomilehto J, Lindstrom J, Eriksson JG, et al. Prevention of type 2 diabetes mellitus by changes in lifestyle among subjects with impaired glucose tolerance. N Engl J Med 2001;344:1343–50.
10. Diabetes Prevention Program Group. Reduction in the incidence of type 2 diabetes with lifestyle intervention or metformin. N Engl J Med 2002;346:393–403.
11. Royal College of Physicians of London (2003)
12. National Health and Medical Research Council of Australia, 2003
13. Healthy Weight, Healthy Lives – toolkit for developing local strategies (2008).
14. WHO Expert Consultation. Appropriate body-mass index for Asian populations and its implication for policy and intervention strategies. Lancet 2004;363:157–63.
15. Bassand J-P. Managing cardiovascular risk in patients with metabolic syndrome. Clin Cornerstone 2006;8Suppl 1:S7–14.
16. Day CP. Genes or environment to determine alcoholic liver disease and non-alcoholic fatty liver disease. Liver Int 2006;26:1021–1028.
17. WHO conference 2008. www.who.int/nutrition/topics/expert_ consultation_wc_whr/en/
18. Toubro S, Astrup A. Dietary weight maintenance: low-fat, high-carbohydrate ad libitum versus calorie counting. Int J Obes 1994;18(suppl 2):123.
19. Toubro S, Astrup A. A randomized comparison of two weight-reducing diets. Calorie counting versus low-fat carbohydrate-rich ad libitum diet. Ugeskr Laeger 1998;160(6):816–20.
20. Hession M, Rolland C, Kulkarni U, et al. Systematic review of randomized controlled trials of low-carbohydrate vs. low-fat/low-calorie diets in the management of obesity and its comorbidities. Obesity Rev 2008:10:36–50.
21. Kahn EB, Ramsey LT, Brownson RC, et al. The effectiveness of interventions to increase physical activity – A systematic review. Am JPreventive Med 2002:22:73–108.
22. Roux L. Pratt M, Yanagawa T, et al. Measurement of the value of exercise in obesity prevention: A cost-effectiveness analysis of promoting physical activity among US adults. Obesity Res 2004;12: A18–A18.
23. Swinburn BA, Walter LG, Arroll B, et al. The green prescription study: a randomised controlled trial of written exercise advice

provided by general practitioners. Am J Public Health 1998;88: 288–91.

24. Sjostrom CD, Lissner L, Wedel H, et al. Reduction in incidence of diabetes, hypertension and lipid disturbances after intentional weight loss induced by bariatric surgery: the SOS Intervention Study. Obes Res 1999;7:477–84.

25. World Health Organization. *Obesity: Preventing and Managing the Global Epidemic*. Technical report 894. Geneva: WHO, 2000: 256.

21 Dietary Management of Obesity: Eating Plans

Janet Franklin

Metabolism and Obesity Services, Royal Prince Alfred Hospital, Sydney, Australia

The changing face of treatment

Obesity has been seen as both a negative and positive situation depending on the times, the environment and the religion [1]. However, around 400 BC Hippocrates observed that the incidence of sudden death, prevalence of menstrual irregularities and infertility were higher in obese people than in the lean. Accordingly, he prescribed treatments such as hard labor, sleeping on a hard bed, eating only once daily, eating fatty food to foster greater satiation and walking naked for long periods. Hippocrates and his successor Galen believed obesity was a sign of personal weakness. By the 15th century obesity treatment consisted of taking lots of baths and eating bulky foods with few calories. Over the next two centuries a more scientific approach to obesity was adopted and the empirically based, moralistic view declined in popularity. At that time it was widely believed that obesity was caused by an imbalance in body chemicals or a mechanical malfunction [2].

During the 18th and 19th centuries, although eating and physical activity were still the focus of treatment, this period also witnessed a resurgence of the moralistic view, which now embraced the roles of eating habits and activity levels in the obese. Treatment generally consisted of advising patients to limit their food choices and to leave the dining area while still hungry. Views of the etiology of obesity were primarily focused on there being physical malfunction, such as Prader–Willi syndrome, and/or a personality weakness [2].

At this time physical anthropometry was performed and a formula was developed for calculating ideal weight (height adjusted) – the Quetelet Index, subsequently known as the Body Mass Index or BMI [2].

During the late 20th century the incidence and prevalence of overweight and obesity spiralled and consequently generated a significant increase in obesity research, focusing on genetics, regulation of food intake, and behavioral treatments [2].

Global treatments in obesity followed similar lines to previous centuries, i.e. urging people to reduce their food intake and increase their physical activity. Psychiatrists also became interested in obesity and offered new ideas about its etiology. Some postulated that obesity resulted from acting out unconscious impulses, reflective of disturbed personality development. However, this has never been scientifically tested and there seems little empiric evidence to support it. In the 1960s and 1970s psychologic assessment was included in the management of obesity; behavior modification targeted to lifestyle changes (based on the learning theory) dominated treatment and achieved reasonable success. Behavior therapy remains a useful adjunct in current weight management programs [2].

Over the last few decades pharmaceutical preparations, very low-energy diets (VLED) and bariatric surgery have also emerged as selective obesity treatments. Surgery for those with greater than grade 3 obesity has been more successful than other forms of treatment but it has attendant risks.

Dietary treatment of obesity

For decades the scientific community has been trying to determine the perfect weight loss diet. Perhaps this is an unrealistic objective, as the etiology of obesity is multifactorial. It logically follows that effective treatment of obesity should be as diverse as its causes. In clinical practice it is highly likely that various approaches will be implemented in order to achieve optimal results in such a large and diverse group and at different stages of their lives.

In reaction to the plethora of commercially available weight loss programs, a task force was established in Michigan, USA, in 1990 which developed guidelines to improve public awareness and education. The guidelines included the following.

Clinical Obesity in Adults and Children, 3rd edition. Edited by Peter G. Kopelman, Ian D. Caterson and William H. Dietz.
© 2010 Blackwell Publishing, ISBN: 978-1-4051-8226-3.

• The weight goal for a patient should be based on personal and family history, not exclusively on height and weight charts.
• Total daily caloric consumption should not be less than 1000 kcal without medical supervision.
• Protein intake should be between 0.8 and 1.5 g per kilogram of goal body weight but no more than 100 g of protein per day.
• Fat should provide 10–30% of the energy in the daily diet.
• A minimum daily carbohydrate intake of 100 g if no medical intervention, but if medically supervized at least 50 g per day should still be consumed.
These guidelines however remain open to wide interpretation.

Energy deficit techniques

An energy deficit diet can be achieved by many means. A 2–4 MJ (500–1000 kcal) deficit from daily intake (i.e. from intakes that are weight maintaining, rather than weight increasing) is thought to lead to approximately 0.5–1 kg weight loss per week [3].

Fixed-energy diets

A fixed-energy diet is one method of achieving an energy deficit. Intake is limited by controlling portion sizes, menu choice and composition. These diets are often around 5 MJ (1200 kcal) for women and 7.5 MJ (1800 kcal) for men, and are considered moderate hypocaloric diets. There is minimal self-monitoring, choice or freedom. Lack of variety and departure from normal eating patterns often result in lack of compliance although many people do find these diets helpful as they reduce decision making and if followed accurately, are successful. Commercial weight loss companies often use this method by supplying prepackaged foods to their consumers. Long-term results are often similar to, if not better than some well-controlled trials [4].

Self-limiting

Another method is to self-limit one or all dietary constituents, e.g. by limiting fat intake or by maintaining 55% carbohydrate in the diet, 30% as fat and 15% as protein, irrespective of caloric intake. This allows the dieter greater flexibility in choosing their food and monitoring their intake. It is often called an *ad libitum* diet. Well-known examples of this type of diet are the National Cholesterol Education, Step 1 and Step 2 programs developed by the American Heart Association. These diets usually lead to a weight loss ranging from 2 to 6 kg and decrease of 2–5 cm in waist measurement over a 1–2-year period [5]. However, the amount of weight loss depends on the pretreatment weight, with heavier adults achieving greater weight loss than their lighter counterparts.

It is postulated that people employing an *ad libitum* diet may maintain weight loss for longer than those who pursue more restrictive diets. Some studies also show adherence to an *ad libitum* diet slows the progression of chronic diseases such as diabetes [6–8].

Low-energy diets (LED)

Low-energy diets provide 3.5–5 MJ (800–1200 kcal) per day and should only be used under medical supervision. As so few kilojoules are consumed it is almost impossible to meet the ideal daily

Table 21.1 Menu plans for different calorie control settings

Meal	3350 kJ (800 kcal)	5000 kJ (1200 kcal)
Breakfast	Cereal 45 g	Cereal 90 g
	180 mL skimmed milk	180 mL skimmed milk
	Multivitamin that contains fat-soluble vitamins and iron	
Morning tea	Apple	Apple
Lunch	1 piece of bread	2 pieces of wholemeal bread
	Chicken 100 g and salad	Chicken 75 g and salad
		200 g diet yoghurt
Afternoon tea	Banana	Nuts 15 g
Dinner	250 mL of low-fat vegetable soup	Meat 90 g
	200 g diet yoghurt	Small potato
		Broccoli 4 florets
		One medium carrot
		Fruit salad 1 cup
Supper	Tea	Tea and plain biscuit

micronutrient requirements, so supplementation is recommended. This can be provided by tablets containing vitamins and minerals or through fortifying the food. Table 21.1 provides examples of these diets. LED achieve better weight loss than *ad libitum* and low-fat diets; over a 14-week period one could expect a 7–13 kg weight loss and a 10 cm reduction in waist measurement. After 12 months weight loss of approximately 6–7 kg is common, and after 2 years the norm is 3.5 kg. However, at 5 years there is often very little change from baseline [9].

As food choices are limited when using low-energy diets, compliance can be high. However, maintaining daily nutrient requirements is often challenging and continuing restriction over time becomes increasingly difficult and therefore weight regain is likely [9].

Partial meal replacement therapy

Partial meal replacement can often be thought of as a LED or a fixed-energy diet. Partial meal replacement means that some of the daily meals (either 1–2 main meals and/or 1–2 snacks) are replaced with supplemented, portion-controlled food. This meal or snack is often a shake or a bar. It has been shown that even when the energy content of meals has been prescribed by dietary professionals who target food type and quantity, the patients who pursue the partial meal replacement method lose as much, if not more, weight than those on professional prescribed therapy, even though the caloric intakes are reported to be similar [10, 11]. It has also been suggested that using partial meal replacement may help people who try to lose weight via low-energy regimens better meet their nutrient requirements [12].

Partial meal replacement appears to have advantages over full meal replacements as they offer participants choice and flexibility in social situations whilst reducing decision making at other times. Although they can be used indefinitely, they lead to slower weight loss than full meal replacements (e.g. very low-energy

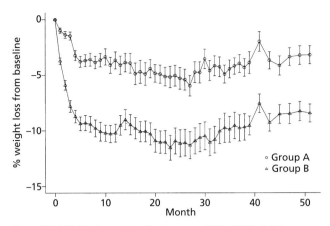

Figure 21.1 Weight loss patterns for those on a 1200–1500 kcal diet over a 4-year period, either with prescribed diet using conventional food (group A) or using two meal replacements and two snacks (group B) for the first 3 months of the study. From months 4 to 51, both groups were put on one meal and one snack replacement. (Reproduced with permission from Ditschuneit [13].)

diets) as they are generally higher in energy. Partial meal replacements are often successful in maintaining weight loss after an initial, intensive period of weight loss (Fig. 21.1) [13]. The amount of weight loss achieved is generally 10–12% in the first 12–16 weeks [14]. This is similar to LED but weight loss may be maintained for longer, e.g. approximately 5.5–6.5 kg after 1–2 years [15]. A meta-analysis by Heymsfield et al. [16,17] compared isocaloric diets using either conventional food or partial meal replacements. This demonstrated that after both 3 months and 1 year, those who used the partial meal replacements lost on average 2.5 kg more than those consuming conventional food.

Very low-energy (calorie) diets (VLED or VLCD)
Very low-energy diets provide approximately 1.7–3.4 MJ (400–800 kcal) per day, and are lower than an individual's resting metabolic rate (RMR). In addition to the energy level, other determinants of a VLED are that it must:
• contain all the RDI for minerals and vitamins, electrolytes and fatty acids
• provide between 0.8 and 1.5 g of high-quality protein/ kg ideal body weight
• be followed for a fixed period
• be different from a person's usual intake.
VLED need to be carefully formulated to prevent complications; they should be medically supervized and followed up regularly. There are several potential complications associated with the use of VLED [18,19] (Box 21.1).

The VLEDs were established after it was found that people who fasted often died suddenly. Although some fasters achieved large amounts of weight loss and reduced hunger, it was a high-risk method of achieving weight loss. Subsequently, it was found that consumption of small amounts of food mitigated the risk of death and importantly, hunger did not increase [18]. VLEDs were originally protein-sparing, modified fasts (PSMF) using wholefoods,

---

Box 21.1 Potential complications associated with the use of VLED

Electrolyte imbalances

Dehydration

Decrease in exercise tolerance

Decreased voluntary physical activity

Cardiac changes

Ketosis*

Nutrient deficiencies

Lethargy, weakness, fatigue*

Light-headedness, dizziness*

Feeling faint on standing

Anemia

Constipation*

Menstrual irregularity*

Hair loss

Muscle cramps

Gastrointestinal upset*

Nausea

Diarrhea

Cold intolerance*

Gout

Gallbladder disease

Dry skin*

Brittle nails

Edema

*Common

---

mostly in the form of game or other lean meats. Now they are mostly provided in liquid form and based on either milk or egg protein.

The VLED should only be used in highly motivated patients, who have tried many other methods or who are high medical risks. VLED should never be attempted by self- initiated dieters. Also, their use should be limited in children, people recovering from severe wounds, those who have a wasting condition, and pregnant or lactating women. People who suffer from psychotic episodes are unlikely to be able to cope with the restrictive nature of VLED (see Box 21.2 for contraindications) [18].

Children should only be prescribed VLED in extreme circumstances, and under medical supervision [20,21]. When VLED are employed it is imperative that optimum protein and caloric consumption occurs in order to maintain growth. VLED have been used successfully in adolescents, but they must be under medical supervision [20,21]. Use of VLED in elderly people is recommended with caution, as the risk of reduced lean muscle mass and the difficulty of balancing medications and food intake may outweigh the potential benefits.

Box 21.2 Quick guide to patient exclusion for VLED

Contraindications

Increased requirements
Pregnancy
Lactation
Illness
Wasting conditions
   Cushing syndrome
   Cancer
   Burns
   Cachexia

Increased medical risk
Recent cardiac disease (last 3 months)
Cerebrovascular disease
   Due to recent accident
   Recent ischemic heart disease
   Transient ischemic heart disease
Underlying renal disease
Underlying hepatic disease
Eating disorders

Used only with medical supervision
Elderly
Children
Insulin-treated diabetics

There appears little benefit in VLED less than 3.2 MJ (800 kcal). Commercially produced VLED generally only provide 1.6 MJ (400 kcal) [19]. A portion-controlled meal could be given in addition to the VLED to achieve 800 kcal daily. This should contain appropriate amounts of protein (1.2–1.5 g protein/ kg ideal body weight (IBW) including the supplementary foods of the program), two cups of low-carbohydrate vegetables and 1–2 teaspoons of oil to stimulate the bile duct and reduce the chance of cholelithiasis.

Thomas Wadden's generally accepted recommendations for the use of VLED are as follows [18,19].
• Medical examinations are necessary before any patient starts on a VLED.
• VLED should only be used as part of a more complex lifestyle modification program, which increases physical activity, reduces the consumption of dietary fat and improves coping skills.
• VLED should only be used when other methods have failed.
• Typically, a program including a VLED comprises:
  – initial 4-week program of 1200 kcal (range 1000–1500 kcal) to help the patient prepare for the restriction and lessen chances of electrolyte loss
  – next 8–16 weeks VLED, consisting mostly of 3–4 drinks of commercially prepared VLED, some vegetables and oil each day

and/or a fiber supplement, 2 liters of fluid and behavioral therapy and a light exercise program
  – next 4 weeks, two meals of the VLED preparation plus one normal meal of low-calorie content, moderate exercise
  – next 4 weeks on one meal of the VLED preparation plus two meals of healthy eating of approximately 1200 kcal, moderate exercise
  – a maintenance phase with follow-up, approximately 1200–1500 kcal and vigorous exercise [19,22].

The above recommendation is based on the view that less severe energy restrictions and the inclusion of a daily meal of conventional foods will produce robust weight loss but avoid dietary deprivation and other factors often associated with weight rebound following VLED treatment [18,19].

Results are rarely as impressive as the caloric deficit suggests. The resting metabolic rate normally drops and the voluntary energy expenditure during physical activity usually falls, so the difference is not as high as one would expect. However, during the active stage 90% of patients generally achieve greater than 10 kg weight loss compared to LED, where only 60% generally achieve this result. The average weight loss for those who maintain the program is approximately 22 kg for women and 32 kg for men. Patients normally regain about 35–50% of their lost weight within 1 year, 10–20% regain all their weight and similar percentages apply to those who maintain their weight loss. Long-term results are generally no better (but no worse either) than other methods of weight loss, particularly LED. However, costs are substantially greater, particularly when medical supervision is required [14]. The major benefit is the rapidity of the weight loss, which may be required preoperatively, for some patients, to enhance mobility or for other medical reasons.

VLED cause diuresis initially which gives people the sense that they are losing weight and in turn improves patients' feeling of success and wellness early in the treatment. Once ketosis has been induced it suppresses hunger and the rate of muscle loss is slowed. Convenience and limited choices are also beneficial to many patients [23]. The average weight loss per week is 1.5–2.0 kg for women and 2.0–2.5 kg for men [18]. Many people claim that the faster the weight loss, the quicker it is regained but this is not necessarily the case. Physiologic (changes in RMR and regulatory hormones), psychologic (fighting against the high restriction) and lifestyle (returning to habitual patterns) factors contribute to rebound weight gain subsequent to the initial, high weight loss [23]. Pharmacotherapy combined with intensive behavioral, dietary and exercise intervention may be needed to maintain weight loss, depending on the individual [23].

If the VLED is repeated, the amount of weight loss achieved is reduced, even if weight regain is close to or above original weight. Weight loss has been achieved for up to 45 months after starting a VLED, but weight loss diminishes dramatically after 12 weeks. For this reason, it is recommended ceasing the VLED at this point. Although attrition rates are reported to be similar to other programs, they could be over 50% in free living conditions [18,24,25].

VLED can be useful for weight maintenance. For example, they have been trialed intermittently, i.e. for 2 weeks every 3 months, or on demand (when weight reaches a certain level) for a period of 2 years. These methods showed that the VLED slowed the progression of weight regain but did not stop overall weight gain [24,25]. Other groups have used it either once daily per week for 15 weeks or for 5 consecutive days every 5 weeks. Both methods showed improved weight loss over a 1500–1800 kcal diet and achieved improved glycemic control [26]. The best maintenance results are achieved when large weight loss occurs during the treatment period in combination with follow-up that includes behavioral therapy and exercise [14,27,28].

Improvement in metabolic syndrome has been demonstrated using a VLED [29]. Glycemic control improves within 1 week of starting the VLED, blood pressure can reduce by 8–13%, total serum cholesterol by 5–25% and triglycerides by 15–50% [18]. Reports of mood improvement may be attributed to accompanying behavioral therapy programs, the weight loss seen, the feeling of control or due to eating higher quality food.

Total fasting

Total fasting is not recommended for weight loss as it leads to large losses of protein, diuresis (fluid loss), kaliuresis (loss of potassium), saluresis (loss of sodium) and other nutrient deficiencies. Loss of muscle mass and the large energy deficit lead to a greater decline in RMR and voluntary physical activity (as lethargy is common). Thus weight regain is likely. There is a high risk of refeeding syndrome when eating is resumed.

Low-fat diets

The relationship between "fat" and "weight gain" remains controversial, as evidence from various studies is inconsistent. The message to eat less fat has been promoted for decades and national nutritional surveys do show an overall reduction in fat intake. However, body weights are increasing. Whether dietary fat intake leads to weight gain seems to depend on the activity patterns of the individual [30–32], and the genetic predisposition to obesity of the individual [33]. Hence these factors may explain why the relationship between weight and fat intake is inconclusive [34,35].

A meta-analysis of intervention trials that compared reduced-fat and normal-fat diets found that the reduced-fat diet enhanced weight loss by 3–4 kg [36], and obese patients who reduced dietary fat by 10% achieved 4–5 kg weight loss [36]. Those who followed *ad libitum* diets achieved small weight losses (2–5 kg) for a brief period, although greater weight loss is achieved by people with initially heavier body weight [37–39]. The meta-analysis demonstrated a dose-dependent relationship between decreased fat intake and weight loss [40] (Fig. 21.2). For every 1% decrease in energy (from fat) there was a 0.28 kg decrease in body weight [36,40,41]. In another meta-analysis no difference was found in weight loss using either a normal-fat or reduced-fat diet [35]. Weight loss of 2–4 kg was achieved by the end of the intervention period and no difference was found in weight maintenance at the end of a 12–18 month follow-up period [35].

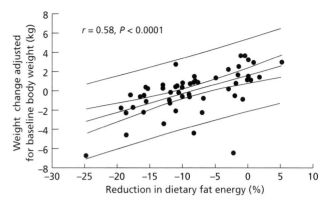

Figure 21.2 A meta-analysis of weight loss in 48 *ad libitum* low-fat diet intervention studies. The relationship between the reduction in dietary fat and weight change adjusted for pretreatment body weight. Each data set represents a study group. (Reproduced with permission from Astrup [40].)

Hence, ultimately there appears to be no significant difference in whether people employ a low-fat or a low-calorie diet to achieve weight loss. There have been reports that low-fat eating is a more palatable way to lose weight, and can often be advantageous with binge eaters [42]. However, long-term studies (minimum 18 months) have not shown any additional benefits [35,38]. Reducing both calories and fat seems to produce significantly greater weight loss compared to just reducing calories [9].

In some instances a decreased fat intake can cause a rise in triglycerides, particularly if the fat has been substituted with carbohydrate. This occurrence appears to be dependent on the type of fat and carbohydrate consumed. By consuming carbohydrates with a low glycemic load and/or having the main fat sources as mono- (MUFA) and polyunsaturated fats (PUFA), the effect seems to disappear or at least be less [43]. A decreased fat intake *per se* can lead to an improvement of triglycerides, particularly if the decreased fat intake is accompanied by a reduction in weight [43,44]. In the long term, there is some evidence to suggest that a low-fat diet helps maintain weight or limits weight gain [34,35,45]. Therefore, low-fat diets are as good as other interventions at reducing weight but are not better.

Moderate-fat diets

Moderate-fat diets can improve an individual's enjoyment of a diet, particularly if the type of fat is manipulated to increase MUFA or PUFA consumption. It can also improve their serum lipid profile, but has minimal impact on weight loss unless a calorie restriction is also in place [43,46]. For instance, when a low-fat, high-carbohydrate diet was compared to a diet of equal hypocaloric value but higher MUFA content, weight loss was identical. The increased MUFA diet did, however, lead to improvements in blood lipids and fasting insulin, even in normolipidemic obese women [47–50]. In a 14-month study comparing a 30% fat diet with a 20% fat diet, the 30% diet achieved greater weight loss, and resulted in a better cardiovascular risk profile than the 20% fat diet. This was thought to be due to better compliance by the 30% group [51]. Another study found that a Mediterranean-style diet of 35% fat had better compliance, a lower attrition rate and greater weight loss at the 18-month and 30-month time points compared to a 20% fat diet [52]. No *ad libitum* dietary intervention study has shown that a normal-fat (30–35%), high-MUFA diet is comparable to a low-fat diet in preventing weight gain [36].

Fat has hedonistic appeal [53–55]. By allowing people to eat slightly more fat than usual, enjoyment and sustainability of a diet are enhanced. The mitigating factor is that less food will need to be consumed in order to lose weight. Eating patterns and compliance become important issues, which reminds clinicians of the need to tailor dietary programs to suit individual needs. It should be noted that often when researchers discuss moderate fat intake, they use 30–33% fat intake but in clinical practice 30% energy from fat is generally considered low fat. To date, there is no evidence to suggest that a high-MUFA diet (>35% of energy from MUFA) is superior to a low-fat diet in promoting weight loss or in the prevention of weight gain. The major benefit is the favorable impact on cardiovascular risk factors [36].

Low-carbohydrate or higher protein diets

A low-carbohydrate diet contains less than 40% of total energy from carbohydrate [56]. A higher protein diet contains over 20% of total energy consumed as protein, and it is very high if the protein content is greater than 30% of the total energy [56].

When consuming lower energy diets, adequate amounts of protein are needed to spare nitrogen and maintain muscle mass, which in turn maintains resting energy expenditure. Often a person's normal diet exceeds the recommended protein intake even at this higher level of consumption, so reduced protein intake is required.

It is widely acknowledged that protein helps to suppress appetite more than fat or carbohydrate. This reduces the amount eaten at subsequent meals and also minimizes the likelihood of snacking. Some evidence suggests that a protein intake of 1.5 g/kg bodyweight and <200 g carbohydrate per day may increase thermogenesis and enhance glycemic control better than a diet that is low in protein and high in carbohydrate [57–61].

High-protein, low-calorie diets are attractive as they induce ketogenesis and initially produce larger weight loss due to fluid depletion and the formation of ketones, which helps to suppress appetite. This in turn promotes reduced caloric intake [61]. It remains controversial whether it is the calorie content or the macronutrient composition that is the major weight loss-inducing factor in low-carbohydrate diets [56,62].

A meta-analysis [62] of 38 studies that compared high- and low-carbohydrate diets conducted for 4 days or more (range 4–365 days) demonstrated that lower carbohydrate diets produced greater absolute weight loss than higher carbohydrate diets (16.9 kg versus 1.9 kg). However, the diets were very heterogeneous. When only the randomized controlled trials and randomized cross-over trials were compared, the difference in weight indicated a trend of greater weight loss with the lower carbohydrate trials, but it was not significantly different (3.6 kg versus 2.1 kg) [62]. It appears that calorie content, initial weight and the duration of the program are better predictors of weight loss than dietary carbohydrate consumption in isolation [62].

There have been concerns that if the protein intake were increased, blood lipid levels would be disrupted or further exaggerated. However, studies have not shown adverse affects on lipid profiles consistently and it is thought that LDL cholesterol is only likely to rise when carbohydrate has been almost exclusively replaced by saturated fat [63]. In most cases there have been improvements in HDL and triglycerides (TG) and no increase in LDL or blood pressure [61,64]. There have been concerns that the increased protein would lead to increased purines (amino acids) and therefore increased uric acid levels (which might cause gout in susceptible people) but there are no studies looking at this to date. Studies have shown that high-protein diets can speed the progression of renal disease in those with diabetes, even if the high-protein diet is only used in the short term [56].

The role of protein in the progression of renal disease remains controversial and further research is needed. More common adverse effects include fatigue (due to a depletion of glycogen), dizziness, headaches or nausea (thought to be caused by sodium loss), constipation, halitosis and muscle cramps, all of which occur more frequently in low-carbohydrate diets compared with conventional weight loss diets [61]. Many low-carbohydrate diets restrict the intake of fruit, vegetables and wholegrains, which provide essential mineral and vitamins and are likely to prevent cancers. They also present a risk of deficiency in vitamins E, A, B6, thiamine, folate, calcium, magnesium, iron, potassium and dietary fiber [65]. Most of the benefits of high-protein diets are short term, as few data exist on long-term outcomes.

One study examined the progression of coronary artery disease in 10 subjects being treated for cardiovascular problems who were prescribed a high-protein diet for 1 year. Average weight loss was 0.6 kg and total cholesterol, LDL, VLDL, TG and fibrinogen levels decreased. An increase in C-reactive protein occurred, indicating an inflammatory or infectious process. Therefore, it seems likely that the high-protein diet was increasing the progression of coronary heart disease in these high-risk patients [66].

High-protein diets may also lead to increased calcium loss. A study conducted on premenopausal women showed there was no effect on calcium retention or biomarkers under controlled conditions [67]. However, another study in adolescents indicated that a short-duration, high-protein diet lead to increased urinary calcium excretion. Over 3 months bone mineral density decreased even with vitamin D and calcium supplementation [68].

High-protein or low-carbohydrate diets (protein 30%) appear to better preserve lean muscle mass in both the obese and pre-obese person in the short term and when low energy requirements exist. They also appear to increase satiety and global pleasure (during energy restriction) and improve lipid profiles but they do not affect kidney function compared to an isocaloric diet with moderate protein content (18%) [69].

Energy density

Energy density is based on the energy content per gram of food. A food is thought to have low energy density if it contains <4 kJ or 1 kcal/g, moderate 4–6 kJ/g (1–1.5 kcal/g) and high if it contains >6 kJ/g (>1.5 kcal/g). Energy density is related mostly to the water, fiber and fat content of the food. Weight loss is often difficult, as individuals generally eat less food which subsequently increases hunger. Hence, prolonging satiety is an important element in dietary compliance and management. Adding bulky, low-energy foods to the diet promotes satiety without adding unnecessary calories. There is some evidence to suggest that the volume of food consumed plays a role in the hunger and satiety process [70]. It has been found that by reducing energy density in the short term, an overall reduction in total calories occurs. This is thought to occur from increased satiety and reduced hunger resulting in decreased total consumption, either per meal or over a few meals [71–75]. Longer term studies show that low energy-dense diets can promote moderate weight loss [75]. In studies lasting longer than 6 months, weight loss was more than three times as great in individuals consuming diets low in fat, high in fiber and low in energy density, versus diets that are only low in fat (−3.4 kg versus −1.0 kg) [75,76]. Often people consuming an *ad libitum* low-fat diet compensate by ingesting more. However, when fiber is added to the diet, therefore adding volume, satiety is increased and physically eating the food becomes more difficult [77–80].

Soups and salads have been shown to be particularly helpful in reducing energy intake [81–84]. One study involving 517 participants, in which 50% were asked to consume soup four times per week over a 10-week period, showed a positive correlation between soup intake and weight loss [85]. The participants who were instructed to eat soup once or twice daily and to restrict total calories were able to maintain their weight better than those who did not consume soup [86]. In a randomized trial 200 overweight or obese subjects were instructed to consume a calorie-controlled diet through an exchange system, by either including two soups per day or consuming two high-energy snacks per day, or with no specific inclusions. At the end of 1 year those who consumed the soups or had no specific inclusion lost approximately 50% more weight than those who ate the high-energy snack [84]. A 2-year observational, follow-up study looked at those who had maintained weight loss or regained lost weight. The results showed that both groups ate similar amounts of food but the weight maintainers consumed a lower energy-dense diet than their counterparts [87]. Another study involving the Danish population, the Danish MONICA study, which reviewed weight change and energy density of the diet over a 5-year period, found that energy density was not related to weight loss but it did contribute to weight gain in women but not men [88]. Men and women from the Framingham offspring cohort were studied to determine if dietary quality (that is, how closely their intake resembled US national dietary guidelines) impacted on weight over an 8-year period. Those who had diets that closely resembled the guidelines gained less weight than those whose diet was considerably different from the recommendations. Although energy density was not addressed in this paper, the results showed that an increase in dietary quality was accompanied by increased fiber consumption but fat and alcohol consumption decreased.

It could be inferred that energy density decreases as diet quality increases [89]. Further, dietary energy density would also decrease if consumers replaced soft drinks or other calorie-rich beverages with water. A retrospective study found that people who consumed water (in preference to higher calorie alternatives) also had a less energy-dense diet and consumed 194 fewer calories (815 kJ) per day. However, it should be noted that the people who drank water were also of high socio-economic status (SES), older and better educated, all situations known to influence other dietary factors [90].

In intervention studies it has been found that energy density of food accounts for about 40% of the variability in energy intake; however, in the free-living situation it probably only accounts for 7% [80]. It is thought that compensatory processes explain this phenomenon, as high-density food is considered more palatable than low-density food, and people learn to have smaller amounts of the higher density and more palatable food than lower density but less palatable food. High-density food is often cheaper, more consistent in taste and quality and is often considered to be a "treat." Its convenience is also attractive to many people [80,91–93].

Hence, evidence shows that augmenting the diet with low-density food enhances weight loss, but only when the food is palatable enough to ensure compliance. Including soups and salads as pre-meals or as snacks and replacing soft drinks with water in the daily diet may assist in avoiding high-energy snacking and meals.

Glycemic index (GI)

The GI ranks a food according to its 0–2 hour effect on postprandial blood glucose levels (BGL). The GI is determined by measuring the area under a blood glucose curve, which is created by plotting the blood glucose levels after ingestion of a food equivalent to 50 g of carbohydrate (Fig. 21.3). This area is compared to a reference food of equal carbohydrate content, either glucose or white bread. This ratio, expressed as a percentage, is the GI of that food [94] (Box 21.3).

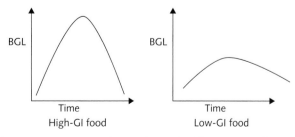

Figure 21.3 Diagrammatic drawings showing the difference in BGL after a food with a high GI and one with a low GI.

Table 21.2 Factors that influence the GI of a food

Factors affecting GI	Comments
Type of starch	Starches have various structures which are digested at different rates. Amylose is slowly digested whereas amylopectin is rapidly digested [95–97].
Type of sugar	Lactose, fructose, sucrose and glucose have variable rates of digestion resulting in GIs between 23 and 100 [98].
Cooking	Cooking changes food's structure. Gelatinization occurs in the carbohydrate after cooking and cooling; this lowers the GI of a food [96,99,100].
Processing	Processing breaks down foods into small particles which enhances digestion, e.g. white flour [99–102].
Other macronutrients	The presence of other nutrients such as fat and protein can lower the GI of a food by slowing its digestion [103].
Acidity	Acidity affects gastric emptying and hence the GI of a food. Hence by adding vinegar, citric acid or other fruits to food, the GI of that food will decline [98,104].
Fiber	Fiber has been shown to slow the rate of digestion, particularly soluble fiber [105].
Food type	Adding certain food groups, e.g. fruit, legumes and wholegrains, can lower the GI of a meal. They can also favorably impact the subsequent meal [106–109].

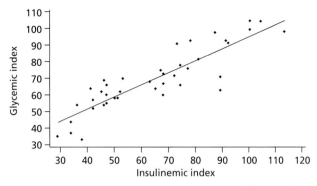

Figure 21.4 Correlation between GI and Insulinemic Index (II) for 43 starchy foods [97].

Box 21.3 Quick guide to classifying GI food

Low <50
Medium 50–70
High >70

The GI of a food varies depending on its rate of digestion so that the faster the digestion, the higher the GI value. There are many factors that will affect the digestion of a food (see Table 21.2) but the only way to determine the GI of a food is to measure it. However, GI is not the only factor that can affect BGL; the amount of carbohydrate present also dictates the response to that food. Harvard University described glycemic load (GL), which considers the amount of carbohydrate in a food in addition to the food's GI. The GL determines the degree of glycemia and insulin demand produced by a serving of the food, as opposed to just the 50 g carbohydrate equivalent.

The obese population is at the greatest risk of developing the metabolic syndrome. This includes dyslipidemia, hyperinsulinemia or severe insulin resistance and hypertension [110]. It has been demonstrated that the consumption of low-GI foods mitigates these risk factors to some degree. Low-GI foods appear to improve blood lipid profile by concurrently decreasing LDL levels and increasing HDL levels. In addition, improved fibrinolytic

activity and reduced risk of myocardial infarction have been demonstrated [111–117].

Many studies have shown that blood insulin levels closely track BGL in most individuals [97] (Fig. 21.4). Significantly, a low-GI diet improves insulin sensitivity, in both those with and without diabetes [112]. One study of obese women who were prescribed a low-GI diet demonstrated that fasting insulin levels declined in parallel with weight loss [118]. However, subsequently it has been found that not all low-GI foods lead to a predicted lower insulin response [97, 119,120]. More work is required before any strong conclusions can be drawn.

There appear to be many benefits associated with using GI and GL to help control BGL and to improve the cardiovascular risk profile in people whose BMI is greater than 23 kg/m^2 [121]. However, it remains controversial as to whether or not GI and/ or GL should be used in weight loss programs *per se*. A meta-analysis of the data has shown that low-GI meals did not lead to significantly lower energy intake (3.5 MJ) compared to high-GI meals (4.1 MJ) nor was there a significant difference in weight loss [122]. In animal studies using a low-GI diet, a decrease in fat deposition can be demonstrated which is not accompanied by depletion of lean muscle mass. However, this has not yet been replicated in human studies [122].

A recent Cochrane review explored the role of low-GI and low-GL diets in weight management and found a small but significant improvement in weight loss and fat mass (~1 kg greater) and BMI (1.3 units) in those who consumed a low-GI diet (compared to a conventional diet). Despite the small weight loss there was an improvement in total and LDL cholesterol. In free-living conditions, those who consumed a low-GI/GL *ad libitum* diet lost as much, if not more, than those who followed a conventional *ad libitum* diet. Unfortunately, only six randomized controlled trials (RCT) involving 202 participants were included in the review. The dietary interventions were relatively short term, ranging from 5 weeks to 6 months, with only two studies having follow-up after the intervention phase of 6 months, both by the same author. Only two of the six RCT included obese participants [123]. Despite these shortcomings, other positive factors such as satiety, palatability, volume, fiber and wholegrains usually occur with low-GL or -GI foods.

In practice, a comprehensive, consistent GI or GL labeling system needs to be implemented in order to avoid consumer confusion and to ensure that consumers are genuinely eating low-GI diets [97,122].

The less restrictive dieting approach

Many people who seek help from weight loss professionals have had a long history of dieting and weight swings. Repeated attempts to lose weight often end in failure when the individual cannot maintain their weight using highly restrictive practices. Some suggest that dieting and being weight obsessed contributes to obesity rather than solving it. Others argue that the detrimental effects of dieting are worse than the weight *per se* and a nondieting approach to health would be more beneficial [124]. It has also been postulated that there are two main forms of dieting: one that relies on external cues, such as food, exercise plans and menu development (the traditional approach), and another that relies on internal cues where the body indicates what and how much to eat through the use of hunger and satiety signals [125]. One such approach is known as Health at Any Size (H@AS). This is based on the premise that an overweight person wants to eat healthily and be active, and by eliminating restrictions and pressures, they would naturally adopt healthier patterns. This would ultimately lead to weight change that was genetically appropriate. The H@AS system also assumes that health is a result of behaviors that are independent of body weight. The person using the system is encouraged to give up dieting and let the body guide them to what it wants and needs. This would lead to a weight that might not be what the medical profession or individual initially would determine ideal but would lead to an improved quality of life.

The supporters of H@AS suggest that dieting has lead to unhealthy practices that have caused people to ignore or not recognize their own hunger cues. Satiety, desire and exercise have traditionally been seen in the context of weight loss, not for enjoyment in themselves [126,127]. Work by Mellin et al. is summarized by Miller and Jacob [128], and shows that nondieting is predicated on mind, body and lifestyle modification. For example, mind skills may involve increasing knowledge of one's feelings and needs, developing appropriate goals, expectations and positive cognitions. Body skills may include minimizing negative thoughts about body weight and understanding the body's weight loss threshold and attending to total body self-care. Lifestyle skills may include learning and responding appropriately to hunger and satiety signals, identifying the tastes of foods and how they make the person feel after consumption, identifying healthy eating habits and participation in daily physical activity for enjoyment and self-restoration [128,129].

As psychologic improvement tends to be the main outcome of H@AS, direct comparisons with other treatment outcomes based on biochemical or anthropometric measurements [128] are problematic. The evidence that traditional methods of weight loss

cause psychologic harm is fairly sketchy and as yet unfounded [128]. Many studies have shown that weight loss is positively correlated with improved quality of life no matter what the method used [130–134]. It is generally accepted that improvements in many medical conditions occur as a consequence of weight loss which is considered one component of quality of life [135] although the improvement in quality of life may not be as great as first thought [136] and it is also widely acknowledged that some medical problems are negatively affected by weight loss [135].

In some cases the nondieting approach (involving less restrictive food choices and exercise) combined with higher calorie choices (1800 kcal) created less weight loss in the short term (2.5 kg versus 5.6 kg) but larger weight losses in the long term (10 kg versus 4.5 kg in 1 year) compared to more traditional weight loss methods (involving restrictive practices, strict 5 MJ (1200 kcal) diet, exercise prescription, stimulus control, self-monitoring and behavioral substitution) [137] (Fig. 21.5). Another study (albeit with a small sample size and no control group) used the nondieting approach and concluded that the participants who were followed up periodically for 2 years experienced weight loss over the total period, rather than initial weight loss followed by weight gain [138]. Other studies that compared highly restrictive practices, e.g. VLED, and conventional higher calorie intake diets showed that although the weight loss was slower, it was better maintained [139].

Some researchers suggest that maintenance of significant weight loss by using traditional methods is unrealistic, as significant energy expenditure via physical exercise is required [128,140]. The H@AS method advocates exercising only to levels that are maintainable in the long term, thereby achieving a weight consistent with achievable habits [128]. A benefit of the H@AS approach is that participants do not feel as though they are on a

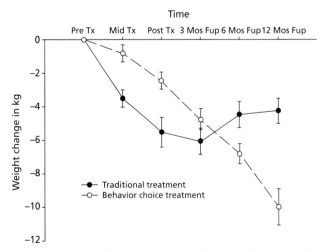

Figure 21.5 Mean weight loss over 12 months of either traditional prescriptive intervention or patient choice approach. (Reproduced with permission from Sbrocco et al [137].)

diet [129,141]. They are encouraged to listen to their bodies and eat to their needs and wants rather than just eating to satisfy the calorie restriction. Long-term empiric evidence shows that individuals who follow a less restrictive plan often consume fewer calories than when they are trying to follow a strict diet [128].

In addition, other factors also need to be considered. The assumption that all obese patients know how to eat a healthy diet following the removal of dietary restrictions is unsubstantiated. Also, for some people, rapid weight loss is essential in order to improve co-existing medical conditions [128]. The American Dietetic Association note that "there may be great variation among individuals in their ability to perceive and act upon internal cues, lengthy interventions may be required to learn to perceive internal signals of hunger and satiety and to develop the trust in themselves to allow these signals to guide food intake" [125].

Irrespective of whether weight loss occurs in patients who follow a nondieting approach or not, other eating-related psychopathology tends to decline. Factors such as restraint eating, bingeing, poor self-image and even depression and anxiety scores are often improved [138,142,143].

H@AS seems to work especially well when combined with a liberal caloric guide, e.g. approximately 1800 kcal. Often these patients have been trapped in the diet cycle (Fig. 21.6) most of their lives and this method can help them to break the repetitive and unsuccessful cycle. It is probably not suitable for individuals who have little understanding of good nutrition, who love high-fat, high-sugar or fatty protein foods, those who think eating extremely large portions is normal and who also report extreme hunger signals. Correcting these attitudes/behaviors should be addressed first before commencing on this style of treatment.

In summary, the H@AS method may be effective for people who:
• have used highly restrictive practices in the past
• have failed at weight loss
• are currently eating reasonably well
• have good nutritional knowledge

• are long-term dieters
• are preoccupied with body weight and eating behavior
• no longer think they can achieve weight loss
• are emotional or nonhungry eaters.
This type of intervention is thought to work if:
• prior to starting the program a comprehensive discussion identifies previous behavior, dietary and exercise patterns so that realistic goals can be set
• enjoyable exercise is included and encouraged for health, body weight control and general well-being
• a behavioral plan based on eating and activity patterns is established, in order to enhance successful outcomes
• a maintenance plan is designed which will help the individual develop skills for maintaining newly developed behaviors [144]. It should be noted that this method has not been tested on a culturally diverse group. Caucasian women comprise the majority of the tested population [128] and a qualified professional is required to administer the cognitive behavioral program, as the H@AS is strongly dependent on cognitive restructuring. Randomized controlled studies, with statically significant numbers of participants, are required in order to validate the H@AS approach.

Meal frequency

The impact of meal frequency on body weight is not as clear as one may expect. Observational data suggest (but this is inconclusive) that an inverse relationship exists between weight and meal frequency [145]. It has also been suggested that people who eat frequently have better internal hunger satiety regularity systems [146]. However, other studies have shown that obese women mostly ate their meals in the afternoon period, and ate more frequently compared to their lean counterparts [147]. Intervention studies suggest that a single meal leads to greater consumption at a subsequent *ad libitum* meal, as opposed to when the same quantity of food is spread over several meals, irrespective of hunger ratings and total insulin secretion (although insulin fluctuations were less in the multi-meal group) [148,149]. The authors suggest that the reduced consumption at the *ad libitum*

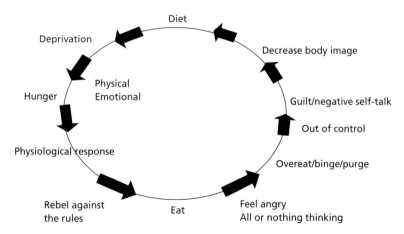

Figure 21.6 The diet cycle. People start a diet because they want to change their body in some way; subsequently they start to feel deprived both physically and emotionally. This deprivation leads them to have increased thoughts about food and display food-seeking behavior; often they feel like they are missing out. Finally they eat. At this point the "all or nothing" thinking starts and they feel guilty. These feelings may lead to overconsumption of food and in some cases, purging behavior. Negative self-talk often follows with statements such as "I am such a bad person," "I have no willpower," which results in poor body image. The cycle repeats, but the person vows that "it will be better this time."

meal may occur as a result of the reduced insulin fluctuations [148,149].

Reduced meal frequency does not appear to lower total insulin secretion (although it may reduce insulin level fluctuations) or total energy expenditure. It does, however, appear to increase LDL and lower HDL cholesterol [150,151]. Even diet-induced thermogenesis does not appear to increase with greater meal frequency [145,152–155].

Changing meal frequency in order to ingest the same amount of food over several meals instead of one meal may be hard for some individuals, as there is a strong genetic influence on predisposition to individual eating patterns. de Castro [156] investigated genetic influences on meal size, meal frequency and meal composition. The study demonstrated that the genetic component explained 44–65% of the variance [156]. However, other contributory factors to food frequency are food availability, food palatability and food density [80,157], and forced eating restrictions [116,158]. All these factors have been shown to lead to increased food intake and, in some individuals, weight gain.

There is little evidence to suggest that meal frequency plays a role in weight loss unless caloric intake is altered. Frequent food intake, consumed at regular intervals, versus a single intake may lead to better intake regulation. The key is for people to eat less food several times a day, and at regular intervals, rather than consume large meals infrequently.

Diets pre- and post- bariatric surgery

Bariatric surgical treatment has been shown to give the best long-term outcomes of any type of weight loss intervention. Hence, in recent years it has become very popular. However, there have been only a few papers looking at dietary intervention and appropriate protocols. There are three main types of intervention:
• gastric restriction reduces the size of the stomach, thus reducing capacity of the stomach so that satiety is achieved sooner
• malabsorptive procedures where part of the stomach and/or the gut is removed to reduce the amount and rate of nutrient absorption
• combination procedure which reduces capacity and decreases absorption.
In all these surgeries, there may be some alterations in satiety brought about by changes in satiety hormones or neural feedback.

The two most common types of bariatric surgery currently are the laproscopically placed band (restriction method) and the Roux-en-Y gastric bypass (RYGB) (combination method).

VLEDs are usually prescribed for 2–6 weeks prior to the banding procedure. This reduces visceral adiposity, fatty liver and liver size which provides easier access to the stomach; it also introduces the patient to restrictive dietary practice, improves any

associated co-morbidities and stops the "last supper" phenomenon [159]. Patients undergoing the other procedures do not normally require specific dietary intervention preoperatively.

Postoperatively patients take clear fluids for 1–2 days, followed by full fluids for 1–2 weeks. Many people stay on the VLED after surgery as they find it easier and receive all nutrient requirements. Generally, most fluids are permissible as long as they can be consumed via a straw, although very high-energy fluids, such as thick shakes, are discouraged. Most people lose weight at this stage but weight loss is not the primary goal. Internal healing and ensuring that the band adheres to the stomach is the postoperative priority in the first month. Over the next few weeks the food consistency can progress from puréed to soft foods [160]. No more than one cup of food per meal should be consumed, and protein intake should be emphasized. The patient may require additional food, depending on their pain, hunger and the type of operation. By the time patients start ingesting solid foods (that is, food that requires chewing before swallowing), they should not be consuming fluids containing calories and soft foods should be avoided. Patients are encouraged to adopt prescribed serving sizes to avoid overeating and to eat only three meals per day but more may be needed if hunger is a problem and the quantity per meal becomes very small [160].

Diet quality can become an issue when small amounts of food are eaten. Protein-containing foods and beverages should be the priority when planning meals, followed by vegetables, fruit, low-fat dairy and wholegrains. Low-fat cooking techniques are important to keep fat content down as the fat content of intake predicts percent of weight loss with restrictive surgical intervention [161]. High-fat and high-sugar foods devoid of nutrients should be avoided. Variety becomes important in satisfying mineral and vitamin requirements and to ensure adequate intake of other lesser known bio-active substances. Individual tolerance levels vary but as restrictions increase, some foods are generally harder to tolerate than others, e.g. most people have problems with stringy meat, white breads or anything that goes "gluggy." Unfortunately, consumption of biscuits and chocolate does not seem to be stopped by the surgical restriction and this is a trap for those who are struggling to keep food down. Eating slowly, taking small bites and chewing the food well are imperative [160]. Some surgeons promote that people with a band around the stomach should limit fluid intake with, and immediately before or after, meals. However, this remains controversial. For other surgery, fluids should not be consumed for 30 minutes before and after the meal [160].

Dehydration, nausea and vomiting and dumping syndrome are common complications due to poor postoperative compliance. They can occur as a result of inadequate fluid intake, overeating, swallowing large pieces of food, stricture or stenosis or eating concentrated amounts of sugar [160]. All symptoms can be managed by changing intake habits, except for stricture or stenosis, both of which need to be treated surgically [160].

Long-term complications can result from poor compliance, restrictions being too tight and serving sizes being too small, or from malabsorption in the intestine. Research on micronutrient deficiencies in bariatric patients over the long term is limited; however, postoperatively patients are advised to take a chewable complete multivitamin [160]. Patients can often become deficient in iron, folate, vitamin B12, calcium, thiamine, vitamin A and other fat-soluble vitamins. Protein deficiency is rare in RYGB and banded patients but occasionally can occur in those who had older bypass surgeries. To consume the recommended daily dose of 60–70 g protein, a supplement may be required [160].

Nonhungry eating, grazing, emotional eating and low moods can all sabotage weight loss efforts, particularly for those with the gastric band. More intense intervention is needed for these patients. Incidental and planned activity is important for greater weight loss notwithstanding the surgical intervention and its importance should be emphasized during routine follow-up counseling sessions [161].

The range of dietary treatments used by the private sector

Slimming clubs

The dietary treatments offered by slimming clubs are conventional, reducing diets with a "twist." Some clubs, such as Weight Watchers, use a form of calorie counting to help the patient control their energy intake. Foods are given "points" based on their energy value and fat content; there are no "forbidden" foods. The client is allowed to eat foods up to the value of a given number of "points", which is calculated on the basis of their body weight (heavier clients being allowed more points). Clients following a Weight Watchers diet are advised to eat a healthy diet and they are allowed a number of "free" foods per day; they also receive "bonus" points for exercise. Other slimming clubs, such as Slimming World (UK), do not use calorie counting. Instead, clients are advised to follow a diet plan made up of different colored days, where, for example, a green day is made up of fruit and vegetables. Each colored day contains a list of "free" foods, healthy extras (which are allowed in moderation), and "sins." Clients are allowed between 5 and 15 "sins" a day – a chocolate bar such as a Mars Bar is 15 "sins" whereas a glass of wine is 5 "sins."

Reviews of commercial weight loss programs showed that the program *per se* had little to do with the participants' weight loss but had everything to do with their compliance [162–164]. There is little available research on commercial weight loss enterprises but the available evidence is not favorable for self- directed, internet-based weight loss programs [165]. Often in the commercial weight loss area the program leaders are people who have successfully lost weight but who do not have any formal training in dietary or exercise matters. Still, there is no reason to believe that the dietary treatments advocated by slimming clubs are less effective than those advocated by health professionals. When Biesalski [166] compared the results from a Weight Watchers study with a clinical study (both performed in Sweden), he found that the

Weight Watchers group had lost significantly more weight than the clinical group at 24 months. This does not lead to the conclusion that obese people who attend slimming clubs fare better than those who attend hospital-run obesity clinics, as different "types" of people pursue different "types" of treatment, but it does indicate that slimming clubs can be effective for some people.

Special diets

There are many special diets which are purported to aid weight loss [167]. Some involve combining certain foods, restricting certain types of food during specific times of the day, or eliminating whole food groups entirely. Essentially, they all involve consuming a low-calorie diet which results in weight loss, but few proponents would admit to such a simple claim. A claim of offering something "different," perhaps by an as yet unknown metabolic pathway, by which the diet produces weight loss is not uncommon. Whatever the claim, it is always compelling. A paper recently published in the *Journal of the American Dietetic Association* found that some popular special diets varied in dietary quality and when tested using the Alternate Healthy Eating Index (which was originally developed by the US Department of Agriculture to identify dietary factors associated with reduced cardiovascular disease risk and subsequently revized by McCullough [168]), many were found to be unhealthy. However, some, such as Weight Watchers, the New Glucose Revolution and Ornish Low Fat Eating, were acceptable [169].

Quackery and "health foods" which claim to aid weight loss

"Health foods" constitute a group of products which from a consumer's perspective straddles the food and medicine fence. In many cases, product advertizing suggests that the product will confer health benefits on the consumer. Of relevance here are the products which claim to assist weight loss. For example, *Healthwatch Newsletter* [170] reported on a slimming product, "Autoslim," which was advertized in 1993 in a British newspaper. The advertizement claimed that the product would "cause steady weight loss day after day" and "your body's metabolism will activate and actually start to burn off excess calories and fat." The metabolic phenomenon was described as a "fat furnace." The product was supplied by postal order only and came with a money back guarantee. It also came with a sheet describing "Newton's special diet plan" in which the customer was allowed to eat unlimited amounts of fresh fruit and vegetables, lean meat and fish, but no white bread, cakes, nuts, sugar, sweets, milk, cheese or fat in any form.

The UK Trading Standards Officer investigated Autoslim, which was found to contain only trivial amounts of some amino acids that are consumed in larger quantities in a normal diet; it would also not significantly affect metabolic rate. The manufacturer was prosecuted for making false claims about the product's efficacy.

There are many other products on the market like Autoslim and health professionals who treat obese patients need to keep abreast of such products so they can provide sound advice to their patients. It is important to report any concerns about the authenticity of slimming or weight loss-related products to the relevant authorities.

Basic principles

Assessment of dietary intake
A first step in making changes is a shared awareness and understanding of the patient's present position. In order to begin education on new eating habits, one must be aware of old habits, regardless of the type of dietary treatment used. Although there are a number of tools which will assess dietary intake [171], the most common methods used in this setting are the diet history and the 7-day unweighed diet diary methods. The 7-day unweighed diet diary is deemed to be the most useful method in this context [172,173]. The patient must be given clear instructions on how to complete the diary, either verbally or, preferably, in written format in the diary provided. Although foods do not need to be weighed, a reasonable description of the types of foods and quantities consumed, in household measures, needs to be given. However, it should be noted that a 7-day unweighed diary can be tedious and for some patients too confronting if used from the first visit in which case the patient rarely completes the diary [173].

How the information collected in diet diaries may be used in the dietary treatment of obesity
The completed diary then becomes the basis for discussion of eating habits. Any changes must be (as far as possible) acceptable to the patient in terms of palatability and practicality, otherwise the patient will not comply with the dietary advice. An understanding of the patient's lifestyle, including financial, time constraints, and cultural issues if appropriate, is also important. The health professional should ensure that any advice would not compromise other aspects of healthy eating [174], such as micronutrient intake, and protein to energy ratio to achieve better nitrogen retention and minimize fat free mass loss [175].

The diary may indicate an erratic eating pattern, with problems such as irregular meals, periods of fasting, excessively restrained eating, frequent snacking, grazing or binge eating [173].

It may be useful to ask for additional information in the diet diary, such as relating mood or circumstances to eating, describing hunger and fullness before and after eating or monitoring physical activity, to help identify areas for behavior change. Many of these factors can be helped by a health professional, in particular a dietitian, but sometimes referral to a clinical psychologist, exercise physiologist or physiotherapist may also be appropriate. Often in complicated cases the additional confounders need to be dealt with before weight loss can be attempted [176,177].

As well as providing a record of reported food intake and eating behavior at baseline, the diet diary can be used throughout management to review and plan for future treatment. A diet diary

encourages the patient to be actively involved in treatment, and to take responsibility for making dietary and other behavior changes. It may also provide an indication of the patient's motivation, ways of improving motivation, and implementing change. It can also be very helpful to the patient to identify their own sabotaging factors.

The problems associated with under-reporting of energy intake by obese clients
A common problem in developing dietary advice for the obese patient on the basis of the reported food and drink consumed is that the energy intake of the reported diet is often significantly less than that estimated from predictive equations for the obese person in energy balance. Predictive equations for obese individuals have been reviewed by Heshka [178] who recommends using those formulated by Fleisch [179] or Robinson [180]. Indeed, there is a wealth of evidence which shows that energy intakes reported by the obese are significantly lower than would be feasible if they were to maintain their level of obesity [181].

Many authors have concluded from this evidence that the obese under-report their habitual energy intake during the study period. This may well be the case, but there is also the possibility that obese patients actively diet when asked to record their food intake and indeed report a true intake of their dieting behavior. Support for this explanation is provided by the frequent (but not published) observation that people often lose weight when they are asked to record their food intake, even when these people are students studying for a nutrition degree. If the low energy intakes reported by obese clients are a result of true dieting behavior, one might predict that if the obese patient were asked to record their food intake for long enough, they would either lose weight (and on this basis one may use continuous recording of food intake in a diary as an adjunct to therapy – see below) or report food intake associated with relapse. Unfortunately, little work around the use of long-term continuous food records in obese patients has been performed.

Regardless of the explanation for the low energy intakes reported by obese patients, the health professional must accept that it may not be possible to obtain a comprehensive record of their food intake from a 7-day diary. If the obese patient is reporting true dieting behavior then the diet which they consume during relapse will remain a mystery, and may be completely different in terms of foods eaten, quantities consumed, and eating behavior compared to the diet they consume while losing weight. It is not sufficiently known if the obese under-report all foods or only selective foods. Limited evidence on under-reporting suggests that the obese tend to under-record food from snacks compared with meals [182–184], and particularly from snacks consumed during the evening [185]. Therefore, since snacks tend to be made up of different foods and drinks and have a different macronutrient composition compared with meals [184], specific under-reporting means that it may be impossible to predict true dietary intake from a 7-day diet diary in an obese patient.

Is it worth assessing food intake in obese patients?

Even with these caveats, it is still useful to use a 7-day diary to assess food intake in obese patients. Apart from gaining an insight into any possible behavioral problems, it also reduces reliance on memory and is a written learning tool.

However, the health professional should also calculate the patient's energy intake from predictive equations since having an estimate of energy intake is useful in calculating the true energy intake which will be required to lose weight; 4200 kJ (1000 kcal) per day below the estimated requirement will normally produce a weight loss of 0.5–1.0 kg per week [186]. A possible scenario (and one which is not uncommon in obesity clinics) may arise whereby the health professional advises the obese patient to consume a diet which contains more energy than that which the obese person reports to consume. Although some patients may be alarmed at such advice, Frost [187] has shown that this approach to formulating dietary advice works well.

In an attempt to improve (i.e. get nearer to the truth) the diet reported in a 7-day diary by obese patients, the health professional could ask additional questions about food intake. Although there are no standard questions or questionnaires which are designed for this specific purpose, one could ask about the frequency (say, per week) of consumption of certain types of foods, e.g. energy-dense foods and take-aways, and cross-reference this information with that in the diet diary. Or one could ask about weekday and weekend variations as weekdays are often more structured and lower in high-energy foods than weekends. Questions around eating behavior may also be helpful, and a question which may be useful is "Do you normally lose weight or gain weight when on holiday". The answers to this question can then be used in helping the obese patient identify triggers for overeating and alter behavior to reduce food intake at home. For example, the obese patient may have reduced their intake as they tend not to overeat with other people around, or perhaps they were preoccupied with other interests and therefore not focusing on food, or they did more exercise on holiday than at home. Indeed, there is evidence to show that many obese individuals do not overeat in public places [188] but do so in private, particularly at home during the evening [189].

Hope for a useable tool to assess true dietary intake comes from two published studies, which have developed food frequency questionnaires that appear to capture realistic energy intakes [190,191].

Setting goals and rate of weight loss

Setting goals is an important part of the weight loss process but these goals must be realistic. Goals should be time specific, small, achievable and behaviorally based. In terms of weight goals, the patients need to have realistic expectations of what they can achieve. For patients with 20 or more kilograms to lose, intermediate weight targets should be set, to reduce the chance of the patient giving up due to the seemingly long and difficult task they have set themselves.

The obese person should also be clear about the expected rate of weight loss. As stated above, if a person consumes 1000 kcal per day less than they would normally eat, then they should lose between 0.5 and 1.0 kg per week. But some people will be disappointed with a weight loss of less than 1 kg a week, and the obese person may give up on a diet because in their view it is not working, whereas in fact it is. Indeed, it has been shown that patients who had unrealistically high initial expected weight loss did not lose weight and consequently dropped out of the program [192]. It has also been shown to lead to greater yo-yo dieting due to setting the individual up to fail [193].

Independent of treatment modality, positive outcome expectations and satisfaction with the treatment have been found to be associated with weight loss [194]. Unrealistic expectations, however, do not limit success with bariatric treatment [195]. It is important to help patients to accept moderate, achievable expectations of weight loss, and to discourage unrealistic goals for the rate of loss and target weight [173].

The impact of information from other sources

It is easy to forget that dietary advice given by the health professional is only part of the information which the patient uses to change eating behavior. Patients present with a wide variation in their baseline knowledge of the energy value of foods; some are real experts and know much more than most health professionals. The advice given by the health professional will be combined with the knowledge that the patient already has, rather than overriding the patient's baseline knowledge, and it is this combined knowledge which will form the basis of change to the diet. The constant and often more compelling background information on dieting from other sources, particularly from media, friends and family, will influence the changes to eating behavior immediately and in the future. Indeed, the patient may request advice from the health professional regarding a specific diet or food that they have heard will enhance their weight loss or make it easier. Regardless of the credibility of reported claims for such diets or foods, it is important that the health professional addresses them seriously and does not dismiss them as "simply ridiculous"; if the patient thought that these claims were ridiculous they would not have asked for advice on them in the first place.

Nutrition in practice

Individual habits, lifestyle, personal needs and health status need to be taken into consideration, as does a person's access to food, their cooking skills, appliances in the home, their financial situation and their motivation. The American Dietetic Association (ADA) [125] position paper emphasizes the need to think about the long-term management of weight rather than short-term losses, paying particular attention to sustainable changes while focusing on overall well-being and not just treatment or prevention of disease. The ADA believes the program should include "training in lifestyle modification with (a) gradual change to a healthful eating style with increased intake of wholegrains, fruit and vegetables; (b) a nonrestrictive approach to eating based on internal regulation of food (hunger and satiety); and (c) gradual increase to at least 30 min of enjoyable physical activity each day" [125].

Changing lifestyle factors still remains the most effective long-term treatment and although the clinician can help with this, it is still the responsibility of the client to maintain changes and achieve the desired outcome [196]. In a recent study in which young adult women were asked what they wanted from a weight loss program, meal planning, cooking, low-fat recipes and stress management were their primary goals [197].

The aim is to help create an energy deficit that achieves weight loss. By taking the above information into account, weight loss programs should include eating patterns, types of food and cooking methods, behavior patterns, emotional/cognitive factors, and exercise. All of this can be gleaned from the food diary and lifestyle history.

Eating patterns

Eating patterns involves the distribution of food, portion sizes, timing and speed of eating [173]. Often the daily ingestion of food is unbalanced and erratic. People will leave large time gaps between meals or skip meals altogether, leading to extreme hunger and food-seeking behavior. Mostly the food sought at this time is convenience food, which is easily accessible, gives instant gratification and comes prepackaged. Convenience foods are mostly of low-satiety, high-energy and high-fat value. When these foods are combined with increased hunger, the individual is predisposed to overconsumption, i.e. eating beyond their energy requirements. If a meal is eaten at this time, often larger portions than normal are consumed in haste, with no adjustment to body satiety cues. Although the number of meals in a day might be low, the total energy intake is often high. Therefore an energy deficit created by skipping a meal or lengthening the time between meals is not achieved. It is best to eat regularly, leaving enough time to become hungry, but not ravenous, between meals. Eating slowly can help one to notice hunger and satiety cues earlier and ultimately leads to decreased consumption. Techniques to slow the pace of consumption include putting the cutlery down between bites, pausing during the meal and chewing food well before swallowing [22].

Other people may eat regularly but consume large portions. An energy deficit could be achieved by reducing the size or composition of the meals. For instance, less food fits on a butter plate compared to a dinner plate but the plate still looks full. Changing the type of food can be helpful; it is harder to overconsume bread that has many grains in it than it is to overconsume white bread, due to its texture and density. Assisting people in recognizing the feeling of satiety rather than being overly full and practicing stopping eating at the point of satisfaction not fullness are useful methods to employ when aiming for portion control.

Food variety has mixed implications for weight management. Variety can enhance compliance as it adds interest and reduces boredom and feelings of deprivation, in addition to helping a person meet their nutritional requirements. But too much choice can lead to overconsumption. It has been shown that cafeteria-style eating leads to higher consumption and weight gain [124,198].

Structured meal plans or meal replacements can help with weight loss. They may help the individual comprehend appropriate portion sizes and reduce confusion around food choice, thus aiding compliance and producing positive early results, which is also motivating [199]. Using grocery lists can yield a similar outcome [9]. However, meal plans need to be flexible enough to accommodate individual social demands, unplanned events and holidays.

Types of foods and cooking methods

The type of food, where it is obtained and how it is cooked are all important issues. The origin provides an indication as to the composition of the food, e.g. take-away foods are often extremely high in fat, salt and energy, whereas home-cooked meals have a greater potential to be lower energy as cooking methods can be manipulated.

Carbohydrate is needed to maintain blood sugar levels and fluid balance. Observationally, higher carbohydrate intake leads to lower BMI and lower waist to hip ratio [200]. The best type of carbohydrate to consume is high-fiber, low-GI foods like wholegrains, fruit and vegetables [43]. Sugar consumed as sugary drinks is more likely to lead to weight gain than sugar ingested in solid forms [5,177,201]. Fiber and water are two other important components of any weight loss diet, especially if protein has been increased. They help avoid constipation (a common side-effect from increased protein and reduced intake), and the fiber adds bulk to the meal. Increased fiber intake has been shown to be associated with lower body weight, fat mass and with BMI irrespective of fat intake [202]. In Australia 30 g of fiber is recommended per day for everyone and international guidelines for diabetes treatment recommend up to 50 g of fiber each day depending on tolerance [203].

Many dieters restrict dairy and meat produce, believing this will help them with weight loss. However, a high proportion of women are anemic and are not meeting their recommended nutrient intakes for calcium. There is no need to eliminate either dairy or meat; they can be included by choosing lower fat versions. Even though some initial research suggested that there was a link between calcium intake, either via supplementation or through dairy products, and weight loss or weight management [204,205], subsequent studies and in particularly a meta-analysis have shown that there was no link between calcium and weight loss or management when confounding factors were taken into consideration [206,207]. Still calcium and dairy intake with regards to weight loss remains controversial.

Alcohol can effect weight management, as there is no body storage capacity for alcohol, it must be oxidized. If energy requirements are met through alcohol alone, any other energy consumed will be stored. Alcohol can lead to increased consumption by affecting restrictive dietary practices by diminishing a person's resolve to limit intake as well as making people hungry. Often the only food available around alcohol is high-energy, high-fat foods such as fried foods, crisps and nuts [208]. However, the role of alcohol in weight gain or loss is complicated; it appears that small amounts have limited effect on weight, moderate amounts lead to increased weight and high consumptions can lead to weight loss. Chronic high-level intake is also associated with nutrient deficiencies and organ damage [209]. Alcohol reduction is usually recommended with obesity treatment for its other associated benefits such as reduced blood pressure and control of gout symptoms [210,211].

Behavioral habits

Self-monitoring and reducing stimuli are two of the most effective dietary behavioral techniques used in obesity treatment today [173]. Self-monitoring, e.g. the food/exercise/mood diary, helps the client become more aware of the type, quantity and pattern of eating [196,212]. Stimulus control involves firstly identifying and then modifying the environmental cues that are associated with a client's overeating or inactivity [196,213]. In the short term people avoid or manipulate problems in their immediate environment; however, over time, living in an obesogenic society may make initiating stimulus control in the wider community near to impossible [199].

Compliance with the program is more important than the program itself. Factors such as flavor, palatability and texture influence patient compliance. Keeping changes close to current habits ensures that the patient will like what they are eating. Gradual change leads to better results in the long term than large changes made all at once [214]. For example, if a person enjoys meat then teaching appropriate cooking techniques (where the meat is trimmed and cooked with no added fat) can reduce energy intake without removing meat from the diet. Adapting frequently used recipes so they contain fewer calories is vital. Helping people focus on the foods they can eat rather than what they should perhaps limit can reassure them that they have options and can still achieve weight loss [215,216].

Prader–Willi Syndrome (PWS): special dietary needs

The PWS was named after Prader, Labhart and Willi in 1956. It is caused by a deletion on the long arm of chromosome 15 and is characterized by failure to thrive in infancy. See Chapter 7. Neonates are hypotonic with insufficient suck and swallow reflexes. An increased appetite occurs during the toddler years. They are developmentally delayed, with intelligence varying between moderate to borderline. They are short in stature, have low lean muscle mass and high percent body fat, particularly in their distal limbs and trunk. Their RMR can be reduced by 20–50% if compared to height and weight respectively. Although

they have the ability to expend as much energy as a non-PWS person, they tend to be less active. Their appetite becomes insatiable and nonselective. It is therefore not surprising that obesity is a consistent characteristic of this condition [217].

Their dietary requirements in infancy should follow normal infant requirements. However, as their appetite grows restrictions are needed. If a person with PWS consumes the same amount of calories as other individuals of the same age and height, they will gain weight. Therefore people with PWS require a low-energy diet to prevent obesity. To lose weight, an individual with PWS requires a diet of 7–9 kcal/cm of height per day and for weight maintenance an energy intake of 8–14 kcal/cm/day is sufficient [218–220]. This applies both for the child and the adult affected by PWS and translates into approximately 600–800 kcal /day for children and 800–1300 kcal for adolescents and adults. To start with, weighing food is necessary so that quantity is determined. Carers need a good understanding of the calorie content of food.

It is generally recommended that the macronutrient composition follows that of a healthy diet. The quality of food is important as quantity is limited, e.g. the protein eaten should be of high biologic value, the carbohydrates high in fiber and low in GI and the fats mostly in the form of MUFA or PUFA rich in omega 3. If a person with PWS follows the diet closely it is important that they take a multivitamin to meet micronutrient requirements. However, dietary compliance is often jeopardized as a person with PWS will seek out food from all sorts of sources such as bins, ground, people, shops (bought or stolen), open bags, unlocked cupboards, refrigerators and well-meaning acquaintances. The more supervision a person with PWS receives and the more consistent their routine, the lower the prevalence of these behaviors.

A person with a PWS child should try to introduce routine and structure. Having meals at the same time every day can help limit tantrums and fights over food.. Having very low–energy foods available can help deal with eating times but amounts should not vary drastically from meal to meal. Fortunately, people with PWS seem to prefer high-carbohydrate to high-fat foods, which helps when trying to find enjoyable low-energy foods for their consumption.

A person with PWS has a constant preoccupation with food even when they appear to be concentrating on something else. They will often scope out rooms too see if someone has been forgetful and left something out that they can reach. They can be very sneaky and will often hide food. Given the insatiable appetite and their need to seek food, locking cupboards and fridges in a home, supervising food preparation areas when in use and clearing away food (even scraps) immediately after finishing are important and necessary. This is often hard if there are people without PWS also living in the home. However, the person with PWS cannot control their desire to eat and no matter how hard you or they try, they will eat food if it is available to them. This problem also extends to the school or work environment where rooms with bags should be locked and bins made inaccessible, tearooms and access to lockers should be limited. The PWS person appreciates these restrictions/strategies as they are often ostracized for their food-seeking actions. Other students may also give PWS students food, particularly if they are not well supervised. Money should be restricted and not managed by the person with PWS as they will generally spend it on food.

Restricting access to food in this way seems to contradict the basic human right of freedom of choice. However, someone with PWS eats not because they lack willpower or have a weak character but because they have a genetic abnormality that leads to uncontrollable and incurable hyperphagia [219]. Restriction helps them to lead a healthy and happy life. Hyperphagia enables them to eat large quantities of food which leads to obesity and most deaths with PWS are due to complications of obesity. The earlier the restrictions are put into place, the easier it is for carers and families to manage those restrictions as the person with PWS ages. If a lot of freedom has been given early on when food-seeking behavior may not be as severe, it is often difficult to then implement the restrictive practices that may be needed as PWS children become adolescents or adults and the food-seeking behavior increases.

Normal, low-energy cooking techniques should be used for this group of people. It again reduces tantrums if everyone at the dinner table is eating the same type and quantity of food. Perhaps portion sizes need to be predetermined. People with PWS love to eat large portions but will eat any food offered to them. For this reason calories should be reduced in as many foods as possible so that the quantity of food offered remains high.

It is important for every person who comes in contact with the individual with PWS to understand the need to restrict food. This can often be difficult, particularly for grandparents and other well-meaning adults. Giving these people information on PWS can help them to understand. If they are still having difficulties, a list of suitable food can help, for example diet versions of soft drinks or air-popped popcorn.

Appetite suppressants do not tend to work in this population. Although there has been some success with the use of VLED, as with any other person, the normal restrictive practices need to be in place to keep weight off in the long term [221].

People with PWS also want independence as they become older but unfortunately, the nature of their condition does not allow them to handle the freedom. This can be a very difficult time for both the family and the person with PWS. Linking in with PWS services, PWS-specific group homes and other community-based programs can make this transition a lot easier. PWS is best managed by a multidisciplinary team [222].

The basic program to follow from childhood [219] is as follows.
• Determine baseline data of the child's caloric intake in relation to weight gain, and express as kcal/cm of height.
• Educate child's primary carer on PWS; for example, suitable diets/foods, caloric content, cooking methods, etc.
• Involve immediate and extended family in the program and necessary changes.
• Control the environment, for example locking cupboards, fridges, etc.

• Educate others who are involved with the child, for example teachers and peers.
• Frequently monitor growth and intake.
• Train the child to accept a food pattern that is compatible, with low caloric diet and regular exercise.
• Maintain changes and programs throughout the child's life.

Maintenance/success

In today's obesogenic society, relapses are common, particularly when people place unrealistic expectations on themselves. We know that weight maintenance is harder after weight loss, and that frequent weight cycling can be damaging to long-term maintenance [223].

Given that the goals during weight maintenance are slightly different from those of weight loss, it is not surprising that a different approach should be taken [22]. Requirements after weight loss are lower than the new body weight might suggest [124]. People believe that if they have been able to maintain their weight at the higher level then they will have no problems maintaining it at a lower level. This is not so. People need to change their habits for life, which often means adhering to some level of caloric restriction indefinitely [124].

What is success? Some have defined it as maintenance of all initial weight loss, or at least 9–11 kg of the original weight loss, a degree of weight loss associated with significant improvement of obesity-related complications [224]. The National Weight Control Registry in America defines success as at least 10% loss of initial body weight which is maintained for at least 1 year [225].

The experience of the people from the registry can help to design appropriate maintenance programs. It was found that 88% of participants in the registry reported restricting intake of certain types of food, 44% limited total quantity, 44% counted calories and 55% used a commercial weight loss program [225,226]. They consumed on average 1381 kcal per day. Only 1% of the group ate diets low in carbohydrate. The average macronutrient profile of the successful dieters can be seen in Figure 21.7. The total group ate approximately 4.9 meals/snacks per day and ate out 3.5

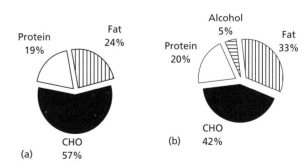

Figure 21.7 Macronutrient composition of successful "dieters." (a) Average diet composition from the National Weight Control Register in the USA. (b) Diet compositions of successful dieters in the UK.

times a week, only once from fast-food outlets. They avoided high-fat, fried foods and used low-fat substitutes. They were also more likely to eat breakfast, eat similarly over weekdays and weekends, limit TV viewing and reported high levels of physical activity [225,227].

Other studies have shown that if cheese, butter, high-fat snacks, fried foods and desserts were eaten less than once per week, the participants were more successful at long-term weight control [228,229] and that reduced consumption of fried potato, dairy products, sweets and meat was positively correlated with weight loss and weight maintenance. Characteristics of a small group of successful and unsuccessful dieters were compared in the UK. The dietary factors in the successful group that were significantly different from the unsuccessful dieters were decreased total energy (achieved through decreased quantity of carbohydrate and fat) and increased percentage of energy from protein. Also, the successful dieters had less emotional eating, were more restrained and less likely to eat in response to external cues [230]. Another interesting result from this study was that successful dieters found their "allowed food" was "good tasting" whereas the unsuccessful

dieters did not always find this [230]. People have also successfully lost weight using low-carbohydrate diets. Those on low-carbohydrate diets generally lost and maintained about the same amount of weight over time compared to people who used other dietary methods. For those on the low-carbohydrate diet, their carbohydrate content increased over time but they kept their energy and fat intake low, limited fast food and did high levels of physical activity, similar to other successful weight loss participants [231]. Astrup, in a review, reports that maintenance is more likely to occur if the individual consumes a low-fat, low energy-dense, moderate-protein diet with only a moderate intake of calorie-containing beverages and does high levels of regular activity [177].

It is widely recognized that people find it hard to stick to changes in the long term. There is a period of high motivation at the beginning of the program but motivation often wanes over time. Clinicians have to be realistic and acknowledge that it is unlikely that dietary intervention alone will maintain weight loss in obese subjects over a period of 2 or more years [232,233].

Sources of recommendations or clinical guidelines in the management of obesity are given in Table 21.3.

Table 21.3 Key documents and information sources on obesity

Toolkits/recommendations/clinical guidelines for health professionals on managing obesity based on systematic reviews of the evidence	
The National Heart, Lung and Blood Institute (NHLBI). *Clinical Guidelines on the Identification, Evaluation, and Treatment of Overweight and Obesity in Adults.*	www.nhlbi.nih.gov/guidelines/obesity/ob_home.ht
A practical guide to The Evidence Report, updated due to be released 2009 Reference: [234]	www.nhlbi.nih.gov/guidelines/obesity/prctgd_c.pdf
The National Heart, Lung and Blood Institute (NHLBI). *Aim for a Healthy Weight* is an excellent interactive website for both health professionals and patients. It lists a number of useful strategies to help treat obesity, based on the Evidence Report. Examples of weight goal records, food substitution ideas and food preparation leaflets, a guide to behavioral change strategies, exercise programs for gradual build-up of activity/fitness are included. Reference: [234,235]	www.nhlbi.nih.gov/health/public/heart/obesity/lose_wt/index.htm
SIGN. *Integrating Prevention with Weight Management* Reference: [236]	
Douketis et al (1999) Periodic health examination, 1999 update: 1. Detection, prevention and treatment of obesity Reference: [237]	http://secure.cihi.ca/cihiweb/products/CPHIOverweightandObesityAugust2004_e.pdf
Spear et al. Recommendations for treatment of child and adolescent overweight and obesity Reference: [238]	http://pediatrics.aappublications.org/cgi/content/full/120/Supplement_4/S254
International Obesity Task Force (IOTF). Excellent website for international information regarding all areas of obesity on a global level.	www.iotf.org
The Autralian and New Zealand Obesity Society. The Asian Pacific region's scientific society that reports on new developments in all areas of obesity research.	www.asso.org.au
Australia's National Health and Medical Research Council have published clinical management guidelines on both adults and children	Adult: www.health.gov.au/internet/wcms/publishing.nsf/Content/obesityguidelines-guidelines-adults.htm Children: www.health.gov.au/internet/wcms/Publishing.nsf/Content/obesityguidelines-guidelines-children.htm
A comprehensive overview of obesity as part of the Health Care Assessment Series. It covers the epidemiologic data, services available and the effectiveness of interventions of the prevention and treatment of obesity in adults and children Reference: [239]	http://hcna.radcliffe-online.com/search/obesity

Table 21.3 *Continued*

The National Audit Office UK published important reports on obesity in 2001 and childhood obesity in 2006 and made a number of health policy recommendations	www.nao.gov.uk
Toolkits/recommendations/clinical guidelines for health professionals on managing obesity NOT based on systematic reviews of the evidence	
DOM UK (Dietitians in Obesity Management UK – specialist interest group of the British Dietetic Association) *The Dietetic Weight Management Intervention for Adults in the One to One Setting. Is it Time for a Radical Rethink?* Reference: [173]	http://domuk.org/wp-content/uploads/2007/11/dietetic-interventionfinalversion301007.doc
International Agency for Research on Cancer (IARC). EPIC Project Faculty of Public Health Medicine *Tackling Obesity: A Toolbox for Local Partnership Action* Reference: [240]	www.iarc.fr/epic/research/obese.html www.pjonline.com/editorial/20000610/articles/**obesity**.html Tel: 0207 935 0243 Email: enquiries@fphm.org.uk
British Heart Foundation (BHF) *So you want to lose weight … for good: a guide to losing weight for men and women.* Publication No M3. BHF Statistics 2006 – Diet, Physical Activity and Obesity Statistics Reference: [241]	https://www.bhf.org.uk/publications/secure/z_index.html
National Obesity Forum (NOF) *Guidelines on management of adult obesity and overweight in Primary Care.* As well as having information for the general public on a healthy approach to weight loss Reference: [242]	www.nationalobesityforum.org.uk
Other useful resources A directory of projects of weight management, compiled by the Department of Health, is available in each Regional Office. Three main themes emerged: that weight loss is rarely maintained, that multicomponent programs are more successful and that regular follow-up is important Reference: [243]	See reference [245].
Clinical Evidence. Relevant sections. A summary of the evidence from systematic reviews, where available, on various health-related topics. National Audit Office (NAO) *Tackling Obesity in England* (2001) *Tackling Child Obesity – First Steps* (2006)	Available via the NELH website: www.nelh.nhs.uk/default.asp www.nao.gov.ukh www.nao.org.uk/publications/nao_reports/00-01/0001220.pdf www.nao.org.uk/publications/nao_reports/05-06/0506801.pdf
WHO *Obesity: Preventing and Managing the Global Epidemic* (2000) Report of the Joint WHO/FAO expert consultation, *Diet, Nutrition and the Prevention of Chronic Diseases* (2003) Reference: WHO, 2000, 2003 [248,249]	www.iotf.org/
Health Development Agency (HAD), now part of National Institute for Health and Clinical Excellence (NICE). On-line evidence base on obesity and its treatments	www.nice.org.uk
Germany's Association of Scientific Medical Societies. Prevention and Management of Obesity 2007	www.uni-dusseldorf.de/www/AWMF/11/050-001.pdf
Cochrane systematic reviews on obesity: Low glycemic index or low glycaemic load diets for overweight and obesity [250] Interventions to prevent weight gain in schizophrenia [244] Low fat diets for the treatment of obesity [34] Interventions for preventing obesity in childhood [245] Interventions for treating obesity in childhood [246] Intervention for improving health professionals management of obesity [247]	Available on Medline and the Nelhi website www.nelh.nhs.uk/default.asp
Organizations dedicated to the scientific study of obesity: The International Obesity Task Force International Association for the Study of Obesity Association for the Study of Obesity The Australian and New Zealand Obesity Society The Obesity Society European Association for the Study of Obesity *Patient-focused organizations/charities:* National Association to Advance Fat Acceptance (NAAFA) The Obesity Awareness and Solutions Trust (TOAST)	www.iotf.org www.iaso.org www.aso.org.uk www.asso.org.au www/naaso.org www.easoobesity.org www.naafa.org/ www.toasthyphen;uk.org.uk/

Conclusion

Although there is little dispute that obesity is due (at least in part) to excess energy intake, best results are usually achieved when energy intake, energy expenditure and emotional issues are all taken into consideration when devising a weight loss program.

References

1. Stunkard AJ, LaFleur WR, Wadden TA. Stigmatization of obesity in medieval times: Asia and Europe. Int J Obes 1998;22(12):1141–4.
2. Bray GA. Obesity: historical development of scientific and cultural ideas. Int J Obes 1990;14(11):909–26.
3. Anonymous. Clinical guidelines on the identification, evaluation, and treatment of overweight and obesity in adults: executive summary. Expert Panel on the Identification, Evaluation, and Treatment of Overweight in Adults. Am J Clin Nutr 1998;68(4):899–917.
4. Lowe MR, Miller-Kovach K, Phelan S. Weight-loss maintenance in overweight individuals one to five years following successful completion of a commercial weight loss program. Int J Obes 2001;25(3):325–31.
5. Astrup A, Buemann B, Flint A, Raben A. Low-fat diets and energy balance: how does the evidence stand in 2002? Proc Nutr Soc 2002;61(2):299–309.
6. Toubro S, Astrup A. Randomised comparison of diets for maintaining obese subjects' weight after major weight loss: ad lib, low fat, high carbohydrate diet v fixed energy intake. BMJ 1997;314(7073):29–34.
7. Tuomilehto J, Lindstrom J, Eriksson JG, Valle TT, Hamalainen H, Ilanne-Parikka P, et al. Prevention of type 2 diabetes mellitus by changes in lifestyle among subjects with impaired glucose tolerance. comment. N Engl J Med 2001;344(18):1343–50.
8. Knowler WC, Barrett-Connor E, Fowler SE, Hamman RF, Lachin JM, Walker EA, et al. Reduction in the incidence of type 2 diabetes with lifestyle intervention or metformin. N Engl J Med 2002;346(6):393–403.
9. Glenny AM, O'Meara S, Melville A, Sheldon TA, Wilson C. The treatment and prevention of obesity: a systematic review of the literature. Int J Obes 1997;21(9):715–37.
10. Ditschuneit HH, Flechtner-Mors M, Johnson TD, Adler G. Metabolic and weight-loss effects of a long-term dietary intervention in obese patients. Am J Clin Nutr 1999;69(2):198–204.
11. Ditschuneit HH, Flechtner-Mors M. Value of structured meals for weight management: risk factors and long-term weight maintenance. Obes Res 2001;9(suppl 4):284S–9S.
12. Noakes M, Foster PR, Keogh B, Clifton P. Meal replacements are as effective as structured weight-loss diets for treating obesity in adults with features of metabolic syndrome. J Nutr 2004;134:1894–9.
13. Flechtner-Mors M, Ditschuneit HH, Johnson TD, Suchard MA, Adler G. Metabolic and weight loss effects of long-term dietary intervention in obese patients: four-year results. Obes Res 2000;8(5):399–402.
14. Tsai AG, Wadden T. The Evolution of very-low-calorie diets: an update and meta-analysis. Obesity 2006;14(8):1283–93.
15. National Healthy and Medical Research Council. Clinical practice guidelines, for the management of overweight and obesity in children and adolescents. Canberra: Department of Communications, Information and Arts, 2003.
16. Heymsfield SB, van Mierlo CAJ, van der Knaap HCM, Heo M, Frier HI. Weight management using a meal replacement strategy: meta and pooling analysis from six studies. Int J Obes 2003;27(5):537–49.
17. Heymsfield SB, Harp JB, Reitman ML, Beetsch JW, Schoeller DA, Erondu N, et al. Why do obese patients not lose more weight when treated with low-calorie diets? A mechanistic perspective. Am J Clin Nutr 2007;85(2):346–54.
18. Anonymous. Very low-calorie diets. National Task Force on the Prevention and Treatment of Obesity, National Institutes of Health. JAMA 1993;270(8):967–74.
19. Mustajoki P, Pekkarinen T. Very low energy diets in the treatment of obesity. Obes Rev 2001;2(1):61–72.
20. Willi SM, Martin K, Datko FM, Brant BP. Treatment of type 2 diabetes in childhood using a very-low-calorie diet. Diabetes Care 2004;27(2):348–53.
21. Willi SM, Wise KL, Welch AS, Key LL Jr. A ketogenic very low calorie diet (VLCD) in the treatment of children with NIDDM + 500. Pediatric Research Program Issue APS-SPR April 1998;43(4):88.
22. Wadden TA. The treatment of obesity: an overview. In: Stunkard A, Wadden T (eds) *Obesity: Theory and Therapy*. New York: Raven Press, 1993:197–217.
23. Delbridge E, Proietto J. State of the science: VLED (very low energy diet) for obesity. Asia Pacific J Clin Nutr 2006;15(suppl):49–54.
24. Lantz H, Peltonen M, Agren L, Torgerson JS. A dietary and behavioural programme for the treatment of obesity. A 4-year clinical trial and a long-term posttreatment follow-up. J Intern Med 2003;254(3):272–9.
25. Lantz H, Peltonen M, Agren L, Torgerson JS. Intermittent versus on-demand use of a very low calorie diet: a randomized 2-year clinical trial. J Intern Med 2003;253(4):463–71.
26. Williams KV, Mullen ML, Kelley DE, Wing RR. The effect of short periods of caloric restriction on weight loss and glycemic control in type 2 diabetes. Diabetes Care 1998;21(1):2–8.
27. Astrup A, Rossner S. Lessons from obesity management programmes: greater initial weight loss improves long-term maintenance. Obes Rev 2000;1(1):17–19.
28. Saris WH. Very-low-calorie diets and sustained weight loss. Obes Res 2001;9(suppl 4):295S–301S.
29. Case CC, Jones PH, Nelson K, Ballantyne CM. Impact of weight loss on the metabolic syndrome. Diabetes 2002;51(suppl 2):A608–A609.
30. Stubbs RJ, Harbron CG, Murgatroyd PR, Prentice Am Covert manipulation of dietary fat and energy density: effect on substrate flux and food intake in men eating ad libitum. Am J Clin Nutr 1995;62(2):316–29.
31. Stubbs RJ, Harbron CG, Prentice Am Covert manipulation of the dietary fat to carbohydrate ratio of isoenergetically dense diets: effect on food intake in feeding men ad libitum. Int J Obes 1996;20(7):651–60.
32. Stubbs RJ, Johnstone AM, Harbron CG, Reid C. Covert manipulation of energy density of high carbohydrate diets in "pseudo free-living" humans. Int J Obes 1998;22(9):885–92.

33. Heitmann BL, Lissner L, Sorensen TI, Bengtsson C. Dietary fat intake and weight gain in women genetically predisposed for obesity. Am J Clin Nutr 1995;61(6):1213–17.

34. Pirozzo S, Summerbell C, Cameron C, Glasziou P. Advice on low-fat diets for obesity. Cochrane Database of Systematic Reviews, 2002(2):CD003640.

35. Pirozzo S, Summerbell C, Cameron C, Glasziou P. Should we recommend low-fat diets for obesity? (Erratum appears in Obes Rev 2003;4(3):185) Obes Rev 2003;4(2):83–90.

36. Astrup A. The role of dietary fat in obesity. Semin Vasc Med 2005;5(1):40–7.

37. Lissner L, Heitmann BL. The dietary fat:carbohydrate ratio in relation to body weight. Curr Opin Lipidol 1995;6(1):8–13.

38. Willett WC. Dietary fat plays a major role in obesity: no. Obes Rev 2002;3(2):59–68.

39. Astrup A, Grunwald GK, Melanson EL, Saris WH, Hill JO. The role of low-fat diets in body weight control: a meta-analysis of ad libitum dietary intervention studies. Int J Obes 2000;24(12):1545–52.

40. Astrup A. The American paradox: the role of energy-dense fat-reduced food in the increasing prevalence of obesity. Curr Opin Clin Nutr Metab Care 1998;1(6):573–7.

41. Yu-Poth S, Zhao G, Etherton T, Naglak M, Jonnalagadda S, Kris-Etherton PM. Effects of the National Cholesterol Education Program's Step I and Step II dietary intervention programs on cardiovascular disease risk factors: a meta-analysis. Am J Clin Nutr 1999;69(4):632–46.

42. Jeffery R, Hellerstedt WL, French SA, Baxter JE. A Randomized trial of counseling for fat restriction versus calorie restriction in the treatment of obesity. Int J Obes 1995;19:132–7.

43. Hung T, Sievenpiper JL, Marchie A, Kendall CWC, Jenkins DJA. Fat versus carbohydrate in insulin resistance, obesity, diabetes and cardiovascular disease. Curr Opin Clin Nutr Metab Care 2003;6(2):165–76.

44. Noakes M, Clifton PM. Weight loss and plasma lipids. Curr Opin Lipidol 2000;11(1):65–70.

45. Kuller LH, Simkin-Silverman LR, Wing RR, Meilahn EN, Ives DG. Women's Healthy Lifestyle Project: a randomized clinical trial: results at 54 months. Circulation 2001;103(1):32–7.

46. Fleming RM. The effect of high-, moderate-, and low-fat diets on weight loss and cardiovascular disease risk factors. Prev Cardiol 2002;5(3):110–18.

47. Zambon A, Sartore G, Passera D, Francini-Pesenti F, Bassi A, Basso C, et al. Effects of hypocaloric dietary treatment enriched in oleic acid on LDL and HDL subclass distribution in mildly obese women. J Intern Med 1999;246(2):191–201.

48. Golay A, Eigenheer C, Morel Y, Kujawski P, Lehmann T, de Tonnac N. Weight-loss with low or high carbohydrate diet? Int J Obes 1996;20(12):1067–72.

49. Low CC, Grossman EB, Gumbiner B. Potentiation of effects of weight loss by monounsaturated fatty acids in obese NIDDM patients. Diabetes 1996;45(5):569–75.

50. Pelkman CL, Fishell VK, Maddox DH, Pearson TA, Mauger DT, Kris-Etherton PM. Effects of moderate-fat (from monounsaturated fat) and low-fat weight-loss diets on the serum lipid profile in overweight and obese men and women. Am J Clin Nutr 2004;79(2):204–12.

51. Azadbakht L, Mirmiran P, Esmaillzadeh A, Azizi F. Better dietary adherence and weight maintenance achieved by a long-term moderate-fat diet. Br J Nutr 2007;97(2):399–404.

52. McManus K, Antinoro L, Sacks F. A randomized controlled trial of a moderate-fat, low-energy diet compared with a low fat, low-energy diet for weight loss in overweight adults. Int J Obes Relat Metab Disord 2001;25(10):1503–11.

53. Drewnowski A. Individual differences in sensory preferences for fat in model sweet dairy products. Acta Psychol 1993;84(1):103–10.

54. Drewnowski A, Brunzell JD, Sande K, Iverius PH, Greenwood MR. Sweet tooth reconsidered: taste responsiveness in human obesity. Physiol Behav 1985;35(4):617–22.

55. Drewnowski A, Greenwood MR. Cream and sugar: human preferences for high-fat foods. Physiol Behav 1983;30(4):629–33.

56. St Jeor ST, Howard BV, Prewitt TE, Bovee V, Bazzarre T, Eckel RH, et al. Dietary protein and weight reduction: a statement for healthcare professionals from the Nutrition Committee of the Council on Nutrition, Physical Activity, and Metabolism of the American Heart Association. Circulation 2001;104(15):1869–74.

57. Erlanson-Albertsson C, Mei J. The effect of low carbohydrate on energy metabolism. Int J Obes 2005;29(suppl 2):S26–30.

58. Claessens M, Calame W, Siemensma AD, Saris WHM, van Baak MA. The thermogenic and metabolic effects of protein hydrolysate with or without a carbohydrate load in healthy male subjects. Metabolism 2007;56(8):1051–9.

59. Scott CB, Devore R. Diet-induced thermogenesis: variations among three isocaloric meal-replacement shakes. Nutrition 2005;21(7–8):874–7.

60. Halton TL, Hu FB. The effects of high protein diets on thermogenesis, satiety and weight loss: a critical review. J Am Coll Nutr 2004;23(5):373–85.

61. Levine MJ, Jones JM, Lineback DR. Low-carbohydrate diets: assessing the science and knowledge gaps. Summary of an ILSI North America Workshop. J Am Diet Assoc 2006;106(12):2086–94.

62. Bravata D, Sanders L, Huang J, Krumholz H, Olkin I, Gardner CD, et al. Efficacy and safety of low-carbohydrate diets: a systematic review. JAMA 2003;289(14):1837–50.

63. Rolls BJ, Bell EA. Dietary approaches to the treatment of obesity. Med Clin North Am 2000;84(2):401–18.

64. Noakes M, Keogh JB, Foster PR, Clifton PM. Effect of an energy-restricted, high-protein, low-fat diet relative to a conventional high-carbohydrate, low-fat diet on weight loss, body composition, nutritional status, and markers of cardiovascular health in obese women. Am J Clin Nutr 2005;81(6):1298–306.

65. Klauer JM, Aronne LJM. Managing overweight and obesity in women. Clin Obstet Gynecol 2002;45(4):1080–8.

66. Fleming RM. The effect of high-protein diets on coronary blood flow. Angiology 2000;51(10):817–26.

67. Roughead ZK. Is the interaction between dietary protein and calcium destructive or constructive for bone? J Nutr 2003;133(3):866S–9S.

68. Tapper-Gardzina Y, Cotugna N, Vickery CE. Should you recommend a low-carb, high-protein diet? (Summary for patients in Nurse Pract 2002;27(4):57) Nurse Pract 2002;27(4):52–3, 5–6, 8–9.

69. Leidy HJ, Carnell NS, Mattes RD, Campbell WW. Higher protein intake preserves lean mass and satiety with weight loss in pre-obese and obese women. Obesity 2007;15(2):421–9.

70. Poppitt SD, Prentice AM. Energy density and its role in the control of food intake: evidence from metabolic and community studies. Appetite 1996;26(2):153–74.

71. Rolls BJ, Castellanos VH, Halford JC, Kilara A, Panyam D, Pelkman CL, et al. Volume of food consumed affects satiety in men. Am J Clin Nutr 1998;67(6):1170–7.

72. Rolls BJ, Roe LS, Meengs JS. Larger portion sizes lead to a sustained increase in energy intake over 2 days. J Am Diet Assoc 2006;106(4):543–9.

73. Ello-Martin JA, Ledikwe JH, Rolls BJ. The influence of food portion size and energy density on energy intake: implications for weight management. Am J Clin Nutr 2005;82(1 suppl):236S–41S.

74. Ledikwe JH, Ello-Martin JA, Rolls BJ. Portion sizes and the obesity epidemic. J Nutr 2005;135(4):905–9.

75. Yao M, Roberts SB. Dietary energy density and weight regulation. Nutr Rev 2001;59(8 Pt 1):247–58.

76. Ello-Martin JA, Roe LS, Ledikwe JH, Beach AM, Rolls BJ. Dietary energy density in the treatment of obesity: a year-long trial comparing 2 weight-loss diets. Am J Clin Nutr 2007;85(6):1465–77.

77. Rolls BJ, Bell EA. Intake of fat and carbohydrate: role of energy density. Eur J Clin Nutr 1999;53(suppl 1):S166–73.

78. Rolls BJ, Bell EA, Thorwart ML. Water incorporated into a food but not served with a food decreases energy intake in lean women. Am J Clin Nutr 1999;70(4):448–55.

79. Kral TVE, Rolls BJ. Energy density and portion size: their independent and combined effects on energy intake. Physiol Behav 2004;82(1):131–8.

80. Stubbs RJ, Whybrow S. Energy density, diet composition and palatability: influences on overall food energy intake in humans. Physiol Behav 2004;81(5):755–64.

81. Himaya A, Louis-Sylvestre J. The effect of soup on satiation. Appetite 1998;30(2):199–210.

82. Rolls BJ, Fedoroff IC, Guthrie JF, Laster LJ. Effects of temperature and mode of presentation of juice on hunger, thirst and food intake in humans. Appetite 1990;15(3):199–208.

83. Rolls BJ, Roe LS, Meengs JS. Salad and satiety: energy density and portion size of a first-course salad affect energy intake at lunch. J Am Diet Assoc 2004;104(10):1570–6.

84. Rolls BJ, Roe LS, Beach AM, Kris-Etherton PM. Provision of foods differing in energy density affects long-term weight loss. Obes Res 2005;13(6):1052–60.

85. Jordan HA, Levitz LS, Utgoff KL, Lee HL. Role of food characteristics in behavioral change and weight loss. J Am Diet Assoc 1981;79(1):24–9.

86. Foreyt JP, Reeves RS, Darnell LS, Wohlleb JC, Gotto AM. Soup consumption as a behavioral weight loss strategy. J Am Diet Assoc 1986;86(4):524–6.

87. Greene LF, Malpede CZ, Henson CS, Hubbert KA, Heimburger DC, Ard JD. Weight maintenance 2 years after participation in a weight loss program promoting low-energy density foods. Obesity 2006;14(10):1795–801.

88. Iqbal SI, Helge JW, Heitmann BL. Do energy density and dietary fiber influence subsequent 5-year weight changes in adult men and women? Obesity 2006;14(1):106–14.

89. Quatromoni PA, Pencina M, Cobain MR, Jacques PF, d'Agostino RB. Dietary quality predicts adult weight gain: findings from the Framingham Offspring Study. Obesity 2006;14(8):1383–91.

90. Popkin BM, Barclay DV, Nielsen SJ. Water and food consumption patterns of U.S. adults from 1999 to 2001. Obes Res 2005;13(12):2146–52.

91. Westerterp-Plantenga MS, Westerterp-Plantenga MS. Modulatory factors in the effect of energy density on energy intake. Br J Nutr 2004;92(suppl 1):S35–9.

92. Drewnowski A, Darmon N. The economics of obesity: dietary energy density and energy cost. Am J Clin Nutr 2005;82(1 suppl):265S–73S.

93. Drewnowski A. The role of energy density. Lipids 2003;38(2):109–15.

94. Wolever TM, Jenkins DJ, Jenkins AL, Josse RG. The glycemic index: methodology and clinical implications. Am J Clin Nutr 1991;54(5):846–54.

95. Kabir M, Rizkalla SW, Champ M, Luo J, Boillot J, Bruzzo F, et al. Dietary amylose-amylopectin starch content affects glucose and lipid metabolism in adipocytes of normal and diabetic rats. J Nutr 1998;128(1):35–43.

96. Jenkins DJ, Jenkins AL, Wolever TM, Vuksan V, Rao AV, Thompson LU, et al. Low glycemic index: lente carbohydrates and physiological effects of altered food frequency. Am J Clin Nutr 1994;59(3 suppl):706S–9S.

97. Bjorck I, Liljeberg H, Ostman E. Low glycaemic-index foods. Br J Nutr 2000;83(suppl 1):S149–55.

98. Trout D, Behall KM. Prediction of glycemic index among high-sugar, low-starch foods. Int J Food Sci Nutr 1999;50(2):135–44.

99. Granfeldt Y, Eliasson AC, Bjorck I. An examination of the possibility of lowering the glycemic index of oat and barley flakes by minimal processing. J Nutr 2000;130(9):2207–14.

100. Ross SW, Brand JC, Thorburn AW, Truswell AS. Glycemic index of processed wheat products. Am J Clin Nutr 1987;46(4):631–5.

101. Brand JC, Nicholson PL, Thorburn AW, Truswell AS. Food processing and the glycemic index. Am J Clin Nutr 1985;42(6):1192–6.

102. Morris KL, Zemel MB. Glycemic index, cardiovascular disease, and obesity. Nutr Rev 1999;57(9 Pt 1):273–6.

103. Trout DL, Behall KM, Osilesi O. Prediction of glycemic index for starchy foods. Am J Clin Nutr 1993;58(6):873–8.

104. Liljeberg H, Bjorck I. Delayed gastric emptying rate may explain improved glycaemia in healthy subjects to a starchy meal with added vinegar. Eur J Clin Nutr 1998;52(5):368–71.

105. Jenkins AL, Jenkins DJ. Dietary fibre, glycaemic index and diabetes. South African Med J 1994;(suppl):36–7.

106. Wolever TM, Jenkins DJ, Ocana AM, Rao VA, Collier GR. Second-meal effect: low-glycemic-index foods eaten at dinner improve subsequent breakfast glycemic response. Am J Clin Nutr 1988;48(4):1041–7.

107. Wolever TM, Jenkins DJ, Josse RG, Wong GS, Lee R. The glycemic index: similarity of values derived in insulin-dependent and non-insulin-dependent diabetic patients.J Am Coll Nutr 1987;6(4):295–305.

108. Wolever TM, Jenkins DJ. The use of the glycemic index in predicting the blood glucose response to mixed meals. Am J Clin Nutr 1986;43(1):167–72.

109. Wolever TM, Jenkins DJ. The use of glycemic index in predicting the blood glucose response to mixed meals. Am J Clin Nutr 1986;43:167–72.

110. Ascott-Evans B. The metabolic syndrome, insulin resistance and cardiovascular disease. Cardiovasc J South Afr 2002;13(4):187–8.

111. Frost G, Dornhorst A. The relevance of the glycaemic index to our understanding of dietary carbohydrates. Diabetic Med 2000;17(5):336–45.

112. Frost G, Leeds AA, Dore CJ, Madeiros S, Brading S, Dornhorst A. Glycaemic index as a determinant of serum HDL-cholesterol concentration. Lancet 1999;353(9158):1045–8.

113. Frost G, Leeds A, Trew G, Margara R, Dornhorst A. Insulin sensitivity in women at risk of coronary heart disease and the effect of a low glycemic diet. Metab Clin Exper 1998;47(10):1245–51.

114. Frost G, Keogh B, Smith D, Akinsanya K, Leeds A. The effect of low-glycemic carbohydrate on insulin and glucose response in vivo and in vitro in patients with coronary heart disease. Metab Clin Exper 1996;45(6):669–72.

115. Frost G, Wilding J, Beecham J. Dietary advice based on the glycaemic index improves dietary profile and metabolic control in type 2 diabetic patients. Diabetic Med 1994;11(4):397–401.

116. Frost G, Pirani S. Meal frequency and nutritional intake during Ramadan: a pilot study. Hum Nutr Appl Nutr 1987;41(1):47–50.

117. Jarvi AE, Karlstrom BE, Granfeldt YE, Bjorck IE, Asp NG, Vessby BO. Improved glycemic control and lipid profile and normalized fibrinolytic activity on a low-glycemic index diet in type 2 diabetic patients. Diabetes Care 1999;22(1):10–18.

118. Slabber M, Barnard HC, Kuyl JM, Dannhauser A, Schall R. Effects of a low-insulin-response, energy-restricted diet on weight loss and plasma insulin concentrations in hyperinsulinemic obese females. Am J Clin Nutr 1994;60(1):48–53.

119. Gannon MC, Nuttall FQ, Krezowski PA, Billington CJ, Parker S. The serum insulin and plasma glucose responses to milk and fruit products in type 2 (non-insulin-dependent) diabetic patients. Diabetologia 1986;29(11):784–91.

120. Liljeberg HG, Granfeldt YE, Bjorck IM. Products based on a high fiber barley genotype, but not on common barley or oats, lower postprandial glucose and insulin responses in healthy humans. J Nutr 1996;126(2):458–66.

121. Liu S, Manson JE, Stampfer MJ, Hu FB, Giovannucci E, Colditz GA, et al. A prospective study of whole-grain intake and risk of type 2 diabetes mellitus in US women. Am J Public Health 2000;90(9):1409–15.

122. Raben A. Should obese patients be counselled to follow a low glycaemic index diet? No. Obes Rev 2002;3:245–56.

123. Low glycaemic index or low glycaemic load diets for overweight and obesity. Cochrane Database of Systematic Reviews, 2007(3):CD005105.

124. Garner DM, Wooley SC. Confronting the failure of behavioral and dietary treatments for obesity. Clin Psychol Rev 1991;11:729–80.

125. Cummings S, Parham ES, Strain GW, American Dietetic Association. Position of the American Dietetic Association: weight management. J Am Diet Assoc 2002;102(8):1145–55.

126. Gaesser GA, Miller WC. Symposium: has body weight become an unhealthy obsession? Med Sci Sports Exerc 1999;31(8):1118–46.

127. Chapman GE, Sellaeg K, Levy-Milne R, Ottem A, Barr SI, Fierini D, et al. Canadian dietitians' approaches to counseling adult clients seeking weight-management advice. J Am Diet Assoc 2005;105(8):1275–9.

128. Miller WC, Jacob AV. The Health at Any Size paradigm for obesity treatment: the scientific evidence. Obes Rev 2001;2(1):37–45.

129. Kausman R, Murphy M, O'Connor T, Schattner P. Audit of a behaviour modification program for weight management. Australian Fam Physician 2003;32(1–2):89–91.

130. Burns CM, Tijhuis MA, Seidell JC. The relationship between quality of life and perceived body weight and dieting history in Dutch men and women. Int J Obes 2001;25(9):1386–92.

131. Dixon JB, Dixon ME, O'Brien PE. Quality of life after lap-band placement: influence of time, weight loss, and comorbidities. Obes Res 2001;9(11):713–21.

132. Dixon JB, O'Brien PE. Changes in comorbidities and improvements in quality of life after LAP-BAND placement. Am J Surg 2002;184(6B):51S–4S.

133. Weiner R, Datz M, Wagner D, Bockhorn H. Quality-of-life outcome after laparoscopic adjustable gastric banding for morbid obesity. Obes Surg 1999;9(6):539–45.

134. Wing RR, Epstein LH, Marcus MD, Kupfer DJ. Mood changes in behavioral weight loss programs. J Psychosom Res 1984;28(3):189–96.

135. Pi-Sunyer FX. National Institutes of Health Technology Assessment Conference. Short-term medical benefits and adverse effects of weight loss. Ann Intern Med 1993;119(7S):722–6.

136. van Hout GC, Boekestein P, Fortuin FA, Pelle AJ, van Heck GL. Psychosocial functioning following bariatric surgery. Obes Surg 2006;16(6):787–94.

137. Sbrocco T, Nedegaard RC, Stone JM, Lewis EL. Behavioral choice treatment promotes continuing weight loss: preliminary results of a cognitive-behavioral decision-based treatment for obesity. J Consult Clin Psychol 1999;67(2):260–6.

138. Mellin L, Croughan-Minihane M, Dickey L. The Solution Method: 2-year trends in weight, blood pressure, exercise, depression, and functioning of adults trained in development skills. J Am Diet Assoc 1997;97(10):1133–8.

139. Paisey RB, Frost J, Harvey P, Paisey A, Bower L, Paisey RM, et al. Five year results of a prospective very low calorie diet or conventional weight loss programme in type 2 diabetes. J Hum Nutr Dietet 2002;15(2):121–7.

140. Tremblay A, Doucet E. Influence of intense physical activity on energy balance and body fatness. Proc Nutr Soc 1999;58(1):99–105.

141. Kausman R. A new perspective to long-term weight management. Is there a better way? Australian Fam Physician 2000;29(4):303–7.

142. Tanco S, Linden W, Earle T. Well-being and morbid obesity in women: a controlled therapy evaluation. Int J Eating Disord 1998;23(3):325–39.

143. Goodrick GK, Poston IW, Kimball KT, Reeves RS, Foreyt JP. Nondieting versus dieting treatment for overweight binge-eating women. J Consult Clin Psychol 1998;66(2):363–8.

144. Miller WC. Effective diet and exercise treatments for overweight and recommendations for interventions. Sports Med 2001;31(10):717–24.

145. Bellisle F, McDevitt R, Prentice AM. Meal frequency and energy balance. Br J Nutr 1997;77(suppl 1):S57–70.

146. Westerterp-Plantenga MS, Kovacs EM, Melanson KJ. Habitual meal frequency and energy intake regulation in partially temporally isolated men. Int J Obes 2002;26(1):102–10.

147. Berteus Forslund H, Lindroos AK, Sjostrom L, Lissner L. Meal patterns and obesity in Swedish women-a simple instrument describing usual meal types, frequency and temporal distribution. Eur J Clin Nutr 2002;56(8):740–7.

148. Speechly DP, Buffenstein R. Greater appetite control associated with an increased frequency of eating in lean males. Appetite 1999;33(3):285–97.

149. Speechly DP, Rogers GG, Buffenstein R. Acute appetite reduction associated with an increased frequency of eating in obese males. Int J Obes 1999;23(11):1151–9.

150. Ziaee V, Razaei M, Ahmadinejad Z, Shaikh H, Yousefi R, Yarmohammadi L, et al. The changes of metabolic profile and weight during Ramadan fasting. Singapore Med J 2006;47(5):409–14.

151. Stote KS, Baer DJ, Spears K, Paul DR, Harris GK, Rumpler WV, et al. A controlled trial of reduced meal frequency without caloric restriction in healthy, normal-weight, middle-aged adults. Am J Clin Nutr 2007;85(4):981–8.

152. Thomsen C, Christiansen C, Rasmussen OW, Hermansen K. Comparison of the effects of two weeks' intervention with different meal frequencies on glucose metabolism, insulin sensitivity and lipid levels in non-insulin-dependent diabetic patients. Ann Nutr Metab 1997;41(3):173–80.

153. Verboeket-van de Venne WP, Westerterp KR, Kester AD. Effect of the pattern of food intake on human energy metabolism. Br J Nutr 1993;70(1):103–15.

154. Verboeket-van de Venne WP, Westerterp KR. Influence of the feeding frequency on nutrient utilization in man: consequences for energy metabolism. Eur J Clin Nutr 1991;45(3):161–9.

155. Wolfram G, Kirchgessner M, Muller HL, Hollomey S. Thermogenesis in humans after varying meal time frequency. Ann Nutr Metab 1987;31(2):88–97.

156. de Castro JM. Genetic influences on daily intake and meal patterns of humans. Physiol Behav 1993;53(4):777–82.

157. Stubbs RJ, Johnstone AM, Mazlan N, Mbaiwa SE, Ferris S. Effect of altering the variety of sensorially distinct foods, of the same macronutrient content, on food intake and body weight in men. Eur J Clin Nutr 2001;55(1):19–28.

158. Lamberg L. Psychiatric help may shrink some waistlines. JAMA 2000;284(3):291–3.

159. Colles SL, Dixon JB, Marks P, Strauss BJ, O'Brien PE. Preoperative weight loss with a very-low-energy diet: quantitation of changes in liver and abdominal fat by serial imaging. Am J Clin Nutr 2006;84(2):304–11.

160. Parkes E. Nutritional management of patients after bariatric surgery. Am J Med Sci 2006;331(4):207–13.

161. Colles SL, Dixon JB, O'Brien PE. Hunger control and regular physical activity facilitate weight loss after laparoscopic adjustable gastric banding. Obes Surg 2008;18(7):833–40.

162. Truby H, Baic S, deLooy A, Fox KR, Livingstone MBE, Logan CM, et al. Randomised controlled trial of four commercial weight loss programmes in the UK: initial findings from the BBC "diet trials". (Erratum appears in BMJ 2006;332(7555):1418.) BMJ 2006;332(7553):1309–14.

163. Dansinger ML, Gleason JA, Griffith JL, Selker HP, Schaefer EJ. Comparison of the Atkins, Ornish, Weight Watchers, and Zone diets for weight loss and heart disease risk reduction: a randomized trial. JAMA 2005;5;293(1):43–53.

164. Lowe MR, Foster GD, Kerzhnerman I, Swain RM, Wadden TA. Restrictive dieting versus "undieting" effects on eating regulation in obese clinic attenders. Addict Behav 2001;26(2):253–66.

165. Tsai AG, Wadden TA, Womble LG, Byrne KJ. Commercial and self-help programs for weight control. Psychiatr Clin North Am 2005;28(1):171–92.

166. Biesalski HK. Essential requirements of long-term treatment of obesity. In: Ditschuneit H, Gries FA, Hauner H, Schusdziarra V, Wechsler JG (eds) *Obesity in Europe 1993*. London: John Libbey, 1994:219–26.

167. Liebermeister H. Novelties and curiosities: miracle diets in the treatment of obesity. In: Ditschuneit H, Gries FA, Hauner H, Schusdziarra V, Wechsler JG (eds) *Obesity in Europe 1993*. London: John Libbey, 1994:263–7.

168. McCullough ML, Willett WC. Evaluating adherence to recommended diets in adults: the Alternate Healthy Eating Index. Public Health Nutr 2006;9(1A):152–7.

169. Ma Y, Pagoto SL, Griffith JA, Merriam PA, Ockene IS, Hafner AR, et al. A dietary quality comparison of popular weight-loss plans. J Am Diet Assoc 2007;107(10):1786–91.

170. Garrow JS. Slimming products: a success in court. Healthwatch Newsletter 1995:8.

171. Bingham S. The dietary assessment of individuals; methods, accuracy, new techniques and recommendations. Nutr Abstr Rev 1987;57:705–42.

172. British Dietetic Association. *Position paper on the treatment of obesity*. London: British Dietetic Association, 1996.

173. Dietitians in Obesity Management DU. *The Dietetic Weight Management Intervention for Adults in the One to One Setting: Is It Time for a Radical Rethink?* London: British Dietetic Association, 2007.

174. Gibney MJ. Are there conflicts in dietary advice for prevention of different diseases? Proc Nutr Soc 1992;51(1):35–45.

175. Garrow JS. The safety of dieting. Proc Nutr Soc 1991;50(2):493–9.

176. Haus G, Hoerr SL, Mavis B, Robison J. Key modifiable factors in weight maintenance: fat intake, exercise, and weight cycling. J Am Dietet Assoc. 1994;94(4):409–13.

177. Astrup A. How to maintain a healthy body weight. Int J Vitam Nutr Res 2006;76(4):208–15.

178. Heshka S, Greenway F, Anderson JW, Atkinson RL, Hill JO, Phinney SD, et al. Self-help weight loss versus a structured commercial program after 26 weeks: a randomized controlled study. Am J Med 2000;109(4):282–7.

179. Fleisch A. Le metabolisme basal standard et sa determination au moyen du "Metabocalculator". Helvi Med Acta 1951;1:23–44.

180. Robinson JD, Reid DD. Standards for the basal metabolism of normal people in Britain. Lancet 1952;1:940–3.

181. Black AE, Goldberg GR, Jebb SA, Livingstone MBE, Cole TL, Prentice AM. Critical evaluation of energy intake using fundamental principles of energy physiology: 2. Evaluating the results of published surveys. Eur J Clin Nutr 1991;45:583–99.

182. Heitmann BL, Lissner L, Osler M. Do we eat less fat, or just report so? Int J Obes 2000;24(4):435–42.

183. Heitmann BL, Lissner L. Dietary underreporting by obese individuals – is it specific or non-specific? BMJ 1995;311(7011):986–9.

184. Summerbell CD, Moody RC, Shanks J, Stock MJ, Geissler C. Sources of energy from meals versus snacks in 220 people in four age groups. Eur J Clin Nutr 1995;49(1):33–41.

185. Beaudoin R, Mayer J. Food intake of obese and non-obese women. J Am Diet Assoc 1953;29:29–34.

186. Garrow JS. *Obesity and Related Disease*. Edinburgh: Churchill Livingstone, 1988.

187. Frost G, Masters K, King C, Kelly M, Hasan U, Heavens P, et al. A new method of energy prescription to improve weight loss. J Hum Nutr Dietet 1991;4:369–73.

188. Coll M, Meyer A, Stunkard AJ. *Obesity and food choices in public places*. Arch Gen Psychiatr 1979;36:795–7.

189. Brandon JE. Differences in self-reported eating and exercise behaviours and actual self-concept congruence between obese and non-obese individuals. Health Values 1987;11:22–3.

190. Lindroos AK, Lissner L, Sjostrom L. Validity and reproducibility of a self-administered dietary questionnaire in obese and non-obese subjects. Eur J Clin Nutr 1993;47(7):461–81.

191. Fricker J, Fumeron F, Clair D, Apfelbaum M. A positive correlation between energy intake and BMI in a population of 1312 overweight subjects. Int J Obes 1989;13:673–81.

192. Bennett GA. Expectations in the treatment of obesity. Br J Clin Psychol 1986;25(Pt 4):311–12.

193. Trottier K, Polivy J, Herman CP. Effects of exposure to unrealistic promises about dieting: are unrealistic expectations about dieting inspirational? Int J Eat Disord 2005;37(2):142–9.

194. Finch EA, Linde JA, Jeffery RW, Rothman AJ, King CM, Levy RL. The effects of outcome expectations and satisfaction on weight loss and maintenance: correlational and experimental analyses – a randomized trial. Health Psychol 2005; 24(6):608–16.

195. White MA, Masheb RM, Rothschild BS, Burke-Martindale CH, Grilo CM. Do patients' unrealistic weight goals have prognostic significance for bariatric surgery? Obes Surg 2007; 17(1):74–81.

196. Poston WS 2nd, Foreyt JP. Successful management of the obese patient. (Erratum appears in Am Fam Physician 2000;62(9):1967.) Am Family Physician 2000;61(12):3615–22.

197. Crawford D, Ball K. What do young women want in their efforts to control their weight? Implications for programme development. Nutr Dietet 2007;64:99–104.

198. Raynor HA, Epstein LH. Dietary variety, energy regulation, and obesity. Psychol Bull 2001;127(3):325–41.

199. Khaodhiar L, Blackburn GL. Obesity treatment: factors involved in weight-loss maintenance and regain. Curr Opin Endocrinol Diabetes 2002;9(5):369–74.

200. Toeller M, Buyken AE, Heitkamp G, Cathelineau G, Ferriss B, Michel G, et al. Nutrient intakes as predictors of body weight in European people with type 1 diabetes. Int J Obes 2001;25(12):1815–22.

201. Astrup A, Raben A. Sugar as a slimming agent? Br J Nutr 2000;84(5):585–6.

202. Slavin JL. Dietary fiber and body weight. Nutrition 2005;21(3):411–18.

203. Katsilambros N, Liatis S, Makrilakis K. Critical review of the international guidelines: what is agreed upon – what is not? Nestle Nutrition Workshop Series Clinical and Performance Program, 2006;11:207–18; discussion 18.

204. Zemel MB. The role of dairy foods in weight management. J Am Coll Nutr 2005;24(6 suppl):537S–46S.

205. Teegarden D. The influence of dairy product consumption on body composition. J Nutr 2005;135(12):2749–52.

206. Trowman R, Dumville JC, Hahn S, Torgerson DJ. A systematic review of the effects of calcium (supplementation on body weight. Br J Nutr 2006;95(6):1033–8.

207. Clifton P. The beginning of the end for the dietary calcium and obesity hypothesis? Obes Res 2005;13(8):1301.

208. Astrup A. Dietary approaches to reducing body weight. Best Pract Res Clin Endocrinol Metab 1999;13(1):109–20.

209. Maillot F, Farad S, Lamisse F. Alcohol and nutrition. Pathol Biol (Paris) 2001;49(9):683–8.

210. Zaninetti-Schaerer A, Guerne PA. Advances in the management of gout. Rev Med Suisse 2007;3(103):734–7.

211. Tejada T, Fornoni A, Lenz O, Materson BJ. Nonpharmacologic therapy for hypertension: does it really work? Curr Cardiol Rep 2006;8(6):418–24.

212. Poston WSC, Hyder ML, O'Byrne KK, Foreyt JP. Where do diets, exercise, and behavior modification fit in the treatment of obesity? Endocrine 2000;13(2):187–92.

213. Lowe MR, Levine AS. Eating motives and the controversy over dieting: eating less than needed versus less than wanted. Obes Res 2005;13(5):797–806.

214. Foreyt JP, Goodrick GK. Factors common to successful therapy for the obese patient. Med Sci Sports Exerc 1991;23(3):292–7.

215. Crombie N. Obesity management. Nurs Stand 1999;13(47):43–6.

216. Lyon X-H, di Vetta V, Milon H, Jequier E, Schutz Y. Compliance to dietary advice directed towards increasing the carbohydrate to fat ratio of the everyday diet. Int J Obes 1995;19:260–9.

217. Butler MG, Theodoro MF, Bittel DC, Donnelly JE, Butler MG, Theodoro MF, et al. Energy expenditure and physical activity in Prader–Willi syndrome: comparison with obese subjects. Am J Med Genet A 2007;143(5):449–59.

218. Hoffman CJ, Aultman D, Pipes P. A nutrition survey of and recommendations for individuals with Prader–Willi syndrome who live in group homes. J Am Dietet Assoc 1992;92(7):823–30, 33.

219. Pipes PL, Holm VA. Weight control of children with Prader–Willi syndrome. J Am Diet Assoc 1973;62(5):520–4.

220. Ho VA, Pipes PL. Food and children with Prader-Willi syndrome. Am J Dis Child 1976;130:1063–7.

221. Bistrian BR, Blackburn GL, Stanbury JB. Metabolic aspects of a protein-sparing modified fast in the dietary management of Prader-Willi obesity. N Engl J Med 1977;296(14):774–9.

222. Eiholzer U, Whitman BY, Eiholzer U, Whitman BY. A comprehensive team approach to the management of patients with Prader-Willi syndrome. J Pediatr Endocrinol 2004;17(9):1153–75.

223. National Task Force on the Prevention and Treatment of Obesity. Weight cycling. JAMA 1994;272(15):1196–206.

224. Goldstein DJ. Beneficial health effects of modest weight loss. Int J Obes 1992;16(6):397–415.

225. Wing RR, Phelan S. Long-term weight loss maintenance. Am J Clin Nutr 2005;82(1 suppl):222S–5S.

226. Wing RR, Jeffery RW. Food provision as a strategy to promote weight loss. Obes Res 2001;9(suppl 4):271S–5S.

227. Raynor DA, Phelan S, Hill JO, Wing RR. Television viewing and long-term weight maintenance: results from the National Weight Control Registry. Obesity 2006;14(10):1816–24.

228. Holden JH, Darga LL, Olson SM, Stettner DC, Ardito EA, Lucas CP. Long-term follow-up of patients attending a combination very-low calorie diet and behaviour therapy weight loss programme. Int J Obes 1992;16(8):605–13.

229. French SA, Jeffery RW, Forster JL, McGovern PG, Kelder SH, Baxter JE. Predictors of weight change over two years among a population of working adults: the Healthy Worker Project. Int J Obes 1994; 18(3):145–54.

230. Kirk SFL. Exploring the food beliefs and eating behaviour of successful and unsuccessful dieters. J Hum Nutr Dietet 1997;10(6):331–41.

231. Phelan S, Wyatt HR, Hill JO, Wing RR. Are the eating and exercise habits of successful weight losers changing? Obesity 2006; 14(4):710–16.

232. Jakicic JM, Wing RR, Winters-Hart C. Relationship of physical activity to eating behaviors and weight loss in women. Med Sci Sports Exerc 2002;34(10):1653–9.

233. Jakicic JM, Clark K, Coleman E, Donnelly JE, Foreyt J, Melanson E, et al. Appropriate intervention strategies for weight loss and prevention of weight regain for adults. Med Sci Sports Exerc 2001;33(12):2145–56.

234. NHLBI. *Clinical Guidelines on the Identification, Evaluation, and Treatment of Overweight and Obesity in Adults.* Available at: www.nhlbi.nih.gov/guidelines/obesity/ob_home.ht

235. NHLBI. *Aim for a Healthy Weight.* Available at: www.nhlbi.nih.gov/health/public/heart/obesity/lose_wt/index.htm

236. SIGN. *Integrating Prevention with Weight Management*. Guideline No 8. Available at: www.sign.ac.uk/

237. Douketis JD, Feightner JW, Attia J, Feldman WF. Periodic health examination, 1999 update: 1. Detection, prevention and treatment of obesity. Canadian Task Force on Preventive Health Care. CMAJ 1999;160(4):513–25.

238. Spear BA, Barlow SE, Ervin C, Ludwig DS, Saelens BE, Schetzina KE, et al. Recommendations for treatment of child and adolescent overweight and obesity. Pediatrics 2007;120(suppl 4):S254–88.

239. Garrow J, Summerbell C. Obesity. In: Stevens A, Raftery J (eds) *Health Care Needs Assessment: The Epidemiologically Based Needs Assessment Reviews*, 3rd series. Abingdon: Radcliffe Medical Press, 2000.

240. Davis AM, Giles A, Rona R. *Tackling Obesity: A Toolbox for Local Partnership Action*. London: Faculty of Public Health Medicine, 2000.

241. BHF. So you want to lose weight … for good: a guide to losing weight for men and women. Available at: www.bhf.org.uk/publications/secure/z_index.html

242. NOF. *Guidelines on Management of Adult Obesity and Overweight in Primary Care*. Available at: www.nationalobesityforum.org.uk/

243. Hughes J, Martin S. The Department of Health's project to evaluate weight management services. J Hum Nutr Dietet 1999;12:1–8.

244. Faulkner G, Cohn T, Remington G. Interventions to reduce weight gain in schizophrenia. Cochrane Database of Systematic Reviews, 2007(1):CD005148.

245. Campbell K, Waters E, O'Meara S, Kelly S, Summerbell C, Campbell K, et al. Interventions for preventing obesity in children. Update in Cochrane Database Syst Rev, 2005;(3):CD001871; PMID: 16034868. Update of Cochrane Database Syst Rev, 2001; (3):CD001871; PMID: 11686999.

246. Summerbell CD, Ashton V, Campbell KJ, Edmunds L, Kelly S, Waters E, et al. Interventions for treating obesity in children. Cochrane Database Syst Rev, 2003(3):CD001872.

247. Harvey EL, Glenny AM, Kirk SF, Summerbell CD. An updated systematic review of interventions to improve health professionals' management of obesity. Obes Rev 2002;3(1):45–55.

248. WHO Consultation on Obesity. Obesity: preventing and managing the global epidemic. WHO Technical Report Series 894. Geneva, 2000.

249. Joint WHO/FAO Expert Consultation. Diet, nutrition and the prevention of chronic diseases WHO Technical Report Series 916. Geneva, 2003.

250. Thomas DE, Elliott EJ, Baur L. Low glycaemic index or low glycaemic load diets for overweight and obesity. Cochrane Database of Systematic Reviews 2007(3): CD005105.

22 Behavioral Treatment of Obesity

Vicki L. Clark, Divya Pamnani and Thomas A. Wadden

Department of Psychiatry, University of Pennsylvania, School of Medicine, Philadelphia, PA, USA

Introduction

Modest weight loss improves many of the health complications of obesity, as demonstrated by the Diabetes Prevention Program (DPP) and the Look AHEAD (Action for Health and Diabetes) study [1,2]. The DPP randomized 3200 overweight individuals with impaired glucose tolerance to: (1) a lifestyle intervention consisting of diet, exercise, and behavior modification; (2) metformin (850 mg bid); or (3) placebo. Patients in the lifestyle intervention lost an average of 7 kg in the first year and were found at 2.8 years to have reduced their risk of developing type 2 diabetes by 58% compared to placebo-treated participants [1]. The Look AHEAD trial assigned 5145 overweight individuals with type 2 diabetes to an intensive lifestyle intervention (similar to the program used in the DPP) or a usual-care condition [2]. At the end of the first year (of this 12-year trial) participants in the lifestyle intervention lost more weight than those in the usual-care group (8.6% versus 0.7% of initial weight) and experienced greater improvements in their diabetes control and cardiovascular risk factors [2]. Other studies have shown improvements in hypertension, sleep apnea, and other weight-related health complications with a loss of 5–10% of initial weight [3–5].

The National Heart, Lung, and Blood Institute (NHLBI) has provided an algorithm to guide the treatment of obesity (see Table 22.1). A program of diet, exercise, and behavior modification is recommended as a first course of treatment for all obese individuals, as well as for individuals who are overweight (i.e. Body Mass Index (BMI) of 25.0–29.9 kg/m^2) and have two or more risk factors. As indicated in Table 22.1, behavior therapy remains an important component of treatment as BMI increases and pharmacotherapy or surgical intervention is prescribed. This chapter describes behavior modification for obesity, which can be used to facilitate adherence to a variety of diet and exercise regimens. We review the components of behavior therapy, examine the short- and long-term results of treatment, and discuss methods to improve long-term weight loss.

Principles of behavior therapy

The goal of behavioral treatment is to help obese patients identify and modify their eating and activity habits. This approach recognizes that obesity is influenced by metabolic and genetic factors [6–8] but holds that recent increases in the prevalence of obesity are attributable primarily to changes in Western nations' eating and activity habits [9]. Therefore, behavior therapy, based largely on learning theories, applies principles of classical and operant conditioning to the regulation of body weight.

According to the principle of classical conditioning, two events will become linked together if they are paired repeatedly [10,11]. The more frequently they are paired, the stronger the association between them will become until eventually, the presence of one event automatically triggers the other. Eating popcorn at the movies is an example. If these events are paired repeatedly, simply entering a movie theater will trigger a craving for popcorn. Behavior therapy seeks to disconnect cues associated with unwanted eating and activity habits. A patient who frequently snacks on high-calorie foods while watching television, for example, might experience an urge to eat whenever he turns the set on. He would, therefore, be encouraged to restrict his food intake to certain places (e.g. kitchen) in order to extinguish the association between watching television and eating.

The principle of operant conditioning is used to promote behavior change by manipulating the consequences of eating and activity choices [10,11]. Behaviors that are rewarded (i.e. reinforced) are more likely to be repeated. For example, an individual who loses 2 lb during the week as a result of recording her food intake will be positively reinforced to continue recording. On the other hand, behaviors that are punished (or followed by negative consequences) are less likely to be repeated. A person, for example,

Clinical Obesity in Adults and Children, 3rd edition. Edited by Peter G. Kopelman, Ian D. Caterson and William H. Dietz.
© 2010 Blackwell Publishing, ISBN: 978-1-4051-8226-3.

Treatment	BMI category					
	<24.9	25–26.9	27–29.9	30–35	35–39.9	>40
Diet, exercise, behavior therapy	–	With co-morbidities	With co-morbidities	+	+	+
Pharmacotherapy	–	–	With co-morbidities	+	+	+
Surgery	–	–	–		With co-morbidities	+

Table 22.1 A guide to selecting treatment.

Guidelines provided by the NHLBI utilize BMI category and the presence of co-morbidities to aid in treatment selection. Table reproduced with permission from reference [22].

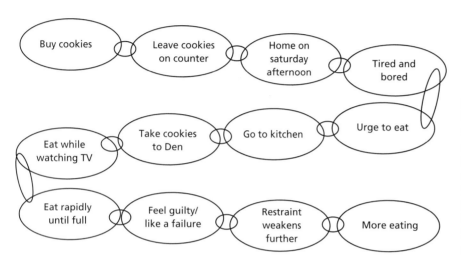

Figure 22.1 A behavior chain, illustrating how one behavior, linked to another, can contribute to an overeating episode. What appears to be an unexpected dietary lapse can be traced to a whole series of small decisions and behaviors. The behavior chain also reveals where the individual can intervene in the future to prevent unwanted eating. Thus, the individual might avoid bringing cookies into the house or at least store them out of sight to reduce impulse eating. (Reproduced with permission from reference [10].)

who increases her activity level by 200 minutes in one week may feel exhausted and fatigued. As a result, she may feel discouraged from continuing her exercise program. If she began with a more modest exercise regimen (e.g. 10 minutes of exercise, 5 days per week) and gradually increased her activity level, she would be less likely to experience negative effects.

Behavior therapy teaches patients to conduct a functional analysis of the antecedent events and consequences of problem behaviors [10]. Such analysis highlights cues that are frequently associated with problem eating and activity behaviors (i.e. times, places, people), thus identifying opportunities for intervention. Problem behaviors are often triggered by a series of events that are linked together in a chain, as illustrated in Figure 22.1 [10]. Mapping the links in a behavioral chain can identify the source of the problem and suggest options for intervention.

Components of behavioral treatment

Behavior therapy provides a very goal-oriented approach to weight loss. Patients are encouraged to set concrete, tangible goals with measurable outcomes [10,11]. They should leave each session with a strategy for how they will achieve their goals. This includes devising a detailed plan of what they will do, when and where they

will do it, and how often. For example, helping patients develop a plan to walk around the neighborhood for 15 minutes on Monday, Wednesday, Thursday, and Saturday evenings, immediately after dinner, is more helpful than simply telling them to increase their physical activity. Patients should set small goals that they can attain in order to maximize feelings of success (which will reinforce their behavior). Small successes build upon each other until patients reach their ultimate goals [10,12].

Behavioral treatment also is typically delivered as a package that includes multiple components such as self-monitoring, stimulus control, diet, exercise, cognitive restructuring, social support, problem solving, slowing the rate of eating, and relapse prevention. Detailed descriptions of these components are available elsewhere [10,13]. The present chapter highlights self-monitoring, stimulus control, and cognitive restructuring. We also discuss interventions for diet and exercise, given that they are the primary targets of behavioral treatment.

Self-monitoring

Self-monitoring is probably the most important component of behavioral treatment for obesity [10,14]. Patients keep detailed records of their food intake, activity, and weight throughout treatment. They initially record the types, amounts, and caloric value of foods eaten. This information is used to help patients reduce their calorie intake by 500–1000 kcal per day. As treatment progresses, patients expand their self-monitoring to include additional data about times, places, and feelings associated with eating [10]. This additional information typically reveals patterns of which patients may not be aware. An individual, for example, may notice that he snacks excessively in the evenings. Another may realize that she often makes poor food choices when upset. Once problem areas have been identified, patient and practitioner work together to develop a plan to tackle the problem behavior.

The importance of self-monitoring has been demonstrated in several studies. Monitoring food intake helps patients reduce their tendency to underestimate how much they eat [15]. Not surprisingly, individuals who regularly keep food records lose significantly more weight than those who record inconsistently [16–19].

Stimulus control

Stimulus control techniques frequently use principles of classical and operant conditioning, described above, to help patients manage cues associated with eating and exercise behaviors. As noted previously, an event can become a cue to eat when it is repeatedly paired with eating. For example, walking into the kitchen often elicits a desire to eat because this room is so strongly associated with food. People rarely experience a food craving when in the attic because of the absence of cues in this area. Many events can prompt a desire to eat. The most obvious are the sight and smell of food. There is truth in the old adage "out of sight, out of mind." Behavior therapy teaches patients to reduce cues to unwanted eating by limiting exposure to problem foods. Patients are also taught to tackle cues related to time, place, and events with strategies such as: (1) limiting the places they eat (at home) to the kitchen or dining room; (2) eating at regular times of day; and (3) refraining from engaging in other activities while eating (such as driving). Food cues are neutralized by disconnecting them from eating.

Stimulus control techniques can also target cues to promote healthy eating and activity habits. A patient might, for example, replace a cookie jar on the kitchen counter with a fruit basket. Another might place his walking shoes by the front door in order to prompt him to exercise. Behavioral treatment aims to decrease negative cues while increasing positive ones [10]. A recent 8-week pilot study found that encouraging patients to use an online grocery shopping and delivery service reduced the number of high-fat foods in the house [20]. There was also a trend (p = 0.08) for the number of grocery deliveries to be associated with weight loss. Future studies are needed to evaluate the long-term impact of interventions designed to improve stimulus control in weight management programs.

Cognitive restructuring

Cognitive theory holds that patients' thoughts determine how they respond to different events. Therefore, negative thoughts can create obstacles to behavior change. A person who thinks, "I've blown my diet. I should just give up," after overeating is likely to respond differently from a person who responds, "I know that wasn't the best choice I could have made, but I am going to stick with my plan for the rest of the day." The catastrophic thinking expressed by the first person is common among individuals attempting to lose weight and can lead patients to abandon their weight control efforts. Cognitive restructuring teaches patients to monitor maladaptive thoughts that may undermine their weight loss efforts, and to replace them with more adaptive thoughts. Rational responses such as, "Just because I ate an extra 300 calories tonight doesn't mean I won't be able to lose weight" are more likely to elicit positive eating and activity habits. Cognitive restructuring is helpful in teaching patients to view a setback as a temporary lapse. The ultimate goal is to determine how lapses occurred and to develop strategies to prevent them. Cognitive techniques also can be used to help patients address body image concerns [21].

Dietary options for weight loss

Weight loss requires the induction of a negative energy balance (i.e. fewer calories are consumed than are expended). It is easier to achieve negative energy balance by reducing calorie intake than by increasing physical activity. Most patients would have to walk approximately 4 miles to induce an energy deficit of 500 kcal. By contrast, the same 500 kcal deficit could be achieved by simply eliminating two 20 oz sugared sodas. Most people find the latter task easier.

Behavior therapy typically encourages patients to decrease their food intake by 500–1000 kcal/d to induce a weight loss of 0.5–1.0 kg/per week, consistent with the recommendations of the NHLBI [22]. Participants are typically instructed to follow a low-fat diet (i.e. fewer than 30% of calories from fat) and a calorie prescription of 1200–1500 kcal/d (for women) and 1500–1800 kcal/d (for men). Behavioral approaches typically support flexibility in food choices, encouraging patients to make changes that they can maintain. Behavioral principles also can be used to facilitate adherence to more structured approaches, including diets using portion-controlled foods or liquid meal replacements, as well as low-carbohydrate and low energy-density diets. This section provides a brief description of each of these approaches.

Portion-controlled foods

Obese individuals tend to underestimate their food intake by 30–50% when eating a diet of conventional foods [15]. This is attributable to misjudging portion sizes, failing to recognize hidden sources of fat or sugar or forgetting about some foods eaten. The use of portion-controlled foods, such as frozen food entrees, takes the guesswork out of calorie counting by providing patients with a fixed amount of food with a known energy content. Jeffery and colleagues compared the weight loss of patients who were prescribed a conventional diet of self-selected foods with that of individuals who were provided with actual foods for five breakfasts and five dinners a week [23]. The second group lost more weight after 6, 12, and 18 months of treatment despite the fact that both groups were prescribed the same calorie goal (approximately 1000 kcal/d). The provision of fixed portions of food appeared to facilitate patients' adherence to their calorie goals.

In a follow-up study, Wing and colleagues randomly assigned women to standard behavior modification plus: (1) no additional treatment; (2) detailed meal plans and grocery lists; (3) meal plans with food provided at reduced cost; and (4) meal plans with free food provision [24]. Results showed that the three latter groups lost more weight than group 1 after 6 months and maintained greater weight losses after 18 months. There were, however, no differences among the three groups that received meal plans. Thus, it appears that the provision of food does not improve outcome more than the structure provided by detailed meal plans. Several other studies also have shown the benefits of using portion-controlled meals [25,26].

Liquid meal replacements

Liquid meal replacements also provide patients a fixed quantity of food with a known calorie content (i.e. 160–220 kcal/serving). They simplify food choices, require little preparation, and are relatively inexpensive compared to a meal of conventional foods. Ditschuneit and colleagues [27] found that patients who consumed liquid meal replacement (e.g. SlimFast) for two meals and two snacks per day lost significantly more weight after 3 months than patients prescribed a conventional diet of self-selected foods (7.8 versus 1.5%, respectively) with an equal calorie value (1200–1500 kcal/d). A follow-up study showed that participants who continued to replace one meal and one snack with meal replacements maintained a weight loss of 11% after 27 months and 8% after 51 months (see Fig. 22.2) [28].

A meta-analysis of six randomized controlled trials found that patients who consumed meal replacements lost an average of 2.5 kg more after 3 months (and 2.6 kg more after 1 year) than participants who consumed diets of conventional foods [29]. In addition, the drop-out rate after 1 year was significantly lower in participants in the meal replacement group.

Recent studies have evaluated the use of meal replacements in the treatment of overweight individuals with type 2 diabetes. Li and colleagues [30] found that patients who used meal replacements lost 4.6% of initial weight in comparison to the 2.3% lost by participants who followed a diet plan based on the American Dietetic Association's (ADA) food exchange system. The use of meal replacements was also associated with greater improvements in glycemic control and reductions in medication prescriptions. Overweight individuals with type 2 diabetes who participated in the Look AHEAD lifestyle intervention group lost

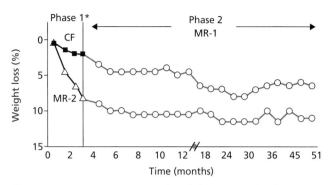

Figure 22.2 Long-term maintenance of weight loss using meal replacements (MR) versus conventional foods (CF) with the same calorie goal. Participants were randomly assigned to MR or CF groups and treated for the first 3 months. Thereafter, CF participants were permitted to replace one meal and one snack with meal replacements, as were individuals in the original MR group. (Reproduced with permission from reference [28].)

8.6% of initial weight during the first year while adhering to a diet that included liquid meal replacements [2].

Low-carbohydrate diets

Low-carbohydrate diets have been a popular topic of investigation in recent years [31–36]. Low-carbohydrate plans, such as the Atkins Diet [37], induce weight loss, in part, by simplifying food choices. During the initial weeks, dieters consume the majority of their calories from protein and fat, limiting carbohydrate to fewer than 20 g/d. Elimination of an entire class of macronutrients facilitates weight loss while the large amounts of dietary protein may satisfy appetite. The high fat content of these diets has raised concerns about the health consequences of low carbohydrate approaches. Several studies, however, have revealed favorable findings.

Two initial studies reported greater weight losses with low-carbohydrate than low-fat diets after 6 months (approximately 7.0 kg versus 3.0 kg, respectively), although there were no significant differences between the diets at 1 year [32]. A recent 2-year trial compared a low-carbohydrate diet to Mediterranean and low-fat diets [36]. The low-fat and Mediterranean groups were given identical caloric prescriptions (i.e. 1500 kcal/d for women and 1800 kcal/d for men) and instructed to restrict their fat intake to 30% and 35% of calories consumed, respectively. The low-carbohydrate condition did not receive any caloric restriction. As shown in Figure 22.3, participants in the low-carbohydrate (4.7 kg) and Mediterranean diet (4.4 kg) conditions achieved significantly larger weight losses than the low-fat group (2.7 kg) at the end of the 2-year intervention [36]. The low-carbohydrate group also had significantly greater reductions in triglycerides and greater improvements in high-density lipoprotein (HDL) cholesterol at 2 years [36]. There were no significant differences in decreases in low-density lipoprotein (LDL). Findings from these and other studies [31,35] suggest that low-carbohydrate diets are an acceptable option for patients who wish to try them.

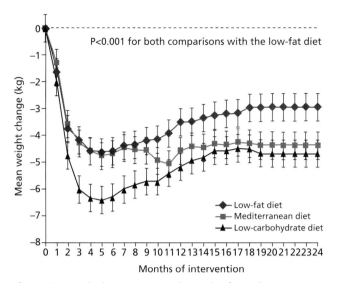

Figure 22.3 Weight change over 24 months on a low-fat, Mediterranean or low-carbohydrate diet. (Reproduced with permission from reference [36].)

Low energy-density diets

Energy density refers to the energy content (i.e. calories) in a given weight (g) of food. The underlying principle of low energy-density diets is that the volume of food consumed, not calorie content, influences satiety [38]. Low energy-density diets aim to minimize the amount of energy in a given weight of food. Energy density can be reduced by replacing fat (e.g. 9 kcal/d) with carbohydrate or protein (e.g. each 4 kcal/d) or by increasing the fiber or water content in foods [39]. Studies have shown that both lean and obese individuals consume fewer calories when allowed *ad libitum* consumption of low energy compared with high energy-density meals [40,41]. The consumption of low energy-density foods (e.g. soup) prior to a meal also reduces calorie intake for the entire meal [42]. To enhance satiety, water must be incorporated into food, rather than being drunk with the meal [43].

A recent study evaluated the efficacy of low energy-density diets for the treatment of obesity [44]. Patients were instructed to reduce fat intake (RF) or reduce fat intake and increase their consumption of water-rich foods, especially fruits and vegetables (RF + FV). Participants in the latter group lost significantly more weight at 6 months (6.7 kg versus 8.9 kg, respectively) and maintained their weight loss at 12 months (7.9 kg) as well as the RF group (6.4 kg), while reporting less hunger [44]. A low energy-density diet, rich in fruits and vegetables, could be an excellent option for patients who feel hungry when dieting. This approach would let them eat more food, while potentially decreasing their calorie intake.

Summary

Dieters can select from a variety of dietary interventions to facilitate the induction of weight loss. As a general rule, a portion-controlled diet will induce weight loss faster than a traditional balanced-deficit diet composed of conventional foods [29]. The choice of a particular approach depends, in large measure, on personal preferences. The most effective diet for long-term weight control is the one a patient can adhere to on a long-term basis [31].

Physical activity for weight control

Physical activity contributes to weight management principally by facilitating the maintenance, rather than the induction, of weight loss. Exercise alone, in the absence of caloric restriction, induces modest weight loss of only 2–3 kg in 4–6 months [22,45]. This is probably due to the difficulty patients encounter in finding the time or motivation to engage in the amount of exercise required to expend enough calories (3500 kcal) to lose 0.5 kg in a week. Physical activity, however, is the strongest predictor of weight loss maintenance [46,47] and it also improves cardiovascular health [48]. Therefore, increasing physical activity is an important goal in the behavioral treatment of obesity. Participants are typically encouraged to gradually increase their energy expenditure throughout treatment until they reach their prescribed physical activity goals. They are instructed to increase both programmed and lifestyle activity.

Programmed activity

Programmed activity refers to planned bouts of aerobic activity such as walking, swimming or biking, usually completed in a discrete period of time (i.e. at least 20–30 minutes) at a moderate intensity level (i.e. 60–80% of maximum heart rate). Patients have traditionally been advised to work towards a goal of exercising at least 150–180 minutes per week (i.e. 30 minutes per day, most days of the week), although research suggests that higher levels of physical activity might be required for successful long-term weight control [49,50], as discussed later in this chapter.

Exercising in short bouts can help reduce barriers to physical activity, such as lack of time, which is commonly identified as a barrier to regular activity. Jakicic et al. [51] randomly assigned patients to complete their exercise in one long bout (40 min) or four short bouts (10 min). Exercise adherence was significantly better in the latter group, and these patients tended to lose more weight than those in the long-bout condition (8.9 kg and 6.4 kg, respectively). Additional studies have shown that adherence is facilitated by having patients complete their activity at home [52,53]. While exercising at a health club is fine for those who enjoy it, exercising at home reduces common barriers including time, transportation, and child care.

Lifestyle activity

Lifestyle activity involves increasing energy expenditure throughout the day, without concern for the intensity or duration of activity. It can be increased by taking stairs rather than escalators, walking rather than riding, and parking farther away. Lifestyle activity, combined with diet, produces weight loss comparable to that induced by programmed exercise plus diet [54,55]. Andersen and colleagues [54] found that participants who engaged in programmed exercise (e.g. attending a 1-hour step-aerobics class three times a week) or lifestyle activity (e.g. increasing movement by 30 minutes a day) lost 8 kg during a 16-week behavioral treatment. There was a trend for the lifestyle participants to maintain their weight loss better than those in the step-aerobics class (p < 0.06).

The use of pedometers to monitor participants' daily steps is an easy and inexpensive method of increasing lifestyle activity. Before treatment, participants typically walk 3000–4000 steps per day. Each week, they increase their step goal until they walk approximately 8000–10,000 steps per day. Pedometers provide immediate feedback about behavior (e.g. walked 200 extra steps by parking farther away from a store entrance) which is reinforcing to patients.

Structure of behavioral treatment

An initial course of behavioral treatment is usually provided in 16–26 weekly sessions. Treatment has a clear start and end date which seems to help participants pace their efforts. Treatment is typically delivered to groups of 10–20 people who start and end treatment together. This approach ensures a high level of social support and continuity of care. Participants assist each other in their efforts to modify eating and activity habits. Group treatment has been shown to be more effective than individual treatment, even among those who preferred the latter approach [56]. Group treatment also is more cost-effective and provides both social support and a healthy dose of competition.

The content of groups is typically guided by a structured protocol such as the LEARN Program for Weight Control [10] or the Diabetes Prevention Program [1]. Sessions begin with a review of patients' food and activity records, followed by discussion of any problems they encountered. The group leader, together with the group members, helps patients identify strategies to overcome barriers to adhering to their eating and activity goals. Therefore, a group format provides patients with extra opportunities to practice problem solving and other skills. A new topic is presented each week by the group leader, typically a dietitian, psychologist, exercise specialist or other healthcare professional. Patients complete behavioral homework assignments in which they apply the techniques they discussed in session.

Short-term weight losses

Previous reviews have shown that patients currently treated by a comprehensive group behavioral approach lose approximately 10 kg (about 10% of initial weight) in 26 weeks of treatment [14]. In addition, about 80% of patients who begin treatment complete it. Thus, behavioral treatment yields very favorable results as judged by the current criteria for success (i.e. a 5–10% reduction in initial weight) proposed by the NHLBI [22], the World Health

Organization (WHO) [57] and the Agricultural Research Service [58].

A comparison of early and more recent behavioral interventions reveals that weight losses have more than doubled over the past 30 years as treatment duration has increased more than threefold. Thus, for example, in 1974 treatment of 8.4 weeks was associated with a mean loss of 3.8 kg, while treatment in 2002 averaged 31.6 weeks and produced a mean loss of 10.7 kg [14]. Although several new components, including cognitive restructuring, have been added to the behavioral approach since the 1970s, the most parsimonious explanation for the larger weight losses is the longer duration of treatment. The rate of weight loss has remained constant at about 0.4–0.5 kg per week.

Improving long-term weight control

The challenge for all obesity interventions is keeping off the lost weight. Without continued treatment, patients typically regain 30–35% of their weight loss in the year following treatment [14] and many return to their baseline weight within 5 years [59]. Factors responsible for weight regain have not been fully identified, despite the frequency with which this problem is observed. Contributors are likely to include compensatory metabolic responses to weight loss that include reductions in resting energy expenditure and leptin, as well as increases in ghrelin and other hormones that regulate eating [60–62]. In addition, patients are confronted daily by a "toxic" environment that explicitly encourages them to consume large quantities of high-fat, high-sugar foods [63]. Weight gain (or regain) appears to be a nearly inevitable response to this environment.

Short-term treatment of 4–6 months clearly is no match for what for most obese individuals is a chronic disorder. Obesity cannot be cured by 6 months of therapy, any more than type 2 diabetes or hypertension can be controlled long term by such brief intervention. This section discusses methods of improving long-term weight control.

Long-term treatment
Numerous studies have demonstrated the benefits of patients continuing to attend weight maintenance classes after completing an initial 16–26-week weight loss program [64,65]. Perri and colleagues [65], for example, found that individuals who attended every-other-week group maintenance sessions for the year following weight reduction maintained 13.0 kg of their 13.2 kg end-of-treatment weight loss, whereas those who did not receive such therapy maintained only 5.7 kg of a 10.8 kg loss. Maintenance sessions appear to provide patients with the support and motivation needed to continue to practice weight control skills, such as keeping food records and exercising regularly. In reviewing 13 studies on this topic, Perri and Corsica [64] found that patients who received extended treatment, which averaged 41 sessions over 54 weeks, maintained 10.3 kg of their initial 10.7 kg weight loss.

A recent study examined several methods of facilitating weight loss maintenance. After completing a 6-month weight loss program that induced an average loss of 8.5 kg, 1032 participants were randomized to one of three 30-month weight maintenance interventions [66]. Participants in a self-directed control group received printed materials that contained diet and activity recommendations and met briefly with a study interventionist at 1 year. Patients in an interactive technology condition received unlimited access to a website that provided information on diet and exercise, as well as other components often included in behavioral treatment programs (e.g. goal setting, problem solving). They were not provided with any individual counseling. A third group received monthly telephone contacts with an interventionist for 5–15 minutes and an in-person, 45–60-minute session every 4 months. Participants in the latter two conditions were instructed to continue to adhere to the recommended diet and to increase physical activity to at least 225 minutes per week in order to maintain or continue to lose weight.

As shown in Figure 22.4, patients in the personal contact group regained less weight than those in the internet technology and self-directed groups (i.e. 4.0, 5.2, 5.5 kg, respectively) after 30 months [66]. These results are comparable to another weight maintenance study that examined participants who had lost at least 10% of their body weight in the prior 2 years. A total of 319 participants were randomly assigned to face-to-face, internet or control interventions. In this 18-month investigation, patients assigned to the face-to-face condition regained less weight (2.5 kg) than participants in the internet (4.7 kg), and control groups (4.9 kg) [67]. These two studies illustrate the benefits of long-term patient–provider contact for facilitating weight maintenance.

Perri and colleagues [68] also demonstrated that long-term therapist contact, provided either by phone or surface mail, significantly improved weight maintenance, compared with no

further intervention. When using telephone calls, the same therapist optimally should contact the patient on each occasion. A study in which patients were contacted by staff members unknown to them failed to improve weight maintenance beyond results of a no-contact group [69].

Importance of physical activity

As mentioned previously, physical activity is the best predictor of weight loss maintenance. Numerous studies have shown that people who continue to exercise regularly after losing weight are more likely to keep off the lost weight [46,70,71]. Recent research has suggested that high levels of physical activity are optimal to facilitate long-term weight control [46,49,50,70,72,73]. A secondary data analysis of the results of a randomized trial, for example, found that obese individuals who exercised >200 min/wk achieved significantly greater weight losses at 18 months than those who exercised <150 min/wk [49]. Members of the National Weight Control Registry (NWCR), a database of individuals who have successfully maintained a weight loss >30 lbs for at least 1 year, reported expending an average of 2621 kcal/week, although there was significant variability among participants [70].

Jeffery and colleagues conducted a randomized controlled trial that compared the benefits of low versus high levels of physical activity [50]. Participants in the high-activity group were instructed to expend 2500 kcal/wk, while those in the low group were prescribed a goal of 1000 kcal/wk. As shown in Figure 22.5, weight losses of the two treatment conditions did not differ significantly at the end of 6 months, during which participants attended weekly group meetings. However, participants in the high-activity group maintained their losses significantly better at both the 12- and 18-month follow-up assessments than did patients in the low-activity group [50]. Activity levels declined, however, after treatment ended, resulting in no differences between groups at the 30-month follow-up [74]. Patients who continued to expend >2500 kcal/wk, across treatment groups,

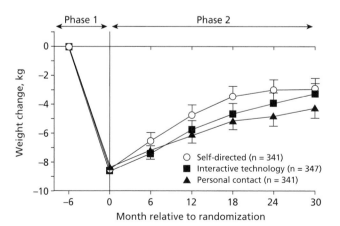

Figure 22.4 Long-term weight loss maintenance among participants assigned to monthly personal contact, unlimited Internet-based intervention (i.e. interactive technology) or self-directed control conditions. (Reproduced with permission from reference [66].)

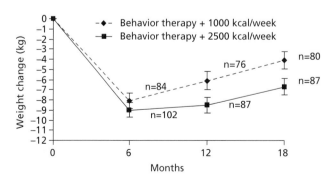

Figure 22.5 Participants prescribed high activity goals (2500 kcal/wk) maintained their weight loss significantly better than those in the low-activity group (1000 kcal/wk) after 18 months. (Reproduced with permission from reference [50].)

maintained a significantly greater weight loss than those who exercised less (12.0 kg and 0.8 kg, respectively).

The mechanisms by which exercise facilitates weight maintenance are not well understood. The simplest explanation is that increased physical activity helps to keep patients in energy balance. Walking 2 or 3 miles a day may help to compensate for occasional dietary indiscretions that are associated with weight regain (in persons who do not exercise regularly). Alternatively, exercise spares the loss of fat-free mass during diet-induced weight loss, an occurrence that could help minimize undesired reductions in resting-energy expenditure [75]. Increased physical activity could be associated with improved mood which, in turn, could facilitate long-term adherence to a low-calorie diet [75]. Regardless of the mechanism of action, the message remains the same: patients should increase their physical activity by whatever means possible, including increasing lifestyle activity and decreasing sedentary behaviors. This latter approach has proven particularly effective in overweight children [76].

Combining behavioral and pharmacologic interventions

The combination of weight loss medications with behavioral treatment provides another option to enhance weight loss maintenance. Lifestyle modification and pharmacotherapy would appear to have different but complementary mechanisms of action [77] which, when combined, could increase weight loss, compared with either approach used alone. Pharmacologic agents modify the internal environment by reducing hunger, cravings or nutrient absorption [78]. Behavioral treatment, by contrast, teaches patients to modify the external environment by, for example, avoiding fast-food restaurants or storing food out of sight in the home [79].

A controlled trial that tested this hypothesis randomized 224 obese individuals to four treatment groups, all 1 year in duration [18]. All participants were prescribed a diet of 1200–1500 kcal per day and were encouraged to exercise for 30 minutes on most days of the week. Participants in the first group (sibutramine alone) received sibutramine (10–15 mg per day), provided during eight physician visits of 10–15 minutes. They were not given any behavioral instruction to help them reach their calorie and activity goals. Two additional conditions received group behavioral treatment without (i.e. lifestyle modification alone) or with sibutramine (i.e combined therapy). A final group received sibutramine (10–15 mg per day) plus brief counseling, provided during eight physician visits of 10–15 minutes (i.e. sibutramine plus brief therapy). These patients also received the treatment manuals provided to participants in the two lifestyle modification conditions, and their physician reviewed their diet and activity records during scheduled appointments.

As shown in Figure 22.6, at the end of the initial phase of treatment (week 18), patients who received lifestyle modification alone and sibutramine plus brief therapy lost significantly more

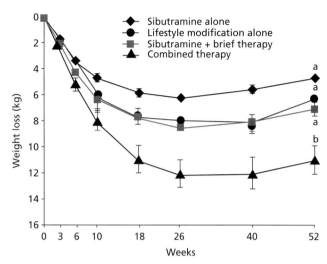

Figure 22.6 Mean percentage reduction in initial weight over 1 year for participants assigned to sibutramine alone, lifestyle modification alone, combined therapy, or sibutramine plus brief therapy. (Reproduced with permission from reference [18].)

weight than those treated by sibutramine alone (8.2%, 7.9% and 5.8% of initial weight, respectively). The combined therapy group lost significantly more weight (10.9% of initial weight) at this time and maintained a significantly greater loss at 1 year than did the other three treatments, which did not differ significantly from each other.

These findings suggest that a combination of medication and behavior therapy may induce and maintain larger weight losses than either approach used alone. Similar results were obtained by James and colleagues who found that patients who received sibutramine plus lifestyle modification maintained a loss of approximately 10% of initial weight at 2 years, as compared to a loss of only 5% for patients who received lifestyle modification plus placebo [80]. Two studies of orlistat, a gastric lipase inhibitor, also obtained good maintenance of weight loss at 2 years in patients who received lifestyle modification plus medication versus lifestyle modification plus placebo [81,82].

Dissemination of behavioral treatment

Behavioral treatment clearly is effective in inducing a loss of approximately 10% of initial weight, and losses of this size are associated with significant improvements in health [1,2]. In addition to its successes, the behavioral treatment of obesity faces several challenges at present. First, treatment must be made more available to the millions of Americans who need to lose weight. Behavioral treatment is offered in academic medical centers that are not readily accessible to many individuals seeking treatment. We briefly discuss two avenues for increasing access to behavioral weight control programs.

Internet and email

The rapid growth of the Internet over the past decade has provided novel opportunities to increase the accessibility of treatment by reducing geographic and transportation barriers. In the first of a series of studies, Tate and colleagues randomized participants to one of two 6-month weight loss programs [83]. An education intervention provided a directory of Internet resources for weight control but no instructions to change eating and activity habits. A behavior therapy intervention provided this component, as well as 24 weekly lessons conducted by email, weekly submission of self-monitoring diaries, and an online bulletin board. Participants in the behavior therapy group lost significantly more weight at 6 months than those in the education group (4.1 kg versus 1.6 kg, respectively). In a 12-month follow-up study, Tate et al. assigned individuals at risk for type 2 diabetes to an Internet weight loss program with or without weekly behavioral counseling, delivered by email [84]. Participants who received counseling lost more weight (4.4 kg) than those who did not have counseling (2.0 kg). These studies clearly demonstrate the benefit of therapist feedback.

A third study conducted by Tate and colleagues evaluated the level of therapist feedback necessary for optimal outcome in an Internet-based weight control program [85]. Patients participated in a 6-month program in which they received: (1) therapist-feedback from a human counselor, (2) computer-automated feedback or (3) no counseling. After 3 months, the human counselor and computer-automated feedback conditions (6.1 kg and 5.3 kg, respectively) were superior to the no counseling group (2.8 kg) but not significantly different from each other. Six months after the beginning of treatment, however, patients in the human counselor group had lost more weight (7.3 kg) than the computer-automated and no counseling groups (4.9 kg and 2.6 kg, respectively). We note that patients in all three groups were encouraged to use meal replacements, which may have been responsible for the greater weight loss observed in this study as compared to the first two.

Finally, a recent study compared a therapist-led Internet program to a commercial, online weight loss program [86]. Patients in the therapist-led condition participated in a 6-month weight loss phase, during which they received weekly online sessions followed by a 6-month weight maintenance phase during which online meetings were held bi-weekly. The commercial program provided a diet and fitness plan based on behavioral weight loss concepts and sent automated feedback messages based on an individual's weight loss. At 1 year, patients in the therapist-led group lost significantly more weight than those in the commercial program (7.8 kg and 3.4 kg, respectively).

These studies, taken together, underscore the importance of participants' completing behavioral assignments (such as keeping records of their food intake and physical activity) and receiving therapist feedback. Educational instruction alone is not sufficient to induce clinically significant weight loss. The studies also suggest that even the most effective Internet interventions are likely to produce only half the weight loss of traditional on-site behavioral programs. However, from a public health perspective, the greater availability of Internet programs may result in this approach having a greater impact on obesity management than traditional clinic- or hospital-based programs that serve so few individuals.

Commercial programs

Commercially available weight loss programs now include many of the components of behavioral treatment described above. Of these, Weight Watchers is by far the largest treatment provider and has been evaluated in three randomized controlled trials [87]. The program provides dietary education and group support in 1-hour weekly meetings at a cost of approximately $14 per visit. Treatment groups may include as many as 100 individuals. Unlike the closed groups used in academic medical centers, in which the same patients attend treatment together each week, Weight Watchers meetings are open to whoever wishes to attend at a given time. This practice makes for ease of enrollment in the program (although it may dilute the continuity of care).

Heshka and colleagues conducted a randomized controlled trial of 426 individuals who were assigned to Weight Watchers or a self-help intervention [88]. Persons in the former group attended weekly Weight Watchers meetings in their local community. (Group leaders did not know that participants were enrolled in a research study.) Those in the self-help condition were provided two 20-minute visits with a registered dietitian, as well as printed materials and other resources. At 1 year, 82% of participants remained in the study, with no differences in attrition between the two groups. Participants assigned to Weight Watchers lost 5.4% of initial weight, compared with 1.6% in the self-help group. At 2 years, losses declined to 3.2% and 0.1%, respectively. Seventy-three percent of participants remained in treatment at this time with no differences in attrition between groups.

A recent randomized controlled trial evaluated a second commercial program, Jenny Craig, in comparison to a usual-care control group [89]. Participants assigned to Jenny Craig attended weekly individual appointments with a consultant. They were also provided with follow-up phone and email contacts and website/message board access. Jenny Craig participants were given individualized caloric prescriptions based on their energy requirements (typically 1200–2000 kcal/d). The usual-care group met with a dietitian at baseline and 16 weeks and was prescribed a 500–1000 kcal/d deficit. Participants assigned to Jenny Craig lost 7.1% of initial weight after 1 year, compared to 0.7% in the usual-care group [89].

These findings suggest that commercial programs, such as Weight Watchers and Jenny Craig, might be an appropriate first step for individuals who have failed to reduce on their own with diet and exercise. A substantial minority of individuals can be expected to lose 5% or more of their initial weight, a loss that could prevent or ameliorate health complications.

Conclusion

As the prevalence of obesity reaches epidemic proportions, the need for effective methods of inducing and maintaining weight loss is evident. This chapter has shown that a comprehensive program of diet, exercise, and behavior therapy facilitates the loss of approximately 10% of initial weight, which is associated with significant health benefits. The maintenance of lost weight remains the challenge to successful weight control. Weight loss maintenance can be improved with the use of structured meal plans and meal replacements, home-based exercise and lifestyle activity, and the use of weight loss medications. Additional research is needed to identify methods of enhancing long-term weight control and increasing its accessibility.

Far greater efforts, however, must be devoted to the prevention of obesity in both children and adults if we are to halt the progression of the obesity epidemic [90]. Ultimately, we must tackle what Brownell has referred to as a "toxic" environment that explicitly encourages the consumption of super-sized servings of high-fat, high-sugar foods, while implicitly discouraging physical activity, as a result of sedentary work and leisure habits [9,90]. While behavioral treatment can assist those who already are obese, there is a pressing need for wide-scale environmental interventions that will reduce the number of individuals who require such treatment.

References

1. Diabetes Prevention Program Research Group. Reduction in the incidence of type 2 diabetes with lifestyle intervention or metformin. N Engl J Med 2002;346:393–403.
2. Look AHEAD Research Group. Reduction in weight and cardiovascular disease risk factors in individuals with type 2 diabetes – one-year results of the Look AHEAD trial. Diabetes Care 2007;30: 1374–83.
3. Blackburn GL. Effect of degree of weight loss on health benefits. Obes Res 1995;3:211S–216S.
4. Goldstein DJ. Beneficial effects of modest weight loss. Int J Obes 1992;16:397–416.
5. Poobalan A, Aucott L, Avenell A, Jung H, Broom J, Grant AM. Effects of weight loss in overweight/obese individuals and long-term lipid outcomes: a systematic review. Obes Rev 2004;5:43–50.
6. Ravussin E, Lillioja S, Knowler WC, Christin L, Freymund D, Abbott WG, et al. Reduced rate of energy expenditure as a risk factor for body weight gain. N Engl J Med 1988;318:467–72.
7. Stunkard AJ, Harris JR, Pederson NL, McClearn GE. The body-mass index of twins who have been reared apart. N Engl J Med 1990; 322:1483–7.
8. Morton GJ, Cummings DE, Baskin DG, Barsh GS, Schwart MW. Central nervous system control of food intake and body weight. Nature 2006;443:289–95.
9. Wadden TA, Brownell KD, Foster GD. Obesity: responding to the global epidemic. J Consult Clin Psychol 2002;70:510–25.
10. Brownell KD. *The LEARN Program for Weight Management 2000.* Dallas, TX: American Health Publishing, 2000.
11. Wadden TA, Crerand CE, Brock J. Behavioral treatment of obesity. Psychiatr Clin North Am 2005;28:151–70.
12. Lutes LD, Winett RA, Barger SD, Wojeik JR, Herbert WG, Nickols-Richardson SM, et al. Small changes in nutrition and physical activity promote weight loss and maintenance: 3-month evidence from the ASPIRE randomized trial. Ann Behav Med 2008;35:351–7.
13. Levy RL, Finch EA, Crowell MD, Talley NJ, Jeffery RW. Behavioral interventions for the treatment of obesity: Strategies and effectiveness data. Am J Gastroenterol 2007;102:2314–21.
14. Wadden TA, Butryn ML, Wilson C. Lifestyle modification for the management of obesity. Gastroenterology 2007;132:2226–38.
15. Lichtman SW, Pisarka K, Berman ER, Pestone M, Dowling H, Offenbacher E, et al. Discrepancy between self-reported and actual caloric intake and exercise in obese subjects. N Engl J Med 1992;327:1893–8.
16. Berkowitz RI, Wadden TA, Tershakovec AM, Cronquist JL. Behavior therapy and sibutramine for the treatment of adolescent obesity: a randomized controlled trial. JAMA 2003;289:1805–12.
17. Wadden TA, Berkowitz RI, Vogt RA, Steen SN, Stunkard AJ, Foster GD. Lifestyle modification in the pharmacologic treatment of obesity: a pilot investigation of a potential primary care approach. Obes Res 1997;5:218–26.
18. Wadden TA, Berkowitz RI, Womble LG, Sarwer DB, Phelan S, Cato RK, et al. Randomized trial of lifestyle modification and pharmacotherapy for obesity. N Engl J Med 2005;353:2111–20.
19. Boutelle KN, Kirschenbaum DS. Further support for consistent self-monitoring as a vital component of successful weight control. Obes Res 1998;6:219–24.
20. Gorin AA, Raynor HA, Niemeier HM, Wing RR. Home grocery delivery improves the household food environments of behavioral weight loss participants: results of an 8-week pilot. Int J Behav Nutr Phys Activity 2007;4:58.
21. Beck JS. *The Beck Diet Solution: Train Your Brain to Think Like a Thin Person.* Birmingham, AL: Oxmoor House, 2007.
22. National Heart, Lung, and Blood Institute. Clinical guidelines on the identification, evaluation, and treatment of overweight and obesity in adults: the evidence report. Obes Res 1998;6:51S–210S.
23. Jeffery RW, Wing RR, Thornson C, Burton LR, Raether C, Harvey J, et al. Strengthening behavioral interventions for weight loss: a randomized trial of food provision and monetary incentives. J Consult Clin Psychol 1993;61:1038–45.
24. Wing RR, Jeffery RW, Burton LR, Thorson C, Nissinoff K, Baxter JE. Food provisions versus structured meal plans in the behavioral treatment of obesity. J Consult Clin Psychol 1996;20:56–62.
25. Hannum SM, Carson L, Evans EM, Canene KA, Petr EL, Bui L, et al. Use of portion-controlled entrees enhances weight loss in women. J Obes Res 2004;12:538–46.
26. Hannum SM, Carson LA, Evans EM, Petr EL, Wharton CM, Bui L, et al. Use of packaged entrees as part of a weight-loss diet in overweight men: an 8-week randomized clinical trial. J Diabetes Obes Metab 2006;8:146–55.
27. Ditschuneit HH, Flechtner-Mors M, Johnson TD, Adler G. Metabolic and weight loss effects of long-term dietary intervention in obese subjects. Am J Clin Nutr 1999;69:198–204.
28. Flechtner-Mors M, Ditschuneit HH, Johnson TD, Suchard M, Adler G. Metabolic and weight loss effects of long-term intervention in obese patients: four-year results. Obes Res 2000;8:399–402.

29. Heymsfield SB, van Mierlo CA, van der Knaap HC, Heo M, Frier HI. Weight management using a meal replacement strategy: meta and pooling analysis from six studies. Int J Obes 2003;27:537–49.

30. Li Z, Hong K, Saltsman P, DeShields S, Bellman M, Thames G, et al. Long-term efficacy of soy-based meal replacements vs an individualized plan in obese type II DM patients: relative effects on weight loss, metabolic parameters, and C-reactive protein. Eur J Clin Nutr 2005:59:411–18.

31. Dansinger ML, Gleason JA, Griffith JL, Selker HP, Schaefer EJ. Comparison of the Atkins, Ornish, Weight Watchers, and Zone diets for weight loss and heart disease risk reduction: a randomized trial. JAMA 2005;293:43–53.

32. Foster GD, Wyatt HR, Hill JO, McGuckin BG, Brill C, Mohammed BS, et al. A randomized trial of a low-carbohydrate diet for obesity. N Engl J Med 2003;348:2082–90.

33. Samaha FF, Iqbal N, Seshadri P, Chicano KL, Daily DA, McGrory J, et al. A low-carbohydrate as compared with a low-fat diet in severe obesity. N Engl J Med 2003;348:2074–81.

34. Stern L, Iqbal N, Seshadri P, Chicano KL, Daily DA, McGrory J, et al. The effects of low-carbohydrate versus conventional weight loss diets in severely obese adults: one-year follow-up of a randomized trial. Ann Intern Med 2004;140:778–85.

35. Tay J, Brinkworth GD, Noakes M, Keogh J, Clifton PM. Metabolic effects of weight loss on a very-low-carbohydrate diet compared with an isocaloric high-carbohydrate diet in abdominally obese subjects. J Am Coll Cardiol 2008;51:59–67.

36. Shai I, Schwarzfuchs D, Henkin Y, Shahar D, Witkow S, Greenberg I, et al. Weight loss with a low-carbohydrate, Mediterranean, or low-fat diet. N Engl J Med 2008;359:229–41.

37. Atkins RC. *Dr. Atkins' New Diet Revolution*. New York: Avon Books, 1998.

38. Rolls BJ, Bell EA. Intake of fat and carbohydrate: role of energy density. Eur J Clin Nutr 1999;53S:S166–S173.

39. Melanson K, Dwyer J. Popular diets for treatment of overweight and obesity. In: Wadden TA, Stunkard AJ (eds) *Handbook of Obesity Treatment*. New York: Guilford Press, 2002: 249–75.

40. Duncan KH, Bacon JA, Weinsier RL. The effects of high and low energy density diets on satiety, energy intake, and eating time of obese and nonobese subjects. Am J Clin Nutr 1983;37:763–7.

41. Bell EA, Rolls BJ. Energy density of foods affects energy intake across multiple levels of fat content in lean and obese women. Am J Clin Nutr 2001;73:1010–18.

42. Flood JE, Rolls BJ. Soup preloads in a variety of forms reduce meal energy intake. Appetite 2007;49:626–34.

43. Rolls BJ, Bell EA, Thorwart ML. Water incorporated into a food but not served with a food decreases energy intake in lean women. Am J Clin Nutr 1999;70:448–55.

44. Ello-Martin JA, Roe LS, Ledikwe JH, Beach AM, Rolls BJ. Dietary energy density in the treatment of obesity: a year-long trial comparing 2 weight-loss diets. Am J Clin Nutr 2007;85:1465–77.

45. Miller WC, Koceja DM, Hamilton EJ. A meta-analysis of the past 25 years of weight loss research using diet, exercise or diet plus exercise intervention. Int J Obes 1997;21:941–7.

46. Klem ML, Wing RR, McGuire MT, Seagle HM, Hill JO. A descriptive study of individuals successful at long-term maintenance of substantial weight loss. Am J Clin Nutr 1997;66:239–46.

47. Wing RR, Hill JO. Successful weight loss maintenance. Ann Rev Nutr 2001;21:323–41.

48. Blair SN, Leermakers EA. Exercise and weight management. In: Wadden TA, Stunkard AJ (eds) *Handbook of Obesity Treatment*. New York: Guilford Press, 2002: 283–300.

49. Jakicic JM, Marcus BH, Gallagher KI, Napolitano M, Lang W. Effect of exercise duration and intensity on weight loss in overweight, sedentary women – a randomized trial. JAMA 2003;290:1323–30.

50. Jeffery RW, Wing RR, Sherwood NE, Tate DF. Physical activity and weight loss: does prescribing higher physical activity goals improve outcome? Am J Clin Nutr 2003;78:684–9.

51. Jakicic JM, Butler BA, Robertson RJ. Prescribing exercise in multiple short bouts versus one continuous bout: effects on adherence, cardiorespiratory fitness, and weight loss in overweight women. Int J Obes 1995;19:382–7.

52. Jakicic JM, Winters C, Lang W, Wing RR. Effects of intermittent exercise and use of home exercise equipment on adherence, weight loss, and fitness in overweight women: a randomized trial. JAMA 1999;16:1554–60.

53. Perri MG, Martin AD, Leermakers EA, Sears SF. Effects of group-versus home-based exercise training in healthy older men and women. J Consult Clin Psychol 1997;65:278–85.

54. Andersen RE, Wadden TA, Barlett SJ, Zemel BS, Verde TJ, Franckowiak SC. Effects of lifestyle activity versus structured aerobic exercise in obese women: a randomized trial. JAMA 1999;281:335–40.

55. Dunn AL, Marcus BH, Kampert JB, Garcia ME, Kohl HW, Blair SN. Comparison of lifestyle and structured interventions to increase physical activity and cardiorespiratory fitness. JAMA 1999;281:327–34.

56. Renjilian DA, Perri MG, Nezu AM, McKelvey WF, Shermer RL, Anton SD. Individual versus group therapy for obesity: effects of matching participants to their treatment preference. J Consult Clin Psychol 2001;69:717–21.

57. World Health Organization. *Obesity: Preventing and Managing the Global Epidemic*. Geneva: World Health Organization, 1998.

58. Agricultural Research Service. Report of Dietary Guidelines Advisory Committee on the dietary guidelines for Americans. Nutr Rev 1995;53:376–9.

59. Dansinger ML, Tatsioni AM, Wong JB, Chung M, Balk EM. Meta-analysis: the effects of dietary counseling for weight loss. Ann Intern Med 2007;147:41–50.

60. Cummings DE, Weigle DS, Frayo RS, Breen PA, Ma MK, Dellinger E, et al. Plasma ghrelin levels after diet-induced weight loss or gastric bypass surgery. N Engl J Med 2002;346:1623–30.

61. Rosenbaum M, Murphy EM, Heymsfield SB, Matthews DE, Leibel R. Low dose leptin administration reverses effects of sustained weight-reduction on energy expenditure and circulating concentrations of thyroid hormones. J Clin Endocrinol Metab 2002;87: 2391–4.

62. Wadden TA, Foster GD, Letizia KA, Mullen JL. Long-term effects of dieting on resting metabolic rate in obese outpatients. JAMA 1990;264:707–11.

63. Brownell KD, Horgen KB. *Food Fight: The Inside Story of the Food Industry, America's Obesity Crisis and What We Can Do About It*. New York: McGraw-Hill, 2003.

64. Perri MG, Corsica JA. Improving the maintenance of weight lost. In: Wadden TA, Stunkard AJ (eds) *Handbook of Obesity Treatment*. New York: Guilford Press, 2002: 357–79.

65. Perri MG, McAllister DA, Gange JJ, Jordan RC, McAdoo WG, Nezu AM. Effects of four maintenance programs on the long-term management of obesity. J Consult Clin Psychol 1988;56:529–34.

66. Svetkey LP, Stevens VJ, Brantley PJ, Appel LJ, Hollis JF, Loria CM, et al. Comparison of strategies for sustaining weight loss: the weight loss maintenance randomized controlled trial. JAMA 2008; 299:1139–48.

67. Wing RR, Tate DF, Gorin AA, Raynor HA, Fava JL. A self-regulation program for the maintenance of weight loss. N Engl J Med 2006;355:1563–71.

68. Perri MG, Shapiro RM, Ludwig WW, Twentyman CT, McAdoo WG. Maintenance strategies for the treatment of obesity: an evaluation of relapse prevention training and posttreatment contact by mail and telephone. J Consult Clin Psychol 1984;52:404–13.

69. Wing RR, Jeffery RW, Hellerstedt WL, Burton LR. Effect of frequent phone contacts and optional food provision on maintenance of weight loss. Ann Behav Med 1996;18:172–6.

70. Catenacci VA, Ogden LG, Stuht J, Phelan S, Wing RR, Hill JO, et al. Physical activity patterns in the national weight control registry. Obesity 2008;16:153–61.

71. Jakicic JM, Otto AD. Treatment and prevention of obesity: what is the role of exercise? Nutr Rev 2006;64:S57–S61.

72. McGuire MT, Wing RR, Klem ML, Seagle HM, Hill JO. Long-term maintenance of weight loss: do people who lose weight through various weight loss methods use different behaviors to maintain their weight? Int J Obes 1998;22:572–7.

73. Schoeller DA, Ravussin E, Schutz Y, Acheson KJ, Baertschi P, Jequier E. Energy expenditure by doubly labeled water: validation in humans and proposed calculation. Am J Physiol 1986;250:R823–R830.

74. Tate DF, Jeffery RW, Sherwood NE, Wing RR. Long-term weight losses associated with prescription of higher physical activity goals. Are higher levels of physical activity protective against weight regain? Am J Clin Nutr 2007;85:954–9.

75. Wadden TA, Vogt RA, Andersen RE, Bartlett SJ, Foster GD, Kuehnel RH, et al. Exercise in the treatment of obesity: effects of four interventions on body composition, resting energy expenditure, appetite, and mood. J Consult Clin Psychol 1997;65:269–77.

76. Epstein LH, Paluch RA, Gordy CC, Dorn J. Decreasing sedentary behaviors in treating pediatric obesity. Arch Pediatr Adolesc Med 2000;154:220–6.

77. Phelan S, Wadden TA. Combining behavioral and pharmacological treatments for obesity. Obes Res 2002;10:560–74.

78. Wadden TA, Berkowitz RI, Sarwer DB, Prus-Wisniewski R, Steinberg C. Benefits of lifestyle modification in the pharmacologic treatment of obesity: a randomized trial. Arch Intern Med 2001;161:218–27.

79. Craighead LW, Agras WS. Mechanisms of action in cognitive-behavioral and pharmacological interventions for obesity and bulimia nervosa. J Consult Clin Psychol 1991;59:115–25.

80. James WP, Astrup A, Finer N, Hilsted J, Kopelman P, Rossner S, et al. Effect of sibutramine on weight maintenance after weight loss: a randomised trial. STORM Study Group. Sibutramine Trial of Obesity Reduction and Maintenance. Lancet 2000;356:2119–25.

81. Sjostrom L, Rissanen A, Andersen T, Boldrin M, Golay A, Koppeschaar H, et al. Randomized placebo-controlled trial of orlistat for weight loss and prevention of weight regain in obese patients. Lancet 1998;352:167–72.

82. Davidson MH, Hauptman J, DiGirolamo M, Foreyt JP, Halsted CH, Heber D, et al. Weight control and risk factor reduction in obese subjects treated for 2 years with orlistat: a randomized controlled trial. JAMA 1999;281:235–42.

83. Tate D, Wing RR, Winett R. Development and evaluation of an Internet behavior therapy program for weight loss. JAMA 2001; 285:1172–7.

84. Tate DF, Jackvoney EH, Wing RR. Effects of internet behavioral counseling on weight loss in adults at risk for type 2 diabetes. JAMA 2003;289:1833–6.

85. Tate DF, Jackvoney EH, Wing RR. A randomized trial comparing human e-mail counseling, computer-automated tailored counseling, and no counseling in an Internet weight loss program. Arch Intern Med 2006;166:1620–5.

86. Gold BC, Burke S, Pintauro S, Buzzell P, Harvey-Berino J. Weight loss on the web: a pilot study comparing a structured behavioral intervention to a commercial program. Obesity 2007;15:155–64.

87. Tsai AG, Wadden TA. Systematic review: an evaluation of major commercial weight loss programs in the United States. Ann Intern Med 2005;142:56–67.

88. Heshka S, Anderson JW, Atkinson RL, Greenway FL, Hill JO, Phinney SD, et al. Weight loss with self-help compared with a structured commercial program: a randomized trial. JAMA 1993;289: 1792–8.

89. Rock CL, Pakiz B, Flatt SW, Quintana EL. Randomized trial of a multifaceted commercial weight loss program. Obesity 2007;15: 939–49.

90. Brownell KD, Horgen KB. Confronting the toxic environment: environmental and public health actions in a world crisis. In: Wadden TA, Stunkard AJ (eds) *Handbook of Obesity Treatment*. New York: Guilford Press, 2002: 95–106.

23 Exercise, Physical Activity and Obesity

Marleen A. van Baak

Department of Human Biology, Nutrition and Toxicology Research Institute Maastricht, Faculty of Health Sciences, Maastricht University, Maastricht, The Netherlands

Introduction

Traditionally, exercise has been recommended as an important strategy for prevention of obesity and as an effective adjunct to its treatment. Much evidence has been accumulated over the past years to strengthen this recommendation, not only with respect to weight management, but also concerning the beneficial effects of exercise on obesity-related morbidities.

More recently, the focus has shifted from exercise to increasing physical activity. Exercise refers to every planned, structured, and repetitive body movement done to improve or maintain one or more components of physical fitness. Physical activity, on the other hand, is any bodily movement produced by the skeletal muscles that results in a substantial increase in energy expenditure over the resting energy expenditure. It includes not only exercise (undertaken with the deliberate intent of improving health or physical performance) and sport, but also other types of daily activities, such as walking or cycling for transportation, occupational activities, domestic chores, leisure activities, etc. Using the term physical activity rather than exercise reflects the notion that activities of normal daily life can also contribute to the increased energy expenditure that is crucial for weight management. The term NEAT (nonexercise activity thermogenesis) has also been introduced, reflecting all energy expenditure above resting energy expenditure excluding exercise. NEAT is therefore the total energy expenditure for physical activity minus exercise [1].

Exercise, physical activity and body weight

In this section the evidence for the importance of regular exercise and high levels of physical activity for weight management, i.e.

the prevention of unhealthy weight (re)gain and the reduction of weight in obese individuals, will be reviewed.

Physical activity and weight gain

Cross-sectional population-based studies usually show a negative correlation between level of physical activity and body mass, but this cannot be taken as proof that less active people gain more weight, because a low level of physical activity may be the consequence rather than the cause of weight gain. The question of cause or consequence is better answered by prospective studies, although problems of reverse causality, measurement error, residual and unmeasured confounding do remain [2].

Reviews of prospective observational studies show no consistent association between the level of physical activity at baseline and subsequent weight gain [2–4]. In children similar mixed results are found and measures of associations are also small [2,5]. There are relatively few high-quality, controlled trials on the primary prevention of weight gain by increasing physical activity in adults [2,6] or children [2,7]. Interventions have been very diverse and often included other components than increased physical activity alone. Moreover, results are inconsistent and therefore have so far provided insufficient evidence for effective intervention programs for primary prevention of weight gain in adults or children by increased physical activity [2].

Physical inactivity and weight gain

Evidence is emerging, mainly from cross-sectional studies, that low levels of nonexercise physical activity (e.g. spontaneous intermittent standing and ambulation) may contribute to weight gain and obesity, independent of levels of leisure-time physical activity [1,8]. Inactive obese individuals spend more time sitting than inactive lean people [9]. This difference is maintained when the obese people lose weight by an energy-restricted diet and the lean people increase weight by overfeeding [9]. Sitting behavior and exercise-based leisure-time physical activity appear to be distinct classes of behavior with distinct determinants and independent risk for disease. Intervention studies, which could provide more conclusive evidence on the role of physical inactivity for weight

Clinical Obesity in Adults and Children, 3rd edition. Edited by Peter G. Kopelman, Ian D. Caterson and William H. Dietz.
© 2010 Blackwell Publishing, ISBN: 978-1-4051-8226-3.

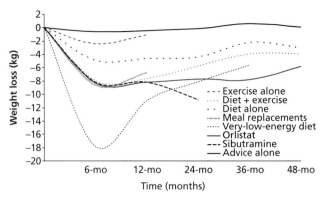

Figure 23.1 Body weight reduction in intervention studies with advice alone, exercise alone, diet alone or the combination of diet and exercise in obese subjects (adapted from Franz et al. [12]).

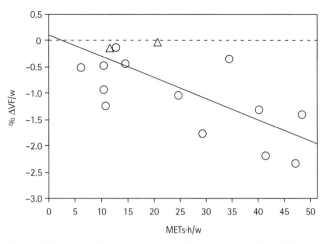

Figure 23.2 Relationship between amount of exercise, expressed as MET h/wk, and change in visceral fat (VF), expressed as percent change per week, in overweight subjects with enlarged visceral fat without concomitant metabolic disorders (adapted from Ohkawara et al.[15]).

gain and its underlying biologic mechanisms, are currently lacking [8].

Exercise and weight reduction

Intervention studies show that overweight and obese adults lose a modest amount of weight on average when they increase their physical activity by exercise. A recent Cochrane review that included randomized controlled trials of exercise in people with overweight and obesity, with a duration of at least 12 weeks and loss to follow-up of less than 15%, identified only two studies meeting these criteria and these had a total of 270 participants [10]. The weighted mean difference in weight loss between the control and exercise group was -2.03 kg (95% confidence interval (CI) -2.82, -1.23) [10]. Catenacci and Wyatt [11] identified 16 trials, some of which were nonrandomized, with over 2000 participants. In agreement with the Cochrane review, most studies showed a weight loss of between 1 and 3 kg. Another meta-analysis compared the weight loss effect of an exercise program with an advice-onlyintervention and found 1.9 ± 3.6 kg more weight loss in the exercise groups after 12 months [12] (Fig. 23.1).

Most studies on the effects of exercise in obesity have focused on body weight. However, obesity is a disease of increased fat mass, therefore the body fat-reducing effect of exercise is more important. Total abdominal fat and visceral fat are reduced by exercise, even in the absence of changes in body mass or waist circumference [13,14]. A dose dependency has been found in obese subjects without metabolic disorders, whereas there was no relationship between amount of exercise and visceral fat loss in subjects with such disorders [15] (Fig. 23.2).

Resistance exercise training has little effect on weight, but tends to increase fat-free mass and reduce fat mass [16–18].

Combined effects of exercise and dietary restriction on body weight

Exercise is almost always prescribed as an adjunct to dietary restriction in weight reduction programs. The combined effects of dietary restriction and exercise training on body weight have

been reviewed extensively [11,12,19] (see Fig. 23.1). Adding exercise training to an energy-restricted diet results in a modest extra weight loss that is small compared to the weight loss attained by the dietary treatment alone. This is to be expected, since most exercise interventions aim to increase energy expenditure by 1000–1500 kcal per week, whereas a caloric deficit of 500–1000 kcal per day is usually induced by energy-restricted diets. Addition of exercise to food restriction produces an average increase in weight loss of about 1.5 kg in overweight and obese subjects. This finding is based on 17 randomized controlled trials with durations of intervention between 4 months and 1 year [11].

Adding exercise to an energy-restricted diet may also help to preserve fat-free mass [16,20]. The meta-analysis by Garrow and Summerbell [16] indicates that for every 10 kg weight loss by diet alone, the expected loss of fat-free mass is 2.9 kg in men and 2.2 kg in women. When the same weight loss is achieved by exercise combined with dietary restriction, the expected loss of fat-free mass is reduced to 1.7 kg in men and women. Resistance exercise may result in a more effective preservation of fat-free mass during a period of energy restriction than endurance training [20,21].

Exercise and weight loss maintenance

Although exercise training results in only modest (extra) reductions of body weight when prescribed alone or in combination with dietary restriction, regular exercise is of crucial importance for successful weight loss maintenance after a period of weight reduction. Most of the evidence comes from nonrandomized weight reduction studies with an observational follow-up. People who successfully maintain weight loss are characterized by high levels of physical activity, low dietary fat and high dietary carbohydrate intake, and regular self-monitoring of weight and food intake [11,22].

A review of weight maintenance studies showed that there is currently very little evidence from randomized controlled trials to support this. When weighted mean weight changes were calculated for 11 randomized studies with an average duration of 20 months (range 12–42 months), the weight regain during follow-up amounted to 0.28 kg/month in the exercise groups and 0.33 kg/month in the control groups [3]. The reason for this relative lack of efficacy in randomized controlled trials may be that the amount of physical activity prescribed in these studies is insufficient and that the long-term adherence to the exercise programs is low.

Exercise and energy balance

In the previous section it has been shown that regular exercise reduces body weight or helps prevent weight (re)gain. It therefore creates a negative energy balance or prevents a positive energy balance. How is this accomplished? Energy expenditure and energy intake represent the two sides of the energy balance equation. Does exercise affect energy balance through effects on energy expenditure or on energy intake, or a combination of the two?

Exercise and energy expenditure

Total daily energy expenditure (24-h EE) can be divided into several components: resting metabolic rate (RMR), which accounts for approximately 60–70% of 24-h energy expenditure; diet-induced thermogenesis (DIT), approximately 10% of 24-h EE; and energy expenditure induced by physical activity or exercise, which is the most variable component and may vary from 15% of 24-h EE in sedentary people, to 30–40% in active people, to even 400% in professional cyclists under extreme circumstances. Acute exercise may affect all three components of 24-h EE. Apart from the acute effects, regular exercise or training may have additional effects. These components are discussed more fully later in this Chapter.

Energy expenditure during exercise in lean and obese individuals

Energy expenditure increases during exercise. During activities such as walking or running at a set speed energy expenditure increases with body mass. There are indications that obese individuals have an inefficient locomotor pattern and thus their energy expenditure at any set speed may be higher than predicted from their body mass [23,24].

Energy expenditure during exercise is often expressed as multiples of resting metabolic rate (METs). It should be realized that average MET values reported in tables, such as the Compendium of Physical Activities [25], are applicable under average conditions and for the average (nonobese) person. Using the MET values in such tables, the energy expenditure of nonweight-bearing activities will be overestimated and that of weight-bearing activities underestimated in obese persons [26,27].

Postexercise energy expenditure

Energy expenditure may remain elevated for up to 48 hours during recovery from acute exercise. The total magnitude of postexercise oxygen consumption (EPOC) depends on the intensity and duration of the exercise performed. Values up to 32 L (or 150 kcal) over 12 hours post exercise have been reported. Dietary restriction lowers EPOC [28]. EPOC is approximately 10% of the energy expended during exercise in overweight and obese men and women and may therefore be responsible for 10% of the weight loss induced by exercise [29].

Training and resting metabolic rate

Although lean body mass accounts for most of the variation in resting energy expenditure, considerable residual variance remains. Several studies have addressed the question of whether exercise training affects this residual variation in RMR, independent of the acute effects of exercise (EPOC) described above. The results of cross-sectional studies comparing untrained and trained individuals are inconclusive. Exercise intervention studies in lean as well as in obese men and women show mixed results with unchanged or increased RMR adjusted for fat-free mass after training. This may be related to the variation in time between the last exercise bout and the measurements of RMR in these studies [30]. Another issue is whether exercise training reduces or even prevents the fall in RMR that is associated with energy-restricted diets. The majority of studies suggest a positive effect, but the evidence is not very strong [31].

In conclusion, exercise training programs generally do not lead to an increase in RMR in lean or obese individuals. The addition of a training program during a period of dietary restriction in obese individuals, on the other hand, may reduce the decrease in RMR accompanying a negative energy balance, most probably through a more favorable ratio between fat mass and fat-free mass loss.

Diet-induced thermogenesis

There is considerable inconsistency regarding the acute effects of exercise and of exercise training on the thermic effect of a meal. Apart from the difficulty of measuring DIT, these inconsistencies may be related to meal size and composition, the timing of the meal and exercise, the intensity and duration of the exercise, and differences in the characteristics of the subjects [32]. The effects of exercise on DIT are likely to be small and will therefore not contribute importantly to exercise-induced changes in energy balance.

24-h energy expenditure

As discussed in the preceding paragraphs, exercise increases energy expenditure during the exercise bout itself and may elevate postexercise energy expenditure. Effects on RMR and DIT, if any, are small. However, from this it cannot automatically be concluded that exercise also elevates 24-h EE, since it is possible that nonexercise physical activity changes because of an exercise bout or training, either in a positive or in a negative direction.

Studies which have measured 24h-EE under free-living conditions with the doubly labeled water technique show that 24h-EE is usually higher during than before endurance training, although the change is not always statistically significant [33,34]. The increase is often greater than expected from the training-related energy expenditure, thus suggesting increased nonexercise energy expenditure [34]. Studies in overweight and obese children and adults show similar trends [35,36].

Exercise and energy intake

The effects of acute and regular exercise on the energy intake side of the energy balance equation have been less extensively studied, probably because of the difficulties associated with the accurate measurement of energy intake.

Blundell and King [37] postulate that no tight coupling between increased energy expenditure by exercise and energy intake exists resulting in weight loss initially. However, a new balance between energy expenditure and energy intake is attained gradually by a combination of behavioral and physiologic adaptations, thus stabilizing body weight (Fig. 23.3). Lean subjects compensate for the energy expended during exercise more readily than obese subjects and body weight reduction with exercise training is therefore more pronounced in obese than in lean persons. However, the variability is large. One of the factors responsible for this variability may be the degree of dietary restraint or disinhibition [38]. Moreover, women tend to adapt energy intake more readily to increases in energy expenditure due to exercise than do men [37].

Another factor that appears to have significant influence is the composition of the diet. Several studies show that larger compensation and even overcompensation of the exercise-induced increase in energy expenditure takes place on a high-fat diet compared to a high-carbohydrate diet [39–41]. These observations are in agreement with the notion that carbohydrate balance is tightly regulated and that replenishment of the carbohydrate stores after exercise requires a larger energy intake on a high-fat than on a high-carbohydrate diet [42]. This finding underlines the importance of being on a relatively low-fat diet during weight loss and weight maintenance.

The classic study by Mayer et al. [43] in male employees of a jute mill in West Bengal, India, who had a wide range of physical activity during work, showed that energy intake was more tightly coupled to the energy demand of the job above the level described as "light work" (Fig. 23.4). In sedentary employees food intake increased inappropriately, resulting in increased body mass. Although this study has major shortcomings in design and analysis, the general conclusion is supported by animal research [44]. Using Mayer's idea that it is harder to maintain energy balance at low levels of physical activity, Hill and Wyatt [45] hypothesized that current levels of physical activity in a large proportion of the

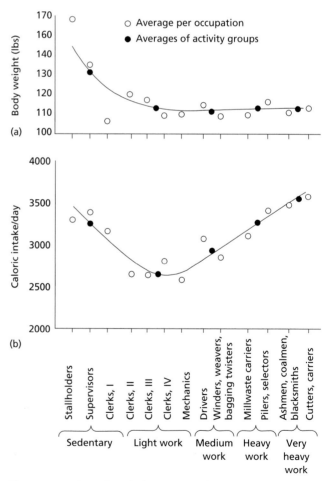

Figure 23.4 Body weight and caloric intake as a function of level of physical activity at work, in an industrial male population in West Bengal (from Mayer et al. [43]).

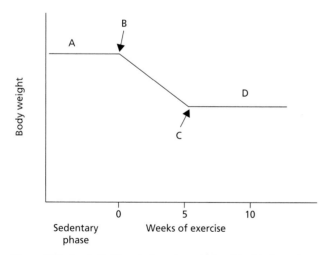

Figure 23.3 Hypothetical impact of exercise on body weight. A indicates the initial steady state, B represents the start of exercise, B to C represents the adjustment period when a higher energy expenditure is not compensated by energy intake; C represents the time at which new forces (behavioral and metabolic) interact to induce a new steady state (D) (from Blundell and King [37]).

population are so low that maintenance of energy balance is impossible without increases in energy balance, thus emphasizing the importance of increasing physical activity for weight control.

Exercise and substrate utilization

Any intervention aimed at inducing weight loss in overweight persons should promote a negative fat balance. Exercise increases energy expenditure and substrate oxidation in skeletal muscles. Fatty acids are an important energy source for the exercising muscles. Moreover, due to depletion of glycogen stores during exercise, fat oxidation is favored following exercise. These combined effects result in increased fat oxidation. Exercise therefore allows fat oxidation to be in balance with fat intake at a lower body fat content [42].

Substrate utilization during exercise

During the first minutes of submaximal aerobic exercise muscle glycogen breakdown is the main source of energy. As exercise continues, blood-borne substrates (glucose and nonesterified fatty acids (NEFA)) become more important. At moderate exercise intensity (65% VO$_2$max) utilization of fatty acids increases and that of carbohydrates decreases with time [46] (Fig. 23.5), which is reflected in a gradual decrease of the respiratory quotient during prolonged exercise at this intensity. During the first hour intramuscular and plasma triglycerides and circulating fatty acids contribute equally to the overall fat oxidation. Thereafter, the reliance on plasma free fatty acids increases progressively with time.

The composition of the substrate mix utilized during exercise depends not only on duration but also on the intensity of exercise. At very low exercise intensity (25% VO$_2$max, comparable to walking) NEFA are the main energy source. As intensity increases, the absolute contribution of plasma glucose and muscle glycogen increases, and that of plasma NEFA decreases [46] (Fig. 23.6). The percentage of VO$_2$max at which absolute fat oxidation (in g/min) is maximal varies between 40 and 63% VO$_2$max across studies, with large interindividual variation within studies. Other factors that influence the substrate mix utilized during exercise are diet, gender and training status (VO$_2$max) [47,48]. The majority of studies report values between 40% and 50% of VO$_2$max for maximal fat oxidation [48–50].

Children show a relatively high contribution of lipid oxidation to energy expenditure during exercise when compared to adults [51].

Substrate utilization during exercise in obesity

Few studies have compared substrate oxidation during exercise in lean and overweight adolescents and adults and results obtained have been equivocal [52–56]. Similar disparities are found with respect to differences in substrate oxidation between lean and obese individuals at rest [57].

A more consistent finding is that the contribution of nonplasma free fatty acids (either from intramuscular or from lipoprotein-derived triglycerides) to total fat oxidation is higher

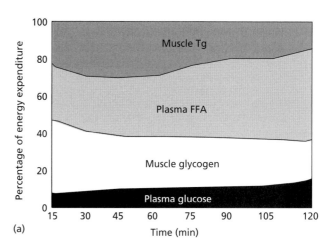

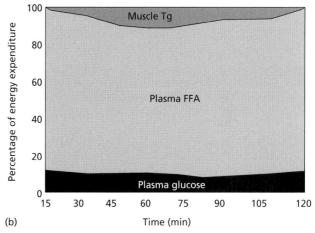

Figure 23.5 Contribution of intramuscular and blood-borne substrates to fuel utilization during prolonged exercise at 65% (a) and 25% (b) VO$_2$max in endurance-trained men (from Romijn et al. [46]).

in obese than in lean individuals [54,55]. In obese adolescents the highest fat oxidation rate is found at approximately 40% of VO$_2$max, which falls into the lower range of values reported for nonobese adults (see above) [56,58].

Acute exercise and 24-h substrate utilization

In the period after a bout of aerobic or resistance exercise, fat oxidation is increased, which allows replenishment of the reduced glycogen stores. Exercise bouts of different intensity, but similar total energy expenditure, have comparable effects on postexercise lipid oxidation [59]. Exercise also has the ability to alter the postexercise partitioning of dietary fat between oxidation and storage towards increased oxidation of fatty acids [60].

To establish the optimal exercise intensity for maximum total fat oxidation, the effects on 24-h fat oxidation need to be studied. Data on this topic are relatively scarce. Exercise, either aerobic or resistance, performed during a 24-h stay in a respiration chamber increased 24-h EE and carbohydrate oxidation, but had no effect on 24-h fat oxidation in lean subjects [61,62]. There was no

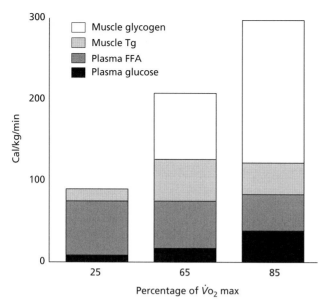

Figure 23.6 Contribution of glucose and free fatty acids (FFA) taken up from blood, from triglycerides in the plasma or stored in the muscle, and from glycogen stored in the muscle to energy expenditure after 30 min of exercise, expressed as function of exercise intensity (from Romijn et al. [46]).

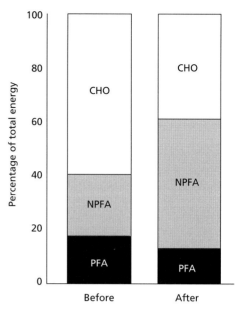

Figure 23.7 Percentage of total energy derived from carbohydrate (CHO), nonplasma fatty acid (FA) and plasma FA fuel sources during prolonged exercise at 63% VO$_2$max before and after 12 weeks of endurance training (from Martin et al. [67]).

difference between aerobic exercise performed at 40% or 70% of VO$_2$max with the same total energy expenditure (400 kcal) [61]. Similar results were obtained for obese men [63]. On the other hand, 24-h fat oxidation during the first days after switching from a low-fat to a high-fat diet is increased by exercise [64,65]. Thus, day-to-day variations in fat intake are less likely to result in a positive fat balance in active individuals.

Exercise training and substrate utilization during exercise

Training, even at exercise intensities as low as 40% of VO$_2$max, reduces utilization of both muscle glycogen and blood glucose during exercise at any given absolute submaximal exercise intensity. This training-induced reduction in carbohydrate oxidation during exercise is compensated for by an increase in fat oxidation. Studies indicate that the main source of this increased fat oxidation may not be adipose tissue lipolysis, but rather intramuscular triglyceride stores [47,66–68] (Fig. 23.7).

Exercise training and substrate utilization in obesity

Data on the effects of exercise training on substrate utilization in the obese are rather scarce. Moderate-intensity exercise training at 70% VO$_2$max enhances whole-body fat utilization under fasting conditions [69] and increases palmitate oxidation in mitochondria isolated from the skeletal muscle of obese persons [70]. Other studies have shown that the combination of weight loss and exercise training increases whole-body fat oxidation in obese individuals, but without an increase in mitochondrial density [54,71], which is the normal adaptive response to this type of exercise training. Instead, the surface area of the inner

mitochondrial membrane was increased by the exercise training [72]. As in lean individuals, exercise training increases fat oxidation during exercise in obese men and women, although the effect may depend on training intensity and fat distribution (as shown in a series of studies by van Aggel-Leijssen and co-workers [73,74]). Low-intensity training also prevented the reduction in fat oxidation induced by weight loss with an energy-restricted diet [75]. Thus, exercise training is able to increase the capacity for fat oxidation in obese individuals although the adaptations responsible for the increased fat oxidation may differ between lean and obese. The optimal training intensity to produce this effect under different conditions and the role of obesity phenotype remain to be established.

Exercise and obesity-related morbidity and mortality

Obesity has been associated with an increased premature mortality and increased risk for chronic diseases, such as type 2 diabetes mellitus, cardiovascular disease associated with dyslipidemia and hypertension, osteo-arthritis and sleep apnea [76]. Regular exercise is known to have beneficial effects on most of these risks.

Insulin resistance and type 2 diabetes mellitus

Insulin resistance is an important feature in the development of glucose intolerance and type 2 diabetes mellitus. An acute exercise bout increases postexercise insulin sensitivity, an effect that is maintained for 48–72 hours. Insulin sensitivity is increased in those skeletal muscles that have been active during the exercise bout. The lowered glycogen content of these muscles after exercise probably plays an important role in determining the insulin response of glucose transport and glycogen synthesis. Incoming glucose is mainly directed to glycogen synthesis and incoming fatty acids to oxidation, and this explains the increased fat oxidation reported after exercise.

Exercise training improves skeletal muscle insulin sensitivity of glucose transport in both insulin-sensitive and insulin-resistant adults with obesity. This is associated with increased expression of GLUT4 and insulin receptor substrate-1 in insulin-resistant muscle [77]. A growing body of evidence suggests that participation in a structured aerobic exercise program also improves insulin sensitivity in overweight youth, even in the absence of changes in body weight [78]. Exercise training also improves glycemic control, even in the absence of weight loss, in patients with type 2 diabetes [79].

The only trial published so far on the effects of exercise training alone on the prevention of type 2 diabetes in high-risk individuals with impaired glucose tolerance, the Da Qing IGT and Diabetes Study, has shown a reduction of the incidence of type 2 diabetes by the exercise intervention [80]. Studies that investigated the role of increased physical activity in the context of a lifestyle intervention that also included weight loss and dietary changes have also reported a reduced risk of type 2 diabetes in subjects with impaired glucose tolerance (IGT) [81,82]. In the Finnish Diabetes Prevention Study an increase in physical activity, as strenuous structured exercise, walking for exercise or lifestyle physical activity, was associated with a reduced incidence of type 2 diabetes, independent of any changes in Body Mass Index (BMI) [83] (Table 23.1).

Thus, regular exercise can reduce insulin resistance and improve glucose tolerance in obesity and type 2 diabetes, and reduce the risk of type 2 diabetes in high-risk populations, even in the absence of changes in weight and/or body composition.

Blood lipids

Exercise training has consistently been shown to increase HDL-cholesterol levels. Reductions in total cholesterol, LDL-cholesterol and triglycerides may also occur with training [84]. Baseline levels of BMI and exercise-induced body weight changes did not modify exercise-induced changes in lipids. However, concurrent diet-induced weight loss potentiates the reductions in LDL-cholesterol, total cholesterol and triglycerides and exercise training may attenuate the HDL reduction with low-fat diets [84].

In sedentary overweight or mildly obese subjects with dyslipidemia, regular exercise improves overall lipoprotein profile [85]. High-amount/high-intensity exercise had significantly more beneficial effects on plasma lipoproteins than low-amount/high intensity or low-amount/low intensity exercise. The beneficial effects on HDL are sustained up to 2 weeks after exercise cessation, but the effects on VLDL and LDL appear to be relatively short-lived [86]. Aerobic exercise training has also been shown

Table 23.1 Relative risk of developing type 2 diabetes during the trial period according to tertiles of change in leisure-time physical activity (LTPA) in the Finnish Diabetes Prevention Program[83]

	Model 1	Model 2	Model 3
Change in total LTPA			
−3.2 (−35 to −0.5)	1	1	1
0.5 (−0.5 to 1.7)	0.47 (0.28–0.79)	0.48 (0.28–0.82)	0.52 (0.31–0.89)
3.8 (1.8–19)	0.26 (0.15–0.47)	0.29 (0.16–0.53)	0.34 (0.19–0.62)
p for trend	<0.001	<0.001	<0.001
Change in moderate-to-vigorous LTPA (≥3.5 METs)			
−1.5 (−13.5 to −0.1)	1	1	1
0.5 (−0.1 to 1.3)	0.78 (0.46–1.33)	0.86 (0.49–1.48)	0.95 (0.54–1.65)
2.6 (1.3–14.4)	0.35 (0.18–0.65)	0.40 (0.21–0.76)	0.51 (0.26–0.97)
p for trend	0.001	0.004	0.037
Change in low-intensity LTPA (<3.5 METs)			
−3.2 (−34 to −1.0)	1	1	1
0.1 (−0.9 to 1.1)	0.83 (0.47–1.45)	0.85 (0.47–1.53)	0.63 (0.34–1.17)
3.1 (1.1–15.0)	0.38 (0.20–0.70)	0.41 (0.22–0.77)	0.36 (0.19–0.67)
p for trend	0.001	0.003	0.001

Data are relative risk (95% CI). LTPA in hours/week. Model 2: adjusted variables in model 1 plus baseline values and changes in dietary intake, total fat, saturated fat, and fiber. Model 3: adjusted for variables in model 2 and baseline values plus changes in BMI.

to reduce plasma triglyceride and tends to increase HDL-cholesterol in obese or overweight children [87].

Blood pressure

A meta-analysis on blood pressure changes associated with endurance exercise training including 72 randomized controlled trials with 3936 participants and showed average systolic and diastolic blood pressure reductions of 3.0 and 2.4 mmHg respectively [88]. Intervention studies in children show similar effects [89]. The reductions were more pronounced in hypertensive subjects (6.9 and 4.9 mmHg) than in the normotensive group (1.9 and 1.6 mmHg). No clear relationships between the blood pressure response and characteristics of the exercise programs (exercise intensity, duration, frequency) were found. The blood pressure-reducing effect of endurance exercise was independent of initial body mass and percent body fat or changes in body weight and composition [88].

Resistance exercise training (12 study groups with 341 participants) caused a significant change in diastolic blood pressure of 3.5 mmHg, and a nonsignificant change in systolic blood pressure of 3.2 mmHg. Most resistance training programs involved dynamic resistance training with variable resistances, numbers of repetitions and number of sets. There was no indication that resistance exercise increased blood pressure [90].

When comparing the effects of a combined intervention including dietary energy restriction and exercise training with the

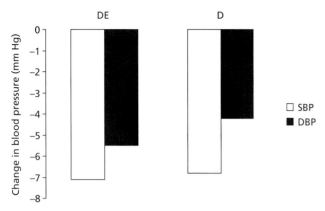

Figure 23.8 Blood pressure reduction in intervention studies with diet alone (D) or a combination of diet plus exercise (DE) in overweight and obese subjects (based on Fagard [91]). SBP, systolic blood pressure; DBP, diastolic blood pressure.

effect of diet alone in 10 randomized trials on blood pressure in overweight subjects, no additional reduction of blood pressure was found over that in exercise trials alone [91] (Fig. 23.8).

Mental health and health-related well-being

It is not fully clear whether obesity is associated with psychopathology or emotional distress in the general population. However, obese patients seeking weight loss treatment often show emotional disturbances, such as depression, binge-eating disorder and disturbed body image [76].

Exercise helps to improve mental health in individuals reporting mood disturbances, including symptoms of anxiety and depression, and in patients with diagnosed depression [92,93]. There are few data to confirm whether this is also the case in obesity. An observational study suggests that higher levels of physical activity and increases in physical activity are associated with improvements in depression and well-being in obese individuals [94]. A randomized study found no effect of exercise training on psychologic well-being or mood states in obese women in the absence of weight loss. Weight loss induced by a combination of diet and exercise significantly improved well-being [95].

Aerobic fitness

Obese individuals have lower aerobic fitness than lean individuals, when fitness is expressed as VO_2max per kg body weight. When VO_2max is adjusted for fat-free mass the difference between lean and obese usually disappears. However, the oxygen consumption during exercise at a submaximal load, such as walking at a certain speed, is higher in obese than in lean when expressed as % VO_2max, thus representing a higher physical stress [96]. Improving aerobic fitness in the obese will therefore have beneficial effects on the physical stress of daily activities.

Regular exercise increases aerobic fitness in lean [92] and obese individuals, independent of changes in body weight [73,74] and

there are no indications that the fitness response to exercise training is modified by increasing adiposity.

Mortality

Although some controversy exists over whether fatness is an independent predictor of mortality, epidemiologic studies quite consistently show that, within each BMI or adiposity category, men and women with a higher aerobic fitness or higher level of physical activity have a lower all-cause mortality risk [97–102].

Exercise recommendations for weight management

Exercise will prevent weight gain, improve weight loss maintenance, reduce the risk of chronic diseases such as type 2 diabetes and cardiovascular diseases, improve mental health and well-being, increase fitness and reduce the risk of premature mortality. Physicians and other healthcare professionals should therefore counsel obese patients to engage in regular exercise as part of their routine practice.

Specific exercise recommendations for weight control have emerged since the 1990s. In 1998 the National Institutes of Health recommended that all adults should set a long-term goal to accumulate at least 30 minutes, or more, of moderate-intensity physical activity on most and preferably all days of the week for weight management. The World Health Organization also adopted this recommendation. However, this recommendation for optimal weight management has been questioned. The amount of physical activity required for weight gain prevention is likely to be higher than this recommended amount [4,26]. It is estimated that 45–60 minutes of moderate-intensity exercise per day are necessary to prevent the transition from overweight to obesity, and 60–90 minutes of moderate-intensity exercise daily (or lesser amounts of more vigorous activity) to prevent weight regain after weight reduction in the obese [26]. In agreement with this, approximately 60 minutes of moderate- to vigorous-intensity activity on most days of the week (while not exceeding caloric intake requirements) are now recommended to help manage body weight and prevent gradual, unhealthy body weight gain in adulthood [103,104].

Currently there is no evidence that exercise intensity has an effect on weight reduction or weight maintenance independent of its contribution to total energy expenditure. However, more vigorous exercise will allow the individual to attain a preset energy expenditure in a shorter time. Two caveats are important: more vigorous exercise is associated with a higher injury risk [104] and it may lead to higher drop-out rates from the program. A careful balance between time restraints and attainment of a sufficiently high total energy expenditure therefore needs to be sought for each individual. The importance of improving aerobic fitness needs to be stressed because this will enable the obese individual to perform a higher workload with less physical stress.

A significant dose–response relationship between amount of exercise, expressed as energy expenditure per week, and body weight reduction has been demonstrated [13]. Suggestions for a dose–response relationship with the total amount of exercise have also been found for several other health parameters [105]. Although the effects of exercise on body weight are related to total energy expenditure rather than exercise intensity, exercise intensity may be important for other health effects of exercise. For instance, it is well known that a minimal exercise intensity is required to improve cardiovascular fitness and that a relationship exists between change in VO$_2$max and exercise intensity. Whether this is also the case for other health effects of exercise is unclear. There is no clear relationship between the blood pressure-lowering effects of exercise and the characteristics of the exercise program [88]. No independent effect of exercise intensity has been found with respect to alterations in the lipoprotein profile [85] but exercise intensity appears to be inversely associated with risk of coronary heart disease, independent of total amount of exercise [106,107]. With respect to insulin resistance, an independent role for exercise intensity cannot be excluded [108].

Thus the question "Which type of exercise training is optimal for the obese patient?" probably does not have one single answer. It depends on the ultimate goal(s) of the training program: is it body weight reduction, fat mass reduction, increased fat oxidation, risk factor reduction or improvement of general fitness, psychologic well-being and health? How fast does one want to attain a certain goal? And interindividual differences in responsiveness to training programs are also likely and complicate the delineation of the program to prescribe. We are only just beginning to see interactions between genotype and the response to exercise training [109–112].

Exercise mode

Dynamic aerobic exercise is usually recommended to improve cardiorespiratory fitness and health and in weight control programs. To attain the high levels of energy expenditure which are important for weight management, activities that employ a large muscle mass are preferred. For the obese especially, nonweight-bearing activities such as swimming or cycling may be appropriate. Addition of dynamic forms of resistance exercise training, although not contributing to body weight loss, may help to enhance muscle mass and muscular strength [113]. Lifestyle approaches to physical activity are often more easily accommodated in the routine of everyday life and the long-term efficacy for weight control and cardiovascular risk reduction is comparable to that of structured exercise programs [114,115].

Exercise prescription

Prescriptions of frequency and duration of exercise sessions are simple and straightforward. The more difficult aspect of exercise prescription is defining and monitoring the intensity of exercise. The intensity of exercise can be prescribed as an absolute intensity (VO$_2$ or MET) or a relative intensity, such as a percentage of the maximal oxygen uptake (% VO$_2$max) or maximal heart rate (% HRmax).

One MET, or metabolic equivalent, represents an individual's energy expenditure while sitting quietly (~3.5 mL O$_2$/kg/min). MET values of selected activities and their classification as light, moderate or vigorous intensity activities are given in Table 23.2. Relative intensities can be classified as shown in Table 23.3.

Since VO$_2$max is difficult to measure in nonlaboratory exercise settings, prescription of exercise intensity is usually based on heart rate (as percentage of measured, but usually estimated, maximal heart rate (% HRmax) or heart rate reserve (% HRR) (= maximal heart rate – resting heart rate) or subjective feelings of exertion (RPE, rating of perceived exertion). This is based on the linear relationship between % HRmax or % HRR and RPE, on one hand, and % VO$_2$max on the other. The relation between % HRmax or % HRR and % VO$_2$max has been found to be similar in lean and obese adults [116]. In normally fit individuals, the classification of activities according to absolute (MET) and relative (% VO$_2$max) intensity categories will be comparable, but in very unfit or very fit individuals they will no longer overlap.

Current recommendations on exercise intensity are usually based on the absolute classification of physical activity intensities, although much of the underlying evidence for these recommendations is derived from exercise training studies using relative training intensities.

Exercise adherence

Drop-out rates from exercise programs are relatively high and the degree of overweight is one of the most consistent predictors of drop-out from an exercise program [117,118]. Unsupervised programs with vigorous-intensity exercise have lower adherence rates [118,119].

Cognitive factors regarding exercise are of critical importance for the success of exercise in weight management. Analysis of prevailing cognitive rules and schemas and, if necessary, intervention should be components of exercise prescription [120].

Little is known about the determinants of adherence to increased physical activity in overweight and obese individuals. Multiple 10-minute exercise bouts per day instead of a single long daily exercise bout, and home exercise, may be associated with better long-term exercise adherence [121,122]. However, further studies in this area are clearly needed.

Exercise risk

Apart from the benefits, exercise may also have risks. The most serious but relatively infrequent risk is that of sudden cardiac death, usually due to underlying atherosclerotic coronary artery disease. Exercise also transiently increases the risk of acute myocardial infarction. The relative risk of both exercise-related myocardial infarction and sudden death is greatest in individuals who are the least physically active and perform unaccustomed vigorous exercise. Sedentary individuals should avoid isolated bouts of vigorous exercise and gradually increase physical activity levels over time [123].

Table 23.2 Energy cost of various physical activities expressed as METs (ratio of work metabolic rate to resting metabolic rate)[104]

Light <3.0 METs	Moderate 3.0–6.0 METs	Vigorous >6.0 METs
Walking, jogging & running Walking slowly around home, store or office = 2.0*	*Walking, jogging & running* Walking 3.0 mph (4.8 km/h) = 3.3* Walking at very brisk pace (4 mph, 6.4 km/h) = 5.0*	*Walking, jogging & running* Walking at very very brisk pace (4.5 mph, 7.2 km/h) = 6.3* Walking/hiking at moderate pace and grade with no or light pack (<10 lb, 4.5 kg) = 7.0 Hiking at steep grades and pack 10–42 lb, 4.5–19 kg = 7.5–9.0 Jogging at 5 mph (8 km/h) = 8.0* Jogging at 6 mph (9.7 km/h) = 10.0* Running at 7 mph (11.3 km/h) = 11.5*
Household & occupation Sitting – using computer, work at desk using light hand tools = 1.5 Standing, performing light work such as making bed, washing dishes, ironing, preparing food or store clerk = 2.0–2.5	*Household & occupation* Cleaning – heavy: washing windows, car, clean garage = 3.0 Sweeping floors or carpet, vacuuming, mopping = 3.0–3.5 Carpentry – general = 3.6 Carrying & stacking wood = 5.5 Mowing lawn – walk power mower = 5.5	*Household & occupation* Shoveling sand, coal, etc. = 7.0 Carrying heavy loads such as bricks = 7.5 Heavy farming such as bailing hay = 8.0 Shoveling, digging ditches = 8.5
Leisure time & sports Arts & crafts, playing cards = 1.5 Billiards = 2.5 Boating – power = 2.5 Croquet = 2.5 Darts = 2.5 Fishing – sitting = 2.5 Playing (most) musical instruments = 2.0–2.5	*Leisure time & sports* Badminton – recreational = 4.5 Basketball – shooting around = 4.5 Bicycling – on flat: light effort (10–12 mph, 15–18 km/h) = 6.0 Dancing – ballroom, slow = 3.0 Dancing – ballroom, fast = 4.5 Fishing from river bank & walking = 4.0 Golf – walking pulling clubs = 4.3 Sailing boat, wind surfing = 3.0 Swimming leisurely = 6.0# Table tennis = 4.0 Tennis doubles = 5.0 Volleyball – noncompetitive = 3.0–4.0	*Leisure time & sports* Basketball game = 8.0 Bicycling – on flat: moderate effort (12–14 mph, 18–21 km/h) = 8.0 Bicycling – fast (14–16 mph, 21–24 km/h) = 10 Skiing cross country – slow (2.5 mph, 3.8 km/h) = 7.0 Skiing cross country – fast (5.0–7.9 mph, 7.5–12 km/h) = 9.0 Soccer – casual = 7.0 Soccer – competitive = 10.0 Swimming – moderate/hard = 8–11# Tennis singles = 8.0 Volleyball – competitive at gym or beach = 8.0

*On flat, hard surface. #MET values can vary substantially from person to person during swimming as a result of different strokes and skill levels.

Table 23.3 Classification of relative intensity of exercise based on 20–60 minutes of endurance training (adapted from American College of Sports Medicine [124])

% HRmax	% VO2max or % HRR	RPE	Intensity classification
<35	<30	<10	Very light
35–59	30–49	10–11	Light
60–79	50–74	12–13	Moderate (somewhat hard)
80–89	75–84	14–16	Heavy
≥90	≥85	>16	Very heavy

VO2max, maximal oxygen uptake; HRR, heart rate reserve (maximal heart rate – resting heart rate); HRmax, maximal heart rate; RPE, rating of perceived exertion (20-point Borg scale).

Although less serious, the risk of falls and musculoskeletal injuries is much larger. Risk of injury increases with obesity, volume of exercise and participation in vigorous exercise, whereas higher fitness and gradual increases in volume over time are associated with reduced injury risk [123].

In the context of risk reduction, obese (and other) individuals with known or suspected cardiovascular, respiratory, metabolic, orthopedic or neurologic disorders should be advised to consult their physician before beginning or significantly increasing physical activity, especially when activities with a vigorous intensity are chosen.

References

1. Levine JA. Nonexercise activity thermogenesis – liberating the life-force. Int J Med 2007;262:273–87.

2. Wareham NJ, van Sluijs EMF, Ekelund U. Physical activity and obesity prevention: a review of the current evidence. Proc Nutr Soc 2005;64:229–47.

3. Fogelholm M, Kukkonen-Harjula K. Does physical activity prevent weight gain – a systematic review. Obes Rev 2000;1:95–112.

4. Erlichman J, Kerbey AL, James W. Physical activity and its impact on health outcomes. Paper 2: prevention of unhealthy weight gain and obesity by physical activity: an analysis of the evidence. Obes Rev 2000;3:273–88.

5. Molnar D, Livingstone B. Physical activity in relation to overweight and obesity in children and adolescents. Eur J Pediatr 2000;159(suppl. 1):S45–S55.

6. Hardeman W, Griffin S, Johnston M, Kimmonth A, Wareham NJ. Interventions to prevent weight gain: a systematic review of psychological models and behaviour change methods. Int J Obes 2000;24:131–43.

7. Campbell K, Waters E, O'Meara S, Summerbell C. Interventions for preventing obesity in childhood. A systematic review. Obes Rev 2001;2:149–57.

8. Hamilton MT, Hamilton DG, Zderic TW. Role of low energy expenditure and sitting in obesity, metabolic syndrome, type 2 diabetes, and cardiovascular disease. Diabetes 2007;56:2655–67.

9. Levine JA, Lanningham-Foster LM, McCrady SK, et al. Interindividual variation in posture allocation: possible role in human obesity. Science 2005;307:584–6.

10. Shaw K, Gennat H, O'Rourke P, del Mar C. Exercise for overweight or obesity. Cochrane Database of Systematic Reviews, 2006, issue 4, art.no. CD003817.

11. Catenacci VA, Wyatt HR. The role of physical activity in producing and maintaining weight loss. Nature Clin Pract Endocrinol Metabol 2007;3:518–29.

12. Franz MJ, VanWormer JJ, Crain L, et al. Weight-loss outcomes: a systematic review and meta-analysis of weight-loss clinical trials with a minimum 1-year follow-up. J Am Dietet Assoc 2007;107:1755–67.

13. Ross R, Janssen I. Physical activity, total and regional obesity: dose-response considerations. Med Sci Sports Exerc 2001;33(suppl):S521–S527.

14. Kay SJ, Fiatarone Singh MA. The influence of physical activity on abdominal fat: a systematic review of the literature. Obes Rev 2006;7:183–200.

15. Ohkawara K, Tanaka S, Miyachi M, et al. A dose-response relations between aerobic exercise and visceral fat reduction: systematic review of clinical trials. Int J Obes 2007;31:1786–97.

16. Garrow JS, Summerbell CD. Meta-analysis: effect of exercise, with or without dieting, on the body composition of overweight subjects. Eur J Clin Nutr 1995;49:1–10.

17. Hunter GR, Wetzstein CJ, Fields DA, et al. Resistance training increases total energy expenditure and free-living physical activity in older adults. J Appl Physiol 2000;89:977–84.

18. Poehlman ET, Denino WF, Beckett T, et al. Effects of endurance and resistance training on total daily energy expenditure in young women: a controlled randomised trial. J Clin Endocrinol Metab 2002;87:1004–9.

19. Miller WC, Koceja DM, Hamilton EJ. A meta-analysis of the past 25 years of weight loss research using diet, exercise or diet plus exercise intervention. Int J Obes 1997;21:941–7.

20. Hansen D, Dendale P, Berger J, van Loon LJC, Meeusen R. The effect of exercise training on fat-mass loss in obese patients during energy intake restriction. Sports Med 2007;37:1–16.

21. Ballor DL, Harvey-Berino JR, Ades PA, Cryan J, Calles-Escandon J. Contrasting effect of resistance and aerobic training on body composition and metabolism after diet-induced weight loss. Metabolism 1996;45:179–83.

22. Wing RR, Hill JO. Successful weight loss maintenance. Annu Rev Nutr 2001;21:323–41.

23. Foster GD, Wadden TA, Kendrick ZV, et al. The energy cost of walking before and after significant weight loss. Med Sci Sports Exerc 1995;27:888–94.

24. Rosenbaum M, Vandenborne K, Goldsmith R, et al. Effects of experimental weight perturbation on skeletal muscle work efficiency in human subjects. Am J Physiol 2003;285:R183–R192.

25. Ainsworth BE, Haskell WL, Whitt MC, et al. Compendium of Physical Activities: an update of activity codes and MET intensities. Med Sci Sports Exerc 2000;32(suppl):S498–S504.

26. Saris WHM, Blair SN, van Baak MA, et al. How much physical activity is enough to prevent unhealthy weight gain? Outcome of the IASO 1st Stock Conference and consensus statement. Obes Rev 2003;4:101–14.

27. Spadano JL, Must A, Bandini LG, et al. Energy cost of physical activities in 12-y-old girls: MET values and the influence of body weight. Int J Obes 2003;27:1528–33.

28. Fukuba Y, Yano Y, Murakami H, Kan A, Miura A. The effect of dietary restriction and menstrual cycle on excess post-exercise oxygen consumption (EPOC) in young women. Clin Physiol 2000;20:165–9.

29. LeCheminant JD, Jacobsen DJ, Bailey BW, et al. Effects of long-term aerobic exercise on EPOC. Int J Sports Med 2007;29:53–8.

30. Speakman JR, Selman C. Physical activity and resting metabolic rate. Proc Nutr Soc 2003;62:621–34.

31. Prentice AM, Goldberg GR, Jebb SA, et al. Physiological responses to slimming. Proc Nutr Soc 1991;50, 441–58.

32. Segal KR. Exercise and thermogenesis in obesity. Int J Obes 1995;19(suppl 4):S80–S87.

33. Toth MJ, Poehlman ET. Effects of exercise on daily energy expenditure. Nutr Rev 1996;54:S140–S148.

34. Westerterp KR. Alterations in energy balance with exercise. Am J Clin Nutr 1998;68(suppl):970S–974S.

35. Blaak EE, Westerterp KR, Bar-Or O, et al. Effect of training on total energy expenditure and spontaneous activity in obese boys. Am J Clin Nutr 1992;55:777–82.

36. Donnelly JE, Hill JO, Jacobson DJ, et al. Effects of a 16-month randomised controlled exercise trial on body weight and composition in young, overweight men and women. Arch Intern Med 2003;163:1343–50.

37. Blundell JE, King NA. Exercise, appetite control, and energy balance. Nutrition 2000;16:519–22.

38. Keim NL, Barbieri TF, Belko AZ. The effect of exercise on energy intake and body composition in overweight women. Int J Obes 1990;14:335–46.

39. Tremblay A, Alméras N, Boer J, et al. Diet composition and postexercise energy balance. Am J Clin Nutr 1994;59:975–9.

40. King NA, Blundell JE. High-fat foods overcome the energy expenditure due to exercise after cycling and running. Eur J Clin Nutr 1995;49:114–23.

41. King NA, Snell L, Smith RD, Blundell JE. Effects of short-term exercise on appetite responses in unrestrained females. Eur J Clin Nutr 1996;50:663–7.

42. Flatt J. Integration of the overall response to exercise. Int J Obes 1995;19(suppl 4):S31–S40.

43. Mayer J, Roy P, Mitra KP. Relation between caloric intake, body weight, and physical work: studies in an industrial male population in West Bengal. Am J Clin Nutr 1956;4:169–75.

44. Oscai LB. The role of exercise in weight control. Exerc Sport Sci Rev 1973;1:103–23.

45. Hill JO, Wyatt HR. Role of physical activity in preventing and treating obesity. J Appl Physiol 2005;99:765–70.

46. Romijn JA, Coyle EF, Sidossis LS, et al. Regulation of endogenous fat and carbohydrate metabolism in relation to exercise intensity and duration. Am J Physiol 1993;265:E380–E391.

47. Coyle EF. Substrate utilization during exercise in active people. Am J Clin Nutr 1995;61(suppl):968S–979S.

48. Venables MC, Achten J, Jeukendrup AE. Determinants of fat oxidation during exercise in healthy men and women: a cross-sectional study. J Appl Physiol 2005;98:160–7.

49. Achten J, Jeukendrup AE. Maximal fat oxidation during exercise in trained men. Int J Sports Med 2003;24, 603–608.

50. Stisen AB, Stougaard O, Langfort J, et al. Maximal fat oxidation rates in trained and untrained women. Eur J Appl Physiol 2006;98:497–506.

51. Aucouturier J, Baker JS, Duché P. Fat and carbohydrate metabolism during submaximal exercise in children. Sports Med 2008;38: 213–38.

52. Kanaley JA, Weatherup-Dentes MM, Alvarado CR, Whitehead G. Substrate oxidation during acute exercise and with exercise training in lean and obese women. Eur J Appl Physiol 2001;85:68–73.

53. Pérez-Martin A, Dumortier M, Raynaud E, et al. Balance of substrate oxidation during submaximal exercise in lean and obese people. Diabetes Metabol 2001;27:466–74.

54. Goodpaster BH, Katsiaras A, Kelley DE. Enhanced fat oxidation through physical activity is associated with improvements in insulin sensitivity in obesity. Diabetes 2003;52:2191–7.

55. Mittendorffer B, Fields DA, Klein S. Excess body fat in men decreases plasma fatty acid availability and oxidation during endurance exercise. Am J Physiol Endocrinol Metab 2004;286:E354–E362.

56. Lazzer S, Busti C, Agosti F, et al. Optimizing fat oxidation through exercise in severely obese Caucasian adolescents. Clin Endocrinol 2007;67:582–8.

57. Houmard JA. Intramuscular lipid oxidation and obesity. Am J Physiol Regul Integr Comp Physiol 2008;294(4):R1111–16.

58. Brandou F, Savy-Pacaux AM, Marie J. Comparison of the type of substrate oxidation during exercise between pre and post pubertal markedly obese boys. Int J Sports Med 2006;27:407–14.

59. Hansen K. Shriver T, Schoeller D. The effects of exercise on the storage and oxidation of dietary fat. Sports Med 2005;35:363–73.

60. Votruba SB, Atkinson RL, Hirvonen MD, Schoeller DA. Prior exercise increases subsequent utilization of dietary fat. Med Sci Sports Exerc 2002;34:1757–65.

61. Melanson EL, Sharp TA, Seagle HM, et al. Effect of exercise intensity on 24-h energy expenditure and nutrient oxidation. J Appl Physiol 2002;92:1045–52.

62. Melanson EL, Sharp TA, Seagle HM, et al. Resistance and aerobic exercise have similar effects on 24-h nutrient oxidation. Med Sci Sports Exerc 2002;34:1793–800.

63. Saris WHM, Schrauwen P. Substrate oxidation differences between high- and low-intensity exercise are compensated over 24 hours in obese men. Int J Obes 2004;28:759–65.

64. Hansen KC, Zhang Z, Gomez T, et al. Exercise increases the proportion of fat utilization during short-term consumption of a high-fat diet. Am J Clin Nutr 2007;85:109–16.

65. Smith SS, de Jonge L, Zachwieja JJ, et al. Concurrent physical activity increases fat oxidation during the shift to a high-fat diet. Am J Clin Nutr 2000;72:131–8.

66. Hurley BF, Nemeth PM, Martin III WH, et al. Muscle triglyceride utilization during exercise: effect of training. J Appl Physiol 1986;60:562–7.

67. Martin III WH, Dalsky GP, Hurley BF, et al. Effect of endurance training on plasma free fatty acid turnover and oxidation during exercise. Am J Physiol 1993;265:E708–E714.

68. Schrauwen P, van Aggel-Leijssen DPC, Hul G, et al. The effect of a 3-month low-intensity endurance training program on fat oxidation and acetyl-CoA carboxylase-2 expression. Diabetes 2002;51: 2220–6.

69. Berggren J, Boyle KE, Chapman WH, Houmard JA. Skeletal muscle lipid oxidation and obesity: influence of weight loss and exercise. Am J Physiol Endocrinol Metab 2008;294(4):E726–32.

70. Bruce CR, Thrush AB, Mertz VA, et al. Endurance training in obese humans improves glucose tolerance, mitochondrial fatty acid oxidation and alters muscle lipid content. Am J Physiol 2006;291: E99–E107.

71. Menshikova EV, Ritov VB, Toledo FG, et al. Effects of weight loss and physical activity on skeletal muscle mitochondrial function in obesity. Am J Physiol 2005;288:E818–E825.

72. Menshikova EV, Ritov VB, Ferrell RE, et al. Characteristics of skeletal muscle mitochondrial biogenesis induced by moderate-intensity exercise and weight loss in obesity. J Appl Physiol 2007;103:21–7.

73. van Aggel-Leijssen DPC, Saris WHM, Wagenmakers AJM, et al. Effect of exercise training at different intensities on fat metabolism of obese men. J Appl Physiol 2002;92:1300–9.

74. van Aggel-Leijssen DPC, Saris WHM, Wagenmakers AJM, et al. The effect of low-intensity exercise training on fat metabolism in obese women. Obes Res 2001;9:86–96.

75. van Aggel-Leijssen DPC, Saris WHM, Hul GB, van Baak MA. Short-term effect of weight loss with or without low-intensity exercise training on fat metabolism in obese men. Am J Clin Nutr 2001;73: 523–31.

76. National Institutes of Health. Clinical guidelines on the identification, evaluation, and treatment of overweight and obesity in adults. Obes Res 1998;6(suppl 2):51S–209S.

77. Henriksen EJ. Effects of acute exercise and exercise training on insulin resistance. J Appl Physiol 2002;93:788–96.

78. Shaibi GQ, Roberts CK, Goran MI. Exercise and insulin resistance in youth. Exerc Sport Sci Rev 2008;36:5–11.

79. Thomas DE, Elliott EJ, Naughton GA. Exercise for type 2 diabetes mellitus (review). Cochrane Database of Systematic Reviews, issue 3, 2006, Art.No. CD002968.

80. Pan XR, Li GW, Hu YH, et al. Effects of diet and exercise in preventing NIDDM in people with impaired glucose tolerance. The Da Qing IGT and Diabetes Study. Diabetes Care 1997;20:537–44.

81. Tuomilehto J, Lindström J, Eriksson JG, et al. Prevention of type 2 diabetes mellitus by changes in lifestyle among subjects with impaired glucose tolerance. N Engl J Med 2001;244:1343–50.

82. Knowler WC, Barrett-Connor E, Fowler SE, et al, for the Diabetes Prevention Program Research Group. Reductions in the incidence of type 2 diabetes with lifestyle intervention or metformin. N Engl J Med 2002;346:393–403.

83. Laaksonen DE, Lindström J, Lakka TA, et al. Physical activity in the prevention of type 2 diabetes. The Finnish Diabetes Prevention Study. Diabetes 2005;54:158–65.

84. Leon AS, Sanchez OA. Response of blood lipids to exercise training alone or combined with dietary intervention. Med Sci Sports Exerc 2001;33(suppl):S502–S515.

85. Kraus WE, Houmard JA, Duscha BD, et al. Effects of the amount and intensity of exercise on plasma lipoproteins. N Engl J Med 2002;347:1483–92.

86. Slentz C, Houmard JA, Johnson JL, et al. Inactivity, exercise training and detraining, and plasma lipoproteins. STRRIDE: a randomized, controlled study of exercise intensity and amount. J Appl Physiol 2007;103:432–42.

87. Kelley GA, Kelley KS. Aerobic exercise and lipids and lipoproteins in children and adolescents: a meta-analysis of randomized controlled trials. Atherosclerosis 2007;191:447–53.

88. Cornelissen VA, Fagard RH. Effects of endurance training on blood pressure, blood pressure-regulating mechanisms, and cardiovascular risk factors. Hypertension 2005;46:667–75.

89. Torrance B, McGuire KA, Lewanczuk R, McGavock J. Overweight, physical activity and high blood pressure in children: a review of the literature. Vasc Health Risk Manag 2007;3:139–49.

90. Fagard RH, Cornelissen VA. Effects of exercise on blood pressure control in hypertensive patients. Eur J Cardiovasc Prev Rehabil 2007;14:12–17.

91. Fagard RH. Effects of exercise, diet and their combination on blood pressure. J Hum Hypertens 2005;19:S20–S24.

92. Surgeon General's Report. *Physical Activity and Health*. Atlanta, GA: US Department of Health and Human Services, 1996.

93. Dunn AL, Trivedi MH, O'Neal HA. Physical activity dose-response effects on outcomes of depression and anxiety. Med Sci Sports Exerc 2001;33(suppl):S587–S597.

94. Foreyt JP, Brunner RL, Goodrick GK, St-Jeor ST, Miller GD. Psychological correlates of reported physical activity in normal-weight and obese adults: the Reno diet-heart study. Int J Obes 1995;19(suppl 4):S69–S72.

95. Nieman DC, Custer WF, Butterworth DE, Utter AC, Henson DA. Psychological response to exercise training and/or energy restriction in obese women. J Psychosom Res 2000;48:23–9.

96. Goran M, Fields DA, Hunter GR, Herd SL, Weinsier RL. Total body fat does not influence maximal aerobic capacity. Int J Obes 2000; 24:841–8.

97. Blair SN, Brodney S. Effects of physical inactivity and obesity on morbidity and mortality: current evidence and research issues. Med Sci Sports Exerc 1999;31(suppl):S646–S662.

98. Haapanen-Niemi N, Miilunpalo S, Pasanen M, et al. Body mass index, physical inactivity and low level of physical fitness as determinants of all-cause and cardiovascular disease mortality – 16 y follow-up of middle-aged and elderly men and women. Int J Obes 2000;24:1465–74.

99. Crespo CJ, Palmieri MR, Perdomo RP, et al. The relationship of physical activity and body weight with all-cause mortality: results from the Puerto Rico Heart Health Program. Ann Epidemiol 2002;12:543–52.

100. Stevens J, Cai J, Evenson KR, Thomas R. Fitness and fatness as predictors of mortality from all causes and from cardiovascular disease in men and women in the Lipid Research Clinics Study. Am J Epidemiol 2000;156:832–41.

101. Farrell SW, Braun L, Barlow CE, Cheng YJ, Blair SN. The relation of body mass index, cardiorespiratory fitness, and all-cause mortality in women. Obes Res 2002;10:417–23.

102. Sui X, LaMonte MJ, Laditka JN, et al. Cardiorespiratory fitness and adiposity as mortality predictors in older athletes. JAMA 2007; 298:2507–16.

103. Fogelholm M, Stallknecht B, van Baak MA. ECSS position statement: exercise and obesity. Eur J Sport Sci 2006;6:15–24.

104. Haskell WL, Lee IM, Pate RR, et al. Physical activity and public health: updated recommendation for adults from the American College of Sports Medicine and the American Heart Association. Med Sci Sports Exerc 2007;39:1423–34.

105. Kesaniemi YA, Danforth Jr E, Jensen MD, et al. Dose-response issues concerning physical activity and health: an evidence-based symposium. Med Sci Sports Exerc 2001;33(suppl):S351–S358.

106. Tanasescu M, Leitzmann MF, Rimm EB, et al. Exercise type and intensity in relation to coronary heart disease in men. JAMA 2002;288:1994–2000.

107. Lee I, Sesso H, Oguma Y, Paffenbarger RS. Relative exercise intensity of physical activity and risk of coronary heart disease. Circulation 2003;107:1110–16.

108. Gill JM. Physical activity, cardiorespiratory fitness and insulin resistance: a short update. Curr Opin Lipidol 2007;18:47–52.

109. Bray MS. Genomics, genes, and environmental interaction: the role of exercise. J Appl Physiol 2000;88:788–92.

110. An P, Borecki IB, Rankinen T, et al. Evidence of major genes for plasma HDL, LDL, cholesterol and triglyceride levels at baseline and in response to 20 weeks of endurance training: the HERITAGE Family Study. Int J Sports Med 2005;26:414–19.

111. An P, Teran-Garcia M, Rice T, et al. Genome-wide linkage scans for prediabetes phenotypes in response to 20 weeks of endurance exercise training in non-diabetic whites and blacks: the HERITAGE Family Study. Diabetologia 2005;48:1142–9.

112. Kilpeläinen TO, Lakka TA, Laaksonen DE, et al. Interaction of single nucleotide polymorphisms in ADRB2, ADRB3, TNF, IL6, IGF1R, LIPC, LEPR, and GHRL with physical activity on the risk of type 2 diabetes mellitus and changes in characteristics of the metabolic syndrome. Metabolism 2008;57:428–36.

113. Jakicic JM, Otto AD. Physical activity considerations for the treatment and prevention of obesity. Am J Clin Nutr 2005; 82(suppl):226S–229S.

114. Dunn AL, Marcus BH, Kampert JB, et al. Comparison of lifestyle and structured interventions to increase physical activity and cardiorespiratory fitness: a randomized trial. JAMA 1999;281: 327–34.

115. Andersen RE, Wadden TA, Bartlett SJ, et al. Effects of lifestyle activity vs structured aerobic exercise in obese women: a randomized trial. JAMA 1999;281:335–40.

116. Miller WC, Wallace JP, Eggert KE. Predicting max HR and the HR-VO$_2$ relationship for exercise prescription in obesity. Med Sci Sports Exerc 1991;25:1077–81.

117. Dishman RK, Sallis JE, Orenstein DR. The determinants of physical activity and exercise. Public Health Rep 1985;100:158–71.

118. King AC, Kiernan M, Oman RR, et al. Can we identify who will adhere to long-term physical activity? Signal detection methodology as potential aid to clinical decision making. Health Psychol 1997;16:380–9.

119. Cox KL, Burke V, Gorely TJ, Beilin LJ, Puddey IB. Controlled comparison of retention and adherence in home- vs center-initiated exercise interventions in women ages 40–65 years: the S.W.E.A.T. study (Sedentary Women Exercise Adherence Trial). Prev Med 2003;36:17–29.

120. Brownell KD. Exercise and obesity treatment: psychological aspects. Int J Obes 1995;19(suppl 4):S122–S125.

121. Jakicic JM, Wing RR, Butler BA, Robertson RJ. Prescribing exercise in multiple short bouts versus one continuous bout: effects on adherence, cardiorespiratory fitness, and weight loss in overweight women. Int J Obes 1995;19:893–901.

122. Jakicic JM, Winters C, Lang W, Wing RR. Effects of intermittent exercise and use of home exercise equipment on adherence, weight loss, and fitness in overweight women. JAMA 1999;282:1554–60.

123. Thompson PD, Buchner D, Pina IL, et al. Exercise and physical activity in the prevention and treatment of atherosclerotic cardiovascular disease. Circulation 2003;107:3109–16.

124. American College of Sports Medicine. The recommended quantity and quality of exercise for developing and maintaining cardiorespiratory and muscular fitness in healthy adults. Med Sci Sports Exerc 1990;22:265–74.

24 Drugs Used Clinically to Reduce Body Weight

George A. Bray

Pennington Biomedical Research Center, Louisiana State University, Louisiana, LA, USA

Introduction

Obesity is often described as an epidemic [1–3]. In this context, it is essential to develop ways of preventing more people from becoming obese but where prevention fails, treatment may be necessary. A number of different strategies have been used to treat obesity, including diet, exercise, behavior therapy, medications, and surgery. Criteria for selecting among these treatments involve evaluating the risks to the individual from obesity and balancing those against any possible problems with the treatment. Since all medications inherently have more risks than do diet and exercise, medications should only be used for people in whom the benefit justifies the risk [4].

This process of evaluation is particularly important when we realize that drug treatment for obesity has been tarnished by a number of unfortunate problems over the years. Since the introduction of thyroid hormone to treat obesity in 1893, almost every drug that has been tried in obese patients has caused undesirable outcomes necessitating its termination. Thus, caution must be used in accepting any new drug for the treatment of obesity unless the safety profile makes it acceptable for almost everyone [4].

Another issue surrounding drug treatment of obesity is the perception that because patients regain weight when drugs are stopped, the drugs are ineffective. Quite the contrary is true. Obesity is a chronic disease that has many causes. Cure, however, is rare, and treatment is thus aimed at palliation, i.e. producing and maintaining weight loss. Physicians do not expect to cure diseases such as hypertension or hypercholesterolemia with medications. Rather, they expect to palliate them. When the

medications for any of these chronic diseases are discontinued, the disease is expected to recur. This means that medications only work when they are used. The same argument applies for medications used to treat obesity [4].

If an individual is to lose weight, he or she must go into "negative" energy balance where the energy consumed as food is less, on average, than the energy needed for daily activities. Thus, the current group of medications can be divided into two broad categories: those that act primarily on the central nervous system to reduce food intake and those that act primarily outside the brain. Wherever the primary site of action may be, however, the net effect must be a reduction in food intake and/or an increase in energy expenditure.

There are currently several drugs available to treat obesity [5–10] (see Table 24.1).

Drugs that reduce food intake primarily by acting in the central nervous system

The drugs considered in this category are sibutramine, phentermine and the other sympathomimetic drugs.

Sibutramine

Sibutramine is a serotonin-norepinephrine reuptake inhibitor that is approved by the US Food and Drug Administration and other international agencies for long-term use. Sibutramine has been evaluated extensively in several placebo-controlled, double-blind multicenter clinical trials lasting 6–24 months and including men and women of all ethnic groups, with ages ranging from 18 years to 65 years, and with a Body Mass Index (BMI) between $27\,kg/m^2$ and $40\,kg/m^2$ [5,7–9,11,12]. In a clinical trial lasting 8 weeks, sibutramine produced a dose-dependent weight loss with doses of 5 mg and 20 mg per day [9]. In a 6-month dose-ranging study of 1047 patients, 67% treated with sibutramine achieved a

Clinical Obesity in Adults and Children, 3rd edition. Edited by Peter G. Kopelman, Ian D. Caterson and William H. Dietz.
© 2010 Blackwell Publishing, ISBN: 978-1-4051-8226-3.

Table 24.1 Drugs Approved by the USFDA for treatment of obesity

Generic name	Trade names	Status	Usual bose	Comments
Drugs approved for long-term treatment of overweight patients				
Orlistat	Xenical	Not scheduled	120 mg three times a day	May have GI side-effects
Sibutramine	Meridia, Reductil	DEA-IV	5–15 mg/d	Raises blood pressure
Drugs approved for short-term treatment of overweight patients				
Benzphetamine	Didrex	DEA-III	25–50 mg one to three times a day	Short-term use only
Diethylpropion	Tenuate	DEA-IV	25 mg tid	Short-term use only
	Tepanil		25 mg tid	
	Tenuate Dospan		75 mg in AM	
Phendimetrazine	Standard release:	DEA-III	35 mg tid before meals	Short-term use only
	Bontril PDM			
	Plegine		105 mg/day in AM	
	X-Trozine			
	Slow release:			
	Bontril			
	Prelu-2			
	X-Trozine			
Phentermine	Standard release:	DEA-IV	18.75–37.5 mg tid	Short-term use only
	Adipex-P			
	Fastin		15–30 mg/d in am of slow-release	
	Obenix			
	Oby-Cap			
	Oby-Trim			
	Zantryl			
	Slow release:			
	Ionamin			

5% weight loss from baseline, and 35% lost 10% or more (Fig. 24.1) [9]. There was a clear dose–response effect in this 24-week trial, and patients regained weight when the drug was stopped, indicating that the drug remained effective when used.

In a 1-year trial of 456 patients who received sibutramine (10 mg or 15 mg per day) or placebo, 56% of those who stayed in the trial for 12 months lost at least 5% of their initial body weight, and 30% of the patients lost 10% of their initial body weight while taking the 10 mg dose [13]. In a third trial in patients who initially lost weight eating a very low-calorie diet before being randomized to sibutramine or placebo, sibutramine (10 mg per day) produced additional weight loss, whereas the placebo-treated patients

regained weight [14]. The Sibutramine Trial of Obesity Reduction and Maintenance (STORM) lasted 2 years and provided further evidence for weight maintenance [15]. Seven centers participated in this trial, in which patients were initially enrolled in a 6-month open-label phase and treated with 10 mg per day of sibutramine. Of the patients who lost more than 8 kg, two-thirds were then randomized to sibutramine and one-third to placebo. During the 18-month double-blind phase of this trial, the placebo-treated patients steadily regained weight, maintaining only 20% of their weight loss at the end of the trial. In contrast, the subjects treated with sibutramine maintained their weight for 12 months and then regained an average of only 2 kg, thus maintaining 80% of their initial weight loss after 2 years [15]. Despite the higher weight loss with sibutramine at the end of the 18 months of controlled observation, the blood pressure levels of the sibutramine-treated patients were still higher than those of the patients treated with placebo.

The possibility of using sibutramine as intermittent therapy has been tested in a randomized, placebo-controlled trial lasting 52 weeks [16]. The patients randomized to sibutramine received one of two regimens. One group received continuous treatment with 15 mg per day for 1 year, and the other had two 6-week periods when sibutramine was withdrawn. During these periods when the drug was replaced by placebo, there was a small regain in weight that was lost when the drug was again resumed. At the end of the trial, the continuous therapy and intermittent therapy groups had lost the same amount of weight.

Some trials have reported the use of sibutramine to treat patients with hypertension. In a 52-week trial involving patients with hypertension whose blood pressure levels were controlled with calcium channel blockers with or without β-blockers or thiazides [17], sibutramine doses were increased from 5 mg to 20 mg per day during the first 6 weeks. Weight loss was significantly greater in the sibutramine-treated patients, averaging 4.4 kg (4.7%), as compared with 0.5 kg (0.7%) in the placebo-treated group. Diastolic blood pressure levels decreased 1.3 mmHg in the placebo-treated group and increased 2 mmHg in the sibutramine-treated group. The systolic blood pressure levels increased 1.5 mmHg in the placebo-treated group and 2.7 mmHg in the sibutramine-treated group. Heart rate was unchanged in the placebo-treated patients, but increased by an average of 4.9 beats per minute in the sibutramine-treated patients.

In two studies, patients with diabetes were treated for 12 weeks or 24 weeks with sibutramine. In the 12-week trial, patients with diabetes treated with sibutramine at 15 mg per day lost 2.4 kg (2.8%), compared with 0.1 kg (0.12%) in the placebo group. In this study, hemoglobin A1C levels decreased 0.3% in the drug-treated group and remained stable in the placebo group. Fasting glucose values decreased 0.3 mg/dL in the drug-treated patients and increased 1.4 mg/dL in the placebo-treated group. In the 24-week trial, the dose of sibutramine was increased from 5 mg to 20 mg per day over 6 weeks [18]. Among those who completed the treatment, weight loss was 4.3 kg (4.3%) in the sibutramine-treated patients, compared with 0.3 kg (0.3%) in placebo-treated patients.

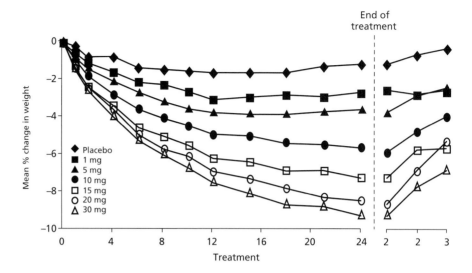

Figure 24.1 Dose-dependent weight loss during 24-week trial of sibutramine. (Reproduced with permission from Bray et al. Obes Res 1999;7:189–98.)

Hemoglobin A1C levels decreased 1.67% in the drug-treated group, compared with 0.53% in the placebo-treated group. These changes in glucose and hemoglobin A1C levels were expected from the amount of weight loss associated with drug treatment.

Sibutramine has also been used in children [19–22]. In a large 12-month long multicenter trial, 498 adolescents ages 12–16 years were randomized to treatment with placebo or sibutramine, 10 mg/d, which could be increased to 15 mg/d in those who had not lost >10% of their body weight by 6 months [21]. After 12 months, the mean absolute change in BMI was -2.9kg/m^2 (-8.2%) in the sibutramine group compared with -0.3kg/m^2 (-0.8%) in the placebo group ($p < 0.001$). Triglycerides, HDL cholesterol, and insulin sensitivity improved, and there was no significant difference in the changes in either systolic or diastolic blood pressure.

Sibutramine has also been studied as part of a behavioral weight loss program. With sibutramine alone and minimal behavioral intervention, the weight loss over 12 months was approximately $-5.0 \pm 7.4 \text{kg}$. Behavior modification alone produced a weight loss of $-6.7 \pm 7.9 \text{kg}$. Adding a brief behavioral therapy session to a group that also received sibutramine produced a slightly larger weight loss of $-7.5 \pm 8.0 \text{kg}$. When the intensive lifestyle intervention was combined with sibutramine, the weight loss increased to $-12.1 \pm 9.8 \text{kg}$ [23].

Sibutramine is available in 5, 10 and 15 mg doses; 10 mg per day as a single dose is the recommended starting level, with titration up or down depending on response. Doses higher than 15 mg per day are not recommended. Of the patients who lost 2 kg (4.4 lb) in the first 4 weeks of treatment, 60% achieved a weight loss of more than 5%, compared with less than 10% in those who did not lose 2 kg (4.4 lb) in 4 weeks. Combining data from the 11 studies on sibutramine showed a reduction in triglyceride, total cholesterol, and LDL cholesterol levels and an increase in HDL cholesterol levels that were related to the magnitude of the weight loss.

Safety

Sibutramine increases blood pressure levels in normotensive patients or prevents the decrease that might have occurred with weight loss. The magnitude of the change may be dose related, so lower doses are preferred. Systolic and diastolic blood pressure levels increased an average of $+0.8 \text{mmHg}$ and $+0.6 \text{mmHg}$, and pulse increased approximately 4–5 beats per minute. Caution should be exercised when combining sibutramine with other drugs that may increase blood pressure levels. Sibutramine is contraindicated in patients with a history of coronary artery disease, congestive heart failure, cardiac arrhythmias or stroke. It should not be used with selective serotonin reuptake inhibitors or monoamine oxidase inhibitors, and there should be a 2-week interval between terminating monoamine oxidase inhibitors and beginning sibutramine. Because sibutramine is metabolized by the cytochrome P450 enzyme system (isozyme CYP3A4), it may interfere with the metabolism of erythromycin and ketoconazole.

Sympathomimetic drugs: pharmacology and efficacy

The sympathomimetic drugs, benzphetamine, diethylpropion, phendimetrazine, and phentermine, are grouped together because they act like norepinephrine. Drugs in this group work by a variety of mechanisms, including the blockade of norepinephrine reuptake from synaptic granules [9].

All of these drugs are absorbed orally and reach peak blood concentrations within a short period. The half-life in blood also is short for all except the metabolites of sibutramine, which have a long half-life. The two metabolites of sibutramine are active, but this is not true for the metabolites of other drugs in this group. Liver metabolism inactivates a large fraction of these drugs before excretion. Side-effects include dry mouth, constipation, and insomnia. Food intake is suppressed either by delaying the onset of a meal or by producing early satiety.

The efficacy of an appetite-suppressing drug can be established through randomized, double-blind clinical trials that show a significantly greater weight loss than in the placebo group and a weight loss that is more than 5% below that with placebo [5,7,11]. Clinical trials of sympathomimetic drugs conducted before 1975 were generally short because it was widely believed that short-term treatment would "cure" obesity. This was unfounded optimism, and because the trials had a short duration and often used a cross-over design, they provided few long-term data. The focus here is on longer-term trials lasting 24 weeks or more that include an adequate control group.

One of the longest clinical trials of drugs in this group lasted 36 weeks and compared placebo treatment with continuous phentermine or intermittent phentermine [9]. Both continuous and intermittent phentermine therapy produced more weight loss than placebo. In the drug-free periods, the patients treated intermittently slowed their weight loss, only to lose weight more rapidly when the drug was reinstituted. Phentermine and diethylpropion are classified by the US Drug Enforcement Agency as schedule IV drugs; benzphetamine and phendimetrazine are schedule III drugs. This regulatory classification indicates the US government's belief that they have the potential for abuse, although this potential appears to be very low. Phentermine and diethylpropion are approved for only a "few weeks," which is usually interpreted as up to 12 weeks. Weight loss with phentermine and diethylpropion persists for the duration of treatment, suggesting that tolerance does not develop to these drugs. If tolerance were to develop, the drugs would be expected to lose their effectiveness, and patients would require increased amounts of the drug to maintain weight loss. This does not occur.

Safety

The side-effect profiles for sympathomimetic drugs are similar [8,9]. These agents produce insomnia, dry mouth, asthenia, and constipation. The safety of older sympathomimetic appetite suppressant drugs has been the subject of considerable controversy because dextroamphetamine is addictive. The sympathomimetic drugs phentermine, diethylpropion, benzphetamine, and phendimetrazine have very little abuse potential, as assessed by the low rate of reinforcement when the drugs are self-injected intravenously by test animals [9]. Sympathomimetic drugs can also increase blood pressure levels.

Drugs approved by the US FDA that reduce fat absorption

Orlistat: pharmacology and efficacy

Orlistat is a potent and selective inhibitor of pancreatic lipase that reduces the intestinal digestion of fat. The drug has a dose-dependent effect on fecal fat loss, increasing it to approximately 30% on a diet that has 30% of its energy as fat. Orlistat has lesser or little effect in subjects eating a low-fat diet, as might be anticipated from its mechanism of action [9].

A number of long-term clinical trials (1–4 years) with orlistat have been published [5,7,11,12]. The first published trial consisted of two parts. In the first year, patients received a hypocaloric diet calculated to be 500 kcal per day less than the patient's requirements (Fig. 24.2) [24]. During the second year, the diet was calculated to maintain weight. By the end of year 1, the placebo-treated patients lost 6.1% of their initial body weight

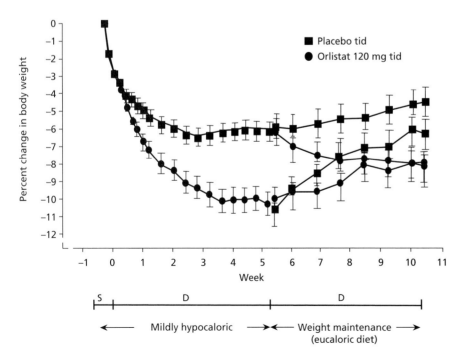

Figure 24.2 Orlistat and body weight. Two-year trial of orlistat versus placebo with a hypocaloric diet. (Reproduced with permission from Sjostrom et al. [24].)

and the drug-treated patients lost 10.2%. The patients were randomized at the end of year 1. Those switched from orlistat to placebo gained weight from −10% to −6% below baseline. Those switched from placebo to orlistat lost weight from −6% to −8.1% below baseline, which was essentially identical to the −7.9% loss in the patients treated with orlistat for the full 2 years.

In a second 2-year study, 892 patients were randomized [25]. One group remained on placebo throughout the 2 years (97 patients), and a second group remained on orlistat (120 mg three times per day) for 2 years (109 patients). At the end of 1 year, two-thirds of the group treated with orlistat for 1 year were changed to orlistat (60 mg three times per day; 102 patients), and the others were switched to placebo (95 patients). After 1 year, the weight loss was −8.7 kg in the orlistat-treated group and −5.8 kg in the placebo group (p < 0.001). During the second year, those switched to placebo after 1 year reached the same weight as those treated with placebo for 2 years (−4.5% in those with placebo for 2 years and −4.2% in those switched to placebo during year 2).

In a third 2-year study, 783 patients remained in the placebo- or orlistat-treated groups at 60 mg or 120 mg three times per day for the entire 2 years [26]. After 1 year with a weight loss diet, the placebo group lost −7 kg, which was significantly less than the −9.6 kg lost by the group treated with orlistat 60 mg three times daily or the −9.8 kg lost by the group treated with orlistat 120 mg three times daily. During the second year, when the diet was liberalized to a "weight maintenance" diet, all three groups regained some weight. At the end of 2 years, the patients in the placebo group were −4.3 kg below baseline, the patients treated with orlistat 60 mg three times per day were −6.8 kg below baseline, and the patients who took orlistat 120 mg three times per day were −7.6 kg below baseline.

The final 2-year trial evaluated 796 subjects in a general practice setting [27]. After 1 year of treatment with orlistat 120 mg three times per day, the orlistat-treated patients (n = 117) had lost −8.8 kg, compared with −4.3 kg in the placebo group (n = 91). During the second year, when the diet was liberalized to "maintain body weight," both groups regained some weight. At the end of 2 years, the orlistat group was −5.2 kg below their baseline weight, compared with −1.5 kg below baseline for the group treated with placebo.

A 4-year double-blind, randomized, placebo-controlled trial with orlistat (XENDOS) treated a total of 3304 overweight patients, 21% of whom had impaired glucose tolerance [28]. The lowest body weight was achieved during the first year, and was more than 11% below baseline in the orlistat-treated group and 6% below baseline in the placebo-treated group. Over the remaining 3 years of the trial, there was a small regain in weight, such that by the end of 4 years, the orlistat-treated patients were −6.9% below baseline, compared with −4.1% for those receiving placebo. The trial also showed a 37% reduction in the conversion of patients from impaired glucose tolerance to diabetes; essentially all of this benefit occurred in the patients with impaired glucose tolerance at enrollment into the trial.

Orlistat has also been used to treat obese children. A multicenter trial tested the effect of orlistat in 539 obese adolescents [29]. Subjects were randomized to placebo or orlistat 120 mg three times a day and a mildly hypocaloric diet containing 30% fat. By the end of the study, BMI had decreased −0.55 kg/m^2 in the drug-treated group but had increased +0.31 kg/m^2 in the placebo group. By the end of the study, weight had increased by only +0.51 kg in the orlistat-treated group, compared with +3.14 kg in the placebo-treated group. This difference was due to differences in body fat. The side-effects were gastrointestinal in origin as expected from the mode of action of orlistat.

Weight maintenance with orlistat was evaluated in a 1-year study. Patients were enrolled if they had lost more than 8% of their body weight over 6 months while eating a 1000 kcal per day (4180 kJ/d) diet. The 729 patients were randomized to receive placebo or orlistat at 30 mg, 60 mg or 120 mg three times per day for 12 months. At the end of this time, the placebo-treated patients had regained 56% of their body weight, compared with 32.4% regain in the group treated with orlistat 120 mg three times per day. The other two doses of orlistat were not different from placebo in preventing the regain of weight.

Patients with diabetes treated with orlistat 120 mg three times daily for 1 year lost −6.5% of their body weight, compared with −4.2% in the placebo-treated group [30–32]. The subjects with diabetes also showed a significantly greater decrease in hemoglobin A1C (HbA$_{1c}$) levels. In another study of orlistat and weight loss, investigators pooled data on 675 subjects from three of the 2-year studies described previously in which glucose tolerance tests were available [33]. During treatment, 6.6% of the patients taking orlistat converted from a normal to an impaired glucose tolerance test, compared with 10.8% in the placebo-treated group. None of the orlistat-treated patients who originally had normal glucose tolerance developed diabetes, compared with 1.2% in the placebo-treated group. Of those who initially had normal glucose tolerance, 7.6% in the placebo group but only 3% in the orlistat-treated group developed diabetes.

Safety

Orlistat is not absorbed to any significant degree, and its side-effects are thus related to the blockade of triglyceride digestion in the intestine [34]. Fecal fat loss and related gastrointestinal (GI) symptoms are common initially, but they subside as patients learn to use the drug. The quality of life in patients treated with orlistat may improve despite concerns about GI symptoms. Orlistat can cause small but significant decreases in fat-soluble vitamins. Levels usually remain within the normal range, but a few patients may need vitamin supplementation. Because it is impossible to tell which patients need vitamins, it is wise to provide a multivitamin routinely with instructions to take it before bedtime. Orlistat does not seem to affect the absorption of other drugs, except aciclovir.

Combining orlistat and sibutramine

Because orlistat works peripherally to reduce triglyceride digestion in the GI tract and sibutramine works on noradrenergic and

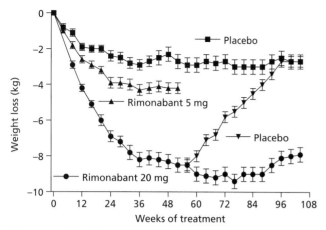

Figure 24.3 Effect of Rimonabant on body weight over 2 years. (Reproduced with permission from Pi-Sunyer et al. JAMA 2006;295:761–775.)

serotonergic reuptake mechanisms in the brain, their mechanisms of action do not overlap, and combining them might provide additive weight loss. To test this possibility, researchers randomly assigned patients to orlistat or placebo after 1 year of treatment with sibutramine [35]. During the additional 4 months of treatment, there was no further weight loss. Thus, we have no data suggesting that combining orlistat and sibutramine is beneficial.

Rimonabant

Rimonabant, a cannabinoid receptor antagonist that blocks the CB-1 receptor, was approved by the European regulatory authorities in 2006, but approval for marketing was withdrawn in October 2008 because of increased risks of psychiatric side-effects, including depression and anxiety (Fig. 24.3).

Drugs that have been used to treat obesity but are not generally approved for this purpose

Fluoxetine and sertraline

Fluoxetine and sertraline are both selective serotonin reuptake inhibitors that block serotonin transporters, thus prolonging the action of serotonin. These drugs both reduce food intake. In a 2-week placebo-controlled trial, fluoxetine at a dose of 60 mg/d produced a 27% decrease in food intake [36]. Both fluoxetine and sertraline are approved by the US FDA for treatment of depression. In clinical trials lasting 8–16 weeks with depressed patients, sertraline gave an average weight loss of −0.45 to −0.91 kg. Fluoxetine at a dose of 60 mg per day (three times the usual dose for treatment of depression) was effective in reducing body weight in overweight patients. A meta-analysis of six studies using fluoxetine showed a wide range of results with a mean weight loss in one study of −14.5 kg and a weight gain of +0.40 kg in another [7]. In the meta-analysis by Avenell et al. [12], the weight loss at

12 months was −0.33 kg (95% confidence interval (CI) −1.49 to 0.82 kg). Goldstein and colleagues reviewed the trials with fluoxetine that included one 36-week trial in type 2 diabetic subjects, a 52-week trial in subjects with uncomplicated overweight, and two 60-week trials in subjects with dyslipidemia, diabetes or both [37]. A total of 719 subjects were randomized to fluoxetine and 722 to placebo. Five hundred and twenty-two subjects on fluoxetine and 504 subjects on placebo completed 6 months of treatment. Weight losses in the placebo and fluoxetine groups at 6 months and 1 year were −2.2, −4.8, and −1.8, −2.4 kg, respectively. The regain of 50% of the lost weight during the second 6 months of treatment with fluoxetine makes this drug inappropriate for the long-term treatment of obesity.

Fluoxetine and sertraline, although not good drugs for long-term treatment of obesity, may be preferred for the treatment of depressed obese patients over some of the tricyclic antidepressants that are associated with significant weight gain.

Bupropion

Bupropion is a norepinephrine and dopamine reuptake inhibitor that is approved for the treatment of depression and for help in smoking cessation. In one clinical trial 50 overweight subjects were randomized to bupropion or placebo for 8 weeks with a blinded extension for responders to 24 weeks. The dose of bupropion was increased to maximum of 200 mg twice daily in conjunction with a calorie-restricted diet. At 8 weeks, 18 subjects in the bupropion group lost −6.2 ± 3.1% of body weight compared to −1.6 ± 2.9% for the 13 subjects in the placebo group (p < 0.0001). After 24 weeks, the 14 responders to bupropion lost −12.9 ± 5.6% of initial body weight, of which 75% was fat as determined by dual-energy X-ray absorptiometry (DXA) [38].

Two multicenter clinical trials, one in obese subjects with depressive symptoms and one in uncomplicated overweight patients, followed this study. In the study of overweight patients with depressive symptom ratings of 10–30 on a Beck Depression Inventory, 213 patients were randomized to 400 mg/d of bupropion and 209 subjects were assigned to placebo for 24 weeks. The 121 subjects in the bupropion group who completed the trial lost −6.0 ± 0.5% of initial body weight compared to −2.8 ± 0.5% in the 108 subjects in the placebo group (p < 0.0001) [39]. The study in uncomplicated overweight subjects randomized 327 subjects to bupropion 300 mg/d, bupropion 400 mg/d or placebo in equal proportions. At 24 weeks, 69% of those randomized remained in the study and the percent losses of initial body weight were −5 ± 1%, −7.2 ± 1%, and −10.1 ± 1% for the placebo, bupropion 300 mg, and bupropion 400 mg groups, respectively (p < 0.0001). The placebo group was randomized to the 300 mg or 400 mg group at 24 weeks and the trial was extended to week 48. By the end of the trial the drop-out rate was 41%, and the weight losses in the bupropion 300 mg and bupropion 400 mg groups were −6.2 ± 1.25% and −7.2 ± 1.5% of initial body weight, respectively [40]. Thus, it appears that nondepressed subjects may respond to bupropion with weight loss to a greater extent than those with depressive symptoms.

Topiramate

Topiramate is approved for treatment of selected seizure disorders. It is a weak carbonic anhydrase inhibitor. Topiramate also modulates the effects at receptors for the γ-aminobutyric acid (GABA$_A$) receptor and the AMPA (α-amino-3-hydroxy-5-methyl-4-isoxazolepropionic acid)/kainate subtype of the glutamate receptor. This drug also exhibits state-dependent blockade of voltage-dependent Na$^+$ or Ca^{2+} channels. These mechanisms are believed to contribute to its antiepileptic properties. The modulation of GABA$_A$ receptors may provide one potential mechanism to reduce food intake, although other mechanisms, yet to be described, may be more important in defining its effects on body weight [41].

Topiramate is an antiepileptic drug that was discovered to promote weight loss in clinical trials for epilepsy. Weight losses of −3.9% of initial weight were seen at 3 months and losses of −7.3% of initial weight were seen at 1 year [42]. Bray and colleagues reported a 6-month, placebo-controlled, dose-ranging study of topiramate. Three hundred and eighty-five obese subjects were randomized to placebo or topiramate at 64 mg/d, 96 mg/d, 192 mg/d or 384 mg/d. These doses were gradually reached by a tapering increase and were reduced in a similar manner at the end of the trial. Weight loss from baseline to 24 weeks was −2.6%, −5%, −4.8%, −6.3% and −6.3% in the placebo, 64 mg, 96 mg, 192 mg and 384 mg groups, respectively. The most frequent adverse events were paresthesias, somnolence, and difficulty with concentration, memory, and attention [43]. This trial was followed by two other multicenter trials. The first randomized 1289 obese subjects to placebo or topiramate 89 mg/d, 192 mg/d or 256 mg/d. This trial was terminated early due to the sponsor's decision to pursue a time-release form of the drug. The 854 subjects who completed 1 year of the trial before it was terminated lost −1.7%, −7%, −9.1%, and −9.7% of their initial body weight in the placebo, 89 mg, 192 mg, and 256 mg groups, respectively. Subjects in the topiramate groups had significant improvement in blood pressure and glucose tolerance [44]. The second trial enrolled 701 subjects who were treated with a very low-calorie diet to induce an 8% loss of initial body weight. The 560 subjects who achieved an 8% weight loss were randomized to topiramate 96 mg/d, 192 mg/d or placebo. This study was also terminated early. At the time of termination, 293 subjects had completed 44 weeks. The topiramate groups lost 15.4% and 16.5% of their baseline weight while the placebo group lost 8.9% [45]. Although topiramate is still available as an antiepileptic drug, the development program to obtain an indication for overweight was terminated by the sponsor due to the associated adverse events.

Zonisamide

Zonisamide is an antiepileptic drug that has serotonergic and dopaminergic activity in addition to inhibiting sodium and calcium channels. Weight loss was noted in clinical trials for the treatment of epilepsy, again suggesting a potential agent for weight loss. Gadde and colleagues tested this possibility by performing a 16-week randomized controlled trial in 60 obese subjects. Subjects were placed on a calorie-restricted diet and randomized to zonisamide or placebo. The zonisamide was started at 100 mg/d and increased to 400 mg/d. At 12 weeks, those subjects who had not lost 5% of initial body weight were increased to 600 mg/d. The zonisamide group lost −6.6% of initial body weight at 16 weeks compared to −1% in the placebo group. Thirty-seven subjects completing the 16-week trial elected to continue for 32 weeks: 20 in the zonisamide group and 17 in the placebo group. At the end of 32 weeks, the 20 subjects in the zonisamide group lost −9.6% of their initial body weight compared to −1.6% for the 17 subjects in the placebo group [46].

Lamotrigine

Lamotrogine is a third antiepileptic drug that has been evaluated for its effects on body weight [47]. In a double-blind randomized placebo-controlled trial, the dose of lamotrigine was escalated from 25 mg/d to 200 mg/d over 6 weeks. The effect on weight loss was compared to placebo treatment over 26 weeks in 40 healthy overweight (BMI 30–40 kg/m^2) adults over 18 years of age. At the end of the trial body weight was marginally lower (p = 0.062) in the lamotrigine-treated group (−6.4 kg) than in the placebo-treated group (−1.2 kg) [48].

Metformin

Metformin is a biguanide that is approved for the treatment of diabetes mellitus. This drug reduces hepatic glucose production, decreases intestinal absorption from the gastrointestinal tract, and enhances insulin sensitivity. In clinical trials where metformin was compared with sulfonylureas, it produced weight loss [9]. In one French trial, BIGPRO, metformin was compared to placebo in a 1-year multicenter study in 324 middle-aged subjects with upper body adiposity and the insulin resistance syndrome (metabolic syndrome). The subjects on metformin lost significantly more weight (1–2 kg) than did the placebo group, and the study concluded that metformin may have a role in the primary prevention of type 2 diabetes [49]. In a meta-analysis of three of these studies, Avenell and colleagues [12] reported a weighted mean weight loss at 12 months of −1.09 kg (95% CI −2.29 to 0.11 kg).

The best trial of metformin for obesity, however, is the Diabetes Prevention Program (DPP) study of individuals with impaired glucose tolerance. This included a double-blind comparison of metformin 850 mg twice daily versus placebo. During the 2.8 years of this trial, the 1073 patients treated with metformin lost −2.5% of their body weight (p < 0.001) compared to the 1082 patients treated with placebo, and the conversion from impaired glucose tolerance to diabetes was reduced by 31% compared to placebo. In the DPP trial, metformin was more effective in reducing the development of diabetes in the subgroup who were most overweight, and in the younger members of the cohort [50]. Although metformin does not produce enough weight loss (5%) to qualify as a "weight loss drug" (FDA criteria require ≥5%

weight loss), it would appear to be a very useful choice for overweight individuals who have diabetes or are at high risk for diabetes. One area where metformin has found use is in treating overweight women with the polycystic ovary syndrome, where the modest weight loss may contribute to increased fertility and reduced insulin resistance [51].

Pramlintide

Amylin is a peptide found in the β cell of the pancreas that is co-secreted along with insulin to circulate in the blood. Both amylin and insulin are deficient in type 1 diabetics where β cells are immunologically destroyed. Pramlintide, a synthetic amylin analog, has a prolonged biologic half-life [52]. It is approved by the US FDA for the treatment of diabetes. Unlike insulin and many other diabetic medications, pramlintide is associated with weight loss. In a study in which 651 subjects with type 1 diabetes were randomized to placebo or subcutaneous pramlintide 60 μg three or four times a day along with an insulin injection, the hemoglobin A1c decreased 0.29–0.34% and weight decreased −1.2 kg relative to placebo [53]. Maggs and colleagues analyzed the data from two 1-year studies in insulin-treated type 2 diabetic subjects randomized to pramlintide 120 μg twice a day or 150 μg three times a day [54]. Weight decreased by −2.6 kg and hemoglobin A1c decreased 0.5%. When weight loss was then analyzed by ethnic group, African-Americans lost −4 kg, Caucasians lost −2.4 kg, and Hispanics lost −2.3 kg, and the improvement in diabetes correlated with the weight loss, suggesting that pramlintide is effective in ethnic groups with the greatest burden from overweight. The most common adverse event was nausea, which was usually mild and confined to the first 4 weeks of therapy.

Exenatide

Glucagon-like peptide-1 (GLP-1) is derived from the processing of the proglucagon peptide, which is secreted by L-cells in the terminal ileum in response to a meal. Increased GLP-1 inhibits glucagon secretion, stimulates insulin secretion, stimulates gluconeogenesis, and delays gastric emptying [55]. It has been postulated to be responsible for the superior weight loss and superior improvement in diabetes seen after gastric bypass surgery for overweight [56,57]. GLP-1 is rapidly degraded by dipeptidyl peptidase-4 (DPP-4), an enzyme that is elevated in the obese. Bypass operations for overweight increase GLP-1, but do not change the levels of DPP-4 [52,58].

Exenatide (Exendin-4) is a 39-amino acid peptide that is produced in the salivary gland of the Gila monster lizard. It has 53% homology with GLP-1, but it has a much longer half-life. Exenatide decreases food intake and body weight gain in Zucker rats while lowering HbA1c [59]. It also increases β cell mass to a greater extent than would be expected for the degree of insulin resistance [60]. Exendin-4 induces satiety and weight loss in Zucker rats with peripheral administration and crosses the blood–brain barrier to act in the central nervous system [61,62]. Exenatide is approved by the US FDA for treatment of type 2

diabetics who are inadequately controlled on either metformin or sulfonylureas.

In human beings, exenatide reduces fasting and postprandial glucose levels, slows gastric emptying, and decreases food intake by 19% [63]. The side-effects of exenatide in humans are headache, nausea, and vomiting that are lessened by gradual dose escalation [64]. Several clinical trials of 30-week duration have been reported using exenatide at 10 μg subcutaneously per day or a placebo [65–67]. In one trial with 377 type 2 diabetic subjects who were failing maximal sulfonylurea therapy, exenatide produced a fall of 0.74% more in HbA1c than placebo. Fasting glucose also decreased and there was a progressive weight loss of 1.6 kg [67]. The interesting feature of this weight loss is that it occurred without lifestyle change, diet or exercise. In a 26-week randomized control trial, exenatide produced a −2.3 kg weight loss compared to a gain of +1.8 kg in the group receiving insulin glargine [68].

Drugs in clinical trial

Serotonin 2C receptor agonists

Mice lacking the 5HT-2C receptor have increased food intake, because they take longer to be satiated. These mice also are resistant to fenfluramine, a serotonin agonist that causes weight loss. A human mutation of the 5HT-2C receptor is associated with early-onset increases in human body weight [69,70]. The precursor of serotonin, 5-hydroxytryptophan, reduces food intake and body weight in clinical studies [71,72]. Fenfluramine [73,74] and dexfenfluramine [75], two drugs that act on the serotonin system but were withdrawn from the market in 1997 due to cardiovascular side-effects, also reduce food intake in human studies. Meta-chlorophenylpiperazine, a direct serotonin agonist, reduces food intake by 28% in women and 20% in men [76]. Another serotoninergic drug, sumatriptan, which acts on the 5-HT1B/1D receptor, also reduced food intake in human subjects [77].

The robust effects of agonists toward the HT-2C receptors in suppressing food intake have stimulated the development of several new compounds. Only one of these has advanced to formal clinical trials. The results of a phase II dose-ranging study for lorcaserin have been presented. A total of 459 male and female subjects with a BMI between 29 and 46 kg/m^2 with an average weight of 100 kg were enrolled in a randomized, double-blind controlled trial comparing placebo against 10 and 15 mg given once daily and 10 mg given twice daily (20 mg/d). During the 12 weeks of the trial the placebo group lost −0.32 kg (88 completers) compared to −1.8 kg in the 10 mg/d dose given once daily (86 completers), −2.6 kg in the 15 mg/d dose (82 completers), and −3.6 kg in the 10 mg twice daily dose (20 mg total) (77 completers). Side-effects that were higher in the active treatment groups than in the placebo group were headache, nausea, dizziness, vomiting, and dry mouth. No cardiac valvular changes were noted [78]. Additional clinical trials are under way.

Cetilistat, a pancreatic lipase inhibitor

Although orlistat, a lipase inhibitor, is already approved for the treatment of overweight, cetilistat, another gastrointestinal lipase inhibitor, is also in development. A 5-day trial of cetilistat in 90 normal volunteers was conducted on an inpatient unit. There was a 3–7-fold increase in fecal fat that was dose dependent, but only 11% of subjects had more than one oily stool. It was suggested that this lipase inhibitor may have fewer gastrointestinal adverse events compared to orlistat [79,80]. A 12-week randomized double-blind clinical trial of cetilistat showed a significantly greater decrease in body weight with cetilistat than placebo (4.1 kg versus 2.4 kg, 120 mg tid). Weight loss with cetilistat was similar to orlistat, but there were fewer gastrointestinal side-effects with cetilistat.

Combinations of drugs that produce weight loss

The first important clinical trial combining drugs that acted by separate mechanisms used phentermine and fenfluramine [81]. This trial showed a highly significant weight loss of nearly 15% below baseline with fewer side-effects by using combination therapy. This combination became very popular [82] but due to reports of aortic valvular regurgitation associated with its use, fenfluramine was withdrawn from the market worldwide in September 1997 [83].

Several other combinations of existing drugs are now under development. One of these is the combination of phentermine with topiramate (Qnexa) with which weight losses of over 10 kg have been reported. A second is a combination of phentermine with zonisamide. A third is the combination of naltrexone with bupropion with which additive weight loss has been noted. Initial data have been published on all these combinations, but longer-term studies are needed to evaluate the potential drug–drug interactions and side-effects produced.

Drugs that increase energy expenditure

There are no effective drugs in this class, although several different molecules have been tested. Most of the early candidates were developed using receptors from experimental animals. When the human β3 receptor was cloned, it was sufficiently different that a new class of compounds were synthesized. The most recent of these molecules developed against the human β3 receptors is a Takeda compound (TAK-677; also AJ-9677 {[3-[(2R)-3-chlorophenyl)-2-hydroxyethyl]propyl]-1*H*-indol-7-yloxy]-acetic acid)}. Although developed against the human receptor, the drug was found to reduce body weight and glucose in experimental animals and to increase uncoupling protein-1 (UCP-1).

A clinical trial with this compound enrolled 65 obese men and women (BMI 33.9 ± 2.1 kg/m^2) in a double-blind randomized placebo-controlled trial lasting 28 days, with subjects assigned to placebo, 0.1 or 0.5 mg twice daily. There was a significant increase in heart rate with the 0.5 mg dose. RMR increased progressively in the treated group, rising by about 7% in the 0.5 mg bid dose and 3% in the 0.1 mg bid dose compared to placebo. There was an acute rise in RMR and pulse rate that was related to plasma levels of TAK-677. Free fatty acids in the plasma also increased with the higher dose of TAK-677. There was no significant change in body weight or body fat during treatment [84].

Which drug to use and when

After the appropriate evaluation and conclusion that a child or adolescent should be treated, the options available should be discussed with the child/adolescent and parent(s). Diet, exercise and lifestyle changes are the first line of treatment. When this has been tried with diligence, and the child/adolescent has failed to respond adequately, the more rigorous therapy of medication can be considered. For individuals who are still expected to gain more height, I dislike using a medication that may slow weight gain for the potential effects it might have on height growth. I thus tend to delay until height growth is complete. For adolescents in whom this is the case, orlistat and sibutramine are the most widely available agents, and both have been shown to be effective in adolescents. Because of the side-effects of orlistat that might become a major embarrassment to an adolescent, I would be inclined to begin therapy with sibutramine.

Conclusion

There are presently comparatively few drugs available for the treatment of overweight patients, and their effectiveness is limited to palliation of the chronic disease of obesity. However, drug development that is now under way is more rapid than in the past, and we anticipate the discovery of safe and effective pharmacologic strategies for the management of obesity and its very serious complications.

Duality of interest statement
The author has received research support from Merck, and has served as a consultant to Sanofi-Aventis, Merck, Schering-Plough, Eli Lilly, Amgen, and Amylin.

References

1. World Health Organization. *Obesity: Preventing and Managing the Global Epidemic.* Geneva: World Health Organization, 1998.
2. NHLBI Obesity Education Initiative Expert Panel on the Identification, Evaluation, and Treatment of Overweight and Obesity in Adults. Clinical guidelines on the identification, evaluation, and treatment of overweight and obesity in adults – the evidence report. Obes Res 1998;6(suppl 2):51S–209S.

3. Ogden CL, Yanovski SZ, Carroll MD, Flegal KM. The epidemiology of obesity. Gastroenterology 2007;132(6):2087–102.

4. Bray GA. *The Metabolic Syndrome and Obesity*. Totowa, NJ: Humana Press, 2007.

5. Padwal R, Li SK, Lau DC. Long-term pharmacotherapy for overweight and obesity: a systematic review and meta-analysis of randomized controlled trials. Int J Obes 2003;27(12):1437–46.

6. Shekelle PG, Hardy ML, Morton SC, et al. Efficacy and safety of ephedra and ephedrine for weight loss and athletic performance: a meta-analysis. JAMA 2003;289(12):1537–45.

7. Li Z, Maglione M, Tu W, et al. Meta-analysis: pharmacologic treatment of obesity. Ann Intern Med 2005;142(7):532–46.

8. Bray G, Greenway F. Pharmacological treatment of the overweight patient. Pharmacol Rev 2007;59:151–84.

9. Bray GA, Greenway FL. Current and potential drugs for treatment of obesity. Endocr Rev 1999;20(6):805–75.

10. Bray GA, Ryan DH. Drug treatment of the overweight patient. Gastroenterology 2007;132 (6):2239–52.

11. Shekelle PG, Morton SC, Maglione M, et al. Pharmacological and surgical treatment of obesity. Evid Rep Technol Assess (Summ) 2004;103:1–6.

12. Avenell A, Brown TJ, McGee MA, et al. What interventions should we add to weight reducing diets in adults with obesity? A systematic review of randomized controlled trials of adding drug therapy, exercise, behaviour therapy or combinations of these interventions. J Hum Nutr Diet 2004;17(4):293–316.

13. Smith IG, Goulder MA. Randomized placebo-controlled trial of long-term treatment with sibutramine in mild to moderate obesity. J Fam Pract 2001;50(6):505–12.

14. Apfelbaum M, Vague P, Ziegler O, Hanotin C, Thomas F, Leutenegger E. Long-term maintenance of weight loss after a very-low-calorie diet: a randomized blinded trial of the efficacy and tolerability of sibutramine. Am J Med 1999;106(2):179–84.

15. James WP, Astrup A, Finer N, et al. Effect of sibutramine on weight maintenance after weight loss: a randomised trial. STORM Study Group. Sibutramine Trial of Obesity Reduction and Maintenance. Lancet 2000;356(9248):2119–25.

16. Wirth A, Krause J. Long-term weight loss with sibutramine: a randomized controlled trial. JAMA 2001;286(11):1331–9.

17. McMahon FG, Fujioka K, Singh BN, et al. Efficacy and safety of sibutramine in obese white and African American patients with hypertension: a 1-year, double-blind, placebo-controlled, multicenter trial. Arch Intern Med 2000;160(14):2185–91.

18. Fujioka K, Seaton TB, Rowe E, et al, for the Sibutramine/Diabetes Clinical Study Group. Weight loss with sibutramine improves glycaemic control and other metabolic parameters in obese patients with type 2 diabetes mellitus. Diabetes Obes Metab 2000;2(3):175–87.

19. Berkowitz RI, Wadden TA, Tershakovec AM, Cronquist JL. Behavior therapy and sibutramine for the treatment of adolescent obesity: a randomized controlled trial. JAMA 2003;289(14):1805–12.

20. Godoy-Matos A, Carraro L, Vieira A, et al. Treatment of obese adolescents with sibutramine: a randomized, double-blind, controlled study. J Clin Endocrinol Metab 2005;90(3):1460–5.

21. Berkowitz RI, Fujioka K, Daniels SR, et al, for the Sibutramine Adolescent Study Group. Effects of sibutramine treatment in obese adolescents: a randomized trial. Ann Intern Med 2006;145(2):81–90.

22. Daniels SR, Arnett DK, Eckel RH, et al. Overweight in children and adolescents: pathophysiology, consequences, prevention, and treatment. Circulation 2005;111(15):1999–2012.

23. Wadden TA, Berkowitz RI, Womble LG, et al. Randomized trial of lifestyle modification and pharmacotherapy for obesity. N Engl J Med 2005;353(20):2111–20.

24. Sjostrom L, Rissanen A, Andersen T, et al. Randomised placebo-controlled trial of orlistat for weight loss and prevention of weight regain in obese patients. European Multicentre Orlistat Study Group. Lancet 1998;352(9123):167–72.

25. Davidson MH, Hauptman J, DiGirolamo M, et al. Weight control and risk factor reduction in obese subjects treated for 2 years with orlistat: a randomized controlled trial. JAMA 1999;281(3):235–42.

26. Rossner S, Sjostrom L, Noack R, Meinders AE, Noseda G. Weight loss, weight maintenance, and improved cardiovascular risk factors after 2 years treatment with orlistat for obesity. European Orlistat Obesity Study Group. Obes Res 2000;8(1):49–61.

27. Hauptman J. Orlistat: selective inhibition of caloric absorption can affect long-term body weight. Endocrine 2000;13:201–6.

28. Torgerson JS, Hauptman J, Boldrin MN, Sjostrom L. XENical in the prevention of diabetes in obese subjects (XENDOS) study: a randomized study of orlistat as an adjunct to lifestyle changes for the prevention of type 2 diabetes in obese patients. Diabetes Care 2004;27(1):155–61.

29. Chanoine JP, Hampl S, Jensen C, Boldrin M, Hauptman J. Effect of orlistat on weight and body composition in obese adolescents: a randomized controlled trial. JAMA 2005;293(23):2873–83.

30. Hollander PA, Elbein SC, Hirsch IB, et al. Role of orlistat in the treatment of obese patients with type 2 diabetes. A 1-year randomized double-blind study. Diabetes Care 1998;21(8):1288–94.

31. Kelley DE, Bray GA, Pi-Sunyer FX, Klein S, Hill J, Miles J, Hollander P. Clinical efficacy of orlistat therapy in overweight and obese patients with insulin-treated type 2 diabetes: a 1-year randomized controlled trial. Diabetes Care 2002;25(6):1033–41.

32. Miles JM, Leiter L, Hollander P, et al. Effect of orlistat in overweight and obese patients with type 2 diabetes treated with metformin. Diabetes Care 2002;25(7):1123–8.

33. Heymsfield SB, Segal KR, Hauptman J, et al. Effects of weight loss with orlistat on glucose tolerance and progression to type 2 diabetes in obese adults. Arch Intern Med 2000;160(9):1321–6.

34. Zhi J, Mulligan TE, Hauptman JB. Long-term systemic exposure of orlistat, a lipase inhibitor, and its metabolites in obese patients. J Clin Pharmacol 1999;39(1):41–6.

35. Wadden TA, Berkowitz RI, Womble LG, Sarwer DB, Arnold ME, Steinberg CM. Effects of sibutramine plus orlistat in obese women following 1 year of treatment by sibutramine alone: a placebo-controlled trial. Obes Res 2000;8(6):431–7.

36. Lawton CL, Wales JK, Hill AJ, Blundell JE. Serotoninergic manipulation, meal-induced satiety and eating pattern: effect of fluoxetine in obese female subjects. Obes Res 1995;3(4):345–56.

37. Goldstein DJ, Rampey AH Jr, Roback PJ, et al. Efficacy and safety of long-term fluoxetine treatment of obesity – maximizing success. Obes Res 1995;3(suppl 4):481S–90S.

38. Gadde KM, Parker CB, Maner LG, et al. Bupropion for weight loss: an investigation of efficacy and tolerability in overweight and obese women. Obes Res 2001;9(9):544–51.

39. Jain AK, Kaplan RA, Gadde KM, et al. Bupropion SR vs. placebo for weight loss in obese patients with depressive symptoms. Obes Res 2002;10(10):1049–56.

40. Anderson JW, Greenway FL, Fujioka K, Gadde KM, McKenney J, O'Neil PM. Bupropion SR enhances weight loss: a 48-week double-blind, placebo-controlled trial. Obes Res 2002;10(7):633–41.

41. Astrup A, Toubro S. Topiramate: a new potential pharmacological treatment for obesity. Obes Res 2004;12(suppl):167S–73S.

42. Ben-Menachem E, Axelsen M, Johanson EH, Stagge A, Smith U. Predictors of weight loss in adults with topiramate-treated epilepsy. Obes Res 2003;11(4):556–62.

43. Bray GA, Hollander P, Klein S, Kushner R, Levy B, Fitchet M, Perry BH. A 6-month randomized, placebo-controlled, dose-ranging trial of topiramate for weight loss in obesity. Obes Res 2003;11(6): 722–33.

44. Wilding J, van Gaal L, Rissanen A, Vercruysse F, Fitchet M. A randomized double-blind placebo-controlled study of the long-term efficacy and safety of topiramate in the treatment of obese subjects. Int J Obes 2004;28(11):1399–410.

45. Astrup A, Caterson I, Zelissen P, et al. Topiramate: long-term maintenance of weight loss induced by a low-calorie diet in obese subjects. Obes Res 2004;12(10):1658–69.

46. Gadde KM, Franciscy DM, Wagner HR 2nd, Krishnan KR. Zonisamide for weight loss in obese adults: a randomized controlled trial. JAMA 2003;289(14):1820–5.

47. Devinsky O, Vuong A, Hammer A, Barrett PS. Stable weight during lamotrigine therapy: a review of 32 studies. Neurology 2000;54(4): 973–5.

48. Merideth CH. A single-center, double-blind, placebo-controlled evaluation of lamotrigine in the treatment of obesity in adults. J Clin Psychiatry 2006;67(2):258–62.

49. Fontbonne A, Charles MA, Juhan-Vague I, et al. The effect of metformin on the metabolic abnormalities associated with upper-body fat distribution. BIGPRO Study Group. Diabetes Care 1996;19(9): 920–6.

50. Knowler WC, Barrett-Connor E, Fowler SE, et al, for the Diabetes Prevention Program Research Group. Reduction in the incidence of type 2 diabetes with lifestyle intervention or metformin. N Engl J Med 2002;346(6):393–403.

51. Ortega-Gonzalez C, Luna S, Hernandez L, et al. Responses of serum androgen and insulin resistance to metformin and pioglitazone in obese, insulin-resistant women with polycystic ovary syndrome. J Clin Endocrinol Metab 2005;90(3):1360–5.

52. Riddle MC, Drucker DJ. Emerging therapies mimicking the effects of amylin and glucagon-like peptide 1. Diabetes Care 2006; 29(2):435–49.

53. Ratner RE, Dickey R, Fineman M, et al. Amylin replacement with pramlintide as an adjunct to insulin therapy improves long-term glycaemic and weight control in Type 1 diabetes mellitus: a 1-year, randomized controlled trial. Diabet Med 2004;21(11): 1204–12.

54. Maggs D, Shen L, Strobel S, Brown D, Kolterman O, Weyer C. Effect of pramlintide on A1C and body weight in insulin-treated African Americans and Hispanics with type 2 diabetes: a pooled post hoc analysis. Metabolism 2003;52(12):1638–42.

55. Patriti A, Facchiano E, Sanna A, Gulla N, Donini A. The enteroinsular axis and the recovery from type 2 diabetes after bariatric surgery. Obes Surg 2004;14(6):840–8.

56. Small CJ, Bloom SR. Gut hormones as peripheral anti obesity targets. Curr Drug Targets CNS Neurol Disord 2004;3(5):379–88.

57. Greenway SE, Greenway FL 3rd, Klein S. Effects of obesity surgery on non-insulin-dependent diabetes mellitus. Arch Surg 2002; 137(10):1109–17.

58. Lugari R, Dei Cas A, Ugolotti D, et al. Glucagon-like peptide 1 (GLP-1) secretion and plasma dipeptidyl peptidase IV (DPP-IV) activity in morbidly obese patients undergoing biliopancreatic diversion. Horm Metab Res 2004;36(2):111–15.

59. Szayna M, Doyle ME, Betkey JA, et al. Exendin-4 decelerates food intake, weight gain, and fat deposition in Zucker rats. Endocrinology 2000;141(6):1936–41.

60. Gedulin BR, Nikoulina SE, Smith PA, et al. Exenatide (exendin-4) improves insulin sensitivity and beta-cell mass in insulin-resistant obese fa/fa Zucker rats independent of glycemia and body weight. Endocrinology 2005;146(4):2069–76.

61. Rodriquez de Fonseca F, Navarro M, Alvarez E, et al. Peripheral versus central effects of glucagon-like peptide-1 receptor agonists on satiety and body weight loss in Zucker obese rats. Metabolism 2000;49(6):709–17.

62. Kastin AJ, Akerstrom V. Entry of exendin-4 into brain is rapid but may be limited at high doses. Int J Obes 2003;27(3):313–18.

63. Edwards CM, Stanley SA, Davis R, et al. Exendin-4 reduces fasting and postprandial glucose and decreases energy intake in healthy volunteers. Am J Physiol Endocrinol Metab 2001;281(1):E155–61.

64. Fineman MS, Shen LZ, Taylor K, Kim DD, Baron AD. Effectiveness of progressive dose-escalation of exenatide (exendin-4) in reducing dose-limiting side effects in subjects with type 2 diabetes. Diabetes Metab Res Rev 2004;20(5):411–17.

65. DeFronzo RA, Ratner RE, Han J, Kim DD, Fineman MS, Baron AD. Effects of exenatide (exendin-4) on glycemic control and weight over 30 weeks in metformin-treated patients with type 2 diabetes. Diabetes Care 2005;28(5):1092–100.

66. Kendall DM, Riddle MC, Rosenstock J, et al. Effects of exenatide (exendin-4) on glycemic control over 30 weeks in patients with type 2 diabetes treated with metformin and a sulfonylurea. Diabetes Care 2005;28(5):1083–91.

67. Buse JB, Henry RR, Han J, Kim DD, Fineman MS, Baron AD. Effects of exenatide (exendin-4) on glycemic control over 30 weeks in sulfonylurea-treated patients with type 2 diabetes. Diabetes Care 2004;27(11):2628–35.

68. Heine RJ, van Gaal LF, Johns D, Mihm MJ, Widel MH, Brodows RG. Exenatide versus insulin glargine in patients with suboptimally controlled type 2 diabetes: a randomized trial. Ann Intern Med 2005; 143(8):559–69.

69. Gibson WT, Ebersole BJ, Bhattacharyya S, et al. Mutational analysis of the serotonin receptor 5HT2c in severe early-onset human obesity. Can J Physiol Pharmacol 2004;82(6):426–9.

70. Nilsson BM. 5-Hydroxytryptamine 2C (5-HT2C) receptor agonists as potential antiobesity agents. J Med Chem 2006;49(14):4023–34.

71. Cangiano C, Ceci F, Cascino A, et al. Eating behavior and adherence to dietary prescriptions in obese adult subjects treated with 5-hydroxytryptophan. Am J Clin Nutr 1992;56(5):863–7.

72. Cangiano C, Laviano A, del Ben M, et al. Effects of oral 5-hydroxytryptophan on energy intake and macronutrient selection in non-insulin dependent diabetic patients. Int J Obes 1998;22(7):648–54.

73. Rogers PJ, Blundell JE. Effect of anorexic drugs on food intake and the micro-structure of eating in human subjects. Psychopharmacology (Berl) 1979;66(2):159–65.

74. Foltin RW, Haney M, Comer SD, Fischman MW. Effect of fenfluramine on food intake, mood, and performance of humans living in a residential laboratory. Physiol Behav 1996;59(2):295–305.

75. Drent ML, Zelissen PM, Koppeschaar HP, et al. The effect of dexfenfluramine on eating habits in a Dutch ambulatory android overweight population with an overconsumption of snacks. Int J Obes 1995;19(5):299–304.

76. Walsh AE, Smith KA, Oldman AD, Williams C, Goodall EM, Cowen PJ. M-Chlorophenylpiperazine decreases food intake in a test meal. Psychopharmacology (Berl) 1994;116:120–2.

77. Boeles S, Williams C, Campling GM, Goodall EM, Cowen PJ. Sumatriptan decreases food intake and increases plasma growth hormone in healthy women. Psychopharmacology (Berl) 1997; 129(2):179–82.

78. Smith SR, Prosser W, Donahue D, Anderson CE, Shanahan W. APD356, an orally-active selective 5-HT2C agonist, reduces body weight in obese men and women: a randomized, placebo-controlled trial. Diabetes Metab 2006;55(suppl 1):A80.

79. Dunk C, Enunwa M, de la Monte S, Palmer R. Increased fecal fat excretion in normal volunteers treated with lipase inhibitor ATL-962. Int J Obes 2002;26(suppl):S135.

80. Kopelman P, Bryson A, Hickling R, et al. Cetilistat (ATL-962), a novel lipase inhibitor: a 12-week randomized, placebo-controlled study of weight reduction in obese patients. Int J Obes 2007; 31(3):494–9.

81. Weintraub M. Long-term weight control: the National Heart, Lung, and Blood Institute funded multimodal intervention study. Clin Pharmacol Ther 1992;51(5):581–5.

82. Stafford RS, Radley DC. National trends in antiobesity medication use. Arch Intern Med 2003;163(9):1046–50.

83. Connolly HM, Crary JL, McGoon MD, et al. Valvular heart disease associated with fenfluramine-phentermine. N Engl J Med 1997; 337(9):581–8.

84. Redman LM, de Jonge L, Fang X, et al. Lack of an effect of a novel beta-3-adrenoceptor agonist, TAK-677, on energy metabolism in obese individuals: a double-blind, placebo-controlled randomized study. J Clin Endocrinol Metab 2007;92(2):527–31.

25 The Management of Obesity: Surgery

Paul E. O'Brien and John B. Dixon

Centre for Obesity Research and Education, Monash University, Melbourne, Australia

Introduction

As obesity becomes identified as the most significant pathogen in the developed world and as obesity-related disease now challenges smoking as the principal contributor to premature death, seeking an effective solution to the obesity epidemic represents our greatest current public health challenge. Prevention is clearly the optimal goal but, with current data indicating progression of the epidemic, effective preventive programs that will impact on the broad community problem are still to come.

Currently there is no nonsurgical method for predictably achieving major weight loss in the obese and maintaining that weight loss for an extended period. Current programs involving diet, behavioral modification, exercise and activity, with or without drug supplementation, are able, at best, to achieve a modest weight loss which is generally sustained only for the duration of the program [1].

In a randomized controlled trial, optimal medical therapy was compared with the bariatric surgical procedure of laparoscopic adjustable gastric banding (LAGB) (Lap-Band, Allergan Health, Irvine, CA) in 80 mild to moderately obese adults over a 24-month period [2]. The surgical group showed significantly greater weight loss, with 22% of initial weight lost and 85% of their excess weight lost compared with the medical group who had 5.5% of their initial weight and 22% of their excess weight lost. There was a greater reduction in the metabolic syndrome in the surgical group (38% to 3%) compared with the nonsurgical group (38% to 24%) with greater improvement in quality of life. There was no difference in the frequency of adverse events.

Surgical methods have been known to achieve substantial and durable weight loss for half a century and yet they have not achieved a significant impact on community health. Only a small fraction of the obese has been prepared to seek the surgical approach to their problem because of the risk of death or complications, the invasiveness and the costs. With the introduction of new techniques, in particular LAGB, and with the application of minimally invasive approaches to all forms of obesity surgery, it is timely to review the range of surgical options and their potential strengths and weaknesses.

The evolution of surgical technique

The initial phase (1950–1970): small bowel bypass

Surgical management of obesity began with the introduction of the jejunoileal bypass (JIB) in the 1950s. In this procedure the proximal jejunum was diverted to the distal part of the gut, leaving a long segment of excluded small intestine and a marked reduction in absorptive capacity. Many variations existed. A typical pattern is shown in Figure 25.1 in which the proximal 35 cm of proximal jejunum was joined end-to-side to the last 10 cm of ileum. The JIB procedure represented the best and the worst of bariatric surgery. Major and sustained weight loss was achieved and there were impressive health benefits, particularly in relation to lipid metabolism. However, it caused serious problems including copious offensive diarrhea, electrolyte imbalances, oxalate calculi in the kidneys and progressive hepatic fibrosis with eventual liver failure and for these reasons was generally abandoned during the 1970s in favor of stomach stapling procedures [3–7].

The middle phase (1970–1990): stomach stapling

The Roux-en-Y gastric bypass (RYGB) operation was introduced by Edward Mason in 1960 [8]. In this procedure the stomach was completely partitioned into a small upper gastric pouch, draining into a Roux-en-Y limb of proximal jejunum of variable length from 40 to 150 cm, and a distal excluded stomach (Fig. 25.2). This procedure provided a hybrid between the malabsorptive approach of JIB and later, more purely restrictive, operations. It has undergone various modifications over the subsequent 40 years and still

Clinical Obesity in Adults and Children, 3rd edition. Edited by Peter G. Kopelman, Ian D. Caterson and William H. Dietz.
© 2010 Blackwell Publishing, ISBN: 978-1-4051-8226-3.

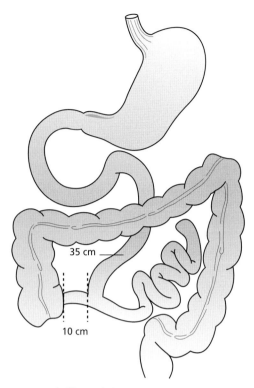

Figure 25.1 Jejunoileal bypass (JIB).

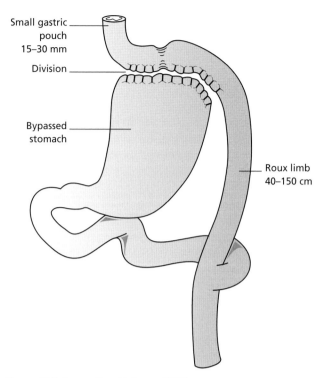

Figure 25.2 Roux-en-Y gastric bypass (RYGB).

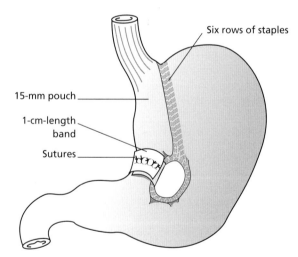

Figure 25.3 Vertical banded gastroplasty (VBG).

serves us well as an effective antiobesity operation. However, its drawbacks of perioperative deaths and significant perioperative and late morbidity, although markedly less threatening than those of JIB, have nevertheless been sufficient to cause most of the obese to stay away.

Dr Mason and his colleague Dr Printen then introduced a purely restrictive operation of gastroplasty in 1973 [9]. The procedure involves partitioning the stomach into a small upper pouch draining through a narrow stoma into the remainder of the stomach. Numerous variations of this procedure have followed, the most significant variant being the vertical banded gastroplasty (VBG) which was first described by Dr Mason in 1982 [10] and is shown in Figure 25.3. It was hoped that this group of operations would provide greater short- and long-term safety and yet retain the power of gastric bypass. Unfortunately, both randomized controlled trials and observational studies have consistently shown that it has failed in both aspirations [11–14].

In the meantime there was a resurgence of malabsorptive surgery with Italian surgeon, Nicola Scopinaro, introducing the biliopancreatic diversion procedure (BPD) [15]. This too has undergone change with time and experience. The basic procedure involves distal gastrectomy, leaving a proximal pouch of 200–500 mL, a 200 cm length of terminal ileum anastomosed to the gastric pouch and the biliopancreatic limb entering at 50 cm from the ileocecal valve (Fig. 25.4) [16]. The most notable remodeling of the procedure is the so-called duodenal switch variant (BPD-DS) proposed by Marceau's group in 1995 [17], in which a

longitudinal gastrectomy enabled retention of the gastric antrum with, hopefully, controlled gastric emptying, and the ileal limb was anastomosed to the proximal duodenum (Fig 25.5). The benefit of this variation remains controversial.

The current phase (1990–present): minimally invasive and adjustable procedures

This phase is characterized by the advent of the LAGB with the particular features of minimal anatomic disturbance,

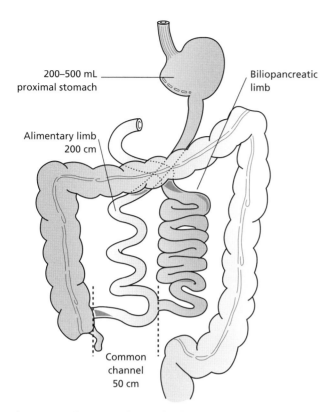

Figure 25.4 Biliopancreatic diversion (BPD).

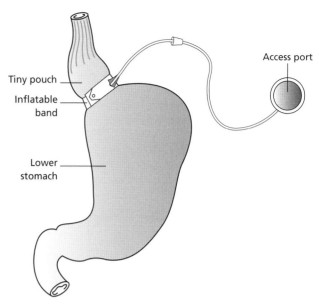

Figure 25.6 Laparoscopic adjustable gastric band (LAGB).

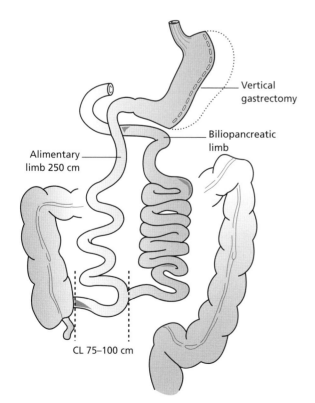

Figure 25.5 Biliopancreatic diversion with duodenal switch (BPD-DS).

adjustability and potential reversibility [18,19]. Also there has been the introduction of a laparoscopic approach to gastric bypass [20] and biliopancreatic diversion [21].

Adjustable gastric banding had first been proposed by two Austrian surgical researchers, Szinicz and Schnapka, in 1982 [22]. The idea was brought into clinical practice by Lubomyr Kusmak in 1986 [23] but did not attract major interest until the the technology that enabled the performance of complex laparoscopic surgical procedures became widespread in the early 1990s. The BioEnterics® Lap-Band® system (LAGB) was specifically designed for laparoscopic placement and was introduced into clinical practice by Mitiku Belachew from Huy, Belgium, in September 1993 (Fig. 25.6). Because of the dual attractions of a controlled level of effect through adjustability and of laparoscopic placement without resection of gut or anastomoses, this has rapidly become the dominant bariatric procedure in all regions of the developed world except, thus far, the USA, where its introduction was delayed by regulatory requirements until June 2001.

Overview of outcomes from bariatric procedures

The most important single outcome in treating obesity is improvement in health. Second, we seek improvement in quality of life. Measuring weight loss itself is inappropriate as a single endpoint. It is measuring the means to the end. Without improvement in the co-morbidities of obesity, the achieving of weight loss is not relevant to community healthcare. However, by tradition, weight loss has been and currently remains the first parameter that is examined and reported. We will stay with this tradition by first reviewing the effectiveness of bariatric surgical procedures in

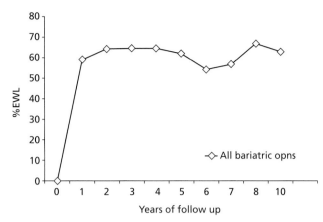

Figure 25.7 Pooled data of %EWL from a systematic review of all bariatric surgical procedures which included an experience of 100 or more patients and at least 3 years of follow-up. (Reproduced with permission from O'Brien et al. [24].)

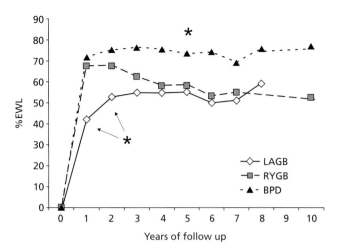

Figure 25.8 %EWL for RYGB, LAGB and BPD from the systematic review. The asterisks indicate a significant difference (p < 0.05). (Reproduced with permission from O'Brien et al. [24].)

causing weight loss and then reviewing the effects on health and quality of life.

Weight loss outcomes from bariatric surgery

Weight loss can be described in different ways, each of which has its advantages and drawbacks. In bariatric surgery % of excess weight lost (%EWL) remains the most common method. For a Caucasian population, excess weight is that weight above Body Mass Index (BMI) of 25. Absolute weight change (in kg or BMI units or % of weight lost) fails to recognize the significance of initial weight as a variable in estimating or comparing effects. Percent of BMI lost (%EBL) is arguably the most relevant to health status and may become preferred but currently lacks broad usage. Most reports provide %EWL, thus allowing comparison between studies.

Reports of short-term weight loss are not relevant when assessing a long-term effect. Ideally, weight loss as an outcome of bariatric surgery should not be considered at less than 5 years follow-up. However, there are surprisingly few reports that can provide such data. In a recent systematic review [24], we restricted our examination to those reports that have included at least 100 patients and that provide at least 3 years of follow-up data, expressing the outcome in the terms of %EWL. Figure 25.7 shows the %EWL over a 10 year follow-up after pooling all bariatric procedures. Figure 25.8 shows the specific patterns of weight loss over the first 10 years for RYGB, LAGB and BPD.

A number of significant observations can be drawn from these figures.
• All the current surgical procedures result in major weight loss with mean values of between 50% and 80% of excess weight lost.
• Biliopancreatic diversion appears to produce the most weight loss and although there are only a small number of reports, these reports indicate a durable effect well beyond 5 years.
• Gastric stapling procedures show good initial weight loss at 1 and 2 years followed by a fading effect clearly evident by 5 years. Interestingly, for a group of operations which have been in use

for more than 30 years and for which there are numerous publications, we could find only three reports which give outcome data beyond 5 years.
• Laparoscopic adjustable gastric banding generates weight loss more slowly than the other procedures but is as effective as gastric stapling procedures at 4 and 5 years (see Fig. 25.8). The adjustability is expected to allow maintenance of the weight loss over a longer period than the nonadjustable gastric stapling operations. As the LAGB procedures were only introduced in 1993, demonstration of the durability of weight loss will take more time.

Changes in health after bariatric surgery

Obesity generates a wide range of illnesses, to the point where it could now reasonably be regarded as the worst pathogen in Western communities. The following is a summary of the changes in a selection of these co-morbidities to illustrate the major health benefits that can be achieved by bariatric surgical procedures. The effects may be achieved through weight loss *per se* or as a result of changes in anatomy and function of the gut.

Type 2 diabetes

Type 2 diabetes mellitus is the paradigm of an obesity-related illness. Multiple studies have documented the benefit achieved by all the current bariatric procedures [25–28]. We have studied 50 patients followed for 1 year after Lap-Band placement [25]. There was a significant improvement in all measures of glucose metabolism with complete remission of diabetes in 32 patients (64%), improvement of control in 13 (26%) and five (10%) were relatively unchanged. Importantly, duration of time with diabetes was a predictor of outcome, indicating that early treatment of obesity is indicated in the newly diagnosed diabetic patient.

On the basis of this time dependency, we recently completed a randomized controlled trial of surgery (Lap-Band) against optimal conventional therapy including very low-energy diets and pharmacotherapy in recently diagnosed (less than 2 years) type 2 diabetes patients [29]. There was remission of diabetes (fasting glucose <7 mmol/L, HbA1c <6.2% while taking no hypoglycemic therapy) in 73% of the surgical group and 13% of the conventional group. The surgical and conventional groups had lost 20.7% and 1.7% of total weight respectively. There were no serious adverse events in either group.

Weight loss protects obese subjects with or without impaired glucose tolerance from the development of diabetes. From a pool of 1300 severely obese subjects whom we have treated by LAGB, 85 patients had impaired fasting glucose. Greater than 90% were found to have normal fasting plasma glucose at 2 years after the operation. For the general community, it is expected that in those with impaired fasting glucose there will be an annual conversion rate to type 2 diabetes of 5–6%. However, none of our patients with insulin resistance have thus far developed diabetes. Furthermore, with a total of more than 4000 patient-years of follow-up of patients without diabetes preoperatively, only a single patient has developed type 2 diabetes. Thus, weight loss following surgery dramatically reduces the risk of developing the disease.

RYGB surgery, the most commonly used procedure in the United States, induces remission of type 2 diabetes in over 80% of cases and appears to have an almost immediate effect on hyperglycemia before significant weight loss has been achieved. The reason(s) for this early effect are likely to be related to the gastrointestinal diversion produced by the bypass procedure. Chyme from the stomach bypasses much of the stomach, duodenum and upper jejunum. Some believe bypass of the duodenum stimulates an incretin effect on the pancreatic β cell stimulating insulin secretion (the foregut hypothesis) [30] and others suggest that the premature delivery of food into the distal small bowel also has an incretin effect, possibly due to glucagon-like peptide-1 secretion from the mucosal L-cells (hindgut hypothesis) [31]. The exact clinical relevance and the durability of this early glycemic control are unknown.

Importantly, the improvement in diabetes following weight loss is related to the dual effects of improvement in insulin sensitivity and pancreatic β cell function [32]. As β cell function deteriorates progressively over time in those with type 2 diabetes, early weight loss intervention should therefore be a central part of initial therapy in severely obese subjects who develop type 2 diabetes. For obese patients with type 2 diabetes, weight loss provides benefit unequaled by any other therapy, and may prove to be the only therapy that substantially changes the natural history of the disease [26,33].

Dyslipidemia of obesity

Increased fasting triglyceride and decreased high-density lipoprotein (HDL)-cholesterol concentrations characterize the dyslipidemia of obesity and insulin resistance [34]. This dyslipidemic pattern is highly atherogenic and the most common pattern associated with coronary artery disease [35]. Weight loss surgery produces substantial decreases in fasting triglyceride levels, an elevation of HDL-cholesterol levels to normal, and improved

total cholesterol to HDL-cholesterol ratio [36–38]. Although elevation of total cholesterol is not a feature of obesity, hypercholesterolemia can be controlled by malabsorptive procedures such as BPD [39] and RYGB [40].

Hypertension

There is evidence of a reduction in both systolic and diastolic blood pressure (BP) following weight loss in association with a bariatric procedure [41]. We have studied the outcome of 147 consecutive hypertensive patients at 12 months after LAGB. Preoperatively, only 17 of these patients had BP within the normal range, all on therapy. Hypertension was present in 130 patients preoperatively; 101 of these were taking antihypertensive medications and the remaining 29 were not on therapy. Mean BP for these patients was 156/97 mmHg prior to surgery.

At 12 months after LAGB, 105 patients had normal BP, 42 remained hypertensive, and only 42 were taking any antihypertensive medication at that time. Mean BP was 127/76 mmHg. From these data, we found that 80 patients (55%) had resolution of the problem (i.e. normal BP and taking no antihypertensive therapy), 45 patients (31%) were improved (less therapy and easier control), and 22 patients (15%) were unchanged [42]. We have demonstrated that the fall in blood pressure is sustained to at least 4 years after surgery but durability of blood pressure reduction over a longer period is uncertain [43].

Ovarian dysfunction, infertility and pregnancy

Obesity, especially central obesity, is associated with ovulatory dysfunction and infertility. In premenopausal women, weight loss significantly reduces active testosterone by reducing total testosterone and increasing the proportion of bound testosterone due to increased sex hormone-binding globulin. This change usually restores normal ovulation and often fertility. Women are advised to use contraception during the very active weight loss phase following LAGB, usually for the first year. However, studies reporting pregnancy after LAGB report unexpected pregnancies in previously infertile women. These studies also report the value of the adjustability of the LAGB, enabling reduction of gastric restriction in early pregnancy to reduce the impact of any hyperemesis and to allow more favorable nutritional conditions for normal fetal development. Weight gain is advised in all pregnancies, with the advised weight gain based on pre-pregnancy BMI. The LAGB provides a mechanism during pregnancy to allow appropriate weight gain, and can be readjusted, if necessary, to prevent excessive weight gain [44]. The Caesarean section rate and the incidence of gestational diabetes and hypertension are also seen to be reduced [45].

Gastroesophageal reflux disease

Gastroesophageal reflux disease (GERD) is more than twice as prevalent in the morbidly obese [46]. Eighty-seven patients who had moderate or severe GERD have been followed for at least 12 months after LAGB. Seventy-three (89%) have had total resolution of the problem, as defined by the absence of symptoms without treatment for the previous month. Preoperative and postoperative pH study and manometry have been performed on 12 of these patients who had severe symptoms preoperatively. The mean DeMeester score was 38 +/− 15 preoperatively and 7.9 +/− 8 at follow-up (p < 0.001). In all but one of these patients symptoms had resolved completely. Others also have demonstrated that a correctly placed LAGB and RYGB both reduce gastroesophageal reflux [47–49].

Symptoms of reflux and heartburn may occur after surgery and indicate obstruction from excessive adjustment or prolapse after LAGB or stomal stenosis after RYGB.

Asthma

There is a positive relationship between asthma and obesity [50]. Certainly, the physiologic changes of obesity on lung function would aggravate asthma. We have reported major improvement, even remission, of asthma following LAGB [51]. Our study demonstrated improvement in all measured aspects of the disease, including symptoms, severity, need for asthma medications (including corticosteroids), and hospital admissions. The asthma severity score fell from 44.5 before operation to 14.3 at 12 months after operation (p < 0.005). It is hypothesized that improved respiratory mechanics and possibly a reduction in gastroesophageal reflux following LAGB may contribute to the improvement in asthma.

Obstructive sleep apnea

A range of sleep disorders is associated with obesity. The most serious of these is obstructive sleep apnea (OSA). Severe obesity is the greatest risk factor for the development of sleep apnea, with a 10-fold increase in prevalence. Excessive daytime sleepiness, a disabling and potentially dangerous condition, is very common in the obese population and is not necessarily related to OSA [52]. There are major improvements in sleep quality, excessive daytime sleepiness, snoring, nocturnal choking, and observed OSA with weight loss following LAGB surgery [53].

Obstructive sleep apnea and other sleep disturbances have been studied in 313 patients prior to LAGB and repeated at 1 year after operation in 123 of the patients. There was a high prevalence of significantly disturbed sleep in both men (59%) and women (45%). Observed sleep apnea was decreased from 33% to 2%, habitual snoring from 82% to 14%, abnormal daytime sleepiness from 39% to 4% and poor sleep quality from 39% to 2%.

Depression

Depression is common in the morbidly obese. Does the presence of obesity cause the person to be depressed or does depression cause the person to eat too much? We have investigated the effect of weight loss induced by LAGB on depression as measured by the Beck Depression Inventory (BDI) [54]. Preoperative BDI on 487 consecutive patients was a mean of 17.7+/− 9.5, a level within the range for moderate depression. Weight loss was associated with a significant and sustained fall in BDI scores with a mean score of 7.8 +/− 6.5 (n = 373) at 1 year after surgery. By 4 years

after surgery, the 134 patients studied had lost 54% of excess weight and had a BDI of 9.6 +/− 7.7. Although a small number remained in the major depressive illness category, the shift of the majority to normal values for BDI strongly indicates that most of the depression of obesity is reactive to the problem of obesity rather than a cause of obesity and is resolved by weight loss.

Changes in quality of life after bariatric surgery

Improvement in quality of life (QOL) is one of the most gratifying outcomes of bariatric surgery. A number of studies clearly demonstrate major QOL improvements following LAGB and other procedures [44,55–58]. We reported a large prospective study of QOL after LAGB, in which we employed the Medical Outcomes Trust Short Form-36 (SF-36). The SF-36 is a reliable, broadly used instrument that has been validated in obese people. In our study, 459 severely obese subjects had lower scores compared with community normal values for all eight aspects of QOL measured, especially the physical health scores. LAGB provided a dramatic and sustained improvement in all measures of the SF-36. Improvement was greater in those with more preoperative disability, and the extent of weight loss was not a good predictor of improved QOL. Mean scores returned to those of community normal values by 1 year after surgery, and remained in the normal range throughout the 4 years of the study. It is significant that patients who required revisional surgery during the follow-up period achieved the same improvement in measures of QOL. Similar improvements in QOL have been demonstrated in patients having LAGB for previously failed gastric stapling [59].

Body image

Studies of appearance orientation and appearance evaluation indicate that the severely obese usually have quite normal pride and investment in their appearance and presentation but they evaluate their appearance as being very poor [60]. Weight loss following LAGB has been shown to produce major improvements in self-evaluation of appearance, although it does not return to community normal levels. The extent of the improvement in appearance is related to the percentage of excess weight loss. The discrepancy between one's pride and investment in appearance and presentation and one's self-evaluation of appearance is lower with weight loss, reducing psychologic stress [60].

The Swedish Obese Subjects (SOS) study

This study is of particular importance because of the large number of patients studied, the long follow-up and the focus on health and survival. It commenced in 1987 with matching of almost 2000 patients seeking obesity surgery with an equal group of severely obese patients who had medical therapy alone. The intention was to follow all patients for at least 10 years. The primary study endpoint was a mortality comparison between the groups and a positive survival advantage for the surgically treated group has recently been demonstrated [61]. There were 129 deaths in the control group and 101 deaths in the surgery group and the hazard ratio adjusted for sex, age, and risk factors was

Table 25.1 Studies of survival benefits of weight loss surgery

Study	Operation	Relative risk	Source of controls
Christou 2004 [82]	RYGB	0.11	Medical
Flum 2004 [83]	RYGB	0.67	Medical
Sjostrom 2007 [61]	Various	0.71	Medical
Favretti 2007 [84]	LAGB	0.38	Medical
Adams 2007 [85]	RYGB	0.40	Community
Peeters 2007 [65]	LAGB	0.28	Community

Box 25.1 Attributes of an ideal bariatric operation

Minimally invasive

Safe

Effective – weight loss, co-morbidities, QOL

Durable – effective over time

Low reoperation rate

Minimal side-effects

Technically feasible

Broadly reversible

Controllable/adjustable

0.71 (p = 0.01). There has been a sustained reduction in the incidence of type 2 diabetes [62] and other cardiovascular risk factors, a reduction in medication needed to treat other cardiovascular risk factors [63], improved health-related quality of life and a reduction in symptoms of depression [64]. Interestingly, there was a return of hypertension after 8 years despite sustained weight loss in the surgical group.

However, the study has several significant weaknesses. It is not a randomized trial and, despite attempts to achieve good matching, there are many significant differences between the groups. Further, gastroplasty, which was the principal surgical procedure used in the study, is now considered obsolete and has been replaced by more effective procedures.

Survival after bariatric surgery

It is now established that bariatric surgery achieves substantial reduction in weight, improvements in many diseases and better quality of life. However, the proof that people live longer as a result has been lacking until recently. There have now been multiple reports, covering a range of bariatric procedures, indicating a survival advantage compared to obese persons who have not had weight loss. The major studies are summarized in Table 25.1. None of the studies was based on a randomization at commencement and none has 100% follow-up. Within those limitations, there is a consistent and generally strong support for a survival benefit.

In Melbourne, 966 patients aged 37–70 who had been treated by LAGB were compared with an obese community group of 2119 persons who were recruited between 1992 and 1994 and who had been followed to June 2005 [65]. There were four deaths in the weight loss cohort and 225 deaths in the control cohort. The weight loss group had a 72% lower hazard of death than the control cohort (hazard ratio (HR) 0.28; 95% confidence interval (CI) 0.10–0.85).

Characteristics of the ideal surgical procedure

Although no alternative treatment for their problem is yet available, very few of the obese in our community are currently seeking surgical treatment. Over the past 10 years, in the USA, an average of less than 80,000 have undergone surgery for weight control each year. On the basis of a prevalence of morbid obesity (BMI > 40) of 8% [66], we can calculate that less than one in 200 of those who have the problem of morbid obesity are seeking a surgical solution each year. Clearly this is not solving a major public health problem and is almost irrelevant in the overall context of treatment strategies. For a surgical treatment of obesity to make an impact, it must become more broadly acceptable to the population at risk.

Box 25.1 lists the characteristics which should be present if surgical treatment is likely to become broadly acceptable.
• Bariatric procedures need to be performed laparoscopically. The patient will require it because they do not want the pain and the scars and the long recuperation. The surgeon will not be able to justify the higher perioperative complication rates.
• They need to be safe, very safe. There should be no "acceptable" level of mortality. Even the 0.5–1.0% that is the norm for RYGB should be regarded as too high.
• It must be effective, not only in achieving weight loss but also improving the co-morbidities of obesity and the quality of life.
• The effects must be durable. They need to last for 5–15 years if they are to be considered worthwhile.
• There should be a low need for revisional surgery. There is no broadly accepted incidence that could be acceptable but possibly a revisional surgery rate of less than 10% during the first 10 years would be a reasonable target.
• There must minimal side-effects. Particularly worrying are the late nutritional side-effects of RYGB and BPD. Why exchange one problem for another?
• With up to 20% of the adult population needing help, an operative procedure has to be able to be done by the broad general surgical group. It must be relatively straightforward or death or complications will ensue.
• Whatever we do today is unlikely to be the best treatment in 20 years time so the procedure should be easily and totally reversible so future options are not excluded.
• Ideally, it needs to be controllable. If the day of the operation is the last chance we have for setting the parameters, it is likely

that, with time, the settings of the procedure will be suboptimal. This does not allow for a durable outcome. The recidivism of the RYGB is a powerful demonstration of this issue.

Each of the current surgical options will now be examined with this list of attributes in mind.

Roux-en-Y gastric bypass (see Fig. 25.2)

Over the past 20 years this operation has represented the gold standard to which other gastric stapling procedures have been compared. There are more short- and medium-term data available on RYGB than other procedures. Several prospective randomized controlled trials have compared the operation with gastroplasty (see Fig. 25.3) and consistently shown better outcomes [11–14] and gastroplasty in its various forms should now be regarded as a superseded procedure.

Key technical features

The procedure has evolved significantly during the past 30 years (see Fig. 25.2). Important aspects of the current technique include the following.

Increasingly the laparoscopic approach is becoming the standard. This approach presents a number of technical challenges for the surgeon resulting in a procedure that is considered to be equal to the most difficult current laparoscopic procedure of esophagectomy [67] and therefore has the potential for a higher mortality and morbidity than the open operation. Nevertheless, the laparoscopic approach is perceived by the patient to be less invasive and preferable. Nguyen et al. performed a prospective randomized trial of the open versus laparoscopic approach to RYGB [68]. They showed improved postoperative respiratory recovery and fewer wound problems in the laparoscopic group. Anastomotic leak rates were similar. Wound problems were more common after open surgery and anastomotic stricturing was more common after the laparoscopic approach.

Total division of the stomach into a very small upper pouch of 15–20 mL from the remainder using the linear cutter form of stapling device is undertaken. The divided stomach reduces the risk of staple line disruption but increases the opportunity for postoperative leaks

A Roux-en-Y loop of proximal jejunum is formed by division of the proximal gut and side-to-side anastomosis of the proximal end to the jejunum to create a Roux length of between 80 and 250 cm. The optimal length of the Roux limb and the benefit of tailoring the length to the individual patient's weight remain to be defined.

The distal end is taken by either an antecolic or retrocolic path to be anastomosed to the gastric pouch. The formation of this anastomosis may involve use of a circular stapler with a 21 mm anvil pass transorally [69], a linear cutter to form a side-to-side anastomosis [70] or suturing a two-layer anastomosis [71].

The stoma size is a further variable, particularly with the laparoscopic approach. With open surgery, a measured stoma of approximately 1 cm was planned. With the laparoscopic approach there is less ability to set the stomal size because of the technical limitations. Discussion of technical details of the gastrojejunostomy and the avoidance or treatment of leaks from this anastomosis remain a major activity at meetings of bariatric surgeons, indicating an unresolved dilemma.

Effects and side-effects

Figure 25.8 shows the weight loss from major reports of RYGB. Other outcomes include a perioperative mortality of 0.3–1%, significant perioperative complications in 5–25% of patients, a median length of stay of 6 days, incisional hernia in up to 24% and a weight loss of 49–62% EWL at follow-up of between 5 and 15 years.

Nutritional problems which include iron deficiency, vitamin B12 deficiency and poor calcium absorption are frequent, and compliance with replacement therapy has been shown to be low, leaving the patient who becomes lost to follow-up vulnerable to deficiency problems. Body composition studies demonstrate an unfavorably excessive loss of lean body weight [72].

Biliopancreatic diversion (BPD) (see Figs 25.4 and 25.5)

Key technical features

The combination of partial gastrectomy and intestinal bypass without a blind loop was created by Nicola Scopinaro in 1979 [15]. His technique involves standard transverse hemigastrectomy, closure of the duodenal stump, division of the small bowel at 200 cm from the ileocecal junction with anastomosis of the distal end to the gastric remnant and end-to-side anastomosis of the proximal end to the distal ileum at 50 cm from the ileocecal junction.

Since 1986, Scopinaro has tailored the size of the gastric remnant to be between 200 and 500 mL, depending on the preoperative weight and a number of patient characteristics and, more recently, has reported tailoring the intestinal lengths on similar grounds [39]. Establishment of the precision or validity of these variations has not been reported.

A prominent variation on the traditional technique is the duodenal switch (BPD-DS) in which there is preservation of normal gastric emptying by performing a longitudinal sleeve gastrectomy, anastomosis of the Roux limb to the proximal duodenum and staple closure of the duodenum beyond this anastomosis [73].

The BPD and its variant can be performed laparoscopically, although with difficulty, and high perioperative mortality has been reported in association with this approach, especially in the superobese [21].

Effects and side-effects

Impressive and durable weight loss is achieved with all variants of the BPD. Marceau reports better weight loss with the BPD-DS when compared to a previous series of BPD [74] but the weight loss in his BPD-DS group is not different from that achieved by Scopinaro without duodenal switch. Recently reported data by Scopinaro relate to patients having the post-1986 variation, which he calls the *ad hoc* stomach (AHS) type of BPD. He reports a remarkable constancy of weight lost with 74%EWL at 2 years (n = 1284) and 78%EWL at 12 years (n = 58) [39]. Hess and Hess have studied multiple variations of intestinal length without establishing a clear difference in outcomes [75]. The relevance of the technical differences with respect to weight loss remain to be established.

The primary mechanism of all forms of BPD is malabsorption, especially of fat. All patients will have foul-smelling stools, generally 2–4 per day, and excessive wind [39]. Whereas fat malabsorption is the aim, malabsorption of protein and micronutrients are the side-effects. Scopinaro measured protein loss in the stool to be an average of 30 g/day, five times the normal value [39], and recommended a daily protein intake of at least 90 g/day to compensate for this. Iron deficiency is expected to occur and anemia occurs in up to one-third of patients at 4 years after surgery if prophylaxis is inadequate [76,77]. All patients need supplemental iron. Because of the low compliance with oral regimens, parenteral replacement is recommended [78]. In addition, supplements of calcium, the fat-soluble vitamins A and D, and water-soluble vitamins are important.

Laparoscopic adjustable gastric banding (see Fig. 25.6)

Key technical features

This procedure has the potential to fulfill the role of ideal bariatric procedure as it satisfies or nearly satisfies all the attributes listed in Table 25.2. It has been designed as a laparoscopic procedure. It could be done by open technique but the safety and the accuracy of placement would suffer as a result. It is safe, 10 times as safe as gastric bypass [79], and remarkably free of significant postoperative complications [80]. It is effective in achieving good weight loss, of the order of between 50% and 60% of excess weight, and there are major improvements in obesity-related co-morbidities and quality of life [42]. With up to 6 years of follow-up data and only 3.6% of patients lost to follow-up, the effectiveness appears to be durable [80]. There is not the progressive fading of effectiveness that was characteristic of gastric stapling procedures. This is presumed to reflect the benefit of adjustability. However, longer follow-up and more studies are required to establish this feature more securely.

A significant weakness of the LAGB has been the need for revisional procedures because of late problems with prolapse, symmetric pouch dilation, erosions and tubing problems. These have been reduced by technical developments and better patient education but there is still an expectation that between 5% and 20% of patients will need revisional procedures.

The procedure is technically feasible for surgeons with competence in laparoscopic abdominal surgery.

Table 25.2 Attributes of an ideal bariatric procedure

Minimally invasive

Safe
Effective – weight loss, comorbidities, QOL
Durable – effective over time
Low reoperation rate
Minimal side effects
Technically feasible broadly
Reversible
Controllable/adjustable

The LAGB can be removed easily by the laparoscopic approach, allowing the stomach to return to its normal configuration. The ability to control the degree of gastric restriction through the adjustability is a unique feature of the LAGB and arguably its greatest attraction.

Effects and side-effects

The LAGB is a very safe procedure with perioperative mortality of less than one in 2000 and a perioperative complication rate of less than 2% [81]. Late difficulties of prolapse, erosions and tubing problems are becoming infrequent but remain a problem.

A summary of the published reports is shown in Figure 25.8. Most are studies of the Lap-Band system. There are several other bands now available but the only other one for which there are any published data is the Swedish adjustable gastric band (SAGB®). It can be reasonably expected that patients will have lost between 50% and 60% EWL by 3 years after operation and that effect remains stable out to 8 years. The benefits to health and quality of life have been impressive and are reviewed above. Inevitably there is some loss of patients to follow-up and it is best practice to assume that these are the least successful. In our study of 700 patients followed for up to 6 years [80], there was a loss to follow-up of 3.6%.

With the LAGB we can offer a very safe procedure with no deaths, a perioperative complication rate of less than 2% and a 5–10% likelihood of needing revisional procedures in the future [81]. The LAGB has been shown to be effective in generating major weight loss and improvement in health and quality of life and the effects are achieved gently through its safe laparoscopic placement and its adjustability.

Sleeve gastrectomy

This is a relatively new option, being the vertical gastrectomy of a duodenal switch procedure, and is now being tested as an independent procedure or as a first stage to duodenal switch in the more challenging patients (see Fig. 25.6). The details of the technique, such as the size of the bougie about which the resection occurs, are not yet settled and there are no reports of follow-up beyond 3 years. The early reports are favorable regarding weight loss and co-morbidity outcomes. However, it carries risk of bleeding and leakage as for other resectional procedures and the perioperative mortality rate is probably not different from RYGB. It is generally anticipated that a further procedure will be required as there is no component of the procedure which stabilizes the size of the residual stomach. It fails on several of the characteristics of the ideal procedure, including safety, durability, adjustability and reversibility. Further experience and medium-term data are needed before it should be considered to be within the established procedures.

Conclusion

All currently available bariatric surgical procedures are effective in achieving substantial loss of weight and improvement in health and quality of life. For the person with severe obesity (BMI > 35), the surgical approach is the only one which can offer a predictable benefit in the short and medium term and should be considered if the obesity is a significant problem to the person.

It is likely that all bariatric procedures will be done laparoscopically as the standard and, on current data, for safety, efficacy and acceptability, the LAGB is the preferred option as a primary bariatric procedure. More long-term data (>5-year follow-up) are needed on all the options and careful randomized controlled trials using each technique optimally and with follow-up of patients for at least 5 years would be very valuable.

References

1. Douketis J, Macie C, Thabane L, Williamson DF. Systematic review of long-term weight loss studies in obese adults: clinical significance and applicability to clinical practice. Int J Obes 2005;29(10): 1153–67.

2. O'Brien PDJ, Laurie C, et al. Treatment of mild to moderate obesity with laparoscopic adjustable gastric banding or an intensive medical program: a randomized trial. Ann Int Med 2006;144:625–33.

3. Jorizzo JL, Apisarnthanarax P, Subrt P, et al. Bowel-bypass syndrome without bowel bypass. Bowel-associated dermatosis-arthritis syndrome. Arch Intern Med 1983;143(3):457–61.

4. O'Leary JP. Hepatic complications of jejunoileal bypass. Semin Liver Dis 1983;3(3):203–15.

5. Corrodi P. Jejunoileal bypass: change in the flora of the small intestine and its clinical impact. Rev Infect Dis 1984;6(suppl 1):S80–4.

6. Parfitt AM, Podenphant J, Villanueva AR, Frame B. Metabolic bone disease with and without osteomalacia after intestinal bypass surgery: a bone histomorphometric study. Bone 1985;6(4):211–20.

7. DeWind LT, Payne JH. Intestinal bypass surgery for morbid obesity. Long-term results. JAMA 1976;236(20):2298–301.

8. Mason EE, Ito C. Gastric bypass in obesity. Surg Clin North Am 1967;47(6):1345–51.

9. Printen KJ, Mason EE. Gastric surgery for relief of morbid obesity. Arch Surg 1973;106(4):428–31.

10. Mason EE. Vertical banded gastroplasty for obesity. Arch Surg 1982;117(5):701–6.

11. Hall JC, Watts JM, O'Brien PE, et al. Gastric surgery for morbid obesity. The Adelaide Study. Ann Surg 1990;211(4):419–27.

12. Pories WJ, Flickinger EG, Meelheim D, van Rij AM, Thomas FT. The effectiveness of gastric bypass over gastric partition in morbid obesity: consequence of distal gastric and duodenal exclusion. Ann Surg 1982;196(4):389–99.

13. Sugerman HJ, Starkey JV, Birkenhauer R. A randomized prospective trial of gastric bypass versus vertical banded gastroplasty for morbid obesity and their effects on sweets versus non- sweets eaters. Ann Surg 1987;205(6):613–24.

14. Sugerman HJ, Londrey GL, Kellum JM, et al. Weight loss with vertical banded gastroplasty and Roux-Y gastric bypass for morbid obesity with selective versus random assignment. Am J Surg 1989; 157(1):93–102.

15. Scopinaro N, Gianetta E, Civalleri D, Bonalumi U, Bachi V. Biliopancreatic bypass for obesity: II. Initial experience in man. Br J Surg 1979;66(9):618–20.

16. Scopinaro N, Gianetta E, Adami GF, et al. Biliopancreatic diversion for obesity at eighteen years. Surgery 1996;119(3):261–8.

17. Marceau P, Hould FS, Simard S, Lebel S, Bourque RA, Potvin M, Biron S. Biliopancreatic diversion with duodenal switch. World J Surg 1998;22(9):947–54.

18. Belachew M, Legrand MJ, Defechereux TH, Burtheret MP, Jacquet N. Laparoscopic adjustable silicone gastric banding in the treatment of morbid obesity. A preliminary report. Surg Endosc 1994; 8(11):1354–6.

19. Belachew M, Legrand MJ, Vincent V. History of Lap-Band: from dream to reality. Obes Surg 2001;11(3):297–302.

20. Wittgrove AC, Clark GW, Schubert KR. Laparoscopic gastric bypass, Roux-en-Y: technique and results in 75 patients with 3–30 months follow-up. Obes Surg 1996;6(6):500–4.

21. Ren CJ, Patterson E, Gagner M. Early results of laparoscopic biliopancreatic diversion with duodenal switch: a case series of 40 consecutive patients. Obes Surg 2000;10(6):514–23; discussion 524.

22. Szinicz G, Schnapka G. A new method in the surgical treatment of disease. Acta Chir Austrica 1982; suppl 43.

23. Kuzmak LI. A review of seven years' experience with silicone gastric banding. Obes Surg 1991;1(4):403–8.

24. O'Brien P, McPhail T, Chaston T, Dixon J. Systematic review of medium term weight loss after bariatric operations. Obes Surg 2006;16:1032–40.

25. Dixon JB, O'Brien P. Health outcomes of severely obese type 2 diabetic subjects 1 year after laparoscopic adjustable gastric banding. Diabetes Care 2002;25(2):358–63.

26. Pories WJ, Swanson MS, MacDonald KG, et al. Who would have thought it? An operation proves to be the most effective therapy for adult-onset diabetes mellitus. Ann Surg 1995;222(3):339–50; discussion 350–32.

27. Rubino F, Gagner M. Potential of surgery for curing type 2 diabetes mellitus. Ann Surg 2002;236(5):554–9.

28. Smith SC, Edwards CB, Goodman GN. Changes in diabetic management after Roux-en-Y gastric bypass. Obes Surg 1996;6(4):345–8.

29. Dixon J, O'Brien PE, Playfair J, et al. Adjustable gastric banding and conventional therapy for type 2 diabetes: a randomized controlled trial. JAMA 2008;299(3):316–23.

30. Rubino F, Forgione A, Cummings D, et al. The mechanism of diabetes control after gastrointestinal bypass surgery reveals a role of the

proximal small intestine in the pathophysiology of type 2 diabetes. Ann Surg 2006;244(5):741–9.

31. Le Roux C, Aylwin SJ, Batterham RL, et al. Gut hormone profiles following bariatric surgery favor an anorectic state, facilitate weight loss and improve metabolis parameters. Ann Surg 2006;243(1): 108–14.

32. Dixon JB, Dixon AF, O'Brien PE. Improvements in insulin sensitivity and beta-cell function (HOMA) with weight loss in the severely obese. Diabet Med 2003;20(2):127–34.

33. Pinkney JH, Sjostrom CD, Gale EA. Should surgeons treat diabetes in severely obese people? Lancet 2001;357(9265):1357–9.

34. Despres J. The insulin resistance-dyslipidemia syndrome: the most prevalent cause of coronary artery disease. CMAJ 1993;148(8): 1339–40.

35. Koba S, Hirano T, Sakaue T, et al. Role of small dense low-density lipoprotein in coronary artery disease patients with normal plasma cholesterol levels. J Cardiol 2000;36(6):371–8.

36. Busetto L, Pisent C, Rinaldi D, et al. Variation in lipid levels in morbidly obese patients operated with the LAP-BAND adjustable gastric banding system: effects of different levels of weight loss. Obes Surg 2000;10(6):569–77.

37. Bacci V, Basso MS, Greco F, et al. Modifications of metabolic and cardiovascular risk factors after weight loss induced by laparoscopic gastric banding. Obes Surg 2002;12(1):77–82.

38. Dixon J, O'Brien P. Ovarian dysfunction, androgen excess and neck circumference in obese women: changes with weight loss (abstract). Obes Surg 2002;12(2):193.

39. Scopinaro N, Adami GF, Marinari GM, et al. Biliopancreatic diversion. World J Surg 1998;22(9):936–46.

40. Brolin RE, Bradley LJ, Wilson AC, Cody RP. Lipid risk profile and weight stability after gastric restrictive operations for morbid obesity. J Gastrointest Surg 2000;4(5):464–9.

41. Sjostrom CD, Lissner L, Wedel H, Sjostrom L. Reduction in incidence of diabetes, hypertension and lipid disturbances after intentional weight loss induced by bariatric surgery: the SOS Intervention Study. Obes Res 1999;7(5):477–84.

42. Dixon JB, O'Brien PE. Changes in comorbidities and improvements in quality of life after LAP-BAND placement. Am J Surg 2002; 184(6B):S51–4.

43. Sjostrom CD, Peltonen M, Wedel H, Sjostrom L. Differentiated long-term effects of intentional weight loss on diabetes and hypertension. Hypertension 2000;36(1):20–5.

44. Dixon JB. Elevated homocysteine with weight loss. Obes Surg 2001;11(5):537–8.

45. Dixon JB, Dixon ME, O'Brien PE. Pregnancy after Lap-Band surgery: management of the band to achieve healthy weight outcomes. Obes Surg 2001;11(1):59–65.

46. Dixon JB, O'Brien PE. Gastroesophageal reflux in obesity: the effect of lap-band placement. Obes Surg 1999;9(6):527–31.

47. Schauer P, Hamad G, Ikramuddin S. Surgical management of gastroesophageal reflux disease in obese patients. Semin Laparosc Surg 2001;8(4):256–64.

48. Balsiger BM, Murr MM, Mai J, Sarr MG. Gastroesophageal reflux after intact vertical banded gastroplasty: correction by conversion to Roux-en-Y gastric bypass. J Gastrointest Surg 2000;4(3): 276–81.

49. Weiss HG, Nehoda H, Labeck B, et al. Treatment of morbid obesity with laparoscopic adjustable gastric banding affects esophageal motility. Am J Surg 2000;180(6):479–82.

50. Young SY, Gunzenhauser JD, Malone KE, McTiernan A. Body mass index and asthma in the military population of the northwestern United States. Arch Intern Med 2001;161(13):1605–11.

51. Dixon JB, Chapman L, O'Brien P. Marked improvement in asthma after Lap-Band surgery for morbid obesity. Obes Surg 1999;9(4):385–9.

52. Vgontzas AN, Papanicolaou DA, Bixler EO, et al. Sleep apnea and daytime sleepiness and fatigue: relation to visceral obesity, insulin resistance, and hypercytokinemia. J Clin Endocrinol Metab 2000; 85(3):1151–8.

53. Dixon JB, Schachter LM, O'Brien PE. Sleep disturbance and obesity: changes following surgically induced weight loss. Arch Intern Med 2001;161(1):102–6.

54. Dixon JB, Dixon ME, O'Brien PE. Depression in association with severe obesity: changes with weight loss. Arch Intern Med 2003;163(17):2058–65.

55. Weiner R, Datz M, Wagner D, Bockhorn H. Quality-of-life outcome after laparoscopic adjustable gastric banding for morbid obesity. Obes Surg 1999;9(6):539–45.

56. Schok M, Geenen R, van Antwerpen T, de Wit P, Brand N, van Ramshorst B. Quality of life after laparoscopic adjustable gastric banding for severe obesity: postoperative and retrospective preoperative evaluations. Obes Surg 2000;10(6):502–8.

57. Balsiger BM, Kennedy FP, Abu-Lebdeh HS, et al. Prospective evaluation of Roux-en-Y gastric bypass as primary operation for medically complicated obesity [see comments]. Mayo Clin Proc 2000;75(7): 673–80.

58. Horchner R, Tuinebreijer MW, Kelder PH. Quality-of-life assessment of morbidly obese patients who have undergone a Lap-Band operation: 2-year follow-up study. Is the MOS SF-36 a useful instrument to measure quality of life in morbidly obese patients? Obes Surg 2001;11(2):212–18; discussion 219.

59. O'Brien P, Brown W, Dixon J. Revisional surgery for morbid obesity – conversion to the Lap-Band system. Obes Surg 2000;10(6):557–63.

60. Dixon JB, Dixon ME, O'Brien PE. Body image: appearance orientation and evaluation in the severely obese. Changes with weight loss. Obes Surg 2002;12(1):65–71.

61. Sjostrom L, Narbro K, Sjostrom CD, et al. Effects of bariatric surgery on mortality in Swedish obese subjects. N Engl J Med 2007;357(8): 741–52.

62. Torgerson JS, Sjostrom L. The Swedish Obese Subjects (SOS) study – rationale and results. Int J Obes 2001;25(suppl 1):S2–4.

63. Agren G, Narbro K, Naslund I, Sjostrom L, Peltonen M. Long-term effects of weight loss on pharmaceutical costs in obese subjects. A report from the SOS intervention study. Int J Obes 2002;26(2): 184–92.

64. Torgerson JS. Swedish obese subjects – where are we now? Int J Obes 2003;27(S1):19.

65. Peeters A, O'Brien P, Laurie C, et al. Substantial intentional weight loss and mortality in the severely obese. Ann Surg 2007;246(6): 1028–33.

66. Calle EE, Rodriguez C, Walker-Thurmond K, Thun MJ. Overweight, obesity, and mortality from cancer in a prospectively studied cohort of U.S. adults. N Engl J Med 2003;348(17):1625–38.

67. Schauer PR, Ikramuddin S. Laparoscopic surgery for morbid obesity. Surg Clin North Am 2001;81(5):1145–79.

68. Nguyen NT, Goldman C, Rosenquist CJ, et al. Laparoscopic versus open gastric bypass: a randomized study of outcomes, quality of life, and costs. Ann Surg 2001;234(3):279–89; discussion 289–91.

69. Wittgrove AC, Clark GW. Laparoscopic gastric bypass, Roux-en-Y-500 patients: technique and results, with 3–60 month follow-up. Obes Surg 2000;10(3):233–9.

70. Schauer PR, Ikramuddin S, Gourash W, Ramanathan R, Luketich J. Outcomes after laparoscopic Roux-en-Y gastric bypass for morbid obesity. Ann Surg 2000;232(4):515–29.

71. Higa KD, Boone KB, Ho T, Davies OG. Laparoscopic roux-en-Y gastric bypass for morbid obesity: technique and preliminary results of our first 400 patients. Arch Surg 2000;135(9):1029–34.

72. Chaston T, Dixon JB, O'Brien PE. Changes in fat-free mass during significant weight loss: a systematic review. Int J Obes 2007;31(5):743–50.

73. Lagace M, Marceau P, Marceau S, et al. Biliopancreatic diversion with a new type of gastrectomy: some previous conclusions revisited. Obes Surg 1995;5(4):411–18.

74. Marceau P, Hould FS, Simard S, et al. Biliopancreatic diversion with duodenal switch. World J Surg 1998;22(9):947–54.

75. Hess DS, Hess DW. Biliopancreatic diversion with a duodenal switch. Obes Surg 1998;8(3):267–82.

76. Brolin RE, Gorman RC, Milgrim LM, Kenler HA. Multivitamin prophylaxis in prevention of post-gastric bypass vitamin and mineral deficiencies. Int J Obes 1991;15(10):661–7.

77. Brolin RE, Gorman JH, Gorman RC, et al. Are vitamin B12 and folate deficiency clinically important after roux-en-Y gastric bypass? J Gastrointest Surg 1998;2(5):436–42.

78. Marceau P, Hould FS, Lebel S, Marceau S, Biron S. Malabsorptive obesity surgery. Surg Clin North Am 2001;81(5):1113–27.

79. Chapman A, Kiroff G, Game P, Foster B, O'Brien P, Ham J, Maddern G. *Systematic Review of Laparoscopic Adjustable Gastric Banding in the Treatment of Obesity*. Adelaide, South Australia: ASERNIP-S Report No 31; 2002.

80. O'Brien PE, Dixon JB, Brown W, et al. The laparoscopic adjustable gastric band (Lap-Band): a prospective study of medium-term effects on weight, health and quality of life. Obes Surg 2002;12(5):652–60.

81. O'Brien PE, Dixon JB. Weight loss and early and late complications – the international experience. Am J Surg 2002;184(6B):S42–5.

82. Christou NV, Sampalis JS, Liberman M, et al. Surgery decreases long-term mortality, morbidity, and health care use in morbidly obese patients. Ann Surg 2004;240(3):416–23.

83. Flum DR, Dellinger EP. Impact of gastric bypass operation on survival: a population-based analysis. J Am Coll Surg 2004;199(4):543–51.

84. Favretti FSG, Ashton D, Busetto L, et al. Laparoscopic adjustable gastric banding in 1,791 consecutive obese patients: 12-year results. Obes Surg 2007;17:168–75.

85. Adams T, Gress RE, Smith SC, et al. Long term mortality after gastric bypass surgery. N Engl J Med 2007;357:753–61.

26 Weight Loss Maintenance and Weight Cycling

Kristina Elfhag and Stephan Rössner

Obesity Unit, Karolinska University Hospital, Stockholm, Sweden

Introduction

Over the last few years a paradigm shift has been observed in the feasibility of long-term weight loss. Clinicians were once satisfied if substantial weight loss could be introduced in patients but realized that relapse was more the rule than the exception because in general the need for weight maintenance strategies was not realized. In this early era Stunkard made the famous quotation: "Most of those who are obese will not go into obesity treatment, most of those who go into treatment will not lose weight and most of those who lose weight will regain it" [1]. This extremely negative view was later challenged when it was realized that weight loss could generally be accomplished in a great number of obese individuals. It also became apparent that the focus had to be shifted much more to weight loss maintenance and prevention of weight regain after the initial treatment period. In addition, it was realized that the amount of weight loss achieved and maintained had to be more realistic.

Our own study in 1985 was one of the first to demonstrate that with standard conventional treatment tools such as diet, exercise and behavior modification, substantial weight loss could be achieved and maintained over a 4-year period [2].

When these patients were reinvestigated 10–12 years later almost all weight loss achieved at the 4-year follow-up had been maintained, as shown in Figure 26.1 [3]. Admittedly, this was a result obtained in a selected group, supervised by a PhD student with an interest, with far more involvement than what could be expected in a routine clinical setting then, and without a control group. However, the study still demonstrated that weight loss maintenance was possible.

Effects of weight loss

In the late 1980s, the focus began to shift and it was realized that weight normalization was an impossible dream. Furthermore, weight normalization was not even necessary for important metabolic benefits to take place. The classic Goldstein meta-analysis in 1992 demonstrated that a 5–10% weight loss was enough to achieve significant improvement in obesity-associated metabolic risk factors, with improved glycemic control, reduced blood pressure and cholesterol levels [4]. Several studies were summarized demonstrating, surprisingly, that as little as 5% weight loss had beneficial health effects. It may indeed seem astonishing that such a small weight loss can improve health. An individual taking part in a weight loss program, by most standards doing quite well and losing weight from 115 to 105 kg, will of course still be obese and may not look much different in appearance, but their health status and metabolic risk factors will have improved markedly. Furthermore, a lower obese body weight has been shown to affect the subjective experience of health-related quality of life positively. Such effects include easier daily functioning, with reduced obstacles to physical mobility and also improvements in the person's general health perception [5,6].

Besides the positive health benefits of a lower body weight, beneficial effects on psychosocial functioning and mental aspects of quality of life have also been demonstrated. Psychosocial functioning has been shown to improve with weight loss. With a reduced body weight, fewer obstacles were perceived concerning activities such as social gatherings, buying clothes, going away for holidays, bathing in public and having intimate relations with a partner [5]. Mental aspects of quality of life, such as mental well-being, are also positively related to reduced body weight. Overall

Clinical Obesity in Adults and Children, 3rd edition. Edited by Peter G. Kopelman, Ian D. Caterson and William H. Dietz.
© 2010 Blackwell Publishing, ISBN: 978-1-4051-8226-3.

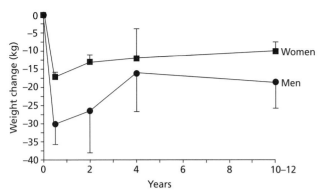

Figure 26.1 Weight loss results and weight loss maintenance in long-term behavioral treatment of obesity (n = 49). (Reproduced with permission from Björvell H, Rössner S. Obese indviduals can achieve permanent weight reduction by means of a behaviour modification program. Lakartidningen 1990;87:2504–47.)

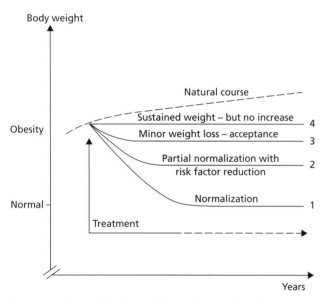

Figure 26.2 Theoretical prediction of the natural course of weight development, and indicators of success in long-term weight reduction programs. (Reproduced with permission from reference [8].)

mood, anxiety and depression have been found to improve with long-term weight loss in some studies using various treatments, although the effect sizes of some of these associations are small [5,7].

Natural weight development

Figure 26.2 illustrates the clinical realities of long-term weight control. As basal metabolic rate decreases with age, in most societies an increase of body weight is observed over time. As an example, our Swedish data would suggest an increase in body weight of 2–3 kg per decade [8]. If this is the situation for the

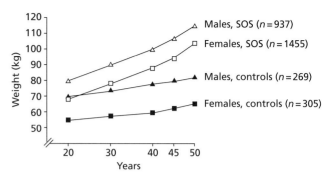

Figure 26.3 Self-reported weight in various age categories. Cross-sectional data from the Swedish Obese Subjects and corresponding controls. (Reproduced with permission from reference [9].)

general public, as exemplified by the Swedish data, the weight development in obese subjects is even steeper.

Figure 26.3 demonstrates the weight trajectory in control subjects in the Gothenburg Swedish Obese Subjects (SOS) study [9]. As can be seen from this figure, for both men and women and all age groups, the weight increase over time is quite pronounced. Taken together, this means that a therapist, working with a patient who can maintain his weight for a significant period of time, has had a certain degree of therapeutic success. A problem, however, is that most therapists, and their patients, will not see this as a treatment success but regard the lack of weight loss as a failure. What is often expected by many is weight normalization, something that would practically never happen in reality. The best therapists and patients can hope for is a result somewhere between curves 2 and 3 in Figure 26.2. This would in clinical reality correspond to a weight loss of 5–10%, but once the nadir has been achieved it is reasonable to assume that unless additional efforts or interventions are made, these curves will again start to slope upwards in parallel with the top line of the figure.

The weight loss plateau

It is interesting that irrespective of treatment, whether diet, exercise, behavior modification or pharmacotherapy, most, although not quite all, treatment programs result in continuous weight loss for about 6 months, after which weight loss plateaus. Thus, whatever method is being used, strategies have to change from the first weight loss period to the maintenance phase. Reassurance, support and acceptance are important components of the treatment, so that the patient understands and hopefully accepts that further weight loss may not take place easily. Although some individuals might find it difficult to accept that weight loss does not continue, the plateau can easily be explained on physiologic grounds. With the reduction in lean body mass, which is an inevitable consequence of any weight loss, the basal metabolic rate will go down and the overall needs of the individual after weight loss are lower [10]. Thus intake and expenditure will balance at a lower level after successful weight loss, and when this takes place, no further weight loss can be expected.

Weight cycling

Weight cycling refers to the repeated loss and regain of weight (although there is no standard definition for weight cycling) [7]. In the early 1990s several studies were published suggesting that weight cycling increased the mortality risk by a factor of 1.5–2.0 [11]. These studies caused distress since they sent out the message that it was better to remain at a higher, stable body weight than to fluctuate over time. Although some of these were adequately performed cross-sectional epidemiologic studies, several subsequent reviews identified problems in their interpretation and weaknesses in their design [12].

It soon became clear that cycling, whether natural or experimental, did not result in permanent alterations of body composition or resting energy expenditure, nor in alteration of fat mobilization. Further critical reviews of the animal literature, where detrimental effects of weight cycling had previously been described, similarly found that in spite of some intriguing results, there was little evidence to support long-standing physiologic effects of weight cycling [13]. In the new millennium there is little physiologic information about the putative role of weight cycling in body weight control.

However, weight cycling still remains a problem, although from another perspective. The present understanding is that weight cycling may pose a problem in successful obesity treatment mainly from the psychologic point of view, as it may be associated with a number of negative factors related to eating behavior.

Weight cycling has sometimes been associated with mental distress and psychopathology [14,15], although others who found no such relationship concluded that weight cycling does not seem to impact psychologic health in an adverse way [16]. Considering the research findings linking weight cycling with distress, mental distress could of course also characterize the person as being more prone to diet and having more difficulties in sustaining the weight lost, rather than it being a consequence of the weight cycling.

More disturbed eating behaviors and a higher prevalence of binge eating have also been noted among weight cyclers [14]. The greater the number of weight loss efforts, the greater was the occurrence or severity of binge eating. However, whether weight cycling causes binge eating or vice versa could not be resolved from these studies.

Patients reporting repeated dietary attempts that would be related to weight cycling have been found to be more prone to regain weight [17,18] but a lack of association between number of previous slimming attempts and weight maintenance has also been reported [19]. Considering the difficulties in maintaining weight loss over time, weight cycling reflects the struggles in controlling the body weight. From this view, weight cycling may be a better alternative than a steady weight gain over time.

The identification of factors associated with weight loss maintenance can enhance our understanding of the behaviors and prerequisites that are crucial in sustaining a lowered body weight. This has implications for the strategies that should be encouraged in treatment, the advice given at the weight maintenance phase, and the selection of persons with a reasonable prospect for long-term success in obesity treatments. We can thus avoid the risk of exposing a patient to additional aversive psychologic consequences of experiencing failure in treatment [20].

Definition and prevalence of weight loss maintenance

Definition

A definition of what constitutes weight loss maintenance must first be considered. Weight loss maintenance implies keeping a weight loss accomplished by treatment interventions or by the patient's own efforts. This would be the general definition shared across studies performed. The specific criteria used, however, differ. Examples of definitions are "achieving an intentional weight loss of at least 10% of initial body weight and maintaining this body weight for at least 1 year" [6] or "losing at least 5% of baseline body weight between baseline and follow-up, and maintaining that weight or less for a further 2 years" [21]. Others have classified "winners" and "losers" based on losing or regaining more than, for example, two Body Mass Index (BMI) points after weight loss [22]. To enable a review of the literature using very different definitions of weight maintenance, we have used a more inclusive definition of weight maintenance that implies an initial weight loss that has been maintained for at least 6 months subsequently.

Another methodologic consideration is that the time of evaluation of weight maintenance can differ. Pretreatment factors determining later weight loss maintenance have the greatest informative value for recommendations on treatment assignment. Sometimes the patients are assessed at the time of discharge from active treatment and further weight change is predicted from these characteristics. Another common approach is to identify retrospectively those who can be classified as successful weight loss maintainers, and to describe the behavioral characteristics of these persons as they manifest at the time of "success." Changes during treatment based on repeated measures have also been analyzed in studying weight maintainers. The latter approaches can give information on the behaviors and strategies that could be encouraged in treatment programs, rather than just focusing on treatment assignment.

In our evaluation of factors affecting weight maintenance, we have included studies with these different methodologic approaches. The studies include patient samples as well as general population samples. With this rather broad inclusion criterion, a fuller description of possible factors in weight maintenance may be derived. Furthermore, as behavioral factors have been considered to be stronger predictors of weight maintenance and regain than physiologic factors, we have focused on the former [6].

Prevalence

Quite optimistic results on weight loss maintenance have been reported from a telephone survey in a US population sample. Weight loss maintenance for 5 years or more was reported by about 25% of those who had deliberately lost at least 10% of their maximum body weight [23]. Looking at patient studies, a median of 15% could be identified as successful weight maintainers in a review of 17 clinical studies. (Weight maintenance was defined as maintenance of the entire weight loss or ≥9–11 kg of the initial weight loss at follow-up periods of at least 3 years [24].) The successful weight maintenance results in the studies reviewed ranged from 0% to 49%. If the patients lost to follow-up were considered failures, then the median success rate was 13%, with a range of 0–35% success [24].

Weight loss goals

It seems common for patients to have unrealistic expectations about the weight loss that will be achieved in treatment. In one study none of the participants achieved the "dream weight" they had hoped for and most of them ended up with a weight loss which before treatment they had considered as a "failure," even though the standard treatment program was well designed and executed [25]. Heavier patients and men had lower target weights [26]. The fact that expectations about the goal weight can be unrealistic has been confirmed in other studies [27]. According to these results, men were more realistic in their approach to what could be achieved with a weight lose regimen than were women.

Weight goals may be one factor in determining if the person will succeed or fail in maintaining a lower body weight [28,29]. Those who maintained their weight were more likely to have achieved their self-determined goal weight. It has been suggested that failure to reach a self-determined weight may affect the person's belief in their ability to control their weight and result in abandonment of weight maintenance behaviors [30]. Modifying weight loss goals therefore seems to be important for subsequent results.

Weight loss patterns

Initial weight loss has been identified as a predictor for later weight loss, and for weight loss maintenance [31–33]. The greater the initial weight loss, the better is the subsequent outcome. This tells us that there is a consistent weight loss pattern from the beginning of the treatment. Initial weight loss can reflect better compliance with the treatment [32]. It has been noted that the findings on initial weight loss challenge the clinical truism that weight loss achieved at a slow rate is better [33].

But according to other results, larger amounts of weight loss during the total intentional weight loss phase have predicted more weight regain [29]. It is still unclear precisely how the early weight loss response predicts long-term outcome and how it should be defined.

The complexity involved in evaluating the predictive value of weight loss patterns can be illustrated by a recent analysis of two long-term clinical trials with orlistat [34]. In this analysis, weight loss of >5% body weight after 12 weeks of diet and orlistat was a good indicator of 2-year weight loss, and other measures such as ≥2.5 kg initial weight loss during the 4-week lead-in [35] and ≥10% weight loss after 6 months did not add significantly to the prediction of the 2-year outcome.

The duration of weight loss has also been studied. The longer the weight loss has been maintained, the better are the chances for further continuation of a lower body weight [6,29]. Subjects who have maintained weight losses for a longer time report that they use less effort in continued weight control [36]. The pleasure derived from controlling weight was not changed over time, suggesting a shift in balance towards overall pleasure in promoting further maintenance of body weight.

Factors affecting weight loss maintenance

Physical activity

Physical activity is related to long-term weight maintenance in many studies [6,21,37,38]. Physical activity can help weight maintenance through direct energy expenditure, and also improved physical fitness which facilitates the amount and intensity of daily activities [39]. Physical activity can also improve well-being, which may in turn facilitate other positive behaviors needed for weight maintenance [40].

Walking is one of the most frequent aspects of physical exercise reported by study participants, and cycling and weight lifting also have some popularity [6]. In the STORM study, leisure activity predicted weight maintenance with sibutramine treatment [32]. Such leisure-time physical activity included time spent walking and cycling, and also implied less time spent watching television. It was suggested these factors can distinguish a sedentary lifestyle from a more active one even better than a measure of sports activity.

A higher number of pedometer-recorded daily steps [41] and other measures including everyday activities [42] have likewise been found among weight maintainers. Impaired physical functioning in daily life, implying limitations in the ability for ambulation, has correspondingly predicted later weight relapse [43]. Perceiving barriers in the life situation for carrying out physical activity has also been related to poorer weight maintenance, whereas confidence concerning exercise may promote long-term weight management [18].

According to one review, the results of physical activity in weight gain are, however, not consistent [44]. Prescribing exercise in experimental designs was, for example, only modestly related to later outcomes. Poor compliance in carrying out the exercise protocol was suggested as one reason for such discouraging results [45].

Dietary intake

Weight loss maintenance is obviously associated with lower total caloric intake [46] and reduced portion sizes [47]. More specifically, it is also associated with reduced frequency of snacks [48] and less dietary fat [6,21,42,48,49].

Reduction of particular food types such as French fries, dairy products, sweets and meat [50] and cheese, butter, high-fat snacks, fried foods and desserts [51] has also been seen in persons successfully maintaining their weight. The importance of including high-quality foods such as fruits and vegetables [48] and healthy eating [52] has also been noted.

Change towards a more regular meal rhythm has been identified as helpful in long-term weight loss [48] and regularly eating breakfast has been reported more often among weight maintainers [37,53]. It is suggested that breakfast can reduce hunger, making the breakfast eaters choose less energy-dense foods during the rest of the day, as well as giving better energy to perform physical activity during the day [53].

Eating patterns

Generally, eating behavior has been evaluated during ongoing treatments. The most common measure of eating behaviors is the Three Factor Eating Questionnaire (TFEQ) [54], which measures eating restraint, disinhibition and hunger. Restraint means trying to resist eating by conscious determination in order to control body weight. Disinhibition measures loss of control over eating, and the hunger scale shows the experience of hunger feelings and cravings for food. Eating restraint is known to be associated with a lower amount of food intake [55] and the restraint increases with successful weight loss in behavior modification treatments [43,56].

For those regaining their body weight, the contrasting pattern, a decrease in eating restraint and increase in disinhibition, has been found [6,57]. This tells us that restraint in food intake leads to less food consumed and thus more weight loss, and that control over food intake is crucial for weight management.

Studies using data on eating patterns somewhat more prospectively, by comparing eating patterns at the time of discharge from treatment in evaluating subsequent weight development, have also been performed. In line with the earlier information on eating patterns, these showed that reduction of disinhibited eating [22] and increase in cognitive restraint [58,59] during active treatment were positive predictors of post-treatment weight reduction and weight maintenance. Higher levels of dietary disinhibition assessed after an intentional weight loss phase [57] or during weight maintenance [41] predict weight regain. More hunger according to the TFEQ at discharge has also been shown to be a negative predictor of post-treatment weight change [22]. This means that more intense hunger and disinhibited eating creates a risk for subsequent overconsumption.

Another study has analyzed pretreatment data on eating behaviors as predictors of weight development after treatment [17]. These results revealed that a high pretreatment score on the TFEQ hunger scale predicted weight regain at follow-up after very low-calorie diet (VLCD) treatment. With more intense hunger initially, long-term success with VLCD treatment is thus less likely. Often, however, the pretreatment TFEQ scores have not provided predictive information on subsequent weight loss [43,56].

On the issue of control over eating behaviors, it has been suggested that more flexible control over eating behavior is associated with weight maintenance, rather than rigid control [60]. Although eating restraint is often reported to be related to weight loss in behavioral treatments, such restraint has also been associated with periods of overeating, and is suggested to be a risk factor for the development of eating disorders [61]. The rigid approach that could be considered a risk factor for a subsequent total breakdown of controls can be described as a dichotomous "all or nothing" approach to weight and eating. It implies extreme behaviors such as attempts to totally avoid sweets and liked foods. The flexible controls are rather characterized by a "more or less" approach that can be adopted as a more long-term task [60]. Regainers have described that during dieting they did not permit themselves any of the food they really enjoyed and therefore felt deprived [37]. Recent research results show that maintaining initial treatment changes towards more flexible control predicts better long-term weight loss results [48] and flexible and rigid controls have been related to lower and higher body weights, respectively [62]. This suggests that rigid controls should not be encouraged in treatment of obese patients, and that flexible controls should rather be supported.

Binge eating

Binge eating is a pronounced problem in obese eating behavior that has been recognized in the last few decades [63]. The prevailing suggested definition of binge eating (binge-eating disorder), although still not a formal diagnosis, includes the consumption of large quantities of food without being in control of this behavior, and also the experience of distress about such binge eating [64]. Binge eating assessed after weight loss has predicted more subsequent weight regain [57]. Gainers had more binge episodes per month in the initial assessment, and had also increased their number of binge episodes at 1-year follow-up. This more profound disturbance in obese eating behavior poses a major problem in weight maintenance. Binge eating has also been related to a history of weight cycling [65], which would reflect prior failures in maintaining weight losses. In obesity surgery, the weight regain after 5 years has been found to be considerably higher in binge eaters than in other patients [66]. However, others conclude that binge-eating status seems to be a weak prognostic indicator of weight regain, and that psychologic dysphoria may be the important factor for such an association [65]. In yet other studies binge eating was not related to long-term weight loss [67]. Such a finding would suggest that although binge eating obviously implies more profound difficulties with eating behavior, the binge eaters could still benefit from standard obesity programs.

Self-monitoring

Self-monitoring means observing oneself and one's behavior. Self-monitoring of body weight and food intake is an important factor in weight loss as well as weight loss maintenance [6,57,68]. Weight maintenance seems to require an ongoing adherence to weight-related behaviors. Regularly weighing oneself is an example of self-monitoring, as is recording food intake. Self-monitoring of food intake is suggested to reflect one component of cognitive restraint known to be important for weight control. It could also be suggested that these patients continue to use self-monitoring strategies that have been learned during the treatment phase [6]. In weight regainers, self-monitoring has been shown to decline with time [57].

Being more aware and vigilant with regard to weight control has likewise been found to characterize weight maintainers [37,69]. The maintainers were, for example, more conscious about their dietary intake and made more conscious decisions with regard to food selection [69]. Maintainers were also more aware that they needed to be conscious of their weight-related behaviors [37]. The regainers, on the other hand, found it too difficult to remain in the state of prolonged consciousness needed to watch themselves over time [69].

Life events and social support

The surrounding environment and the life events facing the person trying to lose and maintain weight can facilitate as well as hamper the outcome. Experiencing stressful life events or rating one's life as stressful has been associated with weight regain [70–72]. In follow-up assessments, the patients who regained weight after treatment reported more psychosocial crises, including major illnesses and bereavements [71], personal or family stress, and a busy schedule [70]. Interviews with successful persons suggest that their maintenance of weight may depend on stable circumstances after the active behavior changes [73]. The critical life events in this study included areas such as family relations and social activities.

Social support is considered as an important aid for weight maintenance [74,75]. Participating in a maintenance support group [70] as well as receiving support from friends [68,76] and having people available for social support [37] have been related to better weight maintenance.

However, according to a systematic review on family involvement in weight control, there are mixed results for a spouse's involvement. Sometimes there is an improved outcome at follow-up, sometimes there are better results for treating the patient alone [77]. In one study weight maintenance was better for women treated together with their spouse, both being targeted for weight loss and social support strategies, whereas the men did better when treated alone [78]. In two other studies including the spouses to provide support (both female and male participants),

weight maintenance was better for the women treated alone [79]. For the men treated alone a better outcome was seen in 1-year maintenance but with no difference at 2 years follow-up [68]. Although support from the social context is often helpful, involvement from a close life partner is therefore not always positive and may for some persons even interfere with long-term outcome. The divergent findings suggest that additional factors in the person's situation determine whether or not the support given by the spouse is helpful for weight maintenance.

Receiving prolonged treatment interventions and continuous professional support in the weight maintenance phase has often been found to improve treatment outcomes [80]. Professional contact may, for example, enhance vigilance and motivation, and provide encouragement and support. Such interventions, however, may be considered a prolonged treatment phase, rather than factors in weight maintenance. A question has been raised whether such long-term interventions may lessen the patient motivation to take responsibility for their lifestyle changes [81]. The alternative view is that support must be given to the patient to accept full responsibility for lifestyle changes from the onset of treatment.

Stress and coping

Stress as an important risk factor has received additional attention. The ability to cope with stress may be crucial for the individual attempting to sustain their weight, rather than the actual number of life changes and circumstances that are stressors [48,82,83].

The research findings on regainers typically describe poor coping strategies. A common definition of coping refers to cognitive and behavioral efforts used to manage external and internal demands that are appraised as taxing or that exceed the person's resources [84]. A common characteristic identified in regainers is that they tend to eat in response to stressful or negative life events and negative emotions that can be evoked by stressors in everyday life [37,82], and they have the tendency to use eating to regulate mood [37,69]. Rather than using direct ways to handle problems in life, it was common to use escape-avoidance ways of coping which typically would include overeating, sleeping more and passively wishing that the problem would vanish [37]. Those likely to regain their weight have also reported seeking more help as a way to cope with dietary lapse, such as seeking help from a friend, spouse or family member, or starting a weight loss program [85]. This finding suggests a lack of self-sufficiency or self-efficacy. Others, however, have shown that help seeking may increase the chances of weight maintenance [37].

Maintainers as compared to regainers have been reported to be able to cope more easily with cravings [86] and to use direct coping in relapse situations [85]. Such direct coping included treating the relapse as a small mistake, recovering and starting to lose weight again, increasing exercise and starting to control food intake [85]. Being active and doing something (anything) rather than being passive in response to an overeating episode, and regaining control quickly, has also predicted better weight maintenance [68]. The maintainers also seem more like to use effective problem-solving skills and confronting ways of coping with demands in life [37,82]. This included finding new solutions, using concepts taught in treatment [82] or using other strategies such as relaxation techniques or even working more [37].

Overeating clearly is an unfortunate coping strategy in obesity, and can reflect the absence of more efficient coping. Having a passive orientation can sometimes represent a less successful approach than finding one's own solutions and being more active. Personality factors can be important in the ability to find coping strategies to be used in various life situations, rather than reverting to old eating habits. Coping capacity has also been shown to increase during treatment of obese patients [86]. The improvements in coping were considered to be general treatment effects as they were not dependent on type of treatment. Greater improvements in coping were found among the patients who had lost most weight. Although coping depends on personality it can thus to some extent be trained. A conclusion from the overall results on coping is that an ability to handle situations by relying on internal resources, involving cognitive abilities, is a crucial factor in weight control.

Attitudes and strategies

Patients who were less prone to attribute the reason for their obesity to medical factors have been shown to be more successful in later maintaining weight loss [52]. Moreover, successful people were more motivated to lose weight for reasons that related to having confidence in oneself, rather than pressures from others or medical reasons. The confidence factors more specifically included increasing self-esteem, liking oneself more and feeling better about oneself [52].

Retrospective studies of successful weight maintainers have shown more concern with weight, shape and appearance in women successfully maintaining a lower body weight [87]. The women were described as having developed a "healthy narcissism" about their appearance and physical condition. In another study pride in appearance was among the top four self-rated factors facilitating weight maintenance, although it did not differ between weight maintainers and weight regainers (the other three factors were regular exercise, low-calorie/low-fat food choices and regular weigh-ins) [70]. Caring about one's appearance and physical condition can thus be important for the motivation to control body weight.

The natural weight increase in female adolescents has also been shown to be somewhat less with higher physical appearance self-esteem, as well as social self-esteem [88]. It is suggested these young women have higher levels of self-efficacy in weight-controlling behaviors. A tendency to evaluate self-worth in terms of weight and shape has, however, also been associated with weight regain [69]. Weight regainers have also been found to see themselves as not just heavy, but also ugly [37]. Yet another study has described that women who had maintained their achieved weight loss were more self-confident and capable of taking responsibility over their lives and assumed responsibility for their

need to lose weight. They had developed their own personally individualized diets, exercise and maintenance plans, and had also become more active outside the home [87]. Personal strategies in weight maintainers have also been described by others [37]. These women used strategies for weight control that were specific to their individual lifestyle. Creating such personally adjusted strategies in weight control could be considered as a sign of psychologic strength and coping ability, as well as an awareness of one's own role in weight control.

Other results agreeing with the notion that taking responsibility for one's life is important for weight development have shown that maintainers attribute their success to their own determination and patience [86]. The specific responses given were often related to having a definitive commitment and making up one's mind.

Motivation

Motivation for weight reduction is one of the most obvious aspects in weight control, and a literature search suggests that many studies do find that a higher pretreatment motivation is related to greater weight loss [89] although a few studies have found no such relationships [90]. In our own search, we found few results on initial motivation with regard to subsequent weight maintenance. In one study, weight regainers, in follow-up assessments, more commonly reported low motivation as an obstacle than the weight maintainers [70]. A test developed to assess weight loss readiness and motivation, the Weight Loss Readiness Test [91], has failed to predict weight loss [89,92] and no data were found on the test related to weight maintenance. Unpublished data from the Weight Loss Readiness Test carried out at our obesity unit revealed no relationship to weight loss or weight loss maintenance (Elfhag & Rössner, personal communication).

Locus of control

The "locus of control" indicates whether a person experiences control over their life as being internal or external. With an internal locus of control, outcomes are perceived to be a consequence of one's own actions, and that it is possible to influence how the future will turn out. An external locus of control indicates perceiving life as being determined by fate, chance or luck, or being under the control of powerful others [93].

There are varying results concerning the relationship between locus of control and weight reduction [94]. Some studies found that an internal locus of control is related to more weight loss, whereas other studies failed to identify a difference between "internals" and "externals" on locus of control. With regard to weight maintenance, some studies have likewise reported that those with an internal locus of control are more successful, interpreted as a better ability to assume full responsibility over one's own actions [94]. A more specific measure of the locus of control over the health [95], was, however, unrelated to weight maintenance [96].

Another specific locus of control scale targeting body weight has also been constructed. The Weight Locus of Control Scale

[97] shows some relationship with weight loss [97] but no information on weight maintenance. More internal control on this Weight Locus of Control Scale has in later research been related to having more confidence in weight loss behaviors whereas external control was related to perceiving external reasons for being overweight, perceiving several barriers to physical activity and being dissatisfied with social support received [98].

Autonomous motivation has predicted more regular attendance at a weight loss program, and also better weight loss maintenance [96]. Such autonomy implies an internal locus of causality for behavior as opposed to controlled behaviors that have an external locus of causality. According to the self-determination theory, the probability that a person will persist with a behavior or not depends on whether they believe the idea for initiating and subsequently continuing to regulate the behavior comes from within themselves [99]. The participants who made their own decision to take part in the program and lose weight were thus more successful.

To conclude, locus of control, or at least some aspect thereof, can sometimes be beneficial for later outcome. An internal locus of control would also have some resemblance to the concept of "self-efficacy" [98] that has received much attention in weight management.

Self-efficacy

Self-efficacy means confidence in one's personal ability to manage life obstacles and accomplish an achievement such as weight loss [100]. Self-efficacy also entails the expectation of success.

Self-efficacy regarding weight loss [101], the ability to handle emotions and life situations [68] and exercise [18] have been related to later weight loss maintenance. Follow-up data on weight maintainers have also shown that they have more confidence in the ability to manage their weight than the weight regainers [70]. With higher self-esteem, weight reduction was furthermore subsequently maintained over a longer period of time [94].

In another study, being more "assured" was found to describe a subset of patients who were more independent and goal directed, had greater self-confidence about weight control, felt they "had what it takes" for weight control and were not prone to giving up easily [102]. These more assured participants retained a lower body weight than the other subgroup described as "disbelievers." These results held only until 2 years post treatment, when the assured had regained just as much as the disbelievers. Being a disbeliever implied a lower faith in the ability to control weight and giving up easily. Moving from being a disbeliever to becoming more assured during treatment was also linked to a more favorable weight loss outcome. This demonstrates that treatment interventions can also strengthen self-confidence during treatment, leading to better outcomes. Improvements in self-efficacy in obesity treatments have also been described by others [103].

Personality

Information on personality characteristics enabling a more comprehensive understanding of the various behavioral manifestations in weight development is so far sparse. Socialization, implying a social orientation, has been positively related to weight loss maintenance in two studies [104,105]. The results on socialization suggest that the patients who were more successful had a greater capacity for close relationships. This means a more complete personality development with regard to relating to other people [106]. In line with this, more perceived initial dysfunctions in social interactions have predicted weight relapse [43].

Higher anxiety and monotony avoidance have been negatively related to weight loss maintenance in one study [104] and have also been found to describe the obese as compared to reference groups, along with more impulsivity [107–109]. This personality pattern has been compared to an impulsivity syndrome with ego weakness, and to drug addiction [104,107]. Others report a profile similar to those found for bulimics and alcoholics, and the possibility of similar personality factors being associated with excessive eating and drinking have been discussed [110].

For weight loss results only, there are some research findings revealing a trend towards psychopathology being associated with poorer weight loss in obesity treatments [111–113]. Cuntz et al. [114] suggested that subsequent "winners" in weight maintenance had more improvements in symptoms of psychopathology during the treatment phase, and that there is some relationship between psychopathology and successful weight reduction. More generally, persons with psychopathology are, of course, considered to be more difficult to treat [115,116]. Dichotomous thinking, implying a simplified "black-and-white" approach, was described as characterizing weight regainers whereas more flexible thinking characterized the maintainers [69]. This would also describe an aspect of personality functioning with more mature thinking and balance in the maintainers.

To summarize, these trends suggest that traits reflecting a more completely developed and integrated personality, including areas such as relating and ego strengths with impulse control and overall better functioning, can imply better chances to maintain the weight loss. In accordance with this psychologic pattern, research has shown that middle-aged women who had stayed slim had better psychosocial adaptation and psychologic health [117].

Depression, mood and psychiatric diagnoses

Depression is a central aspect in obese patients entering treatment, as there is an overlap between obesity and mood disorders [118]. Depression has sometimes been associated with weight regain. More self-reported depressive symptoms at an initial assessment after weight loss have been associated with weight regain, although they did not contribute as a predictor [57] and psychiatric diagnoses seem to interfere with long-term weight control [119]. Lower degrees of depression have been found among those recovering from weight relapses than in those who do not, also suggesting that "successes" in body weight control are related to less depressive symptoms [120].

However, several studies have reported no relationship between depression and weight maintenance [121] or even contradictory findings, with a positive relationship between initial depression and weight loss outcome after gastric bypass [122,123]. Lower initial well-being has also been associated with better weight maintenance in nonsurgical treatments [68,72]. Taken together, some negative impact of depression and more severe dysfunctions, but maybe not overall mood, on weight loss maintenance could be considered. More detailed research is needed on the specific aspects and reasons for initial depression and long-term outcome. One possibility is that being dissatisfied and even experiencing suffering about the present obese condition could promote greater motivation for making changes, whereas more pathology and severe depression disrupt a person's functioning and can interfere with weight control.

Further considerations in research on weight loss maintenance

There is also a need to consider all the critical factors in weight maintenance in an integrated way. Weight control is a very complex process that depends more on changing the whole personal life than on single behaviors. Long-term weight reduction was, for example, better in those who had made five or more behavioral improvements compared to those who had made fewer changes [48]. An interaction among these factors is also likely. The combination of a psychologic and physiologic approach may give us more understanding of the mechanisms in weight loss maintenance [124].

The role of different treatments and the patient–treatment interaction should also be noted. One type of treatment approach can suit some people well, whereas quite another approach would suit others, and this would lead to different patterns concerning maintenance of weight loss. For example, obesity surgery creates quite a different situation for weight maintenance than does behavior modification, and each of these situations may be better suited to patients with different characteristics. One study has shown that patients with substantial weight loss achieved through surgery or nonsurgical means differed in their behaviors to maintain weight losses. The surgical group reported eating considerably more dietary fat and less carbohydrate and protein than the nonsurgical controls, and furthermore had lower levels of physical activity [36]. Another study reported that persons who had chosen liquid formulas through formal programs to reduce their weight relied more on dietary strategies such as counting calories and higher dietary restraint in order to maintain their weight loss, whereas those who lost weight by their own means used more physical exercise and weighed themselves more often to maintain their weight loss [125].

The successful weight maintainer

To summarize the findings on factors affecting weight loss maintenance that we have described, a profile characterizing the "successful weight maintainer" can be suggested. This ideal person starts losing weight successfully quite early in treatment and reaches the self-determined weight loss goals. Our ideal weight maintainer leads an active life with less television watching, and

does more leisure activities such as walking and cycling. He or she is in control over eating behavior and is not overly disturbed by hunger. Food intake is kept at a lower lever, meal rhythm is regular, always including breakfast, and healthy foods are chosen. Snacking is reduced. When cravings occur, they can be dealt with by various mechanisms. If experiencing a relapse, our weight maintainer can handle this in a balanced way without exaggerating it as a detrimental failure. Controls are flexible rather than rigid and there is self-sufficiency and autonomy.

Although personality findings are sparse in the research on weight loss, some conclusions can be inferred from the overall findings in the literature. A consistent pattern emerges where the person likely to succeed in maintaining a lower body weight has a personality functioning with more strengths and stability. Such strengths include a capacity for control and flexible thinking and also the ability to cope with relapse rather than reverting to a more dichotomous, all-or-none thinking. The ability to create and sustain a meal structure and alter food habits can also imply psychologic resources and capacities. Finding coping strategies to handle cravings and stressful situations in life reflects an ability to use creativity and thinking, and come up with one's own solutions. Self-monitoring suggests self-awareness, and self-sufficiency and autonomy would likewise constitute strengths.

Not surprisingly, this ideal weight maintainer has fewer inner afflictions and instability such as mental distress, binge eating and weight cycling but instead more stability of weight patterns, eating and emotions. Support is provided by the social context, although our weight maintainer may prefer to rely on their own solutions. There may be more of an internal motivation for weight loss, with wishes to become more confident and feel better about oneself. A healthy narcissism, implying there is at least some energy invested in oneself, with caring for oneself, one's appearance and physical status, can also be considered as a strength.

The regainer has instead more difficulties in self-management, and less efficient ways of handling obstacles in weight maintenance. It seems that approaching the issue of weight control from a psychologic viewpoint could give a better understanding of obesity behaviors. For a list of factors associated with weight loss maintenance and weight regain, see Boxes 26.1 and 26.2.

Treatment considerations

Long-term weight loss management

In spite of some encouraging effects concerning weight loss maintenance, there are great risks that weight regain will occur once intervention has ceased. Obesity is difficult to treat and the long-term weight loss outcome is generally modest in various types of treatment programs [126,127]. Just as with any other medication, obesity treatment, whether with diet or pharmacotherapy, will only work if the treatment interventions are incorporated and adhered to and the medication is taken. Realization of this problem leads to different views when considering the management of

Box 26.1 Suggested factors associated with weight loss maintenance

Has achieved the self-determined weight loss goal

More initial weight loss

Physically active lifestyle

Regular meal rhythm

Eats breakfast

Less dietary fat, more healthy foods

Reduced frequency of snacks

Flexible control over eating

Self-monitoring

Better coping strategies

Can find ways to handle craving

Self-efficacy

Autonomy

"Healthy narcissism"

Motivation for weight loss: becoming more confident

Box 26.2 Suggested factors associated with weight regain

Fails to reach a self-determined weight goal

Attribution of obesity to medical factors

Sedentary lifestyle

Disinhibited eating

More hunger

Binge eating

Eating in response to negative emotions and stress

Depression

Distress

Poor coping strategies

Escape-avoidance to problem

Passive wishes

Help seeking

Motivation for weight loss: medical reasons, other persons

Personality traits indicating more disturbances

obesity. One view considers obesity as a chronic condition, whereas another view emphasizes the responsibility of the patient.

Obesity as a chronic condition

One trend in understanding the treatment principles for obesity emanates from the realization that obesity is a chronic disease and that it is essential to develop long-term treatment strategies from the beginning of therapy. The typical treatment in the 1980s was a program lasting less than 6 months. Today many standard programs, based on diet, exercise and behavior modification, run for up to 2 years, and some of them for even longer.

It has been claimed that behavioral change can only be achieved if treatment involves a long-lasting training process [60]. Several programs take into account the fact that obese patients need a long time to adjust to a new, healthier lifestyle. In the behavioral modification process, changes are introduced one by one and most patients would start to make the changes in their lives with which it is easiest for them to comply. The experience of our day care unit is that basic behavioral changes such as re-establishing a proper eating pattern with breakfast, lunch and dinner may take a long time to achieve. Training obese patients to eat according to the Swedish so-called plate model, where half the plate is filled with vegetables (raw or cooked), one quarter with a carbohydrate portion (rice, potatoes, pasta, bread) and the last quarter with a protein component (meat, fowl, egg, fish, shellfish, etc.), as recommended by the Swedish Food Agency, may take considerable time to become an inherent part of a new eating style.

Targets in treatment

Accomplishing more regular meals and making better food choices (key elements in behavior modification programs) were also recognized as factors contributing to weight maintenance. Several of the other factors identified are also incorporated in standard behavior modification programs. Such treatments are based on restriction of calories and increased physical activity. Behavioral interventions targeting eating behavior, cognitions and feelings related to food and eating, and self-monitoring of behaviors are also integrated parts of such programs. Recording food intake for several days is an example of training self-monitoring behaviors. Learning to deal with emotions and cognitions that can lead to overeating would imply that new coping strategies are trained. The training of self-control and the handling of situations implying risks for overeating are also stressed [128–130].

This means that the standard programs today are already targeting some crucial factors that seem important for weight maintenance. Some other factors that are not always integrated parts of treatment programs could also be mentioned. To start with, some pretreatment factors could be considered. Special attention may be warranted for patients with pretreatment characteristics such as depression, binge eating, and a history of weight cycling, although there were some conflicting research findings on the role of these factors in weight maintenance. Striving for some positive goals in weight loss, such as feeling better about oneself, rather than starting treatment because of outer pressure could also be addressed before treatment onset.

Modifying unrealistic weight loss goals can be an important initial task in treatment [131]. It is essential that patients and therapists learn to understand that weight loss will hardly ever be up to expectations, and to use this as a starting point for further interventions. This is even more crucial when considering the importance of having a self-determined weight loss goal when it comes to long-term results.

Furthermore, initial weight loss is often related to better long-term results, meaning that the patients likely to succeed can be identified quite early in treatment. A run-in period may even be suggested, and the patients who do not lose weight could be moved to other treatment interventions. This would be cost-effective, as well as sparing the patient a larger disappointment later in time.

In treatment, it seems important that patients should learn how to handle particular stresses in their lives, those which imply a risk for overeating. Providing support for developing self-sufficiency and finding inner strengths, ideas and capacities would be essential for long-term results. Feeling good about oneself, the concept of "healthy narcissism," should also be noted. This could be promoted by acknowledging the importance of feeling more attractive and liking oneself more, and recognizing the enjoyment of taking good care of one's body, appearance and health.

Strategies for long-term treatment

Interventions providing a more long-term perspective are of clinical interest. This does not necessarily mean that patients need to be continuously treated. It would, however, be a challenge to develop more long-term strategies and recommendations. Introduction of weight loss by any standard method such as diet, exercise, behavior modification, VLCD or pharmacotherapy will always be a first step. Strategies that have been less tested in long-term programs could include aspects such as weight loss maintenance with supervized booster sessions, or other means. A pharmacologic agent may be added at a lower dose or given in recurrent cycles. The weight maintenance phase would also include strategies to detect and treat weight relapse immediately, including initiation of pharmacotherapy or other active interventions if weight exceeds a preset threshold. Risk situations may include periods when patients may have less ability to comply with a strict new dietary regimen. Life changes such as starting a new job, getting married or having children, as well as diseases and long-term sick leave are examples of such challenges. Seasonal variations in food intake due to holidays or mood fluctuations, such as those related to seasonal affective disorder (SAD), may also make treatment compliance more difficult.

The role of pharmacotherapy in this long-term strategy is far from clear. Treatment could be given with standard doses when weight exceeds a preset threshold. Intermittent treatment has been found to be effective with sibutramine [132] and could be used to lower the total exposure to a drug, as well as costs. Treatment combinations with drugs with various modes of action, possibly at lower doses, could form an alternative strategy. Drug combination studies as well as head-to-head comparisons are currently scarce [133].

Are long-term interventions necessary for weight maintenance?

As a consequence of the chronic condition approach, many standard programs continue over longer periods of time. It has been argued that such extended treatment periods are of little

benefit to the patient. Finnish therapists have suggested that what is achieved during the first year is all that can be expected and that with extended programs, only attrition problems arise, whereas little else can be gained other than frustration [134]

Another crucial question is whether these interventions can actually lessen the patient's motivation to take responsibility for their lifestyle changes [81]. As treatment of longer duration demands considerable resources, and as the obesity epidemic implies, resources to treat the increasing number of patients referred to obesity clinics are lacking. The cost-effectiveness of programs is becoming more and more crucial. It has been suggested that weight reduction programs lasting 4–6 months can be developed to promote subsequent weight loss maintenance. Supporting the patient's full responsibility for lifestyle changes is then one of the essential components from the onset of treatment.

A less costly weight loss maintenance intervention using the Internet has further been compared to therapist-led interventions; the results showed no difference in weight loss between the groups, although the therapist-led group was more satisfied with their group assignment [135]. Such results suggest that there can be less costly and equally effective ways to promote positive weight development. Long-term weight maintenance was, however, better for the patients who had therapist support [136].

References

1. Stunkard AJ. The management of obesity. NY State J Med 1958; 58:79–87.
2. Björvell H, Rössner S. Long term treatment of severe obesity: four year follow up of results of combined behavioural modification programme. BMJ (Clin Res Ed) 1985;291:379–82.
3. Björvell H, Rössner S. A ten-year follow-up of weight change in severely obese subjects treated in a combined behavioural modification programme. Int J Obes 1992;16:623–5.
4. Goldstein DJ. Beneficial health effects of modest weight loss. Int J Obes 1992;16:397–415.
5. Karlsson J, Sjöstrom L, Sullivan M. Swedish obese subjects (SOS) – an intervention study of obesity. Two-year follow-up of health-related quality of life (HRQL) and eating behavior after gastric surgery for severe obesity. Int J Obes 1998;22:113–26.
6. Wing RR, Hill JO. Successful weight loss maintenance. Annu Rev Nutr 2001;21:323–41.
7. National Task Force on the Prevention and Treatment of Obesity. Dieting and the development of eating disorders in overweight and obese adults. Arch Intern Med 2000;160:2581–9.
8. Kuskowska-Wolk A, Rössner S. Body mass distribution of a representative adult population in Sweden. Diabetes Res Clin Pract 1990;10(suppl 1):S37–41.
9. Sjöström L, Larsson B, Backman L, et al. Swedish obese subjects (SOS). Recruitment for an intervention study and a selected description of the obese state. Int J Obes 1992;16:465–79.
10. James WP. Dietary aspects of obesity. Postgrad Med J 1984;60(suppl 3):50–5.
11. Jeffery RW. Does weight cycling present a health risk? Am J Clin Nutr 1996;63(3 suppl):452S-455S.

12. Muls E, Kempen K, Vansant G, Saris W. Is weight cycling detrimental to health? A review of the literature in humans. Int J Obes Relat Metab Disord 1995;19(suppl 3):S46–50.

13. Read G, Hill J. Weight cycling: a review of the animal literature. Obes Res 1993;1:392–402.

14. Brownell K, Rodin J. Medical, metabolic, and psychological effects of weight cycling. Arch Intern Med 1994;154:1325–30.

15. Foreyt JP, Brunner RL, Goodrick GK, et al. Psychological correlates of weight fluctuation. Int J Eat Disord 1995;17:263–75.

16. Simkin-Silverman LR, Wing RR, Plantinga P, Matthews KA, Kuller LH. Lifetime weight cycling and psychological health in normal-weight and overweight women. Int J Eat Disord 1998;24: 175–83.

17. Pasman WJ, Saris WH, Westerterp-Plantenga MS. Predictors of weight maintenance. Obes Res 1999;7:43–50.

18. Teixeira PJ, Going SB, Houtkooper LB, et al. Pretreatment predictors of attrition and successful weight management in women. Int J Obes 2004;28:1124–33.

19. Hansen D, Astrup A, Toubro S, et al. Predictors of weight loss and maintenance during 2 years of treatment by sibutramine in obesity. Results from the European multi-centre STORM trial. Sibutramine Trial of Obesity Reduction and Maintenance. Int J Obes 2001; 25:496–501.

20. Wooley SC, Garner DM. Obesity treatment: the high cost or false hope. J Am Dietet Assoc 1991;91:1248–51.

21. Crawford D, Jeffery RW, French SA. Can anyone successfully control their weight? Findings of a three year community-based study of men and women. Int J Obes 2000;24:1107–10.

22. Cuntz U, Leibbrand R, Ehrig C, Shaw R, Fichter MM. Predictors of post-treatment weight reduction after in-patient behavioral therapy. Int J Obes 2001;25(suppl 1):S99–S101.

23. McGuire MT, Wing RR, Hill JO. The prevalence of weight loss maintenance among American adults. Int J Obes 1999;23:1314–19.

24. Ayyad C, Andersen T. Long-term efficacy of dietary treatment of obesity: a systematic review of studies published between 1931 and 1999. Obes Rev 2000;1:113–19.

25. Foster GD, Wadden TA, Vogt RA, Brewer G. What is a reasonable weight loss? Patients' expectations and evaluations of obesity treatment outcomes. J Consult Clin Psychol 1997;65:79–85.

26. Foster GD, Wadden TA, Phelan S, Sarwer DB, Sanderson RS. Obese patients' perceptions of treatment outcomes and the factors that influence them. Arch Intern Med 2001;161:2133–9.

27. Linne Y, Hemmingsson E, Adolfsson B, Ramsten J, Rössner S. Patient expectations of obesity treatment-the experience from a day-care unit. Int J Obes 2002;26:739–41.

28. Marston AR, Criss J. Maintenance of successful weight loss: incidence and prediction. Int J Obes 1984;8:435–9.

29. McGuire MT, Wing RR, Klem ML, Hill JO. Behavioral strategies of individuals who have maintained long-term weight losses. Obes Res 1999;7:334–41.

30. Cooper Z, Fairburn CG. A new cognitive behavioural approach to the treatment of obesity. Behav Res Ther 2001;39:499–511.

31. Jeffery RW, Wing RR, Mayer RR. Are smaller weight losses or more achievable weight loss goals better in the long term for obese patients? J Consult Clin Psychol 1998;66:641–5.

32. van Baak MA, van Mil A, Astrup AV, et al. Leisure-time activity is an important determinant of long-term weight maintenance after weight loss in the Sibutramine Trial on Obesity Reduction and Maintenance (STORM trial). Am J Clin Nutr 2003;78:209–14.

33. Astrup A, Rössner S. Lessons from obesity management programmes: greater initial weight loss improves long-term maintenance. Obes Rev 2000;1:17–19.

34. Rissanen A, Lean M, Rössner S, Segal KR, Sjöstrom L. Predictive value of early weight loss in obesity management with orlistat: an evidence-based assessment of prescribing guidelines. Int J Obes 2003;27:103–9.

35. European Agency for the Evaluation of Medical Products, Committee for Proprietary Medicinal Products. *European public assessment report (EPAR)*. London: Xenical, 1998.

36. Klem ML, Wing RR, Chang CC, et al. A case-control study of successful maintenance of a substantial weight loss: individuals who lost weight through surgery versus those who lost weight through non-surgical means. Int J Obes 2000;24:573–9.

37. Kayman S, Bruvold W, Stern JS. Maintenance and relapse after weight loss in women: behavioral aspects. Am J Clin Nutr 1990;52:800–7.

38. Schoeller DA, Shay K, Kushner RF. How much physical activity is needed to minimize weight gain in previously obese women? Am J Clin Nutr 1997;66:551–6.

39. Saris WH. Fit, fat and fat free: the metabolic aspects of weight control. Int J Obes 1998;22(suppl 2):S15–21.

40. Hughes JR. Psychological effects of habitual exercise: a critical review. Prev Med 1984;13:66–78.

41. Fogelholm M, Kukkonen-Harjula K, Oja P. Eating control and physical activity as determinants of short-term weight maintenance after a very-low-calorie diet among obese women. Int J Obes 1999; 23:203–10.

42. Leser MS, Yanovski SZ, Yanovski JA. A low-fat intake and greater activity level are associated with lower weight regain 3 years after completing a very-low-calorie diet. J Am Dietet Assoc 2002;102: 1252–6.

43. Karlsson J, Hallgren P, Kral J, Lindroos AK, Sjöström L, Sullivan M. Predictors and effects of long-term dieting on mental well-being and weight loss in obese women. Appetite 1994;23:15–26.

44. Fogelholm M, Kukkonen-Harjula K. Does physical activity prevent weight gain –a systematic review. Obes Rev 2000;1:95–111.

45. Neumark-Sztainer D, Kaufmann NA, Berry EM. Physical activity within a community-based weight control program: program evaluation and predictors of success. Public Health Rev 1995; 23:237–51.

46. Kathan M, Pleas J, Thackery M, Wallston KA. Relationship of eating activity self-reports to follow-up weight maintenance of obesity. Behav Ther 1982;13:521–8.

47. Jeffery RW, Bjornson-Benson WM, Rosenthal BS, Kurth CL, Dunn MM. Effectiveness of monetary contracts with two repayment schedules on weight reduction in men and women from self-referred population samples. Prev Med 1984;15:273–9.

48. Westenhoefer J, von Falck B, Stellfeldt A, Fintelmann S. Behavioural correlates of successful weight reduction over 3 y. Results from the Lean Habits Study. Int J Obes 2004;28:334–5.

49. French SA, Jeffery RW. Current dieting, weight loss history, and weight suppression: behavioral correlates of three dimensions of dieting. Addict Behav 1997;22:31–44.

50. French SA Jeffery RW, Forster JL, McGovern PG, Kelder SH, Baxter JE. Predictors of weight change over two years among a population of working adults: the Healthy Worker Project. Int J Obes 1994; 18:145–54.

51. Holden JH, Darga LL, Olson SM, et al. Long-term follow-up of patients attending a combination very-low calorie diet and behaviour therapy weight loss programme. Int J Obes 1992;16: 605–13.

52. Ogden J. The correlates of long-term weight loss: a group comparison study of obesity. Int J Obes 2000;24:1018–25.

53. Wyatt HR, Grunwald GK, Mosca CL, Klem ML, Wing RR, Hill JO. Long-term weight loss and breakfast in subjects in the National Weight Control Registry. Obes Res 2002;10:78–82.

54. Stunkard AJ, Messick S. The Three Factor Eating Questionnaire to measure dietary restraint, disinhibition and hunger. J Psychosom Res 1985;29:71–83.

55. Lindroos AK, Lissner L, Mathiassen ME, et al. Dietary intake in relation to restrained eating, disinhibition, and hunger in obese and nonobese Swedish women. Obes Res 1987;5:175–82.

56. Björvell H, Aly A, Langius A, Nordström G. Indicators of changes in weight and eating behaviour in severely obese patients treated in a nursing behavioural program. Int J Obes 1994;18:521–5.

57. McGuire MT, Wing RR, Klem ML, Lang W, Hill JO. What predicts weight regain in a group of successful weight losers? J Consult Clin Psychol 1999;67:177–85.

58. Lejeune MP, van Aggel-Leijssen DP, van Baak MA, Westerterp-Plantenga MS. Effects of dietary restraint vs exercise during weight maintenance in obese men. Eur J Clin Nutr 2003;57:1338–44.

59. Westerterp-Plantenga MS, Kempen KP, Saris WH. Determinants of weight maintenance in women after diet-induced weight reduction. Int J Obes 1998;22:1–6.

60. Westenhoefer J. The therapeutic challenge: behavioral changes for long-term weight maintenance. Int J Obes 2001;25(suppl 1):S85–88.

61. Tuschl RJ. From dietary restraint to binge eating: some theoretical considerations. Appetite 1990;14:105–9.

62. Dykes J, Brunner EJ, Martikainen PT, Wardle J. Socioeconomic gradient in body size and obesity among women: the role of dietary restraint, disinhibition and hunger in the Whitehall II study. Int J Obes 2004;28:262–8.

63. Stunkard AJ. Eating patterns and obesity. Psychiatr Q 1959;33:284–92.

64. American Psychiatric Association. *Diagnostic and Statistical Manual of Mental Disorders (DSM-IV)*. Washington, DC: American Psychiatric Association, 1994.

65. Sherwood NE, Jeffery RW, Wing RR. Binge status as a predictor of weight loss treatment outcome. Int J Obes 1999;23:485–93.

66. Pekkarinen T, Koskela K, Huikuri,K, Mustajoki P. Long-term results of gastroplasty for morbid obesity: binge-eating as a predictor of poor outcome. Obes Surg 1994;4:248–55.

67. Gladis MM, Wadden TA, Vogt R, Foster G, Kuehnel RH, Bartlett SJ. Behavioral treatment of obese binge eaters: do they need different care? J Psychosom Res 1998;44:375–84.

68. Jeffery RW, Bjornson-Benson WM, Rosenthal BS, Lindquist RA, Kurth CL, Johnson SL. Correlates of weight loss and its maintenance over two years of follow-up among middle-aged men. Prev Med 1984;13:155–68.

69. Byrne S, Cooper Z, Fairburn C. Weight maintenance and relapse in obesity: a qualitative study. Int J Obes 2003;27:955–62.

70. DePue JD, Clark MM, Ruggiero L, Medeiros ML, Pera V Jr. Maintenance of weight loss: a needs assessment. Obes Res 1995;3:241–8.

71. Dubbert PM. Physiological and psychosocial factors associated with long-term weight loss maintenance. Miss RN 1984;46:20.

72. Sarlio-Lahteenkorva S, Rissanen A, Kaprio J. A descriptive study of weight loss maintenance: 6 and 15 year follow-up of initially overweight adults. Int J Obes 2000;24:116–25.

73. Tinker JE, Tucker JA. Environmental events surrounding natural recovery from obesity. Addict Behav 1997;22:571–5.

74. Perri MG, Sears SF Jr, Clark JE. Strategies for improving maintenance of weight loss. Toward a continuous care model of obesity management. Diabetes Care 1993;16:200–9.

75. Wolfe WA. A review: maximizing social support – a neglected strategy for improving weight management with African-American women. Ethn Dis 2004;14:212–18.

76. Wing RR, Jeffery RW. Benefits of recruiting participants with friends and increasing social support for weight loss and maintenance. J Consult Clin Psychol 1999;67:132–8.

77. McLean N, Griffin S, Toney K, Hardeman W. Family involvement in weight control, weight maintenance and weight-loss interventions: a systematic review of randomised trials. Int J Obes 2003;27:987–1005.

78. Wing RR, Marcus MD, Epstein LH, Jawad A. A "family-based" approach to the treatment of obese type II diabetic patients. J Consult Clin Psychol 1991;59:156–62.

79. Black DR, Lantz CE. Spouse involement and a possible long-term follow-up trap in weight loss. Behav Res Ther 1984;22:557–62.

80. Perri MG, Sears SF, Clark JE. Strategies for improving maintenace of weight loss. Diabetes Care 1993;16:200–9.

81. Mustajoki P, Pekkarinen T. Maintenance programmes after weight reduction – how useful are they? Int J Obes 1999;23:553–5.

82. Gormally J, Rardin D. Weight loss and maintenance and changes in diet and exercise for behavioral counseling and nutrition education. J Couns Psychol 1981;28:295–304.

83. Grilo CM, Shiffman S, Wing RR. Relapse crises and coping among dieters. J Consult Clin Psychol 1989;57:488–95.

84. Folkman S, Lazarus RS. The relationship between coping and emotion: implications for theory and research. Soc Sci Med 1988;26:309–17.

85. Dohm FA, Beattie JA, Aibel C, Striegel-Moore RH. Factors differentiating women and men who successfully maintain weight loss from women and men who do not. J Clin Psychol 2001;57:105–17.

86. Ryden A, Karlsson J, Sullivan M, Torgerson JS, Taft C. Coping and distress: what happens after intervention? A 2-year follow-up from the Swedish Obese Subjects (SOS) study. Psychosom Med 2003;65:435–42.

87. Colvin RH, Olson SB. A descriptive analysis of men and women who have lost significant weight and are highly successful at maintaining the loss. Addict Behav 1983;8:287–95.

88. French SA, Perry CL, Leon GR, Fulkerson JA. Self-esteem and change in body mass index over 3 years in a cohort of adolescents. Obes Res 1996;4:27–33.

89. Teixeira PJ, Palmeira AL, Branco TL, et al. Who will lose weight? A reexamination of predictors of weight loss in women. Int J Behav Nutr Phys Act 2004;1:12.

90. Edell BH, Edington S, Herd B, O'Brien RM, Witkin G. Self-efficacy and self-motivation as predictors of weight loss. Addict Behav 1987;12:63–6.

91. Brownell KD. Dieting readiness. Weight Control Dig 1990;1:5–10.

92. Fontaine KR, Wiersema L. Dieting readiness test fails to predict enrollment in a weight loss program. J Am Dietet Assoc 1999;99: 664.

93. Rotter JB. Generalized expectancies for internal versus external locus of reinforcement. Psychol Monogr (General and Applied) 1966;80:1–28.

94. Nir Z, Neumann L. Relationship among self-esteem, internal-external locus of control, and weight change after participation in a weight reduction program. J Clin Psychol 1995;51:482–90.

95. Wallston BS, Wallston KA, Kaplan GD, Maides SA. Development and validation of the Health Locus of Control (HCL) Scale. J Consult Clin Psychol 1976;44:580–5.

96. Williams GC, Grow VM, Freedman ZR, Ryan RM, Deci EL. Motivational predictors of weight loss and weight-loss maintenance. J Pers Soc Psychol 1996;70:115–26.

97. Saltzer EB. The weight locus of control (WLOC) scale: a specific measure for obesity research. J Pers Assess 1982;46:620–8.

98. Holt CL, Clark EM, Kreuter MW. Weight locus of control and weight-related attitudes and behaviors in an overweight population. Addict Behav 2001;26:329–40.

99. Deci EL, Ryan RM. *Intrinsic Motivation and Self-Determination in Human Behavior.* New York: Plenum, 1985.

100. Bandura A. Self-efficacy mechanism in human agency. Am Psychol 1982;37:122–47.

101. Rodin J, Elias M, Silberstein LR, Wagner A. Combined behavioral and pharmacologic treatment for obesity: predictors of successful weight maintenance. J Consult Clin Psychol 1988;56:399–404.

102. Dennis KE, Goldberg AP. Weight control self-efficacy types and transitions affect weight-loss outcomes in obese women. Addict Behav 1996;21:103–16.

103. Clark MM, Abrams DB, Niaura RS, Eaton CA, Rossi JS. Self-efficacy in weight management. J Consult Clin Psychol 1991;59: 739–44.

104. Jönsson B, Björvell H, Levander S, Rössner S. Personality traits predicting weight loss outcome in obese patients. Acta Psychiatr Scand 1986;74:384–7.

105. Rydén O, Hedenbro JL, Frederiksen SG. Weight loss after vertical banded gastroplasty can be predicted: a prospective psychological study. Obes Surg 1996;6:237–43.

106. Guntrip H. *Schizoid Phenomena, Object-Relations and The Self.* London: Karnac Books, 1992.

107. Björvell H, Edman G, Rössner S, Schalling D. Personality traits in a group of severely obese patients in two self-chosen weight reducing programs. Int J Obes 1985;9:257–66.

108. Fassino S, Leombruni P, Piero A, et al. Temperament and character in obese women with and without binge eating disorder. Comprehens Psychiatr 2002;43:431–7.

109. Ryden A, Sullivan M, Torgerson JS, Karlsson J, Lindroos AK, Taft C. Severe obesity and personality: a comparative controlled study of personality traits. Int J Obes 2003;27:1534–40.

110. Palme G, Palme J. Personality characteristics of females seeking treatment for obesity, bulimia nervosa and alcoholic disorders. Pers Individ Diff 1999;26:255–63.

111. Barrash J, Rodriguez EM, Scott DH, Mason EE, Sines JO. The utility of MMPI for the prediction of weight loss after bariatric surgery. Int J Obes 1987;11:115–28.

112. Elfhag K, Rössner S, Lindgren T, Andersson I, Carlsson AM. Rorschach personality predictors of weight loss with behavior

113. Rowe JL, Downey JE, Faust M. Psychological and demographic predictors of successful weight loss following silastic ring vertical stapeled gastroplasty. Psychol Rep 2000;86:1028–36.

114. Cuntz U, Leibbrand R, Ehrig C, Shaw R, Fichter MM. Predictors of post-treatment weight reduction after in-patient behavioral therapy. Int J Obes 2001;25(suppl 1):S99–S101.

115. Blanck G, Blanck R. *Ego Psychology: Theory and Practice*, 2nd edn. New York: Columbia University Press, 1994.

116. Kernberg O. *Severe Personality Disorders. Psychotherapeutic Strategies.* New Haven: Yale University Press, 1984.

117. Baghaei F, Rosmond R, Westberg L, et al. The lean woman. Obes Res 2002;10:115–21.

118. McElroy SL, Kotwal R, Malhotra S, Nelson EB, Keck PE, Nemeroff CB. Are mood disorders and obesity related? A review for the mental health professional. J Clin Psychiatr 2004;65:634–51, quiz 730.

119. Jenkins I, Djuric Z, Darga L, DiLaura NM, Magnan M, Hryniuk WM. Relationship of psychiatric diagnosis and weight loss maintenance in obese breast cancer survivors. Obes Res 2003;11:1369–75.

120. Phelan S, Hill JO, Lang W, Dibello JR, Wing RR. Recovery from relapse among successful weight maintainers. Am J Clin Nutr 2003;78:1079–84.

121. Wadden TA, Foster GD, Wang J, et al. Clinical correlates of short- and long-term weight loss. Am J Clin Nutr 1992;56(1 suppl): 271S–274S.

122. Averbukh Y, Heshka S, El-Shoreya H, et al. Depression score predicts weight loss following Roux-en-Y gastric bypass. Obes Surg 2003;13:833–36.

123. Dubovsky SL, Haddenhorst A, Murphy J, Liechty RD, Coyle DA. A preliminary study of the relationship between preoperative depression and weight loss following surgery for morbid obesity. Int J Psychiatr Med 1985;15:185–96.

124. Wing RR. Behavioral interventions for obesity: recognizing our progress and future challenges. Obes Res 2003;11(suppl):3S-6S.

125. McGuire MT, Wing RR, Klem ML, Seagle H, Hill JO. Long-term maintenance of weight loss: do people who lose weight through various weight loss methods use different behaviors to maintain their weight? Int J Obes 1998;22:572–7.

126. Lean ME. Obesity – what are the current treatment options? Exper Clin Endocrinol Diabetes 1998;106(suppl 2):22–6.

127. Wooley SC, Garner DM. Obesity treatment: the high cost of false hope. Journal of the American Dietetic Association, J Am Dietet Assoc 1991;91:1248–51.

128. Allison DB. *Handbook of Assessment Methods for Eating Behaviors and Weight-Related Concerns.* Thousand Oaks, CA: Sage Publications, 1995.

129. Melin I, Rössner S. Practical clinical behavioral treatment of obesity. Patient Educ Counsel 2003;49:75–83.

130. Wadden TA. The treatment of obesity. In: Stunkard AJ, Wadden TA (eds) *Obesity. Theory and Therapy.* New York: Raven, 1993.

131. Rössner S. Factors determining the long-term outcome of obesity. In: Björntorp P, Brodoff BN (eds) *Obesity.* Philadelphia: J.B. Lippincott, 1992.

132. Wirth A, Krause J. Long-term weight loss with sibutramine: a randomized controlled trial. JAMA 2001; 286:1331–9.

133. Neovius M, Johansson K, Rossner S. Head-to-head studies

modification in obesity treatment. J Pers Assess 2004;83(3):293–305.

evaluating efficacy of pharmaco-therapy for obesity: a systematic review and meta-analysis. Obes Rev 2008;9(5):420–7

134. Kaukua J, Pekkarinen T, Sane T, Mustajoki P. Health-related quality of life in obese outpatients losing weight with very-low-energy diet and behaviour modification: a 2-y follow-up study. Int J Obes 2003;27:1072–80.

135. Harvey-Berino J, Pintauro SJ, Gold EC. The feasibility of using Internet support for the maintenance of weight loss. Behav Modif 2002;26:103–16.

136. Harvey-Berino J, Pintauro S, Buzzell P, et al. Does using the Internet facilitate the maintenance of weight loss? Int J Obes 2002;26: 1254–60.

27 Education and Training of Healthcare Professionals

Peter G. Kopelman

St George's Hospital, University of London, London, UK

Introduction

The dramatic increase in the prevalence of overweight and obesity has not been matched by an increase in the amount of education and training provided for health professionals, regardless of their discipline. Too often, health professionals ignore the obvious signs or symptoms of a nutritional disorder within a patient and, if they are overweight, simply instruct the patient to go on a diet. It is therefore not surprising that intervention only comes when medical complications have become apparent. This oversight reflects a poor understanding of nutritional issues and a lack of knowledge and skills about their management. There is limited information provided in both undergraduate and postgraduate training programs and scant attention in specialist medical training. The medical profession's appreciation of the medical consequences of obesity is reflected by the absence of specialist units in most regional hospitals and reluctance to consider pharmacotherapy or surgery for patients most at risk. Since clinical teachers have had little or no training in the subject, they tend not to teach it. As a result, many doctors neglect clinical nutrition through lack of awareness of its potential benefits in the prevention and treatment of disease.

This chapter will first focus on the education of health professionals in nutritional care and then address the deficiencies in training for the management of overweight and obese patients.

Clinical Obesity in Adults and Children, 3rd edition. Edited by Peter G. Kopelman, Ian D. Caterson and William H. Dietz.
© 2010 Blackwell Publishing, ISBN: 978-1-4051-8226-3.

Why is it important to educate health professionals about nutrition?

A health professional's primary role is, by definition, to care for their patients. As a consequence, they need to fully understand the fundamentals of nutritional science and be able to apply these in clinical practice.

It is clear that a substantial proportion of the world's population make imprudent food choices. Increasingly, diets and patterns of food consumption are associated with greater risk of poor micronutrient intake and ultimately deficiencies. The burden of ill health arising from the increased prevalence of overweight and obesity in children and adults, and the substantial increase in risk of co-morbidities such as cardiovascular disease, type 2 diabetes and cancer, are directly related to poor dietary choices and inadequate levels of physical activity. These factors facilitate the following professional roles.

• *Educational:* healthcare professionals are held in regard by the public as providers of authoritative information and advice on food, health and nutrition. Healthcare professionals need to ensure that they remain familiar with up-to-date information about nutritional health. This should be regarded as an essential element of their continuing professional development.

• *Advisory:* health professionals can influence food and nutrition policy in their own hospital setting and within the local community. They should be encouraged to nominate a lead for nutrition and, where appropriate, be involved in nutrition management and the nutrition team. Job plans should reflect the importance of nutrition as a part of weekly duties.

• *Organizational:* health professionals should be encouraged to initiate or contribute to programs on nutrition by working as individuals, through professional societies or other healthcare organizations. Training must include the management of this kind of work.

• *Therapeutic:* high demands are placed on healthcare resources arising from diseases of malnutrition that include overweight and obesity. There is thus an imperative to introduce appropriate screening in order to be able to provide prevention and interventions for those at greatest risk. This responsibility is shared across a wide range of health professionals.

• *Investigatory:* health professionals should be encouraged to consider research into nutritional topics as part of their work. This should include both applied basic and molecular science as well as clinical investigations. Through the provision of research funding for nutrition, governments should acknowledge the importance of such research.

Education and training in nutrition

As a first step there is a need to establish systems which are standardized across all professional groups. These systems should ensure that all those who make up the health professional workforce are appropriately competent to react to the demands of clinical service.

Nutrition fits into every medical discipline. Medical curricula contain a wealth of information relevant to diet and nutrition but generally represent a classic approach through biochemistry and physiology. It remains uncommon for nutrition to be taught as metabolism at the whole-body level, thereby enabling health professionals to understand how function is maintained in health, and disturbed by disease. However, it is generally acknowledged that many recently trained health professionals still have an inadequate knowledge of the nutritional aspects of health promotion and disease treatment.

The need for better training in human nutrition is now recognized in all disciplines of healthcare. In the UK, the Government's Nutrition Task Force, created under the Health of the Nation initiative, published in 1994 a "Core Curriculum for Nutrition in the Education of Health Professionals" that is globally applicable. The curriculum identifies a minimum core of essential knowledge for all health professionals and is divided into three sections.

• *Principles of nutritional science:* to include foods and nutrient, metabolic processes, physical activity, effect of diet and nutrient status on biochemistry and organ function.

• *Public health nutrition:* to include the average diet, lifestyle and risk factors, dietary reference values, nutritional surveillance, education and motivation, food policies and composition

• *Clinical nutrition and nutritional support:* assessment of clinical and functional metabolic state, effect of functional state on nutritional intake and status, effect of status on clinical outcomes.

In each of the three major areas, six bullet points were detailed to make a total of 18 bullet points (see Box 27.1).

The aims of the core curriculum were to enable health professionals to:

Box 27.1 The 18 bullet points covering education and training

Principles of nutritional science
• Diets, foods and nutrients
• Metabolic demand, digestion and absorption, balance and turnover, physical activity, metabolic effects of excess, obesity
• Requirements, essentiality, bio-availability, limiting nutrients, effects of nutritional status on biochemical and organ function
• Adaptation to low nutrient intake, body composition (form and function)
• Assessment of diet and nutritional status
• Physiologic mechanisms that determine appetite, sociologic, psychologic, economic and behavioral aspects of food choice

Public health nutrition
• The average national diet including subgroup differences (e.g. region, gender, ethnic origin), lifestyle, risk factors and epidemiology
• Preconception, pregnancy, breast feeding, infant nutrition, growth and development, aging
• Dietary reference values, dietary recommendations and guidelines, diet and coronary heart disease and stroke, health targets
• Nutritional surveillance and identification of markers of nutritional status
• Achieving change, education, motivation
• Food supply, monitoring, cost/benefit of nutritional interventions, legislation, food labeling and policy

Clinical nutrition and nutritional support
• Assessment of clinical and functional metabolic status
• Anorexia and starvation, response to injury, infection and stress
• Altered nutritional requirements in relevant disease states
• General principles of nutritional support
• Basis of nutrition-related disease, therapeutic diets, weight reduction
• Drug–nutrient interactions

• appreciate the importance and relevance of nutrition in the promotion of good health, and prevention and treatment of disease
• describe the basic scientific principles of human nutrition
• identify nutrition-related problems in individuals and the community
• give consistent and sound dietary advice
• provide appropriate and safe clinical nutritional support, and know how and when to refer to a specialist in clinical nutrition.

To implement the core curriculum, training of health professionals needs to start at an undergraduate/pre-registration level and then continue through into professional training and development.

Undergraduate or pre-registration training

By its nature, nutrition pervades every scientific and clinical discipline. It embraces broader considerations of economics and social interactions. The science of nutrition starts at a cellular level with questions about energy storage and utilization. It permeates through the individual and asks questions about access to food, the adequacy of such food and the environmental impact.

Every opportunity should be taken to introduce nutritional concepts into undergraduate/pre-registration training. Nutrition is a key component of health and illness and should be identified as such by students. There is every reason for students to feel engaged with the science and application of nutrition because good nutrition should be a principle followed by themselves.

There have been advances in teaching nutrition. However, the time allocated in training programs to nutritional issues remains difficult to identify, and information about how well nutrition is incorporated into curricula using problem-based learning as the core method of medical education is not available. This is addressed in the following ways.

• Nutrition should be promoted as a model subject for teaching across the entire undergraduate curriculum and the nutrition being taught should be what a health professional needs to know. Human nutrition can be incorporated as an integrated theme to link basic sciences, clinical and public health aspects of health and disease in the core curriculum.

• Nutrition offers the potential of "horizontal integration" across disciplines as a component of problem-based approaches. Problem-based learning engages students in small groups to investigate and solve clinically based problems presented as case scenarios.

• Nutrition is well suited to project work, particularly for public health nutrition.

• Nutritional screening and assessment should be included as part of the teaching of clinical skills and students should be instructed about relevant practical skills such as the assessment of swallowing.

• Nutritional topics should be assessed at all levels throughout undergraduate/pre-registration training – the objective structured clinical examination (OSCE) provides a practical examination format. OSCEs are a series of examination stations where the student's skills at tackling common clinical problem are observed by an examiner, who marks the student's performance using a structured marksheet.

• An agreed procedure for clinical assessment of the nutritional status of patients should be included as a core skill; this should be part of any routine examination.

• Teaching of nutrition should draw widely on available skills across disciplines, including medicine, pharmacy, dietitics and nursing.

Nutritional education must not stop at the time of graduation but continue through the postgraduation period and into continuing professional development.

Postgraduate and postregistration training – continuing professional development

Postgraduate nutritional training should form a continuum with undergraduate training and lead to an appreciation that nutrition is important in all disciplines of medicine. Health professionals should be motivated to regard nutrition as important in the prevention and management of disease. Much of nutritional learning, whether acquiring knowledge or skills, will be acquired in a work-based setting. The major elements will include:

• assessment of nutritional state and its effect on clinical outcomes

• nutritional requirements in illness and the metabolic effect of injury and infection

• general principles of nutritional support and routes of support

• principles of the dietetic management of nutrition-related disorders.

Regular multiprofessional teaching sessions on nutrition should be included as part of training programs; this should include guidance on nutritional assessment and nutritional requirements in health and disease and an appreciation of nutrition as a determinant of risk. Topics that should be addressed include:

• *undernutrition:* identification of underlying factors and their management

• *overweight and obesity:* identification of patients requiring weight reduction and their management

• *nutritional risk states:* competences in the recognition of suboptimal nutrition that may contribute to risk of ill health

• general principles of nutritional support and the management of starvation.

Health professionals must ensure that a written statement is always made in the clinical notes of patients about their nutritional state as part of the history and physical examination of every new patient. They should be aware of the influence of nutritional status on susceptibility to illness. Every discipline should include an appropriate reference to nutrition in their core curriculum and questions on nutrition should be included in examinations for higher qualifications. Inclusion of questions on nutrition in professional examinations, and incorporation into assessment procedures, are the key to the acceptance of nutrition by teachers and students as an important and valued subject area.

Crucially, clinical teachers must be encouraged to attend training courses on nutrition; education and training in nutrition will only become successful when a multidisciplinary core of staff is established with the necessary experience and teaching skills.

Training in the management of overweight and obese patients

Overweight and obesity are largely preventable through lifestyle changes. The best long-term approach must be their prevention in childhood. An active life course approach will include good infant feeding and nutrition during pregnancy as well as working with adolescents to support healthy physical development of future mothers (and fathers). There are two complementary approaches:

• whole-population approach which aims to reduce the average risk of becoming overweight and obese across the whole population
• individuals at risk approach which aims to identify those at increased risk of becoming overweight and obese and to offer them appropriate advice on how to reduce the risk.

Current literature suggests that many health professionals have inadequate and confused knowledge of best practice in obesity management. Among the nursing and dietetic professions, research has highlighted the limited confidence of these healthcare workers in their ability to assist patients in their attempts to lose weight. Family doctors often fail to recognize obesity as a serious medical condition and commonly recommend weight management only when an accompanying comorbidity is evident. Although the assessment of attitudes towards obesity has been limited, available evidence suggests a very negative approach to the obese, with many health professionals believing its management to be frustrating, time consuming and pointless.

Health professionals should understand the etiology and pathophysiology of increasing body fatness and appreciate the importance of prevention and intervention where the condition is established. They should also acknowledge the familial basis to obesity and bear this in mind when managing the individual patient. Obesity management may be divided into a modular training program to enable health professionals to gain knowledge and skills in a stepwise manner. Importantly, this should also facilitate the acquisition of appropriate attitudes towards patients with the condition. Such programs will include the following topics:

• knowledge and understanding of overweight and obesity
• diet and nutrition
• physical activity
• counseling skills and principles of behavior change
• assessment skills
• therapeutic interventional skills.

An outline of a modular program is provided as an appendix to this chapter.

The aim of such a program is to better equip health professionals with the knowledge, skills and confidence to help obese and overweight patients to implement lifestyle change. It is additionally essential that health professionals are fully aware of when, how and to whom to refer within or outside their multidisciplinary team. Likewise, special groups such as adolescent and childhood obesity, obesity during pregnancy and morbid obesity generally require more specialist input.

The underpinning basis for long-term lifestyle change can be summarized by the "3 E" model approach.
• *Encouragement:* simple methods of encouragement to support individuals to change their lifestyle (including low-calorie foods and increased physical activity). Such opportunities frequently present in a clinical setting.
• *Empowerment:* the process of providing knowledge and skills to help individuals make healthy changes (an educational approach) that include awareness of basic nutritional principles and food shopping skills. It also includes skills to help build confidence and esteem in those with weight problems.
• *Environment:* refers to the totality of the cultural, social, physical and economic environments required to facilitate improvements in lifestyle that include diet and physical activity, thereby making healthy choices easier.

Long-term weight maintenance

Patients who maintain significant amounts of weight loss engage in four behavioral patterns:
• they exercise regularly (1500 kcal or more weekly; for adults, at least 30 min of moderate physical activity each day)
• they weigh regularly (daily)
• they eat a low-fat, low-calorie diet
• they monitor their food intake.

Continuous vigilance appears to be the key. To foster such vigilance, long-term contact by health professionals or support groups is important. Such contact helps maintain motivation, provides encouragement, protects against relapse, and provides further opportunities to learn new skills. Ongoing contact with health professionals can help monitor changes and lapses, provide opportunities to change direction when necessary, and allows referral to new therapeutic options if required. Continuing contact with a well-motivated and trained multidisciplinary health team is the key to long-term success.

Conclusion

Successful management of overweight and obesity requires a structured education program that involves all health professionals and commences at the outset of their training. Health professionals need to be appropriately knowledgeable about the principles of nutrition and nutritional care and be able to apply these principles in practice when managing overweight or obese patients. The implementation of education and training will necessarily involve universities, training colleges for professions allied to medicine, nursing and medical schools, postgraduate medical institutions, health services and governments. However, their longer term success is dependent on the commitment and enthusiasm of present health professionals and all others involved in patient care.

Appendix

Knowledge and understanding of obesity

To cover physiology, genetics, psychobiology, pathophysiology, categorization of obesity types and treatment.

Aims: to enhance awareness and understanding of obesity as a serious medical condition; to extend knowledge and understanding of the etiology of obesity and the physiologic consequences of excess weight; to recognize the medical importance of modest weight loss and maintenance

Learning objectives
• To be aware of worldwide and local obesity prevalence and probable trends for the future.
• To understand the definition and classification of obesity/overweight by BMI.
• To recognize obesity as a chronic disease and to be aware of the medical importance and consequences of overweight/obesity in terms of morbidity and mortality.
• To be aware of the medical complications of obesity and recognize obesity as a risk factor for various co-morbidities.
• To understand the influence of abdominal obesity: definition, visceral fat distribution, subcutaneous fat distribution, clinical assessment.
• To understand the direct and indirect costs of obesity.
• To enhance awareness of the social implications of obesity.
• To consider why obesity should be treated and who should be treated.
• To understand the medical benefits of modest weight loss.
• To increase knowledge of the physiology of weight control and the implication of endocrine, neurologic and gastrointestinal systems.
• To be aware of the multifactorial etiology of obesity.
• To be aware of the importance of realistic weight goals and the concept of weight cycling.
• To understand the role of pharmacotherapy and surgery as adjuncts to lifestyle management in certain selected individuals.
• To increase knowledge of the various local commercial slimming programs.

Skills training
• To be able to calculate and classify BMI.
• To know how to measure and classify waist circumference.
• To know how to assess health risks, cardiovascular risk factors and status.
• To be able to determine realistic weight goals for patients.
• To appreciate the importance of involvement of a multiprofessional team.

Diet and nutrition

To cover nutrition knowledge, dietary manipulation, eating behavior and eating disorders.

Aims: to facilitate understanding and awareness of the role of dietary advice in the management of obesity; to provide a foundation in the dietary knowledge and skills required for best practice in the dietary management of obesity.

Learning objectives
• To increase awareness of the role different macronutrients play in the etiology and treatment of obesity.
• To increase awareness of how patterns of food intake and eating behavior have changed over the last few decades.
• To enhance knowledge of the energy requirements of obese subjects and develop the ability to estimate energy requirements for individual patients.
• To gain insight and understanding into the appropriate non-judgmental approach to helping patients make the required lifestyle changes (linking in with the behavioral change components of the program).
• To understand the function, sources and recommended intakes of macronutrients and relevant micronutrients and how they should ideally be balanced in a healthy diet.
• To be aware of the various dietary assessment methods used.
• To understand the phenomena of energy intake under-reporting and the practical implications this may have in the management of such patients.
• To understand the importance of, and practical strategies to use in, the self-monitoring of food intake.
• To be aware of the importance of matching and tailoring dietary strategies to individual patients and practical techniques to determine such individualized management.
• To increase knowledge of alternative dieting practices, diet trends, myths and misconceptions and the nutritional implications of such practices.
• To understand and develop dietary strategies for eating out, special occasions, etc.
• To enhance knowledge and understanding of food labels in relation to weight management.
• To be aware of the energy content of common foods.
• To increase awareness of dietary considerations among various ethnic groups and vegetarians; knowledge of the nutritional content of various ethnic and vegetarian foods; practical acceptable strategies for manipulating such diets.
• To understand the importance of eating behavior on energy intake and strategies to manage eating behavior (link in with behavior change sessions).
• To be aware of the diagnostic criteria for eating disorders with particular reference to binge-eating disorder and to have an understanding of appropriate referral strategies.

Skills training
• To develop the necessary skills for appropriate assessment of dietary intake in obese individuals.
• To be able to calculate energy requirements of overweight and obese individuals.

• To gain practical experience of how to translate nutritional aims into realistic food changes tailored to the individual patient.
• To be able to interpret the nutritional information on a food label.
• To be able to identify rich food sources of various macro- and micronutrients.
• To be able to judge when a client may be presenting with a significant eating disorder and requires further referral.

Physical activity

Aims: to facilitate understanding and awareness of the role of physical activity in the management of obesity; to provide a foundation in the knowledge and skills required to safely, competently and effectively advise on physical activity in the overweight and obese populations.

Learning objectives

• To understand how activity trends have changed over time.
• To understand the beneficial effect of exercise on risk factors associated with obesity – blood lipids, blood pressure, insulin resistance.
• To be aware of the beneficial psychologic effects of physical activity on mood, self-efficacy, self-esteem and body image.
• To be aware of the lack of importance ascribed by many patients to the role of physical activity in weight management.
• To understand the important role physical activity plays in the prevention of obesity and the maintenance of reduced weight.
• To understand the role of physical activity in weight reduction programs and the combined effects with diet.
• To gain insight into the common barriers to physical activity change and practical strategies for tackling such barriers (link with behavioral management section).
• To increase knowledge of the effects of exercise on 24-hour energy expenditure and postexercise energy expenditure.
• To understand the effects of physical activity on 24-hour energy intake, postexercise energy intake and macronutrient selection.
• To understand the effects of exercise on substrate utilization.
• To be aware of the effects of physical activity on body mass and body composition.
• To understand the different exercise intensities and their effect on metabolism and weight change.

Skills training

• To enhance skills in assessing habitual physical activity in obese individuals.
• To enhance skills in recommending a physical activity program – factors to consider, adherence, risks.

Counseling skills

There is widespread agreement that the interpersonal skills of the health professional, in the way they introduce and recommend behavioral change, contribute significantly to the success of cognitive behavioral treatment (CBT). These generic, interpersonal communication skills help the health professional to maximize the therapeutic effect as they guide, motivate and support the overweight patients in changing their lifestyle. Communication skills are also known as counseling skills, since they are a major feature of counseling training, but it is important to recognize that in the case of CBT, interpersonal skills provide the background for providing treatment, and not the treatment itself.

Aim: to increase awareness and effectiveness of interpersonal interactions in the clinical setting.

Learning objectives

• To be able to create rapport, so that clients feel comfortable and able to communicate their concerns.
• To understand and empathize with the client's position.
• To be able to give advice and guidance in an acceptable, comprehensible and engaging fashion.
• To manage the treatment sessions so that appropriate progress is achieved, and terminate treatment appropriately and sympathetically.
• To maintain or increase clients' self-esteem and self-efficacy, even when treatment outcomes are modest.
• To manage clients in group settings so that participants experience the critical elements of a CBT program while also profiting from insights and support from other group members.

Skills training

• To increase social interaction skills.
• To enhance communication skills.
• To develop treatment management skills.
• To enhance group work skills.

Principles of behavior change

Cognitive-behavioral treatment programs are based on psychologic research that suggests that certain practices are helpful in achieving behavior change. In the classic CBT treatment programme, the approach should be educational, co-operative and empiric, with the therapist and patient working together to discover how best to apply CBT principles in the individual's circumstances.

Learning objectives

• To be aware of the importance of self-monitoring.
• To understand the concept of functional analysis.
• To be aware of the importance of goal setting.
• To understand the value of self-reinforcement.
• To understand the importance of cognitive restructuring.
• To be aware of the role of learned self-control.
• To understand the need for clients to adopt a problem-solving perspective.
• To be aware of the value of recruiting social support for change.

Assessment skills

Aims: to be able to make a comprehensive assessment of overweight and obese subjects to facilitate individualized management; to understand when implementation of treatment may not be appropriate.

Learning objectives
• To be able to assess the client's psychosocial history.
• To be aware of specific issues related to weight loss which should be addressed, e.g. motivation, goals for change, treatment expectations.
• To be able to carry out a comprehensive assessment of dietary intake and eating patterns (linking with nutrition and diet module).
• To be able to assess physical activity.
• To be aware of behavioral contraindications to treatment – bulimia nervosa, psychiatric disorders, major life crisis.

Therapeutic intervention
Aims: to be able to identify the appropriate patient, the appropriate time and type of medical and/or surgical intervention; to be aware of the importance of monitoring patients before, during and after therapeutic intervention.

Learning objectives
• To be aware of the actions of antiobesity drugs, appropriate prescribing and potential adverse reactions.
• To understand the indications and contraindications to the use of antiobesity drugs.

• To understand the principles of drug responsiveness and non-responsiveness and risk/benefit analysis for the use of antiobesity drugs.
• To be aware of the potential for weight regain after cessation of drug treatment and the need to reinforce lifestyle measures to maintain weight loss.
• To understand the principles of surgical treatment for obesity.
• To be aware of the criteria for suitability of obese patients for surgical treatment.
• To understand the preoperative assessment and perioperative monitoring of patients undergoing bariatric surgery.
• To be aware of the need to follow up patients after bariatric surgery on a lifetime basis in a multidisciplinary clinic.
• To be aware of the longer term consequences of bariatric surgery.

Further reading

Department of Health. *Nutrition: Core Curriculum for Nutrition in the Education of Health Professionals*. Health of the Nation series. London: Department of Health, 1995.

The Learn® Program for Weight Management 2000. Available at: www.thelifestylecompany.com

Centers for Obesity Research and Education. Available at: www.uchsc.edu/core

Intercollegiate Course on Human Nutrition (Royal Medical Colleges, United Kingdom). Available at: www.icgnutrition.org.uk

5   Childhood Obesity

28 Childhood Obesity: Definition, Classification and Assessment

Aviva Must and Sarah E. Anderson

Department of Public Health and Community Medicine, Tufts University School of Medicine, Boston, MA; Division of Epidemiology, College of Public Health, The Ohio State University, Columbus, OH, USA

Definition and classification

At its simplest level, obesity in children, as in adults, arises when there is an excess of body fat. Setting a definition of obesity for children that will have utility in a clinical setting presents a formidable task; it is more challenging than in adults for several reasons. Ideally, a definition of obesity for children should accurately reflect body fatness and have cut-off points that predict adverse health. Each of these requirements is difficult to meet in the pediatric population.

Because children are growing, all body compartments are increasing in size, although at variable rates. Thus, any measure of excess weight is a moving target and needs to be tied to age. A further complexity arises because biologic age and chronologic age, although closely correlated, are not interchangeable – a problem that is particularly apparent around the time of puberty, when body composition changes are dramatic. In addition, childhood growth patterns differ by sex.

In adults, Body Mass Index (BMI) cut-off points to define overweight and obesity are based on research that links BMI levels to health risks. In children, the evidence base for definitions is weaker.

BMI-for-age and gender percentiles have been adopted as the basic measure for clinical assessment of obesity in children and adolescents. BMI-for-age and gender is well correlated with adiposity and has been linked to morbidity [1,2]. The American Academy of Pediatrics recommends annual monitoring of BMI in youth [3]. Monitoring of childhood growth using percentile charts is a familiar activity for pediatric health professionals, and BMI growth charts are structured like the weight-for-age and stature-for-age charts. Like any screening tool, BMI-for-age and gender represents a trade-off between precision and accuracy, on the one hand, and ease of use on the other. The use of BMI-for-age and gender to assess childhood obesity is justified by its comparison to criterion measures of body fat. These measures are discussed in the following section.

Measures of body fat

Laboratory measures

In a laboratory setting, in contrast to a clinical or field setting, direct measures of adiposity are possible. Such methods conceptualize the human body as having two or more compartments: a fat compartment and at least one compartment for fat-free mass. Although laboratory body composition analysis methods are more precise than nonlaboratory body composition methods such as anthropometry, they have their own limitations. Whole-body methods of assessing body fat include underwater weighing (hydrodensitometry), isotopic dilution, and dual energy X-ray absorptiometry (DXA). Regional adiposity can be assessed with CT scan, MRI or DXA. Table 28.1 describes these methods and lists some of their advantages and disadvantages when used with children. Although these methods, when applied by trained technicians, provide more accurate measures of body fat than do nonlaboratory methods, none is broadly applicable to clinical use due to the inter-related issues of cost, technical requirements and time, as well as limitations due to their invasiveness, necessity of subject co-operation and for some (like CT scan), associated health risks [4,5]. Furthermore, because they are not widely used, population-based reference data are not available.

Clinical Obesity in Adults and Children, 3rd edition. Edited by Peter G. Kopelman, Ian D. Caterson and William H. Dietz.
© 2010 Blackwell Publishing, ISBN: 978-1-4051-8226-3.

Table 28.1 Strengths and limitations of laboratory methods for assessing body fatness in children and adolescents

Method	Strengths	Limitations	Type
Underwater weighing (hydrodensitometry)	Measures body density Highly reproducible Accurate	Requires high subject compliance. Unsuitable for use in young children Relies on assumption of composition of fat-free mass which is unsystematically influenced by age, sex, and ethnicity	Whole body
Air displacement plethysmography	Measures body density Quick Noninvasive Minimal subject compliance needed	High cost Accuracy in children has not been established Instrument designed for adults Relies on assumption of composition of fat-free mass which is unsystematically influenced by age, sex, and ethnicity	Whole body
Dual energy X-ray absorptiometry (DXA)	Highly reproducible Accurate Quick Minimal subject compliance needed	High cost Slight radiation exposure	Whole body and regional
Total body water – isotope dilution (^{2}H,^{18}O)	Direct measure of body water Provides estimates of fat-free mass, fat mass and percent body fat	High cost Difficult analysis (mass spectrophotometer needed) Relies on assumption of composition of fat-free mass which is unsystematically influenced by age, sex, and ethnicity	Whole body
K^{40} counting	Measure of body cell mass	Shielded room Frightening for children	Whole body
Computed tomography (CT)	Accurate Regional/visceral adiposity can be measured	Exposure to radiation High cost Requires high subject compliance	Regional
Magnetic resonance imaging (MRI)	Accurate Regional/visceral adiposity can be measured No exposure to radiation	High cost Requires high subject compliance	Regional

Nonlaboratory measures

Nonlaboratory measures of body composition assessment refer to methods that are applicable to field and clinical studies. These methods are validated against the laboratory methods summarized above. Bio-electric impedance analysis (BIA) is a nonlaboratory method that has gained widespread use because it is noninvasive (surface electrodes on hands and feet, or feet only) and rapid. BIA is based on electrical resistance, which is inversely related to total body water. Several equations that relate impedance measures to percentage body fat have been published for use in children and adolescents [6–11]. Experience to date suggests caution when applying equations developed in one study population to other groups [1,12].

Anthropometric measures, such as height, weight, circumferences and skinfolds, represent low-cost, minimally invasive measures of nutritional status in general, and of obesity in particular. For children, these measures are moving targets; all will increase with age, and will do so at variable rates.

Weight for height indices

Since the 19th century, various weight-for-height indices have been proposed as measures of relative weight (see Cole [13]). Weight and height can be measured accurately with relative ease. The weight-for-height index that is currently most used is the Body Mass Index, which is calculated as weight in kilograms divided by squared height in meters, or weight in pounds divided by squared height in inches multiplied by 703. See formulas below.

$$BMI = weight\ (kg)/height(m)^2$$

$$BMI = [weight\ (lbs)/height(in)^2] \times 703$$

Other weight-for-height indices differ in the power to which height is raised, but all are proposed to meet two distinct goals: (1) to be maximally correlated with a criterion measure of body fat, and (2) to be minimally correlated with height [14]. In adults BMI meets both goals: it is correlated with adiposity and largely uncorrelated with height. In children, changing relationships between height and weight with age complicate the situation. Whereas in adults, adjusting weight by height raised to the power of 2 best reduces correlation with height, in children the "best" power changes with age, such that for young children it is of the order of two, and around puberty it is closer to three [15]. It would be possible to use Rohrer's Index (weight/height^3) for adolescents during puberty and BMI (weight/height^2) for children, or to have a continually changing exponent across childhood and adolescence. However, for consistency with adult definitions, and because BMI is more strongly correlated with adiposity in adolescence than is Rohrer's Index, BMI is used for assessment of obesity in children and adolescents, as well as adults.

Although BMI is a measure of relative weight and not adiposity, it is correlated with adiposity as measured by skinfold thickness, BIA, and DXA. The correlation of BMI-for-age with percent body fat by DXA in a large sample of children and adolescents from the US, Italy, and New Zealand was approximately r = 0.8, with some variability by child age and sex [16]. Higher correlations have also been reported; in 8–11-year-old children, correlation between BMI and percentage body fat by DXA was 0.92 [17]. However, the relationship between adiposity and BMI is nonlinear, and BMI is more highly correlated with body fat at greater levels of adiposity [18]. It should also be noted that racial-ethnic differences in body fat exist and the validity of BMI to assess adiposity in white and black youth is better established than for other racial-ethnic groups [19–21].

When BMI is calculated for children and adolescents, interpretation must be made in the context of a child's age and gender. In contrast to adults, it is not possible to identify a single BMI cut-point to define obesity in children and adolescents because BMI changes as a child matures. Instead, growth charts based on a large set of reference data are constructed and centile cut-points are chosen as indicative of overweight or obesity. How BMI growth charts are constructed and cut-points chosen is discussed below.

BMI-for-age growth charts

Body Mass Index rises rapidly from birth to about age 2 years, then declines gradually until about age 5.5 years – the adiposity rebound – when it increases again throughout childhood and adolescence. The age at which the adiposity rebound occurs is related to weight status; children with higher BMIs tend to have an earlier adiposity rebound [22].

To construct BMI growth charts, a representative sample of children in the population for which charts are being developed is measured. Then, using the LMS method [23], smoothed curves can be constructed for any centile. BMI-for-age percentile charts for clinical use are available for the UK, France, and the US. The charts for the UK can be obtained from www.health-for-all-children.co.uk. US growth charts (Fig. 28.1) and corresponding LMS values and percentiles are available at www.cdc.gov/growthcharts [24].

Use of BMI growth charts in clinical practice is straightforward after BMI has been calculated. Plotting height and weight on growth charts is a familiar practice in pediatrics and BMI growth charts are used similarly. However, adoption of BMI growth charts by primary care providers has lagged behind other aspects of child growth monitoring [25–28]. Barriers to the use of BMI growth charts in clinical practice are likely to diminish as electronic medical records become commonplace in pediatric primary care settings. This technology facilitates computation of BMI, determination of a child's BMI-for-age centile, and monitoring of a child's BMI-for-age over time.

Disadvantages of alternative weight/height measures

Rather than calculating and plotting BMI to assess obesity, some clinicians determine whether a large difference exists between a child's weight and height centiles [29,30]. The notion is that for a child whose weight-for-age percentile exceeds the height-for-age percentile, excess weight or adiposity is likely. Although there is intuitive appeal to this approach of subtracting weight-for-age centile from height-for-age centile (W-H Index), because it avoids the necessity of calculating BMI, it is not recommended. The W-H Index has the undesirable properties of being only weakly correlated with weight and negatively correlated with height [31].

Weight-for-stature can be used to determine relative weight in children, but it is also not recommended for clinical assessment of obesity. Weight-for-stature compares children of the same height but not necessarily of the same age. BMI-for-age compares children of the same age but not necessarily the same height. In the US, weight-for-stature growth charts are available for children 30–48 inches in height, and approximately 5% of US 5-year-old children are taller than 48 inches [32]. BMI-for-age and weight-for-stature charts are not equivalent with regard to which centile of relative weight an individual child will fall on. Weight-for-stature percentiles tend to be lower than BMI-for-age percentiles, with larger differences between the two approaches at ages 4 and 5 years; between 2 and 3 years of age the difference between percentiles is highly dependent upon the child's height [32].

Defining overweight and obesity: setting a cut-point

Body Mass Index centiles or z-scores are useful to compare relative weight between children or to monitor a child's growth across time, but to use BMI centiles to define obesity, a cut-point must be applied. Although ideally a cut-point to define obesity in children and adolescents would be established based on observed risk for current or future morbidity or mortality relative to BMI, this is not currently possible for three reasons: (1) children and adolescents experience less obesity-related morbidity than adults, (2) long-term health effects of childhood obesity on adult morbidity are mediated through adult obesity, and therefore separating the effect of obesity in childhood from the effect of obesity in adulthood on adult morbidity is difficult, (3) health risk increases progressively with increasing adiposity [33] and a clear threshold, above which level adiposity has deleterious health effects, is not apparent [2,34]. Although a strictly evidence-based process has not been followed, substantial evidence has accumulated to support the validity of the current centile cut-points to define overweight and obesity in children and adolescents.

Having a BMI above the 95th percentile of the US growth reference increases the risk of obesity persistence into adulthood [34,35] and is linked with elevated cardiovascular risk factor levels, such as blood pressure, cholesterol, and blood glucose [2,33]. Recent evidence has linked the US 85th percentile BMI-for-age to obesity persistence throughout childhood [36], elevated levels of cardiovascular risk factors in childhood and adolescence [37] and risk for heart disease in adulthood [38].

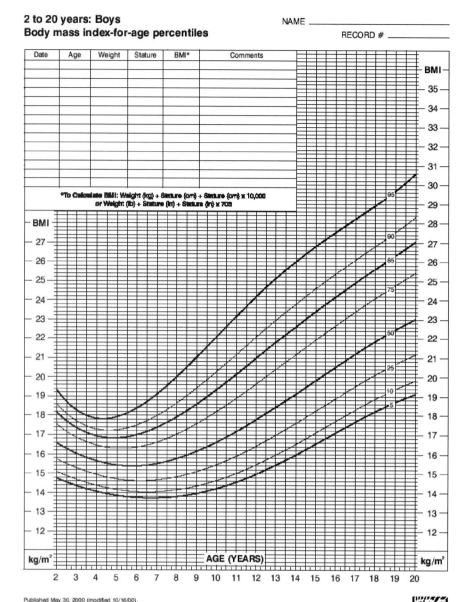

2 to 20 years: Boys
Body mass index-for-age percentiles

NAME _____

RECORD # _____

Figure 28.1 United States BMI-for-age growth charts for (a) boys and (b) girls aged 2–20 years [24].

Reference populations
Country-specific
Body Mass Index reference curves for children and adolescents are available for an increasing number of countries, including, but not limited to, the US [24], France [39], Japan [40], Italy [41], The Netherlands [42] and the UK [43]. An international BMI reference [44] has also been developed and will be discussed in the next section. Although all these reference curves are of similar shape, the location of a particular centile will correspond to different BMI values. In addition, various cut-points have been used to define overweight and obesity depending upon the reference population.

It has been recommended that national BMI references be "frozen" at their current levels [45] to facilitate comparisons within a population across time. Data used to construct the US BMI reference were collected between 1963 and 1980 [46], data for the UK reference were collected in 1990 [43] and data for the Japan reference were collected between 1978 and 1981 [40]; thus these growth references all date from before the rise in the prevalence of childhood obesity.

International
In order to facilitate global comparisons of trends in childhood and adolescent obesity rates [47,48], the International Obesity

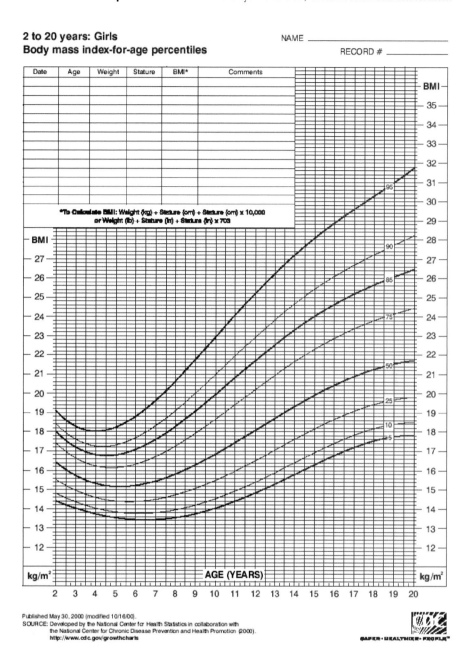

2 to 20 years: Girls
Body mass index-for-age percentiles

NAME _____

RECORD # _____

Figure 28.1 *Continued*

Task Force (IOTF) developed BMI centile curves based on pooled data for children and adolescents aged 2–18 years from nationally representative surveys conducted in Brazil, Great Britain, Hong Kong, The Netherlands, Singapore, and the United States [44]. The IOTF BMI curves were calculated individually for the six national samples, and then averaged. Centiles corresponding to a BMI of 25 and a BMI of 30 at age 18 were fit to the data. That is, these centiles were chosen as extrapolations into childhood of the well-accepted adult BMI cut-points of 25 and 30 to define overweight and obesity respectively. Unlike other pediatric BMI references, the IOTF curves have continuity from childhood into adulthood. Although these international standards are useful to

compare obesity rates in different countries, whether they should be used clinically to classify individual children as overweight or obese is controversial [49–52].

Reference standard comparisons

The choice of centile and reference population will affect the proportion of children and adolescents in a population who are declared overweight or obese. Table 28.2 provides a comparison of BMI values for 9- and 15-year-old boys and girls using the US [24], UK [43], France [39], Japan [40] and IOTF [44] reference curves at cut-points that have been used to classify children and adolescents as overweight or obese. The US 85th percentile, UK

Table 28.2 BMI centiles used to define overweight and obesity from the United States [24], UK[43], France [39], Japan [40]and the International Obesity Task Force [44]. Tabulated are BMI values at the indicated centile by gender at ages 9 and 15 years

	Centile	BMI (kg/m^2)				Centile	BMI (kg/m^2)			
		Age 9		Age 15			Age 9		Age 15	
		Boys	Girls	Boys	Girls		Boys	Girls	Boys	Girls
US	85th	18.6	19.1	23.5	24.1	95th	21.1	21.8	26.8	28.1
UK	91st	19.0	19.8	23.1	24.1	98th	21.0	22.0	26.0	27.0
France	90th	18.0	17.4	22.4	22.5	97th	19.7	19.5	23.8	25.2
Japan	90th	18.6	18.3	22.8	23.2	97th	20.5	19.9	25.2	25.2
IOTF	BMI = 25 at age 18	19.1	19.1	23.3	23.9	BMI = 30 at age 18	22.8	22.8	28.3	29.1

91st percentile, and IOTF centile corresponding to a BMI of 25 at age 18 are broadly equivalent; the France 90th percentile runs at a lower level of BMI, and the Japan 90th centile is intermediate. At the higher obesity definition (US 95th percentile, UK 98th percentile, France 97th percentile, Japan 97th, and IOTF centile corresponding to a BMI of 30 at age 18), the French cut-point has the lowest BMI values and the IOTF has the highest – the US, UK, and Japan references are intermediate.

WHO child growth standards

Between 1997 and 2003, the Multicenter Growth Reference Study was conducted by the World Health Organization (WHO) to develop standards against which to assess child growth from birth to age 5. A large sample of healthy children who were breast fed, of high socio-economic status, and had mothers who did not smoke were studied in six countries. Based on these data, the WHO Child Growth Standards were developed to describe optimal growth in infancy and early childhood [53]. BMI-for-age growth charts were constructed, but recommendations for their use in obesity assessment have not been promulgated at the time of this writing.

It should be noted that the IOTF and country-specific BMI-for-age growth curves described in the previous section provide a growth reference rather than a growth standard. Whereas a growth standard would delineate "optimal" growth, a growth reference describes the population for which it is constructed without any implication that it would be "best" for individuals to follow the pattern of growth depicted.

Children under 2 years of age

The assessment of weight status in children younger than 2 years of age is controversial; however, it is increasingly recognized that prevention of childhood obesity – and therefore obesity assessment – should begin early in life. In general, BMI growth charts start at age 2. An exception is the WHO Child Growth Standards, which include BMI-for-age beginning at birth [53]. As noted above, however, no recommendations for their use in obesity assessment have yet been offered. In the US, the 2007 Expert

Committee on the Assessment, Prevention, and Treatment of Child and Adolescent Overweight and Obesity has suggested that a weight-for-length percentile above the 95th percentile in children under 2 years is indicative of overweight [54]. It should be underscored that research evidence is sparse for the clinical use and interpretation of BMI or weight-for-length percentiles in children under age 2.

Severe obesity

With increasing levels of excess adiposity, the complications of obesity in children become more common and more severe [55,56]. Classification systems for adult obesity include several cut-points above a BMI of 30 to denote higher levels of risk; these are BMI 30–34.9 (obese class I), 35–39.9 (obese class II), and >40 (obese class III) [57]. Like adults, the prevalence of severe obesity in youth appears to be increasing more rapidly than lesser degrees of obesity [58,59]. The 2007 Expert Committee has recommended that the US BMI-for-age 99th percentile be used to define "severe childhood obesity" [54]. The US CDC BMI-for-age growth charts do not include 99th percentile lines; the 97th percentile is the most extreme [60]. Although it is possible to use the LMS values associated with the BMI-for-age growth charts to determine age-specific cut-points for the 99th percentile, the data used to construct the US CDC BMI-for-age growth charts are sparse beyond the 97th percentile and therefore caution is warranted in the interpretation of higher BMI-for-age percentiles [24]. Table 28.3 provides BMI cut-points for the 85th and 95th percentiles of the US growth reference by sex and age. As will be discussed in the second part of this chapter, in a clinical setting it is important to consider the terminology used to communicate with children and parents; use of the term "severe obesity" in a nonresearch context is not recommended.

Terminology

Along with the general agreement about the use of BMI-for-age to identify excess weight in children, consensus terminology is emerging to describe the dual cut-off points to indicate two levels of severity. In the UK, the preferred terminology is overweight

Table 28.3 BMI cut-points by age and sex for overweight (85th percentile) and obesity (95th percentile) from CDC 2000 BMI-for-age growth reference. BMI values tabulated correspond to the midpoint of the child's age in years (e.g. 2.5 years)

Age	Boys		Girls	
	85th	95th	85th	95th
2	17.7	18.7	17.5	18.6
3	17.1	18.0	16.9	18.1
4	16.8	17.8	16.8	18.1
5	16.9	18.1	16.9	18.5
6	17.2	18.8	17.3	19.2
7	17.7	19.6	18.0	20.2
8	18.3	20.6	18.7	21.2
9	19.0	21.6	19.5	22.4
10	19.8	22.7	20.4	23.6
11	20.6	23.7	21.3	24.7
12	21.4	24.7	22.2	25.8
13	22.3	25.6	23.0	26.8
14	23.1	26.5	23.7	27.7
15	23.8	27.2	24.4	28.5
16	24.6	27.9	24.9	29.3
17	25.3	28.6	25.4	30.0

and obesity, comparable to the adult terminology, and the terms "overweight" and "obese" generally signify the 91st and 98th percentiles of the UK90 reference [43]. The same overweight and obesity terminology is used for international comparison with the IOTF growth charts, where the two levels of severity are defined by centiles that extrapolate to adult BMIs of 25 and 30, as described above. In the US, two sets of contradictory terminology are currently in use, with the 85th percentile termed either "at risk for overweight" or "overweight" and the 95th percentile termed either "overweight" or "obesity." The "at risk for overweight" terminology was originally advocated to avoid stigmatizing children, and in recognition of the flaws inherent in defining excess adiposity based on BMI. The terminology proposed by the 2007 Expert Committee is "overweight" and "obesity" [54]. This brings the US in line with the many countries who have developed their own growth references (see Table 28.2) or that have adopted the US or other growth charts. The common language is expected to reduce confusion and communicate the seriousness associated with elevations of BMI in youth.

Screening for obesity with BMI-for-age

This section describes the implications of BMI-for-age definitions in obesity screening. BMI-for-age is correlated with adiposity but is not a direct measure of adiposity. Therefore, irrespective of which centile is used as the cut-point for defining obesity, some youth will be misclassified: either they will be incorrectly classified as obese when they are not "overfat" (false positives) or

they will *not* be classified as obese based on BMI-for-age but will truly be "overfat" (false negatives). There is a trade-off between specificity and sensitivity, and specificity is maximized as the BMI-for-age centile definition becomes more extreme. For example, relative to percentage body fat measured by DXA, the specificity of the US BMI-for-age 85th percentile in children and adolescents was 72.7% and the specificity of the BMI-for-age 95th percentile was 89.4% [61]. Corresponding sensitivities were 98.5% for the 85th percentile and 92.5% for the 95th percentile BMI-for-age [61]. Relative to percentage body fat by skinfolds, the sensitivity and specificity of the US BMI-for-age 95th percentile were compared to the IOTF obesity cut-point in a representative sample of Swiss children (6–12 years old); specificities for boys and girls were uniformly high with either definition (between 96.9% and 99.5%), but sensitivities for the US definition were much higher than for the IOTF definition (91.4% versus 62.2% for boys, 67.9% versus 48.3% for girls) [62]. Reported sensitivities and specificities of BMI-for-age obesity definitions are quite variable and are related to the standard used to define high adiposity [63].

The rationale for maximizing specificity rather than sensitivity of an obesity screening test stems from concern about negative psychologic effects of labeling youth as obese. Use of the 95th percentile of the US BMI reference will keep to a minimum the number of children and adolescents who are classified as obese when they do not have excess adiposity. However, many children with high levels of adiposity have BMIs below the 95th percentile, and would not "screen positive" for obesity. It can be argued that these children, who might benefit from obesity treatment, would be missed. Current US screening guidelines recommend further evaluation if a youth's BMI is between the 85th and 95th percentile and secondary risk characteristics are present [54,64]. In addition, it is assumed that with annual rescreening, children whose level of adiposity is increasing will be identified at a subsequent visit.

The assessment section that follows describes how these cut-points are integrated into comprehensive obesity assessment.

Assessment

The intractable nature of obesity once it is established underscores the necessity of universal obesity screening and assessment within pediatric clinical practice. Identification of overweight and obesity by BMI-for-age percentile should occur as part of the child's physical examination and growth monitoring. Comprehensive assessment includes evaluation of medical risk, lifestyle behaviors that contribute to risk, as well as parent and child concerns and motivation. Figure 28.2 reprints the current schema recommended by the 2007 Expert Committee [54]. The quality of research evidence for each recommendation is included in the 2007 Expert Committee report [54,64–66]. This guidance represents an update and expansion of recommendations published in 1998 [67].

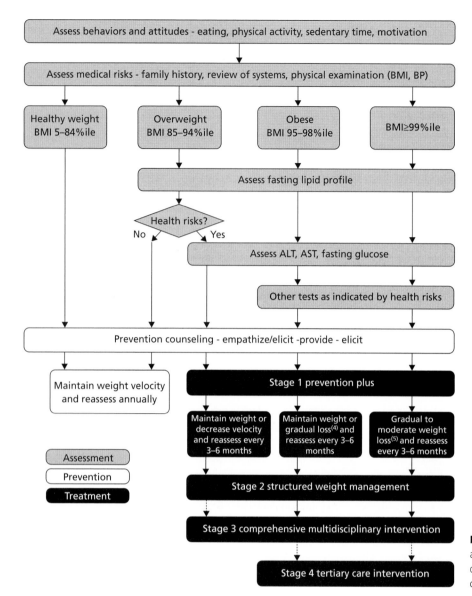

Figure 28.2 Algorithm for assessment, prevention and treatment of childhood obesity (for further details regarding prevention and treatment of childhood obesity, see Chapter 29).

Obesity secondary to other disease states

The vast majority of children who present with obesity will have simple or primary obesity that is not associated with another disease state. Although the line of demarcation is not always clear, obesity that presents with other psychologic problems or accompanies Down syndrome or nonspecific mental retardation is generally considered simple. Obesity due to other pathology is far less common, but these exogenous causes must be ruled out as an early step in assessment. As part of the differential diagnosis, the conditions to be ruled out fall into two main categories: genetic syndromes and endocrinologic abnormalities.

Of the genetic syndromes, Prader–Willi (or Prader–Labhard–Willi) is the most common specific syndrome, with prevalence estimated at one per 10,000–15,000 [68]. Two chromosomal abnormalities seem to account for the syndrome, which presents

with a range of symptoms in addition to obesity, including neonatal hypotonia, orthopedic abnormalities, excessive appetite and hyperphagia, temper tantrums and self-abusive behaviors [69]. Other genetic syndromes that are characterized by obesity occur with far lower frequencies and include Bardet–Biedl, Cohen (or Pepper), Alstrom, Biemond, Laurence–Moon, Borjeson–Forssman–Lehmann, and Carpenter. These all present with other specific symptoms such as specific abnormalities of facial appearance, polydactyly, hypogenitalism or neurologic deficits [70].

Endocrine disorders that present with obesity in childhood include polycystic ovary syndrome (PCOS), Cushing syndrome, hypothyroidism, and growth hormone deficiency. PCOS is commonly identified in obese girls who also have oligomenorrhea. PCOS does not appear to be caused by obesity; rather, it is a sequela of insulin resistance. The other aforementioned endocrine disorders are rare and may be suspected where weight gain is normal but linear growth is poor. These characteristics contrast with simple obesity in which obese children are taller than their peers before puberty. Also exceedingly rare are abnormalities associated with the hormone leptin. Leptin deficiency will be evident as low serum leptin and severe early-onset obesity and hyperinsulinemia. Leptin receptor abnormalities often are accompanied by central hypothyroidism and hypercortisolism as well as delayed sexual maturation [71]. Finally, certain hypothalamic tumors may be associated with obesity. It is important to stress that these conditions are quite rare. In the absence of other clinical signs, a search for genetic, neurologic or endocrine abnormalities is not part of standard diagnostic assessment.

Weight gain may also occur with use of certain medications. Among these, the atypical antipsychotics have received the most attention because the weight gains associated with their use can be substantial. Risperidone, a commonly prescribed neuroleptic, increasingly used to manage behavior in children with autism spectrum disorders, has been associated with weight gain, a side-effect that seems to be most pronounced in youth [72]. Other drug classes, such as antidepressants, mood stabilizers and anticonvulsants, include specific drugs that have been associated with increased weight [73,74]. Corticosteroids, which are used for a wide range of medical conditions, are of particular concern because other side-effects of these drugs include high blood pressure and elevations in blood glucose. Insulin and oral hypoglycemic agents are also associated with excessive weight gain [75].

Medical history, physical examination and laboratory tests

Adverse health effects of obesity affect most of the organ systems of the body. These co-morbid conditions may already be present at the time of assessment, and can be identified as part of the medical history, review of systems or physical examination augmented by laboratory tests. Children and their parents may not recognize symptoms of obesity-related co-morbidities and may not report them unless explicitly asked during the medical encounter. Chapter 29 details the many health consequences of obesity in childhood, and therefore these are considered here only in the context of comprehensive medical assessment.

Immediate health consequences of obesity include sleep, respiratory, and gastrointestinal problems, endocrine disorders, menstrual irregularities, genitourinary problems, skin conditions, orthopedic problems, and psychosocial problems [55,56]. For some of these problems, such as endocrine disorders, diagnosis will depend upon laboratory testing, as discussed below. The presence of several of the most common sequelae may be identified through a careful review of systems, as detailed in the following.

Sleep disorders are common, underdiagnosed, and potentially dangerous. Sleep problems that may be present at the time of obesity assessment include obstructive sleep apnea and disordered sleep [76]. Loud snoring, apnea or general trouble sleeping should be queried. It should be noted that there is emerging research to suggest that short sleep duration is also a risk factor for the development of overweight, operating directly through appetite and satiety centers, or through tiredness which may interfere with physical activity [77]. To the extent that effects exist in both directions, sleep patterns may make behavior change efforts more difficult.

Menstrual abnormalities should be assessed, as they may be indicative of PCOS or hyperandrogenism. Irregular or very scanty menstrual periods may go unreported without specific questioning, especially for those girls who have recently begun menstruating. After ruling out other medical conditions which manifest as irregular menstruation, the diagnosis of PCOS is based on the presence of two or more of the following: amenorrhea or oligomenorrhea, biochemical evidence of hyperandrogenism, and polycystic ovaries identified by ultrasound [78].

Obese children may present with nonspecific abdominal pain, with or without vomiting. This, too, may go unreported without specific questioning of the parent or child. Abdominal pain may be indicative of nonalcoholic fatty liver disease (NAFLD), which is increasingly appreciated as a common co-morbidity of obesity [79]. NAFLD consists of steatosis (increased fat in the liver without inflammation) and steatohepatitis (increased liver fat with inflammation). The latter can progress to hepatic fibrosis, and ultimately to cirrhosis. Diagnostic criteria for NAFLD are not adequately defined [80]; definitive diagnosis requires liver biopsy. Abdominal pain may be reported in association with other common childhood conditions as well, including constipation, gastroesophageal reflux, and gallstones. Gallstones may also be formed as a consequence of rapid weight loss [81].

Certain psychologic disorders may co-occur with obesity and should be routinely assessed as part of medical history taking. Bulimic eating disorders, including binge eating, may be associated with adolescent obesity, particularly in girls [82]. Where discontent about weight is internalized, poor self-esteem may result [83]. Elevated levels of depressive symptoms in overweight children, particularly girls, have been observed in a number of cross-sectional studies [84–86] and accumulating evidence indicates that adolescent obesity may increase risk for depression in women [87,88].

In addition to the full medical history that is part of standard clinical assessment, additional historical items relevant to obesity assessment should be included. Height and weight or obesity status of the biologic and nonbiologic mother and father should be obtained, if possible. The heritability of BMI is estimated to be ~70% [89], underscoring the importance of parental weight status. Parental obesity influences child obesity through *both* heritability of the condition and shared family environment; families share genes as well as eating and activity behaviors and attitudes. Parental overweight is strongly associated with overweight in the young child; its influence appears to dissipate as the child ages, but remains a factor throughout adolescence [90]. More intensive treatment may be indicated when parental obesity is identified. Information on the child's age at obesity onset should be established by review of the growth chart, if available, or by parent report. Overweight onset before age 8 has been linked to persistence into adulthood [91]. When BMI has been monitored and plotted annually, examination of the growth chart provides an objective tool for looking at relative weight status over time. In addition to parental obesity, the medical history may provide important information regarding family history of obesity-related co-morbidities, such as type 2 diabetes, as well as disordered eating and depression. When these conditions are present in family members, the risk for the overweight child is further elevated.

Universal assessment of obesity risk requires assessment of BMI, as well as a few additions to the review of systems and physical examination that are part of routine pediatric practice.

BMI-for-age assessment

Several organizations around the world have developed guidelines for BMI assessment. In the US, the 2007 Expert Committee recommendations start with assessment of age- and sex-specific BMI percentile. The 85th and 95th percentiles are recommended to designate overweight (85th percentile) and obesity (95th percentile). As described in detail above, these cut-offs are statistical definitions, based on an external reference population. The CDC website (www.cdc.gov/growthcharts) contains tables in multiple formats and other supporting materials for calculating BMI percentiles in children using their growth reference. There are several online BMI-for-age percentile calculators as well. The National Obesity Forum (UK) and Scottish Intercollegiate Guidelines Network (SIGN) [92] have also promulgated assessment guidelines based on BMI-for-age. The SIGN guidelines for management of pediatric obesity are evidence based and the quality of evidence for each recommendation is graded.

Accurate measurement of weight and height is needed to calculate BMI. Both height and weight should be measured with the child dressed only in light clothing and without shoes. Large hairstyles can present a challenge for the measurement of height. To minimize risk of embarrassment, weight should be obtained in a private setting and recorded without comment.

All children, regardless of their weight status, should be re-evaluated for obesity every year [3]. The BMI and BMI percentile should be recorded in the medical chart, along with height and weight. Clinicians are encouraged to calculate BMI at all well-child visits and plot the value on a sex-specific BMI-for-age chart. Figure 28.1 displays the US BMI-for-age growth charts for boys and girls, respectively.

Other anthropometric assessment measures

Skinfold thicknesses are a measure of the subcutaneous fat depot and correlate well with overall percentage body fat. Because BMI is a measure of weight adjusted for height, rather than a direct measure of adiposity, assessment of fatness using skinfold thickness has intuitive appeal. However, fatness assessment by skinfolds does not improve the sensitivity or specificity of obesity defined by the 95th percentile BMI-for-age [61]. In addition,

---

> **Box 28.1 Initial screening clinical recommendations for annual assessment of obesity in children and adolescents (US)**
>
> 1. Measure child's weight and height
> 2. Calculate BMI
>
> $$BMI = \frac{Weight(kg)}{Height(m)^2}$$
>
> 3. Plot BMI-for-age on BMI growth chart appropriate for child's sex and determine BMI centile
> 4. Determine if child's BMI is above the 95th percentile (obese), between the 85th and 95th percentiles (overweight), or below the 85th percentile (not overweight)

measuring skinfolds properly requires training to minimize error. These measurements are not recommended as part of routine obesity assessment [64].

Measures of central adiposity

Central adiposity may also be of importance in obesity assessment. As is seen consistently in studies of adults, a central pattern of fat distribution, or abdominal adiposity, is associated with adverse levels of classic cardiovascular risk factors, independent of total fatness or weight status. Greater central adiposity has been associated with elevations in LDL and total cholesterol, triglycerides, and insulin as well as with lower levels of HDL [2,93,94]. Central adiposity is also associated with higher levels of markers of inflammation [95,96] and with higher diastolic and systolic blood pressure [97,98].

Some researchers have suggested that indirect measures of central adiposity, such as skinfold ratios, waist-to-hip ratio, waist-to-height ratio or waist circumference, could be useful additions or alternatives to BMI in early identification of children who would benefit from lifestyle interventions [99]. The criterion measures used to assess abdominal adiposity are MRI, CT scan and regional DXA (see Table 28.1). Anthropometric measures that correlate with abdominal adiposity include waist circumference, waist-to-hip ratio and any one of a number of skinfold ratios, including subscapular:triceps, subscapular + suprailiac:triceps. Of the various anthropometric measures of abdominal adiposity, waist circumference appears to be the best, explaining almost two-thirds of the variance in visceral adipose tissue [100]. Although reference data for waist circumference in children are becoming available from several countries [99,101–104], it is not yet clear what waist circumference adds to the assessment of risk [94,105], which anthropometric measure of central adiposity is most valid or what cut-points should be set [106–108]. For these reasons, assessment of waist circumference is not currently recommended as part of routine screening [66].

Physical examination

The physical examination of the obese child is the same as for all children with a few additional considerations, as detailed in the 2007 Expert Committee report [66]. Vital signs should be assessed in standard fashion. A blood pressure cuff of adequate size so that 80% of the arm is encircled by the bladder of the cuff should be available for the blood pressure measurement. The "white coat" effect may necessitate several blood pressure measurements and/or manual measurement. If repeated measurements exceed the 95th percentile [109], 24-hour ambulatory monitoring should be considered.

The usual examination of the eyes and throat should be supplemented with an examination of the optic disk for papilledema or decreased venous pulsations indicative of pseudotumor cerebri, particularly if frequent headache is reported. The neck should be checked for the presence of goiter, and the pharynx examined for enlarged tonsils. Heart and lung sounds may be difficult to hear in the obese child, so particular attention should be paid to identifying irregular rhythms of the heart or asthmatic wheezing. Palpation of abdominal organs may be difficult; the clinician should be alert to the presence of the enlarged liver associated with steatohepatitis.

The skin should be examined for the presence of acanthosis nigricans, a dark velvety hyperpigmentation usually present in the posterior or lateral folds of the neck, the axillae or joints; keratosis pilaris or skin tags may be indicative of insulin resistance.

Early secondary sexual development and premature pubarche are commonly observed in obese girls. Facial hair, body hair or excessive acne may indicate polycystic ovary disease. Early development of breast tissue in girls and the appearance of gynecomastia in boys is common. Although it is difficult to distinguish fat from breast tissue by visual inspection, palpation allows this differentiation. In boys, fat folds may make the penis appear abnormally small.

The mechanical stress of excess body weight on unfused growth plates and bones may cause orthopedic abnormalities and/or pain. A painful or waddling gait may indicate slipped capital femoral epiphyses, and bowed legs may signal Blount disease. Radiographic studies can confirm these orthopedic problems.

Laboratory assessment

The particular biochemical and radiographic studies recommended as part of assessment depend on the degree of overweight and the nature and presence of risk factors identified by history or physical examination. The 2007 Expert Committee has promulgated two sets of recommendations, one for primary care clinicians and one for subspecialty physicians [66]. In primary care settings, for a child whose BMI falls between the 85th and 94th percentile and who has no other risk factors, a fasting lipid profile is suggested. For children who also have other risk factors, such as family history of obesity-related diseases, blood pressure, lipid levels, fasting glucose levels, and liver function tests (assays for aspartate aminotransferase and alanine amino transferase) should be obtained as well. For children whose BMI exceeds the 95th

percentile, the aforementioned assessments should be obtained, even in the absence of other risk factors. Subspecialists (e.g. endocrinologists, gastroenterologists, orthopedists) who become involved in patient care based on initial medical assessment may consider additional studies and tests [66].

Clinician deportment and choice of terms

Obesity in childhood was dubbed "the dismal condition" by Dwyer and Mayer over 35 years ago [110]. Despite the rising prevalence of obesity, discrimination is widespread: the overweight child is often socially isolated [111] and the target of teasing and bullying by peers [112,113]. Healthcare professionals are not immune to "antifat" bias [114]. Thus, it is not surprising that many overweight children and perhaps their parents have internalized this negative societal reaction.

Clinicians who discuss weight with their pediatric patients and family members should appreciate the importance of an accepting, empathetic nonjudgmental tone. Privacy, confidentiality, and comfort of the physical exam are valued by adolescents [115]. The clinician must recognize that the weight problem may be a highly sensitive and emotionally charged issue, and handle the assessment with care. Every opportunity for enhancing self-esteem and self-acceptance during the medical encounter should be exploited. Further, because obesity runs in families, many parents will be obese themselves and have experienced their own frustrations and negative societal reaction. With adolescents who are trying to assert independence from their parents, navigating the role of the family involvement in weight management is challenging [116]. The advice for healthcare professionals recommended by the National Task Force on the Prevention and Treatment of Obesity [117] is broadly applicable to those who treat children. Some of the adaptations of the physical office space suggested in that report include large-size examination gowns, and large blood pressure cuffs [117].

Although the clinical terms overweight and obesity are recommended for documentation and risk assessment, the words used to describe or talk about the child's weight in the office should be chosen carefully. Most of the terms used to describe excess weight appear to be offensive to obese adults [118]; particularly undesirable for the obese individuals surveyed were the terms fatness, excess fat, obesity and large size. The term "weight" was most preferred. Adolescents prefer the term "overweight" [115]. If weight and lifestyle assessment is to be a positive experience and provide the foundation for successful management and treatment, clinicians are encouraged to avoid potentially offensive terminology.

Lifestyle assessment and family readiness

Rapid assessment tools for diet, activity, and family readiness for behavior change for use in clinical settings are scarce, and fewer have undergone formal validation. Weight management, whether weight maintenance or weight loss, relies on sustained changes in child diet and activity. Broaching these topics with families who are not ready to take them on may be counterproductive. For this reason, patient

Table 28.4 Lifestyle assessment of home, school and family routines, environments, and behaviors

Factors associated with food consumption (energy intake)	Factors associated with activity (energy expenditure)
Frequency and quality of breakfast	Time spent in moderate/vigorous
Frequency of eating food away from	physical activity daily from:
home	structured activity
Take-out/take-away	nonstructured activity
Fast-food restaurants	Routine activity patterns, like walking
Number of meals and snacks	to school
consumed daily	Time spent in sedentary behavior,
Quality of snacks consumed daily	including:
Portions that are large for child's age	viewing television, videos
Amounts consumed of:	playing video games
sugar-sweetened beverages	using the computer
juice	Presence of television/computer in
low-fat and whole milk	child's bedroom
high energy-density/fat foods	Frequency of meals taken in front of
fruits and vegetables	the television
Consumption of meals/snacks while	After-school arrangements
viewing television	Neighborhood safety

and family readiness to make behavioral changes must be evaluated during assessment of the particulars of current diet, eating behaviors, physical activity and sedentary behaviors (i.e. television and video viewing, video games, and computer time).

Table 28.4 provides specific items designed to assess the dietary and activity behaviors currently recommended based on the best available evidence [66].

Dietary assessment

Several aspects of diet represent useful assessment foci as potential intervention targets in clinical settings [66]. For younger children, information should be obtained from the parent or primary caregiver. If a child has multiple caregivers, of course, the accuracy of this information may be compromised. Assessment of frequency with which fruits, vegetables, sweets, salty snacks, fried foods, low-fat milk, whole milk, and soda are consumed will provide an overall picture of food choices, and the likelihood of excess caloric intake. Beverage choice may be an important source of excess calories [119,120]. The frequency of breakfast consumption, meals eaten away from home, and whether meals are eaten "as a family" should be assessed [121,122]. Food eaten or prepared outside the home is more likely to be higher in calories, due to the range of menu offerings, large portion sizes, and because parents are more likely to let their children choose for themselves [123–125]. The information obtained from this assessment may offer useful entry points for discussion and more constructive counseling.

Activity assessment

Activity assessment includes both physical activity and sedentary behavior. Information on structured activity, such as physical

education at school, team sports, lessons or hobbies, should be complemented by information about unstructured time. This includes activities of daily living, such as household chores, walking to school or yard work. Time spent in sedentary behavior, particularly television viewing, should be assessed, given its direct association with overweight [126,127]. Television viewing may influence food intake via satiety cues or through increased exposure to advertised foods [128–131]. The child and parent should be asked about the frequency with which meals are eaten in front of the television [132].

Similarly, time spent playing computer or video games should be assessed. The presence of a television and/or computer in the child's bedroom is also of interest given its relation to time spent viewing [133]. Information on factors which impede or facilitate physical activity should be obtained. Specific knowledge of household structure, neighborhood safety, and who, if anyone besides the child, is at home after school will help the clinician provide realistic suggestions and should make any counseling on these issues more relevant to the child and the family.

Family readiness

Assessment of readiness for change is an essential step in assessment and should be established before initiating obesity therapy [66,134]. Clinical experience supports behavior change theory which suggests that change will not occur until the individual is ready. Attempts at weight management counseling or referral to a weight management program may alienate families who are not ready and/or contribute to the child's negative self-concept. Thus, these attempts may compromise weight management efforts in the future. In the context of childhood obesity, motivation to address a weight problem requires that both the child and the family are ready to tackle the issue with concrete changes.

Motivational interviewing, a client-directed approach borrowed from the treatment of addictive behaviors, reflects the understanding that advice giving should be avoided and may undermine the clinician–patient encounter. Encouraging the patient to actively engage in problem analysis and goal setting increases the likelihood that behavior change will occur [135]. Two short questions are suggested in the clinical encounter [136]:

Box 28.2 Suggested questions to assess family readiness to change

Assess level of child/parent concern:
- Are you concerned about (your/your child's) weight?
- Has (your/your child's) weight caused any problems?

For particular behavior or environmental change targets:
- How important (on a 1–10 scale) is the change in behavior to the child/parent?
- How confident does the child/parent feel in their ability to make the change?

---

(1) how important (on a scale of 1–10) is the change in behavior to the patient, and (2) how confident does the patient feels in his/her ability to make the change? If the parent does not identify high child BMI as important, it is suggested that a conversation focused on specific health-related risks may be more productive. If the problem is identified as important but confidence in behavior change is limited, then a discussion of barriers and strategies to surmount them may be useful [66]. Training programs that teach motivational interviewing skills are available throughout the US and Europe. The clinician should gather additional information to assess the extent to which the child's physical and social environments will impede or facilitate any proposed behavior changes.

Conclusion

The evidence base for childhood obesity assessment guidelines and recommendations continues to be incomplete, as it is largely derived from observational studies, nonanalytic studies (e.g. case reports and case series), and expert opinion. Limitations to the evidence are not a justification for not screening and fully assessing overweight. The emergence of childhood obesity as a major public health problem has stimulated substantial research in this area; thus the research base upon which recommendations are promulgated continues to grow and the quality of studies improves.

Another area of uncertainty is the identification and treatment of overweight and obesity in ever younger children. Some of the rationale for early identification is a result of the difficulty of treating obesity in adolescents, particularly when detrimental eating and activity habits have been reinforced by repetition over many years. The evidence supporting identification of overweight and obesity in preschool age children is accumulating. However, extreme caution is warranted as regards obesity screening in children under age 2 years. The WHO growth charts provide BMI-for-age reference curves for children beginning at birth, but their utility is largely unknown. Similarly, the 2007 Expert Committee on the Assessment, Prevention, and Treatment of Child and Adolescent Overweight and Obesity has recommended that the 95th percentile of the US CDC 2000 weight-for-length growth reference be adopted as a cut-point for identification of overweight in children under age 2.

The significance of central adiposity in children remains an area of substantial research. As described in this chapter, routine assessment of central adiposity in children and adolescents is not currently recommended; the evidence base to support the interpretation and utility of central adiposity screening in clinical pediatric practice is not yet sufficient.

The increased prevalence of childhood obesity has brought with it heightened public awareness of the health consequences of obesity. Annual assessment of obesity in the medical setting communicates to youth and their parents the importance of avoiding excess weight gain. Physicians have the opportunity to capitalize on this awareness and to advocate for healthy eating and physical activity practices within the families they care for and the communities in which they live and work. The increased awareness of the importance of healthy eating and physical activity in obesity prevention should be harnessed to advance social change.

References

1. Pietrobelli A, Faith MS, Allison DB, Gallagher D, Chiumello G, Heymsfield SB. Body mass index as a measure of adiposity among children and adolescents: a validation study. J Pediatr 1998;132(2):204–10.
2. Freedman DS, Dietz WH, Srinivasan SR, Berenson GS. The relation of overweight to cardiovascular risk factors among children and adolescents: the Bogalusa Heart Study. Pediatrics 1999;103:1175–82.
3. Committee on Nutrition. Prevention of pediatric overweight and obesity: policy statement. Pediatrics 2003;112:424–30.
4. Ellis KJ. Human body composition: in vivo methods. Physiol Rev 2000;80:649–80.
5. Goran MI. Measurement issues related to studies of childhood obesity: assessment of body composition, body fat distribution, physical activity, and food intake. Pediatrics 1998;101:505–18.
6. Kushner R, Schoeller D, Fjeld C, Danford L. Is the impedance index (ht2/R) significant in predicting total body water? Am J Clin Nutr 1992;56:835–9.
7. Houtkooper LB, Lohman TG, Going SB, Hall MC. Validity of bioelectric impedance for body composition assessment in children. J Appl Physiol 1989;66:814–21.
8. Deurenberg P, van der Kooy K, Leenen R, Westrrate JA, Seidell JC. Sex and age specific prediction formulas for estimating body composition from bioelectrical impedance: a cross-validation study. Int J Obes 1991;15:17–25.
9. Deurenberg P, Smit HE, Kusters C. Is the bioelectrical impedance method suitable for epidemiological field studies? Eur J Clin Nutr 1989;43:647–54.
10. Deurenberg P, Kusters C, Smit HE. Assessment of body composition by bioelectrical impedance in children and young adults is strongly age-dependent. Eur J Clin Nutr 1990;44:261–8.
11. Sun SS, Chumlea WC, Heymsfield SB, Lukaski HC, Schoeller D, Friedl K, et al. Development of bioelectrical impedance analysis prediction equations for body composition with the use of a multicomponent model for use in epidemiologic surveys. Am J Clin Nutr 2003;77(2):331–40.
12. Phillips SM, Bandini LG, Compton DV, Naumova EN, Must A. A longitudinal comparison of body composition by total body water and bioelectrical impedance in adolescent girls. J Nutr 2003;133:1419–25.
13. Cole TJ. Weight-stature indices to measure underweight, overweight, and obesity. In: Himes JH (ed) *Anthropometric Assessment of Nutritional Status*. New York: Wiley-Liss, 1991:83–111.
14. Cole TJ, Rolland-Cachera MF. Measurement and definition. In: Burniat W, Cole TJ, Lissau I, Poskitt EME (eds) *Child and Adolescent Obesity*. Cambridge: Cambridge University Press, 2003:3–27.
15. Rolland-Cachera MF, Sempe M, Guilloud-Batalle M, Patois E, Pequignot-Guggenbuhi F, Faurad V. Adiposity indices in children. Am J Clin Nutr 1982;36:178–84.

16. Mei Z, Grummer-Strawn LM, Pietrobelli A, Goulding A, Goran MI, Dietz WH. Validity of body mass index compared with other body-composition screening indexes for the assessment of body fatness in children and adolescents. Am J Clin Nutr 2002;75(6):978–85.

17. Dencker M, Thorsson O, Lindén C, Wollmer P, Andersen L, Karlsson MK. BMI and objectively measured body fat and body fat distribution in prepubertal children. Clin Physiol Funct Imag 2007;27:12–16.

18. Freedman DS, Wang J, Maynard LM, Thornton JC, Mei Z, Pierson RN Jr, et al. Relation of BMI to fat and fat-free mass among children and adolescents. Int J Obes 2004;29(1):1–8.

19. Morrison JA, Guo SS, Specker B, Chumlea WMC, Yanovski SZ, Yanovski JA. Assessing the body composition of 6–17-year-old black and white girls in field studies. Am J Hum Biol 2001;13(2):249–54.

20. Shaw NJ, Crabtree NJ, Kibirige MS, Fordham JN. Ethnic and gender differences in body fat in British schoolchildren as measured by DXA. Arch Dis Child 2007;92(10):872–5.

21. Daniels SR, Khoury PR, Morrison JA. The utility of body mass index as a measure of body fatness in children and adolescents: differences by race and gender. Pediatrics 1997;99:804–7.

22. Cole TJ. Children grow and horses race: is the adiposity rebound a critical period for later obesity? BMC Pediatrics 2004;4:6.

23. Cole TJ. The LMS method for constructing normalized growth standards. Eur J Clin Nutr 1990;44(1):45–60.

24. Kuczmarski RJ, Ogden CL, Grummer-Strawn LM, Flegal KM, Guo SS, Wei R, et al. CDC Growth Charts: United States. Hyattsville, MD: National Center for Health Statistics, 2000.

25. Cook S, Weitzman M, Auinger P, Barlow SE. Screening and counseling associated with obesity diagnosis in a national survey of ambulatory pediatric visits. Pediatrics 2005;116(1):112–16.

26. Barlow SE, Dietz WH, Klish WJ, Trowbridge FL. Medical evaluation of overweight children and adolescents: reports from pediatricians, pediatric nurse practitioners, and registered dietitians. Pediatrics 2002;110(1):222–8.

27. Perrin EM, Flower KB, Ammerman AS. Body mass index charts: useful yet underused. J Pediatr 2004;144:455–60.

28. Dorsey KB, Wells C, Krumholz HM, Concato JC. Diagnosis, evaluation, and treatment of childhood obesity in pediatric practice. Arch Pediatr Adolesc Med 2005;159(7):632–8.

29. Hulse JA, Schilg S. Relation between height and weight centiles may be more useful. BMJ 1996;312(7023):122.

30. Mulligan J, Voss LD. Identifying very fat and very thin children: test of criterion standards for screening test. BMJ 1999;319(7217):1103–4.

31. Cole TJ. A chart to link child centiles of body mass index, weight and height. Eur J Clin Nutr 2002;56(12):1194–9.

32. Flegal KM, Wei R, Ogden CL. Weight-for-stature compared with body mass index-for-age growth charts for the United States from the Centers for Disease Control and Prevention. Am J Clin Nutr 2002;75:761–6.

33. Sorof JM, Lai D, Turner J, Poffenbarger T, Portman RJ. Overweight, ethnicity, and the prevalence of hypertension in school-aged children. Pediatrics 2004;113(3):475–82.

34. Whitlock EP, Williams SB, Gold R, Smith PR, Shipman SA. Screening and interventions for childhood overweight: a summary of evidence for the US preventive services task force. Pediatrics 2005;116(1):E125–E44.

35. Guo S, Wu W, Chumlea WC, Roche AF. Predicting overweight and obesity in adulthood from body mass index values in childhood and adolescence. Am J Clin Nutr 2002;76:653–8.

36. Nader PR, O'Brien M, Houts R, Bradley R, Belsky J, Crosnoe R, et al. Identifying risk for obesity in early childhood. Pediatrics 2006;118(3):e594–e601.

37. Zhu H, Yan W, Ge D, Treiber FA, Harshfield GA, Kapuku G, et al. Relationships of cardiovascular phenotypes with healthy weight, at risk of overweight, and overweight in US youths. Pediatrics 2008;121(1):115–22.

38. Baker JL, Olsen LW, Sorensen TIA. Childhood body-mass index and the risk of coronary heart disease in adulthood. N Engl J Med 2007;357(23):2329–37.

39. Rolland-Cachera MF, Cole TJ, Sempe M, Tichet J, Rossignol C, Charraud A. Body mass index variations: centiles from birth to 87 years. Eur J Clin Nutr 1991;45(1):13–21.

40. Inokuchi M, Hasegawa T, Anzo M, Matsuo N. Standardized centile curves of body mass index for Japanese children and adolescents based on the 1978–1981 national survey data. Ann Hum Biol 2006;33(4):444–53.

41. Cacciari E, Milani S, Balsamo A, Dammacco F, De Luca F, Chiarelli F, et al. Italian cross-sectional growth charts for height, weight and BMI (6 to 20 y). Eur J Clin Nutr 2002;56:171–80.

42. Cole TJ, Roede MJ. Centiles of body mass index for Dutch children aged 0–20 years in 1980 – a baseline to assess recent trends in obesity. Ann Hum Biol 1999;26(4):303–8.

43. Cole TJ, Freeman JV, Preece MA. Body mass index reference curves for the UK, 1990. Arch Dis Child 1995;73(1):25–9.

44. Cole TJ, Bellizzi MC, Flegal KM, Dietz WH. Establishing a standard definition for child overweight and obesity worldwide: international survey. BMJ 2000;320(7244):1240–3.

45. Wright CM, Booth IW, Buckler JMH, Cameron N, Cole TJ, Healy MJR, et al. Growth reference charts for use in the United Kingdom. Arch Dis Child 2002;86(1):11–14.

46. Ogden CL, Kuczmarski RJ, Flegal KM, Mei Z, Guo S, Wei R, et al. Centers for Disease Control and Prevention 2000 growth charts for the United States: improvements to the 1977 National Center for Health Statistics version. Pediatrics 2002;109(1):45–60.

47. Prentice AM. Body mass index standards for children: are useful for clinicians but not yet for epidemiologists. BMJ 1998;317(7170):1401–2.

48. Guillaume M. Defining obesity in childhood: current practice. Am J Clin Nutr 1999;70:126S–30S.

49. Reilly JJ. Assessment of childhood obesity: national reference data or international approach. Obes Res 2002;10:838–40.

50. Jebb SA, Prentice AM. Single definition of overweight and obesity should be used. BMJ 2001;323(7319):999.

51. Rona RJ, Chinn S. One cheer for the international definitions of overweight and obesity. Arch Dis Child 2002;87:390–1.

52. Neovius M, Linne Y, Barkeling B, Rossner S. Discrepancies between classification systems of childhood obesity. Obes Rev 2004;5(2):105–14.

53. de Onis M, Garza C, Onyango AW, Martorel lR. WHO Child Growth Standards. Acta Paediatr 2006;450(suppl):1–101.

54. Barlow SE, and the Expert Committee. Expert Committee recommendations regarding the prevention, assessment, and treatment of child and adolescent overweight and obesity: summary report. Pediatrics 2007;120:S164–S92.

55. Daniels SR. Complications of obesity in children and adolescents. Int J Obes 2009;33(suppl 1):S60–5.

56. Must A, Hollander SA, Economos CD. Childhood obesity: a growing public health concern. Expert Rev Endocrinol Metab 2006;1(2):233–54.

57. NHLBI Obesity Education Initiative Expert Panel. Clinical guidelines on the identification, evaluation, and treatment of overweight and obesity in adults: the evidence report. Obes Res 1998;6:51S–209S.

58. Sturm R. Increases in clinically severe obesity in the United States, 1986–2000. Arch Intern Med 2003;163(18):2146–8.

59. Flegal KM, Troiano RP. Changes in the distribution of body mass index of adults and children in the US population. Int J Obes 2000;24:807–18.

60. Centers for Disease Control and Prevention. CDC Growth Charts: United States. 2000. Available from: www.cdc.gov/growthcharts/.

61. Mei Z, Grummer-Strawn LM, Wang J, Thornton JC, Freedman DS, Pierson RN Jr, et al. Do skinfold measurements provide additional information to body mass index in the assessment of body fatness among children and adolescents? Pediatrics 2007;119(6):e1306–13.

62. Zimmermann MB, Gubeli C, Puntener C, Molinari L. Detection of overweight and obesity in a national sample of 6–12-y-old Swiss children: accuracy and validity of reference values for body mass index from the US Centers for Disease Control and Prevention and the International Obesity Task Force. Am J Clin Nutr 2004;79(5):838–43.

63. Neovius M, Rasmussen F. Evaluation of BMI-based classification of adolescent overweight and obesity: choice of percentage body fat cutoffs exerts a large influence. The COMPASS study. Eur J Clin Nutr 2008;62(10):1201–7.

64. Spear BA, Barlow SE, Ervin C, Ludwig DS, Saelens BE, Schetzina KE, et al. Recommendations for treatment of child and adolescent overweight and obesity. Pediatrics 2007;120:S254–88.

65. Davis MM, Gance-Cleveland B, Hassink S, Johnson R, Paradis G, Resnicow K. Recommendations for prevention of childhood obesity. Pediatrics 2007;120:S229–53.

66. Krebs NF, Himes JH, Jacobson D, Nicklas TA, Guilday P, Styne D. Assessment of child and adolescent overweight and obesity. Pediatrics 2007;120:S193–228.

67. Barlow SE, Dietz WH. Obesity evaluation and treatment: Expert Committee recommendations. Pediatrics 1998;102:1–11.

68. Burd L, Vesely B, Martsolf J, Kerbeshian J. Prevalence study of Prader-Willi syndrome in North Dakota. Am J Med Genet 1990;37(1):97–9.

69. Cassidy SB. Prader-Willi syndrome. J Med Genet 1997;34(11):917–23.

70. Chiumello G, Poskitt EME. Prader-Willi and other syndromes. In: Burniat W, Cole TJ, Lissau I, Poskitt EME (eds) *Child and Adolescent Obesity*. Cambridge: Cambridge University Press, 2003:171–88.

71. Yanovski JA. Pediatric obesity. Rev Endocrin Metab Disord 2001;2(4):371–83.

72. Safer DJ. A comparison of risperidone-induced weight gain across the age span. J Clin Psychopharmacol 2005;24:429–36.

73. Taylor DM, McAskill R. Atypical antipsychotics and weight gain – a systematic review. Acta Psychiatr Scand 2000;101(6):416–32.

74. Vanina Y, Podolskaya A, Sedky K, Shahab H, Siddiqui A, Munshi F, et al. Body weight changes associated with psychopharmacology. Psychiatr Serv 2002;53(7):842–7.

75. Pilj H, Meinders AE. Bodyweight change as an adverse effect of drug treatment: mechanisms and management. Drug Safety 1996;14:329–42.

76. Beebe DW, Lewin D, Zeller M, McCabe M, MacLeod K, Daniels SR, et al. Sleep in overweight adolescents: shorter sleep, poorer sleep quality, sleepiness, and sleep-disordered breathing. J Pediatr Psychol 2007;32(1):69–79.

77. Must A, Parisi SM. Sedentary behavior and sleep: paradoxical effects in association with childhood obesity. Int J Obes 2009;33(suppl 1):S82–6.

78. Franks S. Polycystic ovary syndrome. Medicine 2005;33:38–40.

79. Strauss RS, Barlow SE, Dietz WH. Prevalence of abnormal serum aminotransferase values in overweight and obese adolescents. J Pediatr 2000;136(6):727–33.

80. Baker S, Barlow S, Cochran W, Fuchs G, Klish W, Krebs N, et al. Overweight children and adolescents: a clinical report of the North American Society for Pediatric Gastroenterology, Hepatology and Nutrition. Clinical report. J Pediatr Gastroenterol Nutr 2005;40:533–43.

81. Everhart JE. Contributions of obesity and weight loss to gallstone disease. Ann Intern Med 1993;119:1029–35.

82. Friedman MA, Wilfley DE, Pike KM, Striegel-Moore RH, Rodin J. The relationship between weight and psychological functioning among adolescent girls. Obes Res 1995;3(1):57–62.

83. Strauss RS. Childhood obesity and self-esteem. Pediatrics 2000;105(1):e15.

84. Erickson SJ, Robinson TN, Haydel KF, Killen JD. Are overweight children unhappy? Body mass index, depressive symptoms, and overweight concerns in elementary school children. Arch Pediatr Adolesc Med 2000;154(9):931–5.

85. Sjoberg RL, Nilsson KW, Leppert J. Obesity, shame, and depression in school-aged children: a population-based study. Pediatrics 2005;116(3):e389–92.

86. Wardle J, Cooke L. The impact of obesity on psychological well-being. Best Pract Res Clin Endocrinol Metab 2005;19(3):421–40.

87. Anderson SE, Cohen P, Naumova EN, Jacques PF, Must A. Adolescent obesity and risk for subsequent major depressive disorder and anxiety disorder: prospective evidence. Psychosom Med 2007;69(8):740–7.

88. Herva A, Laitinen J, Miettunen J, Veijola J, Karvonen JT, Lasky K, et al. Obesity and depression: results from the longitudinal Northern Finland 1966 birth cohort study. Int J Obes 2005;30:520–7.

89. Allison DB, Matz PE, Pietrobelli A, Zannolli R, Faith MS. Genetic and environmental influences on obesity. In: Bendich A, Deckelbaum RJ (eds) *Primary and Secondary Preventive Nutrition*. Totowa, NJ: Humana Press, 1999:147–64.

90. Whitaker RC, Wright JA, Pepe MS, Seidel KD, Dietz WH. Predicting obesity in young adulthood from childhood and parental obesity. N Engl J Med 1997;337:869–73.

91. Freedman DS, Khan LK, Dietz WH, Srinivasan SR, Berenson GS. Relationship of childhood obesity to coronary heart disease risk factors in adulthood: the Bogalusa Heart Study. Pediatrics 2001;108(3):712–18.

92. Scottish Intercollegiate Guidelines Network. *Management of Obesity in Children and Young People*. Edinburgh: Royal College of Physicians, 2003.

93. Gutin B, Johnson MH, Humphries MC, Hatfield-Laube JL, Kapuku GK, Allison JD, et al. Relationship of visceral adiposity to

cardiovascular disease risk factors in black and white teens. Obesity 2007;15(4):1029–35.

94. Garnett SP, Baur LA, Srinivasan S, Lee JW, Cowell CT. Body mass index and waist circumference in midchildhood and adverse cardiovascular disease risk clustering in adolescence. Am J Clin Nutr 2007;86(3):549–55.

95. Kelly AS, Wetzsteon RJ, Kaiser DR, Steinberger J, Bank AJ, Dengel DR. Inflammation, insulin, and endothelial function in overweight children and adolescents: the role of exercise. J Pediatr 2004;145(6):731–6.

96. Warnberg J, Nova E, Moreno LA, Romeo J, Mesana MI, Ruiz JR, et al. Inflammatory proteins are related to total and abdominal adiposity in a healthy adolescent population: the AVENA Study. Am J Clin Nutr 2006;84(3):505–12.

97. Morrison JA, Sprecher DL, Barton BA, Waclawiw MA, Daniels SR. Overweight, fat patterning, and cardiovascular disease risk factors in black and white girls: the National Heart, Lung, and Blood Institute Growth and Health Study. J Pediatr 1999;135:458–64.

98. Morrison JA, Barton BA, Biro FM, Daniels SR, Sprecher DL. Overweight, fat patterning, and cardiovascular disease risk factors in black and white boys. J Pediatr 1999;135:451–7.

99. McCarthy HD, Jarrett KV, Crawley HF. The development of waist circumference percentiles in British children aged 5.0–16.9 y. Eur J Clin Nutr 2001;55(10):902–7.

100. Brambilla P, Bedogni G, Moreno LA, Goran MI, Gutin B, Fox KR, et al. Crossvalidation of anthropometry against magnetic resonance imaging for the assessment of visceral and subcutaneous adipose tissue in children. Int J Obes 2006;30(1):23–30.

101. Pietrobelli A, Fernandez JR, Redden JT, Allison DB. Waist circumference percentiles in nationally representative samples of black, white, and Hispanic children. Int J Obes 2002;26:S93.

102. Moreno LA, Fleta J, Mur L, Rodriquez G, Sarria A, Bueno M. Waist circumference values in Spanish children – gender related differences. Eur J Clin Nutr 1999;53(6):429–33.

103. Zannolli R, Morgese G. Waist percentiles: a simple test for atherogenic disease. Acta Paediatr 1996;85(11):1368–9.

104. Eisenmann JC. Waist circumference percentiles for 7- to 15-year-old Australian children. Acta Paediatr 2005;94(9):1182–5.

105. Freedman DS, Kahn HS, Mei Z, Grummer-Strawn LM, Dietz WH, Srinivasan SR, et al. Relation of body mass index and waist-to-height ratio to cardiovascular disease risk factors in children and adolescents: the Bogalusa Heart Study. Am J Clin Nutr 2007;86(1):33–40.

106. Maffeis C, Pietrobelli A, Grezzani A, Provera S, Tato L. Waist circumference and cardiovascular risk factors in prepubertal children. Obes Res 2001;9(3):179–87.

107. Taylor RW, Jones IE, Williams SM, Goulding A. Evaluation of waist circumference, waist-to-hip ratio, and the conicity index as screening tools for high trunk fat mass, as measured by dual-energy X-ray absorptiometry, in children aged 3–19 y. Am J Clin Nutr 2000;72(2):490–5.

108. Tybor DJ, Lichtenstein AH, Dallal GE, Must A. Waist to height ratio is correlated with height in US children and adolescents aged 2–18 y. Int J Pediatr Obes 2008;3(3):148–51.

109. National High Blood Pressure Education Program Working Group on High Blood Pressure in Children and A. The fourth report on the diagnosis, evaluation, and treatment of high blood pressure in children and adolescents. Pediatrics 2004;114(2):555–76.

110. Dwyer J, Mayer J. The dismal condition: problems faced by obese adolescent girls in American society. In: Bray GA (ed) *Obesity in Perspective*. Washington, DC: US Department of Health, Education and Welfare, 1973.

111. Strauss RS, Pollack H. Social marginalization of overweight adolescents. Arch Pediatr Adolesc Med 2003;157(8):746–52.

112. Neumark-Sztainer D, Falkner NH, Story M, Perry CL, Hannan PJ, Mulert S. Weight-teasing among adolescents: correlations with weight status and disordered eating behaviors. Int J Obes 2002;26:123–31.

113. Janssen I. Associations between overweight and obesity with bullying behaviors in school-aged children. Pediatrics 2004;113(5):1187–94.

114. Teachman BA, Brownell KD. Implicit anti-fat bias among health professionals: is anyone immune? Int J Obes 2001;25:1525–31.

115. Cohen ML, Tanofsky-Kraff M, Young-Hyman D, Yanovski JA. Weight and its relationship to adolescent perceptions of their providers (WRAP): a qualitative and quantitative assessment of teen weight-related preferences and concerns. J Adolesc Health 2005;37(2):163.

116. Frelut M-L, Flodmark C-E. The obese adolescent. In: Burniat W, Cole TJ, Lissau I, Poskitt EME (eds) *Child and Adolescent Obesity*. Cambridge: Cambridge University Press, 2003:154–70.

117. National Task Force on the Prevention and Treatment of Obesity. Medical care for obese patients: advice for health care professionals. Am Fam Physician 2002;65:81–8.

118. Wadden TA, Didie E. What's in a name? Patients' preferred terms for describing obesity. Obes Res 2003;11(9):1140–6.

119. Mrdjenovic G, Levitsky D. Nutritional and energetic consequences of sweetened drink consumption in 6- to 13-year-old children. J Pediatr 2003;142(6):604–10.

120. Berkey CS, Rockett HRH, Field AE, Gillman MW, Colditz GA. Sugar-added beverages and adolescent weight change. Obes Res 2004;12(5):778–88.

121. Neumark-Sztainer D, Hannan PJ, Story M, Croll J, Perry C. Family meal patterns: associations with sociodemographic characteristics and improved dietary intake among adolescents. J Am Dietet Assoc 2003;103(3):317–22.

122. Siega-Riz AM, Popkin BM, Carson T. Trends in breakfast consumption for children in the United States from 1965–1991. Am J Clin Nutr 1998;67(4):748S–56S.

123. French SA, Story M, Jeffery RW. Environmental influences on eating and physical activity. Annu Rev Pub Health 2001;22:309–35.

124. Young LR, Nestle M. Expanding portion sizes in the US marketplace: implications for nutrition counseling. J Am Dietet Assoc 2003;103(2):231–4.

125. Diliberti N, Bordi PL, Conklin MT, Roe LS, Rolls BJ. Increased portion size leads to increased energy intake in a restaurant meal. Obes Res 2004;12(3):562–8.

126. Gortmaker SL, Must A, Sobol AM, Peterson K, Colditz GA, Dietz WH. Television viewing as a cause of increasing obesity among children in the United States, 1986–1990. Arch Pediatr Adolesc Med 1996;150:356–62.

127. Robinson TN. Reducing children's television viewing to prevent obesity – a randomized controlled trial. JAMA 1999;282(16):1561–7.

128. Matheson DM, Killen JD, Wang Y, Varady A, Robinson TN. Children's food consumption during television viewing. Am J Clin Nutr 2004;79(6):1088–94.

129. Chamberlain LJ, Wang Y, Robinson TN. Does children's screen time predict requests for advertised products? Arch Pediatr Adolesc Med 2006;160:363–8.

130. Bellissimo N, Pencharz PB, Thomas SG, Anderson GH. Effect of television viewing at mealtime on food intake after a glucose preload in boys. Pediatr Res 2007;61:745–9.

131. Halford JC, Boyland EJ, Hughes G, Oliveira LP, Dovey TM. Beyond-brand effect of television (TV) food advertisement/commercials on caloric intake and food choice of 5–7 year-old children. Appetite 2007;49:263–7.

132. Coon KA, Goldberg J, Rogers BL, Tucker KL. Relationships between use of television during meals and children's food consumption patterns. Pediatrics 2001;107(1):e7.

133. Dennison BA, Erb TA, Jenkins PL. Television viewing and television in bedroom associated with overweight risk among low-income preschool children. Pediatrics 2002;109(6):1028–35.

134. Dietz W. How to tackle the problem early? The role of education in the prevention of obesity. Int J Obes 1999;23:S7–9.

135. Emmons KM, Rollnick S. Motivational interviewing in health care settings: opportunities and limitations. Am J Prev Med 2001;20(1):68–74.

136. Rollnick S, Mason P, Butler C. *Health Behavior Change: a Guide for Practitioners*. New York: Churchill Livingstone,1999.

29 Childhood Obesity: Consequences and Complications

Kate Steinbeck

Department of Endocrinology and Adolescent Medicine, Royal Prince Alfred Hospital, Sydney, Australia

The physical and psychosocial consequences of childhood obesity

Obese children and adolescents have ongoing existing medical and psychosocial morbidity and their risks for adult ill health are increased. The rising prevalence of childhood and adolescent obesity has seen increases in obesity-related morbidity and the emergence of conditions that were previously considered relevant only to adult obesity.

The prevalence of many obesity-related morbidities in children and adolescents remains unknown, as most data come from clinical studies in highly selected patient groups. As the prevalence of childhood and adolescent obesity and the percentage of children and adolescents in the heavier weight categories increase, true prevalence data can be obtained from population-based methods.

Consequences of childhood obesity

The consequences of childhood obesity are significant (Box 29.1).

Adult obesity

The first consequence of childhood and adolescent obesity is adult obesity. Tracking studies have used variable definitions of obesity, different length of follow-up and many of the large cohort studies commenced well before the worldwide increase in obesity began. Variable predictions of adult obesity tracking from childhood obesity exist but no study has demonstrated the absence of a relationship.

> **Box 29.1 The consequences of childhood and adolescent obesity**
>
> Adult obesity
> Belonging to an obese family
> Puberty is a risk time for further weight gain
> Fat distribution matters
> Increased adult morbidity and mortality
> Disadvantaged in healthcare provision
> Adverse adult psychologic outcomes
> Failure to be recognized as obese

Earlier studies found that less than a third of obese adults were obese in childhood. More recent studies show that over 75% of obese children remain obese as adults, and that they are more obese than adults with adult-onset obesity [1]. The later in adolescence that overweight persists and the greater the degree of overweight, the more likely it is that an individual will be an obese adult [2]. Less than 2% of obese adolescents will track down to become nonobese [3]. Longitudinal studies cannot distinguish between the influences of genes, environment and social behaviors on the tracking of body weight and other lifestyle habits which impact on obesity, including physical activity and smoking.

Clinical practice point: Do not postpone active intervention in childhood obesity. Spontaneous remission to a normal body weight is unlikely, as our environments become more obesogenic.

Belonging to an obese family

The second consequence of childhood and adolescent obesity is that the child or adolescent is likely to be part of an obese family. There is strong evidence for a significant genetic component to obesity in children and adolescents, from family, twin and adoptee studies [4]. Children of two obese parents have an 80%

Clinical Obesity in Adults and Children, 3rd edition. Edited by Peter G. Kopelman, Ian D. Caterson and William H. Dietz.
© 2010 Blackwell Publishing, ISBN: 978-1-4051-8226-3.

chance of becoming obese [5]. This compares with a less than 10% chance for the offspring of two lean parents. By the age of 17 years, the children of two obese parents are three times as likely to be obese as the children of two lean parents. Genes may not be expressed fully until adulthood but when obesity has been present from childhood, it tends to be more severe. In longitudinal studies in children where parental weights are available and used for their predictive value, parental obesity more than doubles the risk of adult obesity among both obese and nonobese children under 10 years of age [6,7]. This risk is throughout life and will be modified by environment. Obese children under 3 years of age without obese parents appear at lower risk of obesity in adulthood, but among older children obesity is an increasingly important predictor of adult obesity. Obesity-related parental morbidity predicts the presence of cardiovascular risk in their offspring [8]. Children of parents with documented coronary artery disease have significantly higher Body Mass Index (BMI) and cardiovascular risk factors from childhood. These differences become greater in adolescence.

Clinical practice point: The clinical risk of obesity-related co-morbidity in children and adolescents can be predicted by taking a history of weight and weight-related morbidity in first-degree relatives.

Puberty is a risk time for further weight gain

The third consequence of childhood obesity is that the onset of adolescence is not associated with more favorable body composition. Body fatness changes throughout childhood and adolescence [9]. Gender dimorphism for fatness begins before puberty, with girls as young as 4 years having a higher body fat than boys [10]. In all children fat deposition predominates in the first 12 months of life. From 12 months until approximately 4–6 years of age, the percentage of body fat reduces, with lean tissue deposition more marked. There is a reversion of this pattern known as adiposity rebound at 6–10 years of age [11]. This normal physiologic change may be where the term "puppy fat" originates. An earlier age at adiposity rebound has been suggested by some as a risk for later obesity. The timing of this rebound is only apparent in retrospect and it may be an epiphenomenon describing other potentially preventable environmental obesity risks.

Girls show an increase in fat-free mass that slows over adolescence. Boys, in contrast, have a continuing increase in fat-free mass into young adulthood [12]. Total body fat increases with age in adolescent girls and produces the adult gender dimorphism in body composition [13]. Adipose tissue studies parallel clinical observation. The adipocyte size peaks first around 12 months of age, followed by a fall and then a second rise starting from peripuberty. Up to about 10 years of age in lean subjects, most of the increase in fat depot is from increased cell size. The next major increase in fat cell number is at puberty. In obese subjects the number of fat cells increases throughout childhood and adolescence and by the end of puberty they have over twice as many fat cells as the lean subjects [14]. This proliferation can be modified by lifestyle intervention.

Clinical practice point: Puberty is accompanied by major changes in body composition in both sexes. Children will not, however, grow out of their obesity – a concept promulgated by the "puppy fat" myth. Do not postpone intervention in a child or early adolescent who is gaining excess body fat.

Fat distribution matters

The fourth consequence of childhood and adolescent obesity is that it matters where the fat is distributed. Obese children and adolescents show a variation in fat distribution prior to adolescence. Deep visceral fat depots in children, whatever their degree of obesity, are less than those seen in adults. The waist-to-hip ratio is lower in females than in males aged from 6 to 17 years and the ratio falls with age, leveling out at mid-adolescence [15]. Waist circumference measures in childhood track into adulthood. Anthropometric markers of central fat distribution in children correlate with markers of the metabolic syndrome [16]. Whether the waist circumference is a more powerful predictor for cardiovascular risk factors than BMI remains debatable [17].

There are no accepted cut-off points for waist circumference in children and adolescents because the relationship between waist measurement and metabolic complications in children and adolescents remains undefined. Waist circumference percentile charts have been developed for a number of countries [18] and could be used to assess relative risk of central adiposity. For both genders, age-adjusted waist circumference is increasing at a greater rate than age-adjusted BMI [19].

Clinical practice point: Higher waist circumference indicates greater abdominal fat stores and correlates with cardiovascular risk in obese children and adolescents. In the absence of percentile charts, longitudinal change in waist circumference during weight management is a useful clinical tool.

Increased adult morbidity and mortality

The fifth consequence of childhood and adolescent obesity is an increased risk of morbidity and mortality in adulthood. These long-term consequences of childhood and adolescent obesity are difficult to study, because of the time delay between origins of disease and disease appearance. A review of subjects from the third American Harvard Growth Study (1922–1935) demonstrated that for both men and women who had been overweight in adolescence, there was an increased risk of morbidity from coronary artery disease and vascular disease [20]. A retrospective study based on over 13,000 individuals measured as children or adolescents between 1933 and 1945 had similar findings [21]. There was a linear increase in adult mortality with increasing relative weight before puberty for both genders, and for relative weight in adolescent females only. In a Norwegian cohort (1963–1999) of 128,121 adolescents, those in the highest BMI category >85th percentile had a 30–40% increase in all-cause mortality compared to those with a BMI percentile of 25–74th [2]. The results were replicated in the largest cohort study to date in over 250,00 Danish schoolchildren (1930–1976) [22].

As an example from these data, a 13-year-old boy who is 11 kg heavier than the average weight for age has a 33% increase in the chance of a cardiac event before age 60. Whatever the adult weight, overweight in childhood confers higher adult disease risk and the effect of weight is linear. These cohort studies were done before the worldwide increase in childhood obesity, and may underestimate the current adult effects of childhood obesity.

Clinical practice point: Obesity in childhood and adolescence confers a disease risk in adulthood, irrespective of adult weight status. Prevention of obesity is as important as intervention in established obesity.

Cardiovascular disease starts early. Autopsy findings from young subjects in the Bogalusa Study with trauma death demonstrated the presence of fatty streaks and fibrous plaques in the coronary arteries which increased with age, with detectable abnormalities in the 2–15 year age group [23]. There were strongly significant correlations between the presence of cardiovascular risk factors and this atherosclerotic change. Subjects with three or four risk factors had over 30% of the intimal surface of the aorta covered in fatty streaks. In the Muscatine Study, coronary calcification was more prevalent in young adults who as children had elevated cardiovascular risk factors [24]. Increasing body fatness in children is associated with an increase in cardiovascular risk factors (Fig. 29.1).

Risk factor prevalence shows a significant increase with a BMI above the 85th percentile, but children with a BMI above the 95th percentile are 2.4 times more likely to have elevated cardiovascular risk factors, including blood pressure and fasting insulin [1]. The cardiovascular risk associations do not always vary linearly with age: associations for blood pressure and triglyceride tend to be stronger in the younger children, while LDL cholesterol and insulin are stronger in older groups. The strength of the relationship increases from adolescence into young adulthood and the relationship appears stronger among males. Cardiovascular risk factors in parents further predict the presence of such risk factors in their offspring. The Amsterdam Growth and Health Study also demonstrated strong tracking of lipoproteins, hypertension and body fatness, as well as the clustering of such risk factors [25].

Clinical practice point: A fasting lipid profile should be considered in obese children and adolescents, particularly those who have a family history of cardiovascular risk factors. The levels of lipids are unlikely to be at the levels where pharmacotherapy is indicated but these levels can be used as both an indicator of risk and a monitor of successful intervention.

Insulin is an independent risk factor for cardiovascular disease in adults, and insulin resistance also predicts the future risk of type 2 diabetes in adults. Hyperinsulinemia in childhood has been found in several populations known to be at high risk for type 2 diabetes [26]. Hyperinsulinemia is a common finding in childhood and adolescent obesity [27,28] (Fig. 29.2). Hyperinsulinemia is associated with acanthosis nigricans [29], adverse lipid levels and the development of the metabolic syndrome [28]. The relationship between BMI and insulin levels appears nonlinear, with a sharp increase at about the 95th BMI centile. Whether hyperinsulinemia with insulin resistance increases efficiency of fat storage is unclear.

Clinical practice point: The utility of measuring a fasting insulin in clinical practice is debatable as it clusters with other cardiovascular risk factors, particularly as there is no cut-point for diabetes risk. A fasting insulin might be considered in obese children and adolescents, particularly those who have acanthosis nigricans or a family history of type 2 diabetes. It should fall with appropriate weight management.

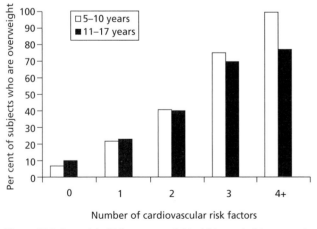

Figure 29.1 Overweight (BMI >95th percentile) in children and adolescents and the number of cardiovascular risk factors (elevated blood pressure, LDL-cholesterol, triglycerides and insulin and low HDL-cholesterol). (Adapted with permission from Freedman et al. [16].)

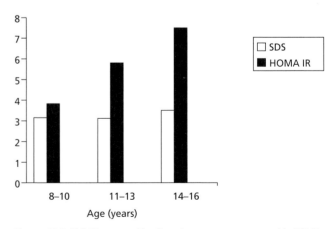

Figure 29.2 BMI SD score and insulin resistance score as measured by HOMA in nondiabetic children and adolescents attending a teaching hospital weight management service. (Johnstone A. Insulin resistance and fitness in overweight children and adolescents. MND thesis, University of Sydney, 2002.)

Disadvantaged in healthcare provision

The sixth consequence of childhood obesity is the difficulties of providing healthcare, particularly in the hospital setting. The main difficulties relate to anesthesia [30], equipment and accommodation, and drug dosage. For anesthesia, obese children and adolescents may have pre-existing abnormal lung function, difficulties in ventilation (especially when supine), and difficulties with both venous access and intubation. Obese children and adolescents admitted for trauma experience more complications and stay longer in the intensive care unit than their lean peers [31]. Standard pediatric equipment may be too small for obese children and adolescents. Hospital furniture may not accommodate body size and in extreme circumstances children may require premature admission to adult facilities, often a very inappropriate placement. Pediatric dosing is carried out on a weight basis. Since the proportion of lean to fat mass in obese children and adolescents is altered, the dosage assumptions may be incorrect. Thus a chance for both therapeutic overdosing and underdosing exists [32]. As an example, there are no clinical algorithms to adjust for higher lean and fat mass or for the change of distribution of lipophilic drugs.

Clinical practice point: Pediatric hospitals should develop protocols to ensure safe management of the obese child or adolescent.

Adverse adult psychologic outcomes

The seventh consequence of childhood and adolescent obesity is adverse psychosocial outcomes in adult life. A study of American women who were obese as adolescents found that they achieved a lower final educational level, had lower incomes and greater rates of poverty and were less likely to marry when compared to peers of lower body weight [33]. Conversely, in a British study, there were no adverse adult outcomes in males who remained obese as adults. However, females with childhood obesity that persisted into adulthood had a higher risk of long-term unemployment and not being partnered [34]. Obesity is not associated with lower intellectual function, as an explanation for poorer personal achievement. These findings represent a high personal cost of obesity with significant societal implications.

Failure to be recognized as obese

A final consequence of overweight and obesity in children and adolescence is that their fatness goes unrecognized by parents [35,36]. Parents underestimate overweight and obesity in their offspring, and are better at recognizing obesity in children not their own [36]. Nearly 90% of parents of overweight 5–6 year olds and two-thirds of parents of overweight older children were not aware that their child was overweight and even when told, the majority displayed a lack of concern about the situation [35]. The consequences of these observations are that parents are unlikely to present their child for weight management and may be affronted if health professionals raise the issue. Reasons for this inaccurate perception include denial, a belief that their child will grow out of their obesity and unfounded concerns about the induction of eating disorders.

Complications of childhood obesity

An important part of the management of childhood and adolescent obesity is the diagnosis and management of current obesity-related co-morbidity. The greater the degree of obesity, the greater the likelihood of multiple obesity-related co-morbidities. Symptoms need to be actively sought. Children may not perceive symptoms as abnormal. Adolescents may be reluctant to discuss symptomatology, due to concerns that it may represent something serious or that they may be ridiculed. The symptoms of some obesity-related co-morbidities may be different in children and adolescents to those in adults. Physical complications may be of minor medical significance but of major importance to the individual (Box 29.2).

Morbidities of minor medical significance

The following complications are morbidities of minor medical significance but of major importance to management. Little research has been directed to these complications and there are no data related to prevalence. These complications will be familiar to those clinicians who manage child and adolescent obesity.

Heat intolerance

Adipose tissue acts as insulation and inhibits the natural dissipation of body heat. Physical activity and muscle use increase superficial skin perfusion and sweating, in order to lose body heat [37]. In child and adolescent obesity, physical activity rapidly increases sweating and perceptions of hotness, together with excessive facial flushing. These events may be the reason why physical activity is avoided or terminated early.

Heat rash and other skin lesions

Overheating and sweating combined with deeper skinfolds increase the likelihood of intertrigo and heat rash in obese

---

Box 29.2 Complications of minor medical significance

Heat intolerance*
Heat rash and intertrigo*
Breathlessness on minimal exertion*
Tiredness*
Musculoskeletal discomfort*
Pseudo-gynecomastia
Male genitalia of small appearance
Cutaneous striae

(*may impact on physical activity in the management of obesity)

children and adolescents. Fungal infections are common in the groin and axilla and under breast tissue in both sexes. Obese children and adolescents have a greater body surface area than their leaner peers and have high perspiration and insensible fluid loss. In clinical practice, obese children and adolescents are frequently described as always thirsty. They often wear loose clothing to hide their body size and shape, which further exacerbates heat-related symptoms.

Breathlessness
In the absence of lung pathology, shortness of breath on exertion is a common morbidity in obese adults. There are no published data to confirm this symptom in children, although it is often observed in clinical practice. Increased respiratory effort will be required at rest because of chest wall mechanics and the situation is worsened by physical activity – another reason why obese children and adolescents avoid physical activity.

Tiredness
Tiredness is a prevalent general symptom in obese children and adolescents. The presence of obstructive sleep apnea should be considered. Tiredness is considered secondary to the increased physical effort of daily lifestyle activity and exacerbated by low levels of physical fitness and exercise tolerance. The presence of depression and of iron deficiency should also be considered [38].

Musculoskeletal discomfort
Obese children and adolescents experience general musculoskeletal discomfort in feet, ankles and calves, exacerbated by physical activity. They display a characteristic walking pattern which includes a longer cycle duration with a prolonged stance period, lower cadence and lower velocity than normal-weight subjects [39]. Gait asymmetry is often apparent.

Foot pronation, or flat feet, is more common in obese children and adolescents, often associated with genu valgus and lax ligaments. A decreased footprint angle and an increased surface area of the foot in contact with the ground are characteristic, as are increased static and dynamic plantar pressures. This functional deformity produces nonspecific joint and ligamentous discomfort and pain [40]. Management involves the use of orthotics, stretching exercises and supportive, enclosed footwear.

Back, knee and hip discomfort are uncommon, even in high grades of obesity, unless there is associated trauma or orthopedic abnormality. Nonspecific discomfort results from the physical forces of excess weight, pronounced lumbar lordosis and gait abnormalities, which in turn increase the risk of falls and soft tissue injury. When injury occurs, symptoms are likely to persist longer in obese children [41]. Obesity impairs functional ability in children [42], is associated with poorer motor skills and contributes to the perception of clumsiness.

Staging of puberty
It is often difficult to clinically assess breast stage in obese children and adolescents and biochemical assessment of gonadal function may be required, particularly if precocious puberty is a concern. Published data suggest that older children and adolescents are competent at self-grading against line drawings of the Tanner stages of pubertal development. Obese girls overestimate breast development by self-assessment in about 40% of cases, higher than for nonobese girls of similar age [43].

Pseudo-gynecomastia in males
A general increase in subcutaneous truncal fat can simulate gynecomastia. Pseudo-gynecomastia is differentiated from true gynecomastia by palpation and ultrasound. The sequelae of pseudo-gynecomastia are psychosocial rather than medical, and the psychologic impact determines surgical intervention. Weight loss may improve appearance.

Small genitalia in males
Obese prepubertal males may have the appearance of an abnormally small penis. The vast majority will have a normal-sized penis, buried in a large pubic fat pad. Appearances will improve with the pubertal increase in penile size. Extreme obesity in boys may compromise micturition when standing. Obesity and true micropenis may co-exist, either as two unrelated conditions or as part of a hypogonadal state such as the Klinefelter or Bardet–Biedel syndromes.

Cutaneous striae
Cutaneous striae, or stretch marks, occur as a result of dermal collagen disruption [44] and are a nonspecific response to rapid deposition of fat. In obesity striae are common, especially during puberty, and are seen over the abdomen and hips. Striae occur in pathologic obesity states such as Cushing syndrome where, unlike in obesity, these are violaceous and combined with other dermal abnormalities such as skin fragility and bruising as a result of the glucocorticoid-induced protein catabolic state. Striae will fade with weight loss and/or stabilization but will not disappear completely.

Recurrent abdominal pain
The nonspecific symptom of recurrent abdominal pain is significantly higher in obese children [45]. Inadequate fruit and vegetable intake, dehydration, constipation and anxiety may all play a role in the absence of organic pathology.

Clinical practice point: There is a high level of chronic physical discomfort in the obese child and adolescent which will impact on lifestyle. This discomfort will often counteract attempts to increase physical activity as part of a weight management program and may further impair self-esteem.

Morbidities of significant medical importance
There is no obesity threshold below which a child or adolescent can be assumed to be free of morbidity. Box 29.3 shows the major medical morbidities of obesity and Figure 29.3 highlights the clinical examination of the obese child or adolescent.

Box 29.3 Significant medical complications present in childhood and adolescent obesity

Cardiovascular
Hypertension
Cardiac muscle abnormalities
Abnormal blood vessel structure and function
Increased heart rate variability

Respiratory
Sleep-disordered breathing
Pickwickian syndrome
Asthma

Endocrine
Type 2 diabetes (and acanthosis nigricans)
Changed onset of puberty
Polycystic ovaries

Orthopedic
Foot pronation
Tibia vara (Blount disease)
Slipped capital epiphysis

Gastrointestinal
Hepatic steatosis
Gastroesophageal reflux
Cholelithiasis

Neurologic
Benign intracranial hypertension

Cardiovascular

Hypertension

Most hypertension in children and adolescents is now essential or primary, rather than secondary to renal disease, and generally clusters with other cardiovascular risk factors [46,47]. Obese children and adolescents have higher blood pressures and higher prevalence rates for hypertension than leaner children, with 30% of obese children and 50% of obese adolescents affected. Prevalence doubles between the 75th and 95th BMI percentiles. Initially, hypertension in childhood obesity is predominantly systolic and may well contribute to their total cardiovascular burden as adults. Age-related percentile charts are required, with arbitrary cut-off points of >90th percentile for high normal blood pressure and >95th percentile for hypertension. The accurate measurement of blood pressure in obese children and adolescents requires the correct blood pressure cuff (width and length). If cuffs are too narrow the reading may be falsely elevated. The width of the cuff bladder should be 40% of the circumference of the mid upper arm.

Cardiac abnormalities

Controlled echocardiography studies in obese children and adolescents show that mean left ventricular mass, ventricular septal and posterior wall thickness and the internal dimension of the left ventricle in diastole are all greater in severely obese children compared to lean counterparts [48]. Echocardiography should be considered in children and adolescents with severe obesity, particularly if they are hypertensive and have additional symptoms such as palpitations, shortness of breath and syncope. A referral for specialist assessment would also be appropriate under these circumstances.

Blood vessel structure and function

Increased intimal-medial thickness and reduced vascular compliance are present in children with diabetes and familial hypercholesterolemia, both known risk factors for early-onset adult cardiovascular morbidity. Obese adolescents also have decreased maximum forearm blood flow and increased forearm vascular resistance [49]. Increased vascular stiffness and endothelial dysfunction are best correlated with abdominal fat and insulin levels [50]. Weight loss will reverse endothelial dysfunction [51] (Fig. 29.4).

The metabolic syndrome

As with adults, there is no single definition of the metabolic syndrome (MS) in children and adolescents. Also, as in adults, this cluster of signs may be an association rather than a syndrome and a cluster which increases the risk of adverse outcomes. Numerous studies have considered the prevalence in pediatric populations using a variety of criteria. Very few children (0–4%) will have the MS when adult definitions are applied [52]. However, the prevalence increases to 39–60% using child-specific definitions for the variables. These rates accord with those of Invitti et al. who described a prevalence of 23% using WHO-derived criteria [53]. If nontraditional cardiovascular risk factors such as plasminogen activator inhibitor type 1, C-reactive protein and interleukin-6 are used, a similar prevalence is achieved. There is a need for better age-related insulin ranges if hyperinsulinemia is to be considered a central component to MS. Brambilla et al. have proposed the use of 10 evidence-based items for the definition of the MS in children and adolescents, of which BMI, the presence of hypertension, waist circumference and acanthosis nigricans are the four clinical indicators [54]. The authors propose that insulin and lipid levels should be excluded until specific age-related reference ranges are available and that impaired glucose tolerance or type 2 diabetes be the only metabolic indicators.

There is evidence that cardiovascular risk factors in children and adolescents can be favorably altered by weight management [55,56]. The percentage loss of body fat or body weight required to improve metabolic risk is about 5–10%. The metabolic improvement in obese children and adolescents is more likely to be significant if there is an exercise component to management. Children maintain this metabolic improvement for some years following intervention [57]. The effect of such metabolic changes on long-term morbidity and mortality is unknown and confirmation would require long prospective trials. Cardiovascular risk factors can be used in the clinical setting to ascertain the effects

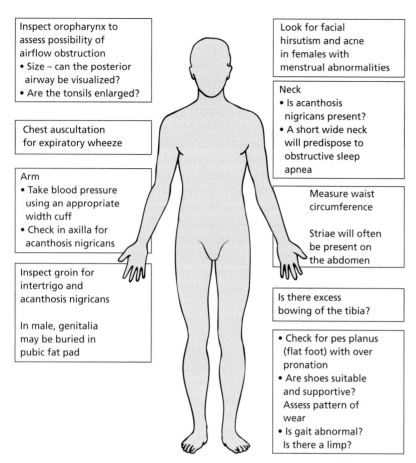

Inspect oropharynx to assess possibility of airflow obstruction
• Size – can the posterior airway be visualized?
• Are the tonsils enlarged?

Chest auscultation for expiratory wheeze

Arm
• Take blood pressure using an appropriate width cuff
• Check in axilla for acanthosis nigricans

Inspect groin for intertrigo and acanthosis nigricans

In male, genitalia may be buried in pubic fat pad

Look for facial hirsutism and acne in females with menstrual abnormalities

Neck
• Is acanthosis nigricans present?
• A short wide neck will predispose to obstructive sleep apnea

Measure waist circumference

Striae will often be present on the abdomen

Is there excess bowing of the tibia?

• Check for pes planus (flat foot) with over pronation
• Are shoes suitable and supportive? Assess pattern of wear
• Is gait abnormal? Is there a limp?

Figure 29.3 Clinical examination of the obese child and adolescent.

of weight management therapy. Metformin could also be considered in the obese, insulin-resistant pediatric patient [58].

Respiratory
Obesity increases the work or effort required to breathe. Mechanical forces such as the weight of the chest wall, increased intra-abdominal fat and narrowing of airways are coupled with diffusion abnormalities. Lung function is altered in obese children [59]. Airway narrowing and increased upper airway resistance, reduced functional residual capacity and reduced diffusion capacity, and ventilatory tiring are common.

Sleep-disordered breathing
Sleep-associated breathing disorders are frequently found in child and adolescent obesity in clinical practice. These disorders include increased airflow resistance in the upper airways, reduction in airflow, regular heavy snoring and multiple, brief cessations of breathing during sleep (apneas) with compensatory arousals.

In clinical cohorts selected for obesity, the prevalence of an abnormal sleep study is between 30% and 50% [59,60]. In one case–control study of children and adolescents recruited from families with and without sleep apnea, obesity is a risk with an odds ratio of over 4.5 [61]. There is also a correlation between the degree of obesity and the severity of the documented sleep disturbance, with 5–10% having severe obstructive sleep apnea and 50% of severely obese children having a degree of central hypoventilation. Adenotonsillar hypertrophy increases the risk of obstructive sleep apnea, as do truncal obesity, a short broad neck and a crowded oropharynx and hyperinsulinemia. Daytime somnolence and tiredness are less commonly reported in children with established obstructive sleep apnea. Neurocognitive deficits (memory, attention and learning performance) present in obese children with sleep-disordered breathing impact on school performance [62].

The diagnosis of sleep-disordered breathing will require an overnight sleep study. Tonsillectomy and adenoidectomy will reduce the symptoms of obstructive sleep apnea in obese children, even in the absence of weight reduction. Paradoxically, tonsillectomy and/or adenoidectomy may be associated with a further increase in BMI [63].

Pickwickian syndrome
The Pickwickian syndrome is present when ventilation capacity cannot be increased to overcome chronic hypoxia and to normalize hypercapnia. It is characterized by severe obesity, hypersomnolence, pulmonary hypertension and right-sided heart failure,

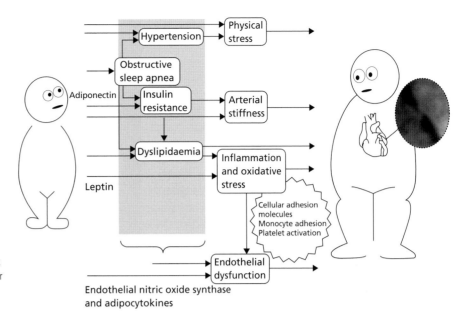

Figure 29.4 Pathophysiologic pathways which link childhood overweight and obesity and cardiovascular disease. (Adapted with permission from Skilton and Celermajer [51].)

polycythemia, daytime hypoxemia and hypercapnia. The syndrome is associated with pulmonary embolism and sudden death in children. It is most likely to be diagnosed in secondary obesity, including hypothalamic hyperphagia syndromes and the Prader–Willi syndrome.

Asthma

While it has been suggested that a causal relationship exists between asthma and obesity in children, not all studies are supportive [64]. Both conditions are increasing in prevalence and associations could be through genetic, immune or mechanical mechanisms [65]. Children who have asthma may be less physically active because of their respiratory condition, thus increasing their risk of obesity. Additionally, drugs used to treat asthma, glucocorticoids in particular, may also increase a child's risk of obesity. There may be other common lifestyle markers or links, especially as the relationship between the two conditions is a recent one.

At least three prospective studies in children show a significant association between obesity and asthma incidence [66]. Using doctor-diagnosed asthma as the criterion, the highest risk for asthma is a family history but a BMI >85th percentile almost doubles the risk [67]. Others have identified female gender as a risk for obesity-associated asthma. In a study of 600 children, females who were obese at 11 years were more likely to have asthma between the ages of 11 and 13 years and more so if they entered puberty early [68]. Obesity in females did not increase the risk of other atopic phenomena which suggests that the etiology of obesity-related asthma may be related to fat mass and possibly its distribution.

Exercise induces a greater frequency and degree of bronchospasm in obese children who are not known to have asthma and it has been proposed that this should be considered a specific obesity-related phenomenon [69]. Obese children who experience shortness of breath and chest discomfort, with physical activity in particular, should be considered for assessment and management of exercise-induced bronchospasm, with a particular emphasis on its prevention. Conversely, weight management in the asthmatic child or adolescent should be considered a key aspect of management.

Endocrine
Type 2 diabetes

In 1996 Pinhas-Hamiel and colleagues described an increase in the incidence of type 2 diabetes in adolescents over the previous decade [70]. The proportion of newly diagnosed patients with type 2 diabetes mellitus (T2DM) rose from 4% to 16% but if the age group of 10–19 years was selected, the figure was 33%. Both obesity and a family history of T2DM are strongly associated with T2DM in children and adolescents. T2DM is associated with excess body weight in 95% of cases, while type 1 diabetes mellitus (T1DM) is associated with excess body weight in only 20% of cases. However, recent data suggest that children with T1DM have become progressively heavier at diagnosis over the past 20 years, and that obese children develop T1DM earlier [71]. This finding suggests that the general population increase in obesity may act as an "accelerator" which contributes to the recognized increase in both T1DM and T2DM in childhood and adolescence. Ethnicity is a strong risk factor for T2DM [72] and indigenous populations are at greater risk of developing T2DM in young age groups [73]. Additional risk factors for the development of T2DM in children and adolescents are female gender and puberty.

Prevalence data for T2DM in children and adolescents are likely to be underestimates because of its insidious onset. The majority of cases are asymptomatic or present with fungal or other skin infections. In a representative sample of 2867 US adolescents, the estimated prevalence of T2DM was 0.41% [74] whereas rates as high as 5% have been found among adolescents in native American populations. This variation may reflect differences in obesity. In an obesity clinic population, 25% of younger obese children and 21% of obese adolescents had impaired glucose tolerance, and undiagnosed diabetes was present in 4% of the adolescents [75].

It is not practicable to perform a standard oral glucose tolerance test in all obese children and adolescents. A fasting blood glucose should be performed in obese children and adolescents from minority groups, those with acanthosis nigricans and those with a family history of diabetes, and puberty should be seen as an additional risk time for development of T2DM. In obesity acanthosis nigricans may be associated with truncal skin tags in the adolescent and it is commonly found around the neck, and in the flexures. The clinical explanation that elevated insulin levels in obesity act through the IGF-1 receptor to cause dermal overgrowth does not explain the predilection for certain areas or certain races. The management is weight loss and the reduction of insulin resistance. Metformin can be used as adjunctive therapy.

The increase in T2DM in childhood and adolescence is expected to bring with it an enormous economic and health service burden as a result of the early development of micro- and macrovascular complications of diabetes [72,76]. There is evolving evidence that the onset and progression of these clinical complications may be particularly rapid when the onset of T2DM occurs early in life. This will mean increasing costs to the young person and the community with blindness and loss of income, early renal failure and dialysis, and even earlier onset of cardiovascular disease. Higher miscarriage rates and the increasing demands for management of high-risk diabetic pregnancy are already being seen.

Lifestyle intervention is the cornerstone of management in T2DM. Adherence to such regimens, particularly when there may be no perceived clinical benefit, is difficult in adolescence. Adolescence is a period of change in lifestyle behaviors with increasing independence from family and reduction in physical activity, particularly in females. Adolescent females require counseling about pregnancy – the risk of fetal abnormalities and overgrowth syndrome with poor control of diabetes, and the requirement for insulin therapy prior to conception. Relatively higher doses of pharmacotherapy are required during puberty. The standard drug therapies in adult T2DM are currently being evaluated in adolescents [77], with the hypothesis that early, intensive reduction in insulin resistance will both improve control and associated co-morbidities and provide much needed evidence for the management of T2DM in youth.

Puberty

Puberty in females
Body weight at both extremes influences time of menarche, menstrual function and fertility. Over the last 10–15 years there has been a decrease in the mean age of menarche, albeit within the normal age range [78]. It is likely that this lowering of menarchal age is associated with the rise in the prevalence of obesity over the same time, with a higher fat mass signaling readiness for sexual maturation. The effect of body weight on early maturation is evident at BMI >85th percentile, with 30% of overweight girls expected to reach menarche before the age of 11 years [79].

Early menarche is associated with earlier onset of sexual activity and its attendant risks. Adolescents who experience earlier menarche are more likely to have depression and substance abuse and eating disorders [80]. Endometriosis and increased severity of dysmenorrhea are more common in young adulthood. Early menarche is a well-established risk factor for breast cancer and has been linked to other cancers, including those of the ovary and thyroid. Cardiovascular disease risks, including hypertension and abnormalities of glucose metabolism, are increased in girls with early menarche independent of body composition [81] and obesity would be expected to further increase the risk profile.

Puberty in males
Overweight boys appear less likely to experience early maturation than their leaner peers [79]. In males lean body mass increases with sexual maturity and boys with a relatively higher lean body mass are the earlier maturers. Increased adipose tissue aromatase activity with conversion of androgen to estrogen in obese boys could impact on sexual maturation at a hypothalamic level.

Polycystic ovarian syndrome
The polycystic ovarian syndrome (PCOS) comprises late menarche, oligomenorrhea or amenorrhea, with hirsutism, acne, abdominal obesity, acanthosis nigricans and insulin resistance [82]. Low birth weight for gestational age, above average birth weight, premature adrenarche, childhood obesity and the metabolic syndrome are all independent childhood risk factors for the development of PCOS. Hyperinsulinemia increases ovarian thecal androgen production and induces the characteristic endocrine pattern of elevated free testosterone. This pattern is increasingly being described in younger obese adolescents, and hyperandrogenism is a feature of obese prepubertal females [83]. Oligomenorrhea or delayed menstruation may be dismissed as normal for adolescents and it may be difficult to distinguish clinically between adolescent anovulation and PCOS [84]. Insulin resistance is seen in at least 50% of adolescents with PCOS [85] and with greater prevalence in obese adolescents with PCOS. PCOS in young adolescents and young adults is associated with infertility and with longer term health risks including the metabolic syndrome, T2DM and early coronary atherosclerosis [86].

Treatment involves a combination of lifestyle changes and pharmacotherapy [87]. There have been no studies demonstrating the efficacy of weight reduction alone in obese adolescents with PCOS. Weight management is an essential component of treatment in PCOS in adolescents, and will also address other cardiovascular risk factors. Ovarian suppression with combined oral contraceptive agents will improve menstrual irregularity and acne and may need to be combined with antiandrogens such as spironolactone or cyproterone acetate to control hirsutism. Cyproterone acetate may cause weight gain. Metformin therapy induces ovulation and improves the endocrine profile in obese adolescents with PCOS [88]. It has the advantage of being weight neutral but adolescents should be warned about its effect on ovulation and contraceptive requirements addressed. Thiozolidinediones as insulin sensitizers and finasteride as an antiandrogen have also been trialed in adults with positive effect but prescribing limitations in many countries affect availability.

Orthopedic

The primary orthopedic morbidities associated with overweight and obesity in children and adolescents are Blount disease [89] and slipped capital femoral epiphysis [90].

Blount disease

Blount disease, or idiopathic tibia vara, is a pathologic bowing of the tibia. All affected older patients are obese, and there is a male preponderance (2:1).

Tibial bowing is initiated by suppression of epiphyseal growth as a result of abnormal pressures causing repetitive trauma to the growth plate. There is then failure to adequately ossify the endochondrium, exacerbated by the adolescent growth spurt. The presentation is knee pain, with slowly progressive clinical deformity. Radiologic examination shows wedging of the epiphysis. Histologic changes include abnormal cellular islands of hyaline cartilage, foci of necrotic cartilage and premature closure of the medial aspects of the epiphysis. The treatment is surgical and if obesity persists, there is a high degree of recurrence, particularly in younger males.

Slipped capital femoral epiphysis (Fig. 29.5)

The presentation for slipped capital femoral epiphysis is hip pain (or referred knee pain) and limitation of movement. The condition may be associated with endocrine disorders, including

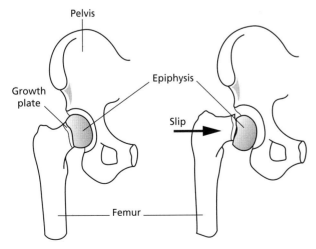

Figure 29.5 Slipped femoral capital epiphysis.

hypothyroidism, and growth hormone therapy for short stature. Obese children present earlier, at a mean age of 12 years (13 years for nonobese) and are more likely to have bilateral slippage (>40% of cases). The clinical threshold for radiologic assessment should be low and the films reviewed by a radiologist with pediatric expertise. If the diagnosis is missed the hip joint will develop early degenerative change. The treatment is surgical. It is important to minimize postsurgical immobility in the obese child or adolescent, in order not to aggravate weight gain.

Gastrointestinal

Gastroesophageal reflux is the most common clinical condition, and hepatic steatosis the greatest long term risk.

Nonalcoholic fatty liver disease (hepatic steatosis)

Nonalcoholic fatty liver disease (NAFLD) is an important obesity co-morbidity in children and adolescents and a growing public health issue [91–93]. The gold standard for the diagnosis of NAFLD is liver biopsy but this is clearly unacceptable as a first-line diagnostic procedure. In clinical practice, hepatic ultrasound and measurement of hepatic transaminases (particularly ALT) are the standard tools [91]. The prevalence of NAFLD diagnosed by ultrasound in obese children and adolescents is between 30% and 50%, and prevalence rises with age. Visceral obesity, the presence of insulin resistance and the metabolic syndrome, and ethnicity increase the risks of NAFLD [93]. The liver is palpable in only a minority of cases and the level of elevation of hepatic transaminases correlates with the degree of fatty liver. There is limited liver biopsy information in children and adolescents and no established criteria for when this should be performed. Fibrosis has been reported in 50–100% of cases in clinical series. In a small percentage of cases, there is clear clinical progression and established cirrhosis has been described in patients as young as 10 years of age. Further prospective studies are required but there is a major public health concern that fat accumulation in the young liver may be particularly damaging.

Little is known of the impact of intervention in hepatic steatosis in children and adolescents, but weight loss of approximately 10% of body weight has been shown to reduce both hepatic size and transaminase levels. The optimal dietary intervention is yet to be defined. Adolescents should be counseled about alcohol intake. Information on pharmacotherapy comes mainly from open-label, uncontrolled trials in children and the list of potentially useful agents includes insulin sensitizers, antioxidants, ursodeoxycholic acid and possibly lipid-lowering agents.

Gastroesophageal reflux

There are no studies of the prevalence or health sequelae of gastroesophageal reflux in obese children and adolescents, although it is well recognized clinically. Children and adolescents will not spontaneously offer symptoms of reflux but identify these when questioned. Weight management, the avoidance of overeating episodes and antacids are the first-line therapy. Proton pump inhibitors are commonly used in pediatric practice and should be prescribed if symptoms persist in order to avoid ulceration. Endoscopy should be considered if symptoms persist. There is a case report of a Nissen fundoplication procedure in an obese 10-year-old male who had pain and apnea that were secondary to reflux and not responsive to medical therapy [94].

Cholelithiasis
In children and adolescents, gallbladder disease is more commonly found in females, but the overall prevalence rate is low (0.13%) [95].Obesity is associated with higher gallbladder volumes in children and adolescents, and obesity and hypertriglyceridemia are common predisposing factors for cholelithiasis. Over 10% of subjects with cholelithiasis will develop pancreatitis. Laparoscopic cholecystectomy is considered the surgical intervention of choice for children and adolescents. Older adolescents who are treated with very low-energy diets may have an exacerbation of underlying gallbladder pathology. An ultrasound should be performed if abdominal pain occurs during this therapy.

Neurologic
Benign intracranial hypertension
Benign intracranial hypertension (BIH) (pseudo-tumor cerebri) is most commonly seen in obese females. There are limited data on the occurrence of BIH in children and adolescents [96] but the condition should be considered particularly in obese adolescent females presenting with persistent headache (in over 90% of cases), visual disturbance and/or papilledema. Younger children present with fewer specific symptoms, including irritability and listlessness. BIH, despite its name, is not benign. Formal visual fields and assessment of visual acuity are mandatory because compression of the optic nerve may lead to visual impairment. Acetazolamide is the mainstay of treatment.

Specific genetic defects
It is beyond the scope of this chapter to consider specific obesity syndromes, such as Prader–Willi, Bardet–Biedl, Alstrom and Cohen. Intellectual disability and short stature with unusual physical stigmata should arouse clinical suspicion. The single gene defects that cause severe, early-onset obesity include leptin deficiency, leptin resistance, pro-opiomelanocortin mutations and proconvertase-1 and peroxisome proliferative-activated receptor γ2 defects. These are all extremely rare. The most common single gene defect is mutations involving the melanocortin-4 receptor. The phenotype includes increased linear growth, increased fat-free mass and severe hyperinsulinemia.

Psychosocial complications of childhood obesity

Research into the psychologic complications of obesity in children and adolescents has often focused on clinical rather than general populations. It is clear in clinical practice that obese children and adolescents suffer distress. Less clear are the psychologic consequences of child and adolescent obesity as there is little

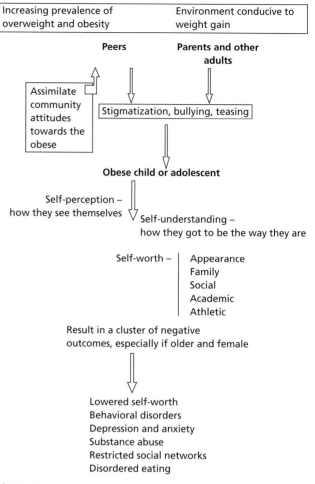

Figure 29.6 The psychosocial world of the obese child and adolescent.

information on long-term psychologic sequelae of childhood obesity. It is likely that the earliest complications or consequences of childhood and adolescent obesity are in the psychologic and social arenas (Fig. 29.6). It is not known how the increasing prevalence of obesity in children and adolescents might impact on societal responses to obesity.

Stigmatization and stereotypes
Stigmatization by the peers of obese children and adolescents is well recognized and is considered in Chapter 3.

How obese children and adolescents feel about themselves
The prejudice and discrimination directed towards the obese are well established by the time children reach primary school. Forty years ago obese adolescents were described as having personality traits that were similar to those seen in persecuted minorities [97]. Low self-esteem and self-worth are common and modified by age, gender, ethnicity and socio-economic status. Study results are also modified by whether it is a population- or clinic-based study, as those presenting for treatment may be more distressed

than those who do not seek help with weight management. Study results are also affected by whether parent or child reporting is used. How self-esteem is measured varies from study to study. It may be a global measure of self-esteem or self-worth or may concentrate on specific areas such as academic performance, body appearance, sporting prowess or social competence [98].

There is little evidence to support the notion that self-esteem is significantly affected in obese preschool children [99]. In primary school children the relationship between self-esteem and body weight is inverse but not strong and many obese children have measures within the accepted range of normal. If a distinction is made between general self-esteem and body self-esteem, relationships between body self-esteem and weight are much clearer, with a trend towards females exhibiting higher body dissatisfaction [100]. While obese primary schoolers have lower self-esteem in relation to physical appearance and athletic competence, they do not seem to differ from their leaner peers in popularity [101]. In this age group parents are often reporters. At least 50% of parents report psychologic distress and difficult behaviors in their obese child [102,103]. Child psychologic distress and difficult behaviors are significantly predicted by maternal psychopathology (particularly that which leads to ineffective parenting styles) and thus there are major implications for clinical weight management.

The inverse relationship between self-esteem and body weight becomes stronger and clearer in adolescents, as pressures of social acceptance, athletic competence and physical appearance become more significant to the individual. Effects of gender and ethnicity become more pronounced [104]. Stress, impairment of physical health, and emotional and social functioning are all more clearly abnormal in obese adolescents [105]. Obese adolescents who exhibit decreasing levels of self-esteem are also more likely to smoke and to drink alcohol than those who maintain self-esteem during adolescence, which may further compromise weight management. High-level physical activity in children and adolescents correlates with self-esteem, but obesity makes such activity difficult [106].

Dissatisfaction with body size and a desire to lose weight are present in young children, particularly in girls. A wish to change body size or shape is found in all weight groups and there is no evidence that obese children or adolescents have a distorted body image. Obese children are more accurate at estimating their real body shape than lean children and express greater dissatisfaction with their body size [107]. Population studies mirror clinical studies, with 30% of obese boys and 60% of obese girls having low appearance self-esteem [108]. Obese children and adolescents are more likely to be bullied but also more likely to be bulliers [109]. They are three times as likely to have clinically meaningful behavior problems [110].

The obese child and adolescent's response to being obese

Younger children will have simplistic views about etiology and possibly believe that obesity is somehow their fault. If their parents are obese they may well incorporate parental views into their belief system. The impact of lifestyle on weight and health will not be understood. Parents report more global impairment of quality of life than do their children, who report only a lower physical quality of life [111]. Children who internalize their obesity (believing that they are responsible for it) score lower on self-esteem measures [112].

Older adolescents may have a better understanding of etiology and future implications, but this does not translate into behaviors necessary for weight control. Many day-to-day behaviors seen in obese children and adolescents are a result of others' behavior towards them. These behaviors include not eating in public (including at school), dressing in loose, cover-up clothing even in hot weather, avoiding situations where they may have to undress in front of others and avoidance of situations where their lack of physical skills will be noted. Obese adolescents particularly have less robust social networks and greater isolation than normal weight peers, which may compound behavioral traits [113].

Are psychiatric disorders more prevalent in obese children and adolescents?

Depression and anxiety would be expected responses in obese children and adolescents. Studies in clinical populations presenting for obesity management consistently demonstrate depression or anxiety disorder (as per DSM-IV criteria) in at least 50% of children and adolescents [114,115]. This is far in excess of the general population. On the other hand, population studies are less consistent in their findings, with the majority reporting no significant differences between the obese and those of normal weight [116,117]. In one prospective study persistence of obesity from childhood to adolescence predicted oppositional defiant disorder in both sexes and depression in males [118].

Childhood and adolescent obesity and disordered eating

Restrained eating and dieting behaviors are already present in preadolescent children [119] and increase with age, female gender and obesity. By adolescence, dieting behaviors are well entrenched, including purging behaviors [120]. In adolescents in the general population, binge-eating disorder (BED) is a risk for obesity, depression and low self-worth [121]. The presence of BED is also a suicide risk with 25% of males and females reporting a suicide attempt [118]. Obese children and adolescents have more emotional and externally cued eating than lean children, with sneaky eating, stealing of food and constant complaints about hunger. Their eating is not driven by hunger alone but is also controlled by restraint (self-imposed eating controls) and by disinhibition (loss of control of intake in the presence of certain cues). Parental eating behaviors influence those of their offspring [122]. High levels of parental restriction and disinhibition – the classic combination for binge eating – increase the likelihood of excessive weight gain in their offspring.

Does treatment of obesity make a difference to psychosocial well-being?

The improvement of self-efficacy and self-competency is a generally accepted approach when working with children in whom behavior change is desired. Such an approach requires that effort is rewarded with some form of success. There is a lack of evidence available on the impact of weight management interventions on psychosocial well-being, although clear improvement has been demonstrated in psychosocial indicators for weight loss camps [123] and residential management programs [124]. Lack of evidence may be due in part to the modest success rates in clinical weight management if weight loss is the primary outcome. A significant risk must exist for the reduction of psychosocial well-being if failure occurs. Thus, in a clinical weight management program, it is advisable to include positive outcome indicators other than weight loss, including improved physical fitness and reduction in body circumferences.

Conclusion

Obesity in childhood and adolescence is not a healthy state and the degree of obesity is proportional to the presence of co-morbidities. Co-morbidities in childhood obesity are likely to be underdiagnosed. This observation is a complex result of failure to perceive the seriousness of the condition, prejudice and stigmatization by health professionals and the inability of children and adolescents to voice symptoms or lack of awareness that symptoms are of significance. Change in associated morbidities is one outcome indicator for successful weight management. Children do not grow out of obesity, and obesity in adolescence is a dangerous situation, as it will persist into adulthood.

References

1. Freedman DS, Khan LK, Dietz WH, Srinivasan SR, Berenson GS. Relationship of childhood obesity to coronary heart disease risk factors in adulthood: the Bogalusa Heart Study. Pediatrics 2001;108: 712–18.
2. Engelund A, Bjorge T, Tverda AL, Sogaard AJ. Obesity in adolescence and adulthood and the risk of adult mortality. Epidemiology 2004;15:79–85.
3. Gordon-Larsen P, Adair LS, Nelson MC, Popkin BM. Five-year obesity incidence in the transition period between adolescence and adulthood: the National Longitudinal Study of Adolescent Health Am J Clin Nutr 2004;80:569–75.
4. Stunkard AJ, Harris JR, Pedersen NL, McClearn GE. The body mass index of twins who have been reared apart. N Engl J Med 1990;322:1483–7.
5. Garn SM, Clark DC. Trends in fatness and origins of obesity. Pediatrics 1976;57:443–56.
6. Whitaker RC, Wright JA, Pepe MS, Seidel KD, Dietz WH. Predicting obesity in young adulthood from childhood and parental obesity. N Engl J Med 1997;337:869–73.
7. Magarey AM, Daniels LA, Boulton TJ, Cockington RA. Predicting obesity in early adulthood from childhood and parental obesity. Int J Obes 2003;27:505–13.
8. Bao W, Srinivasan SR, Valdez R, Greenlund KJ, Wattigney MS, Berenson GS. Longitudinal changes in cardiovascular risk from

childhood to young adulthood in offspring of parents with coronary artery disease. JAMA 1997;278:1749–54.
9. Dugdale AE, Payne PR. Pattern of fat and lean deposition in children. Nature 1976;256:725–7.
10. Byrnes SE, Baur LA, Bermingham M, Brock K, Steinbeck K. Leptin and total cholesterol are predictors of weight gain in pre-pubertal children. Int J Obes 1999;23:146–50.
11. Taylor RW, Grant AM, Goulding A, Williams SM. Early adiposity rebound: review of papers linking this to subsequent obesity in children and adults. Curr Opin Clin Nutr Metab Care 2005;8: 607–12.
12. Mueller WH, Harrist RB, Doyle SR, Labarthe DR. Percentiles of body composition from bioelectrical impedance and body measurements in U.S. adolescents 8–17 years old: Project Heartbeat! Am J Human Biol 2004;16:135–50.
13. Guo SS, Chumlea WC, Roche AF, Siervogel RM. Age and maturity related changes in body composition during adolescence into adulthood. The Fels longitudinal study. Appl Radiat Isot 1998;49: 581–5.
14. Knittle JL, Timmers K, Ginsberg-Fellner F, Brown RE, Katz DP. The growth of adipose tissue in children and adolescents: cross-sectional and longitudinal studies of adipose cell number and size. J Clin Invest 1979;63:239–46.
15. Gillum RF. The association of the ratio of waist to hip girth with blood pressure, serum cholesterol and serum uric acid in children and youths aged 6–17 years. J Chron Dis 1987;40:413–20.
16. Freedman DS, Serdula MK, Srinivasan SR, Berenson GS. Relation of circumferences and skinfold thicknesses to lipid and insulin concentrations in children and adolescents: the Bogalusa Heart Study. Am J Clin Nutr 1999;69:308–17.
17. Savva SC, Tornitis M, Savva ME, et al. Waist circumference and waist to height ratio are better predictors of cardiovascular disease risk factors in children than body mass. Int J Obes 2000;24: 1453–8.
18. Fernandez JR, Redden DT, Pietrobelli A, Allison DB. Waist circumference percentiles in nationally representative samples of African-American, European-American, and Mexican-American children and adolescents. J Pediatr 2004;14:439–44.
19. McCarthy HD, Jarrett KV, Crawley HF. The development of waist circumference percentiles in British children aged 5.0–16.9y. Eur J Clin Nutr 2003;55:902–7.
20. Must A, Jacques PF, Dallal GE, Bajema CJ, Dietz WH. Long term morbidity and mortality of overweight adolescents. A follow up of the Harvard Growth Study. N Engl J Med 1992;327: 1350–5.
21. Nieto FJ, Szklo M, Comstock GW. Childhood weight and growth rate as predictors of adult mortality Am J Epidemiol 1992;136: 201–13.
22. Baker JL, Olsen LW, Sorensen MD. Childhood body mass index and the risk of coronary heart disease in adulthood. N Engl J Med 2007;357:2329–37.
23. Berenson GS, Srinivasan SR, Bao WH, Newman WP, Tracey RE, Wattigney WA. Association between multiple cardiovascular risk factors and atherosclerosis in children and young adults. N Engl J Med 1998;338:1650–6.
24. Mahoney LT, Burns TL, Stanford W. Coronary risk factors in childhood and young adult life are associated with coronary artery calcification in young adults: the Muscatine Study. J Am Coll Cardiol 1996;27:277–84.

25. Kemper HC, van Mechelen W, Post GB, et al. The Amsterdam Growth and Health Longitudinal Study. The past (1976–1996) and future (1997-?) Int J Sports Med 1997;18(suppl 3):S140–50.

26. Rodriguez-Moran M, Guerrero-Romero F. Hyperinsulinemia in healthy children and adolescents with a positive family history for type 2 diabetes. Pediatrics 2006;118:e1516–22.

27. Shalitin S, Abrahami M, Lilos P, Phillip M. Insulin resistance and impaired glucose tolerance in obese children and adolescents referred to a tertiary-care center in Israel. Int J Obes 2005;29: 571–8.

28. Sullivan CS, Beste J, Cummings DM, et al. Prevalence of hyperinsulinemia and clinical correlates in overweight children referred for lifestyle intervention. J Am Dietet Assoc 2004;104:433–6.

29. Sinha S, Schwartz RA. Juvenile acanthosis nigricans. J Am Acad Dermatol 2007;57:502–8.

30. Nafiu OO, Reynolds PI, Bamgbade OA, et al. Childhood body mass index and perioperative complications. Paed Anaes 2007;17: 426–30.

31. Brown CV, Neville AL, Salim A, Rhee P, Cologne K, Demetriades D. The impact of obesity on severely injured children and adolescents. J Pediatric Surg 2006;41:88–91.

32. Sharkey I, Boddy AV, Wallace H, Mycroft J, Hollis R, Picton S. Chemotherapy Standardisation group of the United Kingdom Children's Cancer Study Group. Body surface area estimation in children using weight alone: application in paediatric oncology. Br J Cancer 2001;85:23–8.

33. Gortmaker SL, Must A, Perrin JM, Sobol AM, Dietz WH. Social and economic consequences of overweight in adolescence and young adulthood. N Engl J Med 1993;329:1008–12.

34. Viner RM, Cole TJ. Adult socioeconomic, educational, social, and psychological outcomes of childhood obesity: a national birth cohort study. BMJ 2005;330:1354.

35. Crawford D, Timperio A, Telford A, Salmon J. Parental concerns about childhood obesity and the strategies employed to prevent unhealthy weight gain in children. Public Health Nutr 2006;9: 889–95.

36. He M, Evans A. Are parents aware that their children are overweight or obese? Do they care? Can Fam Physician 2007;53:1493–9.

37. Haymes EM, McCormick RJ, Buskirk ER. Heat tolerance of exercising lean and obese prepubertal boys. J App Physiol 1975;39:457–61.

38. Nead KG, Halterman JS, Kaczorowski JM, Auinger P, Weitzman M. Overweight children and adolescents: a risk group for iron deficiency. Pediatrics 2004;114:104–8.

39. Hills AP, Parker AW. Locomotor characteristics of obese children. Child Care Health Dev 1992;18:29–34.

40. Mickle KJ, Steele JR, Munro BJ. Does excess mass affect plantar pressure in young children? Int J Pediatr Obes 2006;1:183–8.

41. Timm NL, Grupp-Phelan J, Ho ML. Chronic ankle morbidity in obese children following an acute ankle injury. Arch Pediatr Adolesc Med 2005;159:33–6.

42. Riddiford-Harland DL, Steele JR, Baur LA. Upper and lower limb functionality: are these compromised in obese children? Int J Pediatr Obes 2006;1:42–9.

43. Bonat S, Pathomvanich A, Keil MF, Field AE, Yanovski JA. Self-assessment of pubertal stage in overweight children. Pediatrics 2002;110:743–7.

44. Sheu HM, Yu HS, Chang CH. Mast cell degranulation and elastolysis in the early stage of striae distensae. J Cut Pathol 1991;18:410–16.

45. Malaty HM, Abudayyeh S, Fraley K, Graham DY, Gilger MA, Hollier DR. Recurrent abdominal pain in school children: effect of obesity and diet. Acta Paediatr 2007;96:572–6.

46. Rosner B, Prineas R, Daniels SR, Loggie J. Blood pressure differences between blacks and whites in relation to body size among US children and adolescents. Am J Epidemiol 2000;151:1007–19.

47. Sorof J, Daniels S. Obesity hypertension in children: a problem of epidemic proportions. Hypertension 2002;40:441–7.

48. Alpert MA. Obesity cardiomyopathy: pathophysiology and evolution of the clinical syndrome. Am J Med Sci 2001;321:225–36.

49. Rocchini AP, Moorehead C, Katch V, Key J, Finta KM. Forearm resistance vessel abnormalities and insulin resistance in obese adolescents. Hypertension 1992;19:615–20.

50. Tounian P, Aggoun Y, Dubern B, et al. Presence of increased stiffness in the common carotid artery and endothelial dysfunction in severely obese children: a prospective study. Lancet 2001;358: 1400–4.

51. Skilton MR, Celermajer DS. Endothelial dysfunction and arterial abnormalities in childhood obesity. Int J Obes 2006;30:1041–9.

52. Golley RK, Magarey AM, Steinbeck KS, Baur LA, Daniels LA. Comparison of metabolic syndrome prevalence using six different definitions in overweight pre-pubertal children enrolled in a weight management study. Int J Obes 2006;30:1–8.

53. Invitti C, Maffeis C, Gilardini L, et al. Metabolic syndrome in obese Caucasian children: prevalence using WHO-derived criteria and association with non-traditional cardiovascular risk factors. Int J Obes 2006;30:627–33.

54. Brambilla P, Lissau I, Flodmark CE, et al. Metabolic risk-factor clustering estimation in children: to draw a line across paediatric metabolic syndrome. Int J Obes 2007;31:591–600.

55. Reinehr T, Stoffel-Wagner B, Roth CL, Andler W. High-sensitive C-reactive protein, tumor necrosis factor alpha, and cardiovascular risk factors before and after weight loss in obese children. Metab Clin Exper 2005;54:1155–61.

56. Balagopal P, George D, Patton N, Yarandi H, Roberts WL, Bayne E, Gidding S. Lifestyle-only intervention attenuates the inflammatory state associated with obesity: a randomized controlled study in adolescents. J Pediatr 2005;146:342–8.

57. Knip M, Nuutinen O. Long-term effects of weight reduction on serum lipids and plasma insulin in obese children. Am J Clin Nutr 1993;57:490–3.

58. Ambler GR, Baur LA, Garnett SP, et al. Randomized, controlled trial of metformin for obesity and insulin resistance in children and adolescents: improvement in body composition and fasting insulin. J Clin Endocrinol Metab 2006;91:2074–80.

59. Dubern B, Tounian P, Medjadhi N, Maingot L, Girardet JP, Boule M. Pulmonary function and sleep-related breathing disorders in severely obese children. Clin Nutr 2006;2:803–9.

60. Verhulst SL, Schrauwen N, Haentjens D, et al. Sleep-disordered breathing in overweight and obese children and adolescents: prevalence, characteristics and the role of fat distribution. Arch Dis Child 2007;92:205–8.

61. Redline S, Tishler PV, Schluchter M, Aylor J, Clark K, Graham G. Risk factors for sleep-disordered breathing in children. Associations with obesity, race and respiratory problems. Am J Respir Crit Care Med 1999;159:1527–32.

62. Gozal D, Kheirandish-Gozal L. Neurocognitive and behavioral morbidity in children with sleep disorders. Curr Opin Pulmon Med 2007;13:505–9.

63. Soultan Z, Wadowski S, Rao M, Kravath RE. Effect of treating obstructive sleep apnea by tonsillectomy and/or adenoidectomy in children. Arch Pediatr Adolesc Med 1999;153:33–7.

64. To T, Vydykhan TN, Dell S, Tassoudji M, Harris JK. Is obesity associated with asthma in young children? J Pediatr 2004;144: 162–8.

65. Plumb J, Brawer R, Brisbon N. The interplay of obesity and asthma. Curr Allergy Asthma Rep 2007;7:385–9.

66. Ford ES. The epidemiology of obesity and asthma. J Allergy Clin Immunol 2005 115:897–909.

67. Rodriguea MA, Winkleby MA, Ahn D, Sundquist J, Kraemer HC. Identification of population subgroups of children and adolescents with high asthma prevalence: findings from the Third national Health and Nutrition Examination Survey. Arch Pediatr Adolesc Med 2002;156:269–75.

68. Castro-Rodriguez JA, Holberg CJ, Morgan WJ, Wright AL, Martinez FD. Increased incidence of asthma like symptoms in girls who become overweight or obese during the school years. Am J Respir Crit Care Med 2001;163:1344–9.

69. Bibi H, Shoseyov D, Feigenbaum D, et al. The relationship between asthma and obesity in children: is it real or a case of overdiagnosis? J Asthma 2005;41:403–10.

70. Pinhas-Hamiel O, Dolan LM, Daniel SR, Standiford D, Khoury PR, Zeitler P. Increased incidence of non-insulin dependent diabetes mellitus among adolescents. J Pediatr 1996;128:608–15.

71. Betts P, Mulligan J, Ward P, Smith B, Wilkin T. Increasing body weight predicts the earlier onset of insulin-dependant diabetes in childhood: testing the "accelerator hypothesis". Diabetic Med 2005;22:144–51.

72. Ehtisham S, Barrett TG. The emergence of type 2 diabetes in childhood. Ann Clin Biochem 2004;41:10–16.

73. Harris SB, Perkins BA, Whalen-Brough E. Non-insulin dependent diabetes mellitus among First Nations children: new entity among First Nations people of north-western Ontario. Can Fam Physician 1996;42:869–76.

74. Fagot-Campagna A, Narayan KMV, Imperatore G. Type 2 diabetes in children. BMJ 2001;322:377–8.

75. Sinha R, Fisch G, Teague B, Tamborlane WV, Banyas B, Allen K, et al. Impaired glucose tolerance among children and adolescents with marked obesity. N Engl J Med 2002;346:802–10.

76. Pinhas-Hamiel O, Zeitler P. Acute and chronic complications of type 2 diabetes mellitus in children and adolescents. Lancet 2007;369:1823–31.

77. Zeitler P, Epstein L, Grey M, et al. for the TODAY Study Group. Treatment options for type 2 diabetes in adolescents and youth: a study of the comparative efficacy of metformin alone or in combination with rosiglitazone or lifestyle intervention in adolescents with type 2 diabetes. Pediatr Diabetes 2007;8:74–87.

78. Dunger DB, Ahmed ML, Ong KK. Effects of obesity on growth and puberty. Best Pract Res Clin Endocrinol Metab 2005;19:375–90.

79. Wang Y. Is obesity associated with early sexual maturation? A comparison of the association in American boys versus girls. Pediatrics 2002;110:903–10.

80. Stice E, Presnell K, Bearman SK. Relation of early menarche to depression, eating disorders, substance abuse, and comorbid psychopathology among adolescent girls. Dev Psychol 2001;37: 608–19.

81. Remsburg KE, Demerath EW, Schubert CM, Chumlea WC, Sun SS, Siervogel RM. Early menarche and the development of

82. cardiovascular disease risk factors in adolescent girls: the Fels longitudinal study. J Clin Endocrinol Metab 2005;90:2718–24.

82. Rosenfield RL. Clinical review: identifying children at risk for polycystic ovary syndrome. J Clin Endocrinol Metab 2007;92: 787–96.

83. Siklar Z, Ocal G, Adiyaman P, Ergur A, Berberoglu M. Functional ovarian hyperandrogenism and polycystic ovary syndrome in prepubertal girls with obesity and/or premature pubarche. J Pediatr Endocrinol 2007;20:475–81.

84. Rosenfield RL, Ghai K, Ehrmann DA, Barnes RB. Diagnosis of the polycystic ovarian syndrome in adolescence: comparison of adolescent and adult hyperandrogenism J Pediatr Endocrinol 2000;13 (suppl 5):1285–9.

85. Legro RS. Detection of insulin resistance and its treatment in adolescents with polycystic ovary syndrome. J Pediatr Endocrinol 2002;15(suppl 5):1367–78.

86. Shroff R, Kerchner A, Manifeld M, van Beek EJR, Jagasia D, Dokras A. Young obese women with polycystic ovarian syndrome have evidence of early coronary atherosclerosis. J Clin Endocrinol Metab 2007;92:4609–14.

87. Mastorakos G, Lambrinoudaki I, Creatsas G. Polycystic ovary syndrome in adolescents: current and future treatment options. Paediatr Drugs 2006;8:311–18.

88. Glueck CJ, Aregawi D, Winiarska M, Agloria M, Luo G, Sieve L, Wang P. Metformin-diet ameliorates coronary heart disease risk factors and facilitates resumption of regular menses in adolescents with polycystic ovary syndrome. J Pediatr Endocrinol 2006;19: 831–42.

89. Thompson GH, Carter JR. Late-onset tibia vara (Blount's disease). Curr Concepts Clin Orthop 1990;255:24–35.

90. Aronsson DD, Loder RT, Breur GJ, Weinstein SL. Slipped capital femoral epiphysis: current concepts. J Am Acad Orthop Surg 2006;14:666–79.

91. Marion AW, Baker AJ, Dhawan A. Fatty liver disease in children. Arch Dis Child 2004;89:648–52.

92. Patton HM, Sirlin C, Behling C, Middleton M, Schwimmer JB, Lavine JE. Pediatric non-alcoholic fatty liver disease: a critical appraisal of current data and implications for future research. J Pediatr Gastro Nutr 2006;43:413–27.

93. Schwimmer JB. Definitive diagnosis and assessment of risk for non-alcoholic fatty liver disease in children and adolescents. Semin Liver Dis 2007;27:312–18.

94. Lobe TE, Schropp KP, Lunsford K. Laparoscopic Nissen fundoplication in childhood. J Pediatr Surg 1993;28:358–60.

95. Palasciano G, Portincasa P, Vinciguerra V, et al. Gallstone prevalence and gall bladder volume in children and adolescents: an epidemiological ultrasonographic survey and relationship to body mass index. Am J Gastroenterol 1989;84:1378–82.

96. Kessler A, Bassan H. Pseudo-tumor cerebri – idiopathic intracranial hypertension in the pediatric population. Pediatr Endocrinol Rev 2006;3:387–92.

97. Monello LF, Mayer J. Obese adolescent girls: an unrecognised "minority" group? Am J Clin Nutr 1963;13:35–9.

98. French SA, Story M, Perry C. Self-esteem and obesity in children and adolescents: a literature review. Obes Res 1995;3:479–90.

99. Klesges RC, Haddock CK, Stein RJ, Klesges LM, Eck LH, Hanson CL. Relationship between psychosocial functioning and body fat in preschool children: a longitudinal investigation. J Consult Clin Psychol 1992;60:793–6.

100. Hill AJ, Draper E, Stack J. A weight on children's minds: body shape dissatisfactions at 9-years old. Int J Obes 1994;18:383–9.

101. Phillips RG, Hill AJ. Fat, plain, but not friendless: self-esteem and peer acceptance of pre-adolescent girls. Int J Obes 1998;22:287–93.

102. Zeller MH, Saelens BE, Roehrig H, Kirk S, Daniels SR. Psychological adjustment of obese youth presenting for weight treatment. Obes Res 2004;12:1537–8.

103. Decaluwe V, Braet C, Moens E, van Vlierberghe L. The association of parental characteristics and psychosocial problems in obese youngsters. Int J Obes 2006;30:1766–74.

104. Strauss RS. Childhood obesity and self esteem. Pediatrics 2000;105:e111.

105. Doyle AC, Le Grange D, Goldschmidt A, Wilfley DE. Psychosocial impairment and physical impairment in overweight adolescents at high risk for eating disorders. Obes Res 2007;15:145–54.

106. Strauss RS, Rodzilsky D, Burack G, Colin M. Psychosocial correlates of physical activity in healthy children. Arch Pediatr Adolesc Med 2001;155:897–902.

107. Probst M, Braet C, Vandereycken W, et al. Body size estimation in obese children: a controlled study with video distortion method. Int J Obes 1995;19:820–4.

108. Franklin J, Denyer G, Steinbeck KS, Caterson ID, Hill AJ. Obesity and risk of low self-esteem: a statewide survey of Australian children. Pediatrics 2006;118:2481–7.

109. Janssen I, Craig WM, Boyce WF, Pickett W. Associations between overweight and obesity with bullying behaviors in school-aged children. Pediatrics 2004;113:1187–94.

110. Lumeng JC, Gannon K, Cabral HJ, Frank DA, Zuckerman B. Association between clinically meaningful behavior problems and overweight in children. Pediatrics 2003;112:1138–45.

111. Hughes AR, Farewell K, Harris D, Reilly JJ. Quality of life in a clinical sample of obese children. Int J Obes 2007;31:39–44.

112. Pierce JW, Wardle J. Cause and effect beliefs and self-esteem of overweight children. J Child Psychol Psychiatr 1997;38:645–50.

113. Strauss RS, Pollack HA. Social marginalization of overweight children. Arch Pediatr Adolesc Med 2003;157:746–52.

114. Vila G, Zipper E, Dabbas M, et al. Mental disorders in obese children and adolescents. Psychosom Med 2004;6:387–94.

115. Erermis S, Cetin N, Tamar M, Bukusoglu N, Akdeniz, Goksen D. Is obesity a risk factor for psychopathology among adolescents? Pediatr Int 2004;46:296–301.

116. Zametkin AJ, Zoon CK, Klein HW, Munson S. Psychiatric aspects of child and adolescent obesity: a review of the past 10 years. J Am Acad Child Adolesc Psychiatr 2004;43:134–50.

117. Wardle J, Williamson S, Johnson F, Edwards C. Depression in adolescent obesity: cultural moderators of the association between obesity and depressive symptoms. Int J Obes 2006;30:634–43.

118. Mustillo S, Worthman C, Erkanli A, Keeler G, Angold A, Costello EJ. Obesity and psychiatric disorder: developmental trajectories. Pediatrics 2003;111:851–9.

119. Braet C, Wydhooge K. Dietary restraint in normal weight and overweight children: a cross-sectional study. Int J Obes 2000;24:314–18.

120. Field AE, Camargo CA, Taylor CB, et al. Overweight, weight concerns and bulimic behaviours among girls and boys. J Am Acad Child Adolesc Psychiatr 1999;3:754–60.

121. Ackard DM, Neumark-Sztainer D, Story M, Perry C. Overeating among adolescents: prevalence and associations with weight related characteristics and psychological health. Pediatrics 2003;111:67–74.

122. Hood MY, Moore LL, Sundarajan-Ramamurti A, Singer M, Cupples LA, Ellison RC. Parental eating attitudes and the development of obesity in children: the Framingham Children's Study. Int J Obes 2000;24:1319–25.

123. Walker LLM, Gately PJ, Bewick BM, Hill AJ. Children's weight loss camps: psychological benefit or jeopardy? Int J Obes 2003;27:748–54.

124. Braet C, Tanghe A, Decaluwe, Moens E, Roseel Y. Inpatient treatment for children with obesity: weight loss, psychological wellbeing, and eating behaviour. J Pediatr Psychol 2004;29:519–29.

30 The Treatment of Childhood and Adolescent Obesity

William H. Dietz

Division of Nutrition, Physical Activity and Obesity, Centers for Disease Control and Prevention, Atlanta, GA, USA

Introduction

The high prevalence of childhood and adolescent obesity emphasizes the need for both clinical and community-based approaches to prevention and treatment. Throughout this chapter we will use the term overweight to refer to children and adolescents with a Body Mass Index (BMI) between the 85th and 95th percentiles, and obese to refer to children and adolescents whose BMI is ≥95th percentile for individuals of the same age and gender [1]. We will use the term severe obesity to refer to children and adolescents whose BMI is ≥99th percentile for individuals of the same age and gender [2].

Initiation of the therapeutic encounter

Therapy for childhood and adolescent obesity must begin with sensitivity to the social stigmatization that accompanies the disease and the blame and/or shame that sometimes characterizes obesity, particularly severe obesity, within families. Because family influences and attitudes strongly affect the success of obesity management in both children and adolescents, the initial encounter should include at least one parent as well as the affected child or adolescent [3]. Although there has been a suggestion that adolescents may achieve greater weight loss when treated alone [3], an initial interview that includes a parent may disclose significant family issues that must be addressed if therapy is to succeed. In families with younger children, the conversation should begin with open-ended, nonjudgmental questions such as

Clinical Obesity in Adults and Children, 3rd edition. Edited by Peter G. Kopelman, Ian D. Caterson and William H. Dietz.
© 2010 Blackwell Publishing, ISBN: 978-1-4051-8226-3.

"Are you concerned about your child's weight?" or "Has your child's weight caused her any problems?". In adolescents the therapeutic interaction should begin with asking permission to discuss their weight. In one clinical study of severely obese adolescents, only 41% wanted to discuss their weight [4]. Therefore, if a provider raises the issue of weight when the adolescent is not ready to discuss it, the opportunity to build a therapeutic relationship may be compromised. Furthermore, a key decision at the outset of treatment of adolescents is whether to engage the broader family system.

The terms providers use may also interfere with the establishment of a therapeutic relationship. The term "overweight" was preferred over other terms by severely obese adolescents [4]. Like adults [5], few adolescents preferred terms such as obese, big-boned, big or heavy.

Several studies indicate that many parents do not perceive that their child is overweight, and may disagree when their provider tries to convince them that this is so [6–8]. Although the directionality of the association remains unclear, adolescents who have been informed of their weight status were more likely to report that they had altered their diet and were trying to lose weight than patients who had not been informed about their weight [9]. Presumably, parents of overweight children will respond in a similar manner. Rather than debate whether a weight problem exists or not, providers should try to turn the discussion to the parent's concerns about nutrition, physical activity or screen time. Efforts should focus on the identification of areas where providers and families can agree on the need for change, regardless of whether they agree that the child has an existing or emergent weight problem.

Treatment

A variety of challenges exist with respect to the treatment of childhood and adolescent overweight and obesity. Among preschool children, multicomponent clinical and child care programs, with follow-up for more than a year, and programs that involved parents appeared more successful, although the number of studies was limited [10]. A larger systematic review found that most of the intervention studies were of fair to poor quality, and were characterized by small samples and lack of intention-to-treat analyses, and provided limited information on changes in risk factors [11]. The studies could not easily be generalized because of specialized interventions that were not widely available, and because most of the published studies addressed a narrow age range. Furthermore, most of the trials were limited to Caucasian children.

Although these reviews demonstrate a number of gaps in evidence-based clinical interventions, the prevalence of childhood and adolescent overweight and obesity emphasizes the need for therapeutic approaches in primary and tertiary care. In 1997, the need for practice guidelines in the face of a limited science base led to the formation of an expert panel to develop recommendations for the assessment, prevention, and treatment of childhood and adolescent obesity [12]. New trials and developments in practice, as well as the need to update the 1998 recommendations, led the Centers for Disease Control and Prevention, the American Medical Association, and the Health Resources and Services Administration to fund a new expert committee in 2006. In June 2007, this panel delivered its recommendations for the assessment, prevention, and treatment of childhood and adolescent overweight and obesity. Since then, the recommendations have been adopted by a number of major organizations including the American Academy of Pediatrics, the American Heart Association, American Dietetic Association, American College of Sports Medicine, National Association of Pediatric Nurse Practitioners, and the Obesity Society. The recommendations and the rationale for them were subsequently published [1,13]. The new recommendations are consistent with or expand on previously published guidelines from Canada [14] and the United Kingdom [15,16]. As shown in Figure 30.1, approaches common to the care of all overweight or obese patients include the assessment of behaviors, attitudes, and risks. These are considered in detail in Chapters 28 and 29.

The Expert Committee suggested that treatment be divided into four stages, known as prevention plus, structured weight management, comprehensive multidisciplinary intervention, and tertiary care intervention [1,13]. The first two stages are appropriately implemented in primary care settings, whereas the comprehensive approaches required by more severely overweight patients are more appropriate for specialized or tertiary care clinics.

Prevention plus

This approach applies to all overweight children between 2 and 18 years of age, and represents the first stage of treatment. The goals of treatment are to arrest the excessive increase in BMI or to return the BMI to the normal range. The focus of therapy is on increasing fruit and vegetable consumption to five servings a day, elimination of sugar-sweetened beverages, imposing limits on screen time to ≤2 hours/day, and achieving 1 hour of physical activity daily. Emphasis is placed on daily consumption of breakfast, limiting fast food, family meals, and promoting the child's ability to self-regulate their intake.

Structured weight management

Implementation of this approach requires more intensive training and focus on behavior change strategies. The targets are similar to those in prevention plus, but require more family and self-management with more intensive monitoring of dietary intake, screen time and physical activity. In contrast to prevention plus, the goal is modest decrements in BMI as linear growth continues. Weight loss should not exceed 0.5 kg/week for 2–11-year-old children or 1 kg/week for older children and adolescents. Provider training in behavior change strategies such as motivational interviewing, conflict resolution, meal planning and counseling to promote physical activity is recommended.

Comprehensive multidisciplinary intervention

If patients have severe obesity, defined as a BMI ≥99th percentile for children of the same age and gender, and if the approaches outlined above are unsuccessful, more aggressive efforts may be warranted. Therapy for these patients should be directed toward negative energy balance, a structured behavior modification program with monitoring of diet and physical activity patterns, and helping families modify the home environment. The intensity of treatment is also increased, and requires frequent office visits for a minimum of 8–12 weeks. Weight loss goals are identical to those in structured weight management. The use of these therapies requires specialized experiences and a multidisciplinary staff not usually available in primary care settings. Therefore, the use of these approaches should be limited to centers capable of providing specialized multidisciplinary care for severely obese children and adolescents.

Tertiary care intervention

The most intensive care is that required for tertiary care intervention. Patients appropriate to this level of intervention are those with severe obesity or a major complication of their obesity who require more than lifestyle interventions for weight loss. Such patients should first be treated with a comprehensive multidisciplinary intervention, and should be committed to following the regimens outlined below. The specialized experience required for such patients requires a tertiary care facility with a multidisciplinary team familiar with the complications associated with severe obesity and the therapies appropriate for its treatment. As the Expert Committee recommended, "standard clinical protocols for evaluation before, during and after the intervention should be (developed) and followed" [13]. The strategies used in this approach include restrictive dietary therapy, drug therapy or bariatric surgery which are considered below. Few randomized trials of these approaches exist in pediatric patients.

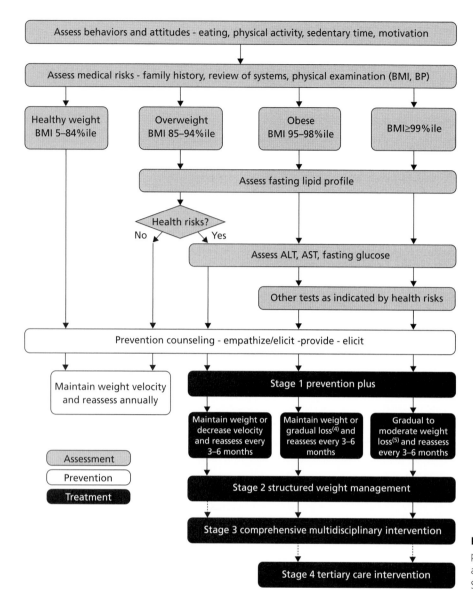

Figure 30.1 Algorithm for the assessment, prevention, and treatment of childhood and adolescent obesity (from reference [13], modified by Scott Gee and used with his permission).

Behavior change strategies

Effective behavior change strategies are essential to success and underlie all four stages of treatment. Family engagement appears to be a key component of therapy, especially among younger patients [17,18]. Furthermore, the engagement of fathers may increase the likelihood of success [19]. Because changes in diet, physical activity or screen time are the family's responsibility, clinicians should elicit from the patient and their family their level of concern about the intake of specific foods, time spent in physical activity, and the quantity and quality of screen time. Furthermore, because what gets measured is more likely to be done, quantification of these targets is essential. For example, reducing sugar-sweetened beverage intake from 16 ounces/day to 8 ounces provides a much more relevant and actionable target than a target of reducing sugar-sweetened beverage consumption without specifying the quantity to be changed.

The successful implementation of these strategies likely depends on provider techniques to help parents and patients change behavior. The oldest and most frequently applied behavioral intervention is behavior modification [20]. This approach relies on a variety of behavioral techniques that have become widely applied, such as self-monitoring, stimulus control, cognitive restructuring, and positive reinforcement to support successes. These strategies and examples of their application to food intake, inactivity or screen time are outlined in Table 30.1 [21].

Behavioral modification approaches were rigorously applied by Epstein in a series of studies of moderately overweight children [17,22,23]. These studies generally involved weekly treatment meetings for periods of 8–12 weeks, and monthly follow-up meetings for 6–12 months after the start of the program. Parents and children met separately, although meetings of a parent and child with a therapist also occurred. The "Stop-light" diet was the

Table 30.1 Behavior change strategies

Behavioral strategy	General principles	Examples
Control the environment To make behavior change easier by reducing cues and opportunities to eat more calories and remain physically inactive, and increasing cues and opportunities to eat fewer calories and become more physically active and less sedentary	Identify existing home/school/family routines or environmental factors associated with increased calorie consumption, inactivity and sedentary behaviors. Help the child/family identify alternative routines or environmental factors to reduce calorie consumption, increase physical activity and decrease sedentary behaviors. Help the child/family prioritize options to those that are most acceptable and easiest to implement. Include these as part of monitoring, goal setting, and rewarding behavior change.	Eliminate sugar-sweetened beverages from the home. Reduce the frequency of eating out and/or fast food. Limit serving sizes by serving onto plates instead of self-service and/or switch to smaller plates to make servings appear larger. Remove high-calorie snacks from the home and replace with fresh fruits and vegetables. Remove television sets from children's bedrooms, budget weekly screen time, and set family screen media rules limiting when, where, and what can be watched/played. Enroll child in an after-school physical activity. Start a new family tradition/routine involving daily or weekly physical activity.
Monitor behavior Necessary to recognize where one is starting from, set goals, assess changes, give and receive feedback, and reward success	Measures must reliably define a baseline level and assess changes over time. Measures should match behavioral goals. Monitoring should be frequent initially and then may become less frequent as the new behaviors are established. May monitor a mix of short- and long-term behavioral goals, including weight changes. If any doubt about continued progress or relapse, reinstitute frequent monitoring.	*Individual behavior* Number of sugar-sweetened beverages consumed daily. Number of meals eaten outside the home and/or fast food meals/week. Number of servings of fruits and vegetables eaten daily. Hours of television watched weekly. Number of days meeting physical activity goals. Weekly measurement of weight. *Environmental changes* Number of sugar-sweetened beverages in the home. Frequency of eating out and/or fast food. Days/week food served to plates and/or use of small plates. Days per week with fruit and vegetables in home. Presence/absence of television in child's bedroom and established screen time limit and family screen time rules.
Set goals	Help family set shorter-term behavior change goals and longer-term weight change goals. To enhance motivation, goals should be challenging but achievable. Goals should be agreed upon by the patient, not set by the provider. Allow the child and family to choose from a selection of possible goals. Limit new goals to one or two at a time. The parent/guardian may set goals for behaviors of their own to help their child lose weight. Goal behaviors must be specific, explicit, unambiguous, and capable of being self-monitored (i.e. if you can't count it, you can't change it).	*Child Individual-level goals* I will drink no more sugar-sweetened beverages. I will eat no more than 1 fast food meal/week. I will eat fresh fruit and vegetables for my after-school snack. I will watch and play less than 7 hours per week of television, videos or DVDs and computer and video games, and only after dinner and all my school work and chores are completed. I will get at least 10,000 steps on my pedometer every day. *Parent individual-level goals* I will praise my child every day he/she achieves a daily goal. I will review behavior monitoring records with my child for 30 minutes every evening. I will walk my child to school at least 3 days/week. *Family environmental goals* Our home will be free of sugar-sweetened beverages in 14 days. We will go out for dinner no more than 1 night/week. All meals will be served on plates. Fruits and vegetables will be available in our home every day. We will remove all televisions from children's bedrooms. We will eat meals without television.

Continued on p. 412

Table 30.1 *Continued*

Behavioral strategy	General principles	Examples
Reward successful behavior change	Both positive and negative responses (rewards and disapproval) should be tied to specific behaviors. Rewards should be given as closely as possible to the completion of the goal behavior. Rewards should be frequent when learning a new behavior and can become less frequent as the new behavior becomes more established. Avoid mixed messages. Rewards and disapproval should be used consistently. Rewards should not be given if the goal was not achieved. The magnitude and/or value of the reward should be consistent with the magnitude of the accomplishment. Large or valuable rewards can be counterproductive. Praise and attention from a parent can be a powerful reward for children. Frequent and specific use of praise and attention should be encouraged. Parents should choose rewards that they are willing and able to give, and also willing and able to not give if the goal is not achieved. Consider "reciprocal contracting" in which parents/guardians reward children for achieving their goals and children reward parents/guardians for achieving their goals [28].	*Praise and attention* "I am proud of you for eating the carrots instead of chips for your snack." Praise tied to a specific behavior is better than the nonspecific "You are such a good child." *Suggested rewards* Activities that the children and the parents/guardians like to perform together (e.g. going skating together). Activities related to the goals, such as going on an active, outdoor excursion, a trip to pick a favorite fruit or vegetables at a local farm, or buying athletic shoes or other sports equipment for accomplishing a physical activity goal. Extra privileges. *Rewards to avoid* Food (especially sweets or other high-calorie foods that are being limited in the diet). Money or items with a specified value (they often lead to expectations and negotiations for greater rewards over time). Expensive material items. Items unrelated to the goals.
Solve problems	Iterative cycles of identifying barriers, identifying potential solutions to overcome the barriers, making plans to implement those potential solutions, and monitoring their success. With some assistance, children and families can identify the most challenging barriers and invent their own strategies to overcome them. Group sessions can provide an opportunity for families to share strategies, successes, and lessons learned with other families facing similar challenges.	*Common barriers requiring problem solving* Resistance to change/sabotage by other family members. Family members who express their love with cooking/food. Eating out in restaurants or at others' homes. Parties and holidays involving food traditions (e.g. birthday parties, Halloween). School meals. After-school hunger. Using eating to cope with stress and anxiety. Neighborhood safety concerns. Transportation difficulties. Perceived limited community resources and opportunities for physical activity. Provider and patient/family have different ideas of what is most important to change.
Parenting skills	Authoritative parenting instead of authoritarian parenting. Support their child's autonomy and self-sufficiency. Model desired behaviors. Monitor and/or supervise their child's behavior. Communicate expectations and consequences clearly. Provide consistent and contingent feedback. Use praise, attention and other rewards to reinforce desired behaviors effectively. Minimize attention for undesired behaviors. Say "no" and set limits when appropriate.	Setting family rules and maintaining a household consistent with healthful behaviors. Parents choose what is available to eat but children choose whether to eat and how much. Saying "no" and setting limits in the best interest of their children's health and well-being. Parents/guardians set their own goals and monitor their own behaviors. Modeling both successful behavior change and coping with unsuccessful attempts to change behavior. All parents/caregivers communicate a consistent message to children. Rewards are provided only when earned. Meeting daily with children to review the day's behaviors, show interest in child's progress and provide a regular opportunity to praise success.

cornerstone of the dietary intervention [24]. This diet classifies foods as green foods which can be consumed freely, yellow foods which can be consumed in moderation, and red foods which are highest in calories and should be consumed rarely and cautiously.

The intensity of the earliest behavior modification programs and the inability to adapt such programs to primary care settings have led to a consideration of other behavior change approaches that providers could use in primary care settings. One of the most recent and promising techniques is motivational interviewing. Motivational interviewing is a technique originally developed for the treatment of addictions, and more recently has been adapted to the treatment and prevention of obesity [25,26]. Motivational interviewing relies on open-ended questions to assess the degree of concern about the child's weight, the child or parent's thoughts about what they might change, and their level of confidence in their ability to change. Efforts are made to tie the parent or patient's interest in change to more fundamental family values. Pediatricians and nutritionists trained in motivational interviewing reported high satisfaction with the use of this counseling approach, and more than 90% of parents queried reported that the pediatrician and nutritionist helped them think about changing their family's eating habits [26]. However, randomized trials of this approach have only recently begun.

A second promising approach is to address parenting style directly. A recent study has shown that when compared to authoritative parenting styles, authoritarian, permissive, and neglectful parenting styles were associated with a higher prevalence of obesity in young children [27]. This finding suggests that interventions that directly address parenting styles may be an effective adjunct to other behavioral interventions. In a study targeting parenting styles, both short-term [28] and long-term [29] weight losses were greater among parents treated in groups than among children treated in groups. In the only study of its type, the Positive Parenting Program [30], developed to provide parents with the parenting skills necessary to change dysfunctional behaviors, was applied to overweight 6–9-year-old children [31]. A parenting group that focused on parenting plus lifestyle modification had a greater decrease in BMI z-score than a waitlist control and a parenting alone group.

Use of aggressive dietary therapy

Although the use of restrictive dietary therapy in severely obese patients was cited by the Expert Committee, its use was not described in detail. Such diets afford rapid weight loss, and are reasonably considered one of the potential therapies employed in tertiary care settings. The only low-calorie diet that has been studied in the pediatric age group is the carbohydrate-free protein-modified fast. Because these diets have received only limited attention, a full description of the carbohydrate-free protein-modified fast is included here to inform tertiary care providers. This diet is not appropriate for application in primary care settings because of the specialized care required. However, it seems reasonable to include some form of aggressive dietary therapy

prior to a trial of pharmacotherapy, and certainly before bariatric surgery is considered. It should be stressed that much of what follows is derived from my research and clinical experience. The literature is too sparse to support a systematic review. Finally, as will be obvious from the references, few recent studies of these diets have been published.

The protein-modified fast (PMF) should be considered for the treatment of the severely obese adolescent who requires tertiary therapy, or for obese children or adolescents for whom rapid weight loss is essential. Major complications that require urgent weight reduction include sleep apnea, pseudo-tumor cerebri, slipped capital femoral epiphysis, and Blount disease. The diet is only appropriate after the more conservative approaches outlined above have failed. I refer to the diet as the protein-modified fast because of the absence of compelling data that a diet free of carbohydrate spares protein better than a diet that contains carbohydrate. For example, in our studies, nitrogen balance was significantly better during a hypocaloric diet containing carbohydrate than an isonitrogenous, isocaloric, carbohydrate-free diet [32,33]. A carbohydrate-free diet and the ketosis that accompanies it putatively blocks hunger, and appears associated with better long-term adherence than a diet that contains carbohydrate. However, this assumption has not been tested in a randomized clinical trial.

Although the elements of the PMF have been described elsewhere [34–36], few articles have described the more practical aspects of its application. In our practice, an essential criterion for eligibility was the demonstrated ability to maintain a stable weight. This stipulation was based on the premise that relapse after substantial weight loss would represent a major setback, and that weight maintenance prior to the diet represented an opportunity to determine if relapse would occur. Additional criteria included normal cardiac function, and the family's agreement to return to the clinic for follow-up visits at 2-week intervals for a 5-month period. We also told families at the outset that rigid adherence was essential, and after they started the diet, failure to adhere to it meant that they would have to discontinue the diet.

Baseline screens included a CBC and differential, electrolytes, calcium, phosphorus, albumin, transferrin, liver enzymes and a 24-hour Holter monitor. Lymphocyte counts, albumin, and transferrin are used to monitor protein nutriture. Liver enzymes were obtained at baseline to identify hepatic steatosis. Mildly abnormal liver enzymes are not a contraindication to the diet, and often normalize after weight loss [37]. Laboratory studies are repeated monthly, except for the Holter monitor, which we repeated every 2 months. In our clinical trials we found no change in albumin, lymphocyte count or transferrin. If decreases occur, protein intake should be increased. A baseline ultrasound of the abdomen to exclude gallstones should be considered, and is required for all patients with abdominal pain or a family history of gallbladder disease. Characteristics of the diet are shown in Box 30.1.

In contrast to adults, in whom losses of nitrogen in the first 2 weeks of the diet are followed by a plateau, approximately 20%

Box 30.1 Components of the protein-modified fast

2.0–2.5 g protein/kg IBW per day

Carbohydrate free

Calcium carbonate, 1000 mg daily

KCL, 30 mEq/d

Multivitamin with minerals daily

48 oz fluid/day

Monitor urine ketones bid

of patients that we [32,33] and others [34–36] studied on diets that contained 1.5 g protein/kg ideal body weight (IBW) appeared to have ongoing nitrogen losses that failed to plateau. Subsequent studies in which we used 2.0–2.5 g of protein/kg IBW/d (Dietz, unpublished observations) were confounded by implausibly positive nitrogen balances, which were largely a consequence of the limitations of the nitrogen balance technique. Additional studies of protein turnover are required to establish the optimum diet to protect body protein stores for weight reduction. However, the lack of careful studies of protein metabolism under hypocaloric conditions in children and adolescents emphasizes the fact that the application of these diets to any but the most severely affected children and adolescents must be considered with care, and they must not be used routinely.

The protein source is lean meat, poultry or fish. In addition, to offer patients some variety, we allowed patients to have up to 3 ounces of cheese or three eggs/day or any combination of the two. This approach made it possible for the patients to have eggs or an omelette for breakfast or a chef's salad for lunch. Diets must be virtually carbohydrate free to induce and maintain ketosis. We also allowed *ad libitum* low-carbohydrate vegetables. However, high-carbohydrate foods such as beans, peas, and eggplant cannot be included. On average, these diets contain approximately 1000–1100 kcal. Although this intake is not considered a very low-calorie diet by adult standards, it represents approximately 30–50% of maintenance calories for normal-weight adolescents. The advantage of these diets is that they induce rapid weight loss, and allow adherence to be monitored through the presence of ketosis.

Patients should monitor their progress daily. Ketonuria occurs within 48 hours and may be accompanied by abdominal discomfort, headache or malaise, but after ketosis develops, these symptoms quickly pass. Ketonuria should be measured and recorded daily, and records reviewed at clinic visits to assure adherence. Constipation occurs in patients with a poor fluid intake or whose vegetable consumption is low. Orthostatic hypotension is also a complication of low fluid intake. When it occurs, supplemental sodium in the form of bouillon may be helpful. Cholelithiasis should be suspected in any patient with abdominal pain, and excluded with an abdominal ultrasound. Despite the absence of carbohydrate, no adverse effects on lipid profiles have been apparent, perhaps because of the substantial weight loss [38,39].

In the initial week of the diet, weight loss may approach 3–4 kg, much of which is attributable to the depletion of body glycogen. Thereafter, weight loss is generally 1 kg/week, depending on the magnitude of the caloric deficit.

The diet should be discontinued in patients who cannot sustain ketosis or who fail to consume the recommended quantity of protein. Patients who report that they cannot sustain ketosis may be consuming excess carbohydrate-containing vegetables or may be consuming additional carbohydrate surreptitiously. The theoretical risk for patients who go in and out of ketosis is that this process may be accompanied by shifts of potassium in and out of cells, and such shifts may increase the risk of a cardiac arrhythmia. In practice, we saw no significant complication associated with patients whose ketosis was irregular. However, surreptitious carbohydrate consumption represents a significant concern, and suggests that the patient may not be an appropriate candidate for the diet or that they may be ready to discontinue the diet. Inability to take either the calcium or potassium supplements is also grounds for discontinuation of the diet, because the early deaths in adults associated with low-calorie diets may have resulted in part from electrolyte abnormalities, as well as a poor source of dietary protein [40–42].

Although we observed no adverse functional or physiologic effects of these diets in over 100 patients we studied or treated, the concern about these early adverse effects as well as the limited experience in adolescents emphasizes the caution with which these diets should be used and the need for careful follow-up. After the successful initiation of the diet, patients should be seen every 2 weeks. The focus of the medical visit is to review the records, which must be brought to each follow-up examination, to assess the patient for complications, and to repeat the biochemical determinations. The history includes a review of adherence, physical activity, ketosis, food and fluid intake, KCl, calcium, and multivitamin intake, weakness, cardiac irregularities, constipation, diarrhea, and abdominal pain. Physical examination should include weight, blood pressure, cardiac auscultation, and palpation of the abdomen. Visits should also focus on whether the family and social environments continue to support this rigorous dietary approach.

Because we lacked any information on the long-term effects of the PMF in adolescents, we were reluctant to continue the PMF for more than 5 months. When the patient had completed the PMF, they were gradually weaned to a diet that contained carbohydrate. We began weaning with the addition of one carbohydrate exchange (approximately 100 kcal) for 2 days, followed by additional carbohydrates at 2–3-day intervals. Ketosis ends promptly. After ketosis ended, KCl was discontinued. When 3–4 carbohydrate exchanges had been added, protein intake was reduced to 1.5 g/kg IBW/day. The gradual weaning approach sustains weight loss after ketosis ends [38]. Patients were warned to anticipate weight maintenance or mild weight gain after the diet ended. Weight gain is attributable to glycogen repletion and emphasizes the need for gradual reintroduction of carbohydrate while a caloric deficit is maintained. Counseling to prevent relapse must be initiated as the end of the PMF nears, and close follow-up is essential thereafter to assure that relapse does not occur.

Although there have been no long-term randomized trials in adolescents, studies in adults have confirmed that more rapid short-term weight loss occurs in low-carbohydrate diets than in low-fat diets [43,44]. However, long-term results of low-fat and low-carbohydrate diets do not differ significantly. These results indicate that the diet alone is unlikely to have a long-term impact on weight without significant attention to weight maintenance following weight loss.

Pharmacotherapy

Although drug therapy plays an increasingly important role in the treatment of obesity in adults, few trials of drug therapy have been conducted in children and adolescents. Only orlistat and sibutramine have been approved for use in children and adolescents. A 12-month randomized trial of sibutramine in obese adolescents demonstrated that its use in combination with behavior therapy was associated with a 2.6 BMI unit greater weight loss than a placebo in combination with behavior modification [45]. Significant improvements occurred in levels of triglycerides, HDL cholesterol, insulin, and diastolic and systolic blood pressure. Although withdrawal from the study because of complications was comparable for both drug and placebo groups, dry mouth, constipation, dizziness and insomnia occurred more frequently in the group treated with sibutramine.

A second large randomized trial compared the effect on weight loss of 120 mg of orlistat three times daily for 12 months to a placebo control in a group of obese adolescents [46]. Behavior modification was employed in both groups to alter diet and exercise patterns. BMI decreased by 0.55 units in the orlistat group, but increased by 0.31 BMI units in the control group. Only diastolic blood pressure was significantly improved when the orlistat group was compared to placebo-treated controls. Six girls treated with orlistat who had a mean weight loss of 17.6 kg developed asymptomatic cholelithiasis identified by ultrasound during the course of the study.

The results of these two studies are compared in Table 30.2. As the table indicates, greater weight loss, as well as greater numbers of adolescents who lost 5% and 10% of their original weight,

occurred with sibutramine therapy. Modest differences between the two trials were also observed in the control groups, perhaps because the intensity of the behavioral interventions also differed.

Several concerns remain with respect to pharmacotherapy. Because most of the subjects in this study had BMIs well above the 95th percentile, a minority achieved sufficient weight loss to achieve a weight less than the 95th percentile. Therefore, although risk factors improved, and more improvement occurred with sibutramine than with orlistat, many of these subjects are still at risk for long-term complications because they remain obese. In order to sustain these weight losses, prolonged drug use for many years may be required, but the efficacy and potential adverse effects of long-term drug use in adolescents remain uncertain. Whether pharmacotherapy for obesity is a cost-beneficial treatment remains uncertain.

Bariatric surgery

Criteria for bariatric surgery for severely obese adolescents were outlined in the United States by an expert committee in 2004 [47] and were reiterated by the Expert Panel on the Assessment, Prevention, and Treatment of Obesity [13]. The recommended criteria for surgery in pediatric patients are shown in Box 30.2. In addition to these criteria, the Expert Panel emphasized the need for such surgery to be performed by surgeons experienced in bariatric procedures, in centers where a team of specialists is available to provide the long-term follow-up necessary for the medical and psychosocial needs of these patients.

The results of bariatric surgery in adolescents have been summarized in an evidence-based review conducted for the Washington State Health Care Authority [48]. The report reviewed 16 published studies that enrolled 494 pediatric patients and concluded that there was moderate evidence that Roux-en-Y gastric bypass (RYGB) and laparoscopic adjustable gastric banding (LAGB) led to sustained and clinically significant weight loss in patients less than 21 years old. Evidence was considered insufficient to provide quantitative estimates of weight loss following bariatric surgery. The evidence indicated that there was a large effect on co-morbid conditions such as hypertension, dyslipidemia, and asthma in some of the studies, but the evidence was

Table 30.2 Comparison of 12-month placebo-controlled randomized trials of sibutramine and orlistat in adolescents[42,43]

Variable	Orlistat placebo	Sibutramine placebo	Orlistat	Sibutramine
Subjects	181	130	352	368
BMI change	+0.31	−1.2	−0.55	−9.4
5% weight loss	16%	21.5%	26%	70%
10% weight loss	4%	6%	10%	46%

Box 30.2 Criteria for bariatric surgery in pediatric patients [44]

Failure of formal 6-month weight loss program

Physical maturity

BMI ≥40 with serious co-morbidities or BMI ≥50 with less severe co-morbidities

Capable of adherence to long-term lifestyle changes

Decision capacity and capable of providing assent

considered weak because of the moderate quality and limited number of studies. Evidence was insufficient to estimate the impact of surgery on quality of life improvement or survival after any bariatric surgical procedure in this age group. No perioperative mortality was reported in the studies reviewed, but one late death was reported in a patient with RYGB. LAGB required reoperation in 9% of cases, but no data were available on the rate of reoperations for RYGB. Protein-calorie malnutrition and micronutrient deficiency were the most frequently reported postoperative complications of RYGB, whereas the most frequent complication of LAGB was band slippage. Severe adverse events after RYGB included pulmonary embolism, immediate postoperative bleeding, gastrointestinal obstruction, and staple line leak.

While promising, these observations indicate that bariatric surgery in pediatric patients must still be approached cautiously and in the context of a multidisciplinary team, because the long-term consequences of surgery remain uncertain.

Adverse effects of rapid weight loss

Approximately 10–25% of obese adults develop gallstones after the initiation of a low-calorie diet [49]. The cholelithiasis that occurred in adolescents who had substantial weight losses in the sibutramine trial suggests that cholelithiasis is also a risk in adolescents with substantial weight loss. Whether gallstones are a consequence of the low-calorie diet or secondary to weight loss remains uncertain. Nonetheless, abdominal pain in adolescents with substantial weight loss from any intervention should prompt an abdominal ultrasound to exclude the possibility of gallstones.

A second important concern that may accompany counseling for obesity is that the patient may develop an eating disorder. However, a recent review indicated that dietary interventions administered by professionals were associated with minimal risks of the development of an eating disorder in overweight children or adolescents [50]. In several of the studies reviewed, no change was noted in tests such as the Eating Disorder Inventory or the Children's Eating Attitudes Test.

Weight maintenance after weight loss

Only one randomized trial of strategies to achieve weight maintenance after weight loss in the pediatric age group has been published [51]. Subjects were 7–12 years old and were randomized to receive no contact (control), behavioral skills maintenance or social facilitation maintenance after 5 months of weight loss therapy. The behavioral skills management intervention focused on a variety of skills such as enhancing motivation, identifying high-risk situations that contributed to overeating or reducing physical activity, and cognitive restructuring. The social facilitation management intervention focused on efforts to build a supportive social network, such as building opportunities for

physical activity with friends and dealing with body image concerns that might impair opportunities for children to engage in physical activity with peers. Both of the weight maintenance intervention groups included weekly 20-minute family treatment and 40-minute sessions for separate child and parent groups for a 16-week period. Twenty months after the end of the weight maintenance interventions, the mean pooled BMI z-scores in the two intervention groups were significantly lower than the mean BMI z-score in the control group. When examined separately, only the social facilitation maintenance group differed significantly from the control group. How these intensive approaches can be translated into effective interventions in primary care remains to be determined.

Care delivery systems

Because obesity among children and adolescents is so prevalent, usual approaches to care based on the traditional patient/provider paradigm are not likely to provide sufficiently widespread solutions to prevention or treatment. As a consequence, attention has begun to focus on the Chronic Care Model [52–56], also known as the Care Model. As originally conceived (Fig. 30.2), the Care Model focused on changes in information systems, decision support, delivery system design, self-management, and a prepared, proactive, practice team. The changes needed to make each of these domains more effective are considered in the following sections.

Information systems

As electronic medical records (EMR) become more commonplace, information systems can be developed to make the collection of information relevant to patient care more efficient. For example, the patient's parent could electronically enter their child's medical, dietary and physical activity histories, and the

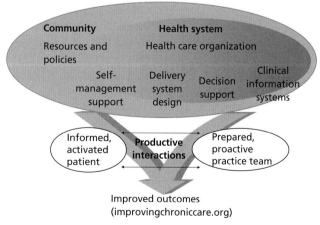

Figure 30.2 The Chronic Care Model[51,52]. Accessed at www.improvingchroniccare.org/index.php?p=The_Chronic_Care_model&s=2).

review of systems, and relevant findings could be flagged by the computer for the provider's review. Measurements of height and weight could also be entered, and absolute and percentile BMI routinely calculated, displayed with previous measurements on a BMI chart and linked to algorithms for care. After the examination, the provider could use the same system to order and review laboratory findings, or provide the family with counseling materials or a list of local resources such as those for physical activity. Few such systems are currently available.

The measurement of BMI is the critical first step in management of childhood obesity. For example, in 13 pediatric practices in Chicago [57], less than a third of obese children and only 5% of overweight children had been identified in the medical record. However, when obese children were identified, screening or referral for co-morbidities was three times more likely than for children whose obesity had not been identified.

In the state of Maine, a network of pediatric practices applied the Chronic Care Model to their approach to the identification, treatment, and prevention of childhood obesity. At the outset of their project, BMI was measured less than 40% of the time. After a systematic effort to focus on obesity that involved the development of an office team, rates of BMI measurement increased to 94% [58]. Other studies have demonstrated that BMI measurements prompt appropriate care [59]

Decision support

Decision support refers to systems or materials that improve the capacity of the provider to deliver care. Lack of demonstrated, reproducible, effective strategies to achieve weight loss is a key gap in decision support.

Two groups have provided novel approaches to support counseling in primary care settings. Kaiser Permanente developed a poster for use in their pediatric examining rooms that focused on increasing fruit and vegetable intake and physical activity, and reducing sugar-sweetened beverage intake and screen time (Fig. 30.3) to "Get more energy." In addition, the poster included a question for families that assessed their readiness to "get more energy." Because weight was not mentioned as a target, the poster could be used for both obesity prevention and control.

The American Academy of Pediatrics chapter in the state of Maine modified this approach in a number of collaborating practices. Their strategy is called "Keep ME healthy: 5-2-1-0 Power Up" (Fig. 30.4) [60]. ME is a play on the abbreviation of Maine, and 5 applies to five fruits and vegetables a day, 2 is for 2 hours or less of television a day, consistent with the recommendations of the American Academy of Pediatrics, 1 is the 1 hour of physical activity recommended daily, and 0 is no sugar-sweetened beverage consumption.

In both cases, these approaches include the strategies recommended by the Expert Panel on the Assessment, Treatment, and Prevention of Childhood Obesity [1,13] and implicitly suggest that multiple targets will be necessary for successful weight control. Furthermore, both approaches have been widely adopted by pediatric practices in Maine. Analyses of the effects of the

application of "Keep ME Healthy" on weight change are in progress (S. Gortmaker, personal communication).

Delivery system design

The historical care paradigm of patient/provider interaction is inadequate to address a problem that affects 18% of children and adolescents in the United States and a growing number of children and adolescents in other countries. Physicians are not generally well trained in behavior change techniques, and rarely have the time to address chronic diseases such as obesity in primary care settings. Although few examples exist, it appears likely that the development of other delivery systems will be required to prevent or treat obesity in primary care. For example, treating children or adolescents in groups rather than individually offers one such potentially efficient approach, as shown in early studies of behavior modification [17,22]. Furthermore, care overseen by a physician but delivered by a nutritionist, nurse practitioner, trainer or psychologist might provide a more efficient and effective use of time for all concerned.

Self-management

Because patients spend most of their time in family, school or community settings and relatively little time with their medical providers, effective family or self-management is essential to care. Although the need for self-management seems obvious, only recently has therapeutic attention begun to focus on helping pediatric patients and families to develop skills necessary to solve problems that exist or arise with respect to food intake or physical activity. The focus on patient/family self-management also requires changes in the paradigm of care delivery [61]. The role of the provider must shift from solving problems for patients to providing patients with the skills to solve problems. This shift involves changes in the ways providers interact with patients, so that patients rather than physicians define the problem, and patients are recognized as those with the experience necessary to describe and solve the problems that impair success.

Prepared, proactive, practice team

The optimal product of the application of the Care Model is a prepared, proactive, practice team. As indicated above, team approaches in primary care settings implemented by a group of pediatric practices in the state of Maine led to rapid improvements in the frequency with which BMI was collected and recorded. However, multidisciplinary team approaches to the delivery of care are not likely necessary, practical or cost-effective to address overweight or more modest levels of obesity in primary care settings. In contrast, the complexity of severe pediatric obesity is likely to require a practice team for the assessment and delivery of care in a tertiary medical setting, and is recommended for the assessment and care of pediatric candidates for bariatric surgery [47].

Limitations of the original Care Model

The prevalence of childhood and adolescent obesity makes it unlikely that clinical approaches alone will resolve the current

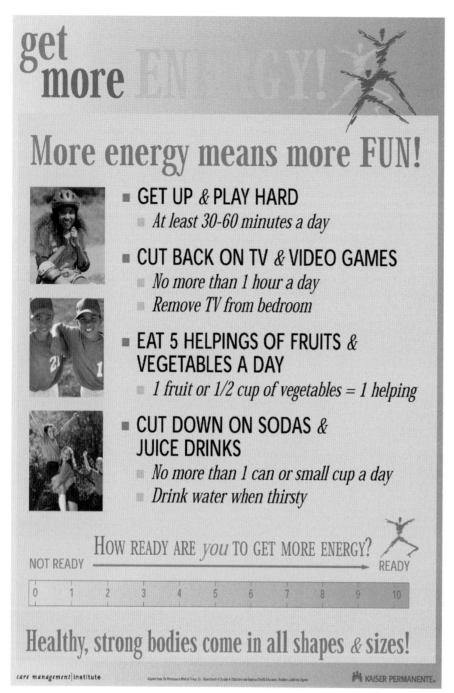

Figure 30.3 The poster used by Kaiser Permanente for addressing the prevention and treatment of obesity in their primary care settings [59].

epidemic. Self- or family management is central to the ability of families to prevent or control childhood obesity. However, because the success of weight management depends as much or more on environmental supports for weight control, complementary changes in the family, school, and community environment are as important as changes in the medical system to achieve successful self-management. Therefore, as shown in Figure 30.5, we accorded the environment as much weight as the medical system in the success of care.

For example, increases in physical activity are more difficult to achieve without easy access to safe recreational facilities. Children are less likely to walk to school if they live in communities that are unsafe or lack sidewalks or crosswalks at intersections. Increases in fruit and vegetable intake to reduce the caloric density of the diet are less likely if neighborhoods lack access to supermarkets or other sources of inexpensive fruits and vegetables. Children dependent on school meals will not likely lose weight if there are no low-calorie choices available in the cafeteria.

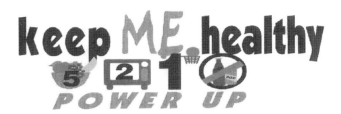

What can YOU do to help keep kids healthy?
Follow the 5-2-1-0 countdown to good health!

5: Eat at least 5 servings of fruits & vegetables on most days
2: Limit screen time to 2 hours or less daily
1: Participate in at least 1 hour or more of physical activity every day
0: Avoid soda & sugar-sweetened drinks; limit fruit juice to half cup or less per day. Instead, encourage water and 3-4 servings/day of fat-free milk.

Figure 30.4 The Keep ME Healthy poster developed by the Maine chapter of the American Academy of Pediatrics [60].

Keep ME Healthy is a joint initiative of the Maine Center for Public Health and the Maine Chapter of the American Academy of Pediatrics. Funded by a grant from the Maine Health Access Foundation.
MAINE CENTER for Public Health

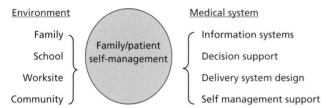

Figure 30.5 Adaptation of the Chronic Care Model for obesity. Family/patient self-management is central to the model. Public health and clinical approaches are essential for successful self-management [61].

The recognition that medical approaches alone represent an inadequate approach to resolving childhood obesity has prompted a number of managed care organizations or insurers to invest in school-based or community interventions to complement their medical efforts. For example, Kaiser Permanente and Blue Cross Blue Shield of Massachusetts have partnered with community or state programs or health departments to foster the environmental changes necessary to the success of clinical programs [62]. Despite the promise of such environmental interventions, few high-quality studies of the impact of such interventions on the prevention or treatment of childhood obesity have been published [18]. Nonetheless, these innovative programs provide important examples of an emerging convergence of clinical and community efforts to address childhood obesity.

Innovations in care

The National Initiative for Children's Healthcare Quality formed a nonprofit Childhood Obesity Action Network in 2006 to share

innovation and advances in care and policy for childhood obesity [59]. One of the first activities of the network was to post the recommendations of the Expert Committee on their website. The network provides an important resource for sharing clinical insights and training.

Conclusion

Treatment for the overweight or obese child or adolescent is an urgent but poorly met need. Few randomized trials of therapy exist and as a result, the literature is insufficient to support a systematic review. Recent recommendations of an Expert Committee on the Assessment, Prevention, and Treatment of Childhood and Adolescent Obesity provide reasonable strategies for treatment, but their efficacy remains uncertain. Even less guidance exists for the treatment of the severely obese child or adolescent. In order to address this widespread problem, the systems of care delivery will need to be improved. Furthermore, successful modification of diets, physical activity, and screen time will require public health approaches that complement clinical interventions.

Disclaimer

The findings and conclusions in this chapter are those of the author and do not necessarily represent the views of the CDC.

References

1. Barlow SE and the Expert Committee. Expert Committee recommendations regarding the prevention, assessment, and treatment of

child and adolescent overweight and obesity: summary report. Pediatrics 2007;120(suppl) S164–S192. Accessed on 2/12/2008 at www.pediatrics.org/cgi/content/full/120/Supplement_4/S/64.

2. Freedman DS, Mei Z, Srinivasan SR, Berenson GS, Dietz WH. Cardiovascular risk factors and excess adiposity among overweight children and adolescents: the Bogalusa Heart Study. J Pediatr 2007;150:12–17.

3. McLean N, Griffin S, Toney K, Hardeman W. Family involvement in weight control, weight maintenance and weight-loss interventions: a systematic review of randomized trials. Int J Obes 2003;27: 987–1005.

4. Cohen ML, Tanofsky-Kraff M, Young-Hyman D, Yanovski JA. Weight and its relationship to adolescent perceptions of their providers (WRAP): a qualitative and quantitative assessment of teen weight-related preferences and concerns. J Adolesc Health 2005;37: 163e9–163e16.

5. Wadden TA, Didie E. What's in a name? Patients' preferred terms for describing obesity. Obes Res 2003;11:1140–6.

6. Mamun AA, McDermott BM, O'Callaghan MJ, Najman JM, Williams GM. Predictors of maternal misclassifications of their offspring's weight status: a longitudinal study. Int J Obes 2008; 32:48–54.

7. Baughcum AE, Chamberlin LA, Deeks CM, Powers SW, Whitaker RC. Maternal perceptions of overweight preschool children. Pediatrics 2000;106:1380–6.

8. Maynard LM, Galuska DA, Blanck HM, Serdula MK. Maternal perceptions of weight status of children. Pediatrics 2003; 111:1226–31.

9. Kant AK, Miner P. Physician advice about being overweight: association with self-reported weight loss, dietary, and physical activity behaviors of US adolescents in the National Health and Nutrition Examination Survey, 1999–2002. Accessed on 2/15/2008 at www.pediatrics.org/cgi/content/full/119/1/e142.

10. Dontrell AA, Sherry B, Scanlon KS. Interventions to prevent or treat obesity in preschool children: a review of evaluated programs. Obesity 2007;15:1356–72.

11. Whitlock EP, Williams S, Gold R, Smith PR, Shipman SA. Screening and interventions for childhood overweight: a summary of evidence for the US Preventive Services Task Force. Pediatrics 2005;116:e125–e144. Accessed on 2/12/2008 at www.pediatrics.org/cgi/content/full/116/1/e125.

12. Barlow SE, Dietz WH. Assessment and treatment of obesity in children and adolescents: recommendations of an expert committee. Pediatrics 1998;102:e29. Accessed 2/12/2008 at: www.pediatrics.org/cgi/content/full/102/3/e29.

13. Spear BA, Barlow SE, Ervin C, et al. Recommendations for treatment of child and adolescent overweight and obesity. Pediatrics 2007;120:S254–S288. Accessed on 2/12/2008 at www.pediatrics.org/cgi/content/full/120/Supplement_4/S254.

14. Lau DCW, Douketis JD, Morrison KM, et al. 2006 Canadian clinical practice guidelines on the management and prevention of obesity in adults and children. CMAJ 2007;176(8 suppl):S1–13. Accessed 4/4/2008 at www.cmaj.ca/cgi/content/full/176/8/S1/DC1.

15. Jain A. *What Works for Obesity? A Summary of the Research Behind Obesity Interventions*. London: BMJ Publishing, 2004.

16. National Institute for Health and Clinical Excellence (NICE). Management of obesity in clinical settings (children): evidence statement and reviews. 2006. Accessed 3/23/2008 at www.nice.org.uk/guidance/index.JSP?action=byID&o=11000.

17. Epstein LH, Valoski A, Wing RR, McCurley J. Ten-year outcomes of behavioral family-based treatment for childhood obesity. Health Psychol 1994;13:373–83.

18. Flynn MAT, McNeil DA, Maloff B, et al. Reducing obesity and related chronic disease risk in children and youth: a synthesis of evidence with "best practice" recommendations. Obes Rev 2006;7(suppl 1):7–66.

19. Stein RI, Epstein LH, Raynor HA, Kilanowski CK, Paluch RA. The influence of parenting change on pediatric weight control. Obes Res 2005;13:1749–55.

20. Brownell KD, Stunkard AJ. Behavioral treatment of obesity in children. Am J Dis Child 1978;132:403–12.

21. Dietz WH, Robinson TN. Overweight children and adolescents. N Engl J Med 2005;352:2100–9.

22. Epstein LH, Wing RR, Koeske R, Andrasik F, Ossip DJ. Child and parent weight loss in family-based behavior modification programs. J Consult Clin Psychol 1981;49:674–85.

23. Epstein LH, Myers MD, Raynor HA, Saelens BE. Treatment of pediatric obesity. Pediatrics 1998;101:554–70.

24. Epstein LH, Squires S. *The Stop-Light Diet for Children*. Boston: Little, Brown, 1988.

25. Resnicow K, Davis R, Rollnick S. Motivational interviewing for pediatric obesity: conceptual issues and evidence review. J Am Dietet Assoc 2006;106:2024–33.

26. Schwartz RP, Hamre R, Dietz WH, et al. Office-based motivational interviewing to prevent childhood obesity. Arch Pediatr Adolesc Med 2007;161:495–501.

27. Rhee KE, Lumeng JC, Appugliese DP, Kaciroti N, Bradley RH. Parenting styles and overweight status in first grade. Pediatrics 2006;117:2047–54.

28. Golan M, Weizman A, Apter A, Fainaru M. Parents as the exclusive agents of change in the treatment of childhood obesity. Am J Clin Nutr 1998;67:1130–5.

29. Golan M, Crow S. Targeting parents exclusively in the treatment of childhood obesity: long-term results. Obes Res 2004;12: 357–61.

30. Families International, University of Queensland/Health Department Western Australia. Triple P. Accessed on 2/23/2008 at www.triplep.net.

31. Golley RK, Magarey AM, Baur LA, Steinbeck KS, Daniels LA. Twelve-month effectiveness of a parent-led, family-focused weight-management program for prepubertal children: a randomized controlled trial. Pediatrics 2007;119:517–25.

32. Dietz WH Jr, Schoeller DA. Optimal dietary therapy for obese adolescents: comparison of protein plus glucose and protein plus fat. J Pediatr 1982;100:638–44.

33. Dietz WH Jr, Wolfe RR. Interrelationships of glucose and protein metabolism in obese adolescents during short-term hypocaloric dietary therapy. Am J Clin Nutr 1985;42:380–90.

34. Merritt RJ, Bistrian BR, Blackburn GL, Suskind RM. Consequences of modified fasting in obese pediatric adolescent patients. I. Protein-sparing modified fast. J Pediatr 1980;96:13–19.

35. Brown MR, Klish WJ, Hollander J, Campbell MA, Forbes GB. A high protein, low calorie liquid diet in the treatment of very obese adolescents: long-term effect on lean body mass. Am J Clin Nutr 1983;38:20–31.

36. Widhalm KM, Zwiauer KFM. Metabolic effects of a very low calorie diet in obese children and adolescents with special reference to nitrogen balance. J Am Coll Nutr 1987;6:467–74.

37. Vajro P, Fontanella A, Perna C, Orso G, Tedesco M, de Vincenzo A. Persistent hyperaminotransferasemia resolving after weight reduction in obese children. J Pediatr 1994;125:239–41.

38. Willi SM, Oexmann MJ, Wright NM, Collop NA, Key LL Jr. The effects of a high-protein, low fat, ketogenic diet on adolescents with morbid obesity: body composition, blood chemistries, and sleep abnormalities. Pediatrics 1998;101:61–7.

39. Sondike SB, Copperman N, Jacobson MS. Effects of a low-carbohydrate diet on weight loss and cardiovascular risk factors in overweight adolescents. J Pediatr 2003;142:253–8.

40. Michiel RR, Sneider JS, Dickstein RA, Hayman H, Eich RH. Sudden death in a patient on a liquid protein diet. N Engl J Med 1978;298:1005–7.

41. Lantigua RA, Amatruda JM, Biddle TL, Forbes GB, Lockwood DH. Cardiac arrhythmias associated with a liquid protein diet for the treatment of obesity. N Engl J Med 1980;303:735–8.

42. Sours HE, Fratalli VP, Brand CD, et al. Sudden death associated with very low calorie weight reduction regimens. Am J Clin Nutr 1981;34:453–61.

43. Samaha FF, Iqbal N, Seshadri P, et al.A low carbohydrate as compared with a low fat diet in severe obesity. N Engl J Med 2003;348:2074–81.

44. Foster GD, Wyatt HR, Hill JO, et al. A randomized trial of a low-carbohydrate diet for obesity. N Engl J Med 2003;348:2082–90.

45. Berkowitz RI, Fujioka K, Daniels SR, et al. Effects of sibutramine treatment in obese adolescents. Ann Intern Med 2006;145:81–90.

46. Chanoine J-P, Hampl S, Jensen C, Boldrin M, Hauptmann J. Effect of orlistat on weight and body composition in obese adolescents: a randomized controlled trial. JAMA 2005;293:2873–83.

47. Inge TH, Krebs NF, Garcia VF, et al. Bariatric surgery for severely overweight adolescents: concerns and recommendations. Pediatrics 2004;114:217–23.

48. Treadwell J, Sun F, Bruening W, et al. Health technology assessment: bariatric surgery for pediatric patients. Accessed on 3/1/08 at www.hta.hca.wa.gov/documents/bariatric_pediatric.pdf.

49. Everhart JE. Contributions of obesity and weight loss to gallstone disease. Ann Intern Med 1993;119:1029–35.

50. Butryn ML, Wadden TA. Treatment of overweight in children and adolescents: does dieting increase the risk of eating disorders? Int J Eating Disord 2005;37:285–93.

51. Wilfley DE, Stein RI, Saelens BE, et al. Efficacy of maintenance treatment approaches for childhood overweight. A randomized controlled trial. JAMA 2007;298:1661–73.

52. Wagner EH, Austin BT, Davis C, Hindmarsh M, Schaefer J, Bonomi A. Improving chronic illness care: translating evidence into action. Health Aff 2001;20:64–78.

53. Bodenheimer T, Wagner EH, Grumbach K. Improving primary care for patients with chronic illness. JAMA 2002;288:1775–9.

54. Bodenheimer T, Wagner EH, Grumbach K. Improving primary care for patients with chronic illness; the chronic care model, part 2. JAMA 2002;288:1909–14.

55. Wagner EH. Chronic disease management: what will it take to improve care for chronic illness? Eff Clin Pract 1998;1:2–4.

56. Wagner EH, Austin BT, Davis C, Hindmarsh M, Schaefer J, Bonomi A. Improving chronic illness care: translating evidence into action. Health Aff (Millwood) 2001;20:64–78.

57. Dilley KJ, Martin LA, Sullivan C, Seshadri R, Binns HJ. Identification of overweight status is associated with higher rates of screening for comorbidities of overweight in pediatric primary care practice. Pediatrics 2007;119:148–155. Accessed on 2/13/2007 at www.pediatrics.org/cgi/content/full/119/1/e148.

58. Maine Youth Overweight Collaborative, Maine Center for Public Health. Accessed on 2/12/2008 at www.MCPH.org/Major_Activities/keepmehealthy.

59. Childhood Obesity Action Network. Accessed on 2/29/2008 at www.nichq.org.

60. Maine American Academy of Pediatrics. Accessed on 2/23/2008 at www.maineaap.org/project_youthoverweight.

61. Bodenheimer T, Lorig K, Holman H, Grumbach K. Patient self-management of chronic disease in primary care. JAMA 2002;288:2469–75.

62. Dietz W, Lee J, Wechsler H, Malepati S, Sherry B. Health plans' role in preventing overweight in children and adolescents. Health Aff 2007;26:430–40.

6 Environmental Policy Approaches

31 Obesity: Global Pandemic

Shiriki K. Kumanyika[1,2], Neville Rigby[2], Tim Lobstein[2], Rachel Jackson Leach[2] and W. Philip T. James[2]

[1] Center for Clinical Epidemiology and Biostatistics, University of Pennsylvania School of Medicine, Philadelphia, PA, USA
[2] International Obesity Task Force, International Association for the Study of Obesity, London, UK

Introduction

The World Health Organization (WHO) convened an expert consultation in 1997 which documented the development of the global epidemic of obesity [1]. This consultation drew upon 2 years of preparatory work led by the International Obesity Task Force (IOTF), which included scientific contributions from all continents. Assessing prevalence and trend data available at that time, the expert consultation identified the need for obesity prevention and management strategies for all regions of the world.

The conclusion that not only the "developed" or "high-income" countries were affected by the obesity epidemic but developed countries undergoing nutrition transition were also faced with a double burden of disease was critical, and reinforced the general finding of the shift in the global burden of disease towards noncommunicable diseases as the major causes of death. In addition, given that obesity as a nutritional problem related to food access, dietary intake and physical activity is mediated by distinct metabolic vulnerabilities which predispose certain populations to greater risk, the consultation emphasized that obesity can become prominent as a health concern while undernutrition persists as a significant problem. This greatly increases the complexity of addressing both obesity and undernutrition issues. The challenge is how to reduce the consumption of excess calories, while also maintaining food supplies and food programs to effectively eradicate hunger and promote appropriate proportional growth in stature and weight during child development [2].

Barely a decade later, the obesity problem has worsened substantially. High levels of obesity threaten the health and longevity of populations, as well as the economies of an ever increasing number of countries. Figure 31.1 illustrates trends in adult obesity in developed countries, with certain limitations. The scale is alarming. The WHO estimates that 1.6 billion overweight people aged 15 and over are affected, including 400 million who are obese, with the projected numbers increasing to 2.3 billion, including 700 million obese, by 2015 [3]. As will be discussed, the estimates and projections for the numbers affected by diabetes, the co-morbidity most closely linked to obesity, are equally alarming, particularly for the Asia-Pacific region.

The characterization of obesity as a "pandemic" – a term once thought of as applying only to infectious diseases – reflects the seeming spread of obesity both within and across countries. The key drivers of the epidemic spread are globalization, urbanization, and economic development. Globalization results from policies that facilitate cross-national interactions by opening borders to link countries through markets, including food markets, media, capital transfers and dissemination of technologic advances [4,5]. Globalization and related aspects of economic development can potentially improve population nutrition and health, e.g. by improving food supplies and helping to eradicate poverty and malnutrition. However, these processes have unfolded in a manner that has the unintended effects of fostering dietary patterns and levels of physical activity that predispose to obesity while not fully addressing issues of food security. The conceptual framework in Figure 31.2 highlights the interplay of economic and social change on the food supply and dietary practices in developing countries with the ultimate paradoxical consequences of increasing malnutrition at the overconsumption and chronic disease end of the continuum and increasing rather than decreasing social inequities [4].

The WHO consultation report emphasized the need to understand and address obesity as a *population* problem rather than one only for individuals, in part because of the scale, with the majority of adults in some countries already overweight or obese.

Clinical Obesity in Adults and Children, 3rd edition. Edited by Peter G. Kopelman, Ian D. Caterson and William H. Dietz.
© 2010 Blackwell Publishing, ISBN: 978-1-4051-8226-3.

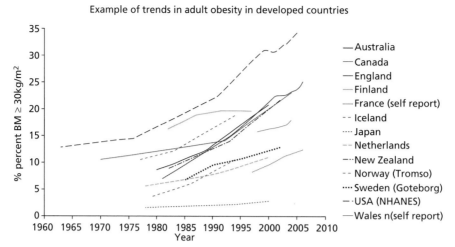

Figure 31.1 Illustrative analysis of trends in obesity in 13 countries. (From Leach R. International Obesity Task Force. www.iaso.org.)
Figure 31.1 is based on available data gathered routinely by the IASO International Obesity Taskforce in its ongoing programme to monitor and analyse prevalence data in relation to the global burden of disease. Data are derived wherever possible from nationally representative measured surveys. Where this is not possible, self reported data, which tend to underestimate prevalence, is indicated. Not all surveys are directly comparable because of differences in methodology, including age ranges. In the case of Norway, limited local data were recalculated. The chart indicates prevalance for BMI ≥ 30 only. In Japan a lower threshold of BMI ≥ 25 is in use, which would suggest a higher prevalence rising from 16.7% in 1976–80 to 24% in 2000, thus suggesting a comparable trend and prevalence of obesity in a more vulnerable Asian population.

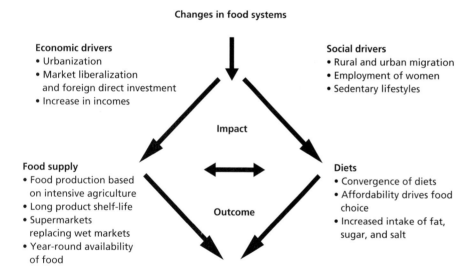

Figure 31.2 Changes in food systems. (From Kennedy et al. [4] with permission.)

Themes related to the need to restore the ability of populations to achieve and maintain an appropriate energy balance have not only been integrated into broader WHO strategies related to improving dietary quality to curb the global increases in cardio-vascular diseases and cancer, but have also become priority aspects of these strategies [6,7]. In essence the "obesogenic" envi-ronment makes it increasingly difficult for individuals to avoid the kind of foods that lead to the gradual accumulation of excess body fat and the same environment makes it difficult to lose excess body fat once acquired. The environments to which individuals are exposed frame the social, economic and cultural parameters which determine how people undertake obligatory as well as voluntary choice behaviors related to eating and physical activity. Key drivers of the epidemic are not accessible to change by individual, community or even national actions in some cases. To break the link between social and economic progress and adverse changes in diet and physical activity [8] will require carefully crafted policy and environmental change based on evaluation and research to identify those measures that are effective without new unintended adverse consequences.

A current or impending scenario in which the majority of people are unable to achieve and maintain a healthy weight is now the context in which all obesity prevention, management and research endeavors occur. In this chapter, we describe further the existing and projected global burden of obesity in adults and children, and review associated health implications, highlighting important methodologic issues related to tracking and understanding the epidemic. The section concludes with a discussion of the causal pathways of obesity at the population level as a framework for subsequent chapters that address specific approaches to environmental and policy changes (see Chapters 32–34).

Scope of the problem

High rates of overweight and obesity have emerged against a diverse array of demographic, ethnic, and economic scenarios and are evident in every region of the world. Awareness of the epidemic has led to increased monitoring of obesity prevalence and trends across and within countries, and to clarifying methodologic issues that influence these comparisons and projecting future trends. In adults, the key indicators are a Body Mass Index (BMI), calculated as weight in kilograms divided by the square of height in meters, of ≥ 25 (overweight) and ≥ 30, respectively. The WHO obtains and reports country-specific data on obesity prevalence [3,9]. Overweight and obesity prevalence data for both adults and children are also compiled by the IOTF, using official data from published and unpublished studies supplemented by national data provided to WHO in some instances [10]. Such data provide an impression of the scope of the problem of obesity, although direct comparisons across countries are complicated by the use of different data collection methods, years, and age ranges for reporting. Note, for example, the footnoted caveats associated with the trend data shown in Figure 31.1. Mean BMI levels are also of interest, although the mean can be misleading in circumstances where both undernutrition and obesity are prevalent and this is the case in some developing countries [4]. The WHO definitions of overweight and obesity for children and adolescents are in flux due to the evolution of reference data that attempt to improve the estimation of what constitutes optimal versus excess weight for a given age, height, and gender [11]. Definitions of obesity in children must take into account the changes in height and body composition of children as they mature.

Adults

The WHO maps in Figures 31.3 and 31.4, obtained from the WHO website, illustrate the scope of the obesity problem worldwide, using prevalence estimates for 2005 and projections for 2015 for males and females, respectively. Gender differences are evident. The emergence of high obesity prevalence is more evident for females than males so that the potential increase by 2015 is less dramatic than on the map for males. The highest levels globally are in the island of Nauru and other Pacific Islands (Micronesia, Tonga, Cook Islands, and Niue). Differences in body composition between Pacific and other populations suggest that BMI may overestimate some related disease risk factors for Pacific Islanders [12]. However, rates of diabetes are also among the highest in the world so that the need for action to address diabetes in Pacific populations is beyond dispute. Although there are large areas in parts of Africa where there are limited data, recent surveys in parts of sub-Saharan Africa indicate that obesity can be a significant factor, and most areas will be affected by 2015 if current trends continue. There is currently evidence to suggest that the prevalence of obesity in countries like Tanzania is rising, at least among women [13]. While earlier surveys indicated that the burden of obesity in East Africa appears to be low, there are rapid changes occurring in urban areas. In South Africa, the prevalence of obesity is already comparable to many Western countries and among African woman, of whom 28.4% were obese in 2003, begins to approach US levels [14].

Table 31.1, which uses the IOTF compilation of country-specific obesity prevalence data, allows a closer look at the situation in a set of countries selected to give a diverse picture across WHO regions. When the data on overweight and obesity prevalence are combined, substantial segments of populations are obese or at risk of moving into the obese range, even where obesity prevalence defined at BMI ≥ 30 is still relatively low. Some populations could soon approach a saturation point when almost all adults are in the overweight or obese range.

Recent trends in the Pacific Islands suggest that obesity prevalence can continue to rise to exceptionally high proportions. The prevalence of obesity among black American women already exceeded 50% when measured in the 2003–2004 survey [15]. This phenomenon of population BMI distributions shifting to the right and becoming wider and flatter around a higher mean BMI was identified by Rose based on groupings of cross-sectional BMI data collected from 52 populations in 32 countries in the INTERSALT Study (Fig. 31.5) [16]. Figure 31.6 shows this rightward shift and flattening of the BMI distribution in data from the US population [17].

Combined overweight and obesity data also characterize the percentage of the population at risk or potentially at risk of obesity-related conditions in Asian populations better than do data based on obesity alone. The combined percentages describe a wider segment of the BMI distribution. Also, there is now a wealth of rigorously collected evidence that the BMI 30 cut-off markedly underestimates obesity-related health risks in Asian populations. At a given BMI level, percentage body fat and the occurrence of type 2 diabetes and obesity-related co-morbidities

Prevalence of obesity, males, aged 30+, 2005

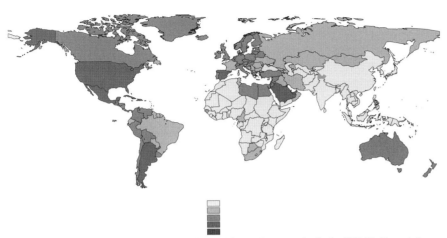

Estimated % of population with BMI ≥30, age-standardized to WHO World population.

Prevalence of obesity, males, aged 30+, 2015

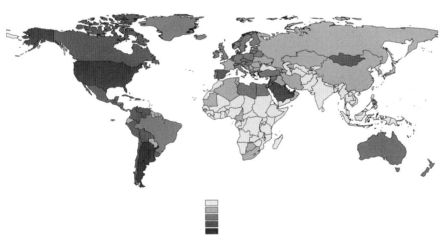

Estimated % of population with BMI ≥30, age-standardized to WHO World population.

Figure 31.3 Estimated global prevalence of obesity in males 30 years and older in the year (a)2005 and (b) 2015.

are higher in Asian-descent populations compared to other populations, i.e. the obesity risk threshold is lower [18–21]. Lower BMI cut-offs and clinical or public health action levels for Asian-descent populations have, therefore, been recommended [19,22]. This is true for Asians living in Asia as well as those who have immigrated to or are born in other countries [23,24].

The BMI-based data do not account for the distribution of body fat, and abdominal obesity is more readily assessed by using waist circumference. Depending on the population and the risk indicator, abdominal obesity may be more indicative of disease

risk than generalized obesity. At the time of writing, the WHO was in the process of developing standardized definitions for abdominal obesity, which may also need to take into account differences in risk among Asian-descent populations and how to cope with such ethnic differences for cross-national comparisons in tracking the epidemic.

The variations in prevalence between countries reflect different starting points for the BMI distributions prevailing at the time the obesity epidemic began to take effect, as well as the nature and intensity of subsequent influences. This differential impact

Prevalence of obesity, females, aged 30+, 2005

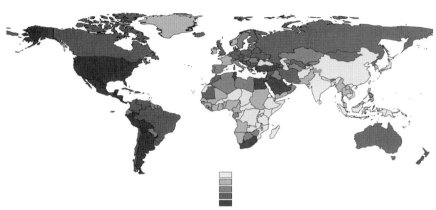

Estimated % of population with BMI ≥30, age-standardized to WHO World population.

Prevalence of obesity, females, aged 30+, 2015

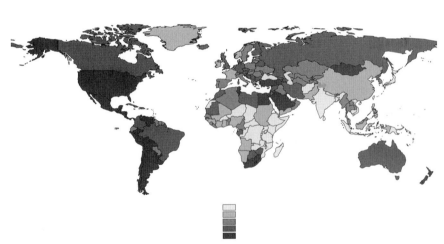

Figure 31.4 Estimated global prevalence of obesity in females 30 years and older in the year (a) 2005 and (b) 2015.

Estimated % of population with BMI ≥30, age-standardized to WHO World population.

of the epidemic is also observed within countries, with some population subgroups having obesity prevalence that is substantially higher than others. Populations sharing the same general environment may vary in socio-economic status and heritable factors influencing exposure to the obesogenic environment and its effects. Obesity prevalence in high-risk groups often predates recognition of the pandemic [25,26] but also shows trends of increase in parallel to increases in the country at large. This applies to aboriginal populations in the United States (Native Americans) and Canada (First Nations), for example [24,27,28].

In the United States, obesity levels in African-American women and Mexican-American men and women were higher than in their non-Hispanic white counterparts in the 1980s, and have tracked upward to remain substantially higher in the most recent national survey data reported [29]. Lower than average risk for obesity may also be defined by ethnicity, e.g. the relatively lower BMI distribution in Asian-descent populations living within the United States [23], although as noted previously, the susceptibility to obesity-related diseases is not low commensurate with the BMI levels.

Table 31.1 International Obesity Task Force estimates of overweight and obesity in adults, selected countries grouped by WHO region

	Year of survey	Age range	Males		Females	
			BMI 25–29.9	BMI 30+	BMI 25–29.9	BMI 30+
WHO Africa Region						
Ghana	1997	25+	17.1	4.6	26.9	20.2
Seychelles	1994	25–64	29.8	8.5	31.6	28.2
South Africa	1998	15+	21.1	10.1	25.9	27.9
WHO Americas Region						
Bolivia (urban)	1998	15–49	–	–	35.2	11.2
Brazil	2001	20–64	31.2	10.7	29.2	13.9
Canada	2004	18+	42.0	22.9	30.2	23.2
Chile (urban)	n/a	25–64	–	15.7	–	23.0
Mexico	2006	20+	42.5	24.4	37.4	34.5
Trinidad & Tobago	1999	20+	29.6	10.7	32.6	21.1
USA	2003–4	20+	39.7	31.1	28.6	33.2
WHO Eastern Mediterranean Region						
Bahrain	1998–89	19+	36.7	23.3	28.3	34.1
Qatar	2003	25–65	34.3	34.6	33.0	45.3
Saudi Arabia	1995–2000	30+	42.4	26.4	31.8	44.0
WHO European Region						
Bulgaria	*2001*	*15+*	*38.8*	*11.3*	*28.8*	*13.5*
Cyprus	1999–2000	25–64	25.1	7.1	26.7	10.2
Czech Republic	1997–98	25+	48.5	24.7	31.4	26.2
England	2006	16+	44.7	24.9	32.9	25.2
France	2006	18–74	41.0	16.1	23.8	17.6
Greece (Attica)	2001–02	20–89	53.0	20.0	31.0	15.0
Iceland	1991–96	18+	47.3	17.0	35.2	18.3
Italy	*2005*	*n/a*	*42.5*	*10.5*	*26.1*	*9.1*
Netherlands	1998–02	20–59	43.5	10.4	28.5	10.1
Poland	2000–01	19+	41.0	15.4	28.7	18.9
Portugal	2003–05	18–64	45.2	15.0	34.4	13.4
Slovakia (CINDI) Trebisov	1998	15–64	57	22	56	28
Spain	1990–2000	25–60	45.0	13.4	32.2	15.8
Sweden (Goteborg)	2002	25–64	43.5	14.8	26.6	11.0
Switzerland (urban)	2000–01	35–74	45.9	14.1	27.6	10.4
Turkey (urban)	2001–02	20+	46.5	16.5	28.6	29.4
WHO South East Asia Region						
India	1998	18+	4.4	0.3	4.3	0.6
Cambodia	2000	15–49	–	–	5.3	0.5
WHO Western Pacific Region						
Australia	2000	25+	48.2	19.3	29.9	22.2
China	2002	18+	16.7	2.4	15.4	3.4
Japan	2000	20+	24.5	2.3	17.8	3.4
New Zealand*	2002–03	35–74	49.6	21.2	35.5	22.1

Italics indicate self-report; * indicates IOTF estimate not available.

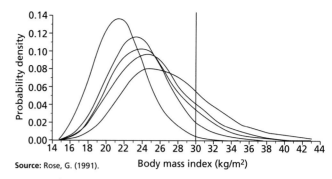

Source: Rose, G. (1991).

Figure 31.5 The shifting distributions of BMI of five population groups of men and women aged 20–59 derived from 52 surveys in 32 countries. (Reprinted with permission of Springer from Rose [16].)

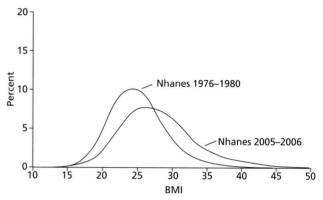

Source: CDC/NCHS, National Health and Nutrition Examination Survey (NHANES).

Figure 31.6 Changes in the distribution of BMI between 1976–1980 and 2005–2006, adults aged 20–74 years, United States. (Source: Ogden et al [17].)

The clustering of high risk by race/ethnicity does not necessarily imply genetic differences, in part because racial/ethnic categories have historical and sociopolitical origins and are often strongly related to socio-economic and other environmental conditions [30,31]. Data to support environmental explanations for ethnic differences in obesity include comparisons of indigenous North American populations living in different circumstances [32] and comparisons for people of African descent living in urban and rural Africa, compared to the Caribbean, the United States, and the United Kingdom [33]. Trends within African-American children suggest relatively greater exposure or response to recent obesity-promoting environmental changes compared to white children [34]. African-American children did not have a higher prevalence of obesity than US white children in the 1960s, but rates have risen more steeply in African-American children [35] and are now notably higher in African-American than in white girls [15]. Gestational environments may be an aspect of the relevant changes, e.g. higher weights of mothers during pregnancy may lead to *in utero* effects or fetal programming, with both genetic and epigenetic influences interacting with an obesogenic food environment [36].

The potential for spread through social norms and interpersonal interactions has also become clearer, with a report from the Framingham Heart Study cohorts in the United States suggesting that social networks defining relationships with others who are obese can have a remarkable influence on one's likelihood of becoming obese [37]. This same concept of social transmission can be extended to characterize the person-to-person spread through globalization of media and markets, e.g. changes in social norms about eating, physical activity, and weight levels resulting from cross-border interactions.

The clustering of high or low risk by social position and the shifts in the direction of associations between social position and BMI levels with societal transitions, even in countries that are relatively homogenous by ethnicity, support this line of reasoning. Gradients of obesity by socio-economic status (SES) were observed, for example, in the MONICA studies of cardiovascular disease in European countries, often the inverse gradient in women that is characteristic of developed countries but also a direct association (obesity increasing with increasing socio-economic status) in some emerging economies and among men [38]. The 10-year comparison showed shifts in these income and education gradients in parallel with societal transitions in these countries so that the inverse gradient – with lowest income populations more obese – began to predominate. The higher risk of obesity among the more advantaged groups is also characteristic of developing countries at certain stages of social and economic transitions, but ultimately also shifts so that higher SES groups have lower prevalence while obesity becomes more noticeable among the poor [39]. However, the impact of the obesity pandemic may be to flatten the gradient of difference on obesity levels according to social position as obesity affects more and more of the population regardless of social position [40, 41].

Children

The societal nature of the obesity pandemic suggests impacts across the life course, and this is evident in country-level data for overweight and obesity in children [42]. For example, in the United States, although levels of overweight and obesity are lower in children than in adults, when plotted together, the slopes of increasing adult and child obesity are remarkably similar [29]. Evidence of pandemic spread in children globally is irrefutable. The prevalence data in Table 31.2, from the IOTF compilation [10], illustrate variation and levels of child obesity by WHO region for a selection of countries similar to that in Table 31.1. Relevant caveats are that child obesity prevalence data are limited overall, and data available are not always representative of the whole country population; as shown, years and age groups reported vary as in the adult data. All data shown in the table use the IOTF reference standard for assessing childhood overweight and obesity and are based on measurements rather than self-report. The IOTF standard is based on reference curves, derived from ethnically and geographically diverse populations, which link child BMI levels to adult obesity cut-off [43].

In Table 31.2, the combined prevalence of overweight and obesity in the range of 30% or 40% is observed in data from

Table 31.2 International Obesity Task Force estimates of childhood overweight and obesity, grouped by WHO region (combined prevalence)

	Year of survey	Age range	Boys	Girls
WHO Africa Region				
Algeria	2003	7–17	6.0	5.6
Seychelles	1999	5,9,12 & 16	9.2	15.8
South Africa	2001–04	6–13	14	17.9
WHO Americas Region				
Bolivia (urban)	2003	14–17	15.6	27.5
Brazil	2002	7–10	23.0	21.1
Canada	2004	12–17	32.3	25.8
Chile	2000	6	26.0	27.1
Mexico	2000	10–17	17	20.7
Trinidad & Tobago	1999	5,6,9 & 10	8.1	8.8
USA	2003–04	6–17	35.1	36
WHO Eastern Mediterranean Region				
Bahrain	2000	12–17	29.9	42.4
Qatar	2003	12–17	36.5	23.6
Saudi Arabia	2002	5–17	16.7	19.4
WHO European Region				
Bulgaria	1998	7–17	18.9	16.1
Cyprus	1999–2000	6–17	25.4	22.6
Czech Republic	2001	5–17	14.7	13.4
England	2004	5–17	29	29.3
France	2000	7–9	17.9	18.2
Greece	2003	13–17	29.6	16.1
Iceland	1998	9	22.0	25.5
Italy	1993–2001	5–17	26.6	24.8
Netherlands	1997	5–17	8.8	11.8
Poland	2001	7–9	13.6	14.7
Portugal	2002–03	7–9	29.5	34.3
Slovakia	1995–99	11–17	9.8	8.2
Spain	2000–02	13–14	35	32
Sweden	2001	6–11	17.6	27.4
Switzerland	2002	6–12	16.6	19.1
Turkey	2001	12–17	11.4	10.3
WHO South East Asia Region				
India	2002	5–17*	12.9	8.2
Sri Lanka	2003	10–15	1.7	2.7
WHO Western Pacific Region				
Australia	2003–04	6–11	23.2	30.3
China	1999–2000	11 & 15	14.9	8.0
Japan	1996–2000	6–14	16.2	14.3
New Zealand	2000	11 & 12	30.0	
Taiwan	2001	6–18	26.8	16.5

* 5–15 years girls.

Only reports reflecting the last 10 years, based on measured rather than self-reported data and using the IOTF cut-offs to define overweight and obesity, are included here. ©IASO, October 2007.

numerous countries. Observed rates in African countries other than South Africa are relatively low, as in adults, but this may change. Gender differences within countries may be minimal or marked. Girls have a notably higher prevalence of obesity than boys in Bahrain and Sweden, whereas boys have a higher prevalence in Greece and Taiwan. The same subgroup issues that were mentioned for adults also apply to data for children. Children in indigenous North American and Australian populations, for example, are at higher risk than the counterpart European-descent populations [44,45]. African-American and Mexican-American children have higher levels of obesity than non-Hispanic white children [15].

Associations of obesity with SES in children have been less consistent than those in adults, in part because studies use different SES indices. A systematic review of this association in school-age children in Western countries, focusing on studies reported from 1989 through 2003, concluded that the association of child obesity with parental education is usually inverse [46]. McLaren's worldwide review of the SES obesity association, cited above, did not include studies of child populations [40]. An analysis of US national survey data found that, while obesity increased in both low- and high-income children aged 12–17, the increase in obesity was greater among low-income relative to high-income children among 15–17-year-old but not 12–14-year-old children [47]. Exposure to and uptake of environmental influences that predispose to excess weight gain differ and may be relatively greater for low-income children at certain ages.

Wang and Lobstein [42] analyzed worldwide trends, based on data published before 2005, for school-age children in 25 countries and preschool children in 42 countries. With some exceptions, e.g. young children in lower income countries, the overall finding was of increased overweight and obesity. This finding is clear in summary estimates and projections of child overweight and obesity prevalence in broad regions for 2006 and 2010 (Fig. 31.7). The component that is obesity varies by region – about one-third in the Americas, less in other regions. US data based on comparable, successive national health and nutrition surveys show striking tripling or quadrupling of obesity prevalence in school-age children and adolescents over the past 3–4 decades [29]. An IOTF analysis of trend data for European children indicated annual increases of 1.3 million per year in the number of overweight and obese children, of which 0.3 million will be obese [48].

Disease burden

The health consequences of obesity are well established (see Chapters 13–19) and affect adults and children globally. Table 31.3, taken from the extensive consideration of the implications of obesity for the global burden of disease [49], quantifies the impact of obesity on several conditions using disability-adjusted life-years, or DALYs, as the indicator. Each DALY reflects 1 year of "healthy life" lost, and therefore includes the burden of disease attributable to high BMI but not likely to be reflected in mortality

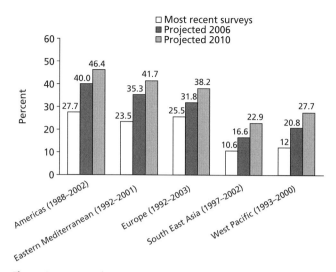

Figure 31.7 Projected increase in childhood overweight (including obesity) by WHO region. Data for children in the WHO African Region were insufficient to project prevalence rates. (Adapted with permission from Wang and Lobstein [42].)

data, e.g. arthritis. Cardiovascular diseases and diabetes are the major causes of disease and disability attributable to overweight and obesity, providing an urgent mandate for controlling the global obesity pandemic. The burden of diabetes risk worldwide, of which 58% is attributed to increases in BMI [49], is quantified in Table 31.4 based on estimates generated by the WHO in collaboration with the International Diabetes Federation [50]. As shown, the number of people affected is expected to double by 2030. The Western-Pacific region (Asia and Australasia) is a critical focal point, representing about half of the total both now and in the future. The extremely high burden of diabetes in this region reflects the population size of India and China, together with the lower BMI risk thresholds for diabetes development and the high burden of diabetes in Pacific populations. Subnationally, other populations with high levels of obesity also require more attention in relation to diabetes, e.g. the aforementioned aboriginal or ethnic minority populations in the United States, Canada, and Australia.

The impact of obesity on cancer deserves attention as well [51]. Based on a systematic review of the world literature on diet, nutrition, and cancer prevention, the World Cancer Research Fund (WCRF) has emphasized the importance of body fatness as a risk factor for cancer development [52]. The WCRF report explains that deaths attributed to cancer are increasing and contribute substantially to the total number of deaths in several countries: for example, 29% of deaths in the US, 18% in Mexico, 20% in Brazil, 33% in the UK, 30% in Poland, 33% in Spain, 44% in Japan, 22% in China, 15% in India, 35% in Australia, 20% in South Africa, and 9% in Egypt. The systematic review found convincing or probable evidence of an increased risk associated with body fatness, abdominal obesity or adult

Table 31.3 Burden of disease in DALYs (000s) from diseases caused by high BMI in adults aged ≥30 years, by subregion

Subregion	Osteo-arthritis	Colon cancer	Postmenopausal breast cancer	Endometrial cancer	Type II diabetes	Stroke	Ischemic heart disease	Hypertensive disease	Total
Africa – D	37	6	2	2	148	110	199	57	564
Africa – E	55	9	14	5	240	188	282	94	887
Americas – A	243	104	77	46	1171	400	1243	195	3479
Americas – B	193	41	40	77	1367	504	892	309	3423
Americas – D	22	5	5	22	164	51	91	62	422
Eastern Mediterranean – B	33	7	6	4	273	84	447	136	990
Eastern Mediterranean – D	70	12	17	6	515	217	865	208	1910
Europe – A	348	185	127	66	876	619	1271	166	3658
Europe – B	176	46	35	37	401	559	1304	306	2864
Europe – C	266	95	66	69	526	1291	2741	208	5262
Southeast Asia – B	85	21	18	7	555	175	406	201	1468
Southeast Asia – D	95	8	20	5	916	309	1156	117	2626
Western Pacific – A	74	31	11	9	224	135	134	11	629
Western Pacific – B	421	104	45	33	1503	1280	1139	709	5234
World	2118	676	486	386	8877	5921	12,170	2780	33,414

DALYs, disability-adjusted life-years.
Letters indicate the Global Burden of Disease mortality strata, as follows.
A. Very low child, very low adult
B. Low child, low adult
C. Low child, high adult
D. High child, high adult
E. High child, very high adultSource: James [49].

Table 31.4 Prevalence of diabetes worldwide in 2000 and projected for 2030, by region (in millions)

	2000	2030	% change
Americas	33	66.8	+202
Africa	7	18.2	+260
Europe	33	48	+145
Middle East	15.2	42	+280
Asia and Australasia	82.7	190.5	+230
Total	171	366	+214

Source: Diabetes Action Now [50].

weight gain for cancers of the breast and colorectum, for example, which appear among the top five causes of cancer in these countries [52].

Children

The consequences of obesity for health and longevity are also affecting children worldwide. The potential lifetime impact of obesity beginning in childhood may be overall much greater than for adult-onset obesity. Obesity in children, especially older children, often tracks into adulthood and the adverse health effects of obesity are cumulative over time if children remain obese. The occurrence of type 2 diabetes is compelling evidence of the potential for obesity to impact lifetime health [45,53]. Lobstein and Jackson-Leach [54], based on a comprehensive analysis for European countries, estimated there were more than 20,000 obese children with type 2 diabetes among the population of some 5 million obese children in the European Union, with 20 times that many showing evidence of impaired glucose tolerance. Kelishadi [55] conducted an extensive, systematic review of obesity levels in association with metabolic syndrome risk factors in developing countries, using studies published between 1950 and 2007. Even considering the limited data and the definitional and methodologic issues affecting the ability to compare across studies, the studies that were identified indicated substantial prevalence of elevated blood pressure and dyslipidemias, with millions of children affected.

Causal pathways

The etiology of obesity involves many factors. Any consideration of causes starts with the deceptively simple observation of a chronic positive imbalance of energy intake over expenditure that is not corrected by metabolism or needed for growth and development. The human body is geared to avoiding hunger and storing fat [1]. The way we live, as a whole, challenges our ability to maintain energy balance. One then asks why this energy imbalance occurs in more and more people and is occurring in all age cohorts, but only in the last few decades and at different levels in different countries and different population groups within countries.

The answer – a conclusion of the 1997 WHO consultation [1] and of numerous subsequent reviews – is that only environmental influences can explain the rapid increases observed in the prevalence of obesity, particularly as these increases have been seen throughout diverse segments of populations and across many different countries worldwide. Obesity levels change as our environments change, whether in Indiana or India. That the increases in BMI affect the entire distribution highlights the broad environmental causation, i.e. the causes are affecting everyone rather than a susceptible minority at the obese end of the continuum, as shown in the US population data in Figure 31.6. In addition, observations that people who immigrate to countries begin to reflect the obesity levels in their new country of residence over time are further evidence for environmental effects [23,56–58]. Within and between societies, obesity varies among subgroups. However, no societal groups appear to be completely resistant to the factors driving body weight levels up over time.

Populations are experiencing profound changes in factors that are conducive to obesity development, chiefly through economic growth and globalization of food markets [1,4,5]. There are many sectors of our political economy that play a role in establishing this causal web of societal influences on obesity at levels extending from the home or workplace all the way through to global trade agreements and the worldwide reach of multinational corporations. With rising incomes and urbanization, dietary patterns that are high in complex carbohydrates and fiber give way to more varied diets that have a higher proportion of fats, saturated fats, and sugars [59–62]. Food production has increased, with concurrent increases in food marketing. Vegetable oils and fats have become cheap commodities, and even people in low-income nations have higher fat consumption than previously. Large shifts towards less physically demanding work have occurred on a worldwide basis in almost all types of occupations, including agriculture. People are also less active because of automated transportation, technology in the home, and passive leisure activities. Few people engage in enough exercise during leisure time to compensate for being inactive in their overall daily routines.

Potential pathways for environment effects and for related environmental and policy changes can be considered using the IOTF causal web shown in Figure 31.8 [59]. This framework illustrates key influences across sectors and levels and suggests where policy instruments (e.g. taxation, regulation, restrictions, subsidies, incentives) can be used to foster changes in these spheres. Relevant potential environmental and policy interventions are discussed in Chapters 32–34.

One can begin at the left, thinking through the various aspects of globalization and trends in development and transnational markets and communication channels, how they cross national borders to impact upon the social structure and the people who

are in equilibrium with that structure. The plane representing national policy and perspectives recognizes that in any given country or region, the effects of global influences will depend on sociocultural history, political systems and many other factors and may permit, dampen or magnify these effects of the societal structure. The vertical listing of sectors recognizes that impacts include but are not felt primarily by the public health or healthcare system. The key societal domains of transportation, commerce, education, social welfare, community development and particularly agriculture are major pathways for factors that influence eating and physical activity. Depending on the influence and on the society in question, where these pathways find targets varies. Some reach directly into homes, e.g. through media channels, while others work through bureaucracies or political structures that have counterparts at national, state or regional, and local levels.

One can also begin at the right of the causal web, with those factors most proximal to the individual (those in the work, school, and home environments) and then move outward to include influences operating at the community level – the systems of transportation, public safety, sanitation, and food production and distribution. The sectors at these first two levels are related, with varying levels of autonomy, to national and regional counterparts, and the national and regional levels in turn are increasingly driven by global marketing, development, and media influences. Working from either direction underscores the critical links between individuals' daily environments for making food and activity choices and the multilevel systems that influence those choices. Hence, although the public health and healthcare sectors may feel the most responsibility to address the problem of obesity, to do this effectively requires working with and through the attitudes, practices, and policy options in the multiple other relevant sectors.

Given the nature, scope, complexity, and inter-related nature of these pathways, it is rare or impossible to generate definitive proof that a particular factor is causally related to obesity. The scientific model that allows us to uncover causation through experiments (randomized controlled trials) in which we manipulate one variable at a time is really not applicable to many environmental pathways. We cannot experiment with society as such – with the economy, with culture and with the environment infrastructure. And when we can experiment with some factors, it is certainly difficult to hold constant what happens in the "control group" and in the surrounding context. Other types of evidence can be useful, when applied appropriately and with an understanding of the limitations [63]

In thinking about evidence that might be informative about where to focus initiatives to reduce population levels of obesity, we raise questions such as:

• Can this factor be related to weight gain?

• Are there clear trends in the expected direction in parallel to changes in obesity?

• Is this factor more prevalent among obese people or population groups?

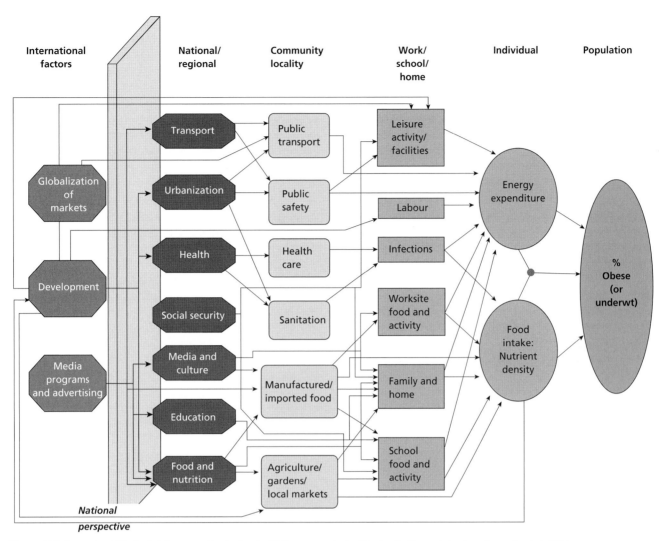

Figure 31.8 International Obesity Task Force causal web of societal influences on obesity. (Reprinted with permission from Kumanyika et al. [59].)

• Can you reduce obesity levels by removing or improving this factor?

Such questions facilitate a logical approach to using the best available evidence to determine whether a factor is likely to hold promise as a target for addressing the epidemic. The following is a brief discussion of three examples that emerge from this thought process related to media environments and use, food marketing, and options for physical activity.

Is the increase in obesity attributable to changes in the media environment, e.g. television, computer games or the Internet?

Television (TV) access is highly prevalent [64] and may be contributing to the obesity pandemic. The theoretical association has several potential mechanisms: TV watching, computer use, and electronic games are sedentary activities that compete with physical activity and are probably not offset by additional physical activity. TV is a major route for food advertising and may stimulate eating of TV-advertised foods or of food in general. A review of 13 cross-sectional and seven longitudinal studies found a relatively consistent association of high levels of TV viewing with higher obesity or weight gain across gender, in minority groups, and in several countries [65].

Can the obesity epidemic be attributed to the amount of food being sold and the way it is marketed?

No one questions whether food intake – specifically overconsumption of calories in relation to expenditure – is in the causal pathway for obesity but it has been quite difficult to show the effect in populations in a way that is convincing with respect to the need for change. It is very difficult to assess subtle changes in caloric intake, and to discover whether an individual is in a prolonged positive energy balance requires simultaneous accurate data on energy expenditure. Hence ascertainment of energy balance as such is beyond the capacity of population surveys.

Explorations of this issue rely heavily on what might be called "circumstantial evidence" to show that people are eating more and, especially, more than they need or can offset by additional physical activity and that food-marketing patterns are partly responsible for this overconsumption [66]. Data from the US Department of Agriculture can be used to demonstrate such circumstantial evidence. The steady increase in the number of calories available per capita parallels the rise in obesity [67]. Even after adjustment for waste, the number of calories available per person exceeds the daily need for most individuals. Other evidence relates to portion sizes of packaged foods and restaurant meals. The upward trend in portion sizes in the US market is legendary and readily observable [68,69]. Consumption of both "fast foods" and soft drinks has received increasing attention in the obesity literature, even in the global market [70–72].

Cost of food is another key issue and one that is especially relevant to the excess of obesity in lower income populations. The food-pricing structure favors high-calorie foods – if one is trying to maximize calories for the dollar [61]. Whether one can actually consume a healthy diet on a limited budget is continually debated, but relates in part to the time available to prepare food and the competing economic activities that are relevant to those, primarily women, who prepare food [4,73]. However, there are ample data to demonstrate that many high-fat or high-sugar foods are readily accessible and available, at relatively low cost and in ready-to-eat forms. Simulations suggest that increases in prices of certain foods could result in a decrease in obesity levels [62]. However, it is also possible that increases in the prices of certain core, nutritious foods could further aggravate patterns that rely on inexpensive, dense sources of calories that may be unintentionally consumed to excess. The potential benefits of having regulations that would limit the marketing of energy-dense foods to children are supported by impressive evidence [66,74,75], and guidelines for such regulations have been developed by the IOTF in collaboration with Consumers International [76].

Can the obesity epidemic be attributed to changes in options for being physically active?

Physical activity patterns across countries are somewhat consistent with patterns of obesity prevalence; overall, they show that car use is more prevalent and walking and cycling are in lower frequency where obesity levels are higher [77]. As already noted, sedentary behaviors such as TV watching are increasing worldwide. Unless people are very active, the potential for decreases or increases in physical activity to influence energy balance is quantitatively less than for changes in food consumption [67]. The upper limit of calories that can be consumed in one meal or day is much higher relative to the upper limit of possible energy expenditure from physical activity on one occasion or per day. The ease of caloric overconsumption is markedly greater than the ability to compensate for such overconsumption by increasing activity.

Decreases in physical activity are critical contributors to changes in energy balance in countries or regions where people may still have relatively high physical activity, e.g. associated with social and economic transitions, including rural to urban migration, but less so where sedentary forms of work and transportation, as well as recreation, have already become entrenched. In such situations, e.g. in high-income countries, changes in the food supply are implicated as the main causes of the epidemic. For example, an analysis of the relative contribution of food-related and activity-related factors to obesity development in countries within the Organization of Economic Co-operation and Development (OECD) found consistent support for the hypothesis that obesity trends in these countries in recent decades are primarily related to changes in food availability and consumption [62]. This does not alter the relevance of attempts to increase physical activity levels in sedentary populations, but reflects the evidence that changes in physical activity may have relatively less impact than food consumption changes in the recent trends. Physical activity can have benefits for overall energy balance behaviors that go beyond their energy expenditure equivalents, i.e. as part of a general picture of lifestyle changes that involve more active pursuits and to displace sedentary pastimes that predispose to overconsumption of high-energy foods and beverages.

The role of sociocultural variables, mentioned earlier in relation to different national perspectives, is critical. In any society or cultural group there may be aspects of traditional foods or food-related rituals that predispose to or protect from overeating, or inactivity, under various circumstances [78,79]. Some cultural practices may be protective and explain partly the within-region variations in the impact of the epidemic on populations living in relatively similar environments (e.g. the long-standing culture of using bicycles, with a supporting infrastructure, may provide protective levels of physical activity in The Netherlands). Cultural attitudes and practices related to body image may influence behavior in relation to obesity. Relevant variables include body image and body size norms and concerns, attitudes and norms about dieting to lose weight, norms about overeating, attitudes and practices related to pregnancy weight gain, physical activity preferences and norms, concepts of social status, e.g. having a car, and social cultural history (or current experience) with hunger and deprivation.

Often cultural influences are invoked as a potential explanation for high levels of obesity in populations that are culturally different, e.g. ethnic minority populations [80]. High levels of obesity in minority populations may be attributed to cultural preferences for high-fat foods or to neutral or positive attitudes about large body size. These factors are probably relevant but can only be understood in light of the environments in which these populations live. Culture interacts with and responds to the environmental context. It is, therefore, useful to focus on *interactions* of cultural attitudes and practices that permit or encourage overeating or inactivity with environments that encourage overeating and discourage or prevent physical activity. For example, there are substantial differences in the environments of African-Americans compared to US whites related to food access and options for physical activity, and the environments of African-Americans are less favorable in these respects [34,81,82]. Food access issues have also been raised with respect to obesity in Pacific populations [83]. Qualitative data from Latinas living in the United States indicate awareness of the environmental disadvantages in the ability to pursue traditional eating and physical activity behaviors that are healthful [84].

Relatively tolerant or even positive attitudes about large body size, which are more common in some populations where high obesity prevalence has been observed for decades, are in part a reaction to perceptions of thinness as indicative of wasting diseases [85,86]. Being somewhat heavy may be considered preferable to being too thin, and healthier, and dieting may seem unnecessary or even risky, leaving one "without anything to fall back on" in case of illness or a food shortage [86,87]. Furthermore, in a population where the prevalence of obesity is longstanding and is very high, e.g. Pacific Island populations, aboriginal populations or African-American women where prevalence of obesity (BMI 30+) among adults may be in the 50–80% range, perceptions of "normal" weight may diverge substantially from clinical or public health standards.

Cultural influences change slowly. Given that all our current eating and physical activity patterns are culturally supported, these influences must be understood in formulating initiatives to reduce population obesity levels. The influence of culture on environment is bidirectional. Cultural attitudes and practices respond to changes in various aspects of the environment. Consider the changes in cultural attitudes and social norms that have followed technologic advances. In this sense, cultural influences are generally not variables to be targeted for interventions but are important to consider when designing initiatives to effect change and for understanding how people respond to interventions.

Conclusion

Obesity considerations now include elements that extend far beyond the clinical domain. Obesity has become a societal problem of populations, not merely of individuals, and has spread to children as well as adults in populations globally. This does not mean that hunger and undernutrition have been conquered. Quite the contrary. These still persist as major nutrition problems in certain regions of the world but co-exist with obesity and chronic disease, which have become the major contributors to the overall global disease burden.

Attempts to ascertain and track trends in obesity prevalence have increased since the global pandemic was recognized by WHO approximately 10 years ago. Although there are many methodologic problems still to be addressed with respect to comparing populations, the available data for adults and children clearly establish that obesity levels are high in some countries in every region of the world, are increasing, and are associated with

alarming levels of diabetes and cardiovascular disease. Perhaps surprising to some, the Asia-Pacific region is the most affected by obesity and diabetes in terms of numbers, and intensified obesity prevention and control initiatives are especially needed in that region.

The reasons for the trends of increased obesity are environmental factors such as globalization, economic changes, and urbanization that have changed the types and quantities of food available and the typical levels of physical activity, resulting in chronic positive energy balance and increases in average body weights. Hence, solutions will involve environmental and policy changes – in multiple sectors of society and at multiple levels – and a greater focus on prevention to provide the supportive environments that may assist individuals to avoid gaining excess weight in the first place. Even with the best treatment strategies, the numbers becoming overweight or obese will overwhelm our capacity for primary care even of secondary conditions such as type 2 diabetes. Thus effective prevention strategies provide the only option for an ultimate long-term solution to the global pandemic.

References

1. World Health Organization. *Obesity: preventing and managing the global epidemic. WHO Technical Report Series 894*. Geneva: World Health Organization, 2000.

2. James WPT, for the Commission on Nutrition Challenges for the 21st Century. Ending malnutrition by 2020. An agenda for change in the millennium. Food Nutr Bull 2000;21(suppl).

3. World Health Organization. WHO Fact Sheet No 311. Facts about overweight and obesity. Available from: www.who.int/mediacentre/factsheets/fs311/en/index.html.

4. Kennedy G, Nantel G, Shetty P. Globalization and food systems in developing countries. A synthesis of country case studies. In: *Globalization of Food Systems in Developing Countries: Impact on Food Security and Nutrition*. FAO Food and Nutrition Paper 83. Rome: Food and Agricultural Organization of the United Nations, 2004.

5. Hawkes C. Uneven dietary development: linking the policies and processes of globalization with the nutrition transition, obesity and diet-related chronic diseases. Global Health 2006;28:2–4.

6. World Health Organization. *Diet, Nutrition and The Prevention of Chronic Diseases*. WHO Technical Report Series 916. Geneva: World Health Organization, 2003.

7. World Health Organization. *Global Strategy on Diet, Physical Activity, and Health*. Geneva: World Health Organization, 2004.

8. Uusitalo U, Pietinen P, Puska P. Dietary transition in developing countries: challenges for chronic disease prevention. In: *Globalization, Diets and Noncommunicable Diseases*. Geneva: World Health Organization, 2002: 6–31.

9. World Health Report. *Primary Health Care Now More Than Ever*. World Health Organization, Geneva, 2008

10. International Obesity Task Force, International Association for the Study of Obesity. Available at: www.iotf.org/database/index.asp

11. de Onis M, Onyango, AW, Borghi E, et al. Development of a WHO growth reference for school-aged children and adolescents. Bull WHO 2007;85:660–7.

12. Rush EC, Goedecke JH, Jennings C, et al. BMI, fat and muscle differences in urban women of five ethnicities from two countries. Int J Obes 2007;31:1232–9.

13. Villamor E, Msamanga G, Urassa W, et al. Trends in obesity, underweight, and wasting among women attending prenatal clinics in urban Tanzania, 1995–2004. Am J Clin Nutr 2006;83:1387–94.

14. South African Demographic Health Survey 2003. Ministry of Health, South Africa. Available from: www.doh.gov.za/facts/sadhs2003/main.html

15. Ogden CL, Carroll MD Curtin LR, et al. Prevalence of overweight and obesity in the United States, 1999–2004. JAMA 2006;295:1549–55.

16. Rose G. Population distributions of risk and disease. Nutr Metab Cardiovasc Dis 1991;1:37–40.

17. Ogden CL, Carroll MD, McDowell MA, Flegal KM. Obesity among adults in the United States. No statistically significant change since 2003–2004. National Center for Health Statistics Data Brief No. 1, November 2007. Centers for Disease Control. Available from: www.cdc.gov/nchs/data/databriefs/db01.pdf

18. Deurenberg P, Deurenberg-Yap M, Guricci S. Asians are different from Caucasians and from each other in their body mass index/body fat per cent relationship. Obes Rev 2002;3:141–6.

19. WHO Expert Consultation. Appropriate body-mass index for Asian populations and its implications for policy and intervention strategies. Lancet 2004;363:157–63.

20. McNeely MJ, Boyko EJ. Type 2 diabetes prevalence in Asian Americans: results of a national health survey. Diabetes Care 2004;27:66–9.

21. Ramachandran A, Snehalatha C, Vijay V. Low risk threshold for acquired diabetogenic factors in Asian Indians. Diabetes Res Clin Pract 2004;65:189–95.

22. Huxley R, James WP, Barzi F, et al, Obesity in Asia Collaboration. Ethnic comparisons of the cross-sectional relationships between measures of body size with diabetes and hypertension. Obes Rev 2008;9(suppl 1):53–61.

23. Lauderdale DS, Rathouz PJ. Body mass index in a US national sample of Asia Americans: effects of nativity, years since immigration and socioeconomic status. Int J Obes 2000;24:1188–94.

24. Tremblay MS, Pérez CE, Ardern CI, et al. Obesity, overweight and ethnicity. Health Rep 2005;16:23–34.

25. Kumanyika S. Ethnicity and obesity development in children. Ann NY Acad Sci 1993;699:81–92.

26. Kumanyika SK. Obesity in minority populations: an epidemiologic assessment. Obes Res 1994;2:166–82.

27. Wilson C, Gilliland S, Moore K, Acton K. The epidemic of extreme obesity among American Indian and Alaska Native adults with diabetes. Prev Chronic Dis 2007;4(1):A06.

28. MacMillan HL, MacMillan AB, Offord DR, et al. Aboriginal health. CMAJ 1996;155:1569–78.

29. National Center for Health Statistics. *Health, United States, 2006 with Chartbook on Trends in the Health of Americans.* Hyattsville, MD: National Center for Health Statistics, 2006.

30. Smelser JN, Wilson WJ, Mitchell F (eds). *America Becoming. Racial Trends and Their Consequences, vol 1.* Washington, DC: National Academy Press, 2001.

31. Fee M. Racializing narratives: obesity, diabetes and the "Aboriginal" thrifty genotype. Soc Sci Med 2006;62:2988–97.

32. Ravussin E, Valencia ME, Esparza J, et al. Effects of a traditional lifestyle on obesity in Pima Indians. Diabetes Care 1994;17:1067–74.

33. Luke A, Cooper RS, Prewitt TE, et al. Nutritional consequences of the African diaspora. Annu Rev Nutr 2001;21:47–71.

34. Kumanyika S, Grier S. Targeting interventions for ethnic minority and low-income populations. Future of Children 2006;16:187–207.

35. Freedman DS, Khan LK, Serdula MK, et al. Racial and ethnic differences in secular trends for childhood BMI, weight, and height. Obesity 2006;14:301–8.

36. McMillen IC, MacLaughlin SM, Muhlhausler BS, et al. Developmental origins of adult health and disease: the role of periconceptional and foetal nutrition. Basic Clin Pharmacol Toxicol 2008;102:82–9.

37. Christakis NA, Fowler JH. The spread of obesity in a large social network over 32 years. N Engl J Med 2007;357:370–9.

38. Molarius A, Seidell JC, Sans S, et al. Educational level, relative body weight, and changes in their association over 10 years: an international perspective from the WHO MONICA Project. Am J Public Health 2000;90:1260–8.

39. Monteiro CA, Moura EC, Conde WL, et al. Socioeconomic status and obesity in adult populations of developing countries: a review. Bull WHO 2004;82:940–6.

40. McLaren L. Socioeconomic status and obesity. Epidemiol Rev 2007;29:29–48.

41. Wang Y, Beydoun MA. The obesity epidemic in the United States – gender, age, socioeconomic, racial/ethnic, and geographic characteristics: a systematic review and meta regression analysis. Epidemiol Rev 2007;29:6–28.

42. Wang Y, Lobstein T. Worldwide trends in childhood overweight and obesity. Int J Pediatr Obes 2006;1:11–25.

43. Cole TJ, Bellizzi MC, Flegal KM, et al. Establishing a standard definition for child overweight and obesity worldwide: international survey. BMJ 2000;320:1240–3.

44. Story M, Stevens J, Himes J, et al. Obesity in American-Indian children: prevalence, consequences, and prevention. Prev Med 2003;37(6 Pt 2):S3–12.

45. Craig ME, Femia G, Broyda V, et al. Type 2 diabetes in indigenous and non-Indigenous children and adolescents in New South Wales. Med J Aust 2007;186:497–9.

46. Shrewsbury V, Wardle J. Socioeconomic status and adiposity in childhood: a systematic review of cross-sectional studies 1990–2005. Obesity 2008;16:275–84.

47. Miech RA, Kumanyika SK, Stettler N, et al. Trends in the association of poverty with overweight among US adolescents, 1971–2004. JAMA 2006;295:2385–93.

48. Jackson-Leach R, Lobstein T. Estimated burden of paediatric obesity and co morbidities in Europe. Part 1. The increase in the prevalence of child obesity in Europe is itself increasing. Int J Pediatr Obes 2006;1:26–32.

49. James WPT, et al. Overweight and obesity (high body mass index). In: *Comparative Quantification of Health Risks Global and Regional Burden of Diseases Attributable to Selected Major Risk Factors.* Geneva: World Health Organization, 2004: 497–596.

50. World Health Organization and International Diabetes Federation. Diabetes Action Now. 2004. Available at: www.who.int/diabetes/actionnow/booklet/en/www.who.int/diabetes/actionnow/booklet/en/

51. Bergstrom A, Pisani P, Tenet V, et al. Overweight as an avoidable cause of cancer in Europe. Int J Cancer 2001;91:421–30.

52. World Cancer Research Fund/American Institute for Cancer Research. *Food, Nutrition, Physical Activity and the Prevention of*

Cancer. A Global Perspective. Washington, DC: American Institute for Cancer Research, 2007.

53. Writing Group for the SEARCH for Diabetes in Youth Study Group, Dabelea D, Bell RA, d'Agostino RB Jr, et al. Incidence of diabetes in youth in the United States. JAMA 2007;297:2716–24. Erratum in: JAMA 2007;298:627.

54. Lobstein T, Jackson-Leach R. Estimated burden of paediatric obesity and comorbidities in Europe. Part 1. The increase in the prevalence of child obesity in Europe is itself increasing. Int J Pediatr Obes 2006;1:33–41.

55. Kelishadi R. Childhood overweight, obesity, and the metabolic syndrome in developing countries. Epidemiol Rev 2007;29:62–76.

56. Goel MS, McCarthy EP, Phillips RS, Wee CC. Obesity among US immigrant subgroups by duration of residence. JAMA 2004;292:2860–7.

57. Himmelgreen DA, Perez-Escamilla R, Martinez D, et al. The longer you stay, the bigger you get: length of time and language use in the U.S. are associated with obesity in Puerto Rican women. Am J Phys Anthropol 2004;125:90–6.

58. Kaplan MS, Huguet N, Newsom JT, McFarland BH. The association between length of residence and obesity among Hispanic immigrants. Am J Prev Med 2004;27:323–6.

59. Kumanyika S, Jeffery RW, Morabia A, et al. Public Health Approaches to the Prevention of Obesity (PHAPO) Working Group of the International Obesity Task Force (IOTF). Obesity prevention. Int J Obes 2002;26:425–36.

60. French SA, Story M, Jeffery RW. Environmental influences on eating and physical activity. Annu Rev Public Health 2001;22:309–35.

61. Drewnowski A. The real contribution of added sugars and fats to obesity. Epidemiol Rev 2007;29:160–71.

62. Bleich S, Cutler D, Murray C, et al. Why is the developed world obese? Annu Rev Public Health 2008;21:273–95.

63. Swinburn B, Gill T, Kumanyika S. Obesity prevention: a proposed framework for translating evidence into action. Obes Rev 2005;6: 23–33.

64. InterMedia. *Children, Youth and Media Around the World – An Overview of Trends and Issues.* 2004. Available from: www.unicef.org/magic/resources/InterMedia2004.pdf)

65. Foster JA, Gore SA, West DS. Altering TV viewing habits: an unexplored strategy for adult obesity intervention? Am J Health Behav 2006;30:3–4.

66. McGinnis JM, Gootman JA, Kraak VI (eds), Institute of Medicine, Committee on Food Marketing and the Diets of Children and Youth. *Food Marketing to Children and Youth. Threat or Opportunity?* Washington, DC: National Academy Press, 2006.

67. Jeffery RW, Harnack LJ. Evidence implicating eating as a primary driver for the obesity epidemic. Diabetes 2007;56:2673–6.

68. Smiciklas-Wright H, Mitchell DC, Mickle SJ, et al. Foods commonly eaten in the United States, 1989–1991 and 1994–1996: are portion sizes changing? J Am Dietet Assoc 2003;103:41–7.

69. Young LR, Nestle M. The contribution of expanding sizes to the US obesity epidemic. Am J Public Health 2002;92:246–94.

70. Schulze MB, Manson JE, Ludwig DS, et al. Sugar-sweetened beverages, weight gain, and incidence of type 2 diabetes in young and middle-aged women. JAMA 2004;292:927–34.

71. Ludwig DS, Peterson KE, Gortmaker SL. Relation between consumption of sugar-sweetened drinks and childhood obesity: a prospective, observational analysis. Lancet 2001;357:505–8.

72. Schmidt M, Affenito SG, Striegel-Moore R, et al. Fast food intake and diet quality in black and white females: the National Heart, Lung, and Blood Institute (NHLGI) Growth and Health Study. Arch Pediatr Adolesc Med 2005;159:626–31.

73. Rose D. Food Stamps, the Thrifty Food Plan, and meal preparation: the importance of the time dimension for US nutrition policy. J Nutr Educ Behav 2007;39:226–32.

74. Hastings G, et al, for the UK Food Standards Agency. *Review of the Research on the Effects of Food Promotion to Children.* Glasgow: Center for Social Marketing, 2003. Available at: www.foodstandards.gov.uk/multimedia/pdfs/promofoodchildrenexec.pdf

75. WHO Forum on the Marketing of Food and Non-alcoholic Beverages to Children. Marketing of food and non-alcoholic beverages to children: report of a WHO forum and technical meeting, Oslo, Norway, 2–5 May 2006. Available at: www.who.int/dietphysicalactivity/publications/Oslo%20meeting%20layout%2027%20NOVEMBER.pdf

76. International Association for the Study of Obesity, International Obesity Task Force and Consumers International. Recommendations for an International Code on Marketing of Foods and Non-Alcoholic Beverages to Children. 2008. Available at: http://consint.live.poptech.coop/shared_asp_files/GFSR.asp?NodeID=97478

77. Transportation Research Board. *Making Transit Work: Insight from Western Europe, Canada, and the United States.* Washington, DC: National Academy Press, 2001.

78. Murcott A. Sociological and social anthropological approaches to food and eating. World Rev Nutr Diet 1988;55:1–40.

79. Mintz SW. *Tasting Food, Tasting Freedom. Excursions into Eating, Culture, and the Past.* Boston: Beacon Press, 1997.

80. Kumanyika SK. Environmental influences on childhood obesity: ethnic and cultural influences in context. Physiol Behav 2008;22:61–70.

81. Taylor WC, Poston WSC, Jones L, et al. Environmental justice. Obesity, physical activity, and healthy eating. J Phys Act Health 2006;3:S30-S55.

82. Grier S, Kumanyika S. The context for choice: health implications of targeted food and beverage marketing to African Americans. Am J Public Health 2008;98(9):1616–29.

83. Evans M, Sinclair RC, Fusimalohi C, Liava'a V. Globalization, diet, and health: an example from Tonga. Bull WHO 2001;79: 856–62.

84. Diaz VA, Mainous AG 3rd, Pope C. Cultural conflicts in the weight loss experience of overweight Latinos. Int J Obes 2007;31:328–33.

85. Brown PJ, Konner M. An anthropological perspective on obesity. Ann NY Acad Sci 1987;499:29–46.

86. Jain A, Sherman SN, Chamberlin LA, et al. Why don't low-income mothers worry about their preschoolers being overweight? Pediatrics 2001;107:1138–46.

87. Baturka N, Hornsby PP, Schorling JB. Clinical implications of body image among rural African-American women. J Gen Intern Med 2000;15:235–41.

32 Obesity and the Environment

Andy Jones and Graham Bentham

School of Environmental Sciences, University of East Anglia, Norwich, UK

The obesogenic environment

Throughout history there have been obese individuals who were often the rich and powerful who could display their wealth as corpulence. What is new about the modern epidemic of obesity is that excessive weight is becoming a mass phenomenon affecting a large and growing proportion of the world's population. This trend started earliest and has gone furthest in affluent societies such as the United States, the United Kingdom and Australia but the direction of travel is unmistakable, with most countries for which reliable data exist showing an increase in obesity [1].

At its most basic, the explanation for these unprecedented trends is beguilingly simply. Hill et al. [1] point out that the increase in weight is the result of a positive shift in the balance between energy intake and expenditure for a substantial number of individuals in the population. They go on to show that substantial increases in weight can result from apparently modest changes in positive energy balance, as long as these are persistent over time. Their study examines high-quality data on body weight for representative samples of the US population at different points in time. This enables them to plot the frequency distribution of weight gain. Some individuals lost weight but more showed an increase which in some cases was very large. What is perhaps surprising is that the average gain over 8 years was only about 2 pounds per year which the authors calculate could be accounted for by a 15 kilocalories per day positive energy balance whilst 90% of the population is gaining 50 or fewer kcal/day. This leads them to the challenging conclusion that relatively modest reductions in food intake or small increases in physical activity would be sufficient to halt the increase in obesity in the US.

Clinical Obesity in Adults and Children, 3rd edition. Edited by Peter G. Kopelman, Ian D. Caterson and William H. Dietz.
© 2010 Blackwell Publishing, ISBN: 978-1-4051-8226-3.

Decisions about food intake and physical activity are taken by individuals who show large differences in attitudes and behavior. These differences, interacting powerfully with genetic factors, exert a major influence on the risk that any individual will become obese [2]. But the increase in obesity has been far too rapid to be accounted for by changes in human nature or genetics which change only slowly. Instead we must look to some widespread, deep-rooted and powerful forces that have tipped the balance of individual behavior towards positive energy balance for much of the world's population.

Our main focus is on the effects of the built environment but we begin by setting this in the context of some broader forces that are key elements of what has been called the obesogenic environment [3]. We begin with a review of how the environment in which humans evolved molded their genetics and physiology and how problems have arisen with the rapid shift to a very different modern world. Next we consider the implications of recent changes in food demand and supply. We go on to review how changes in work, transport and leisure have affected levels of physical activity and thereby energy expenditure. Finally, we look in greater detail at the role of the built environment.

Thrifty genes

Studies of twins and of familial aggregation show the importance of genetic factors in determining individual susceptibility to obesity [4]. Within a given population, genetic factors will exert a major influence on which individuals are obese. However, the increases in obesity that have occurred in many populations have been too rapid to be accounted for by changes in human genetics and must have been the result of changes in the environment interacting with a susceptible genome. A number of commentators [5–8] have sought an explanation for this susceptibility in the contrast between the conditions of life in modern affluent societies and those under which humans as a species have evolved.

Eaton and Eaton [6] emphasize that for most of their evolutionary history, humans have lived as hunter/gatherers acquiring food by hunting animals, fishing and gathering of diverse types of edible materials from the natural environment. Possessing only simple tools, acquisition of the quantities of food necessary for survival would have required high levels of physical activity and therefore of energy expenditure. It is clear that for our ancestors there was a close, obligatory relationship between food energy intake and energy expenditure and that they were typically lean and physically fit. This is in stark contrast to modern affluent societies where abundant quantities of food are available for minimal energy expenditure as physical activity.

Writing more than 40 years ago, Neel [5] was one of the first to recognize that the relationship between our Paleolithic ancestors and their environment may continue to exert an important influence on the health of the modern population. Neel points out that the availability of food would fluctuate with times of abundance and times of scarcity related to factors such as variability in the climate. In times of scarcity, increased levels of physical activity might be needed to acquire a dwindling quantity of food, leading to a state of negative energy balance and an increased risk of malnutrition and death. During these times individuals would become increasingly reliant on their body stores of energy and those with greater stores would tend to have a better chance of survival, especially during famines when those with greater reserves of body fat might be less likely to die of starvation. However, selection might also have been important under less severe, but more common (for example, seasonal) conditions of food shortage [8]. There would have been selection acting via differences in fertility as well as mortality [7]. Famines lead to precipitate declines in conceptions and birth rates but even more modest seasonal variations in food availability are associated with significant reductions in fertility. There would hence be selection for genetic traits that allowed some women to conceive under such conditions when others could not. Acting via both mortality and fertility, there would therefore be selection for genes associated with the tendency to store excess energy as body fat during times of plenty. Neel refers to these as "thrifty genes" and argues that there would be strong selection for such genes during the human species' long evolutionary history as hunter gatherers.

With the development of agriculture from about 12,000 years ago, human control over food supply increased but periodic food crises related to climate, disease, pests and war remained common and so, consequentially, did food crises and the risk of starvation. It is possible that selection pressures may even have intensified. Wells [8] argues that the diversity of sources of food and the ability to migrate in search of food probably made outright famine relatively rare amongst hunter/gatherers. Instead, selection pressures would have been dominated by less severe conditions of food shortage such as those associated with seasonal factors. However, the increased dependence on a narrower range of staple crops and animals and decreased mobility may have served to increase the risk of famine in societies based on agriculture.

Selection for "thrifty" genes has probably been a powerful factor for most of human evolutionary history. However, conditions are very different in modern, affluent societies where the reduction of risk of serious food shortage means that "thrifty" genes no longer provide the biologic advantages they have offered over most of human evolutionary history. Instead, such genes become harmful because they predispose towards obesity in an environment of abundant food available for minimal physical activity and energy expenditure. Neel [5] refers to "A thrifty genotype rendered detrimental by progress." Chakravarty and Booth [9] talk of "… a dissonance between 'Stone Age' genes and 'Space Age' circumstances."

The food environment

Individuals have likes and dislikes that affect what food is consumed but it is a mistake to think of food preferences as being simply a personal matter. The very large differences in diets between countries with similar levels of economic development are testimony to the profound influence of history and culture on what food is regarded as normal. Equally, the changes that have taken place in food-related behavior, such as the increased consumption of convenience food, have their roots in deep-seated social and economic trends as well as in changing personal preferences. What we eat is clearly profoundly affected by what is going on in our society, pointing to important sociologic and economic dimensions of customary diet.

A simple misconception is that obesity has increased because people are eating more. For some individuals this may be the case but for the population as a whole, this appears not to be so. Heini and Weinsier [10] compare changes over time in diet and physical activity using data from a series of large nationally representative samples of the US population. During the period since the 1970s when there has been a large increase in obesity, total energy intake has actually declined. During the same period average fat intake adjusted for total calorie intake has declined significantly. Furthermore, the proportion of the US population consuming low-calorie products increased dramatically from 19% in 1978 to 76% in 1991. They refer to these divergent trends in obesity and fat intake patterns as "the American paradox." Similar evidence of a decline in total calorie intake during a period of rapidly rising obesity has also been shown for Britain [11]. The proportion of fat in the modern British diet has increased compared to 50 years earlier but this rise halted in the 1980s since when there has been evidence of a decrease. Data on trends over time in physical activity are much less complete but nevertheless, both studies conclude that the rise in obesity has been driven mainly by a decline in energy expenditure because of reduced physical activity and more sedentary lifestyles. This does not mean that food intake is irrelevant but the issue is not that we are eating more; it is that we have failed to reduce food consumption by enough to compensate for the decline in energy expenditure, with a resulting shift towards positive energy balance and obesity.

The evidence on the dietary determinants of obesity remains controversial [12] but it points to two factors as important contributors to the observed breakdown of the innate regulation of body weight. These are the energy density of food and portion size, both of which appear to be increasing in the modern diet. Energy density is a measure of the amount of energy in a given weight of food. In an experiment when energy density was manipulated but portion size was held constant, subjects ate similar amounts of food (by weight), irrespective of energy density [13]. Over a 2-day period the energy intake of those offered lower energy-density food was about 30% less than those consuming higher energy-density food, with both groups reporting similar levels of satiety. A number of other studies have produced similar results [14]. Fat content makes an important contribution to the overall energy density of food. Dietary fat is readily stored as body fat and is less satiating than isoenergetic quantities of other nutrients [12]. Combined with the palatability of high-fat food, there is an obvious potential for overconsumption. However, the obesogenicity may not be a product of the fat *per se* but of its high energy density. Sugar is another important contributor to energy density and is commonly added to processed food to increase palatability and improve stability and shelf-life. On the other hand, energy density tends to be lower in foods with more fiber and higher water content. Since food processing often involves a reduction in fiber and water, it can lead to an increase in energy density.

A separate but related issue is that of portion size. For children over 3 years of age and for adults, there is clear evidence that offering large portions leads to eating more [14]. It appears that despite higher intakes, those presented with larger portions do not tend to report increased levels of fullness, suggesting that satiety signals are being over-ridden. Furthermore, it appears that the portion size and energy-density effects are independent of each other, with the highest energy intakes being for those consuming the larger portions of higher energy-dense food.

If the consumption of large portion sizes of energy-dense food does increase the risk of obesity, an important question is why such a diet has become so common in countries such as the USA and the United Kingdom. The Foresight report [15] points to some powerful influences on dietary choice and Drewnowski and Darmon [16] emphasize that many of these involve economics. Perhaps the most fundamental of these is that as incomes have risen, the proportion of total household expenditure devoted to food has fallen and this now stands at about 10% for the United Kingdom. The result is that the overwhelming majority of the population have available to them an abundant supply of palatable food that can meet their energy needs at (relative to incomes) unprecedently low cost. Within the vast array of food that is available to the consumer, it is energy-dense diets characterized by refined grains, added sugars and added fats that provide energy requirements at a lower overall cost than those with larger representation of lean meat, fish, vegetables and fruit [16]. Furthermore, the long-term trends are for the costs of items such as fats and sugars to fall relative to those for fresh fruits and vegetables

[15]. The importance of these economic factors is underlined by the results of a national sample survey of adults in the USA [17] which showed that taste and cost were the main factors influencing food choice, especially for those on lower incomes.

Another major influence on food choice has been the increasing willingness of the population to pay more for the food that they consume in return for greater convenience. Part of the background to this is that rising incomes have allowed an increasing number of people to be able to afford the higher prices of more convenient food. Another factor has been that more women are now in paid employment and thus they have less time available for the preparation of food at home [18]. There are also some important drivers on the supply side emanating from the food industry. Like any other enterprises in a market economy, food companies will seek to expand revenues and profit. However, the severe physiologic constraints on how much food people can consume means that simply producing more food is not a viable path for growth and profitability. There is therefore a powerful incentive to increase revenues by adding value to food in order to persuade consumers to pay more for it. One of the consequences of these diverse forces has been rising sales of convenience foods (ready-meals, take-away food, etc.) that can be consumed in the home without the effort required to prepare meals from raw ingredients [15]. Another has been the increasing frequency of eating out with especially striking increases in the number of meals being consumed in fast-food restaurants [18]. This has important nutritional consequences. Bowman and Vinyard [19] have shown that in a representative sample of American adults, after controlling for age, gender, socio-economic and demographic factors, total energy intake and energy density increased and micronutrient density decreased with frequency of fast-food consumption. Similar results were found in a representative sample of American children and adolescents aged 4–19 years [20]. Controlling for demographic and socio-economic factors, children who ate fast food (in comparison to those who did not) consumed more total energy, more energy per gram of food, more added sugars and fewer fruits and nonstarchy vegetables. The authors conclude that these dietary differences associated with fast-food consumption could plausibly increase the risk of obesity. It has also been shown that portion sizes in the USA have increased over time both within the home and in fast-food restaurants [21].

On balance, there seems to be good evidence that affluent countries such as the USA and the UK have shifted towards a pattern of food consumption that has probably made the regulation of overall energy balance more difficult in the face of a decline in energy expenditure.

Physical activity in work, leisure and transport

Direct evidence on changes over time in physical activity is scarce, particularly for comparisons over longer periods of time. In view of the evolutionary importance of our hunter/gather origins, an important question is how did levels of physical activity then compare with those of typical members of modern, affluent societies? To answer this question, archeologic evidence must be pieced together with data from contemporary hunter/gather populations who are usually restricted to atypical, marginal environments. After reviewing this evidence and acknowledging its limitations, Eaton and Eaton [6] estimate that for Paleolithic humans, energy expenditure as physical activity was probably about 5.4 MJ per day for a composite (males and females averaged) 57 kg individual. They note that this is in line with what is normal for contemporary nonindustrial, physically active populations such as those in rural Africa. It is, however, strikingly higher than the estimate of 2.3 MJ/d for a hypothetic 64 kg male/female contemporary American. This is closely in line with another estimate that energy expenditure from physical activity per unit body mass for contemporary Westerners is about 38% of that for hunter/gatherer ancestors [22]. The authors of this study calculate that for a typical modern American to approximate the total energy expenditure/kg/d of hunter/gatherers would require the addition of the equivalent of a 19 km walk for a 70 kg man to each day's activity level.

What about more recent trends? In 1970, which is before the major recent increase in obesity, American males were 8.7 kg heavier than men measured in 1863 when matched for age and height. Food disappearance data are only available from 1909 onwards but suggest that energy available in the food supply remained broadly constant, pointing to a decline in energy expenditure by physical activity as a plausible explanation for the increase in weight [6]. A novel perspective on estimating historical changes in physical activity is provided by a study from Australia [23]. This compared objectively measured physical activity in two groups of male Australians aged 30–60 years. One comprised workers in modern sedentary occupations. The other group were actors in an historic theme park near Sydney who were employed to play the role of early Australian soldiers, convicts and settlers. These were asked to avoid modern technology as much as possible when they were not working at the park. Both groups wore accelerometers during waking hours for a week and mean activity levels were found to be 1.6 times higher in the historical than the modern group. This difference was calculated to be equivalent to walking an additional 8 km per day. Excluding actors for whom there was evidence of dilution of effect by some use of modern technologies outside work hours increased the contrast in mean activity levels to 2.3 times which is equivalent to walking about 16 km per day. This is closely in line with an estimate of an average decline in energy expenditure in the United Kingdom from World War II to 1995 of about 800 kcal/d [24]. There are no detailed long-term direct measurements to confirm or deny such estimates of a large, and relatively recent, decline in energy expenditure. It is, however, possible to examine some indirect indicators of change in physical activity for important domains such as work, leisure and transport.

The energy expenditure in any activity depends on its frequency, duration and intensity. The importance of work for overall levels of physical activity of the population arises from the involvement of so many people, the long hours and the large variations in energy expenditure in different jobs. Ainsworth et al. [25] give estimates of the rate of energy expenditure for different occupations measured as ratios (MET) of the work metabolic rate to a standard resting metabolic rate. Some examples of METs for traditional heavy manual occupations are coal mining (6.0), working in a steel mill (8.0), and construction (5.5). These are in marked contrast to the estimate of 1.5 MET for typical office work, 2.3 for bar or shop work and 3.0 for light/moderate assembly work. Given these large differences, changes in the occupational structure of the workforce can have a major impact on the overall levels of energy expenditure associated arising from employment.

Reviewing long-term trends in the occupational structure of the USA, Sobek [26] shows that changes have been profound. In 1870, 87% of the workforce were in farming or other blue-collar jobs likely to involve physical labor but by 1990 this had fallen dramatically to only 28%. So in little more than a century America had gone from a situation where the overwhelming majority of jobs involved significant physical labor to one in which the overwhelming majority were sedentary. Looking at this in another way, the odds for being in a sedentary job versus an active one were 17 times higher in 1990 than in 1870. The changes in Great Britain have been no less dramatic. In 1950, 54% of employed persons were in the industrial sectors of agriculture, fishing, mining, manufacturing and construction which are the ones most likely to involve manual labor, whilst in 2006 this had fallen to only 17%. It therefore appears that in countries such as the USA and Great Britain changes in occupational structure related to deep-seated changes in the economy have been sufficient to produce a very marked reduction in the levels of energy expenditure associated with paid employment.

However, this is only part of the story. In addition to these compositional changes, it is likely that widespread mechanization and automation of work will also have produced major reductions in energy expenditure. Taking farming as an example, Ainsworth et al. [25] give a MET of 8.0 for baling hay but only 2.5 for driving a tractor. Milking by hand has a MET of 3.0 whereas milking by machine is 1.5. It therefore seems very likely that changes in occupational structure together with mechanization will have produced very large reductions in energy expenditure related to employment. Direct measurements of changes in physical activity at work are too recent to have been able to capture the potentially large longer term declines but they do show a continuing fall [27,28].

In addition to the obvious direct effect on levels of energy expenditure, these changes in employment have some other, less obvious implications for obesity via their potential interaction with diet and leisure-time physical activity. The requirements for energy balance dictate that high levels of physical activity at work and energy expenditure at work would be accompanied by high levels of energy intake from the diet, favoring characteristics such as high energy density and large portion sizes. Habituation to this type of diet might make it difficult for individuals to adjust to the levels of energy intake required following reductions in energy expenditure at work. There is also evidence that leisure-time physical activity is significantly lower for manual workers than for others in less physically demanding jobs [29,30]. It seems plausible that following heavy physical demands at work, there might be a preference for more sedentary pursuits during leisure hours, although alternative explanations such as income and social and cultural attitudes cannot be excluded. If jobs making heavy physical demands do indeed discourage involvement in physically active leisure, such attitudes could persist even after the levels of physical activity at work have lessened. A culture biased towards high intake of energy-dense foods and low levels of leisure-time physical activity could persist into a new era when energy expenditure in the workplace is much reduced. Given the strong relationships between occupation and social stratification, this could be a factor in the observed association between obesity and social deprivation. There could also be a geographical dimension to this with local concentrations of obesity in areas which formerly had high concentrations of heavy industry such as mining, shipbuilding and steel which then suffered major industrial restructuring and loss of manual jobs [31].

Alongside these changes in paid employment, there is also evidence of a marked reduction in energy expenditure associated with work in the home. Bowers [32] traces some remarkable changes during the 20th century in the time spent by American women on meal preparation and clean-up. In 1900 the average woman spent 44 hours per week on food preparation and clean-up. By 1950 this had fallen to about 20 hours per week and by the end of the century it is estimated that an average of less than 10 hours per week was devoted to food preparation [18,32]. The increased involvement of women in the workforce has been one of the most important influences on these trends. In 1900 only about 6% of married women were in paid employment whereas by 1999 this was over 60%. As the time available for food preparation in the home has shrunk, the widespread availability of appliances such as freezers, microwave ovens and dishwashers has reduced the time and effort needed. The reduction in domestic work associated with food preparation has also been intimately tied up with the increasing availability of convenience food and the growth in eating out.

A fascinating insight into the impact of labor-saving devices on energy expenditure in everyday domestic tasks is provided by data from an experiment by Lanningham-Foster et al. [33]. A sample of healthy men and women were required to carry out standardized clothes washing and dishwashing tasks by hand and using machines. The amount of time taken to complete the task was recorded and energy expenditure was measured using indirect calorimetry. No significant difference was found in the time taken to complete the tasks but there was a significant reduction in energy expenditure when the machines were used. It was estimated that subjects would expend an additional 44 kcal per day by washing their clothes and dishes

by hand rather than using typical domestic machines for these tasks.

As levels of energy expenditure at work have declined, what people do during their leisure time has assumed increasing importance for overall levels of physical activity. One crucial issue is how much time people have for such activities and a recurrent complaint is that the other demands on their time make it difficult for them to take part in physical activities [1,30]. Time spent at work is one important factor and here the trends over time are complex. Over the longer term there has been a decline in working hours for males but some countries, notably the United States, have seen a reversal of this downward trend in recent years [34]. An added complication has been an increasing polarization with an increasing proportion of people working very long hours even in the context of average declines [35]. For women the picture has been dominated by the increasing numbers entering the workforce and for many, increasing hours at work coupled with the continuing demands of child care and other domestic responsibilities will constrain the time they can devote to leisure-time physical activities. The importance of such factors for leisure-time physical activity has been investigated by Burton and Turrell [30]. In a large sample of employed persons aged 18–64 in Australia, these authors showed that leisure-time physical activity was significantly lower for those working longer hours, particularly for males. They also showed that leisure-time physical activity was significantly lower for those with dependent children, with larger effects for women than for men. Consistent with hours at work being a constraint on appropriate levels of leisure-time physical activity is the observation of a positive association between the prevalence of obesity and average hours worked across 21 OECD countries [15].

Notwithstanding questions of time scarcity, another crucial issue is the extent to which in modern, affluent societies such as the USA and UK many individuals are choosing to spend their leisure time in sedentary pursuits rather than those involving more physical activity. Data from the USA show that many Americans are not physically active on a regular basis, with only a minority achieving recommended levels [36]. Similarly, in the UK only about a third of the population are meeting the overall levels of physical activity recommended by the Chief Medical Officer of England [37], although there is some evidence of an upward trend in sports participation in recent years [27]. In addition to the problem of overall low levels of physical activity, there has been particular concern about the amount of time spent watching television and more recently also on other sedentary pursuits such as computer games and time spent online on the Internet. A meta-analysis has shown statistically significant positive associations between body fatness in children and adolescents and both TV viewing and video/computer game use and negative associations with levels of physical activity [38], although the size of the effects were estimated to be relatively small. Further evidence of the impact of such sedentary behaviors was found in a randomized controlled trial in US elementary school children of the effects a 6-month classroom curriculum to reduce television, videotape and video game use [39]. This showed that the intervention group had statistically significant decreases in BMI and other measures of adiposity relative to the control group. Similar positive results for children aged 4–7 years were found in a more recent randomized controlled trial of the "TV Allowance," an automated device that controls and monitors the use of televisions or computer monitors [40]. Children randomized to the intervention group showed greater reductions in the targeted sedentary behavior, reduced age- and sex-standardized BMI and reduced energy intake than the control group. Positive associations between TV viewing and the risks of obesity have also been found in large prospective cohort studies in both the USA [41] and the United Kingdom [42].

One of the obvious ways in which television viewing could increase the risk of obesity is through its effects on overall levels of energy expenditure. Long hours watching television may limit the time available for other activities, involving higher levels of physical activity, and thereby reduce overall levels of energy expenditure. However, there is evidence of an effect on obesity even after adjustment for total energy expenditure [41,42]. A plausible explanation for this is that television viewing increases the consumption of foods that are associated with increased risk of obesity, particularly those that are heavily advertized [43]. Based on an extensive review of the scientific evidence, Coon and Tucker [44] conclude that greater television use is associated with higher intakes of energy, fat, snacks and carbonated drinks and lower intakes of fruit and vegetables.

For most people for most of human history, moving from place to place has meant walking. This is still the case for many poor people today, particularly in rural areas of Africa and Asia where huge numbers of people are on foot collecting water and firewood, going to work in the fields, traveling to market and generally going about their everyday lives. In addition to many other forms of physical exertion, it is estimated that our hunter/gatherer ancestors walked and ran for 5–10 miles daily as they went in search of their food [45]. The invention of the railway in the 19th century was a turning point but undoubtedly the most profound change has been the massive growth of availability and use of private cars in affluent countries. The impact on patterns of travel has been immense, with the latest National Travel Survey for the UK [46] showing that 80% of total distance traveled was by car or van whereas less than 3% was on foot and less than 1% by bicycle. The average distance walked per person fell from 255 miles in 1975–76 to 192 miles in 2003 with the corresponding figures for cycling being 51 and 34 miles. For short distance trips of under 1 mile, walking and cycling are the dominant mode of transport, accounting for 79% of the total and for 34% of those between 1 and 2 miles. However, this declines rapidly with distance with very few longer trips being on foot or by bicycle. The tendency for average lengths of trips to increase [46] is likely to be a further constraint on the viability of these forms of active travel. This in its turn is closely bound up with aspects of the built environment and urban form which are matters to which we now turn.

The built environment

Since the end of the 1990s there has been an increasing research focus on the role of the built environment as a determinant of obesity. This has been partly driven by the development of novel models which suggest routes by which environmental characteristics may influence body weight [47] as well as the advancement of paradigms, such as the social-ecologic theory of health behavior, which proposed that both physical and social environments may influence obesity via their effect of diet and physical activity behaviors [3].

Whilst much has been written about the potential impact of the environment on obesity-related behaviors, existing empiric evidence regarding the importance of environmental factors is patchy [48], with a large amount of the support that is available coming from studies focusing on recreational walking in adults. In part, this may be to do with the relative ease of measuring walking behaviors in an adult population, but the focus ignores the significant potential of other forms of activity. Furthermore, there is a range of yet to be overcome difficulties in understanding the precise environmental determinants of diet and physical activity. One of the most fundamental issues involves the identification of which type of environment, and which components of that environment, may be most influential.

The majority of individuals function in multiple settings, all of which may influence decisions on food consumption and physical activity. Different types of environmental influences may operate across these multiple domains, encompassing not only physical characteristics but also those associated with social, cultural, and policy environments. Research has tended to focus on the environment of the urban residential neighborhood, in large part due to the high availability of data in such localities. As a consequence, the ways in which characteristics of rural environments, or those around workplaces, may be obesogenic is not well understood. A further issue is that many environmental and social characteristics vary together. For example, deprived neighborhoods often have very different structural characteristics to affluent ones. Failure to adequately account for this risks residual confounding whereby apparent associations with environmental components may, in fact, be associated with inadequately controlled social factors. Indeed, the problems of confounding may be serious enough to explain many of the differences reported between published studies. In response, researchers such as Giles-Corti et al. [49] have called for increased specificity in studies and a move towards the development of models that directly link specific components of the built and social environments with those behaviors which may be most expected to be influenced by them.

Despite the current limitations of this research field, the body of evidence suggests that the built environment exerts a clear, although relatively modest, effect on behaviors associated with obesity. Some of the key evidence from which this conclusion is drawn is reviewed here. The studies use a variety of analytic methodologies and are based on data from different sources and collected in various ways, and not all studies are of a comparable quality. Indeed, most of the evidence published to date comes from cross-sectional comparisons where the outcome (for example, a measure of body mass) and hypothesized explanatory factors (environmental characteristics) are measured at the same time. This type of design, whilst the most common, is relatively weak as the coincident measurement of hypothesized cause and effect means it is not possible to determine if observed associations are causal or associated with other unmeasured factors.

Evidence on the built environment and physical activity

It has been widely suggested that an unsupportive environment may play a part in the reduction of community levels of physical activity and has contributed to the rapid rise of obesity levels. Supportive environments have been used as a part of community interventions to change and influence health behaviors like smoking and sexual health; using the environment to promote physical activity could contribute to the potential impact of a community intervention [50].

From the results of a 2005 Sport England review [51], an evidence-informed model of the potential determinants of physical activity was proposed. Key environmental and individual determinants are proposed to interact to achieve two main domains of physical activity, namely transport activity and leisure-time activity. Key elements of neighborhood variables include parks and other green spaces for physical activity, perceived and actual safety, land use and residential density, the provision of facilities to segregate conflicting road users, and neighborhood attractiveness. The model proposes, for example, that increasing opportunities and access to physical activity via safe, high-quality green space will be associated with increased physical activity, although the existence of an association and how this is modified by individual variables requires detailed study.

Many authors have used the concept of walkability to define the pertinent components of the environment to measure. The concept builds upon the work of planners such as Frank Speilberg who have proposed that the design of modern suburban areas is focused on meeting the needs of those wishing to travel by motor vehicle, and they are consequently poorly planned for pedestrians. These ideas have subsequently been developed and empirically quantified by researchers such as Saelens et al. [52] who have shown that more "walkable" neighborhoods, those where more walking is reported, can be differentiated from their less walkable counterparts by a range of structural characteristics including higher residential density, land use mix, street connectivity, esthetics, and safety.

A large number of studies, the majority from the USA and Australia, have examined the associations of environmental perceptions with physical activity. The perceptions of an individual may act as a proxy for the true characteristics of their environment or may be more related to their own underlying attitudes. The environmental variables considered include measures of safety, availability and access, convenience, local knowledge and

satisfaction, urban form, esthetics, and the supportiveness of neighborhoods. The majority of studies amongst adults that have examined the relationship between perceived neighborhood safety or crime come from the USA and most have found no association with overall physical activity or walking [53]. Similarly, studies examining the effect of perceived access to facilities show no consistent pattern of associations [54,55]. The concept of neighborhood "convenience" overlaps with perceived access and availability but it also adds a dimension of willingness to use a facility and hence may indicate, for example, how easily somebody may fit a visit to the park into their daily routine. Here there is a more consistent pattern, with studies generally reporting positive associations for perceived convenience variables with walking. Typical of the findings are those of Sallis et al. [56], and Hovell et al. [57], who undertook a longitudinal study examining the self-reported neighborhood convenience and physical activity status of a random sample of 2053 USA adults. They found a strong association between perceptions of convenience of facilities and levels of walking.

The concept of "urban form" encompasses those particular attributes of the neighborhood that are related to its structure and connectivity [53]. These include residential density, land use mix, connectivity (for example, how easy it is to walk between two points in a neighborhood using pavements), and neighborhood character. A number of studies have examined the association between perceptions of urban form and physical activity although no picture of consistent associations emerges from them. For example, de Bourdeaudhuij et al. [54] found that self-reported vigorous and leisure-time physical activity was not associated with residential density or land use. Saelens et al. [58] constructed a summary variable for neighborhood walkability by merging data on a variety of perceptions including residential density, land use, esthetics, walking/cycling facilities, safety, and crime. They characterized neighborhoods as high or low walkability, and reported that residents of highly walkable neighborhoods had more than 70 minutes of physical activity per week compared to their low-walkability counterparts.

The concept of a "supportive neighborhood environment" for physical activity suggests that combinations of different components of the environment could make it more attractive to physical activity because of the effect of the sum of its parts, rather than the parts alone. This view is supported by ecologic and social cognitive psychologic theories of the environment, with certain environmental features interacting and reinforcing physical activity behavior. However, studies that have attempted to produce a summary measure of supportiveness have generally not shown consistent positive associations with physical activity [59,60]. Nevertheless, in Perth, Western Australia, Giles-Corti and Donovan [61] found that adults who perceived that their neighborhoods had sidewalks and shops within walking distance were more likely to walk for transport and recreation. Amongst 1936 US adults, Sharpe et al. [62] also found that subjects were more likely to achieve recommended levels of walking if they reported well-maintained sidewalks and the presence of safe areas for exercise in their neighborhood, and a study of children aged 6–11 years in six cities in The Netherlands by de Vries et al. [63] found that the children's perceptions of the "activity friendliness" of their neighborhood was the strongest predictor of their overall activity level.

When physical activity amongst infants and adolescents is considered, parental environmental perceptions may be even more important in determining activity levels than those of the subjects, an issue discussed by Carver et al. [64]. In their review of the environmental correlates of physical activity in youth, Ferreira et al. [65] found that parental and school indicators were strong predictors of activity whilst convincing evidence of other environmental factors was not found. Where environmental associations have been found, they are most frequently associated with safety. For example, Weir et al. [66] found that inner-city children in New York were less active the more concerned their parents were about neighborhood safety, although amongst children as young as 10 years of age, Hume et al. [67] found that child perceptions of the safety of their neighborhood could also be used to predict walking frequency. In a sample of children aged between 6 and 12 years, Holt et al. [68] found that children in more walkable areas were more likely to report outdoor play.

Compared to studies of perceptions, fewer works have examined the associations of objectively measured environmental variables with physical activity. Again, most have been conducted in the USA, Australia, and Canada. Environmental variables examined are diverse and typically derived from on-foot audit or observations of the environment, secondary data such as census returns, and geographical information systems (GIS).

Giles-Corti et al. [69] developed an audit tool (POST) to score the attractiveness of public open spaces. They found that residents of Perth with very good access to large, attractive open spaces were 50% more likely to achieve high levels of walking. A cross-sectional study of 6919 adults from eight European countries also found that the level of greenery and vegetation around the home and surrounding environment was associated with the frequency of physical activity [70], although Hillsdon et al.[71] found no evidence of clear relationships between recreational activity and access to green spaces amongst almost 7000 residents of a small English city.

A limited number of studies have created a summary variable for a supportive neighborhood using a combination of secondary and GIS variables. In Canada, Craig et al. [72] constructed a "neighborhood supportive environment score" for walking using 18 different variables for walkability. The summary score was positively associated with walking to work, after controlling for education, income and area poverty. In the USA Pikora et al. [73] also constructed a combined walkability score based on the presence of features in the local neighborhood including safety, esthetics (cleanliness, green space, etc.), function (pavement quality, street width, traffic volume, etc.) and density of destinations such as local amenities and parks. Increased walkability was associated with higher odds of walking for recreation and transport after adjustment for potential confounders. Amongst 2650

Australian adults, Owen et al. [74] also reported a strong independent positive association between weekly frequency of walking for transport and an objectively derived neighborhood walkability index.

The patterns of associations reported in the literature for other objectively measured environmental characteristics such as access to built facilities, parks and public open spaces and measures of urban form are generally inconsistent, although McCormack et al. [75] found a dose–response relationship between access to a mix of destinations and walking, whereby each additional destination within 1500 m of individuals' residences was associated with an additional 11 minutes spent walking per fortnight. Coastal proximity and access have also been associated with leisure-time activity in two studies [61,76]. For example, in Perth, Western Australia, Giles-Corti and Donovan [61] found that access to the beach, assessed at an individual level, was associated with an increased likelihood of exercising vigorously and exercising vigorously at the recommended level.

Most research investigating urban design has shown a relatively modest but positive association between walking and different aspects of design, in particular high land use mix, property density, street connectivity and the accessibility of services [77,78]. A limitation shared with studies of perceptions is that much evidence comes from the USA where urban structure is very different from that found in other countries. Lake and Townshend [79] also caution that one issue that has not clearly emerged from the existing research is whether the mere inconvenience of owning a car in higher density neighborhoods encourages more walking or cycling rather than the driving forces being urban structure itself.

The built environment and diet

The price and availability of food may mediate the relationship between the environment, diet, and obesity. In particular, it could be that the local availability of a range of high-quality foods improves the quality of diets in local populations. For example, Morland et al. [80] found that the presence of supermarkets in an area was associated with a lower prevalence of obesity, and Rose and Richards [81] reported a positive association between proximity to a supermarket, fruit and vegetable intake and diet quality amongst low-income households. However, there are also strong associations between foodstuff provision and deprivation, making it difficult to determine whether any effect of accessibility is causal or due to the confounding influences of deprivation.

Studies in the USA and Canada have generally found that there are disparities between neighborhoods in the price and availability of food, with lower fat and less energy-dense foods being less available and more expensive in poorer communities [82]. Racial differences in the location of supermarkets have also been observed, with Zenk et al. [83] reporting that supermarkets were, on average, 1.15 miles further away for residents of predominantly black compared to white neighborhoods. Unsurprisingly, the diversity of foods available has also been shown to be more restricted in rural compared to urban areas [84].

Outside the USA, the picture regarding social and environmental equalities in foodstuff provision is less clear. Early studies undertaken in the UK during the 1980s and early 1990s suggested that inequalities existed, with high prices and poor availability being associated with areas of deprivation [85]. However, many of these works were small scale. More recent large and empirically robust observational studies have failed to find an independent association between neighborhood retail food provision, individual diet, and fruit and vegetable intake [86,87], differences in food price, availability and access to supermarkets between deprived and affluent areas [88,89], and reasonable availability of a range of "healthy" foods across contrasting urban areas [90]. Indeed, Pearson et al. [87] reported that age, gender and cultural factors influenced fruit and vegetable intake rather than distance to supermarkets.

Although much of the evidence concerning the links between diet and the retail food environment is cross-sectional, two noteworthy studies have evaluated the effects of the introduction of supermarkets in deprived communities. In Leeds, England, Wrigley et al. [91] found there were some small improvements in fruit and vegetable consumption after supermarket introduction in an area, with larger improvements being observed in individuals initially consuming two or fewer portions per day. However, in Glasgow, Scotland, Cummins et al. [92] found little evidence of any effect; fruit and vegetable consumption increased in an area with a new superstore, but notably also increased in a control group, suggesting secular changes in consumption may have been occurring coincidentally.

Eating out accounts for an average of 7.6% of individual energy intakes in Western societies [93], but foods purchased from fast-food outlets and restaurants are up to 65% more energy dense than the average diet [94] and are associated with lower nutrient intakes [95]. There is evidence that individuals who regularly consume these types of foods are heavier than others, even after controlling for confounding factors [96]. Jeffery et al. [97] examined the relationship between access to fast-food restaurants from both home and workplace settings using a telephone survey of 1033 Minnesota residents. They found eating at "fastfood" (takeaway) restaurants was positively associated with having children, a high-fat diet and high BMI and negatively associated with vegetable consumption and physical activity. However, proximity of these restaurants to home or work was not associated with eating at them or with BMI.

A number of studies have shown that the provision of fast-food outlets is generally greater in more deprived areas [98–100]. A study of the relationship between socio-economic deprivation and the location of McDonalds restaurants in England and Scotland found that per capita outlet provision was four times higher in the most compared to the least deprived census output areas [85], and Powell et al. [101] found that fast-food restaurants were more common in predominantly nonwhite areas in the USA. Indeed, Maddock [102] estimated that the prevalence of such outlets explained approximately 6% of the variance in obesity levels recorded between residents of American states.

Given that obesity, once developed, is difficult to rectify, factors affecting food choices amongst children are of particular concern. Austin et al.[103] found that fast-food restaurants in Chicago had a tendency to be clustered around schools, and Powell et al. [104] reported that adolescents living in areas with high densities of convenience stores had an elevated BMI. Nevertheless, the providers of food to be consumed outside the home have also been identified as an important venue for initiatives to improve dietary intake, such as increasing intakes of fruit and vegetables [79]. School environments are receiving considerable attention as they can shape the eating habits of young people, which may continue into adulthood [105]. In New Zealand, Carter and Swinburn [106] found that "less healthy" choices dominated school food sales and concluded that the school food environment was not generally conducive to healthy eating. In the UK, the campaign by television chef Jamie Oliver was one of the driving forces behind the introduction of new nutritional standards in schools in September 2006 [107].

In summary, evidence from the USA suggests that the availability of high-quality and reasonably priced "healthy" food is constrained for those who live in low-income neighborhoods, and that there may be associations between this observation and patterns of poor diet and obesity. Similar findings are not consistently observed elsewhere. This may be due to distinctive social and racial patterns of segregation present in US neighborhoods, particularly if food supplies are particularly sensitive to these factors. However, many of the published research papers are of poor quality, based on cross-sectional associations. There is a need to build the evidence base with high-quality intervention-based studies that examine the effect of interventions that modify food availability rather than simply examine associations at a single point in time.

Conclusions on the importance of the environment as a determinant of obesity

The evidence presented here illustrates how the environment influences levels of physical activity and obesity. It appears that any influences of the environment are critical yet small in magnitude, that the precise mechanisms by which many components may operate are as yet unclear, and the exact environmental components that affect body weight and activity are yet to be identified. At present, it is difficult to determine how appropriate environmental modification may either prevent further increases in the prevalence of obesity or lead to a reversal of trends. Certainly, the evidence base available is limited by the wide variety of study designs, a general reliance on cross-sectional comparisons, and the diversity of findings.

It is noteworthy that the evidence suggests that when the role of the built environment is examined, perceived environmental characteristics show a stronger and generally more consistent association with body weight and dietary behaviors than those that are objectively measured. This suggests that promising future avenues may seek to modify these perceptions so that the environment is seen as a positive facilitator rather than a negative barrier for healthy eating and an active lifestyle. One important, yet unanswered question is whether the environment exerts its greatest effect amongst people for whom exercise is already important, who have confidence to take part in it, and are surrounded by like-minded individuals. Or, if the right kind of environment is built, will people start to change their beliefs, leading to a collective shift in behavior-modifying attitudes? At present, there is no evidence as to whether or not the environment might have a differential effect on people with different levels of physical activity and body weight. Will modifications to the environment lead to the commencement of physical activity in the sedentary, increase activity in the intermittently active or help the already active sustain it? These questions have not been answered.

A further difficulty arises as a result of the problems in capturing the concept of the social norm and modifying that norm. As illustrated by the evidence presented in this chapter, there are evolutionary pressures meaning that humans readily adapt to environments that promote sedentary behavior and poor-quality food choices, and cultures exist where being active and eating "healthy" foods are not top priorities. No matter how good the availability of high-quality food outlets and physical activity opportunities may be in an area, certain individuals may not ever use them. The behavior of such individuals may be the most difficult to modify, yet from a public health point of view such modification may have the greatest impact. Changing behavior at the community level and creating cultures of participation may be the best solution, which raises unanswered questions as to how this might best be done. It is certainly the case that changes to the environment alone are unlikely to solve the problems of current trends in obesity. Successfully tackling these issues will undoubtedly require a range of approaches, and complementary strategies addressing the individual, social, and environmental determinants of activities may be a solution.

References

1. Hill JO, Wyatt HR, Reed GW, Peters JC. Obesity and the environment: where do we go from here? Science 2003;299:853–5.
2. Friedman JM. Obesity in the new millennium. Nature 2000;404: 632–4.
3. Swinburn B, Egger G, Raza F. Dissecting obesogenic environments: the development and application of a framework for identifying and prioritizing environmental interventions for obesity. Prev Med 1999;29:563–70.
4. Friedman JM. A war on obesity, not the obese. Science 2003;299: 856–8.
5. Neel JV. Diabetes mellitus: a "thrifty" genotype rendered detrimental by "progress". Am J Hum Genet 1962;14:353–62.
6. Eaton SB, Eaton SB. An evolutionary perspective on human physical activity: implications for health. Comp Biochem Physiol Pt A 2003;136:153–9.
7. Prentice AM, Rayco-Solon P, Moore SE. Insights from the developing world: thrifty genotypes and thrifty phenotypes. Proc Nutr Soc 2005;64:153–61.
8. Wells JCK. The evolution of human fatness and susceptibility to obesity: an ethological approach. Biol Rev 2006;81, 183–205.
9. Chakravarty MV, Booth FW. Eating exercise, and "thrifty" genotypes: connecting the dots toward an evolutionary understanding of modern chronic diseases. J Appl Physiol 2004;96:3–10.
10. Heini AF, Weinsier RL. Divergent trends in obesity and fat intake patterns: the American paradox. Am J Med 1997;102, 259–264.
11. Prentice AM, Jebb SA. Obesity in Britain: gluttony or sloth? BMJ 1995;311:437–9.
12. Jebb SA. Dietary determinants of obesity. Obes Rev 2007;8(suppl 1):93–7.
13. Bell EA, Castellanos VH, Pelkman CL, et al. Energy density of foods affects energy intake in normal weight women. Am J Clin Nutr 1998;67:412–20.
14. Ello-Martin JA, Ledikwe JH, Rolls BJ. The influence of food portion size and energy density on energy intake: implications for weight management. Am J Clin Nutr 2005;82(suppl):236S–241S.
15. Foresight. *Tackling obesities: future choices – Project Report.* London: Government Office for Science, 2007.
16. Drewnowski A, Darmon N. Food choice and diet costs: an economic analysis. J Nutr 2005;135:900–4.
17. Glanz K, Basil M, Maibach E, et al. Why Americans eat what they do: taste, nutrition, cost, convenience, and weight control concerns as influences on food consumption. J Am Dietet Assoc 1998;98: 1118–26.
18. French S, Story M, Jeffery RW. Environmental influences on eating and physical activity. Annu Rev Pub Health 2001;22:309–35.
19. Bowman SA, Vinyard BT. Fast food consumption of U.S. adults: impacts on energy and nutrient intakes and overweight status. J Am Coll Nutr 2004;23:163–8.
20. Bowman S, Gortmaker SL, Ebbeling CB, et al. Effects of fast food consumption on energy intake and diet quality among children in a national household survey. Pediatrics 2004;113:112–18.
21. Neilsen SJ, Popkin BM. Patterns and trends in food portion sizes, 1977–1998. JAMA 2003;289, 450–3.
22. Cordain L, Gotshall RW, Eaton SB, Eaton SB. Physical activity, energy expenditure and fitness: an evolutionary perspective. Int J Sports Med 1998;19:328–35.
23. Egger GJ, Vogels N, Westerterp KR. Estimating historical changes in physical activity. Med J Aust 2001;175:635–7.
24. James WPT. A public health approach to the problem of obesity. Int J Obes 1995;19:S37–S45.
25. Ainsworth BE, Haskell WL, Whitt MC, et al. Compendium of physical activities: an update of activity codes and MET intensities. Med Sci Sports Exerc 2000;32(9 suppl):S498–S504.
26. Sobek M. Occupations. In: Carter SB, Gartner SS, Haines MR, et al. (eds) *Historical Statistics of the United States. Earliest Times to the Present*, millennium edition, vol 2. New York: Cambridge University Press, 2006: 2–35-2–40.
27. Stamatakis E, Ekelund U, Wareham NJ. Temporal trends in physical activity in England: the Health Survey for England 1991 to 2004. Prev Med 2007;45:416–23.
28. Roman-Vinas B, Serra-Majem L, Ribas-Barba L, et al. Trends in physical activity in Catalonia (1992–2003). Pub Health Nutr 2007;10:1389–95.

29. Kaleta D, Jegier A. Occupational energy expenditure and leisure-time physical activity. Int J Occup Med Environ Health 2005;18: 351–6.

30. Burton NW, Turrell G. Occupation, hours worked, and leisure-time physical activity. Prev Med 2000;31:673–81.

31. Ellis E, Grimsley M, Goyder E, et al. Physical activity and health: evidence from a study of deprived communities in England. J Pub Health 2007;29:27–34.

32. Bowers DE. Cooking trends echo changing roles of women. Food Rev 2000;23:23–9.

33. Lanningham-Foster L, Nysse LJ, Levine JA. Labor saved, calories lost: the energetic impact of domestic labor-saving devices. Obes Res 2003;11:1178–81.

34. Evans JM, Lippoldt DC, Marianna P. *Trends in Working Hours in OECD Countries*. OECD Labor Market and Social Policy Occasional Paper No. 45. Paris: OECD Publishing, 2001.

35. Rones PL, Ilg RE, Gardner JM. Trends in hours of work since the mid-1970s. Monthly Labor Rev 1997;April:3–14.

36. Macera CA, Jones DA, Yore MM, et al. Prevalence of physical activity, including lifestyle activities among adults – United States, 2000–2001. MMWR 2003;52:764–9.

37. Department of Health. *Choosing Activity; A Physical Activity Action Plan*. London: Department of Health Publications, 2005.

38. Marshall SJ, Biddle SJH, Gorely T, et al. Relationship between media use, body fatness and physical activity in children and youth: a meta-analysis. Int J Obes 2004;28:1238–46.

39. Robinson TN. Reducing children's television viewing to prevent obesity. A randomised controlled trial. JAMA 1999;282:1561–7.

40. Epstein LH, Roemmich JN, Robinson JL, et al. A randomised trial of the effects of reducing television viewing and computer use on body mass index in young children. Arch Pediatr Adolesc Med 2008;162:239–45.

41. Hu FB, Li TY, Colditz GA, et al. Television watching and other sedentary behaviors in relation to risk of obesity and type 2 diabetes mellitus in women. JAMA 2003;289:1785–91.

42. Jakes RW, Day NE, Khaw K-T, et al. Television viewing and low participation in vigorous recreation are independently associated with obesity and markers of cardiovascular disease risk: EPIC-Norfolk population-based study. Eur J Clin Nutr 2003;57:1089–96.

43. Robinson TN. Television viewing and childhood obesity. Pediatr Clin North Am 2001;48:1017–25.

44. Coon KA, Tucker KL. Television and children's consumption patterns: a review of the literature. Minerva Pediatr 2002;54:423–36.

45. O'Keefe JH, Cordain L. Cardiovascular disease resulting from a diet and lifestyle at odds with our paleolithic genome: how to become a 21st-century hunter gatherer. Mayo Clin Proc 2004;79:101–8.

46. Department for Transport. *National Travel Survey*. London: Department For Transport, 2007.

47. Ulijaszek SJ. Frameworks of population obesity and the use of cultural consensus modeling in the study of environments contributing to obesity. Economics Hum Biol 2007;5:443–57.

48. Ball K, Timperio AF, Crawford DA. Understanding environmental influences on nutrition and physical activity behaviours: where should we look at what should we count? Int J Behav Nutr Phys Activity 2006;3:33.

49. Giles-Corti B, Timperio A, Bull F, Pikora T. Understanding physical activity environmental correlates: increased specificity for ecological models. Exercise and Sport Science Reviews Exerc Sport Sci Rev 2005;33:175–81.

50. Cavill N, Foster C. How to promote health enhancing physical activity: community interventions. In: Oja P, Borns J (eds) *Health Enhancing Physical Activity*. Berlin: International Council of Sport Science and Physical Activity, 2004.

51. Foster C, Hillsdon M, Cavil N, Allender S, Coburn G. *Understanding Participation in Sport: A Systematic Review*. London: Sport England, 2005.

52. Saelens BE, Sallis JF, Frank LD. Environmental correlates of walking and cycling: findings from the transportation, urban design, and planning literatures. Ann Behav Med 2003;25:80–91.

53. Wilcox S, Bopp M, Oberrecht L, Kammermann S, McElmurray C. Psychosocial and perceived environmental correlates of physical activity in rural and older African American and white women. J Gerontol B: Psychol Sci Soc Sci 2003;58:P329–37.

54. de Bourdeaudhuij I, Sallis J, Saelens B. Environmental correlates of physical activity in a sample of Belgian adults. Am J Health Prom 2003;18:83–92.

55. Huston S, Evenson K, Bors P, Gizlice Z. Neighborhood environment, access to places for activity, and leisure-time physical activity in a diverse North Carolina population. Am J Health Prom 2003;18:58–69.

56. Sallis JF, Hovell MF, Hofstetter CR, et al. A multivariate study of determinants of vigorous exercise in a community sample. Prev Med 1989;18:20–34.

57. Hovell MF, Hofstetter CR, Sallis JF, Rauh MJ, Barrington E. Correlates of change in walking for exercise: an exploratory analysis. Res Q Exerc Sport 1992;63:425–34.

58. Saelens B, Sallis J, Black J, Chen D. Neighbourhood-based differences in physical activity: an environment scale evaluation. Am J Pub Health 2003;93:1552–58.

59. Troped P, Saunders R, Pate R, Reininger B, Addy C. Correlates of recreational and transportation physical activity among adults in a New England community. Prev Med 2003;37:304–10.

60. Suminski R, Carlos Poston W, Petosa R, Stevens E, Katzenmoyer L. Features of the neighborhood environment and walking by US adults. Am J Prev Med 2005;28:149–55.

61. Giles-Corti B, Donovan RJ. Socio-economic status differences in recreational physical activity levels and real and perceived access to a supportive physical environment. Prev Med 2002;35:601–11.

62. Sharpe P, Granner M, Hutto B, Ainsworth B. Association of environmental factors to meeting physical activity recommendations in two South Carolina counties. Am J Health Prom 2004;18:251–7.

63. de Vries SI, Bakker I, Mechelen WV, Hopman-Rock M. Determinants of activity friendly Neighborhoods for Children: results from the SPACE study. Am J Health Prom 2007;21:312–16.

64. Carver A, Timperio A, Crawford D. Playing it safe: the influence of neighbourhood safety on children's physical activity – a review. Health and Place 2008;14(2):217–27.

65. Ferreira I, van der Horst K, Wendel-Vos W, Kremers S, van Lenthe FJ, Brug J. Environmental correlated of physical activity in youth – a review and update. Obes Rev 2006;8:129–54.

66. Weir LA, Etelson D, Brand DA. Parents' perceptions of neighbourhood safety and children's physical activity. Prev Med 2006; 43:212–17.

67. Hume C, Salmon J, Ball K. Associations of children's perceived neighbourhood environments with walking and physical activity. Am J Health Prom 2007;21:201–7.

68. Holt NL, Spence JC, Sehn ZL, Cutumisu N. Neighbourhood and developmental differences in children's perceptions of

opportunities for play and physical activity. Health and Place 2008;14:2–14.

69. Giles-Corti B, Broomhill M, Knuiman M, et al. Encouraging walking: how important is distance to, attractiveness and size of public open space? Am J Prev Med 2005;28(2S2):169–76.

70. Ellaway A, Macintyre S, Bonnefoy X. Graffiti, greenery, and obesity in adults: secondary analysis of European cross sectional survey. BMJ 2005;331:611–12.

71. Hillsdon M, Panter J, Foster C, Jones A. The relationship between access and quality of urban green space with population physical activity. Public Health 2006;120:1127–32.

72. Craig CL, Brownson RC, Cragg SE, Dunn AL. Exploring the effect of the environment on physical activity: a study examining walking to work. Am J Prev Med 2002;23(2):36–43.

73. Pikora TJ, Giles-Corti B, Knuiman MW, Bull FC, Jamrozik K, Donovan RJ. Neighborhood environmental factors correlated with walking near home: using SPACES. Med Sci Sports Exerc 2006;38: 708–14.

74. Owen N, Cerin E, Leslie E, et al. Neighborhood walkability and the walking behavior of Australian adults. Am J Prev Med 2007;33: 387–95.

75. McCormack GR, Giles-Corti B, Bulsara M. The relationship between destination proximity, destination mix and physical activity behaviours. Prev Med 2008;46(1):33–40.

76. Bauman A, Smith B, Stoker L, Bellew B, Booth M. Geographical influences upon physical activity participation: evidence of a "coastal effect". Aust NZ J Pub Health 1999;23:322–4.

77. Frank LD, Schmid TL, Sallis JF, Chapman J, Saelens BE. Linking objectively measured physical activity with objectively measured urban form: findings from SMARTRAQ. Am J Prev Med 2005; 28(2S2):117–25.

78. Doyle S, Kelly-Schwartz A, Schlossberg M, Stockard J. Active community environments and health: the relationship of walkable and safe communities to individual health. J Am Plan Assoc 2006;72:19–32.

79. Lake A, Townshend T. Obesogenic environments: exploring the built and food environments. J Roy Soc Prom Health 2006;126:262–7.

80. Morland K, Diez-Roux ACV, Wing S. The influence of supermarkets and other stores on obesity. Am J Prev Med 2006;30:333–9.

81. Rose D, Richards R. Food store access and household fruit and vegetable use among participants in the US Food Stamp Program. Pub Health Nutr 2004;7:1081–8.

82. Chung C, Myers SL. Do the poor pay more for food? An analysis of grocery store availability and food price disparities. J Consum Aff 1999;33:276–96.

83. Zenk SN, Schulz AJ, Israel BA, James SA, Bao S, Wilson ML. Neighbourhood racial composition, neighbourhood poverty, and the spatial accessibility of supermarkets in metropolitan Detroit. Am J Pub Health 2005;95:660–7.

84. Blanchard T, Lyson T. Access to low cost groceries in non-metropolitan counties: large retailers and the creation of food deserts. Available at: http://srdc.msstaste.edu/measuring/Blanchard.pdf.

85. Cummins S, McKay L, Macintyre S. McDonald's Restaurants and neighbourhood deprivation in Scotland and England. Am J Prev Med 2005;4:308–10.

86. White M, Bunting J, Raybould S, Adamson A, Williams L, Mathers J. *Do Food Deserts Exist? A Multi-Level, Geographical Analysis of the Relationship Between Food Access, Socio-Economic Position and Dietary Intake*. Report to the Food Standards Agency. Newcastle upon Tyne: Institute of Health and Society, 2004.

87. Pearson T, Russell J, Campbell MJ. Barker ME. Do "food-deserts" influence fruit and vegetable consumption? A cross-sectional study. Appetite 2005;45:195–7.

88. Cummins S, Macintyre S. The location of food stores in urban areas: a case study in Glasgow. Br Food J 1999;101:545–53.

89. Cummins S, Macintyre S. A systematic study of an urban foodscape: the price and availability of food in Greater Glasgow. Urban Studies 2002;39:2115–30.

90. Guy C, David G. Measuring physical access to "healthy foods" in areas of social deprivation: a case study in Cardiff. Int J Consum Stud 2004;28:222–34.

91. Wrigley N, Warm D, Margetts B. Deprivation, diet and food retail access: findings from the Leeds "Food Deserts" study. Environ Plan A 2003;35:151–8.

92. Cummins S, Findlay A, Higgins C, Petticrew M, Sparks L. Do large-scale food retail interventions improve diet and health? BMJ 2005;330:6843–4.

93. DEFRA. Family Food in 2004–5. 2006. Available at: http://statistics.defra.gov.uk/esg/publications/efs/005/complete.pdf

94. Prentice AM, Jebb SA. Fast foods, energy density and obesity: a possible mechanistic link. Obes Rev 2003;4:187–94.

95. Burns C, Jackson M, Gibbons C, Stoney RM. Foods prepared outside the home: association with selected nutrients and body mass index in adult Australians. Pub Health Nutr 2002;5:441–8.

96. Cummins S, Macintyre S. Food environments and obesity – neighbourhood or nation? Int J Epidemiol 2006;35:100–4.

97. Jeffery RW, Baxter JE, McGuire MT, Linde JA. Are fast food restaurants an environmental risk factor for obesity? Int J Behav Nutr Phys Activ 2006;3:2.

98. Reidpath D, Burns C, Garrard D, Mahoney M, Townsend M. An ecological study of the relationship between social and environmental determinants of obesity. Health and Place 2002;8:141–5.

99. Block JP, Scribner RA, DeSalvo KB. Fast food, race/ethnicity and income. A geographic analysis. Am J Prev Med 2004;27: 211–17.

100. Macintyre S, McKay L, Cummins S, Burns C. Out-of-home food outlets and area deprivation: case study in Glasgow, UK. Int J Behav Nutr Phys Activ 2005;2:16.

101. Powell LM, Auld CM, Chaloupka FJ, O'Malley PM, Johnston LD. Associations between access to food stores and adolescent Body Mass Index. Am J Prev Med 2007;33:S301–S307.

102. Maddock J. The relationship between obesity and the prevalence of fast food restaurants: state-level analysis. Am J Health Prom 2004;19:137–43.

103. Austin SB, Melly SJ, Sanchez BN, Patel A, Buka S, Gortmaker SL. Clustering of fast-food restaurants around schools: a novel application of spatial statistics to the study of food environments. Am J Pub Health 2005;95:1575–81.

104. Powell LM, Chaloupka FJ, Bao Y. The availability of fast-food and full-service restaurants in the U.S.: associations with neighborhood characteristics, Am J Prev Med 2007;33:S240–S245.

105. Ludvigsen A, Sharma N. *Burger Boy and Sporty Girl: Children and Young People's Attitudes Towards Food in School*. London: Barnado's Foundation, 2004.

106. Carter MA, Swinburn B. Measuring the "obesogenic" food environment in New Zealand primary schools. Health Prom Int 2004;19: 15–20.

107. Department for Education and Skills. *Healthy Living: New School Food and Drink Standards*. London: HMSO, 2006.

33 Obesity: Using the Ecologic Public Health Approach to Overcome Policy Cacophony

Geof Rayner and Tim Lang

Centre for Food Policy, City University, London, UK

Introduction

Although the argument that obesity is a medical and public health problem has won credence in public health circles, that it is a failure of social, economic or public policy has been less often articulated. Taking the example of the UK (although the analysis is potentially applicable to many other societies), this chapter seeks to redress that imbalance by examining the powerful forces engaged in creating obesity within commerce and markets (supply chain factors), within government (the role of the state) and among individuals, families and communities (as consumers or in other capacities). It argues that policy makers must recognize that the rise in obesity represents challenges for all three arenas. The chapter concludes by sketching the parameters of a new ecologic public health approach, which clarifies the different dimensions of existence – physical, physiologic, social and cognitive – in which the obesity drivers exposed by research are manifest. It is proposed that tackling obesity will require an immense and complex concerted effort, analogous to efforts to combat climate change, across all four dimensions by all three sets of forces – supply chains, government and people themselves. Minor adjustments, for example those which appeal solely to individual behavior change, will in contrast produce only minor effects.

Clinical Obesity in Adults and Children, 3rd edition. Edited by Peter G. Kopelman, Ian D. Caterson and William H. Dietz.
© 2010 Blackwell Publishing, ISBN: 978-1-4051-8226-3.

Background

Like others, we see the recent rise in obesity as the result of past decades of societal, technical and ideologic change. The pace and scale of change may only now be gaining attention, but the evidence has been strong for decades [1]. Part of the search for solutions must be the investigation not just of what the drivers of obesity over time have been but how they interact. Too many analyses of obesity are locked into disciplinary "boxes" when, given the complexity and breadth of such drivers – what we refer to refer to here as "interdimensionality" – it's likely that obesity requires a broader interdisciplinary analysis and a sustained, society-wide response. By implication, "quick fixes" or single-factor remedies are unlikely to work.

On a positive note, political processes, globally, regionally and nationally, are beginning to emerge giving due priority to the issue and the severity of warnings. In the UK, after a National Audit Office report and the Chief Medical Officer's clarion call about obesity being a "timebomb," obesity climbed up the national policy agenda [2,3]. A parliamentary inquiry spelled out the complexity of the issues and gave suggestions for direction of travel [4]. All the devolved governments of the UK now have commitments to tackle obesity. In England, after an arguably false start in seeing obesity solely within the area of individual choice, a more integrated obesity strategy – a balance of social determinants and calls for individual behavior change – has emerged [5]. However, even the briefest review of recent trends shows the scale of difficulties and the measure of the forces arrayed against a public health approach to obesity.

In Scotland, childhood obesity is rising rapidly, with levels of overweight and obesity among younger and older children at double the levels that might have been expected on the basis of data for the UK as a whole [6]. Currently in Scotland, 26% of women and 22% of men have a Body Mass Index (BMI) of >30 and 65% of men and 60% of women have a BMI of >25 [7]. Data from the Scottish Health Survey 2003 reported that people living in the most deprived areas were more likely than those in the least deprived areas to be obese or morbidly obese, and morbid obesity was three times higher among women in the lowest-income households than in the highest.

In England, *The Health of the Nation*, the English national strategy for public health introduced by a Conservative government, established a target to reduce the proportion of obese men aged 16–64 in the population from 7% in 1986–87 to 6% in 2005, and obese women from 12% in 1986–87 to 8% in 2005. By 1993, a review by the National Audit Office showed that the proportions of obese men and women in the population had risen to 13% and 16% [8]. By 2003, 22% of men and 23% of women were obese [9]. Childhood obesity in 2–10 year olds has risen from 9.9% in 1995 to 14.3% in 2004. On current trends, 20% of 2–10 year olds, more than 1 million children, will be obese by 2010. The most dramatic predictions for future trends came through the Foresight obesity study, under the auspices of the Government Office for Science. This predicted that by 2050, 60% of men, 50% of women, half of primary school boys and a fifth of primary school girls will be obese [10].

In order to redirect these trends, in 2006 the Labour Government in England, through the Department of Health, began by promoting a new initiative based on social marketing – the use of commercial marketing techniques for noncommercial purposes – called "Small Change, Big Difference." Although this differed somewhat from the US approach to social marketing, focusing heavily on changing individual behavior, it was nevertheless still framed in terms of the personalization of health choices [11]. The Government in England introduced a new obesity target for children but, given the greater sweep of opportunities for intervention by local government, inserted obesity prevention into Local Area Agreements (LAA), the national–local framework for service delivery. One example of an LAA obesity target is for the northern town of Barnsley. Agreed in July 2005, this sets a maximum prevalence target for obesity of 15.5% for children aged 2–10 years [12]. This figure is all the more striking given that the prevalence of obesity in 1984 among 4–12 year olds in England was 0.6% in boys and 1.3% in girls [13]. Other LAA targets relate to precursors of obesity, such as participation in sports or access to free school meals. The implication, perhaps, is that an ambitious target would not be likely to be achieved. By 2007, following the publication of the Foresight report, a revamping of the strategy occurred [5], retaining, in part, an emphasis on social marketing but also much more focused on changing the determinants of obesity, in the words of the accompanying press release, by "support(ing) the creation of a healthy society – from early years, to schools and food, from sport and physical activity to planning, transport and the health service" [14]. This strategy is not considered here, but rather the context in which the strategy has been established.

The figures for most of Europe are not as alarming as for the UK. Nevertheless, they are moving in the same direction. In policy terms, there is maneuvering and "testing" of strength of feeling and options, with ministries of health, pediatricians and others often worried, but politicians in some countries (like Italy) resistant. Targets are also being set but as yet, as in the UK, there are few strong interventions to deliver them. Currently evolving policy frameworks, including that of the European Commission's Obesity Round Table begun in 2004 and subsequently the EU Platform on Diet, Physical Activity and Health, draw on the 1996 Amsterdam Treaty health powers, appear "soft" rather than "hard", and rely on good will and voluntary action more than structural, regulatory or fiscal change [15]. The UK stands in contrast to other European countries because obesity is hardly ever out of the headlines and the issue of obesity is taken seriously by politicians.

The problem of policy cacophony

There are many competing diagnoses of what "really" matters in obesity generation and about the evidence. Different analyses and policy solutions have been developed and proffered, each clamoring for support, funding and adoption. The increasing sophistication of different positions actually adds to the complexity of the policy challenge. For policy makers, many now worried about the cost of obesity (and the spectrum of ailments linked to it, such as diabetes), there is a situation we describe as policy cacophony – noise drowning out the symphony of effort. This cacophony is not helpful because policy makers need coherent directions on which they feel they can deliver. Obesity policy is already weighed down by complexity, accentuated by the multilevel (global, European, national, regional and local) nature of modern systems of governance. It is also shrouded by ideologic fears such as interventions being interpreted as "nanny-ish" or restricting "personal" choices in food and lifestyle. The decline in trust afforded to government, the loss of deference and increasing individualism have propelled the "choice agenda" based upon the assumption that people should make healthier choices for themselves, rather than through government [16].

Compounding this policy cacophony are three other difficulties which this chapter sets out to address. The first is timeframe. Obesity is a problem that has taken decades to develop. Bar sudden external shocks to society, such as a massive oil shortage or steep price rises and food shortages that make eating less or walking a necessity, it's likely to take many years to bring it under control. Yet the political timetable demands quick results. Secondly, there is a difficulty about evidence. What many have described as an epidemic has been open to wide interpretation – and what may seem incontrovertible to many is debated by others. To some extent, part of the obesity policy problem is the evidence, or lack of it. No country has managed to reverse obesity trends, or at least not so far. Yet the rise of obesity is literally visible and the explanation and ways forward are hard to pinpoint. This does not mean we favor disregarding evidence, but rather that we see obesity as a test case for policy changes in advance of perfect evidence. Faint hearts privately muse that obesity is too complex but we see obesity as akin to climate change – complex, yes, and demanding firm action, however hard that might be. The third difficulty is public knowledge and belief, which set the background to government (or for that matter business) confidence that things can and must change. This is the issue of "lock in" or, as economists might say, "path dependency," the tendency for societies to maintain patterns of belief and behavior (organizationally and individually) until some major event resets the default position. Later we look a number of scenarios for how this might occur.

What is the problem – and why?

Why is obesity a problem? Who is it a problem for? Where did it come from? These simple questions have to be asked. Half a century ago, in the years following World War 2, millions of UK citizens and other Europeans went hungry, and obesity as a medical condition appeared little more than a curiosity. These events framed determination on both sides of the Iron Curtain to rebuild agriculture (albeit in different ways) [17–19]. Even just a decade ago, with most of Europe more than adequately fed and EU farming policy consuming almost half of the EU budget, the average politician might have remarked that obesity was an irrelevance. To find a comparable society suffering from obesity meant traveling to the USA.

Until just two decades ago, Britons flattered themselves that the UK, even with its constricted food culture, possessed factors that immunized it from US trends: smaller food portion sizes, cost-conscious purchasing habits, a less car-dominated society, and perhaps too the personal resolve among its citizens to maintain optimal body shape in a social environment less concerned with consumption volume. But the UK, and the rest of Europe, appears to be steadily succumbing to what is sometimes unfairly called the "Americanization" of diet and society: the rise and rise of car culture and other technical "advances" marginalizing daily physical activity; widening distances between homes and work or shops; the overconsumption of food accompanied by its unprecedented, plentiful availability; the culture of clever and constant advertising flattering choice; the shift from mealtime eating to permanent "grazing"; the replacement of water or milk by sugary soft drinks; the rising influence of large commercial concerns framing what is available and what sells; and more [20–23].

Today, the rise in population weight in the UK remains behind US trends, but only as a matter of degree. Copious evidence exists that both adults and children are affected by rising weight. The UK is now one of the leading countries for population weight gain, although there is still considerable variation in trends across the OECD countries, as shown in Table 33.1.

Most worryingly, the biggest national weight increases among children have been in countries such as Greece and Spain or in

Table 33.1 Obese population, % total population, BMI > 30 kg/m²

	1980	1990	2005
Japan (1980, 1990, 2004)	2	2.3	3
Switzerland (1992, 2002)		5.4	7.7
Norway (1995, 2005)		5	9
France (1990, 2004)		5.8	9.5
Italy (1994, 2005)		7	9.9
Netherlands (1981, 1990, 2005)	5.1	6.1	10.7
Sweden (1989, 1997, 2005)	5.5	7.9	10.7
Denmark (1987, 1994, 2005)	5.5	7.6	11.4
Iceland (1990, 2002)		7.5	12.4
Poland (1996, 2004)		11.4	12.5
Belgium (1997, 2004)		11.1	12.7
Spain (1987, 1995, 2003)	6.8	10.3	13.1
Finland (1980, 1990, 2005)	7.4	8.4	14.1
Czech Republic (1993, 2002)		11.3	14.8
Slovak Republic (1993, 2003)		18.9	15.4
Canada (1994, 2005)		12.1	18
Luxembourg (1997, 2005)		14.9	18.6
New Zealand (1989, 1997, 2003)	11.1	17	20.9
Australia (1980, 1989, 1999)	8.3	10.8	21.7
United Kingdom (1980, 1991, 2005)	7	14	23
United States (1976–80, 1988–94, 2003–04)	15	23.3	32.2

Source: OECD Health Data 2007 [24].

the poorer areas of southern Italy, where rates are close to those of the US [25], areas previously justly celebrated for their diet, high in vegetables, pulses and unrefined carbohydrates, culturally close to the land [26,27]. While this needs to be researched, it is possible that a transition to a diet composed of energy-dense foods (high in fat and low in fiber) makes speediest headway in countries that have had high income growth and exposure to more commercialized food pressures. Obesity is emerging in places with previously strong and protective food cultures, with children most at risk.

Although obesity is highly complex, there are some core truths on which thinking can be developed. We suggest the following.
• Obesity isn't just a phenomenon of the UK or the USA. Rates are rising across Europe but there is a particularly worrying acceleration of rates among children [26,28].
• Obesity is known to lead to medical problems, long documented although only formally classified by the World Health Organization (WHO) in 1997 [1].
• Obesity is strongly linked with other social and health inequalities and vulnerabilities, such as social class, ethnicity or genetic factors [29–33].
• There are serious and rising social and financial burdens stemming both directly and indirectly from obesity [34–41].
• Obesity is linked to other societal trends and risks, such as changed food production, falling food prices, motorized transportation and work–home and lifestyle patterns [1,4,15,29,38,42–47].

Policy makers have been slow to recognize the seriousness of the issue, which suggests the public health movement has been slow or ineffective in its advocacy work or that the evidence isn't easily translatable into policy or lacks political champions [48,49].

Remedies based on individual action alone, whether diet plans, surgery or stigma, have limited effectiveness in population terms and often come at a high cost. Part of the difficulty in generating effective policy is having a policy package that will deliver a corrective population-wide shift [26,50,51].

There is a powerful temptation in government to limit actions to a choice-based, personalization approach, in part because this style of intervention is aligned to the commercial sector's own customer management and marketing methods but also because a cross-society approach appears so big in conception that it appears unachievable and failure is assumed [52,53].

Both in the UK and more widely in Europe, and despite some welcome initiatives [11,28], there are, as yet, no comprehensive structures or set of policy models for what to do about obesity. There is as yet no Finland or North Karelia project doing for obesity what that country did for tackling premature diet-related ill health from the 1970s [54]. Europe-wide, we are generally still at the "talking stage" of policy, albeit with some specific initiatives, some mild if inconclusive results, and a variety of targets, rather than well into implementation.

Food companies aren't adequately changing their behavior in response to the request to do so by the WHO under its *Global Strategy on Diet, Physical Activity and Health*. An early review showed that the big food companies were for the most part unconcerned [55]. A more recent review of companies involved in the European Platform on Diet Physical Activity and Health complained that company reporting was "barely adequate" [56].

The complex challenge that obesity raises in terms of governance: who decides which policies?

For all the above reasons, obesity has to be seen as not just a technical, food, physical activity or healthcare problem but a challenge for what sort of society is being built. This is why obesity is beginning to engage social policy interest [57]. The deceptively simple issue of how to encourage physical activity across daily life and modify dietary intake in fact raises complex questions about the need to reshape public policy across a number of areas. These include:

• *agriculture:* because policy affects what is produced and how much
• *manufacturing:* for ingredients, portions and products
• *retail:* for planning, prices, availability and location
• *education:* for health knowledge and food and physical activity skills
• *public procurement:* for determining the healthiness of food choices in institutional or public settings

• *culture:* for the shaping of consciousness around consumption and physical activity
• *trade:* for product pricing and terms of trade
• *economics:* for differential taxation and subsidy of foods
• *environment:* for the walkability of neighborhoods.

Part of the complexity is how to judge what is the appropriate level for policy action and intervention. Who is responsible – local, national or international governance? And how radical or limited should policy be? Small, incremental, publicity-driven (i.e. social market-based) changes might suit the existing balance of policy interests, but what if evidence suggests that a more extensive, co-ordinated, cross-sectoral and interdimensional framework of action would be more effective?

The full extent of the interdimensionality of causation was constructed in the Foresight "obesity map." This resembles a bowl of spaghetti (in fact, a presentation of dynamic flows around energy balance at the center) [10]. Such mapping and analysis support the view, emphasized here, that there may be little pay-off from working on one aspect of obesity without tackling other determinants as well [4]. The challenge is to produce policy analyses and solutions that work *across* policy boxes not just *within* them.

And, again, there is the problem of evidence. Despite the persistent calls for evidence-based policy, obesity illustrates the gap between policy and evidence [58]. How much evidence of prevalence and impact will it take for policy to change? How might that be accumulated and interpreted? Where is the role model (again, Finland's North Karelia project) for obesity that might encourage policy makers not to be fatalistic about obesity? (Might it be Sweden this time? Certainly the debate around obesity in Sweden, contrasted with the UK, suggests that a social consensus for action is far more likely [59].) Is a "beacon country" even possible in a globalizing world? The Finns tell us they could not do today what they undertook 30 years ago; today's policy makers lack the control over media (advertising, lifestyle), agriculture and cultural coherence that they had then. And is modern policy reliance on consumer choice as a driver of change adequate to deal with obesity, especially given the vulnerabilities of social class, sex, age and genetics? Will better food labeling, despite all the attention given to it, have any sustained, positive effect? Or might prices that internalize currently externalized health costs be a better option [60–63]?

These and many such questions explain why obesity is a major challenge not just for European medicine and public health but for governance, the art and practice of government and public as well as private decision making, let alone shifting food supply patterns. It's also the reason why the appeal for policy makers of taking a science-based, though in fact medicalized route of individualized treatment through drugs, therapy and, at the most extreme, bariatric surgery, is still considerable. If obesity is caused by a matrix of factors and policies beyond the health sector, how can health policy makers win sufficient attention to ask other ministers to drive change? There is a risk of appearing to be doing something, by announcing targets unconnected to intervention processes supplemented by a few limited initiatives or projects or providing research grants in pursuit of wonder drugs or technical fixes such as functional foods or nutrigenomics. Obesity prevention could even evolve as a major research and policy intervention "industry," as with drug misuse or tobacco cessation, with mounting expense to the public purse, but unable to deal with the fundamentals. It may only endlessly address symbols and symptoms rather than causes.

Even as the scientific understanding of obesity becomes more sophisticated, the overall policy situation becomes potentially more muddled. The lack of solid evidence can lead to uncertainty over what action to take [4,64,65]. Political leadership in the name of public health is sorely needed. It was effective in kick-starting debate [3] but the extent of change needed requires more than heroics or advice from on high and the breadth of policy change falls beyond the policy expertise of the current cader of public health professionals. It requires an entire culture shift by society, markets and supply chains and government. No wonder obesity is such a thorny problem for policy makers. The public health world's divided and confused messages haven't helped. More policy-oriented research and thinking are needed to help the policy makers [50]. More research is also needed to demonstrate the consequences of leaving the situation to itself.

Culture: the "Cinderella" public health dimension

At its simplest level, obesity policy thinking has to center on the need to tackle diet and lack of physical activity. The scientific endeavor is about unraveling their complex interplay. We have argued elsewhere that the resulting policy focus on biology or social aspects of diet and physical activity has tended to underplay the cultural dimension that bonds diet and physical activity [53,57].

Obesity is the manifestation of inappropriate societal structures framing what people eat and what they do. Such structures are expressed in terms of both physiologic (body) and consciousness (mind) processes, expressed as individual and group behaviors. Western societies have hitherto produced powerful cultural restraints, including personal stigmatization, against overweight or obese people (including the word "obesity" itself). Body weight has therefore risen in defiance of health and appearance norms and media representation [66,67]. While economists have been generally disinclined to value cultural factors, some speculate that new norms are being generated which are resulting in a social accommodation with increasing weight (through a "social multiplier effect"), a situation which is unrelated to food prices [68]. The implication might be that social norms are in conflict between those new norms increasingly accepting of fatness (in the US, termed "fat acceptance") and mass symbolized social aspirations based on social class and celebrity culture which requires thinness. Such a mismatch can occur because while obesity (still)

retains strongly negative associations, the culture of pervasive food marketing, food ubiquity and all-hours snacking and drinking does not [69,70].

Among the conceptual models around obesity, the insightfully termed "Nutrition Transition" [71–77] appears the strongest. It has emerged as a central focus of research and policy thinking in the developing world and within the WHO. However, we think that, despite its strong merits, it deserves to be unbundled. The Nutrition Transition is not one process but, in our opinion, three transitions of:
• diet
• management of, and human interface with, the physical environment
• culture.
These three transitions overlap, combine and amplify each other. We see reduced chances of any obesity policy being effective unless all three are tackled. We therefore argue that policy interventions should be judged from the perspective of these transitions, rather than in some isolated or disconnected way that has the potential allure of inoffensiveness or apparently quick results. The notion of transition implies a strongly historical perspective.

What wins the attention of policy makers? (Is it only monetary costs?)

We restate the question: why is obesity a problem, and for whom is it a problem? The short answer is that obesity is an individual's physiologic and personal problem (which they may see as normal rather than as a problem) that becomes society's problem. Although the media narrative often promotes tales of uncontrolled personal consumption and revels in the sheer visibility of obesity, the issue that consistently wins attention in policy circles is that of costs. Obesity's burden on healthcare, health insurance (in the UK, tax) and pension systems is already under pressure in rich societies and is potentially unbearable for less rich societies.

The USA, as ever, sets the trend. Overweight and obesity afflict respectively two-thirds and one-third of the US population, but a possible one-fifth of US healthcare expenditures will have to be devoted to treating the consequences of obesity in the future [35]. The US Surgeon General notes obesity costing up to 6% of healthcare budgets, a figure now exceeding $100 billion [78]. Obesity is poised to overtake the toll, and health expenditures, associated with tobacco [35]. Over and above direct costs, there is the impact of decreased household incomes, earlier retirement, and higher dependence on state benefits, which overall are likely to exceed the medical costs alone [37]. These trends will be compounded as the weight problems of children and teenagers convert into lifetime disease, mental health and other social costs [79].

Such calculations can be made for Europe too. Obesity was estimated to account for 2% of total French healthcare costs by

1995, long before obesity became a dramatized narrative [80]. In England, the National Audit Office estimated in 2001 that obesity cost the National Health Service (NHS) an annual £480 million (€720 million) and the wider economy a further £2.1 billion (€3.2 billion) [2]. By 2004, that cost was estimated to have risen to £3.3–3.7 billion (€4.95–5.55 billion) for obesity alone and £6.6–7.4 billion (€9.9–11.1 billion) for obesity plus overweight [4]. In The Netherlands, a 2004 study estimated that the proportion of the country's total general practitioner expenditure attributable to obesity and overweight was around 3–4% [81].

Alive to these EU member-state trends, in 2003 the former EC Commissioner for Health and Consumer Affairs cited US evidence as a warning to Europe, stating on one occasion that "[i]t will take nothing short of a behavioral revolution to stop this epidemic in its tracks" [82]. Such statements are welcome signs of political interest, but how exactly is Europe's behavior to be changed dramatically enough? In these societies, is not the consumer sovereign? This is where social marketing's rising appeal lies. It echoes conventional marketing, tailored to socially defined goals [83,84]. Nevertheless, if social marketing represents the market-friendly approach to obesity, its inability to influence the statistical momentum of obesity may mean its nostrums are short-lived. As existing strategies fail and the need for tougher lines of approach becomes more apparent, the advice of the RAND Corporation, the American think tank created by hard-nosed military advisers, which favors stricter controls, such as the restriction and licensing of food outlets, may gain a wider hearing [69,70].

Policy advice: choose your theories carefully

Part of the difficulty of translating evidence into policy stems from cacophony. Obesity can be theorized in various ways and is fissured by significant ideologic distinctions: individual/societal, physiologic/psychologic, economic/cultural, short-/long-termism, and more.

Governments subscribing to the power of individualism tend to propose public health strategies nuanced around consumerist ethics. Hence, again, the attraction of social marketing. Social marketing, which has its core precepts in faulty individual behaviors and beliefs, contains the rhetorically uncomplicated appeal to consumers to make "healthy choices" in the marketplace. While having considerable appeal – using market mechanisms rather than confronting or critically amending markets flows with the ideologic times – even supporters are aware of limitations to its effectiveness [85]. Social marketing isn't a panacea for inaction elsewhere in the policy world. If obesity is framed as an individual problem, the "solution" will be focus on personalized interventions [86]. In circumstances of free information circulation, people "choose" to be overweight simply because they eat too much and do too little [87]. The implication may be that a vastly growing proportion of the population, from their own volition, are "choosing" to gain weight. Indeed, there are US economists

who heartily approve of this conclusion [46]. There is also a flip side to the choice thesis which says that people may indeed be choosing to be overweight but why is this a problem? According to some, obesity is being wildly exaggerated in its significance and anyway is no concern of the state; rather, such "obesity mongering" represents an attempt to mobilize a moral panic [88,89].

Both sets of propositions are deeply flawed. The existence of the diet industry (special foods, diet books, clubs, etc.) and vast numbers of people who say they wish to lose weight and make efforts to do so – minimally counted as one-third of women in the USA or UK at any one time – suggests the very opposite. In 2001 more than half of all Americans attempted weight loss or maintenance through dieting and spent more than $33 billion on products and services [90]. Population weight gain is occurring in conditions of increasing "health consciousness" and enormous personal effort to be slim. There are notable differences between countries in the expression of this trend. For example, North American consumers pay more attention to food labels than their European counterparts but this might only indicate that such information makes little difference to consumption. The underlying point was made earlier: that in many societies, people have gained weight under social and cultural conditions which stress the opposite.

If the focus on individual choice underlying social marketing produces difficulties in analyzing adult obesity, it fails spectacularly for children. While private choices are necessarily part of the total explanatory picture for adults, the well-documented rise in childhood obesity – nationally, regionally and globally – means that such a highly individualized perspective cannot be applied so simply. Children's choices are, for the most part, determined by features of the adult-framed environment encompassing diet, physical activity and culture [91,92]. Of course, there is an answer to this reality too: blame the parents, as many in society – including those who are parents themselves – do [93].

Between individualist perspectives and environmental perspectives – or what we term the ecologic public health approach, discussed later in this chapter – lie a number of other theoretical approaches [52]. Some have been devized explicitly to identify and help us comprehend the determinants of obesity. Some draw on other fields of inquiry. Some are heavily ideologically framed, even when couched in science. Table 33.2 summarizes some of these theories and examines their core arguments, evidence and proposed solutions. The problem for policy makers is that no single theory offers clear-cut solutions.

Policy cacophony: the implications of different models

We view the policy complexity suggested in Table 33.2 as a critical starting place for analysis since the differences between the models helps to explain why obesity is so problematic and why an alternative, unified model is so necessary. Some of the models were devized explicitly to address obesity; others we have imputed

Table 33.2 The policy implications of some key obesity theories

Theory	Core argument	Example of evidence	Implied solutions	Comment
Genetic causation	The predisposition to lay down fat is an evolutionary legacy.	Predisposition by phenotypes is calculable.[94] The GAD2 gene (on chromosome 10, human genome) may interact with and speed up brain neurotransmitters, which then activate part of the hypothalamus, stimulating people to eat [95].	Genomics, gene mapping and nutrigenomics. Functional foods might help play a part in tailoring diets to individual predispositions.	There is a danger of searching for pharmaceutical or bariatric solutions. Technologic solutions are unlikely to resolve societal problems. At best, they are a "sticking plaster" and unaffordable to poor countries.
Economic transition	Lifestyle change is associated with development of a post-industrial consumerist society.	Fatty foods are relatively cheaper than healthy foods.[26, 96] There is a spread of US-style fast foods. There is oversupply of fats and sugars compared to WHO/FAO guidelines [97,98].	Once sufficiently affluent, people will be able to tackle obesity as consumers, choosing or not, as they wish. At the micro level, fiscal measures such as "fat taxes" could be considered. [63]	There is some fatalism that obesity is an inevitable consequence of progress.
Technolog-ical change	Oil as a source of energy is replacing food as source of energy.	Fossil fuels are replacing human/animal motor power [99]. Human physical activity levels decline with societal affluence [46].	Build in more physical energy use into daily life. Design technology to help keep intake in balance with expenditure.	Food companies selling sugary, fatty foods tend to like this theory. They sponsor sports and physical activity while governments promote sports strategies.
Cultural change	Marketing and advertising installs new cultural norms about what and how to eat, and how much to eat.	There has been a worldwide growth in advertising foods and soft drinks. Advertising changes food cultures.[100] Snacking dominates [101].	Social marketing can emulate "business" marketing.	Public health organizations lack sufficient budgets to compete with the food industry. McDonald's and Coca-Cola's marketing budgets are each twice the WHO's full year budget. [55].
Psychosocial	Food choice is intensely personal. Obesity suggests people's well-being is not being met.	Obesity has grown despite cultural obsession with thinness and beauty [66,68,102,103].	Family change. Counselling. This is required both individually and on a mass scale [104].	This has a tendency to become a solution on individualistic rather than population basis.
Obesogenic environment	Obesity is a normal physiological response to an abnormal or inappropriate environment.	Physiology is developed to cope with undersupply, not today's coincidence of over-, mal- and under-supply and decline in energy expenditure [44,105].	Change the physical and dietary environments to allow normal physiologic balance to (re)emerge [50,51].	This approach is arguably the most attuned to social policy thinking.
Nutrition Transition	Rising income leads to dietary changes, leading to shifts in disease patterns.	Many studies in developing countries suggest the transition does occur [74–76].	It's probably too late to prevent rising obesity but education may help.	The Nutrition Transition is a nutrition analysis of cultural, social and technical change.

as shaping the determinants of obesity. Some of the models clearly overlap; others, to use Thomas Kuhn's term, are "incommensurate" [106]. Differences of cause attribution imply differences of strategy and solutions. And, vice versa, different interests are drawn to models that reinforce or suit their predilections. Commercial interests often (but don't always) favor individualized models, just as public health practitioners often (but don't always) favor population-oriented models. Nevertheless, each of the models has a reasoned basis and is backed by different academic, professional, commercial and civic sources. The net result is cacophony, with models competing for policy attention, dominance and funds. This cacophony makes policy makers cautious, demanding stronger evidence. This exposes the fact that evidence

is only part of the problem – equally important is the thinking guiding how evidence is interpreted. In many cases, as the newspaper columns lengthen, the quest for dispassionate inquiry and critical evidence are often eschewed: opinion is enough.

The key question is: which model provides the best, most practical way ahead? Surprisingly, comprehensive answers are scarce [50]. To expect any might even be premature; strategies haven't yet been applied for long enough or extensively enough for evidence of dramatic change to emerge. Even if, for example, a drug is proven to work at the individual level, its impact across the population can't be assumed. Even if a "statin" for obesity emerges, whose responsibility is it to implement a mass prescription: the state, the individual citizen (or civil society as a whole) or companies and the marketplace? Policy viability isn't just a matter of what works, but what works in a manner that governments, business and people will find acceptable.

How good are policy responses so far?

Summary of intervention trials suggests that some limited gains can be made [107]. But, at the important population level, policy responses to obesity have generally been weak. Standing away from the politics, most obesity analysts agree that responses are implicitly fatalist (accepting inevitable rises), palliative or single-factor focused, or else drawn to crisis intervention (*in extremis*, recognizing the efficacy of bariatric surgery) [48]. Variations between countries' obesity rates are variations in speed of generally upward trends, although countries with significant regulation, especially of the food industry, appear to have had less of an increase. While a few societies – again Finland might be mentioned – have made significant efforts to intervene in heart disease [108], so far, obesity has received no such startling population-wide success. While Nordic countries, with their capacity to forge a consensus around a plan of action [59], may be able to mitigate the determinants of obesity, it may take decades for such evidence to emerge. In any case, the social and cultural conditions which might promote success in these countries are not so evident elsewhere.

The few intervention trials in prevention of obesity that focus on children or schools (in Crete, Agita, Sao Paulo, Singapore, Minnesota [26]) give few grounds for unalloyed optimism. Although there is a literature of action on different factors such as price, marketing, education and supply [39], no mass societal policy intervention has taken a "full spectrum" approach [108]. Yet most policy overviews suggest that efforts to combat the epidemic have to be society-wide, extensive and deep [26,107]. In any terms, refurbishment of health promotion and health development is required, demanding significant alteration of supply chains, the routines of daily existence, indeed whole cultures.

The International Obesity Task Force has reviewed possible preventive measures [1,26]. The thinking appears to be that actions can be useful but without overall policy coherence and political drivers, fragmented and atomized initiatives are unlikely to deliver requisite change. What, for example, is the point of a Ministry of Health recommending change in fat consumption if agriculture continues to pour out excess fat, if transport policies make it hard to build exercise into daily life, if trade and economic ministries have policies that cut across or even work against public health efforts?

No wonder health professionals – who are not trained in economics, agriculture or transport policy – feel beleaguered by the subject of obesity. If farm policies produce copious fat and sugar, how can their health promotion (which emerges from the principle of doing what you know and avoiding what you don't know) compensate? If heavy advertising associates soft drinks with fun

and sports, how can social marketing funded by restricted state sources compensate for, let alone defeat, it? And what is the point of forging policy directed mainly (or solely) through governmental agencies such as schools or hospitals (i.e. by public procurement) if no serious obligations are placed on business, or if there is a framework of mutual recrimination? In societies where commercial drivers are deemed of higher value than state action, this policy focus looks myopic; the state sector is being used as a policy "sink." Public health specialists, even ministries, are driven to overglamorize the results of their efforts in order to establish relevance in the debate (and continued funding).

Obesity policy reflects disciplinary and societal fragmentation

European Union member states, like nation-states worldwide, are justly jealous of retaining control over their own public health systems. And some governments are fearful of neoliberal accusations that health interventions constitute what the neoconservative press refers to as the "nanny state," a state that treats its citizens as though they were infants [109]. Yet even in individualistic Britain, where blame is often pointed at parents for having fat children, the parents themselves state that they want support and protection for their children [110]. If the state refuses to apply some protectionist principles, dietary choices will increasingly be set by the rhythm of the marketplace, and this is dominated by large players with massive marketing budgets.

The most heavily marketed foods are those typically associated with weight gain. Key role models in sports, like the Olympics themselves, are sponsored by fast-food and soft drink companies. Coca-Cola and PepsiCo spent respectively $2.2 billion and $1.7 billion on worldwide advertising in 2004, a combined level of spending exceeding the WHO biennial budget for the same period. Put differently, those two companies each spend annually on marketing their products and services about what the WHO spends annually on its entire health work globally [55,111]. This is the financial context for the WHO's *Global Strategy on Diet, Physical Activity and Health* [112,113]. The food industry has long been judged to be collectively enormous, politically well networked, a subtle lobbyist, and major employer. So what chance have public health agencies and arguments with their levers for health? Again, social marketers have an answer: use the weapons of the enemies [114], as if the outcome of the battle of David and Goliath did not depend upon a lucky shot.

The failures of the state, business and consumers

The analysis we have presented so far doesn't single out any one key causal factor. Rather, we have sought to depict a collective, systemic, failure. In Table 33.3, we set out an analysis that links these failures with obesity and the three broad transitions shaping

Table 33.3 Failures and factors shaping obesity in "wealthy societies"

		Factors shaping obesity				
		... alter the two domains shaping obesity		... alter the three transitions shaping obesity		
		Body	Mind	Diet	Physical activity	Culture
Focus of failure	*Markets fail because they ...*	Highlight and oversupply particular taste receptors (sweet and fat) Invest in technical fixes and single-factor solutions	Appeal to pleasure Build brand value over nutritional value Exploit vulnerable groups (e.g. children and low income)	Produce an excess of inappropriate, energy-dense foods cheaply Offer only limited investments in workforce training	Promote fossil-based fuels Glamorize private motor transport rather than expenditure of food-as-energy	Market and mold mass consciousness Overwhelm consumers with energy-dense food and drink as entertainment
	Governments fail because they ...	Adopt inconsistent modes of protection (interventions on sexual protection but not nutrition) Are unwilling to modernize public health scope and capacity	Limit health education to become a minor partner of market information, generating asymmetry of information flow and education	Subsidize overproduction of fat and sugar compared with micronutrient-rich foods Emphasize food safety while semi-abandoning nutrition De-emphasise nutrition and food education	Oversee decline of physical activity (transport, public spaces, sports facilities) Prioritize car use in retail and transport planning	Permit genderized and inadequate food literacy and skills Promote rights of individualized choice Facilitate media transmission by paid marketing Confuse citizenship with marketplace meritocracy (everyone is equal in the market)
	Consumers fail because they ...	Disconnect appetite from need and satiety	Adopt distorted images of body acceptability Accept temporality (short-termism) of choice	Eat a price-led rather than nutrition-led diet Respond individually rather than *en masse* to identity crises about meaning and values	Bow to the ubiquity of the nonenergy-expending material world (e.g. in travel to work/shop/school) Are disinclined to build exercise into daily life	Consume rather than expend energy as the norm of consumer culture Participate in physical activity by proxy (TV sports) Accept inequalities or indulge in victim blaming

it. Table 33.3 conceptually unravels the three interlocking, if differentially paced, transitions suggested earlier in the domains of diet, the physical environment and culture [53]. It represents the distal (distant) forces shaping obesity as, firstly, physiologic (the body) and in consciousness (the mind), alongside the three broad transitions grouped here as changes in diet, physical activity and culture. Policy makers might find it useful to acknowledge three kinds of failure – of markets (all actors throughout the supply chain), government (at all levels and across the range of instruments) and of society or consumers themselves, who ultimately are the actors who eat the food or undertake the activity – recognizing too that individuals who construct their behaviors are members of social groups and in socially regulated settings. Table 33.3 acts as a broad checklist for the range and focus that any policy actions must seek to address.

However, Table 33.3 is a simplification. Failures in the supply chain have occurred due to both market and extra-market factors. In the case of foods, a battery of policy measures that made sense in the 1940s and 1950s (subsidies and policy encouragement to increase output, measured by output per unit of capital or labor) today help create price signals that are inappropriate for health. The Common Agricultural Policy, for instance, has led EU

countries into delivering excessive fats and destruction of fruit [115]. The policy of encouraging the marketization of food supply has been a boon for processed product development and the creation of multiple "niche" food items, but it hasn't built health into the heart of supply [116,117]. Studies have shown how, if agriculture was to meet the dietary guidelines such as those of the WHO or Eurodiet, there would have to be considerable change in what is produced: less sugar, fat, meat, oils, etc. The good news is that northern European societies are emulating southern countries in consuming more fruit and vegetables; the bad news is that the countries of the south are now consuming the fattier, more sugary diets of the north [118,119]. The expansion of the EU eastwards means that the marketing power of the food industry is now focused on these potential growth markets [120].

Governance failure has occurred mainly because public health policy has been marginalized in the face of other priorities (e.g. promoting a successful food industry, raising private funds for education). To some extent, obesity is a jolt to the state about its priorities, just as food safety crises were in the late 1980s. This led to considerable efforts to improve food safety, with some success. A similar push is now required with nutritional health. Children are being exposed to low-quality foods in institutional settings and by the insertion of food marketing and advertising into the interstices of their everyday lives, sometimes in government-approved cause-related marketing projects, although work is now ongoing to address this [121]. On the one hand, there is advice to take more exercise but on the other, transport policies still center on car use. The normalization of car transport to school in place of walking illustrates the point [4]. Walking to school remains in decline, despite "walking bus" initiatives. In its defence, government – and health professionals within it – face a significant delivery challenge compared to food industry advertising or marketing budgets [100].

Turning to consumers, failure here also has to be acknowledged, as it is in many popular explanations for obesity [93]. "No one forces people to eat" can slip into blaming the obese for their obesity and blaming parents for their fat children. An obesity strategy can easily become a problem families (fat families) strategy. People choose the wrong foods and therefore, in effect, choose to be overweight. However, consumer failure might properly be seen as a consequence, at least in part, of the two other forms of failure already considered. That said, there appear to be additionally genetic/evolutionary, social and psychologic dimensions, some of which were considered in several of the models presented in Table 33.2. These might go under the heading of informational, cognitive and behavioral failure, attributes like time-inconsistent preferences, ambivalence, bounded rationality, and projection bias [63]. This is the world of 'treat culture', peer pressure, and pleasure followed by guilt. In such conditions only individuals having higher levels of "social power" are likely to be able to make consistently healthy choices. As noted earlier, patterns of obesity are linked to other societal inequalities and vulnerabilities, whatever the genetic factors [29–31,33]. But that said, and mindful of the dangers of victim blaming, policy makers have to acknowledge that for adults, at least, there is some level of volition involved.

Consumer failure requires policy to re-emphasize both rights and responsibilities within a social framework of action and knowledge. For example, the 19th century witnessed the spread of new behavior rules and shame-based behavior cues linked to the campaigns against infectious (although also "lifestyle-based") diseases of the day. Ordinances against spitting, for example, or the promotion of hand washing occurred in concert with the science-based hygiene revolution. Success did not result from official action or the word of science alone – indeed, it was decades before new hygiene practices were fully accepted by doctors – but through new cheap hygiene products (soap, disinfectants) and their associated marketing [122]. Today obesity policy and practice could usefully draw on the debate about behavior change to promote sustainable consumption [123] or the "happiness" or well-being debate [124]. What is clear is that society is not at a stage whereby antiobesogenic forces outnumber those pulling in the opposite direction: manufacturers' and retailers' messages to eat healthy foods – which should be acknowledged – are drowned out by the bigger budgets (associated with higher margins) devoted to less healthy ranges.

A new policy framework is needed

Having explored why obesity is rising so fast and suggesting that, powerful though it is, the Nutrition Transition is, on its own, inadequate, and that in fact there are three transitions and three forms of failure, what would a new policy framework guiding prevention implementation look like?

We propose that if obesity prevention becomes a genuine policy, engaged with and delivered across government, society and markets and supply chain, its accomplishment will require a paradigm shift, based on principles [125] designed to:
• take a whole-system rather than a partial approach
• reshape not just the physical and dietary environment but also the social and cultural environments
• adopt a long-term strategy by asking what an antiobesogenic environment might look like and then draw out the policy changes needed to deliver it
• recognize the fundamental nature of the challenge posed and give due political priority to building alliances that could overcome the obesogenic social forces (as was done for tobacco in a long 50-year process)
• reformulate the roles of government, markets and consumers to shift them away from reinforcing obesity
• deliver a situation where prevention is the norm, where victim blaming is unacceptable but responsibility not avoided
• engage multisector, multiagency action within and beyond the public health professional discourse.
This combination requires vision with pragmatism, leadership with collective action, along with a new sensibility towards the consumer by the food industry, the media and others; in other words, a new, more "grown-up" perspective on obesity.

What needs to happen in order to deliver this policy framework?

As with climate change, pessimists argue that only a "system shock" such as an oil crisis might shake people out of their cars [99,126]. But even with such "tipping points" – moments when societies agree that enough is enough – strategies are needed to cushion the impact. In place of current "unmanaged" transitions in diet, physical activity and culture, "managed" transitions – as are proposed with climate change policy – are preferable and possible [127,128]. Planning for systemic change requires political will, good evidence, alliances of pro-public health bodies committed to the long-term reorientation of societies, superb organization and commitment, and a long-term perspective. In part, the groundwork for such thinking has already been tabled in the UK by Sir Derek Wanless in his reviews for the Treasury of national healthcare funding and of public health [129,130]. The Wanless reviews presented a "fully engaged" scenario as the optimal basis for action. Carefully couched, this is more radical than it appeared because it actually made the case for demand management in place of "laissez faire." Obesity is nothing if not a problem requiring demand management.

Scenario planning

No one can foretell the future. Britons may start increasing physical activity – following the Dutch, for example – just as they earlier adopted aspects of US-style fast-food and car culture. Escalating oil prices may shock societies into change, as peak oil analysis predicts. Walking or cycling long distances to work and school might become fashionable. Societies and individual citizens might decide to narrow the gap between the very fit and the very fat. If such change does happen, it's likely to be helped by society-wide coalitions pushing, publicizing, researching, sharing successes and failures, and organizing that change. Although some such public health coalitions have emerged, they currently lack momentum and tend to be locked into the professional mode of policy discourse or fascination with one-shot methods (again, social marketing comes to mind) when broadsides are needed.

Scenario planning might help galvanize the necessary intersectoral thinking and work. Taking the current prognosis that obesity is rising, below we present a number of different but plausible policy scenarios. Each of these to some degree implies failure in that it will either perpetuate current obesity levels or marginalize routes to success or result in further complexity. At the end of this review, we present another, more ideal, scenario. It too requires a managed transition.

Policy as usual

This scenario offers continuation of today's small-scale, incremental, piecemeal change. There is investment in endless short-term projects. These offer tantalizing visions of change, building expertise but not transferring to society at large. The result is palliative. Initiatives are encouraged, such as local health and physical education programs, rather than a national advertising moratorium. There are once-a-year sporting activities (fun-runs) rather than policy delivering daily physical activity (biking to school or work daily, subject to weather). Ministers are able to produce reports showing they fund this or that "success" (projects), but society continues to produce divided obesity rates. The paradigm is individualized, personalized, health.

External shock

In this scenario, we envisage extensive and radical change following external shock to society. This comes from an oil crisis or a fiscal crisis over rising healthcare costs. Or an international outcry emerges over childhood obesity. Any of these can deliver a tipping point, and car transport has to be reduced, people use bicycles daily, etc. Policy making requires co-ordinated, cross-cutting themes. Existing institutions are audited for their obesity (health) impact. The drive is for food to be "fuel" rather than using fossil fuels to drive food around the continent of Europe.

Targeting "at-risk" groups

In this scenario, policy makers, for example, abandon any pretence at population health, instead aiming to tackle "at-risk" groups. The poor, the already fat, those with a predisposition, are given ("offered") special programs – therapy, drugs, exercise regimens, Weightwatchers schemes, one-to-one trainers, etc. – mediated, for instance, by healthcare professionals. The incentive to enter such programs is either hard (shame) or soft (enticement and encouragement, in the style of private physical fitness mentoring). The value of this policy scenario is that it focuses preventive expenditure on the social groups that cost most. The problem is that few measures show more than limited success and don't tackle the underlying reasons why these groups are at a higher risk, and therefore don't prevent other people from joining the "high-risk" groups.

Generational focus

In this scenario, policy makers judge that the ideologic complications of tackling adult obesity are too great, despite the emerging focus in government reports on health among the 50-plus. There isn't enough political support. Instead, they focus on children only, assuming that parents are more likely to do things for their children than for others. Radical "walk to school" programs and bans on children's food advertising (and other marketing, e.g. websites, short message texting, product placement) are gained at the European level because they are undertaken in the name of children. In half a century's time, obesity rates fall and the new generation's norms are worked through in a new demographic transition.

Business (almost) as usual

In this scenario, governments abandon state responsibility to shape responses to obesity. The focus here is on individual solutions, serviced by the food and sports industries. Cultural industries sponsor achievers, backing sports "winners," presenting physical activity as something an élite undertakes. Society splits into watchers and doers. Corporate social responsibility becomes the core policy ethos, a substitute for government leadership. Commercial bodies take a lead in offering new product "choices." For example, governments encourage industry-partnered public advertising or social marketing and companies agree only to market what they define as their healthier product ranges.

These are all plausible future scenarios but they all have more or less undesirable features and consequences. More ideal would be a scenario that genuinely delivered population health improvement based upon the principle that healthy food and active society were the mainstream. The problem is that policy makers and public health practitioners are not all that clear about what this might be or even, for that matter, what public health is. In his speech on public health on 26 July 2006, former Prime Minister Tony Blair stated what is possibly the catechism of the modern politician that "questions of individual lifestyle – obesity, smoking, alcohol abuse, diabetes, sexually transmitted disease" were "not, strictly speaking, public health problems at all" [131]. In effect, health was due to lifestyle and choice of lifestyle was personal and individual. It was still important for society to intervene, said Blair, but any intervention had to recognize that every individual was a single point of causation.

Re-specifying what is meant by public health for obesity policy

Obesity, as Mr Blair's statement showed, exposes the weaknesses of public health as a scientific and political force. In large part, it is caused by social change and an image of public health as collective measures of the past. Advances in medical science mean that far more is known about disease, including the role of genetic factors, and more can be done to treat them. Single-factor classifications of disease have given way to multifactoral theories, emphasizing multiple, cross-cutting factors. In part, this acknowledges the fact that the disease burden has shifted. Infectious diseases, while recently undergoing signs of resurgence, have given way to chronic diseases not just among the older part of the population (as predicted by Omran's theory of Epidemiologic Transition [132–134]) but in younger age groups too, with significant growth of noncommunicable diseases (NCD). Even in the case of infectious diseases (HIV and other sexually transmitted infections come to mind), some of the old mechanisms for control and disease management have broken down. If we know more now about disease and disease causation, we appear less able to stop its spread. The dilemma for public health is not just what it doesn't know, but not knowing what it needs to do.

Indeed, much of the contemporary policy debate about obesity is framed by the state supposedly being powerless to know what to do. The litany of arguments about restrictions on governance adds to the policy cacophony. In an age of globalization, it is said, how can levers of influence be pulled? Obesity, being a multifactor disease, is so complex to address. And so on. This analysis is, of course, partly true. Proponents of public health (including Blair in the earlier mentioned speech) tend to look back fondly on eras like the 19th century, when grand social engineering such as Sir Joseph Bazalgette's sewage system for London (tackling the Great Stink) or individual heroic public health interventions such as Dr John Snow at the Broad Street pump (tackling cholera) were not only possible but effective [135,136]. But romance shouldn't cloud our judgment [49]. Even then, the policy context was furiously complex, with class interest-led politics deeply entrenched, opposition to action immense (as in the case of Bazalgette) and citizen rights far fewer. It could even be argued, to follow from former Prime Minister Blair's thinking, that these measures were not, strictly speaking, public health responsibilities either; rather, they were due to industrialization, population growth and urbanization. Much of the problem of thinking about public health therefore follows from locking in its meaning to any one era, any one set of methods or activities, or any one set of professional groups [137].

We are more optimistic about what can be done today, but it means rethinking what public health encompasses, from the physical engineering of the environment – the principal achievement of the Victorians – to our proposals to reshape the social, economic and cultural environment today. Part of our analysis is that if the dynamics sketched in Table 33.2 are followed through, clear actors can be discerned, with realms of influence. The 2001 National Audit Office, 2003 Health Select Committee and 2007 Foresight reports all mapped many of them [2,4]. But the fact remains that public health requires a stronger mandate and champions. The term "public health" is used to denote a population condition, an activity, a set of disciplines, a profession (or rather competing professions), an infrastructure, a set of policies, laws, a philosophy, even a movement. Given this fragmentation of meaning, methods, institutional forms and profile, it is not surprising that public health is poorly represented in government, misunderstood, and only momentarily achieves some limited degree of power during perceived emergencies (avian and swine flu being the latest). Advocates of public health as we are, we nonetheless think that obesity requires a return to basics. Currently, public health in the UK can be thought of as composed of action on (at least) three essential elements

Health protection encompasses all forms of disease prevention in terms of its control and regulatory elements. In the UK health protection in its institutional forms was boosted by the creation of the Health Protection Agency (HPA). However, the purview of the HPA is limited to infectious diseases, hazards or bioterrorism preparedness, while health protectionism in terms of NCD is diffused through a variety of bodies, some of which don't even have health in their remit. The Food Standards Agency does; Ofcom, for example, doesn't, yet it regulates advertising which, though not a magic bullet, some critics argue is nonetheless a not insignificant factor in the cultural transition or systematic framing of mass consciousness indicated in Table 33.3. Unsurprisingly, from a health perspective, the regulatory aspects of the control of the determinants of NCD is poor.

Health development (sometimes called health promotion) is the promotion of healthy communities. In professional forms, these span school nursing to health visiting. Increasingly, the focus is on the role of local authorities in obesity strategy (through, as noted, LAAs, but also through healthy schools, health scrutiny functions, etc.). In its institutional form, the establishment of a national program of health development, with its focus on putting good health evidence into practice, occurred through the Health Development Agency (HDA), now part of the National Institute for Health and Clinical Excellence (NICE).

Health education involves the promotion of what the WHO calls "health literacy"; in other words, the creation of a population informed about its health and how to maintain it. Health education has been progressively weakened in its institutional forms both nationally (the Health Education Council/Authority became the HDA and then merged into NICE) and locally (most health education departments in NHS primary care trusts have withered). Health education has given way to the rival theory of social marketing – to the delight of the advertising industry, which switches between formulating campaigns for crisp manufacturers to activities on behalf of the Department of Health. Social marketing now has the status of an unquestionable strategy – because no other option is perceived to be left.

These streams have also been conceptualized in terms of the "three domains of public health" by the UK's Faculty of Public Health [138]:
• *health protection*: clean air, water, food; infectious diseases; radiation; environmental health protection, etc.
• *health and social care quality*: service planning, clinical effectives and governance; research, etc.
• *health improvement*: reducing inequalities; employment; housing; lifestyles; etc.

Valuable as this latter model is, it lends itself to a professional-centric and NHS/primary care-based approach to public health, with the Director of Public Health role at its core. 139]. In practice, despite the copious energies of many departments of public health, and in some cases the establishment of joint local authority/NHS appointments and the shift to a more local authority focus of work, it is easier to work within boundaries than across them and far easier to research or document problems than to deal with them. The other side of the equation has been the relative deskilling of local authorities in public health, which in the past has interpreted the term as something to do solely with the NHS rather than local government, despite the fact that local government, for more than a century, *was* public health.

The deeper reality is that the societal transitions referred to earlier – diet, the physical environment, and culture – which once produced, in conditions of erratic but generally spreading economic benefit, a serendipitous relationship with health improvement have now turned against public health. The convergent streams of economic, state, science and civil society activities which underpinned the hygiene revolution have petered out. A conventional model of public health may be adequate for many things, but it is quite inadequate to deal with the complexity exposed by obesity, which requires societally systemic, population-wide change [48].

In its place, we propose a more fundamental analysis, which addresses the long-term societal transitions in diet, physical activity and culture, the multilevel nature of causation and the disparate range of levers needed for change. This model seeks the convergence of traditions in natural ecology and human ecology, drawing upon an understanding that human health is based upon secure foundations in the natural world and, vice-versa, that natural ecology requires social institutions and human behavior to build in new rules for planetary protection.

This approach has the advantage of seeing agents outside conventional public health as key agents for (and barriers to) change. Too often, obesity interventions are conceived of as the responsibility of a few public health professionals, when in fact it requires much wider, cross-sectoral, interdimensional and concerted action [3]. This doesn't mean that local actors are irrelevant. On the contrary, we suggest they need more power and resources. People won't be able to alter diets or take more exercise unless these goals are primary drivers at the local level. It also means that local actions cannot merely be "commissioned" from higher points in the "delivery chain" in a downward cascade of governance but that governance is conceived as inherently multilevel and cross-organizational (engaging markets and civil society) with correspondingly flexible frameworks of responsibility and action. The box-ticking era of public health must therefore draw to a close.

Towards an ideal scenario for public health success

The failures of market, government and consumers presented in Table 33.3 need to be recast in order to deliver success by changing diet and physical activity. At the heart of the obesity problem is the simple fact of mismatch between energy input and output. As Fogel has pointed out, rapidly industrializing Britain in the early 19th century, then the richest country in the world, didn't achieve the average calorie supply now present in low-income economies until past the middle of the 19th century [140]. Today, calories can be purchased almost infinitely more cheaply. Fogel notes that in 1800 the supply of calories per equivalent adult male available for work was about 848 per day; today a Mars "Duo" bar provides almost 500 calories for 50 pence ($1). Cheap calorie foods and soft drinks are spreading worldwide. Although much of the world still suffers dietary insufficiency, as the Food and Agriculture Organization (FAO) and the WHO have shown, there is a systemic oversupply of fat, particularly in Europe and North America (see Table 33.4) [113]. The rest of the world is following behind. Like markets – indeed through markets – obesity is being globalized.

Re-engineering the world of food – merely one component of the new task – requires, we think, the recategorization of public health within four dimensions of human existence:
• the physical world, by which we mean the world of nature and transformed nature – the built environment, urbanization – and the extractive relationship with the environment, i.e. nature as the reserve on which human existence draws
• the physiologic world, by which we mean the importance of the bodily processes that transform food – not just calories but micronutrients too – into bodily manifestation; the food can either be expended or translated into "thermodynamic overload", i.e. obesity
• the social world, by which we mean organized human relationships and all the societal institutions (administration, the economy) that frame how humans live
• the cognitive world, by which we mean the interpretive structures within the human mind – what European philosophy calls the "lifeworld" – that are necessarily personally experienced and yet have meanings that others may share.

Table 33.4 Trends in the dietary supply of fat

Region	Supply of fat (g per capita per day)				
	1967–1969	1977–1979	1987–1989	1997–1999	Change between 1967–1969 and 1997–1999
World	53	57	67	73	20
North Africa	44	58	65	64	20
Sub-Saharan Africa[a]	41	43	41	45	4
North America	117	125	138	143	26
Latin America and the Caribbean	54	65	73	79	25
China	24	27	48	79	55
East and South-East Asia	28	32	44	52	24
South Asia	29	32	39	45	16
European Community	117	128	143	148	31
Eastern Europe	90	111	116	104	14
Near Est	51	62	73	70	19
Oceania	102	102	113	113	11

[a]Exctudes South Africa.
Source: WHO/FAO [86].

This four-part distinction helps reform what is meant by public health. The oft-quoted modern definition of public health is that it is: "[t]he science and art of preventing disease, prolonging life and promoting, protecting and improving health through the organized efforts of society" [141].

We propose a modification. In an era that is having to face the consequences of mining nature, the material infrastructure for human health has to be recognized. In an era of massive culture shifts, when product marketing saturates the human consciousness, health education is largely the domain of the private, self-interested forces.

So, in place of the common definition of public health, we believe that the true art and science of what we would rather term "ecologic public health" is:

"to comprehend the composite interactions between the physical, physiologic, social and cognitive worlds that determine health outcomes in order to intervene, alter and ameliorate the population's health by shaping society and framing public and private choices to deliver sustainable planetary, economic, societal and human health."

This approach allows policy makers in "health" to link actions with others focused on apparently different policy problems and objectives. This "ecologic public health" perspective, drawing upon thinking in natural ecology and human ecology, is closely aligned to the policy goal of sustainable development, grouped around the core foci of society, economy and environment [142].

In Table 33.5, we present a forward-looking set of indicative goals for each of the three domains indicated in Table 33.3:

markets (supply chains), government (state) and the public (consumers). Each of these needs to be translated into practical terms, which is a separate task. Whereas in Table 33.3 we linked the failures in terms of three transitions of diet, physical activity and culture representing the evolution and interpretation of obesity as a policy problem to date, we now propose that future policy might more usefully be cast around the four, more fundamental, dimensions of existence emerging from our discussion of the dimensions underpinning what is meant by public health: the physical, physiologic, social and cognitive. For each of these, policy makers must consider which actors – in supply chain, society and government – are needed to deliver change both within the four dimensions and across them, and on what terms they could deliver change across the other sectors.

The criticism of this approach is that it might take public health policy away from practicality into abstraction. We would argue, conversely, that the test of practical strategies and interventions, in toto, is the capacity to address these different dimensions of existence. Ecologic public health is not just a perspective but a framework for policy testing. Current policies are failing because they don't cover the range and depth of interventions needed. Policy making has to move beyond the realm of tick boxes and unrealistic targets and, instead, face the world of real power, culture, consumption and the well-springs of consumption. More realistic targets should promote cultural change processes and other change processes linked to more sophisticated target setting. Similarly, the determinants of health must also be understood as working at multiple levels and dimensions and across multiple policy terrains.

Policy about obesity must engage with economic drivers, not just the costs of obesity. Dietary change is shaped as much by the affordability of and mixed messages on a healthy diet as it is by the financial implications of national (or European) farming policy that currently troubles government. The Treasury's desire to reform the Common Agricultural Policy is likely to win more support if other member states see it as health oriented, tapping into the WHO European Region's summits on obesity, which culminated at Istanbul in November 2006 [143].

Our point is that the new policy on obesity has to cover the entire terrain, or continued drivers in one dimension might undermine positive action in others. Thus, children should not only be provided with school meals (tackling the physiologic dimension directly) but also introduced to the culture of food and the means by which food is produced (the social dimensions of institutions which produce and manufacture foods and the cognitive dimension of norms and expectations about food). Equally, social marketing, more correctly seen as more rigorously applied health education (oriented at the cognitive), should not disseminate "healthy" beliefs about food or physical activity without allowing "regulators" (who might be schools as well as parents) to have the power and the incentives to block "antisocial marketing." Of course, policies have to address the means of access to healthier, affordable food or promote the normalization of physical activity into everyday life; but this aim, if taken

Table 33.5 Ideal indicative actions to shape healthy and sustainable futures

		... altering the four dimensions of existence to reshape diet and physical activity			
		Material world (nature)	**Physiologic world (body)**	**Social world (human relationships)**	**Cognitive world (mind and experience)**
Focus of success	*Making markets work for health by ...*	Linking profitability to healthier food ranges Making food acquisition costs reflect environmental externalities Reducing reliance on fossil fuels to encourage physical activity in daily life Ensuring health targets are built into wastage reduction targets Making environmental indicators meaningful for obesity policy	Changing price signals of food to favor fruit and vegetables Shopping more often for less to burn energy from food rather fuel Promoting smaller portion sizes Farmers producing less fat/sugar/meat/dairy products	Promoting good, wholesome food to all, but especially to low-income social groups Aligning companies' success with consumer health Accepting restrictions on the commoditization of relationships in food marketing Promoting only self-regulation that works for health	Agreeing not to target children Supporting honest consumer information Promoting more flexible and diverse social role models
	Making governments work for health by ...	Making it secure to walk or bicycle to work/school/leisure Aligning sustainable consumption targets with public health targets Incorporating health into food industry sustainability strategy targets Using planning functions to routinize physical activity	Setting incentives for better-quality food for all socio-economic groups and ethnic minorities Focusing subsidies to promote healthier food ranges Using public procurement and other fiscal measures to manage demand Setting and paying for high standards of public sector catering Ensuring Public Service Agreements and Local Area Agreements fully reflect government obesity targets	Setting minimum income standards for a sustainably produced, wholesome diet Ensuring all citizens have a requisite level of food choosing, sourcing and preparation, and general food literacy Supporting the strengthening of social rituals when people bond through food Redefining what is acceptable and unacceptable (norms)	Setting clear, long-term cultural goals Helping educate "taste" to be more discriminatory Changing desirability of foods and behavior by fiscal measures such as aligning taxation of marketing expenditures with the health properties of food and drink Providing more remedial support for overweight people
	Making the public live healthily by ...	Demanding an extension of "defensible" public space beyond home and protected malls, etc. Enabling children to play in streets and parks Getting out of their homes more to reclaim civic space Accepting fewer parking spaces for cars	Altering the composition of their diets Building exercise into daily life to promote energy balance Creating new cultures of daily activity, e.g. accepting less car use	Using food as an affirmative social engagement Eating together Establishing overt social norms that support people to be of health-desirable weight and incentivize healthy weight	Accepting the need to eat less unless they exercise more Being more health-discerning about when, how often and what to eat Being prepared to redefine parental responsibility for long-term benefit rather than short-term "peace"

seriously, implies a radical move away from the ideology of "choice" (i.e. to establish a life consumption pattern based upon heavily advertized foods), particularly in the case of children.

Who should be responsible for policy and process coordination? The rapid and continuous upward trend of obesity exposed by Foresight might demand that new policy is led from the higher reaches of government but, if so, it should also be "owned" by everyone. It is a long-term vision that requires copious political resources and some financial resources. The point must be to catalyze new forms of leadership but of the many rather than the few, engaging people who currently feel powerless or who don't understand that obesity is a shared societal problem ("everyone's business") that breaks down policy segmentation and genuinely seeks the participation of the public. If recent policy making around smoking (which does, for the most part, pass the ecologic public health test) provides a model, it also provides a warning. Addressing obesity in British society also runs up against intransigent social and economic divisions.

Conclusion

The argument presented here is the need to tackle not just the manifestations of obesity but the forces that shape it. This chapter has tried to reconceptualize the basis on which attempts to tackle obesity are and could be made. We have suggested that obesity is the public health equivalent of climate change. This is a striking analog in at least five respects. First, failure to act at an early stage is already having immense and undesirable consequences. Second, the policy discourse about obesity – vibrant though it is among the problem-watchers – is not yet being matched by requisite, measurable changed direction of travel by society, governments and economy. Third, obesity is being normalized, even as the trends accelerate and the evidence grows. Fourth, as Jain has remarked, the environmental determinants remain misunderstood and under-researched, while policy drifts towards individualized responsibility [48]. Fifth, there is a danger that the political moment to act radically and coherently will be missed, and that the possibility of reversing population obesity will be lost. A tipping point will have passed – both adiposally and metaphorically. Already too many actors and institutions feel powerless.

In sum, we think it highly unlikely that obesity rates in any society will be reversed by small steps, reliance on single solutions being offered in conditions of policy cacophony, as outlined earlier, or by unwarranted emphasis on either community change or individualized change with limited societal support. From our analysis, obesity change is more likely to be delivered by "big thinking, many changes." Coherence and optimism are needed, with firm political leadership across government, supply chains and civil society.

On an optimistic note, it should be stressed that many governments worldwide, led by health ministries, are beginning to realize the scale of the obesity challenge. The climate change analogy has been accepted by the Foresight Obesity Report [10] and subsequently by the UK Secretary of Health prior to the publication of the government's new cross-governmental obesity strategy [144]. However, as this chapter has noted, while elected health officials may "get the point," other departments of government may not. Indeed, they may see themselves as partners to, and indeed defenders of, industries which are implicated in producing the problem. Economic departments have, until recently, had a tendency to see "health" as expenditure on healthcare, but this reflex is beginning to be shifted by initiatives such as Wanless's "fully engaged scenario," by the costing of the impact of climate change [145] and the realization that food supply chains must be rebuilt around sustainable development [146].

Obesity is hardly the only challenge in the early 21st century. From the ecologic public health perspective offered here, investment in prevention and building capacity will have pay-offs not just in massive reductions to healthcare costs but also by turning broader societal costs into higher well-being and quality of life, including the capacity to address the bigger questions of climate change. However, the resolution of policy cacophony does not,

in the final analysis, depend on new research, new information or even new strategy. The biggest challenge for politicians, public health and for society at large is to know the sort of future they collectively want to construct and then apply a coherent strategy to achieve it.

References

1. WHO. *Obesity: Preventing and Managing the Global Epidemic*. Report of a WHO Consultation. WHO Technical Series No. 894. Geneva: World Health Organisation, 2000.
2. National Audit Office. *Tackling Obesity in England*. London: Stationery Office, 2001.
3. Donaldson L. *Annual Report of the Chief Medical Officer for England 2002*. London: Department of Health, 2003.
4. Health Committee of the House of Commons. *Obesity. Third Report of Session 2003–04*, vol 1. HC 23–1. London: Stationery Office, 2004.
5. Department of Health and Department for Children. *Healthy Weight, Healthy Lives: A Cross Government Strategy for England*. London: Stationery Office, 2008.
6. Lang T, Dowler E, Hunter D. *Review of the Scottish Diet Action Plan: Progress and Impacts 1996–2005*. Report 2005/2006 RE036. Edinburgh: NHS Scotland, 2006.
7. Scottish Executive. *Scottish Health Survey 2003*. Edinburgh: Scottish Executive, 2005.
8. National Audit Office. *Health of the Nation: A Progress Report*. HC 458 1995/96. London: Office of the Comptroller and Auditor General, 1996.
9. Department of Health. *Health Profile of England*. London: Department of Health, 2006: 112.
10. Foresight. *Tackling Obesities: Future Choices*. London: Government Office of Science, 2007.
11. Department of Health. *Health Challenge England – Next Steps for Choosing Health*. London: Department of Health, 2006: 40.
12. Department of Health. *Local Area Agreements and Local Public Service Agreements*. London: Department of Health, 2005.
13. Chinn S, Rona RJ. Prevalence and trends in overweight and obesity in three cross-sectional studies of British children, 1974–94. BMJ 2001:322:24–6.
14. Department of Health. *Government announces first steps in strategy to help people maintain healthy weight and live healthier lives*. London: Department of Health, 2008. Available at: www.gnn.gov.uk/environment/fullDetail.asp?ReleaseID=347137&NewsAreaID=2&NavigatedFromDepartment=False (accessed 23 January 2008).
15. Commission of the European Communities. *Promoting Healthy Diets and Physical Activity: A European Dimension for the Prevention of Overweight, Obesity and Chronic Diseases*. Green Paper, COM(2005) 637 final. Brussels: CEC, 2005.
16. Hewitt P. Public engagement. Speech by Rt Hon Patricia Hewitt MP, Secretary of State for Health, 23 June 2005. London: Department of Health, 2005.
17. Dunman J. *Agriculture: Capitalist and Socialist*. London: Lawrence and Wishart, 1975.
18. Brandt K. *The Reconstruction of World Agriculture*. London: George Allen and Unwin, 1945.
19. Body R. *Agriculture: The Triumph and the Shame*. London: Temple Smith, 1982.

20. Schlosser E. *Fast Food Nation: What the All-American Meal is Doing to the World*. London: Allen Lane, 2001.

21. Critser G. *Fatland: How Americans Became the Fattest People in the World*. London: Penguin, 2003.

22. Brownell KD, Horgen KB. *Food Fight. The Inside Story of the Food Industry, America's Obesity Crisis, and What We Can Do About It*. Chicago: Contemporary Books, 2004.

23. Kuchler F, Golan E. Is there a role for government in reducing the prevalence of overweight and obesity? Choices Magazine (publication of the American Agricultural Economics Association), 2004.

24. Organization for Economic Cooperation and Development. *OECD Health Data 2007*. Paris: Organization for Economic Cooperation and Development, 2007.

25. Maffeis C, Consolaro A, Cavarzere P, et al. Prevalence of overweight and obesity in 2- to 6-year-old Italian children. Obesity 2006:14(5): 765–9.

26. Lobstein T, Baur L, Uauy R, et al. Obesity in children and young people: a crisis in public health. A report to the World Health Organisation. Obes Rev 2004:5(suppl 1).

27. Robertson A, Tirado C, Lobstein T, et al. *Food and Health in Europe: A New Basis for Action*. Copenhagen: World Health Organisation Regional Office for Europe, 2004.

28. James WPT, Rigby NJ, Leach RJ, et al. Global strategies to prevent childhood obesity: forging a societal plan that works. *A discussion paper prepared for the Global Prevention Alliance McGill Integrative Health Challenge October 26–27, 2006*. London: International Obesity Task Force/International Association for the Study of Obesity, 2006.

29. Gordon-Larsen P, Nelson MC, Page P, et al. Inequality in the built environment underlies key health disparities in physical activity and obesity. Pediatrics 2006;117(2):417–24.

30. Gordon-Larsen P, Adair LS, Popkin BM. The relationship of ethnicity, socioeconomic factors, and overweight in U.S. adolescents. Obes Res 2003:11(1):121–9.

31. Pickett KE, Kelly S, Brunner E, et al. Wider income gaps, wider waistbands? An ecological study of obesity and income inequality. J Epidemiol Commun Health 2005;59(8):670–4.

32. Wang Y, Zhang Q. Are American children and adolescents of low socioeconomic status at increased risk of obesity? Changes in the association between overweight and family income between 1971 and 2002. Am J Clin Nutr 2006:84(4):707–16.

33. Zhang Q, Wang Y. Using concentration index to study changes in socio-economic inequality of overweight among US adolescents between 1971 and 2002. Int J Epidemiol 2007;36(4):916–25.

34. Rayner G, Rayner M. Fat is an economic issue: combatting chronic diseases in Europe. Eurohealth 2003;9(1, Spring):17–20.

35. Sturm R. The effects of obesity, smoking, and drinking on medical problems and costs. Health Aff 2002;21(2):245–53.

36. Sturm R, Ringel J, Andreyeva R. Increasing obesity rates and disability trends. Health Aff 2004;23(2):1–7.

37. Yach D, Stuckler D, Brownell KD. Epidemiologic and economic consequences of the global epidemics of obesity and diabetes. Nat Med 2006:12(1):62–6.

38. Cutler DM, Glaeser EL, Shapiro JM. Why have Americans become more obese? J Econ Perspect 2003;17(3):93–18.

39. Oxford Health Alliance Working Group. *Economic Consequences of Chronic Diseases and the Economic Rationale For Public And Private Intervention*. Oxford: Oxford Health Alliance, 2005.

40. Hughes D, McGuire A. A review of the economic analysis of obesity. Br Med Bull 1997;53(2):253–63.

41. Lang R. An economic analysis of obesity on wages. Working Paper Series 1. Social Science Research Network, 2002.

42. James WP, Rigby TN, Leach R. The obesity epidemic, metabolic syndrome and future prevention strategies. Eur J Cardiovasc Prev Rehab 2004;11(1):3–8.

43. Institute of Medicine of the National Academies. *Preventing Childhood Obesity: Health in the Balance*. Washington, DC: Institute of Medicine of the National Academies, 2004.

44. Hill JO, Peters JC. Environmental contributions to the obesity epidemic. Science 1998:280(5368):1371–4.

45. Saelens BE, Sallis JF, Black JB, et al. Neighborhood-based differences in physical activity: an environment scale evaluation. Am J Pub Health 2003:93(9):1552–8.

46. Lakdawalla D, Philipson T. *The Growth of Obesity and Technological Change: A Theoretical and Empirical Examination*. NBER Working Paper No. 8946. New York: National Bureau of Economic Research, 2002.

47. Campbell KJ, Crawford DA, Salmon J, et al. Associations between the home food environment and obesity-promoting eating behaviors in adolescence. Obesity 2007;15(3):719–30.

48. Jain A. Treating obesity in individuals and populations. BMJ 2005;331:1387–90.

49. Editorial. The catastrophic failures of public health. Lancet 2006;363(9411):745.

50. Swinburn B, Gill T, Kumanyika S. Obesity prevention: a proposed framework for translating evidence into action. Obes Rev 2005; 6:23–33.

51. Swinburn B, Egger G. Preventive strategies against weight gain and obesity. Obes Rev 2002;3:289–301.

52. Lang T, Rayner G. Obesity: a growing issue for European policy? J Eur Soc Policy 2005;15(4):301–27.

53. Rayner G, Hawkes C, Lang T, et al. Trade liberalisation and the diet transition: a public health response. Health Prom Int 2006;21(suppl 1):67–74.

54. Puska P, Tuomilehto J, Nissinen A, et al. (eds) The North Karelia Project: 20 years results and experiences. Helsinki: National Public Health Institute and World Health Organisation Regional Office for Europe, 1995.

55. Lang T, Rayner G, Kaelin E. *The Food Industry, Diet, Physical Activity And Health: A Review of Reported Commitments and Practice of 25 of the World's Largest Food Companies*. London: City University Centre for Food Policy, 2006.

56. Hallsworth M, Ling T. *The EU Platform on Diet, Physical Activity and Health: Second Monitoring Progress Report*. Cambridge: RAND Corporation, 2007.

57. Lang T, Rayner G. Food and health strategy in the UK: a policy impact analysis. Political Q 2003;74(1):66–75.

58. Marmot M. Evidence based policy or policy based evidence? BMJ 2004;328(7445):906–7.

59. Roos G. Media debate on obesity prevention in the UK and Sweden. Scand J Nutr 2005;49(1):38–9.

60. Jacobson MH, Brownell KD. Small taxes on soft drinks and snack foods to promote health. Am J Public Health 2000;90:854–7.

61. Leicester A, Windmeijer F. *The "Fat Tax": Economic Incentives to Reduce Obesity*. London: Institute for Fiscal Studies, 2004.

62. Marshall T. Exploring a fiscal food policy: the case of diet and ischaemic heart disease. BMJ 2000;320:301–5.

63. Strnad J. *Conceptualizing the "Fat Tax": The Role of Food Taxes in Developed Economies*. Palo Alto, CA: Stanford Law School, 2004.

64. Petticrew M, Whitehead M, Macintyre SJ, et al. Evidence for public health policy on inequalities: 1: The reality according to policymakers. J Epidemiol Commun Health 2004;58:811–16.

65. Whitehead M, Petticrew M, Graham H, et al. Evidence for public health policy on inequalities: 2: Assembling the evidence jigsaw. J Epidemiol Commun Health 2004;58:817–21.

66. Offer A. Body weight and self-control in the United States and Britain since the 1950s. Soc Hist Med 2001;14(1):79–106.

67. Himes SM, Thompson JK. Fat stigmatization in television shows and movies: a content analysis. Obesity 2007:15(3):712–18.

68. Burke MA, Heiland F. *Social Dynamics of Obesity*. Washington, DC: Brookings Institution, 2006.

69. Farley T, Cohen D. *Prescription for a Healthy Nation: A New Approach to Improving Our Lives by Fixing Our Everyday World*. Boston: Beacon Press, 2005.

70. Cohen D. A desired epidemic: obesity and the food industry. Washington Post, 2007.

71. Caballero B, Popkin BM (eds) *The Nutrition Transition: Diet-Related Diseases in the Modern World*. New York: Elsevier, 2002.

72. Drewnoski A, Popkin BM. The Nutrition Transition: new trends in the global diet. Nutr Rev 1997;55:31–43.

73. Popkin BM. Urbanisation, lifestyle changes and the nutrition transition. World Dev 1999;27(11):1905–15.

74. Popkin BM. The Nutrition Transition in low-income countries: an emerging crisis. Nutr Rev 1994;52:285–98.

75. Popkin BM. The Nutrition Transition and its health implications in lower income countries. Public Health Nutr 1998;1(1):5–21.

76. Popkin BM. The Nutrition Transition in the developing world. Dev Policy Rev 2003;21:581–97.

77. Popkin BM. An overview on the nutrition transition and its health implication: the Bellagio Meeting. Public Health Nutr 2001;5(1A):93–103.

78. US Department of Health and Human Services. *The Surgeon General's Call to Action to Prevent and Decrease Overweight and Obesity, 2001*. Washington, DC: US Department of Health and Human Services Public Health Service, 2001.

79. Witt L. Why we're losing the war against obesity. Am Demogr 2003;25(10):27–31.

80. Levy E, Levy P, Le Pen C, et al. The economic cost of obesity: the French situation. Int J Obes Relat Metab Disord 1995;19(11):788–92.

81. Kemper HC, Stasse-Wolthuis M, Bosman W. The prevention and treatment of overweight and obesity. Summary of the Advisory Report by the Health Council of The Netherlands. Netherlands J Med 2004;62(1):10–71.

82. Byrne D. EU and the obesity epidemic. Eurohealth 2003;9 (1 Spring):16–17.

83. California Department of Health Services, Cancer and Nutrition Section. *California 5 a Day*. Sacramento, CA: Department of Health Services, 2005.

84. Baranowski T, Cullen KW, Nicklas T, et al. Are current health behavioral change models helpful in guiding prevention of weight gain efforts? Obes Res 2003;11(90001):23S–43.

85. Carroll A, Craypo L, Samuels S. *Evaluating Nutrition and Physical Activity Social Marketing Campaigns: A Review of the Literature for Use in Community Campaigns*. Davis, CA: Samuels and Associates

and the Center for Advanced Studies in Nutrition and Social Marketing, University of California at Davis, 2000: 60.

86. Weber Shandwick. *Obesity: Challenges and Implications for Europe*. London: Weber Shandwick Worldwide and International Business Leaders' Forum, 2004.

87. Rothschild M. Carrots, sticks and promises: a conceptual framework for the management of public health and social issues behaviours. J Marketing 1999;63(October):24–37.

88. Campos P. *The Obesity Myth: Why America's Obsession with Weight is Hazardous to Your Health*. New York: Gotham Books, 2004.

89. Campos P, et al. The epidemiology of overweight and obesity: public health crisis or moral panic? Int J Epidemiol 2006;35(1):55–60.

90. Blumenthal SJ, Hendi JM, Marsillo L. A public health approach to decreasing obesity. JAMA 2002;288(17):2178.

91. Strauss RS, Knight J. Influence of the home environment on the development of obesity in children. Pediatrics 1999;103:e85.

92. Ebbeling CB, Pawlak DB, Ludwig DS. Childhood obesity: public-health crisis, commonsense cure. Lancet 2002;360(9331):473–82.

93. Lightspeed Research. *Global survey reveals parents are to blame for child obesity*. London: Lightspeed Research, 2006.

94. Comuzzie AG, Allison DB. The search for human obesity genes. Science 1998;280(5658):1374–7.

95. Boutin P, Dina C, Vasseur F, et al. GAD2 on chromosome 10p12 is a candidate gene for human obesity. Public Library of Science, 2003.

96. Lobstein T. Suppose we all ate a healthy diet … ? Eurohealth 2004;10(1):8–12.

97. Irz X, Shankar B, Srinivasan C. *Dietary Recommendations in the Report of a Joint WHO/FAO Expert Consultation on Diet, Nutrition and the Prevention of Chronic Diseases (WHO Technical Report Series 916, 2003): Potential Impact on Consumption, Production and Trade of Selected Food Products: Report for the International Federation of Agricultural Producers and Institute for European Food Studies*. Reading: University of Reading Department of Agricultural and Food Economics, 2003: 59.

98. Irz X, Srinivasan CS. Impact of WHO dietary recommendations on world sugar consumption, production and trade. Eurochoices 2004;3(2):24–5.

99. Leggett J. *Half Gone: Oil, Gas, Hot Air and the Global Energy Crisis*. London: Portobello Books, 2005.

100. Hastings G, Stead M, Macdermott L, et al. *Does Food Promotion Influence Children? A Systematic Review of the Evidence*. London: Food Standards Agency, 2003.

101. Nielsen SJ, Popkin BM. Patterns and trends in food portion sizes 1977–1998. JAMA 2003;289(4):450–3.

102. Lupton D. *Food, the Body and the Self*. London: Sage, 1996.

103. Orbach S. *Hunger Strike: the Anorectic's Struggle as a Metaphor for our Age*. London: Faber and Faber, 1986.

104. Stunkard AJ, Wadden TA (eds) *Obesity: Theory and Therapy*. New York: Raven Press: 1993.

105. Egger G, Swinburn B. An "ecological" approach to the obesity pandemic. BMJ 1997;315(7106):477–80.

106. Kuhn TS. *The Structure of Scientific Revolutions*. Chicago: University of Chicago Press, 1970.

107. Summerbell CD, Waters E, Edmunds LD, et al. Interventions for preventing obesity in children. Cochrane Reviews, 2005, Issue 3.

108. Prättälä R, Roos G, Hulshof K, et al. Food and nutrition policies and interventions. In: Mackenbach J, Bakker M (eds) *Reducing Inequalities in Health: A European Perspective*. London: Routledge, 2002: 104–24.

109. Cockett R. *Thinking the Unthinkable: Think-Tanks and the Economic Counter-Revolution, 1931–1983.* London: HarperCollins, 1994.

110. Business in the Community. Responsible marketing to children: exploring the impact on adults' attitudes and behaviour. In: *Marketplace Responsibility Research.* London: Business in the Community, 2005.

111. World Health Organization. *WHO Program Budget 2002–2003: Performance Assessment Report.* Geneva: World Health Organization, 2004: 12.

112. World Health Organization. *Global Strategy on Diet, Physical Activity and Health.* 57th World Health Assembly. Geneva: World Health Assembly, 2004.

113. World Health Organisation/Food and Agriculture Organisation. *Diet, Nutrition and the Prevention of Chronic Diseases.* Report of a Joint WHO/FAO Expert Consultation. WHO Technical Report No 916. Geneva: World Health Organisation/Food and Agriculture Organization of the United Nations, 2003.

114. Hastings G. *Social Marketing: Why should the Devil have All the Best Tunes?* London: Butterworth Heinemann, 2007.

115. Elinder LS. *Public Health Aspects of the EU Common Agricultural Policy: Developments and Recommendations for Change In Four Sectors: Fruit and Vegetables, Dairy, Wine and Tobacco.* Östersund: Swedish National Institute of Public Health, 2004.

116. Heasman M, Mellentin J. *The Functional Foods Revolution: Healthy People, Healthy Profits?* London: Earthscan, 2001.

117. Lang T, Rayner G. *Why Health is the Key to Farming and Food.* Report to the Commission on the Future of Farming and Food chaired by Sir Don Curry. London: UK Public Health Association, Chartered Institute of Environmental Health, Faculty of Public Health Medicine, National Heart Forum and Health Development Agency, 2002.

118. Schmidhuber J, Traill BW. The changing structure of diets in the European Union in relation to healthy eating guidelines. Public Health Nutr 2006;9(5):584–95.

119. Alexandratos N. *The Mediterranean Diet in a World Context.* Paper for the Vth Barcelona Congress on the Mediterranean Diet. Rome: Food and Agriculture Organization, 2004.

120. Euromonitor. *The New Europe: Marketing Opportunities in the Enlarged EU.* London: Euromonitor, 2007.

121. Hawkes C. *Marketing Food to Children: the Global Regulatory Environment.* Geneva: World Health Organization, 2004.

122. Mokyr J. *The Gifts of Athena: Historical Origins of the Knowledge Economy.* Princeton, NJ: Princeton University Press, 2002.

123. Jackson T, Michaelis L. *Policies for Sustainable Consumption: A Report to the Sustainable Development Commission.* London: University of Surrey/University of Oxford, 2003.

124. Layard R. *Happiness: Lessons from a New Science.* London: Allen Lane, 2005.

125. Paulus I. *The Search for Pure Food.* Oxford: Martin Robertson, 1974.

126. Lang T. Food control or food democracy: re-engaging nutrition to civil society, the state and the food supply chain. Public Health Nutr 2005;8(6A):730–7.

127. Huynen M, Maartens P, Hilderlin HBM. The health impacts of globalisation: a conceptual framework. Globaliz Health 2005;1(1):14–26.

128. Loorbach D, Rotmans J. Managing transitions for sustainable development. In: Olshoorn X, Wieczorek AJ (eds) *Understanding Industrial Transformation: Views from Different Disciplines.* Dordrecht: Springer, 2006.

129. Wanless D. *Securing Our Future Health: Taking a Long-Term View.* London: HM Treasury, 2002.

130. Wanless D. *Securing Good Health for the Whole Population.* London: HM Treasury, 2004.

131. Blair T. *Our Nation's Future: Public Health.* Speech by the Prime Minister on healthy living. Nottingham, July 26, 2006, Available from: www.number-10.gov.uk/output/Page9921.asp.

132. Omran AR. The epidemiologic transition: a theory of the epidemiology of population change. Milbank Mem Fund Q 1971;49(4): 509–38.

133. Omran AR. The epidemiologic transition theory: a preliminary update. J Trop Pediatr 1983;29:305–16.

134. Omran AR. The epidemiologic transition theory revisited thirty years later. World Health Stat Q 1998;51:99–119.

135. Porter D. *Health, Civilisation and the State. A History of Public Health from Ancient to Modern Times.* London: Routledge, 1998.

136. Halliday S. *The Great Stink of London: Sir Joseph Bazalgette and the Cleansing of the Victorian Capital.* Stroud: Sutton, 1999.

137. Rayner G. Multidisciplinary public health: leading from the front? Public Health 2007;121(6):449–54.

138. Griffiths S, Jewell T, Donnelly P. Public health in practice: the three domains of public health. Public Health 2005;119(10):907–13.

139. Faculty of Public Health. *Public Health and the Role of the Faculty.* London: Faculty of Public Health, 2005.

140. Fogel RW. *Nutrition, Physiological Capital, and Economic Growth.* Washington, DC: Pan American Health Organization and Inter-American Development Bank, 2002.

141. Acheson D. *Public Health in England.* Report of the Committee of Inquiry into the Future Development of the Public Health Function. London: Department of Health, 1998.

142. HM Government. *Securing the Future: Delivering UK Sustainable Development Strategy*, Cm 6467. London: HM Government, 2005.

143. World Health Organization European Region. *European Charter on Counteracting Obesity.* Copenhagen: World Health Organization European Region, 2006.

144. Johnson A. Together we can beat obesity. The Times, 2008.

145. Stern N. *The Economics of Climate Change: The Stern Review.* Cambridge: Cambridge University Press, 2007.

146. Rayner G, Barling D, Lang T. Sustainable food systems in Europe: policies, realities and futures. J Hunger Environment Nutr 2008;3(2):145–68.

34 A Comprehensive Approach to Obesity Prevention

Boyd Swinburn[1] and A. Colin Bell[2]

[1] School of Exercise and Nutrition Sciences, Deakin University, Melbourne, Australia
[2] University of Newcastle, Wallsend, New South Wales, Australia

The obesity epidemic

Treating obesity as an epidemic

Taking a step back from people with obesity problems to look at populations with obesity problems gives one a very different view of the likely causes of and solutions to this major health challenge. For populations, the role of genes fades into the background and the role of the economic, environmental and social changes becomes dominant. The patterns of change of obesity prevalence within a population over time and between populations tell us a great deal about the nature of the epidemic.

In the high-income countries of Western Europe, North America and Australasia, the epidemic started to increase rapidly over the 1980s and 1990s, whereas in middle-income countries, it has increased more recently. Even in some of the poorer countries, it is overtaking undernutrition in prevalence rates [1]. In the early stages of the epidemic, the effects are seen predominantly in middle-aged people, women, urban dwellers, and the higher socio-economic (SES) groups. These are the first population subgroups influenced by the environmental drivers of obesity – cars, labor-saving devices, passive entertainment and recreation choices, high-fat foods, and high-sugar drinks.

As the time passes (and the population's economic prosperity increases), the obesity prevalence rates in men increase to match those in women in parallel with reductions in occupational physical activity due to mechanization. The SES gradient reverses (especially in women) as lower-income people gain access to the "obesogenic" forces in the environment and education about the

need for healthy eating and regular physical activity slows the rate of weight gain in the higher SES groups. The urban/rural gradient also reverses as agriculture and horticulture become mechanized and the urban populations take on healthier eating and activity patterns.

The major trend now being seen in many countries is increasing prevalence rates among children [2]. The specific obesogenic factors for children that are on the increase include marketing of energy-dense foods and beverages to children, concerns about the safety of neighborhoods, both parents (or the solo parent) working so that children spend their after-school time inside the house (so-called "latchkey" kids), and electronic and computer games.

One way of viewing obesity at a population level is through the classic epidemiologic triad. The triad was originally used as a model for combating infectious diseases and was later applied to injuries and some noncommunicable diseases [3]. It is eminently applicable to obesity and helps to define the different nature of the determinants of obesity and potential strategies for action [4]. All corners of the triad are, of course, interconnected.

The "Agent" is the final common pathway and for infectious diseases it is the infecting organism. For obesity, it is chronic positive energy imbalance. The energy intake "vectors" or carriers of passive overconsumption of total energy [5] are largely energy-dense foods (mainly high-fat foods), energy-dense beverages (high sugar, fat or alcohol), and large portion sizes [6]. The vectors of low energy expenditure are two types of machines – those that reduce the energy cost of work or transport (e.g. electric appliances, cars) and those that promote passive recreation (e.g. television, computers).

The "host" factors include age, gender, genetic make-up, physiologic factors (e.g. hormonal status, metabolic rate), behaviors, and personal attitudes and beliefs. The "environmental" factors can be considered in four different categories – the physical environment (what is available), the economic environment (the

Clinical Obesity in Adults and Children, 3rd edition. Edited by Peter G. Kopelman, Ian D. Caterson and William H. Dietz.
© 2010 Blackwell Publishing, ISBN: 978-1-4051-8226-3.

financial factors, both income and costs), the policy environment (the rules), and the sociocultural (society's attitudes, beliefs, perceptions and values) [7].

The real drivers of the current obesity epidemic are economic – the profit generated from changing environments and vectors in such a way as to make life easier, more convenient, and more enjoyable for people. Obesity has, therefore, been described as a "commercial success" but an "economic failure" because the market is giving people short-term gratification and long-term obesity, making it a market failure in classic economic terms [8]. This model helps to explain the changing obesity prevalence in the following way: changes in the environments and vectors are driven by powerful motives of improving people's lives and making money. People respond to these changes by largely changing their "default" behavior choices based on what is easy, what is desirable (which is influenced by marketing) and what everyone else is doing. These changes are creating the increasing prevalence of obesity over time. On top of that, the natural variation in host characteristics (mainly biology and behavior) creates most of the differences between individuals and on top of that, the natural variation in different cultures and physical environments probably creates most of the differences in obesity prevalence between populations.

The concept of genetic susceptibility to weight gain would be familiar to most people – a person with a "high dose of fat genes" will gain more weight than a person with more "lean genes" in an obesogenic environment. The classic experiment that demonstrated this was the Quebec overfeeding study in identical twins [9]. Over a period of 3 months, participants were overfed by 1000 kcal/day for 6 days a week for 3 months. Under these identical, closely controlled obesogenic conditions, all participants gained weight (not surprisingly) but some gained much more than others (the range was +4.3 kg to +13.3 kg, Fig. 34.1).

Identical twins tended to gain similar amounts of weight, suggesting that much of this variation in weight gain could be genetically based.

Building on this concept of susceptible individuals in obesogenic environments, one could also consider some cultures to be more susceptible (or resilient) than others. A particular culture might have hospitality traditions that place a high value on hosts overproviding foods (especially high-status, fatty foods) and on guests overeating the offered food. There may also be a low cultural value placed on adults (especially women) being physically active. Therefore, a person from this cultural background would be more predisposed to weight gain than someone from another culture with different traditions such as a high vegetable-based diet and belief systems about the benefits of regular physical activity and overall balance in life.

Furthermore, people may be socio-economically predisposed to weight gain. In high-income countries, there is a consistent trend, especially in women, for people with low income or low educational attainment to have higher prevalence rates of obesity [10]. In addition, there is some evidence for a vicious cycle between SES and obesity such that one begets the other [11]. So people from low-income families could be considered economically and/or educationally predisposed to obesity.

These broader concepts of predisposition to obesity (genetic, cultural, economic, educational) help to explain the wide variation in body sizes between individuals when they all seem to have dietary and physical activity habits that are not particularly extreme. People generally make similar default behavioral choices to those around them, but put on weight at different rates. This is why it is important to tackle both the behaviors and the wider environment in its broadest sense.

To reverse the obesity epidemic, therefore, will require both individual- and population-based approaches. The individual approaches focus on the host and are largely educational, with some medical and surgical options for those with established obesity. The population-based approaches also try to influence the hosts (mainly through health education and social marketing campaigns), but in addition try to influence the vectors and environments as well.

What are the main drivers for making the environment less obesogenic? The economic driver of making a profit can make some aspects of the environment less obesogenic such as making low-fat food items and private gyms more readily available. However, this will only achieve so much. For more major and sustained changes, the drivers will need to be enlightened policy and public attitudes and beliefs. Indeed, "market failure" is a well-recognized trigger for government intervention to use policies to change the ground rules and hopefully tip the balance back in favor of population well-being [8]. Policies that promote active transport over car transport, reduce the heavy marketing of energy-dense foods to young children, change the foods available at school canteens, and increase the recreation space in neighborhoods will create sustainable environmental changes.

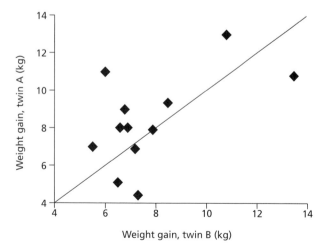

Figure 34.1 Weight gain in response to an identical overfeeding dose (6000 kcal/week for 3 months) in identical twins. (From Bouchard et al. [9].)

Changes in the public's knowledge, attitudes and beliefs will translate into consumer demands for less energy-dense foods and beverages, housing in neighborhoods with good public transport and recreation spaces, improved school food and so on. Such changes in public demand may take a long time but when they do occur, they tend to be long-lasting and powerful. A parallel example has been the increasing public demand and expectations for smoke-free public environments.

Lessons from other epidemics

A degree of success has been achieved in controlling several epidemics of infectious and noninfectious causes of death in many high-income countries and some general principles can be extracted and applied to the obesity epidemic [12]. The key components of the control of these epidemics can be classified as host (h), vector (v) and environment (e).

Reductions in morbidity and mortality from tobacco have been achieved through a multipronged approach including taxation (e), smoke-free legislation (e), education and quitlines (h), regulations (e) on labeling and warnings (v). Cardiovascular diseases have also decreased in response to improved healthcare (h), reduced saturated fat content of meats and low-fat dairy options (v), education on diet and physical activity (h), regulatory framework (e) for nutrient labeling on foods (v), and tobacco control (above).

The road toll has been reduced by social marketing campaigns and driver education (h), regulations and laws on drink driving, seat belts, driver licenses (e), median barriers and improved roads (e), improved car safety (v), and changes in public attitudes (e). Reduced mortality from cervical cancer has mainly involved population-screening programs and surgical treatment (h). Reductions in sudden infant death syndrome (SIDS) have been achieved mainly through education (h). Control of the HIV AIDS epidemic has involved substantial education (h), medical care (h & v), changes in social attitudes (e), increased availability of condoms and needle exchange/disposal systems (v), and blood screening (v). The melanoma mortality rates are no longer rising in countries like Australia, probably due to the increased awareness of the need for sun protection (h), local authority policies on shade provision (e), school policies on hats (e) and the widespread availability of devices like sunscreen, hats with neck protection, and shade cloth to block UV light (v).

The successes in controlling these epidemics have been achieved in the face of substantial barriers including: strong commercial interests (tobacco, dairy industries), social taboos (social marketing about sex), fashion (suntanned skin), unknown cause (SIDS), huge and increasing rates (heart disease), addiction (smoking), traditions and habits (butter and full-fat milk), and social attitude norms (drinking and driving, smoking in enclosed public spaces) [13]. The barriers for preventing obesity are no less formidable, but the strategies for surmounting them have been well tested in these other epidemics.

The main lessons learned from these prevention programs that could be applied to the obesity/diabetes epidemic are: taking a

more comprehensive approach by addressing all corners of the triad; increasing the environmental (mainly policy-based) initiatives; increasing the "dose" of interventions through greater investment in programs; exploring opportunities to further influence the energy density of manufactured foods (one of the main vectors for increased energy intake); developing and communicating specific, action messages; and developing a stronger advocacy voice so that there is greater professional, public and political support for action.

A comprehensive approach to obesity prevention

What is a comprehensive approach?

A comprehensive approach to obesity prevention is one that simultaneously addresses as many of the underlying behavioral and environmental causes of obesity as possible. The underlying premise is that single-strategy approaches such as public education about healthy choices [14] or single-setting approaches such as a school-based program [15,16] will be insufficient to achieve the "intervention" dose required to reverse the current trends in obesity. Theoretically, the approach with the greatest likelihood of effect is one that encompasses multiple strategies (such as social marketing, policy change, environmental change, management of current overweight and obesity), in multiple settings and sectors, across both sides of the energy balance equation [17].

Within such a comprehensive approach, influencing the environment to make healthy choices the easy choices has to be central. The environmental causes of obesity are often difficult to conceptualize and therefore influence. To support this process, we have previously described a systematic approach to classifying and scanning obesogenic environments [7,18]. The ANGELO framework (Analysis Grid for Elements Linked to Obesity) for dissecting environments is shown in Figure 34.2.

Large or macroenvironments that can influence obesity include industries, services or infrastructures such as transport systems, the media, and food production, manufacturing, distribution and marketing industries. Microenvironments are the settings where people gather, particularly those involving food and/or physical activity. Examples include homes, schools, churches, clubs and neighborhoods. Within both macro- and microenvironments, different types of environment can be identified. We define these environments as physical (what is or is not available), economic (the financial factors), policy (the rules) and sociocultural (society's attitudes, perceptions, beliefs and values). Using this ANGELO framework, a group of informed stakeholders can readily "scan" the relevant environments and identify specific elements for prevention strategies.

The combination of these potential interventions should be included in a multisetting, multistrategy prevention program determined by local relevance, likely impact, changeability and resource constraints. Setting-specific delivery is also pragmatic and needs to be guided by those with the relevant expertise. For

Environment type \ Environment size	Microenvironment (settings) Food	PA	Macroenvironment (sectors) Food	PA
Physical	What is available?			
Economic	What are the financial factors?			
Policy	What are the rules?			
Sociocultural	What are the attitudes, beliefs, perceptions and values?			

Figure 34.2 The ANGELO framework (Analysis Grid for Elements Linked to Obesity) used to "scan" the environment for barriers and facilitators to healthy eating and physical activity (PA).

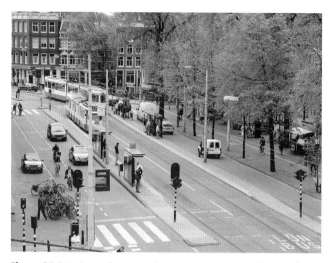

Figure 34.4 An Amsterdam street showing the majority of the lanes are for "active transport" – walking, cycling, public transport – with only one lane for cars.

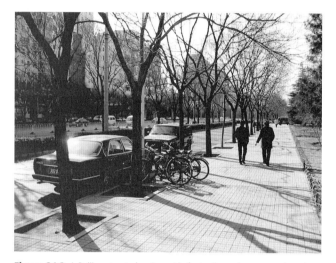

Figure 34.3 A Beijing street, showing wide footpaths and a separate lane for bicycles and parked cars only.

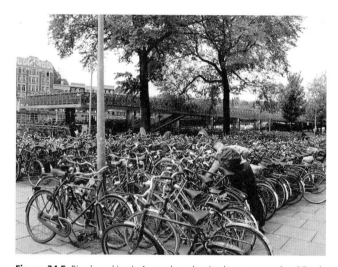

Figure 34.5 Bicycle parking in Amsterdam, showing large areas and multilevel parking building next to the railway station for parking bicycles.

example, teachers know most about schools and what they can deliver, parents know about home-based strategies and their local environment.

To be effective, obesity prevention strategies require government support at a national level to combat macroenvironmental influences that are obesity promoting and to encourage those that are obesity preventing. For example, countries such as China (Fig. 34.3) and The Netherlands (Figs 34.4, 34.5) have a tradition of active transport with a transport infrastructure and culture that promotes bicycles and public transport as well as cities with mixed land use and high population densities [19]. Their challenge is to preserve and extend these structures and cultures in the face of an increasing pressure for private car transport.

Countries like the US and Australia, on the other hand, are faced with the monumental long-term task of trying to retro-fit their current car-dominated culture and infrastructure towards an environment that is more conducive to active transport

[20,21]. For example, most suburbs that have been built in the last 50 years have been designed for car travel almost exclusively with poorly interconnected looping street patterns (Fig. 34.6).

The characteristics of a comprehensive approach thus include support for obesity prevention at a macroenvironment level (in most cases through international, national, and state initiatives), engaging multiple settings at a community level, applying multiple strategies within each setting and focusing on populations who have most to gain from prevention efforts (e.g. children) and the most to lose from nonintervention (e.g. low-income and other high-risk groups). Supporting activities for interventions are also needed, such as: ongoing monitoring of overweight and obesity and its determinants; training programs to increase the

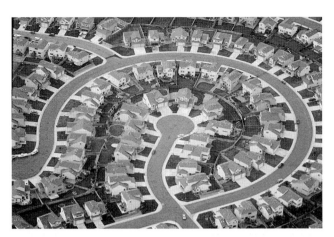

Figure 34.6 Suburban planning designed for car transport. Very few intersections or cross-connections between streets means that a pedestrian has to walk long distances between places that are relatively close.

capacity of the public health workforce to manage obesity prevention; co-ordination of activities and demonstration projects; and a national communication campaign to promote consistent action-orientated messages to the public.

One way of creating action at a community level is through the development of community demonstration programs where obesity prevention efforts can be concentrated and quantified. The selection of communities for demonstration sites is important. The community needs to be large enough to contain sufficient population and settings for population, yet small enough to be manageable. Ideally, the involved community organizations should have good, functioning relationships between them and have some influential champions who can spearhead the efforts. Having good access to communications channels (e.g. local paper and radio, school newsletters, etc.), intervention expertise (e.g. in nutrition, health promotion, social marketing) and evaluation expertise is important.

Within communities or demonstration areas, schools, early childhood care centers, neighborhoods, fast-food environments, sport and recreation clubs, religious organizations and individual households are settings that can make changes to their policy, economic, physical or sociocultural environment to prevent obesity. Because we are still at the stage of demonstrating the impact of this type of approach, the effect and cost-effectiveness of each of these actions need to be closely evaluated. Health services need to complement these community setting activities with a range of obesity management options for those children who are already overweight and obese (see below). These services are in short supply in Australia and other developed countries and urgent investment is needed.

Priority target groups

Who should be the priority groups for obesity prevention action? Once obesity becomes well established in the adult population, one could argue that it is too late for prevention efforts. However,

these people will be contributing the most to the obesity-related burden in the short and medium term, and obesity management should be focused on the high-risk individuals and subpopulations (such as those at risk of diabetes) [22]. The primary prevention efforts, on the other hand, should be targeted to populations prior to the expected large increases in obesity prevalence. This includes those living in low-income countries [23] and children and adolescents [24]. Additional reasons for focusing on children include: they have less control over their own food and physical activity choices; they are more dependent on their environments and are more susceptible to its influences (e.g. television advertizing); they are at the formative stage of life where many lifelong habits are being developed; there is a duty of care for adults and society to provide the best possible environment for children. This last point is an important argument for gaining political and community support for obesity prevention programs and is central to the Sydney Principles – a set of principles to guide national and transnational action on changing food and beverage marketing practices that target children [25].

Role of clinical management programs in reducing obesity prevalence

The evidence for the effectiveness of obesity management programs, particularly for children, has not kept up with the obesity epidemic. Available studies in school and clinical settings suggest conventional behavioral modification approaches to reducing energy intake (dietary changes) and increasing energy expenditure (physical activity) that involve the child's family have the best chance of success [26,27]. Pharmacologic treatment may be an option in some situations but experience is understandably limited in this area. Theoretically, if an obesity management program is integrated into a comprehensive community-based program (as outlined above) it should increase the chances of long-term success, but this has not been tested. The constraints of the systems that govern clinical care (especially the funding systems) usually do not allow clinicians sufficient time to measure, let alone fully manage overweight children and their families even if they have the skills and training to do so. Community-based management programs run by other health professionals could provide clinicians with the "effector arm" to deliver much of the education, counseling and follow-up.

Rose and Day [28] have suggested that the best way to reduce the prevalence of conditions like obesity is to shift the whole distribution curve of the Body Mass Index (BMI) to the left. Evidence that such a population approach works comes from efforts to reduce blood cholesterol levels in North Karelia, Finland, between 1972 and 1992 [29]. The whole distribution curve of cholesterol levels shifted to the left and corresponded with substantial declines in coronary heart disease mortality. Since 1992 and the advent of widespread prescribing of lipid-lowering drugs, the high cholesterol end of the distribution has been remarkably flattened, further shifting the population mean levels to the left. This indicates the potential of combined population approaches and effective clinical management to

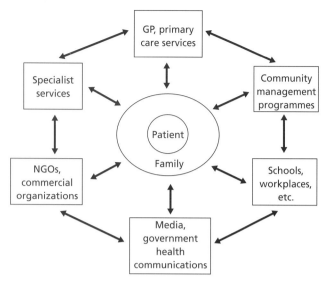

Figure 34.7 Multiple sources of information and support for overweight patients and their families.

substantially reduce the incident rates of disease. Unfortunately, tackling obesity is at about the same stage that tackling high cholesterol levels was 30 years ago – few proven long-term strategies at both population and clinical levels.

We are therefore at the stage where research into effective prevention and treatment options is paramount. However, there are already many people with overweight and obesity who are in need of treatment. This is particularly true for two groups of patients: those who already have (or are at high risk of) obesity complications such as diabetes and sleep apnea, and children and adolescents because of the associated psychosocial problems, strong tracking of obesity into adulthood [30] and long-term health outcomes associated with obesity [27].

There are multiple potential sources of information and support for weight management (Fig. 34.7). Apart from commercial organizations, most options are not well developed. Settings-based promotion of nutrition and physical activity (in schools, workplace, etc.) and communication programs (social marketing) from government agencies, which would form the basis of a comprehensive obesity prevention program, are in their infancy. Community-based weight management programs led by trained professionals such as school nurses, practice nurses or teachers are also an option that needs to be developed, especially for the management of overweight and obesity in children and adolescents where there is a reluctance by parents to medicalize the problem [31]. As the prevention programs and community-based management options develop, the need for strong links between the provider groups will become paramount (see Fig. 34.3). In particular, general practitioners will need to link with community-based management programs as part of their referral network. Specialist services are clearly important for difficult cases where significant medical or psychologic problems are part of the cause or consequence of obesity.

Demonstration site case study – the Colac Be Active, Eat Well program

By focusing funding, training programs, management programs, research expertise and other resources into a whole community as a demonstration site, programs can be developed and evidence gathered about effectiveness and sustainability. This protects the intervention activities from becoming so big that they are unwieldy and difficult to manage and maximizes the chances of achieving a sufficient intervention dose. Such a demonstration site for childhood obesity prevention was established in Colac, South-Western Victoria, Australia, a rural township with a population of approximately 11,000 people, 2 hours by car from Melbourne. The Victorian Department of Human Services funded the implementation program over 4 years as well as the support and evaluation components run by Deakin University. The philosophy behind the intervention was one of community capacity building which builds the structures, resources and skills within the community to develop and implement their own programs to promote healthy eating and physical activity [32,33].

The formative parts of the project, from the establishment of a working group to starting the implementation of an action and marketing plan, took about a year. The first step was to establish networks between community workers, teachers, health professionals, local government and others with an interest in obesity prevention. These networks took shape around a local steering committee which included representatives from local government, Colac Area Health and Deakin University which was providing intervention and evaluation support. A series of training workshops was held to build the knowledge and skills of physical activity and nutrition promotion in the networks and increasing their capacity to plan, market, run and evaluate intervention programs. A key feature of the planning process was using the ANGELO framework to help members of the community identify opportunities for change in their own settings and prioritize these based on likely impact, relevance and changeability. This formed the basis of a 10-point action plan which included objectives around capacity building and communications as well as specific behavioral changes such as reducing television viewing and increasing fruit consumption [34].

Having reached a critical mass of "obesity prevention" capacity (resources secured, key stakeholders engaged and trained, a community action group operating successfully), the action plan could be progressed. The target population selected was children aged 2–12 years and their parents and carers and the target settings were homes, schools, preschools, neighborhoods, primary care and fast-food outlets. A social marketing plan was developed following a specific training workshop on the topic. The program brand "Be Active, Eat Well" with its by-line "Making it easy" (Fig. 34.8) provided the umbrella under which four linked messages were developed to coincide with the action plan – more active play after school, less TV; more fruit every day, fewer packaged snacks; more water, fewer sweet drinks; more active transport to and from school, less car transport. The strategies to

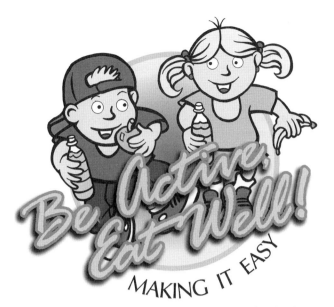

Figure 34.8 Logo from the "Be Active, Eat Well" project in Colac, Victoria.

publicize the messages included paid and unpaid coverage in the local paper, school newsletters, local radio, posters around town, and so on.

Close evaluation is essential for demonstration programs. Each objective of the action plan had an associated evaluation outcome and each strategy was linked with process evaluation measures. There were four linked surveys undertaken before and after 3 years of intervention.

• *Children:* weight, height, waist and lunchbox contents
• *Parents:* computer-assisted telephone interview on the child's eating and physical activity patterns, aspects of the home environment (e.g. family television viewing patterns), aspects of the local neighborhood (e.g. perceived safety for children riding bikes and walking)
• *School:* an environmental audit of the school in relation to physical activity and nutrition
• *Town:* an environmental audit of the town in relation to physical activity and nutrition (e.g. fat content of hot chips, available playgrounds, etc.).

The comparison group was a group of similar schools randomly selected from the rest of the Barwon-South Western region as part of a regional monitoring program (see section on monitoring). Reinforcing the value of a comprehensive approach to obesity prevention with a full evaluation, we found after 3 years of community-based action in Colac that the intervention had significantly reduced unhealthy weight gain [35]. Children from Colac gained about a kilogram less in weight and 3 cm less in waist circumference compared with the comparison group. Interventions included reducing sweetened drinks, increasing active play after school and increasing the healthiness of foods available at school canteens and interestingly, there did not appear to be a particular behavioral change that stood out

as being primarily responsible for the impact on weight and waist measurement.

Collaborative networks for community-based action

Several other whole-community interventions have been established in Victoria [36], New South Wales [37], South Australia [38] and Queensland [39]. These sites are linked into a collaborative network across the country to share knowledge, experience, measurement tools and so on in an effort to maximize the learning and knowledge translation from these demonstration projects. The advantages of such a network lie not just in economies of scale but in getting the necessary variation across communities to measure effectiveness, ensuring it is the local experts who are the main contributors to the design and implementation of the interventions and achieving broader monitoring of secular trends in obesity prevalence. Other advantages are that it allows local innovative ideas to be evaluated and it contributes to a groundswell of public action to reduce childhood obesity. Within a country, therefore, a set of networked whole-community demonstration projects could be a vital catalyst and advocate for broader national action on reducing childhood obesity.

Specific settings and sectors

Influencing homes and parents

Many of a child's physical activity and eating behaviors are learned in the home, making the home or family environment a vital setting for preventing childhood obesity. Children's eating patterns are shaped in the family environment by food availability and accessibility, parental role modeling, television viewing and child–parent interactions [40]. Children's activity patterns and sedentary behaviors are also shaped by the family environment [41]. For example, parent participation in physical activity has significant positive influences on physical activity in children [42]. Children in Australia watch an average of 23 hours of television per week at home [43] and other studies have shown that the home environment, especially having television sets in children's bedrooms and the lack of family rules, is associated with higher television viewing hours [44].

Opportunities for influencing the family environment are limited, however, because it is difficult to access. There is also a danger that interventions directed only at the home may encourage the prevailing but counterproductive attitude that parents and children should be held solely responsible for childhood obesity. The mass media are probably the most important way to access parents and families and to deliver action messages in relation to making the home environment less obesogenic [45]. Other opportunities to influence homes are through the contact that schools, preschools, sports clubs, churches and other settings have with parents and families. Small trials which targeted reductions in television viewing showed significant reductions in unhealthy weight gain [46,47] but these have yet to be replicated across populations.

The school (and preschool) settings

Schools, and increasingly preschools and daycare, are key settings for promoting healthy weight because they have contact with virtually all children throughout a substantial part of childhood and adolescence. This includes children at the highest risk of obesity, for example those from low-income families. One approach that can be used for school-based obesity prevention is the Health-Promoting Schools model [48] that employs multiple strategies across the whole school environment. For obesity prevention, this could include: policies on physical activity and nutrition; physical structures and spaces that promote active play and sport; incorporating nutrition and expanding physical education in the curriculum; teacher training; parent and community support; linking with local government to promote active play; increased availability of healthy choices in school food services; water fountain provision; and an expanded use of specialist teachers, especially for physical education in primary schools.

Many studies contribute to the evidence for school-based obesity prevention, including a limited number of randomized controlled trials [49]. In general, school-based programs are eminently achievable, are well received by stakeholders, and have proven successful in influencing dietary and physical activity knowledge and behavior as well as health behaviors beyond those that were originally planned. Few, however, have demonstrated any long-term impact on weight. Some of the earlier short- to medium-term studies produced decreases in childhood obesity [46,50,51]. More recently, school-based approaches with a stronger community base have shown promising results [52,53].

An explanation for some studies showing changes in physical activity and eating behavior but little change in weight is likely to be that children do not spend all their time in school. A significant proportion of their energy intake and energy expenditure occurs in other settings. For example, in Australia, 37% of children's daily energy intake is consumed in the school environment on a school day, but only 16% of energy is consumed in the school environment over the period of a year when holidays and weekends are taken into account [54].

Schools are attractive as a setting for interventions for a variety of reasons: they provide access to most children for an extended period; synergies are possible between education goals and health promotion; they provide an avenue through which parents can be reached; and they are highly symbolic for the community and can take a lead in creating healthy behavior patterns in children [55]. The limitations are that schools often have enough on their plates without stretching their resources to accommodate interventions, the contribution health can make to helping staff achieve education outcomes is often not well articulated and therefore underestimated, and they are only one of many settings that influence children's weight.

Active neighborhoods

The available trend data for children in North America, Europe and Australia indicate that there has been little change or modest increases in moderate or vigorous activity, sports participation, and physical education at school [56–59]. The only area of physical activity with clear decreases over the last couple of decades is in active transport – particularly to and from school. Nevertheless, ongoing efforts are needed to ensure that the local environments are conducive to physical activity and that these are promoted, because the potential benefits are substantial. One estimate from a systematic review [60] indicates that exposure to an environment that is supportive of physical activity could produce a 20–25% increase in the number of people exercising for at least 30 minutes three or more times each week.

Environmental factors that influence physical activity at a neighborhood level include access to and density of recreation facilities (and the upkeep of the facilities), safety, street design, housing density, land use mix, availability of public transport and pedestrian and bicycle facilities [61]. Interventions focusing on these areas may include policies, regulations and guidelines that support and promote active recreation and transportation, awards and funding support for local governments, facility improvements, monitoring programs and communications to increase active transport, active play and recreation. With appropriate support, local governments have the structures, skills and experience in working with the community and the environment to be able to action many of these activities [62].

In Britain, 50% of children aged 4–11 years were driven less than a mile to school on a regular basis, a distance that is easily walked [63]. Similarly, most children at a New Zealand school traveled to school by car even though their preferred method of travel was walking [64]. Therefore, one strategy that can be adopted relatively quickly is promoting active transport (walking, cycling), especially to and from school [65].

Fast-food outlets and vending machines

A growing body of evidence links rising obesity prevalence with increasing fast-food consumption [66]. Australian household expenditure on take-aways and snacks increased from 10.5% to 18% between 1984 and 1994 [67] and increasing alongside expenditure has been the size of the fast-food meal. Chain outlets practice "Supersizing" which is likely to promote overconsumption of high-fat foods and high-sugar drinks (a large Big Mac meal (4796 kJ) contains 37.6 % more energy and 29% more fat than a small Big Mac meal (3485 kJ) but only costs 20.6% more). Moreover, fast-food outlets tend to cluster in low-income areas, potentially promoting increased consumption among those most at risk of obesity. Reidpath et al found the density of fast-food outlets in low-income neighborhoods to be 2–3 times that of high-income neighborhoods [68]. Fast food also has a higher total fat and saturated fat content than food prepared at home [69,70]. In Australia this is largely because the deep-frying oils that are high in saturated fatty acids (SFAs) (tallow and palm oil) are the least expensive.

Significant reductions in fat intake can be achieved simply by modifying deep-frying practices, and this has important implications at a population level [71]. Components of interventions aimed at reducing saturated and total fat consumption include training programs for best practice deep frying, regulations on training as well as monitoring the amount and type of fat in fast foods (similar to food safety regulations), communication of the nutrition content of fast food to customers (i.e. extending food labeling regulations to include fast food), levying of the SFA content of frying fats (to neutralize the price incentive of high SFA fats), collaboration with industry to reduce supersizing and increase healthy options, and, limiting the density of fast-food outlets. Some of the large fast-food chains are now offering a range of healthier choices, but many of these are still under trial to see if they are commercially viable. Other chains, unfortunately, are not making any real effort to improve the healthiness of their products.

Of course, fast-food outlets are not the only source of energy-dense foods outside the home. A typical 362-item vending machine, for example, contains 5.5 kg of sugar, 4.4 kg of fat and more than 380 MJ. The vast majority of items in vending machines are high in sugar and/or fat and for those vending machines sited within healthcare facilities or in sports and recreation centers, there is a clear dissonance between the *raison d'etre* of those facilities and the food environments they provide in the way of vending machines. Another example of "nutritional dissonance" is graphically illustrated at a zoo where the Western lowland gorilla consumes an appropriate diet of fruit, leafy green veg, skim milk and protein-rich "primate" cake (grains, cereals, peanuts) while the primates visiting the zoo are served an inappropriate diet of energy-dense snacks and fried foods at the zoo cafeteria (Figs 34.9, 34.10). Government food and nutrition policies which require healthy food environments in those facilities under government control or government funded would provide tangible leadership, much in the same way that hospitals and government offices were among the first places to go smoke free. The Health Department in NSW has heeded this call and is progressively rolling out policy requiring healthier choices in health facilities.

Other community settings

A comprehensive approach to obesity prevention should also encompass interventions in other settings or areas, as appropriate. These include early childhood care and education settings, clubs, and churches or other religious communities.

Interventions in early childhood care settings aim to provide environments and education activities that promote healthy food choices and regular active play and to increase parents' and carers' knowledge and skills in nutrition and physical activity. Components of the intervention may include policies on food and active play, curricula on nutrition and motor skills, staff training, and guidelines and monitoring on food service and environments for active play. In a recent review, two of five prevention programs in preschool children showed anthropometric changes, with suggestions that longer term, multicomponent approaches might be more successful [72]. The effect of food policy improvements on behavior change has not been quantified but curriculum-based approaches have been associated with

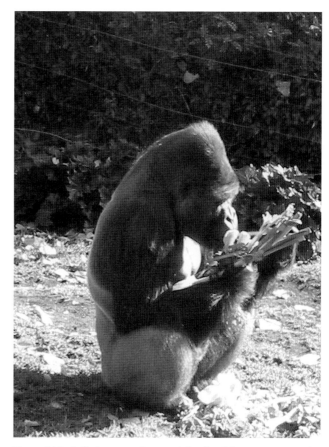

Figure 34.9 Gorilla in a zoo eating a specially tailored diet to ensure optimal health.

increased familiarity with and consumption of fruits and vegetables [73].

For many people, churches and other religious institutions are the center of community life and have been successfully used as a setting for weight loss in Pacific Islands and African-American communities [74,75]. We found that a nutrition and exercise intervention program was successful in arresting weight gain in adult members of a Samoan church community in New Zealand but that in the absence of wider environmental change, the weight was regained in the long term [76].

The settings that support antenatal/postnatal care are important for promoting breast feeding which may be protective against unhealthy weight gain and a number of other childhood illnesses [77]. Several large-scale, longitudinal studies have suggested a protective effect of exclusive breast feeding against the development of obesity in later childhood [78,79] with an estimated population attributable fraction of 15% for breast feeding in the development of obesity. However, some of this effect size may be due to confounding factors such as the body size and SES of the mothers and this now appears to be the case as a recent large randomized controlled trial in which substantially increased breast feeding made no difference to childhood adiposity [80].

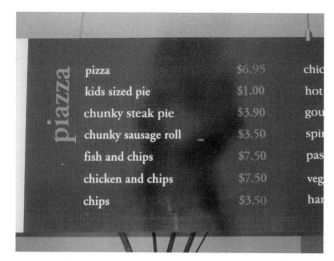

Figure 34.10 Cafeteria menu in the zoo to feed the visiting primates with high-fat, unhealthy food.

The built environment

Within the built environment, the land development patterns (i.e. public transport and pedestrian oriented versus car orientated) and the mode of transport investment (i.e. public transport, walking and cycling paths versus highways) are closely inter-related and between them they have a profound effect on physical activity levels [81]. Public transport can be categorized with walking and cycling as "active transport" because of the regular short walking trips included in the use of public transport. In car-dominated societies, only a minority of trips are walking or cycling (for example, in the US it is about 10%) and most of them are for recreation purposes rather than transportation to a destination, whereas in several European countries, walking plus cycling trips equal or exceed car trips [81]. This probably explains part of the differences in obesity prevalence rates between the continents. In a study from China, where cycling is still the most common form of transportation, the acquisition of a motorized vehicle doubled the odds of becoming obese [19].

While there is an opportunity (largely unrealized) to ensure that new urban/suburban developments are conducive to active transport and active recreation, so much of the current built environment is car orientated. For these existing communities, a long and expensive process of "retro-fitting" the appropriate structures and urban forms to promote physical activity will be needed. Higher density developments, greater mix of land use (a balance between residential and commercial), pedestrian- and cycle-friendly street design, greater investment in public transport, and the designation of streets and areas in the central business districts as car free are all options to achieve this [81,82]. Influencing attitudes towards active transport is also an important part of gaining shifts in modes of transport use because attitudes may be as strongly associated with car transport as land use characteristics [83].

If the environment is conducive to active transport, a mass marketing approach appears to be able to influence long-term behaviors. In Perth, Australia, simple marketing of the active transport options to each household in a suburb resulted in 14% less car travel and increased use of walking, cycling and public transport [84]. Changes were most marked for short journeys and were sustained over 2 years. Modest shifts in transport mode multiplied by the large volumes of short journeys where active transport is an option can result in important increases in physical activity for the population.

The design of buildings also influences incidental activity. In particular, stairs seem to have evolved from a design feature (often with central prominence) and a means of moving between floors to a hidden, locked security risk for use as a fire escape only. Several studies have shown that when stairs are a viable option to taking a lift or an escalator, a prompt sign at the bottom increases the use of the stairs [85].

The food supply
Food distribution and pricing

Food supply interventions aim to increase or decrease the availability and accessibility of certain types of foods. Some programs, such as the school fruit and vegetable scheme in the UK, have been evaluated and found to have some effect on increasing consumption (about a half a serving per day) on the targeted students, although this higher intake was not sustained in the children after they became ineligible for the program [86]. The wider development and promotion of energy-dilute, micronutrient-dense products, or the gradual reformulation of existing high-volume, energy-dense snack foods, such as potato crisps, are options for promoting healthy eating that are under the control of the food industry. Small changes in the fat content of high-volume products have significant potential to provide health benefits at a population level.

Fiscal strategies such as levies can be used to modify prices to influence consumption. Levies are rarely applied to improve population health but this potential exists. Theoretical models have been developed to predict changes in consumption and health outcomes [87,88] but what is really needed is empirical data to demonstrate an effect. Eighteen states in the US apply soft drink levies, which are too small to affect consumption but raise substantial revenue [89] and in Australia, levies currently apply to milk and sugar to raise revenue to support primary producers in the dairy and sugar cane industries [90]. Revenue raised through levies could potentially be used to fund public health nutrition programs.

Food labeling interventions

Full nutrition information panels on foods have been or are being introduced by regulation in many countries. In the US, about two-thirds of people report using nutrition panels [91] and this appears to significantly influence food choices [92]. The impact of mandatory nutrition panels on the formulation and reformulation of manufactured foods may also be significant but it is not well documented. Mandatory nutrition information panels are a key strategy to improve the nutrition status of populations;

however, they need to be complemented by other strategies that will influence the food choices of low-income and less educated consumers [93].

Nutrition "signposts" are signals (such as logos) at point of choice which indicate to the consumer that a food meets certain nutrition standards. An example is the "Pick the Tick" symbol program run by the National Heart Foundations in Australia and New Zealand. They make identifying healthier food choices simpler for consumers and are frequently used by shoppers when choosing products [94]. In addition, the nutrition criteria for the products serve as *de facto* standards for product formulation and many manufacturers will formulate or reformulate products to meet those standards [95]. Energy density criteria are needed for low-fat products.

Health and nutrition claims are closely regulated because of the potential for misleading information and need to be backed by appropriate scientific evidence [96]. About a quarter to a third of new products launched into the market each year in the US carry a nutrition claim [92] but the consumer understanding of these claims is clearly mixed [97] and for some restrained eaters, "low-fat" or "low-calorie" claims can become an unconscious message to eat more of the product [98]. In some manufactured products, the fat is removed so that a low-fat claim can be made but it is replaced with sugar such that the energy density remains unchanged [99]. This negates the impact of low-fat products for preventing weight gain.

Food marketing targeting young children

Heavy marketing of energy-dense foods and beverages to children, especially through television advertizing, has been implicated as a causal factor in increasing obesity. The fat, sugar and energy content of foods advertized to children is extremely high compared to their daily needs and most of the foods advertized fall into the "eat least" sections of the recommended dietary guidelines [100,101]. Exposure to advertizing has been shown to increase children's requests for advertised products [102,103] and that young children have a limited ability to understand advertizing intent [104].

Television advertizing to children under 12 years has not been permitted in Sweden since commercial television began over a decade ago although television channels broadcast into Sweden from elsewhere have diluted the impact of the ban in Sweden. Norway, Quebec and now the UK also have significant restrictions on television advertizing to children [105]. A set of principles (the Sydney Principles) has been developed to guide action on restricting food and beverage marketing of all forms to children under 16 years and there is a growing call for an international enforceable code to implement such regulations [25].

The justification for policies or regulations to restrict food marketing directed at young children cannot rest on a proven cause and effect link between such marketing and childhood obesity because no such direct evidence exists. There is, however, a substantial amount of indirect evidence of an important linkage, including the continued huge investment in marketing (especially through television advertizing) by companies selling fast food, soft drinks and other energy-dense products [106]. The potential impact of 13 childhood obesity interventions has been modeled to provide a sense of their relative population health impacts and cost-effectiveness [107]. Bans on television advertizing turned out to be the most effective and cost-effective of the interventions and this was because of its wide reach (all children affected rather than just a few from program-based interventions) and the regulations would be very inexpensive to implement.

Role of the media
Mass media campaigns

Social marketing of healthy eating and physical activity lifestyles is an essential element of any comprehensive program for obesity prevention. Although information, education and communication strategies alone generally do not change behavior over the long term, they are vital for raising awareness, increasing knowledge, and changing intentions [108]. Some changes in behavior can be seen from mass media campaigns in certain circumstances, such as during a campaign on physical activity participation [109] or if the message is highly specific and action oriented, such as changing from high-fat to low-fat milk [110].

A sustained media campaign backed by programs, policies and other sources of information and support would be a central component of a comprehensive approach to obesity prevention. Experience from campaigns on road safety campaigns, quitting smoking, sun protection, safe sex and the like can be translated into a similar program for obesity prevention.

Unpaid media, lobbying

The most cost-effective way to influence change is through lobbying decision makers (usually politicians). Lobbying is big business in the corporate world and comparatively, public health advocates are neophytes with tiny budgets. However, the issues promoted by public health advocates often resonate with the community and the opportunities to get significant unpaid press coverage are often substantial. A well-organized public lobby group can keep an issue bubbling in the media and put pressure on decision makers in this way. For childhood obesity, there is little in the way of such public movements, although individually most parents are anxious to provide healthy environments for children (including safer streets, less advertizing of junk foods, and better school food). Advocacy groups such as the Center for Science in the Public Interest [111] now have a strong focus on food, and an innovative Internet-based parents' advocacy group called the Parents' Jury [112] is now a strong voice for parents calling for improved food and physical activity environments for Australian children.

Building the evidence

What type of evidence is needed?

There is no shortage of evidence on obesity. Unfortunately, most of it is related to genes, metabolism, and biochemistry or it is

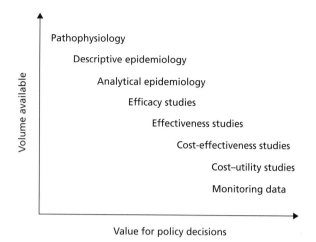

Figure 34.11 The inverse relationship between the volume of evidence available and its value to policy makers.

descriptive epidemiology. The evidence that is desperately needed is around the effectiveness of interventions. There appears to be almost an inverse relationship between the volume of evidence available and its utility to decision makers (Fig. 34.11). Monitoring data to show comparative trends in obesity and its determinants plus data on cost-effectiveness or cost utility (i.e. the cost per disability-adjusted life-year saved), to show where future investments should be made, are probably the two most useful types of information for decision makers.

How much evidence is needed for action?

Evidence-based medicine (EBM) has been developed as an aid to decision making at the clinical level by making the evidence upon which decisions are made explicit, transparent and as unbiased as possible. The EBM movement has moved into other areas so that evidence-based health promotion, health policy, and health communication are now being demanded but the processes and models for reaching the population equivalent of EBM are not well developed. Randomized controlled trials (the backbone of EBM) are rarely available or even possible at the population level. Other frameworks have been developed that take account of the broader types of evidence needed for obesity prevention [113]. The processes for taking the evidence and adding in other issues such as feasibility, cost, acceptability, and equity to develop priorities for action are also being developed [107]. These are the equivalent processes for clinical medicine that take place inside the doctor's head (the evidence is weighed up with other patient factors, costs, and external factors to reach a clinical action decision).

In many instances, action is needed before sufficient evidence of effectiveness is available and in these instances, it is extremely important to fully evaluate any programs or policies. With a vulnerable population, such as children, there is a strong case for taking a highly precautionary approach so that there is a low threshold for action to prevent harm. The precautionary principle has been borrowed from environmental action when considering potential action to protect the environment in circumstances of high uncertainty of outcome [114]. The battle over the high volume of television advertizing for junk foods that is targeted at children is a classic case for invoking the precautionary principle so that regulations are put in place to reduce the advertizing even in the absence of unequivocal evidence that it is doing any harm.

Role of monitoring in obesity prevention

Monitoring is crucial for assessing prevalence and showing trends. In addition to providing trend data, monitoring also allows appropriate benchmarking where a jurisdiction, such as a local government authority, can compare its results with other similar jurisdictions. Monitoring data can also be used to evaluate the impact of community interventions and health promotion programs in demonstration areas. This would, in the long term, be a key strategy for the sustainability of programs and actions by schools, local governments, regions, states and other participants. For obesity prevention, the key indicators should include obesity prevalence data and where possible, determinants at the individual level (such as knowledge, attitudes, and behaviors) and the environmental level (such as school food policies and canteen sales, funding for active transport options, and the presence of footpaths and bike tracks).

However, very few countries have systems in place for regularly monitoring the height and weight of children and most rely on widely spaced national surveys or occasional local surveys for trend information. Only three national or state monitoring systems have been described. As part of a broad set of obesity prevention programs, the State of Arkansas legislated a BMI measurement program in 2003–04 for school students that included an individual report card that went to parents and aggregate report cards for schools and districts [115]. Texas has a monitoring system for fourth, eighth and 11th graders [116], and the UK began a national monitoring system in 2005 [117]. Lack of strong policy backing and funding partly explains the relative absence of monitoring but there are other explanations. In Australia, sensitivities related to taking the measurements, consent processes, difficulties in providing appropriate feedback to children or parents about body size, uncertainty around BMI definitions of overweight and the lack of clinical interventions with demonstrated effectiveness for overweight and obese children also play a role and are currently being debated [118].

Research needed to build the evidence on prevention

The research base underpinning population-based obesity prevention is very small. A substantial investment is needed to boost knowledge in this area so that strategies are much better informed. The foundational research needs to be evaluation of community-based demonstration programs that test multiple prevention strategies in varied environments. The outcome of interest should be BMI, and other individual characteristics and behaviors along with household, neighborhood, school and community factors should be measured as explanatory variables. Recognizing that factors beyond the control of the community also influence obesity, policy-relevant research on the macroenvironmental and sociocultural influences is also needed. For example, we don't fully understand the influence of food advertizing on obesity. Neither are we well informed about how cultural practices in the home, community or business may influence food choice or physical activity. The economic case for obesity prevention needs to be researched in a much more complete way so that we are able to present a balance sheet to government that outlines the cost of the obesity epidemic and also the savings if particular interventions are introduced. We also need to carefully consider how to fund this type of evidence building and taxing energy-dense foods and technology that promotes sedentary behavior should be considered a realistic option.

Other key areas of research include the relationships between social and environmental factors (including SES) and physical activity and nutrition behaviors, the needs and issues of at-risk populations (such as low-income groups, indigenous communities) and effective options for management of currently overweight children.

Conclusion

Multiple strategies (educational, policy, fiscal, environmental changes, social marketing) in multiple settings (homes, schools, workplaces, neighborhoods, etc.) will be needed along with enlightened policies at the macro level (regulations of television advertizing directed at young children, policies promoting active transport, etc.) to reduce the burden of obesity. Integrating obesity management programs with prevention programs is also likely to achieve the synergies needed to deal with both the current and future problem of overweight and obesity.

References

1. World Health Organization. *Obesity: Preventing and Managing the Global Epidemic. Report of a WHO Consultation.* Geneva: World Health Organization, 2000.
2. Lobstein T, Bauer L, Uauy R. Counting the costs: the physical, psychosocial and economic consequences of childhood obesity. Obes Rev 2004;5:4–32.
3. Haddon W Jr. Advances in the epidemiology of injuries as a basis for public policy. Pub Health Rep 1980;95(5):411–21.
4. Egger G, Swinburn B. An "ecological" approach to the obesity pandemic. BMJ 1997;315(7106):477–80.
5. Blundell JE, King NA. Over-consumption as a cause of weight gain: behavioural-physiological interactions in the control of food intake (appetite). Ciba Found Symp 1996;201:138–54.
6. Kral TV, Roe LS, Rolls BJ. Combined effects of energy density and portion size on energy intake in women. Am J Clin Nutr 2004;79(6): 962–8.
7. Swinburn B, Egger G, Raza F. Dissecting obesogenic environments: the development and application of a framework for identifying and prioritizing environmental interventions for obesity. Prev Med 1999;29(6 Pt 1):563–70.
8. Moodie R, Swinburn B, Richardson J. et al. Childhood obesity – a sign of commercial success but market failure. Int J Pediatr Obes 2006;1(3):133–8.
9. Bouchard C, Tremblay A, Despres JP, et al. The response to long-term overfeeding in identical twins. N Engl J Med 1990;322(21): 1477–82.
10. Ball K, Crawford D. Socioeconomic status and weight change in adults: a review. Soc Sci Med 2005;60(9):1987–2010.
11. Stunkard AJ. Socioeconomic status and obesity. In: Cadwick DJ, Cardew G (eds) *The Origins and Consequences of Obesity*. Chichester: Wiley, 1996: 174–93.
12. Swinburn B. Sustaining dietary changes for preventing obesity and diabetes: lessons learned from the successes of other epidemic control programs. Asia Pacific J Clin Nutr 2002;11(suppl 3): S598–606.
13. A.D.A.M. Inc. Atherosclerosis diagram. Available from: http://health.yahoo.com/health/encyclopedia/000171/i18020.html.
14. Jeffery RW, French SA. Preventing weight gain in adults: the pound of prevention study. Am J Pub Health 1999;89(5):747–51.
15. Sahota P, Rudolf MC, Dixey R, et al. Randomised controlled trial of primary school based intervention to reduce risk factors for obesity. BMJ 2001;323(7320):1029–32.
16. Sahota P, Rudolf MC, Dixey R, et al. Evaluation of implementation and effect of primary school based intervention to reduce risk factors for obesity. BMJ 2001;323(7320):1–4.
17. Flynn MAT, McNeil DA, Maloff B, et al. Reducing obesity and related chronic disease risk in children and youth: a synthesis of evidence with best practice recommendations. Obes Rev 2006;7:7–66.
18. Swinburn B, Egger G. Influence of obesity-producing environments. In: Bray GA, Bouchard C (eds) *Handbook of Obesity – Clinical Applications*, 2nd edn. New York: Marcel Dekker, 2004: 97–114.
19. Bell AC, Ge K, Popkin BM. The road to obesity or the path to prevention: motorized transportation in China. Obes Res 2002;10:277–83.
20. Craig CL, Brownson RC, Cragg SE, et al. Exploring the effect of the environment on physical activity: a study examining walking to work. Am J Prev Med 2002;23(2 suppl):36–43.
21. Bell AC, Garrard J, Swinburn B. Active transport to work in Australia: is it all downhill from here? Asia Pacific J Pub Health 2006;18(1):62–8.
22. Knowler WC, Barrett-Connor E, Fowler SE, et al. Reduction in the incidence of type 2 diabetes with lifestyle intervention or metformin. N Engl J Med 2002;346(6):393–403.
23. Bell AC, Popkin BM. The epidemiology of obesity in developing countries. In: Johnston FE, Foster GD (eds) *Obesity, Growth and Development*. London: International Association for Human Auxology, Smith Gordon, 2001.
24. Robinson TN. Population-based prevention for children and adolescents. In: Johnston FE, Foster GD (eds) *Obesity, Growth and Development*. London: International Association for Human Auxology, Smith Gordon, 2001.
25. International Association for the Study of Obesity. International Obesity Taskforce. Available from: www.iotf.org/sydneyprinciples/.
26. Epstein LH, Valoski A, Wing RR, et al. Ten-year follow up of behavioural family based treatment for obese children. JAMA 1990;264:2519–23.

27. Berkowitz RI, Lyke JA, Wadden TA. Treatment of child and adolescent obesity. In: Johnston FE, Foster GD (eds) *Obesity, Growth and Development*. London: International Association for Human Auxology, Smith Gordon, 2001.

28. Rose G, Day S. The population mean predicts the number of deviant individuals. BMJ 1990;301(6759):1031–4.

29. World Health Organization. *World Health Report 2002: Reducing Risks, Promoting Healthy Life*. Geneva: World Health Organization.

30. Magarey AM, Daniels LA, Boulton TJ, et al. Predicting obesity in early adulthood from childhood and parental obesity. Int J Obes Relat Metab Disord 2003;27(4):505–13.

31. Wilkenfeld R, Pagnini D, Booth M. *The Weight of Opinion: Perceptions of School Teachers and Secondary Students on Child and Adolescent Overweight and Obesity*. Sydney: NSW Centre for Overweight and Obesity, 2007.

32. Hawe P, Noort M, King L. Multiplying health gains: the critical role of capacity-building within health promotion programs. Health Policy 1997;39:29–42.

33. Smith BJ, Tang KC, Nutbeam D. WHO health promotion glossary: new terms. Health Prom Int 2006;21(4):340–5.

34. State Government of Victoria, Department of Human Services. Go for Your Life: Information for Professionals. Available from: www.goforyourlife.vic.gov.au/hav/articles.nsf/pracpages/Be_Active_Eat_Well?Open.

35. Friedrich MJ. Researchers address childhood obesity through community-based programs. JAMA 2007;298(23):2728–30.

36. Deakin University Faculty of Health, Medicine, Nursing and Behavioural Sciences. WHO Collaborating Centre for Obesity Prevention. Available from: www.deakin.edu.au/hmnbs/who-obesity/ssop/ssop.php.

37. NSW Health. Good for Kids, Good for Life. Available from: www.goodforkids.nsw.gov.au/.

38. Government of South Australia. Eat Well, Be Active: community programs. Available from: www.health.sa.gov.au/PEHS/branches/health-promotion/hp-eat-well-be-active.htm.

39. Queensland Government. Eat Well, Be Active. Available from: www.eatwellbeactive.qld.gov.au/eatwellbeactive/default.asp

40. Campbell KJ, Crawford DA, Salmon J, et al. Associations between the home food environment and obesity-promoting eating behaviors in adolescence. Obesity 2007;15(3):719–30.

41. Davison KK, Birch LL. Childhood overweight: a contextual model and recommendations for future research. Obes Rev 2001;2(3):159–71.

42. Trost SG, Sallis JF, Pate RR. Evaluating a model of parental influence on youth physical activity. Am J Prev Med 2003;25(4):277.

43. Zuppa JA, Morton H, Mehta KP. Television food advertising: counterproductive to children's health? A content analysis using the Australian Guide to Healthy Eating. Nutr Dietet 2003;60:78–84.

44. van Zutphen M, Bell AC, Kremer PJ, et al. Association between the family environment and television viewing in Australian children. J Pediatr Child Health 2007;43(6):458–63.

45. Huhman ME, Potter LD, Duke JC, et al. Evaluation of a national physical activity intervention for children: VERB Campaign, 2002–2004. Am J Prev Med 2007;32(1):38–43.

46. Robinson TN. Reducing children's television viewing to prevent obesity: a randomized controlled trial. JAMA 1999;282(16):1561–7.

47. Gortmaker SL, Peterson K, Wiecha J, et al. Reducing obesity via a school-based interdisciplinary intervention among youth: Planet Health. Arch Pediatr Adolesc Med 1999;153(4):409–18.

48. World Health Organization. *Regional Guidelines: Development of Health Promoting Schools – A Framework For Action*. Geneva: Regional Office for the Western Pacific, 1996.

49. Campbell K, Waters E, O'Meara S, et al. Interventions for preventing obesity in childhood. A systematic review. Obes Rev 2001;2(3):149–57.

50. Flores R. Dance for health: improving fitness in African American and Hispanic adolescents. Pub Health Rep 1995;110(2):189–93.

51. Manios Y, Kafatos A. Health and nutrition education in elementary schools: changes in health knowledge, nutrient intakes and physical activity over a six year period. Pub Health Nutr 1999;2(3A):445–8.

52. Economos CD, Hyatt RR, Goldberg JP, et al. A community intervention reduces BMI z-score in children: Shape Up Somerville first year results. Obesity 2007;15(5):1325–36.

53. Taylor RW, McAuley KA, Barbezat W. APPLE Project: 2-y findings of a community-based obesity prevention program in primary school age children. Am J Clin Nutr 2007;86(3):735–42.

54. Bell AC, Swinburn BA. What are the key food groups to target for preventing obesity and improving nutrition in schools? Eur J Clin Nutr 2004;58(2):258–63.

55. Bell AC, Swinburn B. School canteens: using ripples to create a wave of healthy eating. Med J Aust 2005;183(1):5–6.

56. Eisenmann JC, Katzmarzyk PT, Tremblay MS. Leisure-time physical activity levels among Canadian adolescents, 1981–1998. J Phys Activ Health 2004;1(2):154–62.

57. Salmon J, Timperio A, Cleland V, et al. Trends in children's physical activity and weight status in high and low socio-economic status areas of Melbourne, Victoria, 1985–2001. Aust NZ J Pub Health 2005;29:337–42.

58. NSW Health. SPANS: NSW School Physical Activity and Nutrition Survey. Available from: www.health.nsw.gov.au/pubs/2006/spans/index.html.

59. Samdal O, Tynjala J, Roberts C, et al. Trends in vigorous physical activity and TV watching of adolescents from 1986 to 2002 in seven European Countries. Eur J Pub Health 2007;17(3):242–8.

60. Kahn EB, Ramsey LT, Brownson RC, et al. The effectiveness of interventions to increase physical activity. A systematic review. Am J Prev Med 2002;22(4 suppl):73–107.

61. Saelens BE, Sallis JF, Frank LD. Environmental correlates of walking and cycling: findings from the transportation, urban design, and planning literatures. Ann Behav Med 2003;25(2):80–91.

62. King AC, Bauman A, Abrams DB. Forging trandisciplinary bridges to meet the physical inactivity challenge in the 21st century. Am J Prev Med 2002;23(2 suppl 1):104–6.

63. Sleap M, Warburton P. Are primary school children gaining heart health benefits from their journeys to school? Child: Care, Health Dev 1993;19(2):99–108.

64. Collins DC, Kearns RA. The safe journeys of an enterprising school: negotiating landscapes of opportunity and risk. Health Place 2001;7(4):293–306.

65. Tudor-Locke C, Ainsworth BE, Popkin BM. Active commuting to school: an overlooked source of childrens' physical activity? Sports Med 2001;31(5):309–13.

66. Binkley JK, Eales J, Jekanowski M. The relation between dietary change and rising US obesity. Int J Obes 2000;24(8):1032–9.

67. Jones V. *Takeaway Food Project Triennial Report (1996–1999)*. Sydney: National Heart Foundation of Australia (NSW Division), 2000.

68. Reidpath DD, Burns C, Garrard J, et al. An ecological study of the relationship between social and environmental determinants of obesity. Health Place 2002;8(2):141–5.
69. Lin B-H, Frazao E, Guthrie J. *Away-from-Home Foods Increasingly Important to Quality of American Diet*. Washington, DC: Food and Rural Economics Division, Economic Research Service, US Department of Agriculture, 1999.
70. Ashton B, Hughes R. *Takeaway Food Project Report Number 1: A Review of Public Health Nutrition Intelligence of the Takeaway Food Sector.*Queensland: Queensland Health, The Heart Foundation (Qld division), Griffith University, 2000.
71. Morley-John J, Swinburn B, Metcalf P, et al. Fat content of chips, quality of frying fat and deep-frying practices in New Zealand fast food outlets. Aust NZ J Pub Health 2002;26(2):101–7.
72. Bluford DAA, Sherry B, Scanlon KS. Interventions to prevent or treat obesity in preschool children: a review of evaluated programs. Obesity 2007;15(6):1356–72.
73. Edmunds L. Evaluation of the Grab 5! project to increase fruit and vegetables in primary school age children. Available from: www.grab5.com.
74. Simmons D, Thompson CF, Volklander D. Polynesians: prone to obesity and type 2 diabetes mellitus but not hyperinsulinaemia. Diabet Med 2001;18(3):193–8.
75. Kumanyika SK, Charleston JB. Lose weight and win: a church-based weight loss program for blood pressure control among black women. Patient Educ Couns 2002;19(1):19–32.
76. Bell AC, Swinburn BA, Amosa H, A nutrition and exercise intervention program for controlling weight in Samoan communities in New Zealand. Int J Obes 2001;25:920–7.
77. Oddy WH. Breastfeeding and asthma in children: findings from a West Australian study. Breastfeeding Rev 2000;8(1):5–11.
78. Armstrong J, Reilly JJ. Breastfeeding and lowering the risk of childhood obesity. Lancet 2002;359(9322):2003–4.
79. Dietz WH. Breastfeeding may help prevent childhood overweight. JAMA 2001;285(19):2506–7.
80. Kramer MS, Matush L, Vanilovich I, et al. Effects of prolonged and exclusive breastfeeding on child height, weight, adiposity, and blood pressure at age 6.5 y: evidence from a large randomized trial. Am J Clin Nutr 2007;86(6):1717–21.
81. Frank LD, Engelke P. *How Land Use and Transportation Systems Impact on Public Health: A Literature Review of the Relationship Between Physical Activity and the Built Form*. Report to the Centers for Disease Control and Prevention. Atlanta, GA: Georgia Institute of Technology, 2001.
82. Crawford J. *Carfree Cities*. Utrecht: International Books, 2000.
83. Kitamura R, Mokhtarian PL, Laidet L. A micro-analysis of land use and travel in five neighborhoods in the San Francisco Bay area. Transportation 1997;24:125–58.
84. Western Australian Government. TravelSmart (Transport). Available from: www.travelsmart.transport.wa.gov.au
85. CDC. Guide to Community Preventive Services. Available from: www.thecommunityguide.org/home_f.html
86. Ransley JK, Greenwood DC, Cade JE, et al. Does the school fruit and vegetable scheme improve children's diet? A non-randomised controlled trial. J Epidemiol Commun Health J Epidemiol Commun Health 2007;61:699–703.
87. Mytton O, Gray A, Rayner M, et al. Could targeted food taxes improve health? J Epidemiol Commun Health 2007;61: 689–94.
88. Schroeter C, Lusk J, Tyner W. Determining the impact of food price and income changes on body weight. Journal of Health Economics, J Health Econ 2008;27(1):45–68.
89. Jacobson MF, Brownell KD. Small taxes on soft drinks and snack foods to promote health. Am J Pub Health 2000;90(6): 854–7.
90. Gordon J. Bevy of levies. The Sunday Age, September 15, 2002; Sect. 8.
91. French SA, Story M, Jeffery RW. Environmental influences on eating and physical activity. Annu Rev Pub Health 2001;22: 309–35.
92. Weimer J. *Accelerating the Trend Toward Healthy Eating. America's Eating Habits: Changes and Consequences*. Washington, DC: USDA, 1999: 385–401.
93. Wang G, Fletcher SM, Carley DH. Consumer utilization of food labeling as a source of nutrition information. J Consum Aff 1995;29(2):368.
94. Noakes M, Crawford D. The National Heart Foundation's "Pick the Tick" program. Consumer awareness, attitudes and interpretation. Food Australia 1991;43(6):262–6.
95. Young LR, Swinburn B. The impact of the Pick the Tick food information programme on the salt content of food in New Zealand. Health Prom Int 2002;17(1):13–19.
96. Schneeman B. FDA's review of scientific evidence for health claims. J Nutr 2007;137:493–4.
97. van Trijp HCM, van der Lans IA. Consumer perceptions of nutrition and health claims. Appetite 2007;48(3):305–24.
98. Miller DL, Castellanos VH, Shide DJ, et al. Effect of fat-free potato chips with and without nutrition labels on fat and energy intakes. Am J Clin Nutr 1998;68(2):282–90.
99. Seidell JC. Prevention of obesity: the role of the food industry. Nutr Metab Cardiovasc Dis 1999;9(1):45–50.
100. Institute of Medicine. *Food Marketing to Children and Youth. Threat or Opportunity?* Washington, DC: National Academy of Sciences, 2006.
101. Hastings G, Stead M, McDermott L, et al. *Review of the Research on the Effects of Food Promotion to Children*. Glasgow: Centre for Social Marketing, University of Strathclyde, 2003.
102. Borzekowski DL, Robinson TN. The 30-second effect: an experiment revealing the impact of television commercials on food preferences of preschoolers. J Am Dietet Assoc 2001;101(1):42–6.
103. Robinson TN, Saphir MN, Kraemer HC, et al. Effects of reducing television viewing on children's requests for toys: a randomized controlled trial. J Dev Behav Pediatr 2001;22(3):179–84.
104. Oates C, Blades M, Gunter B. Children and television advertising: When do they understand persuasive intent? J Consum Behav 2001;1(3):238–45.
105. Hawkes C. *Marketing Food to Children: The Global Regulatory Environment*. Geneva: World Health Organization, 2004.
106. Morton H. The television advertising of foods to children: a case for regulation? Multidisciplinary approaches to food choice. Adelaide: Adelaide Conference on Food Choices, 1996.
107. Haby MM, Vos T, Carter R, et al. A new approach to assessing the health benefit from obesity interventions in children and adolescents: the assessing cost-effectiveness in obesity project. Int J Obes 2006;30(10):1463–75.
108. Beaudoin CE, Fernandez C, Wall JL, et al. Promoting healthy eating and physical activity: short-term effects of a mass media campaign. Am J Prev Med 2007;32(3):217–23.

109. Huhman M, Potter LD, Wong FL, et al. Effects of a mass media campaign to increase physical activity among children: year-1 results of the Verb Campaign. Pediatrics 2005;116: e277–e84.

110. Reger B, Wootan MG, Booth-Butterfield S. Using mass media to promote healthy eating: a community-based demonstration project. Prev Med 2009;29(5):414–21.

111. Center for Science in the Public Interest. Available from: www. cspinet.org.

112. The Parents Jury. The Parents Jury: your voice on food and activity. Available from: www.parentsjury.org.au/.

113. Swinburn B, Gill T, Kumanyika S. Obesity prevention: a proposed framework for translating evidence into action. Obes Rev 2005;6(1):23–33.

114. Tickner J, Raffensperger C, Myers N. *The Precautionary Principle in Action: A Handbook*. Lowell: Lowell Centre for Sustainable Production, Science and Environmental Health Network.

115. University of Arkansas for Medical Sciences. *Year Three Evaluation: Arkansas Act 1220 of 2003 to Combat Childhood Obesity*. Little Rock, AR: Fay W. Boozman College of Public Health, 2006.

116. Hoelscher DM, Day RS, Lee ES, et al. Measuring the prevalence of overweight in Texas school children. Am J Pub Health 2004;94(6): 1002–8.

117. Crowther R, Dinsdale H, Rutter H, et al. *Analysis of the National Childhood Database 2005–2006*. A Report for the Department of Health by the South East Public Health Observatory on behalf of the Association of Public Health Observatories: Oxford: South East Public Health Observatory, 2006.

118. O'Dea JA. Prevention of childhood obesity: 'First do no harm'. Health Edu Res 2005;20(2):259–65.

Index

Index

Index

Index

Index